Little, Brown's Paperback Book Series

Basic Medical Sciences

Boyd & Hoerl	Basic Medical Microbiology
Colton	Statistics in Medicine
Hine & Pfeiffer	Behavioral Science
Kent	General Pathology: A Programmed Text
Levine	Pharmacology
Peery & Miller	Pathology
Richardson	Basic Circulatory Physiology
Roland et al.	Atlas of Cell Biology
Selkurt	Physiology
Sidman & Sidman	Neuroanatomy: A Programmed Text
Siegel, Albers, et al.	Basic Neurochemistry
Snell	Clinical Anatomy for Medical Students
Snell	Clinical Embryology for Medical Students
Streilein & Hughes	Immunology: A Programmed Text
Valtin	Renal Function
Watson	Basic Human Neuroanatomy

Clinical Medical Sciences

Clark & MacMahon	Preventive Medicine
Eckert	Emergency-Room Care
Grabb & Smith	Plastic Surgery
Green	Gynecology
Gregory & Smeltzer	Psychiatry
Judge & Zuidema	Methods of Clinical Examination
MacAusland & Mayo	Orthopedics
Nardi & Zuidema	Surgery
Niswander	Obstetrics
Thompson	Primer of Clinical Radiology
Wilkins & Levinsky	Medicine
Ziai	Pediatrics

Manuals and Handbooks

Alpert & Francis	Manual of Coronary Care
Arndt	Manual of Dermatologic Therapeutics
Berk et al.	Handbook of Critical Care
Children's Hospital Medical Center, Boston	Manual of Pediatric Therapeutics
Condon & Nyhus	Manual of Surgical Therapeutics
Friedman & Papper	Problem-Oriented Medical Diagnosis
Gardner & Provine	Manual of Acute Bacterial Infections
Iversen & Clawson	Manual of Acute Orthopaedic Therapeutics
Massachusetts General Hospital	Diet Manual
Massachusetts General Hospital	Manual of Nursing Procedures
Neelon & Ellis	A Syllabus of Problem-Oriented Patient Care
Papper	Manual of Medical Care of the Surgical Patient
Shader	Manual of Psychiatric Therapeutics
Snow	Manual of Anesthesia
Spivak & Barnes	Manual of Clinical Problems in Internal Medicine: Annotated with Key References
Wallach	Interpretation of Diagnostic Tests
Washington University Department of Medicine	Manual of Medical Therapeutics
Zimmerman	Techniques of Patient Care

Little, Brown and Company
34 Beacon Street
Boston, Massachusetts 02106

Medicine
Essentials of Clinical Practice

Medicine

ESSENTIALS OF CLINICAL PRACTICE

SECOND EDITION

EDITED BY

ROBERT W. WILKINS, M.D.
Professor of Medicine (Emeritus),
Boston University School of Medicine;
Consultant, University Hospital, Boston

NORMAN G. LEVINSKY, M.D.
Wade Professor and Chairman,
Division of Medicine, Boston University
School of Medicine; Physician-in-Chief
and Director, Evans Memorial Department
of Clinical Research, University Hospital, Boston

ASSOCIATE EDITORS

Jay D. Coffman, M.D.
Cardiovascular Diseases

Alan S. Cohen, M.D.
Rheumatology and Immunology

Daniel Deykin, M.D.
Hematological Disorders

Raymond D. Koff, M.D.
Gastrointestinal Disorders

William R. McCabe, M.D.
Infectious Diseases

James C. Melby, M.D.
Endocrinology

Gordon L. Snider, M.D.
Respiratory Disorders

LITTLE, BROWN AND COMPANY   BOSTON

Notice

The indications and dosages of all drugs in this work
have been recommended in the medical literature
and conform to the practices of the general medical
community at Boston University School of Medicine.
The medications described do not necessarily have
specific approval by the Food and Drug Administration for use in the situations and dosages for which
they are recommended. The package insert for each
drug should be consulted for use and dosage as
approved by the FDA. Because standards for usage
change, it is advisable to keep abreast of revised
recommendations, particularly those concerning new
drugs.

Contents

Preface

Every textbook should have a purpose and should aim at a particular audience. The purpose of the second edition of MEDICINE is to present a lucid account of those aspects of internal medicine that are essential for clinical practice. It is aimed primarily at medical students. Contributing authors were asked to select for detailed discussion topics in their fields that they felt should be understood and remembered by every American medical student. The editors then attempted to integrate the contributions into a textbook whose size and style would make it attractive to students who wish to read systematically while taking their principal course in general internal medicine. Therefore, we have not compiled a comprehensive reference work, several of which are already available. This book, about one-third the length of such reference texts, represents selectivity based on the premise that students should focus on the essentials. Those seeking more extensive information will find guidance to the detailed literature through the review articles cited in the bibliographies.

Although we have concentrated upon medical students, we believe that the text will also be of value to several other groups, both physicians and paramedical professionals. The incredibly rapid growth of medical knowledge forces us all to read more selectively nowadays. General internists and family practitioners may find this book a useful review, while subspecialists may wish to read parts of it to assuage their guilt about areas of internal medicine that they may have neglected while staying abreast in their own fields.

This second edition has been substantially revised. Several sections have been largely rewritten and every chapter has been thoroughly updated to include concepts developed during the six years since the first edition. As a product of the Division of Medicine at Boston University, the book reflects the clinical and scientific attitudes of individual members of our faculty. As in the first edition, the editors have not tried to homogenize any differences, preferring to allow each writer's individuality and special interests to enliven the book. The authors are all subspecialists, and each has selected from his field of expertise the topics he believes to be of greatest interest and importance. It remains our belief that the recent growth of knowledge precludes the writing of successful textbooks by generalists, particularly in a field as broad as internal medicine.

This book presents individual topics as they are encountered by an experienced practicing clinician. Many clinical situations develop as problems of an organ system. For example, when a patient has a persistent cough, the clinician usually thinks about disorders of the organs possibly involved. Hence, respiratory infections are discussed in the section on respiratory diseases. To describe them in a general section on infections would assume that the clinician has prior knowledge of the specific causative agent, knowledge which is rarely available when he first evaluates a patient. On the other hand, many infections are multisystemic in clinical presentation. These are covered in a new separate section on systemic infectious diseases. In short, in this edition we have attempted to follow clinical practice, instead of insisting upon either an organ or an etiologic approach. Strong emphasis on the scientific basis of medical practice, part of the tradition of Boston medicine, is represented by appropriate aspects of pathophysiology in each section. However, a book of this scope could include only those aspects immediately relevant to clinical problems.

A final word to the student reader. Internal medicine is exciting: it challenges the emotions and the mind with an endlessly varying series of human contacts and with intellectually stimulating problems. At the outset of your career, you may wonder if you can meet the challenge. We trust that our text will help you over the early hurdles. We also hope that you will come to share the feelings of our first editor, Chester Keefer, who said, "I'd rather see a disease or syndrome I've never seen before than play golf, go to a show, read a book, listen to music, or anything else pleasurable I can think of. It gives me more pleasure to make a rare, but correct, diagnosis than to make a hole in one. The thing about medicine is that I love it." Enjoy yourselves!

R.W.W.

N.G.L.

Acknowledgement

The editors are grateful to Mrs. Patricia Simonson, Assistant to the Chairman, for graciously organizing and prodding recalcitrant or dilatory authors and editors. Without her efforts this volume might not have been completed — at least in this decade.

Contributing Authors

Bruce F. Bachus, M.D.
Instructor in Medicine, Boston University School of Medicine; Staff Physician, Pulmonary Section, Veterans Administration Hospital, Boston

Chapter 14

Madeline Bachta, M.D.
Clinical Associate, Department of Dermatology, Boston University School of Medicine; Assistant in Dermatology, University Hospital, Boston

Chapter 5

D. Frank Benson, M.D.
Professor of Neurology, Boston University School of Medicine; Associate Chief, Department of Neurology, Veterans Administration Hospital, Boston

Chapter 62

Merrill D. Benson, M.D.
Associate Professor of Medicine, Indiana University School of Medicine; Chief, Rheumatology Section, Indianapolis Veterans Administration Hospital, Indianapolis; formerly Assistant Professor of Medicine, Boston University School of Medicine, and Chief, Allergy-Immunology Clinic, Boston City Hospital

Chapter 45

Daniel S. Bernstein, M.D.
Associate Clinical Professor of Medicine, Boston University School of Medicine; Associate Visiting Physician, University Hospital, Boston

Chapter 61

Neil R. Blacklow, M.D.
Professor of Medicine and Microbiology, University of Massachusetts Medical School; Chief, Department of Infectious Disease, University of Massachusetts Hospital, Worcester

Chapters 6, 8, 11, 39

Kenneth D. Brandt, M.D.
Professor of Medicine, Indiana University School of Medicine; Head, Department of Rheumatology, Indiana University Medical Center, Indianapolis

Chapter 46

Mark J. Brauer, M.D.
Assistant Professor of Medicine, Boston University School of Medicine; Acting Director of Hematology and Director of the Blood Bank, Boston City Hospital

Chapter 50

Jerome S. Brody, M.D.
Associate Professor of Medicine, Boston University School of Medicine; Chief, Pulmonary Section, University Hospital and Boston City Hospital

Chapters 16, 23, 24

Edgar S. Cathcart, M.D.
Associate Professor of Medicine, Boston University School of Medicine; Program Director, Arthritis Section, University Hospital, Boston

Chapter 46

Aram V. Chobanian, M.D.
Professor of Medicine and Director, Cardiovascular Institute, Boston University School of Medicine; Visiting Physician, Boston City Hospital and University Hospital, Boston

Chapter 26

Sanford Chodosh, M.D.
Associate Professor of Medicine, Boston University School of Medicine; Director, Sputum Laboratory, Boston City Hospital

Chapter 20

Jay D. Coffman, M.D.
Professor of Medicine, Boston University School of Medicine; Chief, Peripheral Vascular Section, University Hospital, Boston

Chapter 27

Alan S. Cohen, M.D.
Conrad Wesselhoeft Professor of Medicine, Boston
University School of Medicine; Chief of Medicine
and Director, Thorndike Memorial Laboratory,
Boston City Hospital

Chapter 46

Sidney R. Cooperband, M.D.
Professor of Medicine and Microbiology, Boston
University School of Medicine; Visiting Physician,
University Hospital, Boston

Chapter 44

William G. Couser, M.D.
Associate Professor of Medicine, Boston University
School of Medicine; Associate Visiting Physician,
University Hospital, Boston

Chapter 53

Frank F. Davidson, M.D.
Assistant Professor of Medicine, Boston University
School of Medicine; Assistant Visiting Physician,
University Hospital, Boston

Chapters 19, 23

Daniel Deykin, M.D.
Professor of Medicine, Boston University School of
Medicine; Chief of Medicine, Veterans Administration
Hospital, Boston

Chapter 52

Charles P. Emerson, M.D.
Former Chief of Hematology and Professor
Emeritus of Medicine, Boston University School
of Medicine

Chapter 49

Robert G. Feldman, M.D.
Professor of Neurology and Pharmacology, Boston
University School of Medicine; Chairman, Depart-
ment of Neurology, University Hospital, Boston

Chapter 62

S. Edwin Fineberg, M.D.
Assistant Professor of Medicine, Boston University
School of Medicine; Co-Program Director, Clinical
Research Center, Boston City Hospital

Chapter 59

Athanasios P. Flessas, M.D.
Adjunct Associate Professor of Clinical Medicine,
Boston University School of Medicine; Chief of
Cardiology, NIMTS Hospital, Athens, Greece

Chapter 28

Jules Friedman, M.D.
Instructor in Neurology, Boston University School
of Medicine; Director, Oto-Neurology Unit,
University Hospital, Boston

Chapter 62

Edward A. Gaensler, M.D.
Professor of Surgery and Physiology, Boston
University School of Medicine; Visiting Surgeon
(Thoracic), University Hospital, Boston

Chapter 17

Nelson M. Gantz, M.D.
Assistant Professor of Medicine, Boston University
School of Medicine; Infectious Disease Section,
Boston City Hospital and University Hospital, Boston

Chapters 6, 8, 11, 63

Richard Alan Gleckman, M.D.
Assistant Professor of Medicine, Boston University
School of Medicine; Staff Physician, Infectious Disease
Section, Veterans Administration Hospital, Boston

Chapter 7

Lauran D. Harris, M.D.
Associate Professor of Medicine, Boston University
School of Medicine; Associate Visiting Physician,
University Hospital, Boston

Chapter 34

John A. Hermos, M.D.
Assistant Professor of Medicine, Boston University
School of Medicine; Gastroenterology Section,
Medical Service and Co-Medical Director, Substance
Abuse Unit, Veterans Administration Hospital,
Boston

Chapters 3, 36

William Hollander, M.D.
Professor of Medicine and Biochemistry, Boston
University School of Medicine; Visiting Physician
and Director, Section of Hypertension and
Atherosclerosis, University Hospital, Boston

Chapter 25

William B. Hood, Jr., M.D.
Professor of Medicine, Boston University School of
Medicine; Chief, Cardiology Section, Boston City
Hospital

Chapter 31

David C. Hueter, M.D.
Assistant Professor of Medicine, Boston University
School of Medicine; Assistant Visiting Physician and
Head, Cardiac Graphics Laboratory, University
Hospital, Boston

Chapter 33

Paul Kaufman, M.D.
Associate Professor of Psychiatry, Boston University
School of Medicine; Assisting Visiting Physician,
University Hospital, Boston

Chapter 2

M. Anees Khan, M.D.
Assistant Professor of Medicine, Boston University
School of Medicine; Director, Tuberculosis Clinic,
Boston City Hospital

Chapter 13

Michael D. Klein, M.D.
Associate Professor of Medicine, Boston University
School of Medicine; Staff Cardiologist, University
Hospital, Boston

Chapter 32

Raymond S. Koff, M.D.
Associate Professor of Medicine, Boston University
School of Medicine; Chief, Hepatology Section,
Veterans Administration Hospital, Boston

Chapters 41, 43

Philip Kramer, M.D.
Professor of Medicine, Boston University School of
Medicine; Chief, Gastroenterology Section,
University Hospital, Boston

Chapters 37, 38

Simmons Lessell, M.D.
Professor of Ophthalmology, Neurology, and
Anatomy, Boston University School of Medicine;
Director, Department of Ophthalmology,
Boston City Hospital

Chapter 62

Robert M. Levin, M.D.
Associate Professor of Medicine, Boston University
School of Medicine; Associate Director, Boston City
Hospital Medical Service

Chapter 60

Paul A. Levine, M.D.
Assistant Professor of Medicine, Boston University
School of Medicine; Staff Cardiologist, University
Hospital, Boston

Chapter 32

Norman G. Levinsky, M.D.
Wade Professor and Chairman, Department of
Medicine, Boston University School of Medicine;
Physician-in-Chief, University Hospital, Boston

Chapters 53, 54

Christopher Longcope, M.D.
Associate Professor of Medicine and Director,
Endocrine Outpatient Clinic, Boston University
School of Medicine; Senior Scientist, Worcester
Foundation for Experimental Biology, Shrewsbury,
Massachusetts

Chapter 57

William R. McCabe, M.D.
Professor of Medicine and Microbiology, Boston
University School of Medicine; Chief, Infectious
Disease Section, University Hospital, Boston

Chapters 6, 8, 11, 39, 63

James C. Melby, M.D.
Professor of Medicine, Boston University School of
Medicine; Head, Section of Endocrinology and
Metabolism, University Hospital, Boston

Chapters 55, 56

Herbert Mescon, M.D.
Professor and Chairman, Department of Dermatology,
Boston University School of Medicine; Chief of
Dermatology, University Hospital, Boston

Chapter 5

Aaron Miller, M.D.
Associate Research Professor of Medicine, Boston
University School of Medicine; Chief of Hematology,
Veterans Administration Hospital, Boston

Chapter 48

Thomas A. O'Gorman, M.B., M.R.C.P.I.
Assistant Professor of Medicine, Boston University
School of Medicine; Research Fellow in Gastro-
enterology, Peter Bent Brigham Hospital, Boston

Chapter 35

Wlademir Pereira, M.D.
Assistant Professor of Medicine, Boston University
School of Medicine; Staff Physician, Pulmonary
Section, Veterans Administration Hospital, Boston

Chapters 10, 24

Burton J. Polansky, M.D.
Associate Professor of Medicine, Boston University
School of Medicine; Chief of Medicine and Cardiology,
Brockton Hospital, Brockton, Massachusetts

Chapter 29

Sander Robins, M.D.
Assistant Professor of Medicine, Boston University
School of Medicine; Assistant Chief, Gastroenterology
Section, Veterans Administration Hospital, Boston

Chapter 36

F. C. A. Romanul, M.D.
Professor of Neurology, Boston University School
of Medicine; Chief, Section of Neuropathology,
University Hospital, Boston

Chapter 62

Isadore N. Rosenberg, M.D.
Professor of Medicine, Boston University School of
Medicine; Chairman, Division of Medicine,
Framingham Union Hospital, Framingham,
Massachusetts

Chapter 58

Thomas J. Ryan, M.D.
Professor of Medicine, Boston University School of
Medicine; Chief, Cardiology Section, University
Hospital, Boston

Chapters 28, 30

Elihu M. Schimmel, M.D.
Associate Professor of Medicine, Boston University
School of Medicine; Chief, Gastroenterology
Section, Veterans Administration Hospital, Boston

Chapter 42

Stephen H. Schneider, M.D.
Thorndike Fellow in Endocrinology and Metabolism,
Boston University School of Medicine and Boston
City Hospital

Chapter 59

Charles J. Schwartz, M.D.
Assistant Professor of Medicine, Boston University
School of Medicine; formerly Director, Gastro-
intestinal Laboratory and Endoscopy Unit,
University Hospital, Boston

Chapters 37, 38

Donald M. Small, M.D.
Professor of Medicine and Biochemistry, Boston
University School of Medicine; Chief, Biophysics
Section and Visiting Physician, University Hospital
and Boston City Hospital

Chapter 40

Gordon L. Snider, M.D.
Professor of Medicine, Boston University School
of Medicine; Director of Pulmonary Medicine,
University Hospital, and Chief, Pulmonary
Section, Veterans Administration Hospital, Boston

Chapters 9, 13, 14, 20, 21, 22

Martin L. Spivack, M.D.
Associate Professor of Medicine, Boston University
School of Medicine; Chief, Infectious Disease
Section, Veterans Administration Hospital, Boston

Chapter 12

William P. Steffee, M.D., Ph.D.
Assistant Professor of Medicine, Boston University
School of Medicine; Director, Clinical Nutrition
Unit, University Hospital, Boston

Chapter 4

Albert L. Sullivan, M.D.
Assistant Professor of Medicine, Boston University
School of Medicine; Assistant Visiting Physician
and Hematologist, University Hospital, Boston

Chapter 51

Jacob Swartz, M.D.
Professor of Psychiatry and Associate Dean for
Admissions, Boston University School of Medicine;
Visiting Physician, University Hospital, Boston

Chapter 2

Lilia Talarico, M.D.
Assistant Professor of Medicine, Boston University
School of Medicine; Assistant Visiting Physician
and Hematologist, University Hospital, Boston

Chapter 52

Judith L. Vaitukaitis, M.D.
Professor of Medicine and Physiology, Boston
University School of Medicine; Chief, Section of
Endocrinology and Metabolism, Boston City
Hospital

Chapters 55, 57

Lewis R. Weintraub, M.D.
Associate Professor of Medicine, Boston University
School of Medicine; Chief, Hematology Section,
University Hospital, Boston

Chapter 47

Michael E. Whitcomb, M.D.
Assistant Professor of Medicine and Chief, Pulmonary
Section, Ohio State University School of Medicine,
Columbus; formerly Assistant Professor of Medicine,
Boston University School of Medicine, and Chief,
Pulmonary Section, University Hospital, Boston

Chapters 15, 18

Robert W. Wilkins, M.D.
Professor of Medicine (Emeritus), Boston University
School of Medicine; Consultant, University Hospital,
Boston

Chapter 1

Some General Considerations

1

Clinical
Internal Medicine

Robert W. Wilkins

Internal medicine offers the physician a wide choice of activities and contacts: He can practice, teach, or do research, either singly or together; he can enter administration, public health, or group practice; or he may select combinations of interests, duties, and locations that suit his background and training. Most internists settle on clinical practice, which requires a personal commitment to patients, responsibility for their care, and tolerance for their foibles. If the physician can accept these or, preferably, get positive satisfaction from them, he is well suited for the life of a clinician.

Functions of the Clinician

DIAGNOSIS

The three traditional functions of the clinician are diagnosis, prognosis, and treatment. Diagnosis is the most honored; to be confirmed in a difficult diagnosis is one of the great satisfactions in clinical medicine. Diagnosis requires knowledge and skill, persistence and thoroughness, and above all, an open mind. "Once thought of, the diagnosis was easy" is a cliché, but the greatest source of error is a wrong mental set, established on initial impression or superficial evidence.

Students may be impressed by the way an experienced clinician "senses" a new case. There is nothing mysterious about the process, although often it is so automatic as to be almost unconscious. It requires the acquisition and the mental and written notation of every available scrap of information about a patient. This gathering of data may begin even before the patient is seen, when he first calls on the telephone or walks down the corridor to the office. The good clinician is interested in the pitch and timbre of the voice, the choice of words and expressions, the slap of the gait. On first seeing the patient, he notes for future reference the patient's apparent age, race, coloring, posture and carriage, state of consciousness and attention, degree and nature of discomfort, and the like. These become the basis for

the questions to be asked in the history-taking interview.

Obviously, it is necessary to obtain an accurate history, skillfully elicited, carefully interpreted, and critically evaluated. A good history is usually more valuable in diagnosis than the physical examination or even than extensive laboratory studies. Young physicians, however, especially those recently in academic hospitals, tend too often to reverse the relative importance of these diagnostic procedures.

The value of the history is proportional to its accuracy and completeness. While every physician knows this, not every physician is able and willing to obtain a correct, detailed account. Too often the excuse is made, "The patient is a poor historian," when in fact the physician is at fault. In questioning a patient, the physician must accomplish two objectives: (1) convince the patient of the importance and relevance of the questions being asked, and (2) establish the complete sequence of events leading up to the present illness. The physician begins with the circumstances and details of the chief complaint — these are what the patient wants to discuss first, and the physician must concern himself with them even when other more serious problems may be apparent.

The skilled doctor quickly gains the patient's confidence, while at the same time making an appraisal of the patient's reliability. He does not necessarily believe all the patient says, and he is alert to what the patient may be trying to conceal. However, he recognizes that a patient may simply have forgotten many details of the history and may be able to recall them if repeatedly pressed for them, sometimes with the family's help.

As the history-taking proceeds, the doctor begins to formulate tentative ideas about the diagnosis. These ideas should be merely possibilities to be explored, and if not confirmed, set aside. The good diagnostician does not play hunches or jump to conclusions that might set up a mental block. Since he cannot follow every lead and order every conceivable laboratory test and diagnostic procedure, the physician should formulate a plan based upon the more plausible hypotheses.

In terms of the diagnosis, one of the most helpful features of any disease is the evolution of its course.

3

While an occasional case may be diagnosed at first sight, most are not so diagnosed but become clarified only as the course of the disease unfolds. Therefore, repeated interviews, laboratory studies, and clinical observations have to be made until the correct diagnosis is apparent. Time charts and diagrams depicting the waxing and waning of symptoms, signs, and laboratory findings help enormously in this process, not only in dramatizing and clarifying the disease, but also in assuring thoroughness and careful attention to detail.

The superior diagnostician is always thorough. It has been said, "The skilled consultant does a rectal"; this means that he does personally whatever another busy doctor may have neglected to do. He also asks questions that may have been forgotten, such as "Have you been in a foreign country?" and "Have you worked in an industrial plant?" The expert takes the time and trouble to look for obscure clues; he is meticulously thorough.

PROGNOSIS

The second duty of the clinician is to give a prognosis. The patient is entitled to know not only what ails him, but also what it is liable to do to him. When a doctor does not know the diagnosis or the prognosis, he should say so honestly, and ask for more time or the help of a consultant. No physician loses the respect of his patient by saying, "I don't know, but I'll try to find out."

Some knowledge of statistics is often helpful in making a prognosis, even though a given patient may defy statistics. In explaining the risks, for example, of an operation, the doctor may say, "Now if we took 100 cases like yours, 95 (or whatever the percentage might be) would recover." But statistics on the relation of factors such as age, sex, and race to prognosis do not account for many other variations among patients, much less for important factors such as complications, prior illnesses, essential vigor, and the will to live.

The importance of a prognosis to the patient is often overlooked, particularly by someone who has never been very ill himself. Patients often fear the worst and need to hear a doctor express hope, if not confidence that they will recover. It is not only the possibility of dying that concerns patients (often they ignore or deny that), but also the burden on the family, the financial costs, or the disruption of home life or of business that a period of invalidism would entail. The physician should therefore advise the patient and the family as tactfully and as wisely as he can, so that they can prepare for what is to come. He should also reassure the patient who is afraid that he cannot stand up to suffering and disability that he will be able to do so with the doctor's help.

TREATMENT

More effective therapeutic agents have been developed in this century than in all times past. Insulin, vitamins, antibiotics, and antihypertensives are some of the drugs that have revolutionized medical care. But we are still in the early stages of the development of scientific therapy; not even the surface has been scratched in some critical fields, such as cancer and atherosclerosis, because we still do not know enough about the basic causes of health and disease. As a result, only a few treatments bring about cure; many effective treatments are palliatives to be continued, often indefinitely.

There is an ancient device that is still effective therapeutically — the use of the physician himself. Patients really mean it when they say, "It makes me feel better just to talk to you, Doctor." In this connection it is important for the patient to do most of the talking while the physician listens attentively and sympathetically. The positive and the negative powers of suggestion have been scientifically demonstrated in numerous double-blind studies of drugs and placebos. Most physicians are fully aware that a blank pill given with the suggestion that it will be helpful will have statistically significant beneficial effects. However, they are not as aware that even a strong medication given with the suggestion that it will have no effect, or the opposite effect, will indeed often have the suggested action. Therefore, the physician should never assume a flat or negative attitude about treatment. To tell a patient, "Nothing can be done for you" is not only cruel, it is false. Something can always be done: The physician can use cheerfulness, hope, and reassurance as positive therapeutic agents.

Suggestion is the most common form of psychotherapy. Psychiatrists readily admit that generalists and internists can and should do most of the counseling and psychotherapy for the patients in their practices. Psychotherapy requires listening to the patient in an unhurried, interested, and optimistic manner; asking questions that indicate a sincere and intelligent understanding; and offering reassurance. Reassurance is given more by one's manner than by one's words, and expressions of encouragement and confidence are better than complicated explanations. Provided it is used to supplement modern scientific drugs and procedures, supportive psychotherapy makes the physician maximally effective in treatment (see the chapter on Medical Care and the Emotional Life of the Patient).

The Doctor-Patient Relationship
The attitude of the physician toward his patients should be one of polite and friendly concern. As a professional man he should maintain decorum and not engage in excessive familiarity. His interest should be primarily intellectual, objective, and calm. He should never become deeply involved emotionally with the patient, which would cloud his judgment and could lead to intolerable pressures. Nor should he accept as patients persons with whom he is already emotionally involved. These include the doctor's own family, relatives, and close friends.

The physician's fee has both a therapeutic and a protective value: It ensures the maintenance of a professional relationship, obligating the doctor to the patient financially; it also symbolizes the value of the physician's services. The considerate physician will discuss his fees with his patients, either when they ask for an appointment or at the beginning of the first visit. The amount should be and usually is determined by local custom, with allowances for the patient's financial circumstances. When fees are questioned, they should be explained and they should be moderated if they cause hardship. More and more

physicians are insisting on paying fees for their own and their families' medical care and are buying insurance so that their colleagues will accept such payments.

The Patient's Family
Physicians are familiar with "hospitalization neuroses," in which patients become so dependent on the hospital and its personnel that they must be literally pushed out. The same basic neurosis can occur at home. Physicians should be tolerant in this situation, and they should not upbraid or even criticize the patient but rather should encourage and praise any progress, remembering that invalidism is insidious, particularly when an insurance company is paying the bills. The family of such a patient may need special attention. The overtired, anxious housewife may require a sedative, or the whole family may have to be relieved by moving the patient temporarily out of the home. The doctor should allay any guilt the family members may feel about this, and keep them fully informed, particularly if the patient is in danger of dying; this will prepare the family for the blow, and also will enable them to make any religious arrangements they wish.

When a patient dies, the physician must pronounce him dead. There need be no hurry about this, and the physician should be sure. Above all, he must never make a remark in the patient's presence, even if he believes the patient to be dead (or unconscious), that he would not make if the patient were fully conscious. The doctor must inform the family; he does so gently, offering such comfort as he can. As soon as he tactfully can, he should request permission for a postmortem examination. He should explain to the family the value of knowing whether or not any familial or contagious disease was present.

Good physicians do not attempt to preserve life at any and all cost of pain, grief, and money. Modern techniques of maintaining respiration and circulation in an otherwise "dead" body make it necessary to redefine death. Doctors should help lawyers, ministers, and other public leaders to face the difficult decisions involved.

Health Conservation

Another function of medicine, but one often neglected by practitioners, is the prevention of disease,
that is, the conservation of health. Barely touched
upon in many medical schools, this subject may be
neglected in the training of interns and residents
unless the hospital arranges for them to follow
patients on an extended ambulatory basis. Social,
economic, and geographic factors are all important
in maintaining health in a community. Lately, political interests have become involved in health care,
creating numerous problems for the medical profession. Physicians today must concern themselves with
chronic care of the old and young, with periodic
health examinations, and with the prevention of disease. They must look at the costs as well as the values
of various health services, and at new ways of providing them. Physicians are becoming less afraid of the
old clichés against "socialized medicine."

The Profession

Internal medicine is an honorable and proud profession. It imposes obligations upon its members to
behave ethically toward both patients and colleagues.
In the simple words of the golden rule, ethical behavior means doing to others as you would have them do
to you. If, in spite of trying to live by this rule, one
offends a colleague, one should apologize voluntarily
and not wait for the colleague to demand an explanation. On the other hand, the physician should not
be too sensitive, and certainly not paranoid about
slights or insults from his colleagues; they are among
his best friends, and he should take every opportunity
to exchange favors and ideas with them. The good
physician welcomes consultations; when he is not
sure of himself, he requests a consultant, realizing
that both he and the patient may benefit. Even when
he is quite sure of himself, the good physician is
happy to have a consultant if the patient wants one.
The safe physician is not the one who is always sure
of himself, but the one who asks for help when he
is not.

Continuing Education

The clinician learns from his cases because he lives by
them, studies for them, reviews the literature relating

to them, attends meetings to learn more about them,
discusses them with his colleagues, and publishes
reports on them. The clinician's practice stimulates
him to continue to educate himself. The best self-
educational device I know is the file of a busy
generalist who keeps careful records on the diagnosis,
laboratory data, clinical course, and relevant published articles on each case in his practice. Most
doctors have files of journals and reprints; the difficult thing is to find time to read them. One way is to
set aside a regular time every day (at breakfast, for
instance) for such reading.

No physician can know it all today; no one can be
an authority on every medical subject. Nonetheless,
all can learn and all can teach. Modern medical education should be continual, mutual, and reciprocal.
It is done best in a teaching hospital, where all diagnoses are questioned daily and treatments are frequently modified. It takes both courage and humility
for the established practitioner to do this, but it pays
great rewards. A doctor who is never checked on may
be dangerous — at best he becomes out of date; also
he loses much of the enjoyment of medicine, that
which comes from learning more and more about it.

But a physician should know more than medicine.
As a highly educated man he should be well informed
on many subjects, such as literature, arts, music,
public affairs, and politics. Osler's habit of doing
"outside reading" in bed is a good one; it takes one's
mind off the day's work and prepares one for restful
sleep. Practiced a few minutes every night, it also
provides an astonishing amount of information and
pleasure.

Diversion

Every physician needs to "get away" regularly. He
deserves the equivalent of at least one full day off a
week. In that time he should do only what is completely recreational, in the sense that it "re-creates"
him. It may, but need not have considerations of
usefulness, and it should be what he truly enjoys and
gives him peace. Fishing, golf, tennis, sailing, and
other sports are the obvious hobbies, but if one likes
to work with his hands, he can do tinkering, painting,
sculpture, carpentry, or gardening. If outside reading
is a hobby, he may collect books; or he may prefer

antiques, art, records, stamps, rocks, or anything that fascinates him. He may want to get away from people entirely on his days off, or he may wish to see different people in different relationships. If he has talents in civic affairs or in politics, he may get satisfaction from participating or leading in these areas. Physicians always have been and presumably always will be leading citizens. As such, they should play active roles in the welfare of their communities.

2

Medical Care and the Emotional Life of the Patient

Jacob Swartz and Paul Kaufman

Physicians are concerned for the most part with the care of patients who are ill. Therefore they may overlook the normative, homeostatic, and adaptive devices that all people use in coping with life, particularly psychological life. Physicians need a basic background knowledge of personality development in order to understand the emotional and psychological problems of their patients.

General Considerations of Personality Development

The development of human personality is complex and varied, and the significance of many of its determinants is not completely known. Constitutional and biologic elements, internally engendered instincts and drives, environmental factors, and historical realities all exert powerful influences. Equally important in determining later adaptations are the early experiences of the individual in the nuclear or surrogate family. It is likely that the paradigm for all future interpersonal relationships is dependent on the extent to which the child develops a confident, trusting, and loving relationship with confident, trusting, and loving parents. This fact is crucial in understanding a patient's responses to illness and health; it is also crucial in understanding the responses of the patient to the physician, and, indeed, in understanding the responses of the physician to the patient as well.

Growth and development involve conflicts between the gratification of one's own instincts, drives, wishes, and needs on the one hand, and, on the other, the wishes, needs, and demands of other people and society. A simple example of the conflict between personal wishes and societal requirements is the toilet training of the child. Children can be observed to take a good deal of pleasure and pride in the waste products of their bodies. However, society, through the family, requires that the child take the wishes of others into account and perform these functions in a particular place and a particular time. No matter

how enlightened and considerate toilet training is — as indeed it should be — it is nevertheless alien to the "natural" wishes of the child. The child acquiesces in order to retain the approval and love of the parent. Nevertheless, later attitudes concerning autonomy, response to authority, and feelings about one's own body have important roots in such issues.

We do not experience instincts directly, and in fact the mediation that goes on between our internal wishes and external reality is frequently not known to us — at least not directly — but forms in concert a large and important aspect of mental functioning that is termed the *unconscious*. The term *ego* has been applied to the great mediator of the personality, and although its adaptive functions will be emphasized here, it does in fact serve many other functions. Motility, perception, intellectual functions, perception of self, and certain derivative aspects of what comes to be known as conscience are all ego functions. It is particularly important to understand that the ego is also the great agency of compromise within the personality. It is the ego that unconsciously arranges compromises between instinctual expression, demands of conscience, and requirements of reality. Often enough, these compromises are effective, but in some instances the best compromise that the personality can achieve leads to symptom formation, as in hysterical conversion or obsessional thinking, or in the expression of conflicts through physical illness. For the most part the mediating and adaptive functions of the ego become automatic and repetitive and result in set patterns of behavior that characterize the way one deals with work, friends, problems, successes, and failures. Maladaptive responses are known as *neuroses* and *personality disorders*. The most grave instances of serious personality disorganization are the *psychoses,* in which major distortions of reality occur. However, adaptive responses by and large go unnoticed because they are the means by which people cope with their daily lives. If it is not already clear, it might be well to state specifically that although the major foundations for psychological development are laid in infancy and childhood, growth and adaptation are lifelong psychological processes and are by no means either completed or ended during the early years.

ADAPTATION AND THE LIFE CYCLE

The human personality passes through successive phases of development, and although the various milestones of infancy, childhood, latency, and adolescence are of central importance, the maturational epochs of postadolescent life are no less significant. Some of these postadolescent phases will now be discussed.

Work

Both the significance of work and one's adaptation to the work situation are important to most people. For those who work in an area related to their own major interests, work is both an important source of self-esteem and an important means of self-expression. Unhappily for many people, this is not always true, but they do get from work the satisfaction of being independent, having a sense of accomplishment, or of supporting oneself and one's family. The work situation itself typically involves relationships with others, including superiors, fellow employees, and subordinates for whose work one is responsible. The response of an individual to each of these relationships tends to be repetitive of earlier relationships. Thus, one person gets along poorly with his employer because he is constantly rebelling against authority and so is angry or hostile. Another person may be anxious, fearful, or overly submissive. Relationships with fellow employees tend to repeat former sibling and peer relationships, so that some people are intensely competitive, others feel constantly cheated, while still others assume a protective attitude. Some people in positions of authority are excessively demanding and critical; others are not firm enough. Thus there is a great variety of possible responses to the work situation, and indeed some people seem to have little or no stress at work. The physician who is aware that work requires a new mode of adaptation and who has some understanding of the personality of the patient and of the typical modes of response to work can be helpful when the patient takes a new job or has difficulties in the current work situation. Furthermore, concern or dissatisfaction with work may be manifested in bodily complaints such as tachycardia, palpitation, excessive fatigue, or insomnia, as well as in excessive alcoholic intake. A patient's work may be of concern in yet another way to a physician who is asked to determine whether or not the patient can work or should return to work after an illness.

Early Adult Life

Another phase of the life cycle with far-reaching implications for happiness and unhappiness or for illness and health is the time when a person chooses a mate and decides to establish a family. The choice of a spouse is determined both by conscious factors such as mutual attraction and interests, and by various unconscious factors, present and past. In order to establish a lasting relationship, a man must be sufficiently free of attachment to his mother so that the feelings that flow from that early relationship can appropriately be invested in another female. Similarly, the woman must be sufficiently free of attachment to her father to be able to establish an enduring relationship to a male peer. This time of life can be very stressful, and a number of relationships may be tested before the definitive relationship is established. The disruptions of such close relationships may be painful and may be accompanied by loss of self-esteem and other unpleasant effects. The very process of making a decision may itself produce stress and may come to the physician's attention through symptoms or complaints such as anxiety, inability to make decisions, fears of inadequacy or of sickness, or a sudden, sometimes inexplicable attraction to still another person when the decision has already been made.

Marriage and family life present the necessity for another series of adaptations, namely, to the realities of living together and the daily give and take. Although sexual problems are a feature of some unhappy marriages, such problems are not at all uncommon in marriages that otherwise appear to be harmonious. Certainly the rearing of children is a maturational task that brings both gratification and stress. Assumption of the role of parent is particularly significant because the parent is now confronted through the child with a repetition of earlier relationships to parents and siblings and a revival of the memories, feelings, and conflicts of childhood. Neither the new father nor the new mother can effectively undertake this responsibility if either has the feeling that he or she is still a child who cannot deal with a helpless, dependent infant. The physician who understands these adaptational tasks is neither surprised nor dismayed by them and views the responses of the patient as taking place on a continuum of personality development in which the patient will do more or less well. The physician will recognize the patient's verbalized or nonverbalized concerns about daily marital living and will assist the patient to cope with them.

Midlife

For our purposes, midlife can be considered as the time when the pressures of child rearing have somewhat lessened. The children are now young adults, at various stages of independence and separation from the family. For the wife and mother who has not previously sought full-time employment outside the home, this is a period when she may do so, or she may return to previous creative interests that may have been carried on part time or suspended. For men and women whose work or careers outside the home are major activities, this is usually the time of life when the highest levels of employment or promotion are reached and when considerable satisfactions of status and recognition may be achieved. By the same token, this is also a time when there are particular vulnerabilities. The nature and degree of vulnerability will be dependent on earlier experiences and previously established repetitive patterns. At this time many people face the reality that further advancement, promotion, or reward in some form will not be forthcoming. There are numerous other potential sources of disappointment or loss: Parents or older family members may be lost through illness and death; grown children leave home for school or work, or to establish families of their own. Although these events may bring some compensations, they may also cause feelings of separation and emptiness. Parents are particularly vulnerable when they have had certain conscious or unconscious expectations — particularly unrealistic expectations — of how their children would turn out, the kind of work they would do, and the kind of people they would marry.

Specifically for women, at this time of life there is a gradual cessation of the reproductive function

with the physiologic and psychological events that comprise the menopause. Women whose feelings about themselves are significantly invested in physical attractiveness may find the menopause difficult. Certainly the physician can be exceedingly helpful in explaining that menopause does not have an adverse effect on sexual responsiveness and that, in fact, with the children leaving home, there are opportunities for the renewal of intimacy and closeness.

Although no clear and identifiable events can be called menopause in men, the "midlife syndrome" is no less common. Men who have put great store in physical attractiveness or physical strength are vulnerable as the years leave their mark. Some men attempt to deny or to ward off recognition of the passage of time by an increased competitiveness with younger men or attempts at self-reassurance about sexual potency by a series of affairs. Another variant of the same theme for both men and women is a regression to immature and inappropriate behavior in the mistaken view that one can in that way be young again. Not uncommonly, depressive feelings are experienced in response to lessened vigor or to a disappointment. Some patients may displace these feelings by having a disability, illness, or accident that inexplicably does not become resolved but leaves the patient with what is viewed as an incapacity attributable to external or physical causes.

Another midlife crisis is the issue of retirement for those who have been employed full time outside the home and for whom work is and has been the central theme of life. Enforced retirement because of age is particularly difficult because age does not necessarily reflect one's vigor or capacity for work. Certainly the physician can be extraordinarily helpful in preparing patients for retirement because, even under the best of circumstances, there tend to be feelings of loss of status or strength, of being discarded, and of being unwanted. It is likely that physicians will have to make a special effort to understand feelings about retirement because what physicians call retirement for themselves usually means a shift to another aspect of the profession. This is not the case with retirement in industry or from other careers, so that the feelings that physicians have about retirement are not necessarily those generally felt by others.

Aging

The process of aging and one's responses to it involve a complex set of both sociocultural and individual factors. Ours is a youth-oriented society in which, despite some changing attitudes, the aged are not viewed in a particularly attractive light. Older people are generally viewed as ill, dependent, physically unattractive, and somehow different in their needs and aspirations from younger people. In fact, the aged, like the young, wish to be well regarded, want a continuation of established relationships and opportunities to establish new ones, and wish to be listened to and respected as worthwhile individuals. The anatomic and physiologic changes of age cannot be denied, but the responses to these changes as well as to the inevitable losses of family and friends tend to be dealt with in the same ways a person has used as adaptive and coping responses during his earlier life. It has been said appropriately that the older person is not different from what he or she was as a younger person but rather is more as he was. Illness and a greater dependency on younger members of the family, or on society if family support is not available, do indeed occur. However, this is not characteristic of all old people, and it is likewise a myth that the aged are typically neglected and abandoned by their families. Families are particularly troubled and have feelings of guilt when their older family members cannot be cared for at home because of problems of psychological or physical ill health. The physician is frequently asked for assistance in weighing the realities involved in such a decision.

Death

Finally, of course, there is the matter of death. In a sense it is inappropriate to discuss "adaptation" to death, because we have no awareness of our own death. Most human beings make life tolerable simply because they have an element of denial concerning personal death. That is not to say that attitudes about death do not need changing for, just as with aging, such changes are slowly taking place. Our whole culture, however, denies death; in particular, it avoids viewing death as the final phase of the life cycle. Death therefore is invariably attributed to external causes, which is true in a way, but it is more

true that death is an inevitable part of the biologic process of evolution. Although the physician cannot change attitudes toward death, either those of the individual patient or of the family, when death is imminent or takes place, the physician's task remains one of helping the patient to cope with it. This task includes keeping anxiety, discomfort, and pain at tolerable levels and making the end of life as dignified as the circumstances will permit.

Personality Assessment

THE INTERVIEW

The interview conducted by a physician is a traditional part of the doctor-patient relationship and serves a variety of purposes, some of which are more apparent to both participants than others. Although the giving of information by the patient in response to the physician's specific queries is an important aspect of the interview procedure, it would be simplistic to regard this as the only feature of the interview, or even in many instances as the most important part of it.

The fact that the interview serves many functions simultaneously requires the physician to be well versed in its various uses and meanings if its full benefits are to be derived and possible harm to the doctor-patient relationship averted. Much of what the patient remembers and reacts to in the encounter with the physician centers around the interview, which is broadly defined to include all verbal and nonverbal communications. Thus one important consideration in the initial interview or history-taking procedure is that the groundwork for the future doctor-patient relationship is being established.

Patients vary enormously in their previous experiences with helping figures, including parents and physicians; these experiences influence the patient's expectations regarding the physician. The physician cannot assume that a trusting relationship will develop spontaneously. The patient's present attitudes and feelings, as well as past experiences, especially medical experiences, will need to be assessed if impediments are to be understood adequately and removed.

Another goal of the initial interview is the establishment of an atmosphere in which the patient can tell the physician things that are difficult to talk about but that are of great concern to the patient, and often are essential for the doctor's diagnosis and management. Fear, guilt, shame, and embarrassment are some of the feelings that can inhibit the patient. Frightening fantasies surrounding certain symptoms, such as unusual bleeding, for example, can result in denial, in which the patient fails to mention the symptom with the childish idea that if the doctor does not know, or if nothing is noted or said, then all will be well. The extent to which the physician can help the patient regard him as nonjudgmental, genuinely listening, and interested — but without undue investment in only learning relevant facts, will dictate the patient's capacity to tell the physician even what he most fears. It is useful for the physician to treat all revelations with an evenhanded interest and concern, with no special emphasis or reaction that might unduly influence the patient as he talks about himself.

The interview may also serve to convey information from the doctor to the patient, but this depends on the doctor-patient relationship in terms of mutual trust, the doctor's recognition and management of the patient's anxiety, and a correct assessment of the patient's adaptive modes and patterns of behavior. All these factors can influence what the patient hears and understands the doctor to say, and thereby how he will participate in the doctor's diagnostic and therapeutic procedures. Thus, if the doctor-patient interaction is good, the interview can provide considerable benefit; it can alleviate anxiety and allow the patient to function at a more mature level.

The interview will also affect whether the patient will convey new information to the doctor both as it is remembered and as it develops during the course of an illness and its management. Feelings of awe or fear of the doctor can inhibit the patient; failure by the doctor to recognize the patient's assets and accomplishments sufficiently can aggravate the regressive tendencies that are present in all seriously ill persons and can result in inappropriately clinging behavior by the patient.

The interview should be conducted so that patients can convey even their fantasies about their conditions. The often unrealistic ideas of patients about the meanings and implications as well as the causes of illness can affect the subsequent course of the doctor-patient relationship and the degree of recovery, if, for example, illness is fantasized as a deserved punishment. Compliance in taking medications, accepting referrals for surgery, or participating in painful and frightening diagnostic procedures is influenced by the patient's ideas, which, because they may be frightening, embarrassing, or even childish, are often not expressed openly by the patient, especially if the physician seems disinterested. Meaningful reassurance of patients requires knowledge of their often unspoken and at times relatively unformulated imaginings that underlie their more adult, directly expressed ideas and thoughts. Reassuring comments, therefore, can often fail in their intent, if the patient does not tell the doctor what is really feared and when the doctor therefore does not know about these fears and cannot give the patient appropriate reassurance.

A physician ought to develop an understanding of the patient's characteristic patterns of behavior and prior modes of adaptation, especially when under stress. The characteristic defenses and actions used by the patient to minimize anxiety and fear will aid in predicting reactions to new and possibly frightening developments. Not only the types of relationships that the patient has found most supportive in the past, but also those that have created most difficulty, will be of special interest to the physician. An important supplement to historical data is an accurate observation of the patient's emotional response to the physician himself; this observation serves as a portent of future relationships with physicians and others.

Mental Status
As the physician listens to the patient, he also conducts a mental status examination. This examination is performed almost entirely during the routine history-taking procedure, and only incidentally through a separate, formal set of questions. Quite detailed determinations of intellectual ability, orientation, and memory can be made simply as part of the inquiry about the patient's present illness and life history. In addition to noting the usual categories of behavior — orientation, perceptual and cognitive

function, emotional response, and thought content — the doctor observes how the patient reports information about his problems. Avoidance, embarrassment, or agitation can indicate areas of conflict, areas of special concern or anxiety, and even areas too frightening for the patient to mention.

Techniques

Interviews may be conducted in a variety of settings, some by choice and some by necessity, as at the bedside in a busy ward. In any setting, the fundamental principle is that the physician devote himself entirely to the patient during the time of the interview. Actions such as drawing the curtains and making certain that both participants are physically as comfortable as possible and able to hear each other, that interruptions will not occur, and that both participants have been adequately identified to each other by name and role are all necessary in creating an atmosphere of trust. The professional and unique nature of the transaction is reassuring to the patient and is underlined by attention to such details.

The purpose of the interview should be made clear to the patient, who may not be certain what to expect. The interviewer should help the patient start talking about what he feels is uppermost and most pressing. An attempt to elicit information in a preconceived order will often get the interview off to a bad start, because the patient may quickly decide that the physician does not really want to hear his most important concerns. Therefore, one should begin the interview with the broadest, least directive queries, which are designed to facilitate the patient's confidence that he can say anything and that he will be listened to with interest. Such open-ended or relatively nondirective questioning also protects the physician against premature conclusions derived from intuition or hunches developed before all the information is available. Patients can be directed to a remarkable degree to give a history that fits whatever condition the interviewer may have prematurely diagnosed. In any area, questions should be utilized to allow the freest possible response. For example, when the physician becomes interested in learning about the patient's past relationships with other physicians, rather than asking something like "Did you

get along well with your previous doctor?" which both suggests to the patient that he is being asked for a value judgment and also may carry with it a somewhat authoritarian air requiring a conditioned response, a better question might be, "What has your experience been with physicians?"

The associational pattern — the relationship of one group of thoughts and verbalizations to the next as the patient speaks spontaneously — can often provide clues about areas of conflict, misconception, and characteristic responses to anxiety. The detection of the patient's preoccupations as manifested by unusual thought content, formal thought disorder, and even underlying disorganization can often be facilitated by the encouragement of spontaneous speech and the avoidance of questions that can be answered with one or two words or a phrase, especially early in the interview. As the interview progresses the questions may become increasingly specific and directive, and the interviewer begins to make hypotheses to be tested.

Patients may need encouragement to speak freely. The best encouragement is evidence that the interviewer is listening carefully and with interest. Occasional paraphrases of what the patient is saying or requests for clarification indicate to the patient that active listening is occurring.

Empathy

Empathy is a critical tool in the interview. The physician attempts to place himself in the patient's position, to feel what the patient feels, to experience the same circumstances; if a physician is successful at this, the patient will feel understood and the physician will have a better idea of how to be helpful in psychologically supporting the patient. The ability to follow the affective thread and to confront the patient gently with the important feelings being elaborated will also help the patient speak more freely and develop a sense of being heard. Summary statements should be made at natural shifts in the interview and the patient should be invited to make additions or corrections.

Interview Behavior

The behavior of the interviewer can either facilitate or inhibit the flow of the interview. Looking the patient directly in the eye, avoiding distracting mannerisms, and occasionally nodding or saying "aha" are useful and necessary. The taking of notes is a somewhat controversial item; many physicians feel that note taking should be kept to a minimum, as for example, the occasional jotting down of material that might otherwise be forgotten. What is to be avoided is giving the patient the impression that he or she is merely dictating to someone who is writing down each word rather than someone who is listening thoughtfully and carefully, trying to understand the meaning of what is said, and responding in a nonjudgmental, interested way. With practice, the interviewer learns to exert a gentle pressure on the patient that can help the patient to say what needs to be said and to experience the relief and alleviation of anxiety that usually accompanies the feeling of having really told a potentially helpful person things that are most upsetting and frightening.

Illness and Hospitalization

THE PSYCHOSOMATIC POINT OF VIEW
It is unlikely that any medical student or any prospective internist will be unfamiliar with the discussion that is to follow; rather the hazard is that the material may be thought of as so familiar that the physician need not attend to it. Most patients seek a physician who is grounded in basic science, skilled in scientific diagnostic skills, knowledgeable about the old and the new in therapeutics, and in addition is compassionate and knowledgeable about human beings. The psychosomatic point of view in medicine, while in some ways as old as medicine itself, nevertheless has come to represent over the past few decades the idea that physiologic and emotional responses are not disparate, but rather are part of the total response of the human organism to stress, be it internal or external in origin.

Some psychosomatic phenomena are simple and well known, such as the tachycardia of fright or excitement, the blush of embarrassment. More complex are the psychosomatic propositions that in many instances disease does not have a single cause, but that a multiplicity of factors enter into the circumstances under which a patient will develop symptoms,

consider himself to be ill, and be viewed as ill by others. Angina pectoris and myocardial infarction are certainly disorders in which the pathologic physiology has been repeatedly demonstrated. At the same time the frequency of these disorders is higher in patients with a certain constitutional background, a certain type of bodily configuration, and a certain emotional style with which they approach the tasks of everyday life. Still another aspect of psychosomatic medicine refers to specific disease entities such as peptic ulcer, bronchial asthma, and ulcerative colitis in which psychological and physiologic factors are frequently inextricably bound together.

Whereas issues of etiology continue to be complex, the concept of loss or the threat of loss is held to be more and more important in the setting in which patients develop physical illness. Grief itself, the most commonly experienced response to a loss that takes place in reality, is accompanied by physical symptomatology. Prolonged grief that has been poorly resolved and feelings of having been beaten or having given up in life, of having reached a dead end, or of having losses that are less obvious to others but that nonetheless symbolize loss of personal status, competence, or respect have all been implicated in the circumstances in which diseases such as ulcerative colitis and rheumatoid arthritis, among others, begin or become exacerbated.

ACUTE ILLNESS
Reactions to illness vary with both the past personal experience of the patient and the nature of the illness. Anxiety that is minimal on the occasion of routine visits to the physician increases when there are worrisome diagnostic problems or illnesses that raise the possibility of pain, disability, or threat to life. The degree of anxiety and the manner in which it is handled will depend on childhood experiences with illness, the specific meaning of illness to the patient, and the total personality structure of the patient. In some instances the mechanism of denial is prominent, as evidenced by the continuation of a taxing work schedule, smoking, and overeating in the face of a myocardial infarction.

It is helpful to recall the usual response when a child becomes ill. There is concern, the child becomes for that period of time the focus of parental attention, performance of his usual tasks is waived, special privileges may be granted, inducements are offered for cooperation in the medical regimen and, in sum, were it not for the discomforts of the illness, a climate of gratification and solicitude prevails. This is not to say that it should be otherwise; it is only to clarify some aspects of the adult response to illness. Some regression takes place during illness in the adult as a side effect of the bed rest, medication, diet, and interruption of daily routine that is prescribed. The adult has to have the capacity to accept this regression and not to feel particularly disturbed because it is reminiscent of childhood. It is in instances of family conflicts, dissatisfaction with work, or interpersonal difficulties of one kind or another that the dependency and gratification of illness may be unconsciously sought as a solution to conflict. Perhaps it is an expression of the patient's hostility when an illness is prolonged or when a puzzling disability ensues that is inconsistent with the physical findings. In other instances, issues of litigation or compensation may be involved. All in all, these instances illustrate the phenomenon of secondary gain from illness. It must be understood that these phenomena are not conscious or deliberate on the part of the patient, so that for the physician to respond with anger or retaliation toward the patient is neither appropriate nor helpful. The sources of conflict must be identified in discussions with the patient; then in a manner that is not accusatory, but tactful and firm, the patient is encouraged to resume activity.

For other patients illness has quite another meaning. Their childhood experiences may not have been in any way like those previously described; rather illness in such instances may have been equated with punishment for wrongdoing, or it may have been seen as weakness or merely as something painful or shameful. Under such circumstances illness in the adult will evoke feelings of shame, guilt, or fear of punishment.

CHRONIC ILLNESS
There are differences in the responses of patients to acute illness, just described, and the responses to chronic illness. Chronic illness confronts both physician and patient with a situation for which there is

no definitive cure and in which symptoms or disability may persist indefinitely. The attitudes and the feelings of the physician are important in the management of such patients. It is with such patients that the physician's wish to be helpful is often frustrated. Furthermore, with many illnesses it is not possible to keep the patient from taking a downhill course; this causes discouragement on the part of both patient and physician. Under these circumstances the physician has to accept the limitations in his capacity to be definitively helpful and the chronicity of the patient's symptoms, illness, and disability. Optimal management of chronic illness certainly requires attempts at alleviation of discomfort, but it also requires that the climate of care be such that the patient will utilize his strengths and capabilities to the fullest degree so that problems of excessive dependency either on the physician or on the family are minimized.

PROBLEMS OF HOSPITALIZATION
Hospitalization adds a new dimension to the patient's concerns. Again, it is well for the physician to keep in mind that the hospital and hospitalization have different meanings for physician and patient. To the physician the hospital is a familiar place where he is known and feels comfortable; it certainly does not frighten him. The patient may have had previous unpleasant hospital experiences, and even if not, he associates hospitals with serious illness, absence from work and home, expense, a large number of medical personnel, and an equally large number of poorly understood procedures. The regression that usually takes place to some extent in the face of illness can be expected to be even more pronounced in the hospital. No matter how careful are the efforts to avoid it, the hospital setting fosters dependency, and patients have differing responses to it. Some patients become more demanding than usual, and the infantile sources of their verbalizations and actions are not hard to discern. They make excessive demands or insist upon attention when there may be other priorities for the personnel; they may demand excessive medication. Such patients can be so irritating that they militate against their own best interests. Conversely, some patients are angry, hostile, and dissatis-

fied about almost everything that goes on in the hospital. Basically both the dependent behavior and the hostile behavior are manifestations of the patient's anxiety. The hospital situation stirs up long-standing conflicts about dependence and independence, about activity and passivity. For the hostile patient who feels that he is being pushed around, ways can be found to help him be more active in the decisions made about him. Choices should be explained and offered to the patient whenever possible, and certainly about such matters as selection of diet, requirements about going to sleep, and continuation of mental work in the hospital.

Threat of Death and Dying

Among the most trying tasks with which the physician is confronted is that of dealing with the feelings and reactions of the patient in whom a diagnosis of a fatal disease is first suspected or later established. The threat of death is frightening to the patient and distressing for the physician. Under few circumstances is it more important that the physician have an understanding of the patient's personality and therefore some idea of how to deal with the many problems that will be involved. Responses to the threat and to the fact of dying are so varied that no single policy or approach can be recommended except, of course, the policy that whatever is told should be factual. Nor can the patient's expressed wishes or instructions prior to such an illness be taken completely at face value. Experienced internists are familiar with the fact that what the patient may discuss during the annual interview and physical examination when the patient is in good health does not necessarily apply to what the patient wants to be told or does not want to be told when faced with a life-threatening illness. There are patients whose personalities and life-styles are such that they make it clear that they wish an open, step-by-step clarification of diagnosis, treatment, and prognosis. There are patients at the other extreme who apparently deny the implication of the procedures, the treatment, and the physical decline; however, it would be an error to conclude that they therefore have no knowledge of what is happening to them. There are still other patients who manage best by assimilating

what is happening in a gradual manner so that global denial is not operative. Certainly families have to be given all the facts as well as some guidance in those instances in which the family takes the position that all medical facts be kept from the patient; this is not really possible, and to attempt to do so only adds unnecessary evasion, silence, and loneliness to the patient's burden.

The mechanism of denial is operative in both illness and health, and it is on the basis of the doctor-patient relationship that optimal use will be made of it. It is unwise to overwhelm the mechanism of denial with more information than the patient can tolerate. On the other hand, the physician should not avoid discussions with the patient out of a concern that the patient will be too upset or will make excessive demands. The physician can be guided by the extent to which the patient undertakes those reasonable medical measures that are necessary to prolong life and alleviate suffering. Some patients do so without necessarily discussing the specific meaning of the medical regimen with the physician. As long as the patient is behaving in this manner, the physician can be reasonably confident that the patient understands what is going on whether the patient verbalizes it or not. Of course, no matter what the patient's response turns out to be, a sustaining, supportive relationship with the physician is of crucial importance until the end.

Diagnosis and Treatment

DIAGNOSIS

Diagnosis in psychiatry is unfortunately not simple; on the one hand there are reasonably well delineated syndromes to which labels are applied, and on the other hand there are many individualized reactions that are best diagnosed by a description of the behavior combined with an understanding of its symbolic meaning and historical determinants. Today diagnoses may be based on differential responses to treatment modalities as, for example, unipolar and bipolar affective disorders, or neuropsychological phenomenology such as "reactive" and "process" schizophrenia. Diagnosis serves a variety of purposes, such as providing the basis for effective treatment, predicting the course of a given condition, and communicating meaningfully about the patient.

Broadly speaking, psychiatric symptom complexes can be understood as the organism's attempt to adapt to psychological change or stress, in much the same way that consolidation of the lung in certain types of pneumonia is the organism's response to the stress of the etiologic agent. The number of adaptations that actually become sufficiently malfunctional in character to be labeled illnesses, which create difficulties for the patient and his relationships with others or cause severe subjective discomfort, is reasonably limited and can usually be readily ascertained. If the functioning personality is conceptualized as an ongoing compromise between forces, managed by a psychological structure called the ego, one can look for the source of a difficulty by examining the nature of the forces being dealt with. The inner needs of the individual, such as the management of aggression, of sexuality, of dependence, of autonomy, or of security, are those that often play a role in the difficulties encountered in medical practice. Maintenance of self-esteem and feelings of being effective, competent, lovable, and worthy are also important. External change must be integrated; factors such as physical disability, physical and physiologic changes in adolescence, economic reversals, or new or lost relationships all create circumstances requiring new compromises and adjustments which at times can be maladaptive and extreme.

The organism's capacity to monitor and deal with change adequately may be directly affected if the function of the brain tissue is impaired for any reason. When this happens acutely, the response is delirium. Changes persisting over a long period of time result in dementia.

Psychosis
The distinction between *psychosis* and *neurosis* is one that often troubles clinicians. Psychoses involve more severe impairments of personality functioning, to the extent that patients in the acute phase are unable to deal with the usual obligations of their everyday lives, including working effectively, fulfilling familial roles, and maintaining fulfilling relationships with those close to them. Psychotic individuals suffer from some impairment of their ability to think in a logical and coherent fashion, and they usually have an impairment in their emotional responses, either quantitatively in terms of the degree of emotional experiences, or qualitatively in terms of the appropriateness of the emotion to the underlying thought content. Of most practical importance is the fact that the psychotic patient suffers a significant inability to assess reality adequately. Another way of stating this is that the psychotic patient has an impairment of the capacity to distinguish his own thoughts and fantasies from his perception and understanding of his environment, so that the latter becomes distorted and may be responded to inappropriately. It should be emphasized that a diagnosis of psychosis does not in itself imply that the patient is totally incapacitated, that the patient is unable to care for himself, that the patient must be hospitalized, or that emergency measures are required to deal with him. Indeed, many patients who are chronically schizophrenic, for example, lead reasonably productive lives and are well able to care for themselves; nevertheless, even such patients are quite impaired in comparison to their full functional capacity were they well.

Neurosis
Neurotic problems do not generally involve a major incapacity to assess and respond to reality, nor do they usually involve a thinking disorder, although certain dissociative states may temporarily involve both. Neurosis manifests itself clinically in two ways, which are not mutually exclusive. Characteristic patterns and traits that are not usually experienced by the patient as "something wrong" and that do not usually bring him to the physician with a resulting chief complaint may interfere with the patient's ability to interact with others and to adjust flexibly and maximally to new situations; thus these traits may adversely affect interpersonal relationships. Such fixed patterns and traits under the impact of additional stress, together with the appearance of more discrete neurotic symptoms, constitute one broad category of neurotic difficulty. An example would be the person with an obsessive-compulsive personality who is characteristically rigid and inflexible in opinion, experiences little pleasure, is preoccu-

pied with details, is unusually parsimonious and concerned about issues of control, and who tends to lead life in as predictable and patterned a way as possible; such a person may, when faced with an unavoidable new situation calling for a new series of responses, develop symptoms of anxiety, obsessional thoughts or compulsions, or marked exaggeration of his preexistent character traits to the extent that his family, friends, or physician find him difficult. Patterns of behavior and specific character traits of course typify all personalities and are not usually considered "neurotic" unless they are relatively fixed, predictable, and from a practical point of view eventually lead to difficulties in adjustment that bring the patient to seek help, albeit often without any direct complaint about psychological or emotional problems. This type of disturbance is considered a personality disorder.

Neurosis or psychoneurosis is characterized by symptoms that are experienced by the patient as such. Underlying the formation of neurotic symptoms is anxiety, which is experienced by all neurotic patients to one extent or another. The anxiety neurosis, for example, is characterized by pervasive anxiety which is interposed with episodes of more acute panic. Conversion symptoms, on the other hand, which are understood as a way of solving a psychological problem to avoid anxiety (as are all neurotic symptoms), are often characterized by very little or no anxiety at all that can be detected clinically. The development of neurotic symptoms, unlike the personality disorders that are usually long standing, is usually rather discrete and occurs in response to an often identifiable precipitant, such as an alteration in an important relationship. Neurotic symptoms can be understood as both exaggerated and relatively maladaptive responses on the part of the personality in an effort to solve a problem. It is important for the physician to remember, however, that the nature of the problem is not in the patient's conscious awareness and that the emergence of such knowledge is avoided because it is fraught with so much anxiety that a symptom has developed. It is also relevant here to emphasize that although the patient with the neurotic symptom is aware that *something* is the matter, he may often characterize

the difficulty in medical terms and not have any understanding of the psychological nature of his symptoms. Patients suffering from anxiety attacks will often arrive at emergency rooms complaining that they are having "heart attacks." They point to the palpitations, diaphoresis, dizziness, and other physiologic manifestations of anxiety as evidence that they are having severe physical illness and then will insist that that is the reason they are so frightened. Patients with conversion symptoms may have similar rationalizations, and depressed patients will often acknowledge that they are depressed but will attribute their unhappy feelings to the very physiologic manifestations that are part of the depressive syndrome. Even to acknowledge that the symptom is a manifestation of underlying emotional conflict may for some patients involve considerable amounts of anxiety and in itself be avoided.

PSYCHIATRIC CONSULTATION

Although a number of patients will refuse referral for psychiatric evaluation or treatment under almost any circumstances, the number can be minimized by giving attention to a few basic principles. Patients tend to feel a sense of rejection under these circumstances, especially those emotionally ill patients who are sensitive to these issues anyway. If the internist implies either overtly or covertly that the referral constitutes an attempt to get rid of a troublesome patient who is not really sick, the problem becomes worse. The physician, of course, must examine his own attitudes toward such patients carefully in order to avoid this conscious or unconscious bias. It is suggested that physicians become acquainted with one or two psychiatric colleagues with whom they develop a working relationship over a period of time so that they may refer patients more confidently, having a good idea of just what the patient can expect, what the physician can expect, and a reasonable confidence that the patient will be competently evaluated and treated. If the internist feels this sense of confidence, it is more likely that he will convey it to the patient and that the referral will be easier. In most instances the internist should specifically state his intention to continue to follow the patient and to maintain an interest in the future course of events, and when at all appropriate, to treat the patient collaboratively with the psychiatrist.

The referral is more likely to succeed if it is offered as a positive recommendation with positive indications. A statement that indicates to the patient that the internist cannot find *anything* the matter and is therefore sending the patient to a psychiatrist is much more likely to result in the patient's seeking another internist's opinion rather than accepting the referral. If the internist has indeed made a diagnosis such as anxiety neurosis or depression, with supporting evidence based on the examination to substantiate the diagnosis, and indicated to the patient that the matter is taken seriously, the patient will more readily understand that the referral is made on clinical rather than on personal grounds.

A description of what the patient can expect when he sees the psychiatrist will also be helpful. The referring physician should be aware that many patients are very frightened of losing control of themselves, or of the idea that they might be "going crazy." Such patients are often apprehensive about expressing these concerns, so that once the suggestion of referral has been made, the physician should give the patient every opportunity to express as many inquiries and questions as come to mind about the condition and the referral. This will allow the physician the opportunity to convey factual information that is reassuring and will tend to reduce the anxiety connected with frightening and unrealistic fantasies. The physician should do his best to help the patient understand that his complaints are based on a legitimate, bona fide illness and are not simply manifestations of "weakness" or "all in his head," and therefore unreal or unworthy of respect. Indeed, the referral is much more likely to succeed if the physician can convey the same type of concern, sympathetic interest, and respect for the patient that he would if he were referring the patient to a hematologist for a workup of a blood dyscrasia.

The question of confidentiality is also important. Patients may feel quite ashamed of having to see a psychiatrist. Indeed, there is some realistic basis for the belief that such treatment can result in bias or prejudice against the patient in a number of situations. Thus it is often useful for the physician to address himself specifically to this issue and to state quite candidly what it is that he will discuss with the psychiatrist about the referral, and whether this will be in the form of a written letter or a telephone conversation. It is also useful to inform the patient about the nature of future communication between the psychiatrist and the internist. Because the physician is often viewed as a parental figure, patients may want assurance that certain material confided to the psychiatrist will not be relayed back to the referring physician. This is a point that must be clarified by discussion, with both the patient and the psychiatrist.

MANAGEMENT OF VARIOUS PSYCHIATRIC DISORDERS

The Schizophrenic Patient

The schizophrenic patient may come to the attention of the internist either as a patient who is relatively stable or as one who is in an acute psychotic episode representing the onset or the exacerbation of the illness. (The management of the acutely psychotic patient will be discussed later in this chapter.) The chronically ill patient may be recognized from his mental status. Peculiarities of affect, thought content, or progression of thought, bizarre or unusual fantasies, and unusual relationships to the physician such as distant or suspicious attitudes in which the physician feels somehow left out of the patient's consideration are all, at times, characteristic of schizophrenic patients. The presence of secondary symptoms such as delusions and hallucinations may be harder to detect; these symptoms are, of course, not necessary to the diagnosis but help to confirm it, along with the other more primary symptoms. Many chronically schizophrenic patients, however, especially if in reasonably good remission, can appear to be quite psychologically intact, so that the physician may have to rely on the history. Unfortunately, many patients are quite ashamed of having had psychiatric treatment or hospitalization. They may be concerned that the physician will not take their physical complaints seriously but will dismiss them as manifestations of an emotional illness. Such patients may not acknowledge, even on direct questioning, having a history of mental illness, at least during the initial interview. After the doctor-patient relationship has been established it becomes easier for the patient to acknowledge such prior difficulties. It should be emphasized that patients who are currently being treated by psychiatrists or at mental health facilities, or even those taking antipsychotic medications, may neglect to tell a physician whom they consult for a physical illness of this fact. The likelihood of the patient's giving this information is certainly increased if the physician takes the patient's complaints seriously and has an index of suspicion that allows him to make inquiries tactfully and in such a way as to allay the patient's concern that the information may in some way be used against him.

Once the diagnosis of a chronic schizophrenic process has been made, there are certain considerations that may influence the course of the doctor-patient relationship. Such patients often have difficulty in giving adequate histories, and it may well be that, with the patient's permission, another member of the family should be interviewed. Moreover, the patient may find it uncomfortable, even frightening, if his physician is unduly friendly and warm, and may do better when the doctor is not overly hearty but provides a well-structured relationship and a business-like setting for the medical transaction. These patients may also be somewhat distrustful or suspicious, or even hostile. This can best be dealt with first by acknowledging the patient's concern, then by providing in a direct way the factual information relevant to the situation in even more complete form than might be the usual practice, and then listening to and responding to the patient's questions and reactions.

Schizophrenic patients may have unusual or bizarre ideas as to the nature of the processes underlying their physical complaints; special efforts may have to be made to emphasize the realistic aspects of the situation. If diagnostic procedures such as cardiac catheterization or thoracentesis are planned, it is of particular importance that the physician spend enough time with the patient to make sure the procedure is fully understood and has not been incorporated into a delusional context, lest the patient at the last minute become panicky or refuse the procedure. It should be emphasized that by and large chronically ill schizophrenic patients do remarkably

well when physical illness supervenes, and the physician should not presume that the patient will respond adversely. It is especially important not to convey to the patient such a presumption, but to regard both the chronic psychotic process and the current treatment procedures as simply aspects of the patient's medical history and medical status.

Patients who are taking antipsychotic drugs such as phenothiazines may present special problems. The phenothiazines can potentiate other drugs, especially those that produce hypotension or analgesia. These drugs may have long-term, untoward side effects such as dyskinesia, manifested by twitching of the mouth and facial muscles. Untoward side effects present a problem in the differential diagnosis. Moreover, a large number of patients suffer an exacerbation of schizophrenia within weeks to months of the cessation of drug therapy, and this factor must be taken into account as the physician prescribes treatment or writes hospital orders.

A history of schizophrenic episodes does not mean that the patient is currently chronically psychotic; indeed, many such patients are for all practical purposes free of any evidence of a continuing schizophrenic disorder. Nevertheless, a sudden alteration of the patient's mental status should certainly alert the physician to the possibility of a recurrence of the illness.

The Patient with Organic Brain Syndrome
Any adult patient who undergoes noticeable change in his mental functioning must be evaluated in relation to the possibility of impairment of brain tissue function. The presenile dementias may present initially as a variety of neurotic symptoms, and the changes can be quite subtle. For example, an individual who had been unusually bright and perceptive in one area and who over a period of time begins to have only the usual amount of capacity or ability in this area may be suffering from one of the presenile dementias, a brain tumor, or one of the myriad of systemic illnesses in which the primary symptoms are related to personality function. If there is an impairment of brain tissue function, careful examination should reveal some deficit of intellectual functioning, although in the early stages this may be sufficiently

minimal as to be missed. If the physician has sufficient index of suspicion, however, he may wish to
pursue this to the extent of referring the patient for
psychological testing. The utilization of cognitive
or intelligence tests combined with tests involving
visual motor coordination can often reveal early
signs of chronic brain dysfunction before the more
gross changes in the mental status become evident.
Many systemic diseases that can cause impairment of
brain tissue function with concurrent alterations of
personality and intellectual capacity are susceptible
to treatment, with either arrest or remission of the
psychological and intellectual changes, as for example
in combined systems disease, central nervous system
syphilis, or normal pressure hydrocephalus. Therefore, any indication from the patient or from his
relatives of alteration in the characteristics of the
personality must be taken seriously and should not
be presumed to be caused by neurotic difficulty.

The Patient with Anxiety
The various somatic manifestations of anxiety are
often presented to physicians by patients as their
chief complaint. Palpitations, sweating, a tight feeling in the chest, diarrhea, and frequency of urination
are examples. Anxiety is the response to conflict
within the personality; its source by definition is
unknown to the patient, which distinguishes it from
fear, in which the threat is known. As mentioned
before, anxious patients often insist that their concern arises from preoccupation with the physiologic
concomitant of the anxiety.

Anxiety can present as a relatively mild agitation
or as severe panic. The principles of management are
essentially the same in both instances: A thorough
history, physical examination, and definite diagnosis
are most helpful. A calm physician who carefully
attempts to help the patient explore the events and
feelings surrounding the onset of the episode can
usually help the patient to feel more at ease quickly.
It is then equally important to outline a plan for
further evaluation and treatment if the patient is to
continue to feel reassured. If the anxiety is severe
and incapacitating, the physician may wish to refer
the patient for psychiatric consultation and initiate
treatment with one of the minor tranquilizers such as

chlordiazepoxide (15–100 mg/day) or diazepam
(6–40 mg/day). These medications are among the
most widely prescribed and do have definite antianxiety effects; however, their use is still somewhat
controversial. Some psychiatrists are concerned that
the chronic ingestion of these substances can produce
not only an emotional dependency but a physiologic
one to the extent that withdrawal symptoms can
occur if the drugs are stopped after prolonged high
dosage. The routine prescription of these medications may serve to convince the patient further that
his symptoms have an organic basis and thus may
interfere with the possibility that a more lasting
ameliorization of the condition could be achieved
through psychological treatment. Another problem
associated with the use of these drugs is that for some
busy physicians they serve unwittingly in lieu of a
fuller doctor-patient relationship that would encourage the patient to ventilate and clarify the nature of
the concerns producing the anxiety symptoms. Such
a doctor-patient relationship can perhaps in the long
run be more efficacious than continued utilization of
medication. Nevertheless, if these tranquilizers are
used judiciously, with an understanding of the problems involved, they can be very helpful in dealing
with acute, time-limited, anxiety-producing situations
and in helping patients function better in situations
in which the anxiety is disruptive.

The Depressed Patient
The recognition and management of depression is of
necessity a part of virtually every physician's practice. Depression is the syndrome of response to loss.
The loss may be of an important relationship, of a
physical capacity, of attractiveness, of a sense of the
possibility of future accomplishments and pleasures,
of a sense of oneself as a worthy or good person, or
of the capacity to feel competent and to deal effectively with a number of situations that a person encounters in life.

The internist will find that many depressed
patients do not present with depression as the chief
complaint. Patients have a tendency to frame their
concerns in the particular metaphor that is suitable
to the person they are consulting as a potential source
of help. Thus depressed people who turn to their

ministers may often experience their difficulties in religious or moral terms; those seeking the help of psychologists or psychiatrists may frame their problem in more psychological terms; those going to practitioners of internal medicine will often have physical complaints. Very often the physician is confronted with a patient whose chief complaint is one of fatigue, digestive disturbance, sleep disturbance, appetite disturbance, or a lack of interest in sexual activity. Further inquiry may elicit the fact that the patient has a lack of enthusiasm and vitality, an inability to enjoy previously pleasurable pursuits, irritability, a fear of being alone, and perhaps even crying spells and feelings of hopelessness and despair. The mood disturbance, as with anxiety, may be understood by the patient as a response to the physiologic disturbances accompanying the depression, and the patient may have difficulty in acknowledging that he or she is undergoing a primarily emotional disturbance. However, as the history taking progresses and the symptoms are elaborated, the physician will begin to suspect the diagnosis of depression as he integrates the history and complaints with the observed mental status and thought content of the patient. Indications of depression are feelings of helplessness, inability to master a situation, pessimism, references to lowered self-esteem, and indications that the patient feels that nothing ever goes right. In more severe instances the patient is preoccupied with nothing but feelings of guilt and unworthiness. Often the interviewer is able to clarify the precipitant of the depression, although it may not be consciously connected with the symptoms by the patient. Inquiry into prior reactions to loss and separation may be helpful in establishing the diagnosis, as is a history of early unfulfilled needs, which can result in a depressive tendency in some people. A thorough physical examination with careful attention to the patient's complaints is useful.

After the physician has completed the examination a discussion with the patient about the diagnosis and the reasons for reaching it, including a discussion of any apparent precipitant, will often be met with considerable relief and an acknowledgment of depression by the patient. More severe or psychotic depressions are usually quite obvious; the patient may come to the physician with somatic delusions and other similarly bizarre complaints, and there is a discernible thought disturbance. It is the large group of patients whose primary problem is depression but who present with physical complaints who represent the greatest diagnostic challenge.

The Suicidal Patient

Once the diagnosis of depression is suspected, the physician is obligated to consider the degree, if any, of suicidal risk. Patients who successfully commit suicide have often seen physicians within the previous 6 months. To some extent this may be explained by the fact that some such patients do indeed have severe physical illnesses that precipitate the suicide. However, potentially suicidal patients usually visit a physician in the hope of obtaining some help with problems that appear to them to be otherwise insoluble, but which are not a matter of physical illness.

Suicidal behavior should be thought of as being on a continuum with so-called gestures at one end, where the patient has little, if any, real suicidal intent but feels there is no other way to deal with a situation than by making a suicidal attempt; at the other end of the continuum, the patient is absolutely determined to do away with himself without any apparent ambivalence. The majority of patients fall somewhere between these two extremes and frequently attempt to seek help. However, their plea for help is often disguised; it almost seems as if the patient is testing the helping person by unconsciously saying that if the patient is really loved, his dilemma will be detected without his having to verbalize it. Furthermore, many patients are very ashamed of their suicidal wishes because they consider them a violation of ethical or religious doctrine and are therefore reluctant to reveal them, although they very much want someone to assist them. Although there are certainly indirect ways of detecting suicidal intent, such as hearing the patient speak in a way that indicates he or she does not plan to continue existence for any length of time, it is probably necessary in almost every case to confront the patient gently with the concern about suicidal intent. Since the contemplation of suicide is usually a frightening and upsetting state of mind, most patients appreciate this concern and are then able to discuss their suicidal thoughts. It is certain that an obviously depressed patient who absolutely and flatly denies having any suicidal ideation must be considered a risk, either because the denial may break down suddenly or because the patient may be deliberately misleading the physician out of concern about being prevented from carrying out his intent.

If the patient acknowledges suicidal ideation, assessment of the degree of risk will determine his management, which may consist either in continued treatment by the physician, referral to a psychiatrist on an emergency or routine basis, or immediate hospitalization. Although the degree of risk is difficult to determine, there are some guidelines. Inquiry should be made into the precise nature of the suicidal thoughts; one wishes to know if they are pervasive, or only occasional and fleeting. The degree to which the suicidal impulses are structured and precise is important, in that an occasional unstructured thought about not going on is probably of less immediate risk than a fixed preoccupation with specific means of doing away with oneself, such as taking an overdose of pills that are available in the household. Has the patient set a time limit or determined a specific date? The patient's ideas as to what the outcome of his suicide would be, both in terms of the patient and those around him, can be helpful in assessing the risk as well. Any overt action whatsoever that points toward performing the suicidal act is considered an ominous portent and may be as indirect as simply driving a few blocks out of the way on the trip home after work to see if one can jump off the bridge, or as specific as purchasing a gun. If the patient has in any way translated fantasy and thought into actual motor activity, the risk of suicide must be considered more acute. An important aspect of assessment is for the physician to empathize with the patient and to answer, as the patient might, the question of whether there is any reason to continue living and whether there is anyone in the patient's life who would wish him to continue to live.

Numerous statistical findings about suicide may be of some value in thinking of the general problem of suicide but they are probably not too helpful in deciding what to do about an individual patient. For example, the incidence of suicide increases with age; suicide is much more common among alcoholics; women attempt suicide more frequently than men; men succeed in killing themselves more often than women. Delirious patients are at high risk for suicide. Patients who are to be hospitalized because of the risk of suicide must not be left alone once that decision is made, since there is a distinct increase in the likelihood of suicide during the interval after leaving the physician's office and before arriving at the hospital.

Patients who have attempted suicide are often seen by physicians for treatment of the resulting condition, which may range from a minor wrist laceration to an almost lethal comatose state resulting from a huge overdose of a central nervous system depressant. An important principle of management is to take all suicide attempts seriously, no matter how trivial they might seem. The reasons for the attempted suicide must be explored; attention only to the management of the medical complications is insufficient and dangerous. The patient who has attempted suicide must be evaluated; in the presence of continued suicidal intent, psychiatric consultation should be obtained. The patient must be assured that the physician will initiate a definite plan of management of the problem that precipitated the attempt. If this is not done, the next attempt may be lethal even if the first was relatively benign. The underlying "plea for help" must be attended to, even though the patient is sometimes willing to give the physician an anxiety-alleviating denial of any further need for concern. A substantial number of successful suicides have been preceded by unsuccessful attempts.

MANAGEMENT OF PSYCHIATRIC EMERGENCIES
Acutely disturbed patients may be brought to the physician's office by relatives, or they may be seen in the emergency room or on the wards of general hospitals. Although patients suffering major acute psychiatric decompensation frequently bring attention to themselves through unusual and conspicuous behavior, the physician should be aware that serious disturbance can go relatively unnoticed in cases in which the patient withdraws and ceases active, overt interaction with his environment.

The differential diagnosis of acutely disturbed mental functioning may at times be difficult but is of major importance. The most important initial differentiation should be a decision as to whether or not there is evidence of impairment of brain function. The nature of the initial management will vary considerably, depending on the underlying condition.

The Delirious Patient

Delirium is defined as an acute brain syndrome without permanent destruction of nervous tissue. It is caused by a metabolic defect and may have a variety of etiologies that involve either increased demands for nutriment due to high fever, an impairment of nutrition to the brain, direct impairment of tissue function as in infection, or additional demands for integration of new perceptions overtaxing an already stressed cortex. Usually social factors contribute simultaneously to the syndrome. The hallmark of delirium is fluctuation in the level of consciousness. The earliest manifestation is often a disturbed sleep pattern accompanied by fear and restlessness. This syndrome gradually increases, and the patient becomes confused and may begin to hallucinate and develop delusions and illusions. As the syndrome progresses, the panic that the patient experiences may result in impulsive suicidal attempts. Exhaustion, stupor, coma, or death can supervene if the underlying disturbance in the metabolism of the brain is not corrected. Although many delirious patients are overtly agitated and disturbed, often loudly so, it should be remembered that another manifestation of delirium may be an increasing withdrawal that may be misinterpreted as the patient's simply being quiet and cooperative.

The patient's mental status often varies considerably from one time to the next, especially early in the onset of the syndrome. The patient may be reasonably alert and intellectually intact during the day but will become confused and bewildered in the evening. Careful examination will reveal that the patient is disoriented, initially as to time, later to place, and finally to person. There is an impairment of the ability to think abstractly and to grasp the meaning of perceptions and reach proper conclusions. Memory is disturbed, although early in the syndrome efforts may

be made to deny that fact. The patient's incapacity to understand the meaning of perceptions leads to misinterpretations that are sometimes acted upon, as when the patient calls to friends or relatives whom he thinks are talking together in the hall, or when he gets up in the middle of the night to go to work. Hallucinations are often frightening; they tend to be visual in character and relatively fleeting. The patient has great difficulty in learning and thus cannot be expected to understand explanations.

The most common problem in the differential diagnosis of delirium is to distinguish it from an acute schizophrenic episode. However, the impairment of cognition, memory, and orientation found in an acute brain syndrome, or in chronic brain syndrome for that matter, is not characteristic of schizophrenia. The relatively fleeting and unstructured nature of both the delusions and the hallucinations is more characteristic of delirium, especially hallucinations of visual and tactile senses, and the fluctuation in the level of mental functioning is much more characteristic of delirium. The patient's history may be of help (although it can also be misleading). Patients who have had prior schizophrenic episodes may, of course, become delirious under certain circumstances.

When the diagnosis of acute brain syndrome has been made, an active search must be undertaken to determine the etiology so that adequate measures can be instituted. Supportive treatments, including adequate hydration, are most important in the interim. An adequately lighted room with a minimum of extraneous stimuli is indicated. The continued presence of one person, who helps the patient with acute brain syndrome to remain as oriented as possible by constantly reminding him of the date, time, and place and explaining carefully the meaning of events, can reduce the apprehension and restlessness. A multiplicity of personnel and an overly complex environment can exacerbate the condition. Obviously, as many medications as possible should be eliminated, starting with those that are known to have depressive effects on the central nervous system. The anxiety should be treated by medications that have as little depressive effect as possible; therefore, the utilization of the group of drugs exemplified by chlordiazepoxide is generally considered most useful. This medication can be given in dosages of 50 to 100 mg intramuscularly at 4- to 6-hour intervals but should not exceed 300 mg in 24 hours, and the dosage should be lowered as soon as possible. Treatment should continue until the syndrome is well under control. Care must be taken to protect the patient from suicide.

The Acute Schizophrenic Patient

The patient suffering from an acute schizophrenic reaction will often exhibit bizarre behavior. The patient's speech may be moderately to extremely incoherent and difficult to follow. The affect may be peculiar and not appropriate to the situation. The patient often has a perplexed and preoccupied air, and the answers to questions may be seemingly irrelevant and unresponsive. Unlike the delirious patient, however, the schizophrenic is oriented as to time and place, has intact recent memory, and maintains the ability to perform basic intellectual functions such as calculations. It may be difficult for the examiner to determine these factors, and considerable time may be needed in interviewing the patient to become aware that the patient is indeed oriented and has intact memory. Direct questioning is sometimes the least effective way of making this determination; the intactness of these functions more often becomes apparent as one listens to the patient talking about himself and the events surrounding his difficulties.

In the acute schizophrenic reaction, delusions may be apparent as well as hallucinations in virtually all sensory spheres, although auditory ones are the most common. The patient may appear to be listening to voices during the interview, and it may be difficult to obtain his attention. Comments and explanations aimed at orienting the patient do not have the momentary beneficial effect that one sees in delirium, nor is there the characteristic diurnal variation seen in the early stages of delirium. On the other hand, time spent with the patient in a quiet, reassuring, and nonthreatening atmosphere may result in increasingly coherent communication. One can frequently obtain a history from the patient's friends and relatives of a period of days, weeks, or even months of increasingly bizarre behavior and thought processes preceding the patient's contact with the physician.

The initial management of schizophrenic patients will depend on several factors, including the presence or absence of suicidal or homicidal preoccupation, the patient's capacity to care for himself, the presence or absence of social support for the patient in the community, and when available, the recommendations of a consulting psychiatrist. The diagnosis of an exacerbation of a schizophrenic process or of an initial acute schizophrenic reaction in most instances warrants psychiatric consultation and referral for treatment, either on an outpatient basis or in a hospital. The initial management of such patients usually consists of antipsychotic medications from either the haloperidol group or the phenothiazine group, combined with supportive psychotherapy and often the presence of a supportive environment in the hospital.

The Manic Patient

The patient experiencing an acute manic attack will be hyperactive, extremely verbose, and euphoric (or angry if his activities are inhibited). There is a diminution of sleep and a preoccupation with grandiose fantasies and plans, and the patient is markedly overactive and talkative. In more extreme form, the patient may be in an acutely excited state. Patients who are manic lack awareness of the social and economic consequences of their activities, which may cause extreme embarrassment and economic hardship or may even bring them into contact with law enforcement agencies. The patient often assumes an attitude of great intimacy with the physician and may become angry if not responded to in a similarly overfriendly way. Although outpatient therapy with haloperidol, chlorpromazine, or lithium can at times be undertaken when there is sufficient environmental support, it is generally necessary to hospitalize these patients to protect them from the consequences of the psychosis. It may be difficult to convince a manic patient of the necessity for hospitalization; a face-saving rationalization is occasionally helpful in this regard. Psychiatric consultation is suggested, and on occasion involuntary hospitalization may be indicated. Since mania in some patients can very quickly become severe depression, all such patients must be carefully monitored.

The Violent Patient

Occasionally the physician is confronted with a patient who is extremely angry or violent; this behavior can be very frightening to the physician who feels a responsibility to "do something." It is important to remember that such patients are themselves usually fearful about losing control of their aggressive impulses. The physician should arrange the interview under conditions in which anxiety about safety is minimal. Telling the patient that one is concerned can be helpful, as can conveying to the patient the insight that the patient, too, must be worried about losing control, and describing the measures that will be taken to help prevent this eventuality. Every effort should be made to help the patient convert his anger into verbalizations. If additional measures are necessary, the patient may be asked to take some medication. As a last resort, the patient may have to be physically subdued and intramuscular medication administered in the form of phenothiazines (chlorpromazine, 50 mg). No attempt should ever be made to subdue a patient if there is any chance that it will not be successful. Sufficient security personnel should be present so that restraint can be applied quickly and without harm to the patient or to those attempting to help him. A variety of conditions can underlie extreme anger and violent feelings and behavior, and it is necessary to investigate these conditions through adequate history taking, a physical examination, and laboratory tests, which may often include electroencephalography. Paranoid states, paranoid schizophrenia, certain forms of seizures, dissociative states, and intoxication with alcohol and other drugs are some of the conditions that can result in threatened or actual violence.

Medical Psychotherapy

THE DOCTOR-PATIENT RELATIONSHIP

To understand the doctor-patient relationship, one must be aware of the multiplicity of factors that enter into the shaping of it. Cultural and societal attitudes have for centuries placed the physician in a unique position as a person with special duties, powers, and responsibilities. To this combination of culture and myth is added the personal experience of the individual who learns early in life that parents give comfort and care for their children during illness. Then, too, part of the way in which human beings feel about themselves includes fantasies of omnipotence and invulnerability which, during illness, are readily displaced onto the physician with the hope and wish that thereby the invulnerability will be preserved. On the other hand, a patient's early experiences with illness and with physicians may have been frightening, unpleasant, and painful, thus leading to a fear of the repetition of such experiences. This set of fantasies and expectations on the part of the patient may considerably affect his relationship with the physician even before patient and physician meet.

People generally, and patients in particular, readily displace onto the person of the physician — a parental figure after all — their own feelings, attitudes, and expectations toward parents and other authority figures. This is the phenomenon known as transference. It is ubiquitous, it has conscious and unconscious elements, and it is bipolar; that is, the feelings about the physician can be positive or negative, and there will usually be elements of both. If we keep in mind that this phenomenon has its origins in the feelings of the child for the parent, we will be better able to understand some manifestations of transference that may become troubling when not properly managed. Thus a patient may become aware of the development of sexual feelings for the physician. Such a feeling may or may not be verbalized, but there are clues to it in any event. If the physician keeps in mind that these feelings originate in the past and are displaced onto him or her, the physician will find it possible to maintain a professional attitude and will feel neither unduly flattered nor particularly inclined to participate in unprofessional conduct. In the instance of negative feelings, the physician should, of course, determine that the patient's anger has no basis in reality, and then should initiate brief discussions with the patient for the purpose of maintaining the relationship but not necessarily for the purpose of proving who is right and who wrong. A common source of negative feelings is related to fees. Many physicians continue to feel uncomfortable about the fact that fees are involved and will not discuss fees directly with the patient; this is a frequent source of misunderstanding that can be prevented and corrected by treating the fee as an integral and open part of the relationship.

The fact that feelings are invested in the physician creates a setting in which medical psychotherapy can take place. The psychotherapy begins with the initial interview in the context of a relationship which, if properly managed, can represent to the patient a partial repetition of the relationship that was experienced or hoped for from kindly and interested· parents and family. The physician may represent to the patient a person who, for one of the few times in the patient's life, listens in a noncritical and nonjudgmental way. It is of course of paramount importance that the physician develop the capacity for this noncritical and nonjudgmental stance. Following the initial interview and the history taking, the physical examination in itself is also an important psychotherapeutic tool when it is conducted in a dignified and unhurried manner, thus imparting to the patient the fact that he is being taken seriously.

It is not possible to indicate specifically under what circumstances it is appropriate for the internist himself to undertake the psychotherapeutic management of the patient and under what circumstances psychiatric referral is indicated. We have discussed in an earlier section circumstances under which psychiatric consultation is appropriate. In general, internists prefer to refer patients whose symptoms or disorders are primarily psychogenic and who will require prolonged, intensive treatment. By and large, the internist can undertake psychotherapy with patients whose emotions are playing a significant role in the illness for which the internist is treating them, with patients who are under some stress in connection with a phase of the life cycle described earlier, and with patients whose lives are such that a supportive relationship with an understanding physician will be helpful in the treatment of what is almost invariably an admixture of emotional and physical disorder. Patients requiring intensive treatment may need interviews of considerable length, but psychotherapeutic sessions of 15 to 20 minutes are also effective if properly managed, and they fit realistically into the internist's working schedule.

TECHNIQUES OF PSYCHOTHERAPY

There are a number of psychotherapeutic techniques that physicians utilize in their daily work; these techniques can be systematically utilized with a patient who is in need of some assistance with a troubling life situation. Thus, *ventilation* refers to that technique in which we encourage the patient to tell his story without any particular probing. Even if the verbalized concerns refer to conflicts or stresses that cannot be alleviated, we are all familiar with the fact that it is sometimes helpful simply to share one's burden with another person – in this instance the physician – who will be neither critical nor judgmental. *Abreaction* has the same meaning and the same function.

Corrective information is a psychotherapeutic technique that is particularly appropriate to the role of the physician. There are considerable areas of misconception and misinformation about illness and health for both conscious and unconscious reasons. The physician is in a particularly strategic position to be helpful to the patient simply by virtue of his knowledge about myths, misconceptions, and facts.

Universalization and *generalization* are important and commonly used psychotherapeutic techniques; they utilize the fact that there are experiences that many people have in common. Feelings of anxiety or depression may be reduced if the physician is able to point out to the patient that what the patient is experiencing has been experienced by many people under similar circumstances. For instance, feelings of guilt are an almost universal experience on the part of the bereaved when a close friend or relative has died. The feelings of guilt are usually inappropriate because they are not related to the fact of death, yet the bereaved feels guilty because medical care was not instituted earlier, or because an apology was not offered for an unintentional slight. Pointing out to the patient that such feelings are a part of the grieving process and are widely experienced is useful in psychotherapy.

Although *reassurance* is a widely discussed and widely utilized psychotherapeutic principle, it is likely that its use is not properly understood. The most common error in its utilization occurs when the well-intentioned physician reassures the patient prematurely – that is, reassuring comments are made *before* the patient's fears or fantasies have been verbalized. Under such circumstances the patient does not feel particularly reassured because he has not yet had the opportunity to express (hence, to realize) his concerns. In a similar vein, it is unwise to give reassurance under circumstances in which the outcome is in doubt, because mistrust and confusion will be added to the patient's anxiety if the reassurance turns out to be either premature or incorrect.

The Physician as a Person

Everything we have discussed and described in the preceding material applies to the physician as well as to the patient. The physician is as vulnerable as all other human beings; in fact, there is evidence that medicine is a stressful profession. Medicine itself is demanding, and it is practiced by individuals who are demanding of themselves and of those around them. Longitudinal studies have been made of the lives of physicians. Many have had troubled developmental years that left them vulnerable to the stresses of their work. For instance, physicians themselves are notoriously poor patients; they delay seeking medical assistance for themselves and for their families, and they frequently are somewhat less than conscientious in adhering to the therapy that is prescribed. There is evidence that physicians have serious emotional problems for which they do not seek help. Thus, physicians have the highest suicide rate of any identifiable population group in the United States, and the incidence of narcotics addiction is also higher among physicians than in any other identifiable group in this country. The incidence of alcoholism among physicians is on the increase, as is the incidence of marital disruption.

To some extent these facts are surprising, because the other side of the coin is that medicine is a gratifying profession that most practitioners have voluntarily chosen. Patient care is demanding, however, and the physician must be aware of his or her feelings about those demands and toward patients, which may not be remarkably different from the feelings that patients have toward physicians. Accordingly, the physician must recognize the need for time away from work, for time with family, and for support from family, friends, and colleagues.

Perhaps it is belaboring the obvious, but it is nevertheless worthwhile to state specifically that physicians should have regular health evaluations as other patients do. Furthermore, when a physician is the patient, the assumption should not be made that the illness, the procedures, and the therapeutic plan are understood or will necessarily be followed. When it comes to emotional stresses, either of practice or of personal life, the physician may be particularly sensitive about seeking outside help. This is especially true for physicians who are well known in smaller communities where the need for privacy and confidentiality is somewhat harder to observe. Under such circumstances a reasonable approach is the sharing of concerns with a trusted colleague and a request for confidentiality, if more formal psychotherapy is not available. Certainly when psychotherapy is available it should be utilized. The principles of ventilation, universalization, generalization, reassurance, and support, as well as psychiatric consultation and treatment, should be recommended to the physician as to any other patient when it is so indicated. Finally — and wholly apart from the physician's need to accept appropriate measures for his or her own personal health — self-understanding and an awareness of the place of both the intellect and the feelings of patients and of oneself are an indispensible part of the armamentarium of the physician.

Bibliography

Abram, H. S. Psychological response to illness and hospitalization. *Psychosomatics* 10:218, 1969.

Anderson, W. H., and Kuehnle, J. C. Strategies for the treatment of acute psychosis. *J.A.M.A.* 229:1884, 1974.

Berezin, M. Psychodynamic considerations of aging and the aged: An overview. *Am. J. Psychiatry* 128:1483, 1972.

Castelnuevo-Tedesco, P. *The Twenty-Minute Hour: A Guide to Brief Psychotherapy for the Physician.* Boston: Little, Brown, 1965.

Enelow, A. J., and Swisher, S. N. *Interviewing and Patient Care.* New York: Oxford University Press, 1972.

Gould, R. The phases of adult life: A study in developmental psychology. *Am. J. Psychiatry* 129: 521, 1972.

Havens, L. L. Recognition of suicidal risks through the psychologic examination. *N. Engl. J. Med.* 276:210, 1967.

Kahana, R. J., and Bibring, G. Personality Types in Medical Management. In N. E. Zinberg (Ed.), *Psychiatry and Medical Practice in a General Hospital.* New York: International Universities Press, 1964. P. 108.

Kaufman, M. R., Franzblau, A., et al. The emotional impact of ward rounds. *Mt. Sinai J. Med.* 23:782, 1956.

Kubler-Ross, E. *On Death and Dying.* New York: Macmillan, 1970.

Lidz, T. *The Person: His Development Throughout the Life Cycle.* New York: Basic Books, 1968.

Poser, C. M. The presenile dementias. *J.A.M.A.* 223:81, 1975.

Schwab, J. J. *Handbook of Psychiatric Consultation.* New York: Appleton-Century-Crofts, 1968.

Shader, R. I. (ed.). *Manual of Psychiatric Therapeutics.* Boston: Little, Brown, 1975.

Szasz, T., and Hollender, M. A contribution to the philosophy of medicine: Basic models in the doctor-patient relationship. *Arch. Intern. Med.* 97:585, 1956.

3

Drug and
Alcohol Dependence

John A. Hermos

With the widespread availability and use of psycho-active and analgesic drugs and alcohol in the United States, the practicing physician is frequently called upon to diagnose dependence on these substances and to initiate treatment. Areas of drug and alcohol dependence that are particularly relevant to the practice of medicine will be discussed in this chapter. An example of a drug dependence problem encountered in medical practice is illustrated in the following case history.

A 54-year-old man was admitted to a medical ward for severe leg pains and paresthesia. Six years earlier, diabetes mellitus had been diagnosed, and he now complained of polyuria and a 35-pound weight loss. He had continued his 20-year habit of drinking a pint of vodka or Scotch daily, and he was taking up to 20 aspirin tablets daily for his pains. Diabetic mono-neuropathy and polyneuropathy were diagnosed, and he was treated with insulin, vitamins, and sedatives. In addition, the following analgesics were ordered and administered for pain:

Day 1. Acetaminophen (Tylenol) 600 mg q4h as needed
Day 2. Propoxyphene (Darvon) 100 mg q4h as needed
Day 5. Oxycodone (Percodan) 1 tablet q4h as needed
Day 12. Oxycodone (Percodan) 2 tablets q4h as needed
Day 14. Pentazocine (Talwin) 50 mg q4h as needed
Day 17. Pentazocine (Talwin) 50 mg q3h as needed
Day 22. Pentazocine (Talwin) 100 mg q4h as needed
Day 23. Meperidine (Demerol) 100 mg q4h as needed
Day 29. Hydromorphone (Dilaudid) 4 mg q4h as needed

After being discharged from the hospital the patient took excessive amounts of Dilaudid, up to twenty 4-mg tablets daily, with no appreciable relief of his pain. Moreover, he was frequently lethargic and irri-table and caused severe disruptions of his family's life. (He had stopped drinking alcohol.) He was read-mitted to the hospital for the persistent pains, his narcotic addiction was recognized, and he agreed to attempt detoxification from the narcotic in a drug-dependence treatment unit. Detoxification was

accomplished with methadone over a 2-week period, after which he expressed confidence that he could tolerate his pain without using drugs. Shortly after discharge, however, he resumed using large doses of narcotics and sedatives by obtaining prescriptions from several different physicians, and his home life deteriorated further. He was readmitted after an overdose of sedatives, entered the drug treatment program for the second time, and remained in the program for long-term rehabilitation. Psychological evaluation indicated a high degree of hypochondriasis, depression, cynicism, and hostility toward authorita-tive figures (physicians, for one), as well as severe manipulative behavior. His pain greatly worsened during periods of stress and depression. Treatment was directed toward enabling the patient to gain insight into his behavior; providing alternative meth-ods for dealing with his pain, depression, and tension; reestablishing his family relationships; and returning him to work. He has continued in outpatient treat-ment and is seemingly coping with the vicissitudes of work, marriage, and his medical illness without resort-ing to addicting drugs or alcohol. His prognosis, far better than before, is still guarded.

Several points are noteworthy in this case: The patient readily switched from alcohol dependence to drug dependence given the appropriate situation. While being treated on the medical ward he rapidly developed tolerance to narcotic analgesics and liber-ally used all of his medications that were ordered on an "as needed" basis. Relieving the patient's pain became a more important therapeutic goal for his physicians than understanding the nature of his pain and his behavior. In addition to the medical com-ponents of his addiction (tolerance and physical dependence), the patient suffered severe personal consequences. Psychological evaluation, although per-formed subsequent to his drug addiction, indicated personality characteristics that no doubt contributed to his addiction. Relapse occurred shortly after he was medically detoxified. Finally, after intensive rehabilitative treatment, his prognosis improved.

Terminology
The pharmacologic agents capable of producing alter-ations in mood, behavior, or perceptions are the principal drugs of abuse or addiction in this country. In this discussion, these drugs will be classified as follows: (1) narcotic analgesics or opiates, (2) cen-

tral nervous system depressants, including alcohol, (3) central nervous system stimulants, (4) hallucinogens, and (5) cannabis. The principal drugs in these categories and the major signs of intoxication, overdose, and withdrawal are listed in Table 3-1. Nicotine and caffeine, two important and widely used substances that may indeed produce dependence, will not be discussed.

It is often difficult to ascertain whether drugs or alcohol are being taken in a socially or medically acceptable manner and for psychologically sound reasons, or whether a pattern of consumption represents misuse or abuse. Clearly any use of narcotics, depressants, or stimulants, either unprescribed or in an amount and frequency that produces intoxication, represents drug abuse, even in the absence of overt social, psychological, or physical deterioration. When alcohol is used by a person on repeated occasions in order to "escape" or to "relieve tension" by getting drunk, this represents alcohol abuse. But what of the husband, father, and good provider who drinks half a case of beer or more on weekends because he "enjoys his beer"; or the person who takes prescribed opiate analgesics every 6 to 8 hours for chronic, severe pain syndromes? In such cases, the amount of substance consumed may be excessive, but deleterious consequences relating to this use may be minimal.

Certain signs allow for a more objective appraisal of drug or alcohol abuse. When the user perceives that continual use of the substance is necessary for him in order to function satisfactorily, he is *psychologically dependent* on or *habituated* to that drug. When, after repeated use, a given dose of a drug produces less of an effect, *tolerance* has developed. Tolerance may develop as a result of enhanced drug metabolism (drug-disposition or metabolic tolerance) or as a result of central nervous system adaptation to the drug (cellular, pharmacodynamic, or behavioral tolerance). *Cross tolerance,* to a variable degree, will occur between drugs in the same categories. Chronic, excessive use of the narcotic analgesics and of the central nervous system depressants produces *physical dependence,* and their continued use is necessary to prevent a *withdrawal* or *abstinence syndrome.* Within the same general categories of drugs are variable degrees of *cross dependence,*

wherein one drug (e.g., chlordiazepoxide) will alleviate the withdrawal symptoms and signs of another (e.g., alcohol).

The precise definition of *addiction* is debatable, but the concept is reasonably clear. Drug or alcohol addicts will demonstrate tolerance to the pharmacologic agent used and will be psychologically and physically dependent on this agent. Moreover, the compulsive use of the substance and the compulsive need to obtain it will result in deterioration of the user's personal, family, social, or vocational life and in his physical or psychological health. Unfortunately, an additional feature of addiction is the great tendency to relapse after drug withdrawal.

Classification of Drugs

NARCOTIC ANALGESICS
The narcotic analgesics, or opiates, are comprised both of natural drugs derived from opium from the poppy plant *Papaver somniferum,* and of synthetic drugs with essentially similar pharmacologic properties. As the most effective pain relievers used, opiates have the well-known characteristics of producing euphoria or a "high." Indeed, the analgesic and euphoric effects of opiates are closely related, if not the same. The recent identification of opiate receptors and endogenous peptides that bind to these receptors in the brain has generated great interest. Extension of these discoveries will very likely increase our understanding of pain, pain relief, and opiate addiction.

Patterns of Abuse
Heroin, injected intravenously ("mainlining"), subcutaneously ("skin-popping"), or intranasally ("snorting") is the main street drug of the narcotic addict. Heroin is approximately three times as potent an analgesic as morphine on a milligram basis; it more readily crosses the blood-brain barrier, and with intravenous use it produces a faster high. The availability of heroin on the market has important epidemiologic consequences; not only are the cost and purity of the drug affected, but also the number and types of users. When heroin was plentiful in Vietnam there were many users but relatively few became addicted; most users had no underlying character disorders and did

Table 3-1. Principal Drugs of Abuse and Addiction

Classification and principal drugs		Signs of intoxification[b]	Signs of overdose[b]	Signs of withdrawal[b]
Narcotic analgesics (opiates)				
Morphine	10.0[a]	Euphoria	Coma	Irritability
Diacetylmorphine (heroin)	3.0	Drowsiness	Pinpoint pupils	Tachycardia
Methadone (Dolophine)	7.5–10.0	"Nodding"	Depressed respirations	Hypertension
Hydromorphone (Dilaudid)	1.5	Miosis	Hypotension	Dilated pupils
Oxycodone (Percodan)	10–15	Constipation	Hypothermia	Rhinorrhea
Meperidine (Demerol)	80–100	Urinary retention	Pulmonary edema	Lacrimation
Codeine	120	(Needle or track marks)	(Needle or track marks)	Piloerection
Pentazocine (Talwin)	30–50		Diagnosis: Analysis of urine; response to narcotic antagonist	Abdominal cramps
Propoxyphene (Darvon)	200			Nausea, vomiting
				Diarrhea
				Muscle spasms
CNS depressants (sedatives, hypnotics, minor tranquilizers)				*Early*
Barbiturates (Amytal, Tuinal, Nembutal, Seconal)		Drowsiness	Stupor, coma	Anxiety
Ethyl alcohol		Ataxia	Depressed respirations	Anorexia
Glutethimide (Doriden)		Incoordination	Sluggish pupillary response, initially constricted, then dilated	Insomnia
Methaqualone (Quaalude)		Slurred speech	Reflexes: hyperactive to diminished	Tremulousness
Meprobamate (Miltown, Equanil)		Emotional lability	Diagnosis: Analysis of blood	Hallucinations
Methyprylon (Noludar)		"Disinhibitory" effects		Tachycardia
Chlordiazepoxide (Librium)				Diaphoresis
Diazepam (Valium)				Seizures
Chloral hydrate				*Late* (Delirium tremens)
				Disorientation
				Fever, tachycardia
				Agitation
CNS stimulants				
Amphetamines (Benzedrine, Dexedrine, Methedrine, Preludin)		Alertness	Agitation	No definite physical dependence
Cocaine		Hyperactivity	Psychosis	There may be confusion, depression, or suicide
Epinephrine		Anorexia	Delirium	
Strychnine		Tachycardia	Fever	
		Aggression	Convulsions	
		Psychosis	Diagnosis: Analysis of blood	

Hallucinogens			
D-Lysergic acid diethylamide (LSD, acid)	Hallucinations	Panic	No definite physical dependence
Mescaline (peyote)	Exaggerated senses	Psychosis	There may be
Dimethoxy-methylamphetamine (DOM, STP)	Disordered perceptions	Suicide	Confusion
Phencyclidine hydrochloride (PCP, Serynl)	Panic		Depression
Psilocybin (mushrooms)	Psychosis		Suicide
Possibly: High doses of *Cannabis* (marijuana, hashish)	Suicide		

aEquivalent analgesic doses in milligrams.
bIndividual signs or symptoms may be variably present or may depend on the particular drug used.

not return to drug use in this country. With plentiful heroin supplies, the nonaddicted users appear to be important in the spread of heroin use to peers. Conversely, with limited supplies and high costs, the users will represent a hard-core population of addicts whose rehabilitation will be generally poor. In the mid-1970s there were an estimated 400,000 to 600,000 heroin users in the United States

"Medical" narcotic addicts comprise two groups. First, physicians, nurses, pharmacists, and others in the health field have higher rates of narcotic addiction than the general population, in part as a result of their familiarity with and access to drugs. Second, patients with chronic pain syndromes (for example, chronic pancreatitis, low back pain, or recurrent headaches) may become dependent on narcotics following excessive chronic use of prescription analgesics, and will continue to obtain repeated prescriptions either from one or many physicians. Often these patients are depressed and derive secondary gains from their chronic pain syndromes. A well-recognized syndrome is narcotic addiction in the patient with alcohol-induced chronic pancreatitis; typically, this patient has stopped drinking alcohol, but is using a narcotic analgesic instead. It is frequently difficult to determine if such a patient is having episodes of pancreatitis or is merely maintaining an addiction.

Intoxication, Tolerance, and Physical Dependence
The reader is referred to standard pharmacology texts for detailed descriptions of the pharmacologic actions of the narcotic analgesics. For the drug abuser, the important intoxicating effect of opiates is the resultant calm or euphoric feeling. Moreover, the intravenous injection of heroin will produce a warm, pleasant sensation known as a "rush" or "thrill," and the preference for heroin over other opiates appears to be due to this initial rapid effect. With repeated doses, tolerance develops within several days and substantially increases the effective analgesic, intoxicating, and lethal doses. Whereas enhanced drug metabolism occurs to a minor degree, tolerance develops mainly by central nervous system cellular adaptation. Physical dependence after narcotic use depends on a number of factors: the dose and duration of use, the duration of action of the narcotic, and the criteria for diagnosing withdrawal signs and symptoms. Following ordinary analgesic doses of morphine for 1 to 2 weeks, virtually no withdrawal signs will occur, whereas if high doses are given over even a few days withdrawal signs may occur on cessation of the drug.

When opiate use is terminated in a dependent person, withdrawal symptoms will begin at 4 to 12 hours, peak at 24 to 48 hours, and last for several days. Initially, the patient may display purposeful symptoms, may complain of anxiety, irritability, nausea, pain, or abdominal cramps, and may plead or bargain for treatment. Objective signs, which accompany or shortly follow these symptoms, include dilated, sluggishly reactive pupils, lacrimation and rhinorrhea, elevated pulse and blood pressure, piloerection, vomiting, and diarrhea. In severe, untreated withdrawal, muscle spasms (which might produce involuntary jerking of the legs; thus, "kicking the habit") and convulsions (rarely) may occur. Untreated, "cold turkey" withdrawal is not associated with mortality unless terminated by suicide. The easiest explanation for the signs of withdrawal is a neurologic "rebound hypersensitivity" manifested by signs opposite to those produced by the drug: for example, dilated for constricted pupils; lacrimation and rhinorrhea instead of dry mucous membranes; abdominal cramps and diarrhea instead of constipation; irritability instead of calmness.

Objective signs of withdrawal should be present before treatment is started. Oral methadone is an effective drug for treating withdrawal; its duration of action is 12 to 24 hours, and when the daily dosage is tapered, it leaves only mild, albeit prolonged, withdrawal symptoms. An initial dose of 10 to 15 mg will alleviate most withdrawal symptoms and signs, following which a detoxification schedule can be implemented.

Overdose
Acute poisoning with heroin, morphine, or other opiates is characterized by coma, depressed respirations, and pinpoint pupils. Additional signs are cyanosis, muscle flaccidity, hyporeflexia, hypothermia, and occasionally pulmonary edema. The presence of "track" or needle marks will be helpful in

reaching a diagnosis, and a positive urine analysis for opiates, although delayed, will confirm the diagnosis. In such cases a complete toxicology screening is necessary, since the patient may have used several drugs. The dosage of opiate that causes severe poisoning is highly variable, depending primarily on the tolerance of the individual. In nonaddicts parenteral doses of morphine greater than 30 mg may produce severe respiratory depression, whereas some addicts may tolerate doses of several hundred milligrams or more.

Treatment requires two approaches: (1) supportive measures with intensive medical and nursing care, and (2) use of a narcotic antagonist. The antagonists utilized are naloxone hydrochloride (Narcan), 0.4 mg given intramuscularly or intravenously and repeated at 2- to 3-minute intervals for up to three doses, or nalorphine (Nalline), 5 mg given intravenously at 15-minute intervals as needed. Such treatment will inevitably improve respiratory function in opiate poisoning, confirming the diagnosis, and it may precipitate withdrawal symptoms.

Medical Complications
Aside from overdose or acute reactions to heroin, the medical complications of heroin use result not from the drug itself but from the intravenous or subcutaneous injection of contaminants, primarily infectious organisms. Localized infections or inflammation, skin abscesses, cellulitis, and phlebitis occur frequently. In heroin users, acute or subacute bacterial endocarditis can involve any heart valve and is caused by any of the usual offending organisms, but heroin users seem particularly susceptible to right-sided valvular lesions with *Staphylococcus aureus.* Septicemia, with joint, bone, or central nervous system infections, may occur without an obvious endocardial infection. Pulmonary complications include abscesses and pneumonia, as well as granulomas caused by the foreign bodies used to adulterate heroin. Rarely, syphilis or malaria may be transmitted by injection, and drug addicts appear more susceptible to tetanus than is the general population.

Parenterally transmitted viral hepatitis represents an important index of heroin use in a community or country. Heroin users may report several distinct episodes of acute hepatitis and may develop chronic persistent or chronic aggressive hepatitis following hepatitis infections. Approximately 5 percent of chronic heroin users will be positive when tested for hepatitis B surface antigen (see Chap. 41).

Overdose with heroin, either accidental or resulting from suicidal or homicidal intent, is an important cause of death among addicts. Moreover, acute heroin reactions occur, which are manifested by fever, pulmonary edema, cyanosis, diffuse intravascular coagulation with bleeding, coma, or sudden death; these reactions may represent, in part, reactions to adulterants. The heroin addict has many other general medical problems relating to poor nutrition and poor personal habits: dental hygiene is often extremely poor; tuberculosis infections occur commonly; and venereal diseases are common, although it is noteworthy that a false-positive serologic finding may occur in persons using heroin or methadone. In summary, chronic heroin users present a number of medical problems, some of which are recognized as direct and others as indirect consequences of heroin addiction.

CENTRAL NERVOUS SYSTEM DEPRESSANTS
The category of central nervous system (CNS) depressants includes a large number of commonly used drugs and substances, including the sedative-hypnotics and minor tranquilizers, with liability for profound abuse and addiction. All these drugs have the common effect of producing generalized, reversible depression of the central nervous system, and all can produce severe intoxication and potentially fatal poisoning. Many of the pharmacologic effects of ethyl alcohol are similar to those of the CNS depressant drugs, and both cross tolerance and cross dependence exist between alcohol and these drugs. Because of its overwhelming social and medical importance, special consideration will be given to the problem of alcohol abuse.

Patterns of Abuse
The short-acting and medium-acting barbiturates are the CNS depressants most frequently abused, either through illegal acquisition of drug supplies or through unwarranted use of prescribed medication. In addi-

tion to the barbiturates ("downs," "reds," or "yellows") there is widespread abuse of glutethimide (Doriden), methaqualone (Quaalude), meprobamate (Miltown, Equanil), and diazepam (Valium) within the drug culture. Survey data from drug treatment programs indicate that barbiturates and other CNS depressants are the primary or secondary drug of abuse in 15 to 25 percent of drug addicts seeking treatment. These drugs, including alcohol, are the most common substances associated with overdoses. The use of depressant drugs, either alone or in combination with alcohol, stimulants, or occasionally narcotics, is increasing dramatically in teenagers and young adults. Within the population of persons chronically addicted to CNS depressants are many with underlying psychopathology, particularly depression, anxiety neurosis, or frank psychosis.

Intoxication, Tolerance, and Physical Dependence
Standard textbooks of pharmacology should be consulted for detailed descriptions of the pharmacology of the CNS depressant agents. For those who use these drugs to achieve intoxication, the effects include generalized sluggishness, difficulty with thought and speech, memory impairment, incoordination, and emotional lability. Personality traits and feelings that may be ordinarily suppressed, such as anger, aggression, sexuality, sadness, or loneliness, may be expressed as a result of the disinhibitory effects of the intoxicating drug.

Tolerance to and physical dependence on these drugs have been studied most extensively with the barbiturates. Tolerance develops by two mechanisms: drug disposition tolerance through increased metabolism by hepatic enzymes, and pharmacodynamic tolerance through currently unknown mechanisms of adaptation in the brain. Whereas substantial tolerance develops to the sedative and intoxicating doses of barbiturates, little if any occurs to alter the lethal dose. Thus with increasing blood levels the dangerous effects of barbiturates in tolerant and nontolerant individuals become similar. The type and dose of barbiturate used will determine the development of physical dependence. A withdrawal syndrome will occur after only several days' use of short-acting barbiturates in high doses. Conversely, longer-acting

barbiturates may be used in low or moderate doses for prolonged periods without overt evidence of physical dependence when the drug is discontinued. The characteristic features of the CNS depressant abstinence syndrome, which are listed in Table 3-1, are essentially similar to those of alcohol withdrawal. Seizures are particularly common in untreated barbiturate withdrawal, occurring in 50 to 75 percent of cases, and are often followed by frank delirium tremens. The goal of detoxification is to prevent seizures and delirium by administering a CNS depressant that will suppress the major signs and symptoms of early withdrawal. This drug may be the same sedative that the patient had been using or one that exhibits a cross dependence. The daily dose of the drug is then slowly reduced over a period of a week or longer. Treatment of frank delirium tremens is discussed in the section on withdrawal from alcohol.

Overdose
Since little tolerance develops to the coma-producing and lethal doses of the CNS depressants, severe poisoning or overdose with one or more of these drugs represents an important problem for both the addicted and nonaddicted user. The depressant effects of these substances are additive, if not synergistic; for example nonlethal doses of alcohol and barbiturates, when combined, may cause death. The duration and the depth of coma depend on the offending drug, its mode of detoxification, and the blood level achieved. The diagnosis of sedative drug poisoning is made from the combined signs of unresponsiveness, normal or sluggishly reacting pupils, absent oculovestibular response, hyporeflexia or areflexia, depressed respirations, and hypotension. Toxicology screening of a blood sample will determine the offending drug or drugs and their serum concentrations. In contrast to narcotic poisoning, there are no useful pharmacologic antagonists that safely reverse the effects of depressant substances; thus successful treatment rests on early and intensive medical and nursing care. Emphasis is placed on instituting a patent airway, cautious oxygenation, assisted ventilation, positional pulmonary drainage, endotracheal suction, intravenous hydration, possible use of pressor agents, and detection and treatment of

infections. If the drug was taken only a few hours before admission, gastric lavage is indicated. Forced diuresis and alkalization of the urine will increase the renal excretion of all the barbiturates; hemodialysis is indicated for patients in a prolonged coma caused by the long-acting barbiturates. For specific signs and treatment of poisoning for each of the large number of available depressant drugs, physicians should consult toxicology and pharmacology textbooks, the *Physicians' Desk Reference,* and Poison Control Centers. Following successful treatment of a sedative overdose, psychiatric evaluation is indicated for the patient to determine the need for further observation and care.

CENTRAL NERVOUS SYSTEM STIMULANTS

Amphetamines ("ups," "bennies," "dexes," or "pep-pills") and cocaine are the major CNS stimulants used for psychotropic effects. Recent surveys indicate widespread use, although not necessarily chronic abuse, of amphetamines. Close to 10 percent of young men recently surveyed in the United States had used these stimulants on one or more occasions. Among chronic drug abusers, amphetamines are frequently used orally in combination with alcohol, barbiturates, or other CNS depressants (poly-drug users); or they are used intravenously by "speed freaks" and some heroin addicts. In some cases, the initial use of stimulants is for the purpose of dieting or for remaining awake to study or work, but tolerance to the anorectic and analeptic effects develops after a week or more of continued use. Cocaine may also be used intravenously, but it is taken mostly by intranasal sniffing. In the 1970s, cocaine may be one of the more commonly used and profitable of the illicit drugs in the United States. When it is used infrequently, there may not necessarily be deleterious effects.

The pharmacologic effects of the stimulants, both central and peripheral, include tachycardia, hypertension, increased cardiac contractility, bronchodilatation, alertness, anorexia, and insomnia. In severe intoxication, the user may exhibit aggressive, agitated, paranoic, or psychotic behavior, with possible convulsions and cardiovascular collapse. Hyperactive individuals may exhibit a paradoxical calming effect

from amphetamines. The chronic stimulant (amphetamine) abuser is usually thin and suffers the debilitating effects of deprivation of sleep and nutrition. Tolerance and psychological dependence are major features of stimulant abuse, but true physical dependence does not appear to develop with either amphetamines or cocaine. Nevertheless, detoxification of these patients requires attentive psychological support, reassurance, and often judicious use of tranquilizers. Other than their use in severely hyperactive children, there are no justified medical indications for the chronic use of CNS stimulants.

HALLUCINOGENS

Although the peak use of hallucinogens (psychedelics, psychotomimetics) occurred with great attendant publicity in the late 1960s, use of these "mind-expanding" drugs continues in certain drug-using populations. These drugs, listed in Table 3-1, have no human medical indications, and it is illegal to manufacture or sell them. Lysergic acid diethylamide (LSD, "acid") is the most commonly used hallucinogen, although the animal tranquilizer phencyclidine (Serynl, PCP, "angel dust") has widespread use also. The "trip" from hallucinogens includes heightened sensations, altered perceptions, and detachment, and may result in extreme anxiety, panic, or a psychotic reaction. Associated physical findings are dilated pupils, tachycardia, hypertension, fever, hyperreflexia, and tremor. Tolerance to the effects of these drugs develops, but there are no predictable withdrawal symptoms. However, withdrawal, like the "bad trip," may be characterized by agitation, depression, or psychotic reactions and requires reassurance ("talking-down") and possibly treatment with a tranquilizer such as diazepam. Phenothiazines should be avoided in these patients since adverse reactions between these drugs and certain hallucinogens have been reported.

CANNABIS

Marijuana and hashish, of which Δ-9-tetrahydrocannabinol (THC) is the major active principal, do not fit within any of the preceding categories of drugs; however, they clearly have intoxicating effects that alter mood, perceptions, and behavior. These substances, particularly marijuana, are smoked by a broad spectrum of young adults: marijuana in home-made cigarettes (joints), and hashish in pipes. The majority of those who smoke marijuana do so infrequently in certain social settings, and they use no other psychoactive drugs except for alcohol. However, the chronic user who smokes to intoxication is likely to seek similar effects from alcohol and other drugs.

The major psychoactive effects of cannabis are an enhanced or altered perception, especially of time; disinhibitory effects; detachment; and variable mood changes including euphoria, anxiety, or depression. High doses may induce frank hallucinations, paranoia, or psychotic behavior. Physical dependence does not occur, and there are no reports of fatal poisoning. Numerous adverse physical effects from marijuana have been described but not confirmed. It is reported that chronic, heavy use is associated with inflammation of the upper and lower respiratory tract, and possibly with decreased respiratory function.

ALCOHOL

Ethyl alcohol is a mood-changing drug of the sedative-hypnotic or CNS depressant type and is potentially habituating. The essential features of "alcoholism" and of an "alcoholic" include (1) compulsive, uncontrolled drinking to intoxication; (2) pharmacologically, tolerance and physical dependence; (3) chronicity of abuse, with a high tendency to relapse; and (4) deterioration of effective functioning and health. In addition to these features, use of the term *problem drinking* broadens the spectrum of alcoholism. This term implies frequent episodic drinking to intoxication, generally caused by and leading to significant personal or social problems.

That some authorities have identified alcoholism as a disease has evoked considerable controversy. Briefly, the disease concept implies that biologic or psychological factors, or both, cause certain individuals to be unable to control their alcohol consumption; hence loss of control of alcohol consumption is basic to the disease concept. Examination of this concept has yielded equivocal results. Most hereditary studies have failed to define an inherited susceptibility to alcoholism in humans. However,

results from a recent adoption study in Denmark indicate that having an alcoholic biologic parent enhances the chance of future alcoholism in offspring even when the children are raised totally by nonalcoholic adoptive parents. Despite the existence of national, ethnic, and familial differences in the prevalence of alcoholism, racial and ethnic differences in rates of alcohol metabolism have not been established. In this regard, cultural differences both in drinking habits and in attitudes toward acceptable and unacceptable drinking behavior probably have the major influence on the prevalence of alcohol abuse within countries, ethnic groups, communities, and families. Although many alcohol addicts and problem drinkers demonstrate character disorders, neuroses, or psychoses, a predictable premorbid "alcoholic" or "addictive personality" has not been defined.

As a general working hypothesis, it is probable that certain psychological, biologic, and sociocultural factors enhance both the likelihood of problem drinking and the development of tolerance for and psychological dependence on alcohol in certain individuals, but that learned or conditioned behavior plays the essential role in the habituating process. When frank addiction to alcohol occurs, physical dependence and additional psychological and social factors (e.g., hopelessness, loss of self-respect, loss of job and family) perpetuate the uncontrolled drinking. Problem drinking does not necessarily progress into alcohol addiction, however, and remissions from both problem drinking and addiction do occur.

Patterns of Abuse

The principal alcoholic beverages are (1) beer, fermented from barley malt, 3 to 8% alcohol by volume; (2) table wine, fermented from grapes, 12% alcohol; (3) dessert wine, 2 to 13% sugar, 20% alcohol; (4) liqueur, up to 50% sugar, 20 to 55% alcohol; and (5) distilled spirits (fermented from a variety of grains and then distilled), 35 to 70% alcohol. Distilled spirits, inexpensive table wines, and beer are the principal alcoholic beverages consumed by alcoholics in this country. Surveys by the National Institute of Alcohol Abuse and Alcoholism (NIAAA) estimate that of those of drinking age in the United States, 42 percent are nondrinkers (defined as being total abstainers or drinking only negligible amounts), 31 percent are light drinkers (averaging less than ¼ ounce of absolute alcohol daily), 18 percent are moderate drinkers (averaging up to 1 ounce daily), and 9 percent are heavy drinkers (averaging more than 1 ounce of absolute alcohol daily). In this latter category of about 14 million people over 18 years old, 9 million are estimated to be problem drinkers and addicts. It is estimated that the 14 million heavy drinkers consume 70 percent of the alcoholic beverages sold in this country.

Some segments of the population seem particularly at risk to develop alcohol abuse problems: examples are Indians on reservations, young Irish-American men who live in cities, and blacks in ghettos. For some groups, drinking problems are minimal, including Jews, despite a high percentage of drinkers, and practicing Mormons, who have strict codes against drinking. The prevalence of alcohol use and problem drinking is rising among teenagers and young adults: Close to 40 percent of twelfth-grade boys drink alcoholic beverages once a week or more; 20 percent of men age 18 to 21 are classified as heavy drinkers; and men age 21 to 24 have the highest numbers of alcohol-related problems. A profile analysis of the men in the United States with the greatest risk for problem drinking has been derived from the national surveys. Such a man is under 25 years of age; of low socioeconomic status; a resident of or immigrant to a large city; either separated, divorced, or single; and without religious affiliation or not attending a church. In addition, a man with childhood disjunctions (e.g., from a broken home) and with one or more alcoholic parent is at high risk to develop alcohol abuse problems.

The estimated costs of alcohol abuse in lives and dollars are impressive: 20,000 to 30,000 deaths a year are directly attributable to alcoholic liver disease; approximately one-half (25,000 to 30,000) of all traffic fatalities yearly and one-third of violent deaths are alcohol related; alcoholism costs an estimated $10 billion in lost work time to industry and government yearly; and health, welfare, and property costs for alcoholics and their families amount to $5 billion yearly.

Intoxication

The relationships among alcohol ingestion, blood alcohol concentration, and signs of intoxication are variable and depend on rates of ingestion, absorption, and metabolism and on the specific pharmacodynamic tolerance of the individual. Alcohol is more rapidly absorbed from the small intestine than from the stomach; thus conditions that delay gastric emptying (food in the stomach, high alcohol concentrations in the stomach, sedative drugs) or that enhance gastric emptying (carbonated beverages, partial gastric resection with gastrojejunostomy) affect the rate of alcohol absorption accordingly. Ninety to 98 percent of absorbed alcohol is oxidized by the liver to acetaldehyde by an alcohol dehydrogenase-NAD mediated reaction and by a microsomal ethanol oxidizing system (MEOS) in the smooth endoplasmic reticulum. The approximate rate of oxidation is 10 ml or 0.8 gm of absolute alcohol per hour.

In the nonhabituated drinker, alcohol concentrations of 20 to 100 mg per 100 ml are associated with mild muscular incoordination and disinhibitory effects with changes in mood and behavior; 100 to 200 mg per 100 ml with incoordination, prolonged reaction time, slurred speech, and ataxia; 200 to 400 mg per 100 ml with amnesia and marked incoordination; and above 400 mg per 100 ml with stupor, coma, respiratory depression, and possibly death. A serum concentration greater than 150 mg per 100 ml is the usual legal definition of intoxication. Tolerance in a chronic heavy drinker will be manifested both by increased rates of alcohol metabolism by the liver (metabolic tolerance) and by decreased CNS manifestations at elevated blood alcohol concentrations (pharmacodynamic tolerance). Even in the chronic alcohol addict, however, only moderate tolerance develops to the respiratory depressant and lethal levels of blood alcohol. Relatively little is known regarding the physiologic and psychological mechanisms that enhance the development of tolerance in certain drinkers; advancing this knowledge is an important goal for investigators in the field of alcohol abuse.

Withdrawal Syndromes

Abrupt cessation of alcohol intake following intoxication for two or more weeks will generally result in overt withdrawal symptoms. *Minor or early withdrawal,* occurring within the first 48 hours, is characterized by variable degrees of tremor, tachycardia, hypertension, hyperventilation, diaphoresis, anxiety, insomnia, bad dreams, anorexia, nausea, and vomiting. Hallucinations, usually visual, may occur during early withdrawal, but the patient is oriented with only mild confusion. *Seizures* ("rum fits") usually occur in the first 48 hours during early withdrawal and may be indistinguishable from generalized epileptic convulsions. Approximately 5 to 10 percent of untreated alcohol addicts develop frank *delirium tremens,* which occurs from 2 to 7 days into the withdrawal period. Delirium tremens is characterized by profound disorientation, agitation, fever, diaphoresis, and labile pulse and blood pressure. The average duration of delirium tremens is 2 days, and the mortality is 1 to 5 percent. Older patients and those with concurrent infections, high fevers, alcoholic hepatitis, pancreatitis, or traumatic injuries have a higher mortality associated with delirium tremens than do those without these complications. Physiologic mechanisms that have been proposed as contributing to the early withdrawal syndrome include hyperventilation with respiratory alkalosis and cerebral hypoxia, hypomagnesemia, and abnormal hypothalamic-pituitary-adrenal function with increased end-organ sensitivity to hormonal stimuli. Intense anxiety contributes to the clinical findings of early withdrawal in some patients. It is not known why only certain patients progress into delirium tremens, and the underlying pathophysiologic mechanisms are poorly understood. Some investigators postulate that delirium tremens is related to a marked increase in REM sleep, which previously had been suppressed during chronic alcohol use.

The goals of treatment of early withdrawal are to prevent withdrawal seizures and delirium tremens and to provide symptomatic relief, particularly a restful sleep. All alcoholic patients should receive thiamine during the initial phase of treatment to prevent acute Wernicke's encephalopathy. Only minimal controversy remains as to whether or not sedation given during early withdrawal actually prevents delirium tremens. Most controlled studies and the

experience from detoxification centers and psychiatric units in which relatively healthy patients are treated indicate that the incidence of delirium tremens can be reduced with medical detoxification. Chlordiazepoxide hydrochloride (Librium) and diazepam (Valium) are commonly used for alcohol detoxification. In the first 24 hours, from 100 to 400 mg of chlordiazepoxide in 25- to 100-mg doses may be given to the otherwise healthy patient; the daily dose is then reduced in the ensuing 4 to 5 days to complete detoxification. The half-life of chlordiazepoxide, diazepam, and most other sedatives is prolonged twofold to fourfold with concomitant overt hepatocellular disease. Moreover, injudicious use of sedatives is a major cause of hepatic coma in patients with cirrhosis; thus sedatives may have to be withheld or used at reduced doses with such patients. The addition of phenytoin sodium (Dilantin), 300 mg daily, is reported to reduce seizures during withdrawal in alcoholics with a prior history of seizures, regardless of their etiology. Because magnesium deficiency is common in alcoholics and may contribute to neuromuscular irritability, parenteral magnesium sulfate is occasionally used. Evidence supporting its efficacy is lacking, however, and magnesium deficiency alone does not explain the withdrawal syndrome. Treatment by reassuring personnel in a calm atmosphere is of great benefit to the anxious patient withdrawing from alcohol.

The goals of treatment of delirium tremens are (1) to identify and treat concurrent medical or traumatic illnesses; (2) to maintain hydration and administer vitamins and nutrients parenterally; and (3) to achieve a state of calm that prevents the agitated, confused patient from harming himself and others and allows time for diagnosis and treatment of other disorders. X-rays of the skull, a lumbar puncture for cerebrospinal fluid examination, and a full fever evaluation are usually necessary. Intravenously administered diazepam or rectally administered paraldehyde are effective in inducing and maintaining a state of calm in the agitated patient with delirium tremens.

Medical Complications
The wide variety of alcohol-related medical disorders,

which are discussed in detail in other chapters in this text, are listed below:

Neurologic and muscular disorders
Peripheral neuropathy
Organic brain syndromes
Wernicke's encephalopathy
Korsakoff's psychosis
Cerebellar ataxia
Withdrawal syndromes — minor, seizures, delirium tremens
Intoxication — impaired coordination, judgment, reaction times
Myopathy

Hepatic and gastrointestinal disorders
Liver diseases — fatty liver, alcoholic hepatitis, cirrhosis
Pancreatitis — acute, chronic
Gastritis — acute hemorrhagic, chronic atrophic
Nonspecific diarrhea
Oropharyngeal, laryngeal, and esophageal carcinoma

Hematologic disorders
Folate deficiency anemia
Iron deficiency anemia secondary to gastrointestinal blood loss
Leukopenia, impaired granulocyte function
Thrombocytopenia
Impaired clotting factors in liver disease

Cardiac disorders
Alcohol and beriberi cardiomyopathy

Metabolic disorders
Hypoglycemia
Hypertriglyceridemia
Hyperlactacidemia and hyperuricemia
Ketosis
Hypomagnesemia
Hypophosphatemia
Hypoalbuminemia

Pulmonary disorders
Aspiration pneumonia
Increased risk of tuberculosis, bacterial pneumonia

Dermatologic disorders
Rhinophyma, rosacea

Infestations
Cutaneous ulcers

Traumatic events
Head trauma, fractures
Automobile and pedestrian accidents
Violent injuries and deaths

Pharmacologic actions
Drug interactions with alcohol

Alcohol-related hepatic and neurologic diseases are the most common and most severe medical consequences of chronic alcohol abuse. The interrelations between alcohol ingestion and nutritional factors in the pathogenesis of liver and other organ system diseases are complex and remain poorly understood. However, most recent studies indicate the importance of the direct toxic effects of alcohol (and possibly of its metabolic product, acetaldehyde) on the liver and other organ systems. The search for congeners in alcoholic beverages that produce chronic or acute organ toxicity has not been particularly fruitful, although the increased concentration of iron in some wines may cause excessive iron deposition in the liver in the presence of alcoholic cirrhosis, and cobalt in some beers may contribute to a cardiomyopathy.

Alcohol has important interactions with a large number of commonly used drugs. Ingestion of alcohol together with other sedative-hypnotics results in additive, and possibly synergistic, CNS depressant effects. These effects appear to result from delayed hepatic metabolism of either the alcohol or the other sedative drug due to competition for microsomal oxidizing enzymes in the smooth endoplasmic reticulum. Conversely, when a chronic alcoholic becomes alcohol-free, metabolism of some sedative drugs and of warfarin and phenytoin is enhanced, presumably by prior induction of microsomal oxidizing enzymes. Alcohol may potentiate the hypotensive effect of hypotensive agents by causing direct vasodilatation, and it may also potentiate the hypoglycemic effects of insulin and oral hypoglycemic agents by interfering with hepatic glyconeogenesis. Alcohol and aspirin both facilitate hydrogen ion back diffusion in the gastric mucosa and may potentiate each other in causing acute hemorrhagic gastritis. The absorption

of thiamine and folic acid, and probably of other
water-soluble nutrients, is impaired with high concentrations of alcohol in the gut. Thus, these and other
alcohol-drug interactions may interfere with either
the efficacy or the safety of prescribed medications.

Treatment of Drug and Alcohol Dependence

Drug and alcohol abusers represent a heterogeneous
group of people from a wide variety of social and
cultural environments. Although specific psychological characteristics that might predict substance abuse
have not been defined, a great deal of psychopathology, character disorders, and sociocultural deprivation
exists within this population. It is likely that substance abuse initially develops as learned or conditioned behavior; that is, the user is "rewarded" by the
effects of the drug (e.g., relief of tension, anger, pain,
depression), which is taken in response to internal or
external stimuli. However, the important factors that
contribute to early drug or alcohol abuse may be
supplemented by new psychological, physical, and
social factors that maintain the habit. Therefore,
treatment cannot be confined solely to elucidating
the psychodynamics of the individual addict but must
also be directed toward practical aspects of the
addict's behavior and life-style.

The ultimate goals of treatment are to return to
society a person who is drug-free or alcohol-free,
emotionally stable, introspective, and capable of
establishing honest interpersonal relations. Additional
goals include "straight" or "sober" friends and activities, and a productive job or educational pursuits.
The principles for treatment of drug and alcohol
dependence are essentially similar, although special
modes of therapy exist for each. There are two
major phases of treatment: *detoxification* or withdrawal from the addicting substances, and *rehabilitation* or continued treatment. Specific methods for
medical detoxification have been described previously.
Detoxification is best accomplished in a drug-free and
alcohol-free setting with medical, psychological, and
peer-group support. Little if any rehabilitation therapy can be accomplished if the patient is still taking
drugs or drinking alcohol.

For drug addicts who are motivated for treatment,
effective rehabilitation may take place in drug-free

therapeutic communities that utilize group therapy
and methods of behavioral modification. The general
thrust of such treatment is to encourage clients to
deal honestly with their feelings and with the substan-
tive issues in their lives, and to effect changes in attitudes and behavior. Comprehensive drug treatment
will also provide family, vocational, educational, and
legal services to facilitate reentry of the individual
into society. For the opiate addict enrolled in a
methadone maintenance program, methadone is
administered in a daily dose sufficient to decrease the
desire for and block the euphoric effect of heroin.
The success of some addicts maintained on methadone
in terms of work, education, and cessation of criminal
activities has been impressive, but many others continue to use illicit drugs. Some develop an intense
psychological dependence on methadone, which
makes subsequent detoxification extremely difficult.
The utility of narcotic antagonists that block the
euphoric effects of heroin and prevent physical
dependence is currently being investigated.

In urban settings, various treatment facilities and
modalities are generally available to the problem
drinker or alcohol addict who is well motivated.
Ideally, treatment should be long term and comprehensive, the primary goal being indefinite sobriety.
Some of the associated medical, psychological, and
social problems presented by alcoholics and some
specific modes of therapy that are effective are outlined in Table 3-2. Committed membership in Alcoholics Anonymous (AA) fills many of the emotional
and social needs of problem drinkers, in addition to
providing strong structural support to the goal of daily
sobriety. For some patients disulfiram (Antabuse) is
an effective adjuvant to outpatient treatment for alcoholism. Disulfiram interferes with the aldehyde dehydrogenase-NAD mediated oxidation of acetaldehyde,
and when alcohol is ingested causes a pronounced rise
in blood acetaldehyde associated with headache,
dizziness, nausea, vomiting, flushing, and often hypotension. Some physicians and programs favor the use
of antidepressants or tranquilizers for patients who
have substantial depression or anxiety contributing to
drinking; however, the effectiveness of these forms of
therapy is debatable. Unfortunately, well-controlled
evaluations of programs and of specific modes of

Table 3-2. Common Problems Associated with Alcohol Abuse and Treatment Modalities

Problem	Treatment modality
Pathologic intoxification; potential harm to self or others	Protective custody; overnight facility
Withdrawal syndromes	Detoxification at home, detoxification center, or hospital
Related medical or psychiatric illnesses; severe neurologic or physical impairment	Hospital or outpatient care; chronic institutionalization; nursing home or home care
Behavioral, psychological, or emotional problems	AA; counseling; individual or group therapy; behavioral modification; psychodrama; transactional analysis; assertiveness training; meditation; antidepressants; tranquilizers
Family, vocational, financial, or legal problems	Family counseling and therapy; Al-anon; Alateen; social services; legal services; job training; industrial alcoholism programs
No place to live; difficult reentry into society; no sober friends; no leisure time activities	Halfway houses; AA; drop-in centers; resocialization activities

therapy are difficult to obtain, and many problem drinkers stop drinking or markedly improve their drinking habits without formal treatment. However, many well-motivated patients who actively participate in treatment that is logical and positive in its approach benefit substantially from the adjustments made in their lives to achieve sobriety. A concerted national effort is being made to educate the American public to identify alcohol as a potentially harmful and habituating substance, to recognize problem drinking, and to deal with it openly. Such an effort is important and is worthy of support from the medical profession.

Suggestions to Young Physicians in Managing Drug- and Alcohol-Dependent Patients

The physician has important but limited responsibilities in managing alcohol- or drug-dependent patients. Generally it is not the goal, nor is it within the capabilities, of most practicing physicians to be the sole provider of definitive, long-term treatment for these patients. Nevertheless, the physician must use diagnostic and therapeutic skills, must seek appropriate referrals and consultations, and must remain sympathetic and objective in his dealings with these patients. The following suggestions may be helpful to those who will be treating alcohol- and drug-dependent patients in their medical training and practices.

1. Be able to recognize and manage the intoxication, overdose, and withdrawal symptoms caused by the common addicting drugs and by alcohol.
2. Be able to recognize and manage the medical complications associated with drug and alcohol abuse.
3. Be able to diagnose substance abuse through a careful history of the medical, personal, and social consequences of excessive alcohol or drug consumption. However, even the most carefully and tactfully obtained history may fail to detect substance abuse in a patient who is unwilling to deal with the problem.
4. Make appropriate referrals to counselors, social workers, clinics, professional or voluntary agencies, or physicians that specialize in the treatment of alcohol-dependent or drug-dependent patients. Know what resources are available in your hospital and community.
5. In treating drug-dependent patients, avoid situations in which the patient can alter your treatment plans. Set firm rules regarding dosage and the time of administration of medications. Avoid orders for analgesics and tranquilizers (if necessary) on an "as needed" basis; such orders encourage bargaining by the patient, reward drug taking for relief of pain or tension, and may contribute to the development of tolerance.

6. Be sympathetic to the patient with a drug or alcohol problem and avoid being judgmental or demeaning. However, attempts to change the behavior of the unmotivated patient rarely succeed and often trap the well-meaning physician in a compromised role of trying to save the patient who does not want to be saved. Advise the patient objectively of your assessment of the severity of his drug or alcohol problem, recommend treatment, and seek appropriate consultations or referrals.

Bibliography

Alcohol and Health. First Special Report to Congress. Washington, D.C.: U.S. Department of Health, Education, and Welfare, 1971.

Alcohol and Health, New Knowledge. Second Special Report to Congress. Washington, D.C.: U.S. Department of Health, Education, and Welfare, 1974.

Greene, M. H., Nightingale, S. L., and DuPont, R. L. Evolving patterns of drug abuse. *Ann. Intern. Med.* 83:402, 1975.

Jaffe, J. H. Genesis of Drug Use and Dependence. In L. S. Goodman and A. Gilman (eds.), *Pharmacological Basis of Therapeutics* (5th ed.). New York: Macmillan, 1975. P. 284.

Mendelson, J. H. Biologic concomitants of alcoholism. *N. Engl. J. Med.* 283:24, 71, 1970.

Nightingale, S. L., Dormer, R. A., and DuPont, R. L. Inappropriate prescribing of psychoactive drugs. *Ann. Intern. Med.* 83:896, 1975.

Seixas, F. A. Alcohol and its drug interactions. *Ann. Intern. Med.* 83:86, 1975.

Sellers, E. M., and Kalant, H. Alcohol intoxication and withdrawal. *N. Engl. J. Med.* 294:757, 1976.

Thompson, W. L., Johnson, A. D., and Maddrey, W. L. Diazepam and paraldehyde for treatment of severe delirium tremens, a controlled trial. *Ann. Intern. Med.* 82:175, 1975.

Victor, M., and Wolfe, S. M. Causation and Treatment of Alcohol Withdrawal Syndrome. In P. G. Bourne and R. Fox (eds.), *Alcoholism, Progress in Research and Treatment.* New York: Academic, 1973. P. 137.

4

Clinical Nutrition

William P. Steffee

Nutrition means different things to different people. To the lay public, nutrition implies food supplies, food additives, or food preparation. To most dietitians, nutrition signifies an understanding of the basic food substances, the recommended daily allowances of calories and vitamins, and suitable modifications of these allowances for various individuals. To epidemiologists, nutrition suggests the search for cause-and-effect relationships between diet and patterns of disease. To world planners, nutrition is expressed in terms of factors such as the political interaction of populations, malnutrition, and world agriculture.

To many physicians, the term *nutrition* calls to mind some of the above factors, but too often physicians fail to assess their patients' nutritional needs, even when intensive nutritional support is most necessary. Although the human body is an extremely adaptable organism, capable of responding to severe stress, it must always be maintained by adequate nutritional support. Therefore, a physician's understanding of nutrition should include a clear conception of how the human body utilizes energy substrates and amino acids to support its metabolic and protein synthetic needs, particularly when under stress, as well as an appreciation of the role of various hormones, vitamins, and minerals.

Requirements for Energy, Amino Acids, and Essential Compounds

The body is in constant need of energy substrates, amino acids, and other essential substances that must be provided either by the diet or by release from storage areas within the organism. Most patients seen in hospitals in the United States have sufficient storage reserves to tide them over the ordinary infectious and traumatic occurrences to which they are exposed. There are others, however, who have consumed all reserves of energy substrates and amino acids because of prolonged or recurrent illness and must therefore rely on their physician to supply these requirements.

ENERGY

The basal energy expenditure of the adult body is somewhere between 1000 and 2000 kilocalories (kcal) per day, depending on body size and metabolic rate. The increased demands induced by various forms of exercise have been assessed. Unfortunately, the requirements placed on the organism by trauma or disease, or both, have not been as clearly defined. Fever alone has been estimated to increase energy demands by as much as 8 percent above basal requirements for each degree of elevation in temperature. Major surgical trauma will increase glucose consumption twofold. Daily caloric intakes in the range of 4000 to 5000 kcal are necessary to allow the spontaneous closure of a cutaneous fistula from the gastrointestinal tract. In severe trauma and sepsis, a caloric requirement as great as 10,000 kcal per day has been found to be necessary in order to begin to reverse the catabolic effects on body protein stores.

It should be obvious that reliance on the daily intravenous provision of 2 liters of 5% dextrose in water (100 grams of dextrose, or 350 kcal) for its protein-sparing effect is totally inadequate for a healthy adult, let alone for a patient with increased demands induced by stress. Should the stress be relatively short-lived and the subject have sufficient reserves, he will survive. However, a patient nutritionally depleted or with severe stress, or both, may not survive.

The average energy stores of a 70-kg man are presented in Table 4-1. Note that adipose tissue represents an exceptional amount of potential energy even in the nonobese subject. However, only when total starvation is permitted to evolve will the energy stored in adipose tissues be utilized efficiently. The hormone insulin performs many functions relative to energy homeostasis; one of the most effective functions is its antilipolytic effect, which insulin has at relatively low plasma concentrations. Thus a continuous infusion of 5% dextrose, with its resultant stimulation of pancreatic insulin production, may effectively inhibit the release of free fatty acids from adipose tissues and at the same time fail to meet caloric demands. Very little carbohydrate is stored as a potential energy supply. Hepatic and muscle glycogen can account for only 700 to 800 kcal.

Table 4-1. Potential Energy
Stores of a 70-kg Reference Man

Body tissue	kg	kcal
Adipose	15	135,000
Glycogen-muscle	0.120	480
Glycogen-liver	0.070	280
"Protein"	6	24,000

Protein is not "stored" to any degree because all proteins in the body serve a specific function. In the 70-kg man only about 6 kg of skeletal and visceral protein can be sacrificed for the supply of energy before death ensues. The most obvious clinical indication of protein loss is wasting of skeletal muscle. If protein loss is allowed to progress, a concomitant loss of visceral protein can lead to a self-destructive cycle in which the increasing protein loss causes additional stress, loss of organ function, failure to adapt to stress, and eventual death.

Many tissues actually prefer noncarbohydrate substrates, such as free fatty acids and ketone bodies, as energy sources. These tissues include skeletal and cardiac muscle, the renal cortex, and any other tissues amply supplied with mitochondria. The central nervous system, if allowed to adapt to total starvation, can convert to the use of ketone bodies as an energy source; otherwise, it relies primarily on glucose as the preferred energy substrate. Other tissues that are either not endowed with ample mitochondria (such as erythrocytes, leukocytes, and the renal medulla) or are insufficiently supplied with oxygen (fibrocytes in the relatively avascular area of wound healing) are obligatory metabolizers of glucose. It is important to note that fatty acids cannot be converted to glucose. Therefore, when glucose from external sources is not sufficient, it must be obtained by the process of gluconeogenesis. The principal substrate for gluconeogenesis is derived from protein.

AMINO ACIDS AND PROTEINS
Proteins are necessary for nearly all biochemical reactions to occur. In addition, all proteins have a finite life span, ranging from minutes to years. In general, the more adaptive a biochemical response, the more rapidly its regulating protein is altered either in amount or function. This ability to adapt is usually based on the rapid turnover of a protein (synthesis and degradation). Estimates of total body protein turnover in a state of health are in the range of 3 to 4 gm/kg/day; this rate is undoubtedly increased during times of stress. (Think of how much protein synthesis is required to maintain a white blood cell count of 20,000 per milliliter when the total life span of the polymorphonuclear leukocyte is only 8 to 10 hours.) As part of the adaptive response, proteins are degraded and their amino acids are transported to sites of synthesis of other protein molecules. Since this process does not operate at 100 percent efficiency, many amino acids must be degraded and "lost" as a result. In addition, other amino acids are degraded to gluconeogenic precursors when the demands for glucose are not being met by glycogen. In a state of health, these two processes result in the loss of about 0.4 gm of protein per kilogram of body weight per day. If the protein is replaced by dietary sources, nitrogen balance will be maintained. (Published recommended minimal intakes of mixed quality proteins are 0.57 gm/kg/day; these requirements are increased during growth, pregnancy, and lactation. The average American adult acquires approximately 1 gm/kg/day.)

In stress, protein losses are accelerated through both of the processes just described. A negative nitrogen balance after infection or trauma is well documented. When a patient is thus rendered catabolic, one usually thinks of "sparing" his protein with adequate calories, and indeed this must be accomplished. Also it is most important that amino acids (including the eight essential amino acids) be supplied in amounts necessary to permit protein synthesis to take place. This process is depicted diagrammatically in Figure 4-1, which shows that a net loss of protein mass can result from both an accelerated catabolism and an impaired synthesis.

If adequate protein synthesis is not permitted, critical protein structures will be degraded but not replaced. The effects will be reflected clinically by decreased striated muscle (including intercostal and cardiac musculature), lowered plasma concentrations of albumin and transport proteins, decreased wound

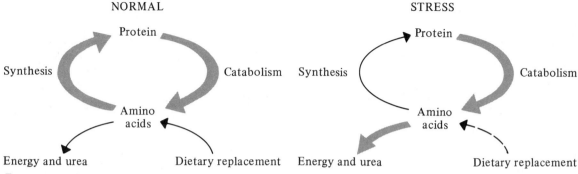

NORMAL

Protein

Synthesis   Catabolism

Amino
acids

Energy and urea   Dietary replacement

STRESS

Protein

Synthesis   Catabolism

Amino
acids

Energy and urea   Dietary replacement

Figure 4-1. The central role of protein turnover.

healing, and depressed immune responsiveness with resultant susceptibility to infection.

VITAMINS AND TRACE ELEMENTS

Vitamins are, as named, essential for vital body functions. They will not be discussed individually or in detail here because many articles relating to vitamin deficiency and nutritional states have been published. The important data relating to the various vitamins are presented in Tables 4-2 and 4-3.

In general, the water-soluble vitamins are utilized as cofactors for many biochemical reactions and are not stored to any great degree. Their requirements are in many instances related to the metabolism of other nutrients. Their deficiencies become clinically manifest in a number of weeks or months; an exception is vitamin B_{12}, which is stored in the liver in amounts sufficient to last up to three years, provided liver disease is not present. In contrast, the fat-soluble vitamins act more in the manner of hormones. An example is the renal conversion of vitamin D from 25-hydroxycholecalciferol to 1,25-dihydroxycholecalciferol, which is dependent on adequate amounts of parathyroid hormone. Fat-soluble vitamins are generally stored for periods of months to years; if used to excess, they can lead to toxicity.

The essentiality of trace elements is slowly being clarified, as is their relation to other disease entities (e.g., chromium to atherosclerosis). Deficiencies of two elements, copper and zinc, have been found to create defined clinical syndromes, which include poor wound healing and decreased resistance to infections. This finding has been particularly true in

patients undergoing long-term therapy with total parenteral nutrition. Lack of other minerals, such as iron and iodine, can precipitate the well-known syndromes discussed elsewhere in this book.

ESSENTIAL FATTY ACIDS

Linoleic and arachidonic acids are necessary for the formation of prostaglandins and are essential in the diet since they cannot be formed in adequate amounts by the human body. Their absence creates a deficiency state characterized by a scaling dermatitis and anemia. Of interest is the evidence that sufficient amounts can be obtained daily by rubbing as little as 7 gm of safflower or corn oil into the skin. If at all possible, however, essential fats should be administered by the oral route.

The Concept of Gut Failure

Malnutrition results from a failure of organ function. An insufficient intake of food itself can lead to "functional" gut failure, in that the organ designed to absorb nutrients becomes unable to do so; this is the classic concept of malnutrition by dietary deprivation. However, many patients suffer from true organ failure. For example, acute outlet obstruction of the stomach secondary to ulcer disease results in a decreased delivery of nutrients to the absorptive surface of the small intestine. Ileus, following operative manipulation within the abdomen, is a frequent though transient cause of gut failure. In most such short-term episodes, a sufficient reserve of nutrients is available to tide the patient over.

A "short-gut" syndrome, secondary either to segmental inflammatory disease or surgical removal,

Table 4-2. Water-soluble Vitamins

Vitamin	Source	RDA[a]	Lability	Absorption
Thiamine	Grains Meats Nuts Legumes	0.5 mg/ 1000 kcal	Heat pH	Duodenum and upper small bowel. Rate limited (15 mg/day)
Riboflavin	Meats Dairy products Green, leafy vegetables	0.6 mg/ 1000 kcal	Light	Small intestine
Niacin	Tryptophan Meats Whole grains Legumes	4.4 mg or equivalent[b]/ 1000 kcal	....	Small intestine
Pantothenic acid	Liver; Meats Grains Vegetables Peanuts Eggs	5−10 mg/day	Heat Acid	Small intestine
Pyridoxine	Meats Potatoes Cereals Lentils Bananas	2 mg/day	Heat	Small intestine
Biotin	All foods, esp.: Organ meats Mushrooms Peanuts	....	Raw egg whites (avidin)	Small intestine
Folic acid	All foods, esp.: Liver Leafy vegetables Fruits	400 μg/day	Heat	Proximal third of small intestine
Cyanocobalamin	Meats	3.0 μg/day	Heavy metals Oxidation Reduction	Combines with intrinsic factor for ileal absorption
Ascorbic acid	Vegetables Fruits	60 mg/day	Heat Oxidation Drying Aging	Small intestine

[a] 1974 *Recommended Daily Allowances* (8th ed.), National Academy of Sciences.
[b] 60 mg dietary tryptophan is equivalent to 1 mg of niacin.

Active Form	Primary site of action	Deficiency syndrome	Laboratory evaluation
Thiamine Pyrophosphate	Enzymes of carbohydrate metabolism	Beriberi Polyneuritis Cardiomyopathy	Erythrocyte transketolase
Flavin mononucleotide (FMN), Flavin adenine dinucleotide (FAD)	Biologic oxidation reactions	Glossitis, cheilosis Stomatitis Corneal vascularization	Microbiologic assay
Nicotinamide-adenine dinucleotide (NAD), Nicotinamide-adenine dinucleotide phosphate (NADP)	Oxidation reduction reactions	Pellagra Dermatitis Diarrhea Dementia	Urine N'-Methylnicotin-amide
Coenzyme A Acylcarier protein	Carbohydrate metabolism Lipogenesis Lipolysis	GI distress Paresthesia	Microbiologic assay
Pyridoxal 5-phosphate	Transamination Decarboxylation	Cheilosis, glossitis CNS symptoms	Tryptophan load (urine xanthenuric acid)
Biotin	Carbohydrate reactions	Dermatitis CNS symptoms	. . . .
Tetrahydrofolic acid derivatives	DNA synthesis Methyl donor	Macrocytic anemia Glossitis	Microbiologic assay Radioassay
5'-Deoxyadenosyl cobalamin Methylcobalamin	DNA synthesis Methyl donor Myelin synthesis	CNS symptoms Peripheral neuropathy Macrocytic anemia Glossitis	Radio assay
Ascorbic acid	Hydroxylation reactions	Scurvy Hemorrhages Hyperkeratosis	Plasma ascorbic acid

Table 4-3. Fat-soluble Vitamins

Vitamin	Source	R.D.A.	Absorption	Storage	Active form
A	Carotenoids in yellow vegetables Whole milk Egg yolk Fish liver oils Liver	5,000 IU	Small intestine	Liver	Retinol Retinal
D	Fortified milk Fish liver oils	400 IU	Small intestine	Liver	1,25-Dihydroxychole-calciferol
E	Vegetable oils Leafy vegetables Wheat germ	15 IU[a]	Small intestine	Liver Adipose tissue	α-Tocopherol
K	Peas Cereals Green, leafy vegetables Gut microorganisms	200 IU[b]	Small intestine	Liver	Phylloquinone (K_1) Menaquinone-n (K_2)

[a]Related directly to amounts of dietary polyunsaturated fatty acids.
[b]Not clearly defined; approximately 50 percent supplied by intestinal flora.

may produce prolonged malnutrition. Diffuse and chronic involvement by an inflammatory process such as extensive regional enteritis may eventually cause clinical malnutrition. The most obvious form of complete gut failure is acute infarction of the entire small intestine by occlusion of the superior mesenteric artery, a condition incompatible with life unless an alternative means of providing nutrition is accomplished. This concept is presented graphically in Figure 4-2.

For any specific disease entity a decreased nutrient intake or an increased nutrient loss will shift the organism toward greater malnutrition. Decreased intake may be secondary to conditions such as anorexia, nausea, and vomiting or to comatose states. Very often in a hospital setting the decreased intake is iatrogenic, as in repetitive withholding of meals for the performance of diagnostic tests, for example, or prolonged reliance on only 5% dextrose in water for energy supply. Of equal importance is the increased nutrient loss that occurs in malabsorption syndromes,

drug-induced diarrhea, intestinal fistulas, or loss through extensive burned areas of skin. In most instances the premorbid nutritional state has been adequate to maintain the expression of malnutrition at a subclinical state. If, however, the patient is nutritionally at risk and deprivation is maintained for a critical period of time, malnutrition becomes clinically manifest. Therapy — that is, the provision of adequate nutrition — shifts the entire process in the opposite direction.

As in renal failure, a complete spectrum of gut failure can be found, from normal to completely afunctional. The condition may exist as pregut, gut, or postgut failure (the last is seen in diabetes mellitus, in which nutrients, although absorbed, are not utilized). Clinical gut failure often requires a longer time to develop than renal failure and can be modified by more nebulous factors such as appetite. What is needed, clinically, is a good biochemical test to assess gut dysfunction, such as the inulin and creatinine clearance tests in renal failure.

Principal mode of action	Deficiency syndrome	Toxicity syndrome	Laboratory evaluation
Rhodopsin in vision Glycopeptide synthesis	Night blindness Xerophthalmia Keratomalacia Hyperkeratosis	Fatigue Abdominal pain Headaches Night sweats	Colorimetric determination
Transport of intestinal Ca^{++} Mobilization of bone Ca^{++}	Rickets (children) Osteomalacia (adults)	Hypercalcemia	Biologic assay
Antioxidant of fatty acids	Depends on species; Disorders of reproductive, muscular, nervous, and vascular systems Bleeding disorders Hemorrhagic disease of newborn	. . . .	Biologic assay
Synthesis of clotting factors II, VII, IX, X	Bleeding disorders	. . . .	Prothrombin time

It should be recognized that the function of the gut itself becomes markedly reduced as protein-calorie malnutrition progresses. The gut and its appended exocrine organs are among the more active protein synthesizers in the body. The mucosa of the small intestine sloughs and regenerates approximately 1×10^{12} cells each day. Such regenerative capabilities are dependent on adequate amounts of both protein and energy. As protein-calorie malnutrition develops, the gut itself becomes less able to absorb nutrients, and at some critical point it becomes functionally unable to recover by the simple reinstitution of oral nutrients. Even marginal atrophy of the gut has serious therapeutic implications because it decreases the patient's ability to absorb nutrients during the early phases of oral hyperalimentation. At such a time parenteral nutrition becomes mandatory.

The Syndrome of Protein-Calorie Malnutrition
Most physicians believe that protein-calorie malnutrition exists only among children in underdeveloped countries. When the diet is deficient in protein but is marginal in total calories, the syndrome of *kwashiorkor* is found. If both protein and calories are deficient, total starvation, or *marasmus,* develops. The two conditions are at opposite ends of a continuum; most individual cases fall somewhere between these extremes, and the syndrome is referred to collectively as protein-calorie malnutrition (PCM).

Protein-calorie malnutrition exists commonly in adult American patients. The most blatantly obvious marasmic is the patient suffering from the long-term effects of carcinoma. Less obvious are patients with small bowel bypass surgery for morbid obesity who develop liver dysfunction and muscle wasting similar to that seen in kwashiorkor, or patients maintained on overzealous protein restriction as in therapy for chronic renal or hepatic failure. Any patient who for any reason is provided with inadequate calories and protein for prolonged periods will develop some degree of PCM, which in turn will affect almost all organ systems.

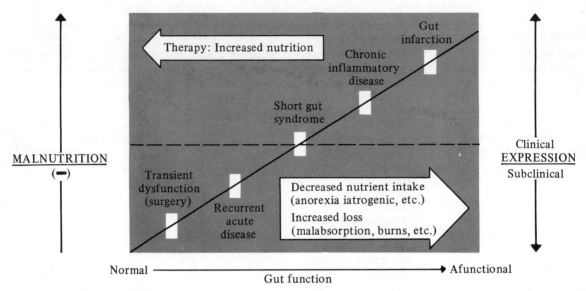

Figure 4-2. The concept of gut failure.

EFFECTS ON STRIATED MUSCLE

Skeletal muscle atrophies in hospitalized patients for one of two reasons. The first is the atrophy of disuse, which will develop in many bedridden patients regardless of their nutritional state. The second condition results from the use of existing body proteins to supply both energy substrates and the amino acids for necessary endogenous protein synthesis to occur. Weakness of the muscles of locomotion may become apparent only when rehabilitation measures are instituted. Loss of intercostal and diaphragmatic muscles limits the ability of the patient to breathe and cough adequately, the effects of which, though insidious, may be disastrous. Cardiac muscle is also wasted. This wasting of cardiac muscle can be documented by decreased voltage on an electrocardiogram, and it may play a significant role in the patient's ability to recover from coexistent cardiac disease.

EFFECTS ON "VISCERAL" PROTEIN

Decreased function of the gut itself has been discussed. Evidence of impaired hepatic function is seen early in the course of PCM and is manifested primarily by a fall in the plasma albumin concentration. Fat frequently accumulates in the liver, and eventually other evidence of impaired function, such

as elevated hepatic enzymes, jaundice, and prolongation of the prothrombin time, can be found.

Concentrations of other transport proteins are commonly decreased; prominent among these is plasma transferrin, with a coincident fall in serum iron levels. This process in itself may play a significant role in the development of anemia in patients with PCM. In many instances the "anemia of chronic disease" merely reflects PCM.

Neutropenia as well as a decrease in erythropoiesis is often present with PCM and most likely reflects a generalized failure of bone marrow protein synthesis. Total circulating lymphocytes are generally decreased. In addition, suboptimal transformation of lymphocytes in response to antigenic stimulation is evident and may be expressed clinically by a failure of the cell-mediated immune response to occur after skin testing with tuberculin, mumps, or dinitrochlorobenzene (DNCB) antigens.

The effects of any of the above complications of PCM on recovery from other serious illnesses, though often not clear-cut, are more than incidental. Associated multiple vitamin deficiencies may also complicate the picture (see Tables 4-2 and 4-3). Because PCM symptoms are often difficult to separate from those of the primary disease, and, similarly, because the benefits of nutritional therapy are frequently difficult to assess, the physician must always give the patient the benefit of any nutritional doubt.

TREATMENT

Intensive nutritional support has come to be known as hyperalimentation. It can be administered by either the oral or the parenteral route or both, parenteral alone being more correctly referred to as total parenteral nutrition.

Oral Hyperalimentation

If at all possible a functional gut should be utilized in hyperalimentation. One of the major obstacles in providing optimal oral nutrition to a hospitalized patient revolves around the problems of hospital diets. Many times suboptimal nutrition results from unsatisfied taste preferences, cold meals, inadequate assistance at mealtime, insufficient time to eat, and a disinterested or overworked nursing staff. Every effort should be made to correct such problems; however, in many instances one has to resort to the use of a liquid diet to provide total nutrition. Usually the oral route is acceptable, but in some cases the only assurance that a patient will receive optimal support is the insertion of a small feeding tube. A pediatric-size tube may be used, or if prolonged use is anticipated, a small, flexible Silastic tube can be inserted into the stomach and remain almost unnoticed by the patient.

The main groups of liquid diets with representative examples are presented in Table 4-4. There are three main types: general diets, formula diets, and chemically defined or elemental diets. In addition, other formulations that are not designed to provide total nourishment can be administered as caloric or amino acid supplements. These formulations are particularly useful if sodium, potassium, or both must be restricted, since they are generally absent from these supplements.

A few general comments can be made about liquid diets. Most are formulated to provide approximately 1 kcal per milliliter, mainly in the form of carbohydrate with the percentage derived from fat ranging from as little as less than 1 percent (just sufficient to provide essential fatty acids) to nearly 50 percent.

The fat is most often included as vegetable oils; however, some formulations incorporate medium chain triglycerides. Protein content can vary as much as threefold. It is important to consider protein quality, especially if it is provided in limited amounts. A protein of high biologic value means, in essence, that almost all the amino acids administered are utilized for protein synthesis. Egg albumin and lactalbumin (milk) are examples in which approximately 95 percent of the administered protein is incorporated. In most instances in which vegetable protein is used, more than 50 percent is degraded and excreted as nonutilized nitrogen. Almost all liquid diets provide an excess of the recommended daily allowances of vitamins and minerals, since very little is known of the body's requirements under conditions of stress.

The more preparation a given diet requires, the more it costs; thus the chemically defined diet is by far the most expensive. Also, the more complex a diet, the worse it generally tastes. Attempts are and should be made to improve the flavor of these products; some of them are not premixed, and therefore it may be necessary to order flavoring along with a liquid diet if any degree of patient acceptance is expected.

General Diets. General diets attempt to provide all major food groups in a liquid form. The caloric and protein sources are exactly what one would eat otherwise: meat, vegetables, fruit, and milk. The residue, that is, the amount of cellulose fibers, is high in these diets, causing the patient to have frequent bowel movements. A possible advantage of general diets is that they provide many trace elements not routinely added to more refined formulas.

Formula Diets. Formula diets are essentially the same as baby formulas and are generally prepared by the same manufacturers. In most instances the base for the formula is whole milk. The protein found in milk is of high biologic value and is therefore probably better utilized for synthetic demands than the protein in the general formulas. Unfortunately, formulas with a milk base also provide significant amounts of lactose. This disaccharide requires lactase

Table 4-4. Selected Examples of Liquid Diets[a]

| Characteristics | Formula | | | | | | | | | | | |
| | General | | | | | | | Chemically defined[b] | | | | |
	Formula 2	Compleat-B	Nutri-1000	Meritene	Sustacal	Isocal	Ensure	Vivonex	Vivonex-HN	Flexical	Precision-LR	Precision-HN
Calories/cc	1	1	1	1	1	1	1	1	1	1	1	1.3
Protein gm/liter	34	38	31	55	60	34	37	21	42	19	24	42
Protein source	Beef Egg Milk	Beef Milk Vegetable	Milk	Milk	Milk Casein Soy	Casein Soy	Casein Soy	L-Amino acids	L-Amino acids	Casein Hydrolysate	Egg Albumin	Egg Albumin
Fat % total kcal	49	36	47	30	20	39	32	1.3	0.33	30	0.7	0.3
Fat source	Corn oil Beef fat	Corn oil Beef fat	Soy oil Coconut oil	Vegetable oils	Soy oil	Soy oil Mct oil	Corn oil	Safflower oil	Safflower oil	Soy oil Mct oil	Vegetable oils	Vegetable oils
mOsm/kg	....	468	500	560	625	350	374	500	844	725	590	580
Na/k[c] mEq/liter	19/54	68/40	22/39	40/43	39/53	22/33	31/33	37/30	34/18	15/38	36/27	51/28
Residue	High	High	Medium	Medium	Medium	Medium	Medium	Low	Low	Low	Low	Low
Producer	Cutter	Doyle	Syntex	Doyle	Mead Johnson	Mead Johnson	Ross	Eaton	Eaton	Mead Johnson	Doyle	Doyle

[a] Examples selected are based on availability at University Hospital, Boston University Medical Center. The inclusion or exclusion of a product does not imply endorsement.

[b] Note that only Vivonex and Vivonex-HN meet the strict criteria of a "chemically defined" diet.

[c] Be aware that the sodium and potassium content is often the most limiting factor in many clinical situations.

for its degradation, an enzyme that is not present in adequate amounts in patients who have not consumed milk for a prolonged period of time. Consequently, when these formulas are administered the lactose may not be degraded, resulting in clinical symptoms such as gas and diarrhea. A patient need not have classic lactase deficiency to exhibit such symptoms, which can be prevented by starting with a diluted formula and gradually increasing its concentration. As an alternative, certain formulas use only the casein from milk as a protein source. Casein, combined with a soy-based protein, provides a total protein source of relatively high biologic value.

Chemically Defined Diets. Chemically defined diets have been designed for cases in which digestive enzyme production or the intestinal absorbent surface, or both, are limited. When ordinary diets containing whole proteins, polysaccharides, and complex lipids are administered, they usually stimulate the production of large amounts of enzymes and other substances from the stomach, duodenum, pancreas, and liver. These substances are necessary for the digestive breakdown of complex foods to their simple molecular elements. In clinical situations such as acute or chronic pancreatitis, inflammatory bowel disease, or gut dysfunction from any prolonged illness, one assumes that by eliminating these digestive steps greater absorption of the "elemental" compounds is promoted. Therefore, nitrogen is provided in the form of free amino acids, either as a protein hydrolysate or as synthetic amino acids. These amino acids are generally mixed according to the pattern found in egg albumin, a protein of high biologic value. Carbohydrates are usually provided as glucose or sucrose. Fats are generally kept at a minimum.

The two primary disadvantages of chemically defined diets are their high cost and their osmolarity. Since these diets contain mostly very small molecules, they have great osmolarity; when they enter a gut unadapted to their absorption, water moves into the gut lumen faster than the cells can move the small molecules into the circulation and results in a relatively large flux of liquids through the intestine, leading to diarrhea. The intestinal cells will eventually adapt, however, and diarrhea can be prevented if

initially the diets are given slowly and in a diluted form. The concentration may then be gradually increased.

The advantages are that these diets are generally well tolerated and leave essentially no residue after their absorption. For this reason they are sometimes used for preparation of the gut prior to surgical procedures. It should be recognized that patients on such diets will have bowel movements reduced to a minimum, and they should be reassured concerning this fact.

Total Parenteral Nutrition
Possibly the greatest single stimulus to the recent resurgence of interest in clinical nutrition has been the development of safe and effective methods for total parenteral nutrition (TPN). Its use has been described in most all disease entities. A major complication of TPN is sepsis; however, sepsis can be kept to a minimum when a team of highly trained personnel, which usually includes a physician, nurse, nutritionist, and pharmacist, is used to administer the procedure.

TPN is indicated in any case in which an adequate intake of nutrients is not possible via the gastrointestinal tract. It is contraindicated when septicemia is either present or imminent, since a venous catheter can easily be "seeded" with microorganisms. The catheter is inserted into a high flow vessel, such as the superior vena cava, because the high osmolarity of the solution (usually 1,800 mOsm/liter) will cause inflammation and eventual sclerosis of a more peripheral vein.

TPN Solutions. TPN solutions must be prepared in the pharmacy in a laminar flow hood to reduce the incidence of contamination, which includes the addition of additives. Because these solutions are ideal culture media, any violation of strict sterile techniques can result in a septic infusion.

Calories are generally provided as 25% dextrose; however, the concentration may be increased if total fluid administration must be restricted. Intravenous fats (10% emulsions) have been used in Europe but have only recently been approved for use in the United States. The higher molecular weight of fat emulsions (and thus the lower osmolarity) will allow their infusion via a peripheral vein. The value of intravenous fats during the early phases of acute trauma, when the specific demand for glucose is high, is questioned.

Amino acids were originally provided in TPN solutions as an acid hydrolysate of protein. The effective amount of protein that could be administered by these solutions was decreased by their considerable content of incompletely hydrolyzed, short-chain peptides. In addition, the administration of some hydrochloric acid with the amino acids was one reason for the metabolic acidosis caused in many patients. More recent formulations of synthetic amino acids have had the dual benefit of increasing the utilization of administered protein and reducing the incidence of metabolic acidosis.

The continuous infusion of glucose and the concomitant rise in insulin levels result in a flux of glucose into the cells. The glucose is accompanied by phosphate for the initial phosphorylation steps. As a result, serum concentrations of phosphorus can decrease to symptomatic levels. This effect can be alleviated by the addition of phosphate to the amino acid solutions. Other electrolytes will also have to be added, depending on the amounts added to the solution by the manufacturer.

Water-soluble vitamins are added daily, and in most instances fat-soluble vitamins are added once or twice weekly. The latter may be given daily; however one must be aware of potentially toxic levels.

A deficiency of trace elements, particularly copper and zinc, has been documented in cases of prolonged TPN. In some institutions these compounds are added to the solution; however, they can be provided by means of biweekly plasma transfusions. Essential fatty acid deficiencies have also been described; this deficiency can be prevented by the use of intravenous fat emulsions.

Complications. The complications of TPN are shown in the following list:

Sepsis (bacterial, fungal)
Catheter complications
  Misplacement
  Hemorrhage
  Pneumothorax
  Severed catheter tip
Air embolus
Hyperosmolar, nonketotic hyperglycemic coma
Rebound hypoglycemia
Metabolic acidosis
Hypophosphatemia

Sepsis is the most common and potentially the most troublesome complication. Meticulous care of the catheter site, with rigid prohibition of use of the line for any other purpose (e.g., central venous pressure) will keep this complication to a minimum, particularly in infections caused by *Candida albicans*. Catheter complications otherwise can be avoided by careful attention to the proper principles of insertion of subclavian and, in some cases, internal jugular lines.

Hyperosmolar, nonketotic, hyperglycemic coma can result when circulating glucose levels are permitted to rise above the renal threshold. As glucose is lost in the urine, free water clearance is increased, leading to dehydration of the patient and eventually to coma; therefore accurate measurements of urinary glucose must be performed several times daily. If significant glucosuria occurs, insulin (crystalline zinc) should be administered subcutaneously in appropriate amounts. Once the need is defined, insulin can be added to the solution. Frequent monitoring of electrolytes (including calcium, phosphorus, and magnesium) should be performed.

Obesity

DEFINITION AND INCIDENCE
Obesity may best be defined as an excess of adipose tissue above the norm, although many factors must be considered in attempting to establish the norm. Body weight by itself is not especially useful. Obviously, a lineman of a professional football team may be big but is not necessarily obese. One must, in addition, allow for height and body build. Age is yet another factor, in that lean body mass decreases with advanced age. In females the effect of estrogen on fat distribution should also be considered. Most practicing physicians assess obesity by insurance

tables that relate "ideal weight" to age, sex, and body frame. The data for these tables have been collected from a multitude of physicians with an extreme diversity of interests and therefore are subject to considerable error. They are, however, probably the most representative guide available.

Most physicians accept a weight of greater than 20 percent above the norm as an indication of "massive obesity." At the extreme end of the spectrum is the clinical syndrome of alveolar hypoventilation, cyanosis, periodic respirations, right ventricular hypertrophy and failure, and polycythemia — the so-called pickwickian syndrome. Less secure is the diagnosis of "morbid obesity," a term now frequently used to justify extreme surgical procedures for obesity.

The incidence of adult obesity (20 percent above ideal weight) in the general U.S. population has been determined by the U.S. Public Health Service to be in the range of 25 to 45 percent. Socioeconomic status, reflecting a great number of coincident factors, has been demonstrated to influence the expression of the syndrome, with an inverse relationship being noted. In one study, the incidence of obesity among women of a lower socioeconomic status was 37 percent, falling to only 2 percent among those of the highest status; similar though less marked relationships existed among males.

ETIOLOGY OF OBESITY

Fat accumulates in adipose cells when the intake of energy substrates exceeds their expenditure. Most people develop obesity simply as a result of this basic consideration, that is, they eat too much in comparison to the amount of exercise they perform. The percentage of patients having documented hormonal imbalance (e.g., hypothyroidism, Cushing's syndrome) is by comparison exceedingly small. Whereas animal models have demonstrated specific causes of obesity, these causes are obscure in human patients. For example, several strains of genetically induced obesity have been produced in rodents, but such patterns are not clear in humans. Disturbance of midbrain satiety centers, produced either by surgical ablation or by gold thioglucose administration, creates obesity in experimental animals; this finding has

led some investigators to propose the hypothesis that disturbances of endogenous satiety control mechanisms are at least in part responsible for the development of human obesity. Again, very little concrete evidence has accumulated to support this hypothesis.

In 1970 it was proposed that obese human subjects have more adipocytes than normal subjects have, implying that overfeeding during a critical neonatal period promoted proliferation of these cells. The further implication, of course, has to be that the resultant increased number of cells somehow influences the deposition of fat in later life. There is considerable evidence that the size of an adipocyte influences its behavior, especially in relation to its sensitivity to insulin, and would explain in part the elevated insulin levels and the relative insulin resistance seen in obese subjects. However, there is as yet no concrete evidence to support the adipocyte proliferation hypothesis for the etiology of obesity, regardless of how attractive it might be to those who want a "fait accompli" reason for their condition.

Psychological factors are most likely of extreme importance in the development of obesity. There is little question that many people turn to eating as part of their defense mechanisms to combat anxiety. Eating habits, which sometimes reach bizarre proportions, are also of obvious significance. Recent work in the area of behavior modification as a mode of therapy clearly supports such a hypothesis. Man's reactions to external cues from his environment tend to override endogenous controls of satiety and hunger.

Regardless of the complexity of the underlying causative factors, obesity is one of the most prevalent forms of malnutrition and presents the practicing physician with a challenging and at times frustrating therapeutic experience.

EFFECTS OF OBESITY ON HEALTH

The effects of obesity on the health of patients with the pickwickian syndrome are clear. It is also true that many chronic diseases of advancing age are associated with an excess of body weight. Some indices of disease such as hyperlipemia and abnormal glucose tolerance are indeed improved by weight reduction. It is not clear, however, whether the actual progression of any disease has a causal relationship with obesity.

A tenfold increase in the incidence of hypertension was noted in subjects of the Framingham study who were more than 20 percent over ideal weight. There is little conclusive evidence, however, that a cause-and-effect relationship exists — that obesity in itself causes hypertension. Similarly, from the same experience, angina pectoris and sudden death were more common in obese persons, but no significant correlation existed between obesity and actual myocardial infarction. Hypercholesterolemia appears to develop during periods of weight gain, although it is not significantly associated with stable obesity. Such a positive correlation should be of concern to those patients who repeatedly go on "crash diets" and then regain lost fat by recurrent overeating. This correlation exists, of course, because there is a highly significant relationship between hypercholesterolemia and coronary artery disease. To summarize, whereas the effects of obesity per se on the cardiovascular system are unclear, there are definite risks to life from both hypertension and increased lipids, two conditions that are positively correlated with excessive weight.

Diabetes mellitus occurs with increasing incidence with advancing age, as does obesity. In addition, as mentioned previously, obese subjects may exhibit an abnormal response to administered glucose, presumably secondary to an increased resistance of the enlarged adipose cell to the effects of insulin. Such relationships create a large nebulous area in which it is exceedingly difficult to separate the diabetic from the obese patient. Certainly the reversion of carbohydrate metabolism toward normal after weight reduction must be of value regardless of the exact diagnosis.

The effects of obesity during pregnancy are debatable. There is ample evidence that many pregnant women eat far more than their minimally increased caloric expenditure would warrant and so become obese. This effect has led to efforts both by the public and by the profession to limit weight gain in pregnant women, with the hope of preventing problems of parturition (e.g., toxemia, mechanical problems) as well as the ill effects of obesity on general health. On the other hand, overconcern carried to the point of providing an inadequate caloric intake during pregnancy may play a role in the excessive infant mortality in the United States, which is presumably secondary to the high incidence of low-birth-weight (and thus high-risk) infants born in this country. Appropriate control of weight gain during pregnancy should be of value to both mother and child.

TREATMENT OF OBESITY

In addition to the medical complications of obesity, the sociologic and cosmetic stigmas placed on an obese person in our society are intense. This is reflected in the constant promulgation of "magic cures" in the lay media. In spite of dramatic presentations of exceptional cases, the record of almost all dietary means of weight reduction, legitimate or ridiculous, is indeed dismal. Regardless of how complex the underlying etiologic factors of obesity may be, a single basic premise for weight reduction always holds true: caloric intake must be reduced to a level less than expenditure. It should also be remembered that the manner in which body weight is decreased may be of greater harm than the syndrome of obesity itself.

Drug Therapy

There is no drug that will specifically mobilize fat from adipose stores at rates faster than those at which fat is laid down. Similarly, there is no drug that will inhibit the conversion of excess energy substrates to storage triglycerides. The drugs in use to treat obesity fall into two main classes: anorectics and hormones. The anorectic drugs, primarily the amphetamines and metamphetamines, are effective in reducing appetite in many patients. In carefully controlled studies, however, approximately one-third of patients demonstrate no effect of amphetamines on weight reduction, another one-third respond equally to a placebo, while the remaining one-third will lose weight. Unfortunately, weight loss has been exceedingly small in studies in which these drugs are the primary form of therapy. Any potential benefit of anorectics must be measured against the drug dependence that most certainly can occur with this form of therapy.

Thyroid hormone is very effective in the therapy of obesity resulting from hypothyroidism. Other forms of hormonal therapy for obesity are not effective. Most conspicuous is the use of human chorionic gonadotropin (HCG) obtained from the urine of pregnant women. Although many treatment centers in the country use this therapy for obesity, there is no documented evidence that it is beneficial. The weight loss that does occur probably results from the patient's adherence to the 500-kcal diet that usually is prescribed coincident with the use of the hormone.

Diet Therapy

Most often a physician responds to a request for help with weight loss by prescribing a 1000-kcal diet with no pills, and placing the burden on the patient to adhere to the strict diet. This type of dietary therapy used by itself is notoriously unsuccessful. In recent years, there has been some interest in total starvation programs, especially for those with "morbid" obesity. Of benefit is the nearly complete loss of appetite that occurs coincident with a rise in plasma ketone levels. Unfortunately there are other complications, including hyperuricemia, hypokalemia, and cardiac arrhythmias. Some investigators claim that they can generate a ketotic state and conserve lean body mass by allowing only small amounts of high biologic value protein. Regardless of the mode employed, starvation is a potentially dangerous form of therapy that should be performed only under guidance by trained personnel, and then for only the most life-threatening forms of obesity.

Surgical Methods

Surgical methods, primarily jejunal-ileal bypass procedures, are presumably reserved for only the most morbidly obese. When all but approximately 30 cm of small bowel is bypassed, the gut responds to almost all food intake with diarrhea. The patient learns to avoid foods that cause diarrhea and rapidly loses weight. Unfortunately, patients have a tendency to level off at a weight still considered to be obese, even though much lower than that existing prior to treatment. They also develop fatty infiltrates of the liver, probably as a result of protein malnutrition.

Jejunal-ileal bypass is hazardous and has caused fatalities; it should not be used.

Group Therapy

Several organizations have been formed to deal with obesity. Two of the most recognized are TOPS (Take Off Pounds Sensibly), a nonprofit organization, and Weight Watchers, a profit-making corporation based in New York City; the statistics for the latter are not public. TOPS has generated statistics that are as valid as those of any form of therapy extant. Not only is weight lost by the participants, but a significant number are able to maintain their losses.

Behavior Modification

The most promising method now emerging for treating obesity is one in which the multiplicity of social and environmental influences is recognized, and an attempt is made to have the patient deal with them. A combination of group instruction and individualized counseling to change eating and exercise habits has been initially successful. Whether or not this form of therapy will result in prolonged benefits has yet to be evaluated.

Bibliography

Cahill, G. F. Physiology of insulin in man. *Diabetes* 20:785, 1971.

Fischer, J. (ed.). *Total Parenteral Nutrition.* Boston: Little, Brown, 1976.

Goodhart, R. S., and Shils, M. E. (eds.). *Modern Nutrition in Health Disease* (5th ed.). Philadelphia: Lea & Febiger, 1974.

Lee, H. A. (ed.). *Parenteral Nutrition in Acute Metabolic Illness.* New York: Academic, 1974.

Mann, G. V. The influence of obesity on health. *N. Engl. J. Med.* 291:178, 1974.

Munro, H. N. General Aspects of the Regulation of Protein Metabolism by Diet and by Hormones. In H. N. Munro and J. B. Allison (eds.), *Mammalian Protein Metabolism.* Vol. 1. New York: Academic, 1964. P. 381.

National Research Council, Food and Nutrition Board. *Recommended Dietary Allowances* (8th ed.). Washington, D.C.: National Academy of Sciences, 1974.

Owen, O. E., and Reichard, G. A., Jr. Fuels con-
    sumed by man: The interplay between carbo-
    hydrates and fatty acids. *Prog. Biochem.
    Pharmacol.* 6:177, 1971.
Stunkard, A. J. Environment and obesity: Recent
    advances in our understanding of regulation of
    food intake in man. *Fed. Proc.* 27:1367, 1968.
Waterlow, J. C. The Assessment of Protein Nutrition
    and Metabolism in the Whole Animal, with
    Special Reference to Man. In H. N. Munro
    (ed.), *Mammalian Protein Metabolism.* Vol. 3.
    New York: Academic, 1970. P. 325.

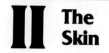

II The Skin

5

Dermatology in the Practice of Internal Medicine

Herbert Mescon and Madeline Bachta

The purpose of this chapter is to give an overview of the skin problems commonly encountered in medical practice. These problems include both cutaneous manifestations of internal diseases and some of the more prevalent primary cutaneous disorders.

Dermatologic diagnosis is based on careful visual examination of the entire skin in good light, palpation of lesions, and knowledge of the terms used to describe lesions: a *macule* is a flat (nonpalpable) spot; a *papule* is a small (less than 5 mm) elevation of the skin; a *nodule* is a large (more than 5 mm) elevation; a *vesicle* is a small blister (up to 5 mm) filled with clear fluid; a *bulla* is a large blister; a *pustule* is a blister containing pus; a *crust* is the deposition of dried blood, sebum, or exudate; *scales* are dry, white plates of horny material resulting from shedding of the most superficial layer of skin; an *ulcer* is a deep depression in the skin resulting from loss of epidermis extending into the dermis; an *erosion* is similar to an ulcer, but more superficial; a *patch* is a large macule; and a *plaque* is a large (usually more than 1 to 2 cm), circumscribed, flat-topped elevation of the skin.

When dermatologists use the word *eczema,* it is a description of a kind of dermatitis but not a specific diagnosis; however, pediatricians frequently use the term as a synonym for atopic dermatitis (see later in this chapter, under Hypersensitivity and Allergic Diseases). Furthermore, whereas eczematous dermatitis can have several different appearances, it almost always causes pruritus. Acute eczematous skin is red, swollen, and moist with a serous exudate; vesicles and erosions may also be present. As resolution occurs, the skin becomes less red (it may take on a violaceous color) and becomes scaly. At this point, the eczema usually heals. In some individuals, however, persistent rubbing or scratching may lead to a lichenified stage, in which the skin is thickened (indurated), its lines exaggerated, and sometimes its color hyperpigmented.

Diagnostic laboratory procedures in dermatology are generally easy to perform and harmless; some examples are skin scrapings for microscopic examination for fungi or scabies mites, culture for bacteria or fungi, Wood's lamp examination, and punch biopsy. The relative ease of obtaining objective evidence to support one's clinical impression demands frequent use of these techniques.

Cutaneous Manifestations of Systemic Disease

METABOLIC DISORDERS

Diabetes
Both specific and nonspecific skin lesions are seen in diabetes. Cutaneous ulcers may occur as a consequence of either microangiopathy or neuropathy, or both. Furunculosis (staphylococcal-induced, red, painful nodules, progressing to pus formation) is seen with great frequency in diabetes, as is cutaneous candidiasis (moniliasis) (page 70). Diabetics may develop red or red-brown papules on the pretibial skin, which progress to hyperpigmented, atrophic scaling areas. This condition is called diabetic dermopathy and is thought to be related to microangiopathy. Xanthomas may occur from secondary hyperlipidemia. *Diabetic bullous dermopathy* refers to the spontaneous appearance of bullae, usually on the extremities. Case reports so far offer conflicting evidence on the relation of these lesions to the duration of the disease and to microangiopathy or neuropathy. Yellow-brown plaques with overlying superficial atrophy, telangiectasia, and occasional spontaneous ulceration are called necrobiosis lipoidica (diabeticorum). These plaques are usually seen on the shins but may appear elsewhere; their appearance may precede the clinical diagnosis of diabetes. Up to 85 percent of all cases of necrobiosis are associated with either the eventual development of diabetes or a definite family history of the disease. The histology is usually suggestive and may be diagnostic.

Hypothyroidism
Generalized myxedema is manifested classically by dry, waxy, nonpitting edema. The face is characterized by swollen lips and a thick nose. The hair is dry, lusterless, and may be sparse; the nails are friable. There may be xanthomas with hypercholesterolemia.

Localized myxedema generally occurs as a pretibial plaque and is usually associated with preceding hyperthyroidism and exophthalmos (see Chap. 58). (Localized myxedema may also be associated with euthyroid and hyperthyroid states.) Minute, localized, or *papular myxedema* may occur in euthyroid persons; it is characterized by tiny, waxy papules arranged in lines or groups. Histologically, all three types of myxedema have the same characteristic mucinous material scattered throughout the dermis. Generalized myxedema responds readily to thyroid hormone; the other types do not.

Hyperthyroidism

The skin is usually warm and flushed. Spoon nails (Plummer's nails) occasionally occur in hyperthyroidism, as well as in iron-deficiency anemia; the distal ends of the nails become loose and grow upward, resulting in a spoonlike shape. *Vitiligo* (patchy loss of pigment) occurs in 6 percent of hyperthyroid patients.

Other Endocrine Diseases

The skin findings of acromegaly, Addison's disease, and Cushing's disease are adequately described in Chapter 56. Female virilization, manifested on the skin as acne and hirsutism (growth of coarse hair on the face and trunk), is seen in both benign and malignant adrenal and ovarian tumors.

Amyloidosis

Amyloid deposits in the skin cause clinical lesions both in *primary systemic amyloidosis* and in *localized cutaneous amyloidosis.* In *secondary systemic amyloidosis,* amyloid deposits rarely result in clinical skin lesions. However, some chronic skin diseases (e.g., stasis ulcers) can cause secondary amyloidosis. Yellow-brown translucent papules (especially facial), nodules, and plaques are found in primary systemic amyloidosis. Localized forms include lichen amyloidosis, characterized by aggregates of yellow-brown papules, usually on the shins; macular amyloidosis, characterized by macular hyperpigmented patches, usually on the lower extremities; and isolated amyloid tumors. All three types have the same microscopic picture on biopsy. The histochemical demonstration of amyloid in skin biopsies for diagnosis of amyloidosis is simple, but it must be well controlled to be valid. Green birefringence in alkaline Congo red sections is one of the most reliable findings.

Porphyria

Porphyrias are disorders of porphyrin metabolism, usually inherited (see Chap. 37). Uroporphyrins and coproporphyrin I or III (or both) are usually present in abnormal amounts in urine or feces or both; they can usually be detected in urine by red-pink fluorescence under Wood's (ultraviolet) light following acidification and extraction with chloroform. *Congenital erythropoietic porphyria* is characterized by the production of porphyrins in bone marrow and causes the teeth and marrow to appear red when viewed in ultraviolet light. It may be lethal at an early age. *Erythropoietic protoporphyria* is a milder form in which photosensitivity is the chief skin sign, often manifesting itself by the development of large bullae following exposure to sun. Exposure to sunlight should, therefore, be reduced to a minimum.

Acute intermittent porphyria, a very serious disease, may be precipitated by alcohol or medications — sulfonamides, Sedormid (2-isopropyl-4-pentenoylurea), and barbiturates — and may be accompanied by abdominal or neurologic symptoms. *Chronic porphyria* (porphyria cutanea tarda) is characterized by bullous, photosensitive skin lesions and may be accompanied by hepatic, gastrointestinal, or neurologic symptoms (variegate or mixed types). Hepatotoxic chemicals, food, and drugs should be avoided.

Gout

Gout is a disturbance of purine metabolism that may manifest itself by palpable subcutaneous nodules (tophi) of the ears, fingers, or other areas. Tophi have a diagnostic histologic picture and may also show microscopic urate crystals (see Chap. 35).

Urticaria Pigmentosa

Urticaria pigmentosa, also known as mastocytosis, may have a spectrum of involvements. Mast cells release histamine and also possibly heparin in man. Mastocytosis may involve only the skin with multiple tumors, as in most childhood cases; these patients have a good prognosis. When the disease has an adult onset it may be more serious, involving not only the skin but also the viscera and bones. Stroking the yellow-tan papular or macular skin lesion causes release of histamine and wheal formation (urtication). In adults histamine released into the circulation may cause flushing, headache, diarrhea, and hypotension; codeine or polymyxin B may cause such a histamine release, producing a similar acute systemic reaction. A skin biopsy stained for mast cells is diagnostic when positive. If bone lesions are present, the mast cells may also be found in aspirated biopsy specimens. Urinary tests will reveal an increase in histamine. Urticaria pigmentosa may be distinguished from the carcinoid syndrome (argentaffinoma), which is caused by serotonin and bradykinin release into the circulation with flushing and fainting, by the finding of increased 5-hydroxyindolacetic acid in the urine in argentaffinoma.

Calcinosis Cutis

There are two types of calcinosis cutis, both usually diagnosed by x-ray or biopsy. One type occurs with normal blood calcium levels and is usually associated with local inflammatory lesions; 50 percent of these cases occur in patients with systemic scleroderma or dermatomyositis. This type of calcinosis cutis can also be seen without a systemic disease when it occurs at sites of infection, scars, or epidermal cysts. The second type occurs in patients with elevated blood calcium levels associated with various metabolic disturbances such as hyperparathyroidism, chronic osteomyelitis, high vitamin D ingestion, and rarely malignancy.

Hyperlipidemias

The biochemistry and cardiovascular complications of hyperlipidemias are discussed in Chapter 26. Hyperlipidemias may be manifested on the skin by yellow-orange xanthomas. There are several different clinical types of xanthomas. *Plane xanthomas* are simply yellow plaques containing lipids; they may occur anywhere. *Xanthelasmas* are plane xanthomas on or near the eyelids; only about half the patients with xanthelasmas, and only occasional patients with plane xanthomas, have a disorder of blood lipids.

Palmar xanthomas are a form of plane xanthoma (on the palms). *Secondary plane xanthomas* are most commonly seen with familial type III hyperlipidemic disease, myeloma, or biliary cirrhosis. *Eruptive xanthomas* are clusters of red-yellow papules that occur on the buttocks, posterior thighs, and body folds. They are seen with rapid elevations of plasma triglyceride levels and thus may occur in association with types I, III, IV, and V hyperlipidemias. The most common cause of eruptive xanthoma is uncontrolled diabetes mellitus. When the lesions of eruptive xanthomas coalesce, they form nodules called *tuberous xanthomas*. *Tendon xanthomas* occur with types II and III hyperlipidemic disease. Xanthomas can be easily diagnosed both clinically and histologically; determination of the specific lipoprotein abnormality must be made biochemically.

COLLAGEN-VASCULAR DISEASES

A discussion of the cutaneous manifestations of collagen-vascular diseases is found in Chapter 46.

NONDIAGNOSTIC SKIN LESIONS ASSOCIATED WITH INTERNAL MALIGNANCY

Various nonspecific rashes, usually of the erythema multiforme type, may be associated with and apparently result from internal malignancy. Often a rash will be precipitated by radiation therapy of a large tumor. A generalized exfoliative dermatitis (scaling and redness) or a persistent erythema multiforme in a patient over 60 years old must be considered to be caused by malignancy until proved otherwise.

Dermatomyositis

Dermatomyositis is often manifested by red-purple discoloration and edema of the skin, usually involving the face and especially the periorbital area (heliotrope sign); it is associated with weakness and aching of involved muscles. In approximately 25 percent of cases there is an associated internal malignancy which sometimes may not become manifest for several months. A careful survey to uncover any existing tumor must therefore be instituted in every case.

ACANTHOSIS NIGRICANS

Acanthosis nigricans is characterized by velvety, verrucous, hyperpigmented lesions usually extending over a sizable area of the axillae, groins, neck, or genitals. The juvenile type is usually benign. The adult type is associated in about 50 percent of patients with internal malignancy, usually of the stomach, intestines, or uterus. The lesions can also be seen in markedly obese patients with endocrine disease; the condition is then referred to as pseudo-acanthosis nigricans. This condition may regress when the obesity is brought under control.

Herpes Zoster

Most physicians readily recognize herpes zoster (shingles): clusters of vesicles, on erythematous bases, in a dermatome distribution. An occasional vesicle is found outside the affected dermatome. Herpes zoster is quite common, and it is not always painful (particularly in younger patients). Most cases of localized herpes zoster are not related to malignancy and occur in relatively healthy people. Lymph nodes draining the region are frequently palpable as a result of inflammation; this does not necessarily signify lymphoma. Zoster is clearly more common in some kinds of patients than in the general population; in a recent study, 25 percent of patients with Hodgkin's disease, 8.7 percent of other lymphoma patients, and only 1.2 percent of patients with solid tumors were affected. Malignancy is a more serious consideration when more than about 20 vesicles are found outside the affected dermatome (generalized zoster).

SARCOIDOSIS

When the internist suspects sarcoidosis, he should inspect the skin carefully. Cutaneous sarcoidosis has many different morphologies, from hypopigmented macules to violaceous plaques. Biopsy should reveal the presence of noncaseating granulomas. A distinctive syndrome of cutaneous sarcoidosis is lupus pernio, in which violaceous papules and nodules are found on the nose, cheeks, and earlobes. Skin lesions in sarcoidosis are frequently responsive to local steroid therapy.

NEUROCUTANEOUS DISORDERS

Neurofibromatosis

Neurofibromatosis may affect the skin, the viscera, or the bones. The earliest skin signs are large, light brown macular lesions called café au lait spots. These spots are also seen in otherwise normal persons; however, when the lesions are larger than 1.5 cm and occur in multiples, there is increased correlation with systemic neurofibromatosis. These brown areas usually have a smooth border, in contradistinction to the ragged, unilateral tan spots of Albright's syndrome (see Chap. 46). Nodular and pendulous fibromas or neurofibromas may be present in the skin.

Sturge-Weber Syndrome

The Sturge-Weber syndrome is the association of facial hemangiomas with hemangiomas of the leptomeninges of the cerebral cortex. Seizures and mental retardation may occur.

Tuberous Sclerosis

Tuberous sclerosis is the triad of adenoma sebaceum (fibrous papules and nodules in a facial butterfly distribution), epilepsy, and mental retardation. The disease usually presents in childhood. Other cutaneous markers are subungual fibromas and hypopigmented macules in the shape of ash leaves ("ash-leaf" spots).

PURPURA

Purpura can occur as a manifestation of hypersensitivity and also of venous stasis, hypergammaglobulinemia, macroglobulinemia, embolic phenomena (e.g., bacterial endocarditis), scurvy, and platelet deficiency. Multiple laboratory tests may be necessary to classify a given lesion.

PYODERMA GANGRENOSUM

Pyoderma gangrenosum is an ulcerative condition of the skin having undermined edges and a violaceous halo. About one-half the cases are related to ulcerative colitis or regional ileitis; in these instances the course of the skin disease usually parallels that of the bowel disease, and effective treatment of the bowel disease may cause regression of the skin lesions. Other associations include rheumatoid arthritis and the dysproteinemias. However, patients who are otherwise normal may have pyoderma gangrenosum. The skin lesions respond to systemic steroids. Unless the process is in the healing phase, attempts at grafting usually result in failure. Occasionally a new lesion of pyoderma gangrenosum may develop at the donor site of the graft.

General Considerations

PRURITUS

Patients with internal malignancies (especially lymphomas) may have considerable pruritus as a manifestation of their tumor. However, pruritus is a common nonspecific symptom (see the following general discussion).

Pruritus (itching) is the most common symptom of skin disease, occurring in 50 percent of dermatologic patients. Usually it is associated with local skin disease; however, internal malignancy, uremia, diabetes mellitus, and liver disease (especially cholestatic) may also be accompanied by generalized pruritus. Itching is an outstanding symptom of some primary generalized skin diseases that might escape recognition by an internist (e.g., scabies, dermatitis herpetiformis). Other common causes of itching are excessive washing and the compulsive use of potentially irritating grooming agents (deodorants, astringents, perfumes).

The perception of itching is controlled by the central nervous system and can be influenced considerably by emotional stress. When a patient is tired or upset, the same itch stimulus results in much greater subjective pruritus. When an organic cause, such as Hodgkin's disease or uremia, or a drug eruption is present, efforts should be instituted to remove or diminish the underlying cause. As palliatives, the sedatives, the tranquilizers, or the antihistamines in large doses — for example, tripelennamine (Pyribenzamine), 25 to 100 mg every 3 hours — are often helpful. The corticosteroids used either locally or systemically will tend to reduce inflammation and thus reduce itching. Simple cooling agents such as cold water applied locally will help replace the harmful itch sensation with a less irritating cooling one.

PSYCHOGENIC SKIN DISORDERS

Tension may cause increased palmar and plantar sweating. Occasional patients under psychogenic stress may excoriate themselves out of all proportion to, or even in the absence of, any underlying organic disease (neurotic excoriations). Other patients have delusions of parasitosis, and some even inject materials into their skin (factitial dermatitis) or pull out their hair (trichotillomania). These patients must be seen and may need treatment by a psychiatrist.

HAIR LOSS

Hair loss *(alopecia)* and pigmentation changes are interesting diagnostic problems, since they represent any of a number of systemic or primary cutaneous diseases. Hair growth in man is characterized by a resting (telogen) and a growing (anagen) stage. Hair cycles are not synchronous; that is, one hair in an area may be in the growing stage, another at rest, and still another ready to fall out. Conditions of stress, such as severe infection (e.g., pneumonia or typhoid fever), severe emotional stress, rapid weight loss, or an exacerbation of systemic lupus erythematosus, may interfere with hair growth and result in a greater number of hairs going into a slower growth or a resting phase and then falling out in a few weeks. Usually the follicle still has the potential to regrow hair within a few months *(transient alopecia)*. The puerperium is a common period for such increased hair loss, but hair growth usually returns to normal within six months. The antimitotic agents used in cancer therapy, or even simple heparin, may temporarily (and either partially or totally) interfere with hair growth so that hairs fall out or become narrowed and break. Other causes of transient hair loss include infections (secondary syphilis or superficial fungi); physical damage, such as traction from hair styling (tight ponytails); and low-dose x-irradiation. Clinically, transient alopecias may show slight inflammation, but not atrophy; histologically all the hair-bearing structures (follicles) are intact.

Hereditary baldness in males is at present untreatable. Since its appearance depends on the presence of testosterone, it does not occur in eunuchs, who were castrated before the hereditary trait would normally manifest itself. However, in eunuchs with a strong hereditary history of baldness, testosterone administration will result in irreversible hair loss. Females may also have irreversible thinning of the hair on a hereditary basis.

Some types of scalp disease with hair loss lead to considerable scarring and loss of follicles so that hair loss is irreversible; examples include pyogenic infection, fungal infection with a marked inflammatory component (kerion), plaques of discoid lupus, localized scleroderma, and malignant tumors.

SKIN COLORATION (PIGMENTATION)

Skin coloration is determined by the depth and amounts of pigment (that is, hemoglobin and melanin) in the skin and by their absorption and reflection of light. In general, skin tends to transmit the red wavelengths of light and to reflect the blue wavelengths. Therefore, transilluminated tissue appears red, as when a flashlight placed in the mouth is seen through the cheeks. It must be remembered that in general skin temperature is related to total skin blood flow, which is determined by the deeper, nonvisible arterioles that impart very little color to the skin. The color of the skin usually depends on the amount of blood in the superficial subpapillary venous vessels; this blood may or may not be flowing rapidly. Thus one can have a cool, red skin in frostbite, and a warm skin, which may or may not be red, in hyperthyroidism. Melanin pigment appears brown at the surface in reflected light, but it looks bluer and blacker the deeper its location. Hemoglobin appears redder the closer it is to the surface, and bluer the deeper it is; thus petechiae usually look red, whereas hematomas have a blue to purple appearance. Oxygenated blood appears redder than that containing reduced hemoglobin; therefore, patients with high levels of carboxyhemoglobin appear cyanotic.

Increased melanin in the skin may result from a variety of local skin diseases – for example, local inflammation, ultraviolet burn, bites, and prolonged scratching. Systemically, melanin production or distribution (or both) is under the control of the melanocyte-stimulating hormone (MSH) of the pituitary gland (see Chap. 55). In pregnancy, when pituitary output is high, there is increased pigmentation of nipples and nevi. In Addison's disease, with diminished cortisol production and consequently less suppression of the pituitary, there is increased MSH output and resultant hyperpigmentation. Following severe surgical stress or debility, when the adrenal glands are perhaps exhausted, there is also increased MSH output with hyperpigmentation. In panhypopituitarism the skin is quite pale.

Various metals deposited in the skin may cause changes in the skin color; for example, the blue-gray color of argyria is caused by silver, the tan-to-brown color of chrysiasis by gold. In hemochromatosis, iron is deposited in the tissues and may be demonstrated in the skin in about one-third of the cases. These metals also tend to cause increased melanin production when deposited locally in the skin.

Phenylketonuria (PKU), a metabolic disorder in which there is a congenital defect in the conversion of phenylalanine to tyrosine, a precursor of melanin, causes pallor of the skin. The disease can easily be discovered in newborn infants by suitable urine tests, which are compulsory in some states. Restriction of dietary phenylalanine will often prevent the mental deficiency (phenylpyruvic oligophrenia) that may be associated with PKU.

In *jaundice* the skin is yellow as a result of excess bilirubin. In *ochronosis,* a derangement of tyrosine metabolism, the skin overlying the cartilaginous areas (ears, nose) is bluish due to deposits of homogentisic acid, and the alkaline or alkalinized urine turns black on standing (alkaptonuria) (see Chap. 46). Coloration of skin may also be influenced by the ingestion of certain foods in excess (carrot juice, carotenemia; tomato juice, lycopenemia).

When deeply pigmented persons have inflammation in the skin, its resolution may be accompanied initially by either hyperpigmentation or hypopigmentation. The pigment can be expected to return to normal after several months. This condition is different from *vitiligo,* a spontaneous loss of melanocytes leading to patches of absolute pigment loss. Hyperthyroidism, adrenocortical insufficiency, and pernicious anemia are more prevalent in vitiligo patients than in the general population. Sometimes patches of vitiligo become repigmented; more often they do not. The only available treatment at present, topical or oral psoralens with standard ultraviolet irradiation or sun exposure, is time consuming and not consistently effective.

Common Skin Diseases

PSORIASIS

Psoriasis is one of the most common skin diseases; it is also one that may cause sufficient disability to require hospitalization. It is usually manifested by silvery-scaled erythematous lesions on the scalp, elbows, knees, and sacrum, but it may involve any or all of the skin, including the nails, where thickening, pitting, and whitening may occur. Less than 10 percent of patients have joint involvement of a type formerly considered to be rheumatoid, but now believed to be distinct; in general, it improves when the psoriasis improves. The cause of psoriasis is unknown, although psychological stress seems to make it worse. Most patients have remissions in time following local therapy, which may include topical steroids, tar preparations, and salicylic acid compounds.

Psoriasis is not life-threatening, but in severe cases it may cause such disability from the skin involvement alone that systemic therapy is necessary. Although the disease usually responds to large doses of corticosteroids, the complications of this medication and the flare-ups occasionally encountered upon its withdrawal have resulted in its being rarely used. Antimetabolites (e.g., methotrexate given intramuscularly or orally in low doses) tend to slow down the accelerated epithelial turnover rate of the skin from 4 days in psoriasis toward the normal 28 days, and thus usually lead to improvement. Control can usually be attained with low enough doses (20 to 25 mg weekly of methotrexate) so that leukopenia, thrombocytopenia, nausea, and diarrhea are seldom encountered; nevertheless, patients should be closely observed for these complications. However, presently available data strongly suggest that chronic low-dose methotrexate treatment increases the risk of cirrhosis of the liver. A careful review finds no increased tumor incidence in methotrexate-treated psoriatic patients, as contrasted with the increased incidence of tumors observed in some patients on chronic cytotoxic therapy. Azaribine has been used to treat psoriasis when methotrexate has failed or has been contraindicated. Recent series, however, have reported a number of thrombovascular and neurologic complications; thus azaribine should be reserved for patients who are severely disabled by psoriasis. A newly developed treatment for psoriasis — oral administration of methoxsalen followed by exposure to high-intensity, long-wave ultraviolet light (black light) —

appears very promising. Little toxicity has been encountered with short-term use; long-term toxicity is unknown.

ACNE VULGARIS

Acne vulgaris is a disease usually involving the large pilosebaceous units of the face. The initial noninflammatory lesions are comedones, which are follicular impactions of keratin, lipid, and bacteria. The inflammatory lesions (or papules and pustules) result from the rupture of the follicular wall with subsequent escape of the follicular contents. The sebum is unique in that it contains a large percentage of fatty acids. The fatty acids are initially esterified, but free fatty acids are formed in the follicular canal, probably by follicular bacteria. It has been shown that the free fatty acids are exceedingly irritating and are likely the chief inflammatory agents in acne. Acne becomes evident during the endocrine changes of puberty because the sebaceous glands, which are under the control of androgens, undergo great enlargement at that time. Corticosteroid acne is probably caused by the androgenic properties of the corticoid hormones.

Newer systemic approaches to acne therapy include the use of antibiotics and estrogenic hormones. The antibiotics, especially tetracycline, are effective in reducing the concentration of free fatty acids, probably as a result of their activity against the primary follicular organism, *Corynebacterium acnes.* Antibiotics often produce this effect with dosages as low as 250 mg per day. Estrogen in a large daily dose — that is, approximately 0.1 mg ethinyl estradiol or its equivalent — decreases the amount of sebum formed. However, such doses of estrogen should be given only to women and only in a cyclic fashion, as for suppression of ovulation. Both estrogens and antibiotics owe their effectiveness to a decrease in the amount of available irritating material — in the former instance, a decrease in the total sebum pool; in the latter instance, a decrease in the amount of free fatty acids.

Topical treatments such as vitamin A acid, benzoyl peroxide, and salicylic acid aim at reducing formation of comedones. Currently attempts are being made to formulate effective antibiotic preparations for topical use in acne.

ACNE ROSACEA

Acne rosacea is clinically similar to acne vulgaris; patients have red papules and pustules, usually confined to the central face. In rosacea, however, telangiectases are present, whereas comedones are absent. Acne rosacea also differs from acne vulgaris in that patients tend to be middle-aged rather than adolescent; no hormonal influences have been observed; sebum secretion rates are normal; and histologically the follicles are uninvolved. Rosacea responds well to low-dose oral tetracycline (250–750 mg daily).

SEBORRHEIC DERMATITIS

Seborrheic dermatitis is a greasy, scaling, erythematous eruption that appears in the scalp, behind the ears, on the midforehead, eyebrows, eyelids, nasolabial folds, presternal area, interscapular area, and occasionally in the axillae and the inguinal area. Low-potency topical steroids (e.g., 1% hydrocortisone cream 2 to 3 times daily) achieve control readily.

FUNGUS INFECTIONS

Superficial fungal infections (involving epithelium only) are basically of three types: (1) *Candida albicans (Monilia),* (2) dermatophyte *(Epidermophyton, Trichophyton, Microsporum),* and (3) *Pityrosporon. Candida albicans* is a regular inhabitant of normal skin, particularly near body orifices. It may multiply and cause clinical disease under special circumstances, such as (1) prolonged apposition of wet skin surfaces (the groin of an incontinent, bedridden patient, or the body folds of an obese person who sweats profusely); (2) diminished host resistance (steroid therapy, immunodeficiency disease, diabetes); and (3) alterations of normal flora (administration of broad-spectrum antibiotics). In candidiasis one sees bright red, scaling patches with satellite papules and pustules on the skin; on the mucous membranes one sees thick white plaques overlying erosions. Scrapings of skin usually show pseudohyphae and spores microscopically.

Dermatophyte infections have many different clinical pictures, since the group encompasses several genera and host responses are variable. Common manifestations of infection include fissuring under the toes, a well-demarcated, hyperpigmented, scaling eruption in the groin, and red, annular, scaling lesions. Microscopic examination of skin scrapings shows long, thin, branching, septate hyphae. The word *tinea* is a clinical term referring to an eruption caused by superficial fungi; it does not imply a specific etiologic agent. Tinea capitis, tinea cruris, tinea unguium, and tinea manum simply refer to superficial fungal infections of the scalp, groin, nails, and hand respectively. Like *C. albicans,* most dermatophytes grow best on moist skin; therefore reduction of moisture by using powder or wearing loose clothing that allows for ventilation is excellent both for treatment and for prophylaxis of mild disease. A number of topical antibiotics (amphotericin B, haloprogin, tolnaftate) are effective against dermatophytes. Groin rashes may be caused by *Candida,* dermatophytes, or simply inflammation resulting from maceration and prolonged contact with sweat, urine, or soap residues. Drying the skin is helpful in all instances; specific therapy should be directed toward a specific diagnosis.

Pityrosporon causes tinea versicolor, a disease with pink, tan, or white (usually one color in one person) scaling patches, mostly on the upper trunk. Short, broad hyphae and clumps of spores are seen microscopically. Since *Pityrosporon* resides only in the superficial epidermis, the most common treatment consists in peeling the lesion away with keratolytic agents such as sodium thiosulfate or salicylic acid.

DEEP MYCOSES

Blastomycosis, coccidioidomycosis, paracoccidioidomycosis (South American blastomycosis), actinomycosis, sporotrichosis, cryptococcosis (torulosis), histoplasmosis, and chromoblastomycosis are diseases that may either have skin lesions only or may be systemic When there are skin lesions, the organisms can be either cultured from the lesion or seen in biopsy specimens, or both. Special stains may be necessary.

In patients with lymphomas and in patients on long-term corticosteroid therapy in whom immune mechanisms are reduced, systemic fungal disease is not uncommon, including central nervous system involvement. Under these circumstances, even a fungus that is ordinarily nonpathogenic — for example, *Rhizopus,* the common bread mold — may grow in the spinal fluid or lungs.

WARTS

Warts can occur on any part of the body surface; in all instances they are caused by the same papovavirus. *Plantar warts* are so named because they occur on the plantar surface of the foot. Most warts resolve spontaneously if left untreated; they may, however, persist for many years and can present such a cosmetic and occasionally functional problem that patients demand treatment. Furthermore, genital warts are infectious and most patients prefer not to transmit them to others. Since a specific antiviral therapy is not available, treatment is directed at destroying the tissue that the virus parasitizes without damaging the normal skin. Application of chemical agents (e.g., salicylic acid, trichloracetic acid, podophyllin), sharp excision, electrodesiccation, and freezing are all reasonably effective. Freezing with liquid nitrogen is currently popular; it is quick, less painful than some other modalities, and seems less likely to damage normal tissue.

Calluses and corns are frequently mistaken for plantar warts. Calluses are merely thickened skin overlying pressure points, and corns are localized deeper callosities. Skin marking lines are clearly visible over the entire surface of such lesions, whereas plantar warts interrupt the skin marking lines. When paring warts, one may frequently see pinpoint blood vessels just below the surface of the involved skin.

HYPERSENSITIVITY AND ALLERGIC DISEASES

The clinical skin manifestations of hypersensitivity and allergic diseases are discussed briefly here; the mechanisms of these diseases are discussed elsewhere (see Chap. 45).

Contact dermatitis presents as an eczematous eruption. The diagnosis is made most often by correlating the patient's history and the distribution of lesions; for example, a person may consistently have eczema on the dorsa of his toes whenever he wears a particular pair of shoes. There are two types of contact dermatitis: (1) *allergic,* mediated by immune mechanisms, and (2) *primary irritant,* caused by direct damage to the skin by irritating substances (e.g., alkaline or acidic solutions that result in activation of the mediators of inflammation). Morphologically, the two types are indistinguishable.

Drug eruptions may have any morphology. The most common patterns are generalized maculopapular and generalized urticarial eruptions. Vesicular, bullous, and pustular reactions also occur. *Fixed drug eruptions* are localized eczematous patches that heal with hyperpigmentation, but recur in the same place with repeated systemic administrations of the offending agent. The same drug may give rise to different types of lesions in different individuals; for example, penicillin may cause hives in one patient and a fixed drug eruption in another. In a patient who is taking multiple medications, it may be very difficult to single out the cause of a rash. Information about the types and incidence of rashes produced by the commonly administered drugs is available; this helps the physician to make an educated guess. The ideal treatment is to stop the medication. When an eruption lasts longer than 2 weeks after cessation of the suspected drug, one must consider other possibilities.

Atopic dermatitis (atopic or infantile eczema) is a common and distinctive clinical entity. Its etiology is unclear. It is discussed in this section because ingestion or inhalation of any of a number of substances (presumably allergens) can cause exacerbation in some individuals. Usually IgE levels are markedly increased with severe dermatitis. The disease also clusters in families with hay fever and asthma. It begins in infancy as red, erosive, weeping, crusted patches, usually seen on the face and the diaper area. Later the dermatitis becomes more papular and involves the face and flexor surfaces, especially the anterior neck, popliteal, and antecubital fossae. In adolescents and adults, lichenification of flexor surfaces is prominent. These individuals almost always have dry, itchy skin and react even to seemingly minor irritants (e.g., frequent hand washing) with an eczematous dermatitis.

NEOPLASMS

Only a selected few of the more common or interesting neoplasms are discussed here.

Hemangiomas of the skin in children, especially the port-wine stain type, are occasionally associated with visceral lesions which, if they involve the brain, may give rise to a variety of neurologic syndromes. In the elderly, however, it is not uncommon to see small (1 to 5 mm), multiple, cherry-red hemangiomas without clinical significance. Spider angiomas are hardly tumors and may be present in normal persons, but they are found in large numbers in patients with liver disease and in pregnant women. Rarely spider or even frank angiomas may be seen on a hereditary basis associated with similar lesions of the nasal and oral mucosa, which sometimes hemorrhage (Rendu-Osler-Weber familial hereditary telangiectasia).

Actinic keratoses (also called senile or solar keratoses) are found on sun-exposed surfaces of fair-skinned persons in middle and old age. Clinically they are scaling, sometimes erythematous, patches with a gritty texture. Histologically they are carcinoma in situ, but they progress very slowly. The physician may elect to wait and watch for changes suggesting carcinoma, or he may treat the patient at the initial diagnosis with fluorouracil cream, freezing, or electrocautery. *Bowen's disease* is a patch of red, crusted skin. Histologically, it is also carcinoma in situ; however, when the term *Bowen's disease* is used, it implies severe dysplastic changes and, usually, occurrence on covered areas of skin. At one time a retrospective study at the Armed Forces Institute of Pathology found a correlation between Bowen's disease and internal malignancy. A more recent prospective study disputes this observation.

Squamous cell carcinoma of the skin is a dysplastic epithelial tumor with dermal invasion. Clinically it may be an ulcer with a red, indurated border or a verrucous nodule with or without ulceration. Lesions arising in sun-exposed skin rarely metastasize; lesions arising in chronic ulcers, radiation scars, or in arsenical keratoses are more aggressive. *Basal cell carcinoma* is also an epithelial tumor with dermal invasion; the tumor cells resemble those of the basal epidermal layer, hence the name. Clinically the lesions are ulcers with a translucent, pearly border and telangiectasia. These lesions grow slowly and locally, and only rarely metastasize. They are much more common in light-skinned, blue-gray-eyed people exposed to considerable sun over a period of years.

Mycosis fungoides is a pleomorphic lymphoma that is primary in the skin. Initially it is characterized by generalized eczematous dermatitis, then by indurated, violaceous, scaling plaques, and later by cutaneous, lymphatic, and visceral tumors. Mycosis fungoides has been a topic of great interest recently because it is one of the few T cell malignancies (see Chap. 51). Patients maintain intact delayed hypersensitivity until very late in the course of the disease. Because the disease is so uncommon, its natural history is unclear. It is not even known whether any treatment affects the overall course of the disease; therefore, unless patients are in a controlled prospective study, it is unwise to do more than to attempt palliation and symptomatic relief. Patients may survive a few to many years. Useful palliative agents include topical steroids, topical nitrogen mustard, electron beam, and any of a number of cytotoxic agents.

All *pigmented lesions* require careful examination because they range from benign (seborrheic keratosis) to highly malignant (malignant melanoma). *Seborrheic keratoses* are greasy, scaling, pigmented lesions that have a "stuck-on" appearance; their edges can easily be lifted by a fingernail or a blade. They are actually benign epithelial proliferations, not melanocytic tumors. *Pigmented nevi* (moles), which result from clusters of nevus cells (melanocytes) in the dermis or at the dermal-epidermal junction, are macules or papules. The overlying epidermis is usually smooth. Their color is generally uniform in a given lesion, although different nevi can range from blue to pink (no melanin produced). Their outlines are regular. "Bathing trunk" nevi (moles involving an area of skin about as large as that covered by a bathing suit) are known to have a high malignancy potential; thus serious consideration should be given to their complete excision. Guidelines for dealing with a smaller congenital lesion (present at birth) are not yet firmly established, again because the natural history is unclear.

Malignant melanomas are pigmented macules, papules, or nodules. Variations in pigment, serpiginous outlines, an erythematous halo, spontaneous ulceration, and satellite lesions are ominous signs of melanoma. When a patient states that he has observed any change in a pigmented lesion that appears clinically benign, it is still reasonable to perform a biopsy. Available evidence shows that the prognosis is not altered by a biopsy performed just prior to definitive treatment, and malignant melanomas diagnosed early (atypical melanocytes confined to epidermal and upper dermis) have 90 to 95 percent ten-year survival rate.

Bullous Diseases

Pemphigus, pemphigoid, and dermatitis herpetiformis are blistering diseases with a low incidence but a high morbidity and mortality. Recent immunofluorescent studies suggest that antigen-antibody binding in the skin is important in these diseases and helps to characterize each of these clinical problems.

Pemphigus vulgaris is a severe blistering disease with a mortality of more than 50 percent when untreated. Clinically the disease is characterized by vesicles or bullae of varying sizes on the skin or mucous membranes. Large amounts of fluid and protein can be lost when the bullae rupture and leave erosions. The broken-down skin is a portal of entry for bacteria, and sepsis is the most common cause of death. Corticosteroids alone or in combination with cytotoxic agents frequently control the basic disease; however, complications of the high steroid doses that are sometimes necessary may be fatal. The diagnosis is objectively supported by finding (1) intraepidermal vesicles with acantholytic cells on routine hematoxylin and eosin staining of skin biopsies of fresh vesicles; (2) serum positive for *intercellular* epithelial immunofluorescence; and (3) skin positive for direct immunofluorescence.

Pemphigus foliaceus is a more benign form of the disease and is characterized primarily by extensive scaling. Rarely it may change to pemphigus vulgaris. Immunofluorescent studies again are positive.

Pemphigoid is a chronic subepidermal bullous disease usually seen in elderly persons. Mucous membranes are infrequently involved. The disease is less often fatal than pemphigus. Direct and indirect immunofluorescent studies consistently show deposits at the basement membrane. *Benign mucous membrane pemphigoid* is a bullous disease involving the mucous membranes of the eyes and mouth, resulting often in blindness but usually not in death. The vesicles are subepidermal. Immunofluorescent studies have been inconsistent.

Dermatitis herpetiformis is characterized by clus-

ters of intensely pruritic vesicles in a symmetrical distribution, mostly on the shoulders, elbows, scapular areas, and buttocks. It rarely causes systemic problems, but before effective treatment (sulfapyridine and dapsone) was available, patients were miserable because of the tormenting itch. On hematoxylin and eosin stained sections, subepidermal blisters filled with neutrophils or eosinophils are seen. Deposits of IgA are found in patches at the dermal papillae. A number of cases exist of association of dermatitis herpetiformis with adult celiac disease.

Systemic Manifestations of Cutaneous Disease

Both generalized eczematous dermatitis and generalized bullous dermatitis may have significant noxious systemic effects. Large amounts of water and protein are lost through the skin, and vasodilation in an inflamed area can cause considerable shunting of blood to the skin surface, with cooling of the body. Chills are common, and occasionally hypothermic shock occurs. In rare instances high output cardiac failure may appear. Conversely, dermal infiltration with inflammatory cells can interfere with the functioning of sweat glands, and the resultant lack of cooling may cause patients to have fever of 38 to 39°C (101 or 102°F). Finally, acute renal tubular necrosis has been described in a severely ill psoriatic patient with no other disease (presumably secondary to water loss).

Bibliography

Allen, G. E., and Hadden, D. R. Bullous lesions of the skin in diabetes. *Br. J. Dermatol.* 82:216, 1970.

Andersen, S. L. C., et al. Relationship between Bowen disease and internal malignant tumors. *Arch. Dermatol.* 108:367, 1973.

Bailin, P. L., et al. Is methotrexate therapy for psoriasis carcinogenic? *J.A.M.A.* 232:359, 1975.

Braverman, I. M. *Skin Signs of Systemic Disease.* Philadelphia: Saunders, 1970.

Brownstein, M. H., and Helwig, E. B. The cutaneous amyloidoses. *Arch. Dermatol.* 102:8, 1970.

Bruinsma, W. *A Guide to Drug Eruptions.* Princeton, N. J.: Excerpta Medica Amsterdam, 1973.

Cantwell, A., and Martz, W. Idiopathic bullae in diabetics. *Arch. Dermatol.* 96:44, 1967.

Demis, J. D., et al. *Clinical Dermatology.* Hagerstown, Md.: Harper & Row, 1975.

Fitzpatrick, T. B., et al. *Dermatology in General Medicine.* New York: McGraw-Hill, 1971.

Fitzpatrick, T. B., and Walker, S. A. *Dermatologic Differential Diagnosis.* Chicago: Year Book, 1962.

Fleischmajer, R., et al. Familial hyperlipidemias. *Arch. Dermatol.* 110:43, 1974.

Graham, J. H., and Helwig, E. B. Bowen's disease and its relationship to systemic cancer. *Arch. Dermatol.* 80:133, 1959.

Keefer, R. A., et al. Azaribine therapy for psoriasis. *Arch. Dermatol.* 111:853, 1975.

Kurwa, A., et al. Concurrence of bullous and atrophic skin lesions in diabetes mellitus. *Arch. Dermatol.* 103:670, 1971.

Lever, W. F., and Schaumburg-Lever, G. *Histopathology of the skin.* Philadelphia: Lippincott, 1975.

Lutzner, M., et al. Cutaneous T-cell lymphomas: The Sezary syndrome, mycosis fungoides, and related disorders. *Ann. Intern. Med.* 83:534, 1975.

McDonald, C. J. Guidelines for use of azaribine in treatment of psoriasis. *Arch. Dermatol.* 112:388, 1976.

Mihm, M. C., Jr., et al. Early detection of primary cutaneous malignant melanoma. *N. Engl. J. Med.* 289:990, 1973.

Mihm, M. C., et al. The clinical diagnosis, classification and histogenic concepts of the early stages of cutaneous malignant melanomas. *N. Engl. J. Med.* 284:1078, 1971.

Parrish, J. A., et al. Photochemotherapy of psoriasis with oral methoxsalen and longwave ultraviolet light. *N. Engl. J. Med.* 291:1207, 1974.

Paslin, D. A. The effect of biopsy on the incidence of metastases in hamsters bearing malignant melanoma. *J. Invest. Dermatol.* 61:33, 1973.

Schimpff, S., et al. Varicella-zoster infection in patients with cancer. *Ann. Intern. Med.* 76:241, 1972.

Shapiro, H. A., et al. Liver disease in psoriatics — an effect of methotrexate therapy? *Arch. Dermatol.* 110:547, 1974.

Shuster, S., and Marks, J. *Systemic Effects of Skin Disease.* New York: Appleton-Century-Crofts, 1970.

Tobias, H., and Auerbach, R. Hepatotoxicity of long-term methotrexate therapy for psoriasis. *Arch. Intern. Med.* 132:391, 1973.

Zacarian, S. A. *Cryosurgery of Tumors of the Skin and Oral Cavity.* Springfield, Ill.: Thomas, 1973.

III Systemic Infectious Diseases

6

Bacterial and Viral Diseases

Nelson M. Gantz, Neil R. Blacklow,
and William R. McCabe

Whenever feasible, infections that involve primarily
a single organ system have been described under that
system in other chapters of this book. Some generalized infections are difficult to classify under a specific organ system; in addition, certain general principles of diagnosis and treatment are applicable to
every infection, regardless of the primary site of
involvement. For these reasons, this chapter is
devoted to infections in general, and to the specific
infections not easily classified by site of predominant
involvement. These guidelines also have made it
necessary to include a few diseases in this chapter
that are related to each other only by their infectious
causes.

Diagnosing Infections

GENERAL PRINCIPLES

Adequate therapeutic agents are now available against
most bacterial infections, but optimal therapeutic
results depend on the isolation and identification of
the etiologic agent. This does not mean that therapy
must always be withheld until the infecting organism
has been isolated and identified, but only that adequate diagnostic specimens should be obtained prior
to the institution of therapy.

Specific therapy is not available for most viral
infections. Nevertheless, an etiologic diagnosis should
be sought in selected cases both for prognostic and
epidemiologic purposes, and for the detection of
those few viruses that may be amenable to specific
therapy. Such studies should not be routine in every
illness of suspected viral etiology, however, because
of the time and expense entailed. Attempted isolation and identification of the etiologic agent, or serologic tests demonstrating a significant antibody rise
(fourfold or greater) against a suspected agent, are
the laboratory procedures most commonly employed
for the diagnosis of viral diseases (see the section on
Viral Isolation). Such examinations are unavailable
or impractical for some viral infections, the diagnosis

of which must be based solely on clinical or pathologic findings (e.g., infectious hepatitis). By contrast,
effective therapy is available for rickettsial diseases,
and the considerable morbidity and fatality rates in
such infections make their early identification and
treatment important.

METHODS OF DIAGNOSIS

Stains

Microscopic examination of stained smears of purulent discharges, sputum, urine, pleural and peritoneal
exudates, cerebrospinal fluid, and occasionally petechiae and peripheral blood is of inestimable value for
obtaining prompt diagnosis of bacterial infections and
instituting early therapy. Appropriate Gram stains
alone may be diagnostic, and these should be obtained in all patients with abscesses, wound infections, pneumonia, or lesions in which anthrax, gas
gangrene, or tetanus is suspected. When meningitis is
suspected, Gram's stains of sediment from centrifuged
spinal fluid are of paramount diagnostic importance.
Stains for acid-fast bacilli and fungi in sputum or in
drainage fluids from cutaneous sinuses or other
lesions can often circumvent the delay in obtaining
cultural evidence of these diseases. However, in
general, stained stool preparations are of no value in
patients with bacterial gastrointestinal infections
because the etiologic agents are indistinguishable
morphologically from normal flora. By contrast, in
the diagnosis of enterocolitis caused by *Staphylococcus aureus,* stained preparations of stools or rectal
swabs are helpful since these organisms are not frequently seen in stained normal fecal specimens.
Similarly, a preponderance of polymorphonuclear
leukocytes among the cells in stool specimens suggests a bacterial rather than a viral cause of diarrheal
illness (see Chap. 39).

Cultures

Although the attending physician himself may not
specifically identify the bacteria, he must recognize
the indications for culture, submit the most appropriate clinical material, and recognize the capabilities
and limitations of available bacteriologic procedures.
The assistance of the physician in ensuring the proper
collection and delivery of specimens, and in alerting

the bacteriologist to diagnostic suspicions or to the prior use of antibiotic therapy, is rewarded by an increased frequency of positive bacteriologic diagnoses.

It is advisable to obtain blood cultures from all patients with fever, especially patients with febrile illnesses without localizing signs. Physicians seeing patients outside the hospital may not find this feasible, and in these instances blood cultures may be delayed in less seriously ill patients until the clinical features of the illness become clarified. In general, the more cryptic the illness, the greater is the indication for extensive bacteriologic investigation. A minimum of two or three blood cultures, taken at intervals of 1 to 2 hours, should be obtained. In more urgent situations, this interval may be shortened to 15 minutes. The optimal time for obtaining blood cultures is immediately before a chill or rise in temperature, but such timing is rarely possible. Ten milliliters of venous blood should be obtained by strict aseptic technique for addition of 5 ml to each of 100 ml of aerobic and anaerobic broth culture medium.

Cultures should also be obtained from any site exhibiting inflammation. Sources such as the throat or pharynx, sputum, urine, stool, bone marrow, furuncles, and abscesses should be cultured when they appear to be involved in an infection. Every effort must be exerted to obtain fluid from involved serous cavities for Gram's stain and culture when pleural, pericardial, joint space, peritoneal, or meningeal infections occur that are associated with the oropharynx, sinuses, mastoids, or the respiratory, gastrointestinal, and female genital tracts. Anaerobic bacteria do not grow in the presence of oxygen, and specimens for anaerobic culture should be collected and transported to the laboratory in special oxygen-free containers or in prereduced media. Since anaerobic bacteria constitute a major portion of the flora of the oropharynx, large bowel, and female genital tract, particular care must be taken to ensure that specimens collected for anaerobic culture are not contaminated by the normal bacterial inhabitants in these sites. For this reason, it is fruitless to perform anaerobic cultures on sputum; transtracheal aspirates are required for attempts to identify anaerobic bacteria causing pulmonary infection. Anaerobic cultures should not be obtained routinely in all infections, but only when there is reasonable suspicion of anaerobic infection. Certain clinical clues — the site of infection, a putrid odor of exudate or pus, and inability to culture aerobic pathogens from obvious sites of infection — should suggest cultures for anaerobic bacteria.

Interpretation of cultural reports requires a knowledge of the normal body flora and may be difficult on occasion. Contamination from the skin may result in a falsely positive blood culture, but dismissal of a positive culture as being the result of contamination requires that a searching clinical appraisal first be made and repeated cultures be done, since almost every known microorganism may produce serious infections under the proper conditions. Similarly, staphylococci may be found in the sputum of patients with pneumococcal pneumonia; streptococcal carriers may have viral or diphtheritic pharyngitis; and *Salmonella* carriers can acquire viral enteritis.

Viral Isolation

A wide variety of specimens — sputum, feces, pharyngeal and rectal swabbings (in appropriate holding media), blood, urine, spinal fluid, vesicle fluid, biopsy material, exudates, and postmortem material — may be submitted for viral examination. These specimens should be appropriate for the disorder under consideration. Specimens should be adequately preserved until they reach the laboratory (information regarding the technique should be obtained from the laboratory). Most specimens are best held at −70°C; alternatively, they may be kept in an electric deep freeze at −20°C, in a freezing compartment at −10°C, or in a refrigerator at 4°C in this order of preference. Clotted blood should be stored at 4°C to minimize hemolysis, or better, it should be separated and the serum and the clot frozen, if the latter is to be submitted for viral or rickettsial isolation. A brief history listing the date of onset of the illness and pertinent clinical, laboratory, and epidemiologic findings should also be submitted to assist the virologist in determining which of the variety of host systems for viral isolation and which serologic procedures will be most efficacious.

The specimens, usually with antibiotics added to inhibit bacteria and yeasts, are inoculated into susceptible animals, fertile eggs, or suitable tissue cultures. These are examined or tested at intervals for changes indicative of viruses such as histologic lesions, inclusion bodies, or viral antigens. In tissue culture systems the presence of virus is indicated by a cytopathogenic effect, by adsorption of red cells (hemadsorption), or by inhibition of growth of a subsequently added challenge virus (interference). Final identification of the isolated agent is demonstrated by the use of a specific antiserum to inhibit the pathologic changes ordinarily induced by the agent (for example, the identification of poliovirus type 1 is made by the inhibition of the cytopathogenic effects of the "unknown" agent when antiserum to poliovirus type 1 is added).

Isolation of a virus from sources such as the pharynx or feces during an illness suggests, but does not prove, an etiologic association; the agent may merely represent persistence of virus from another recent infection. The antibody response to a virus during illness indicates that infection with the agent was concomitant with the illness and is strong presumptive evidence for an etiologic relation to the virus. The presence of clinical findings known to be caused by a given agent in association with the isolation of the agent, or an antibody response to the agent, or both, provides additional evidence of its etiologic involvement. Isolation of an agent or demonstration of an antibody response from several patients during an outbreak of illness also strengthens the evidence of a causal relationship. Recovery of virus from a parenteral source during an illness is strong proof of cause, and when this source is the site of the disease (e.g., spinal fluid in meningitis), the relationship may be regarded as established.

Serologic Studies
Serologic studies are important adjuncts to etiologic diagnosis of bacterial infections but are rarely diagnostic during the clinical illness. Diagnostic antibody responses during the course of an illness are usually observed only in typhoid or paratyphoid fever, brucellosis, tularemia, infectious mononucleosis, coccidioidomycosis, histoplasmosis, some rickettsial infec-

tions, and *Mycoplasma pneumoniae* pneumonia associated with cold agglutinins. In other infections, antibody response is not measurable until the convalescent stage of the disease. Single determinations of antibody titers are of little value; both acute phase and convalescent phase serum specimens should be obtained for comparison.

Histologic Examinations
The histologic study of involved tissues is primarily of value for identification of tuberculous, mycotic, or nonbacterial causes of fever. Aspiration biopsy of the liver is particularly valuable in establishing a definite etiologic diagnosis in disseminated tuberculosis, since sputum smears and cultures are often negative in this disease. Pleural biopsy is often of value in cases of tuberculous pleural effusion.

Direct microscopic examination of smears made from scrapings of lesions, or from secretions or excretions, may give information concerning possible viral etiology. Thus, cytoplasmic inclusions in cells from scrapings of the base of vesicular lesions are indicative of variola or vaccinia, whereas multinucleated giant cells and cells with intranuclear inclusions are characteristic of infection with herpes simplex or varicella-zoster virus. Conjunctival scrapings may reveal the basophilic inclusions of trachoma or inclusion conjunctivitis. Similar inclusions may be seen in cervical smears when the cervix is infected with inclusion conjunctivitis virus. Characteristic multinucleated giant cells may be found in the patient's urine and nasal secretions early in the course of measles. Also, cytomegalic inclusion cells in the urine are pathognomonic of infection with human cytomegalovirus.

Retrospective diagnosis of certain viral infections may be made on the basis of characteristic histopathologic lesions; for example, Negri bodies (cytoplasmic inclusions) are diagnostic of rabies. Distinctive pathologic lesions may also be seen in various other viral disorders including cytomegalic inclusion disease, poliomyelitis, and yellow fever.

Skin Tests
Dermal hypersensitivity often develops during a number of infections and may persist for years (see Chap. 45). Intradermal inoculation of an appropriate

antigen may provide a rapid and simple method of determining previous exposure to such agents. A positive reaction is characterized by erythema and induration, usually 1 cm or larger, reaching maximum size within 2 days. This test may be useful when coccidioidomycosis, histoplasmosis, tuberculosis, cat-scratch disease, brucellosis, or trichinosis is suspected. In actuality, skin tests are of relatively little diagnostic value and may lead to an increase in circulating antibody levels that can cause confusion when more specific serologic studies are subsequently attempted. The major use of skin tests is for the recognition of patients with prior infection with tuberculosis who are at risk of reactivation.

The Rickettsial Diseases
The rickettsiae are intermediate between bacteria and viruses. Like bacteria, they possess metabolic activity and are sensitive to broad-spectrum antibiotics (especially tetracyclines and chloramphenicol). Like viruses, however, they require living cells for growth. In nature, these agents are usually transmitted to man by various arthropods (see, however, Q Fever).

CLASSIFICATION
The rickettsial diseases are classified into the following groups on the basis of their clinical, epidemiologic, and immunologic features:

1. Typhus group. This group includes epidemic (louse-borne) typhus, Brill-Zinsser disease (recrudescent typhus), and murine (flea-borne) typhus.
2. Spotted fever group. This group includes various regional tick-typhus fevers such as Rocky Mountain spotted fever; also rickettsialpox.
3. Scrub typhus.
4. Q fever.
5. Trench fever.

The incubation period for rickettsial diseases ranges from about 3 to 14 days. Clinically, these disorders are characterized by an acute influenzalike syndrome, intractable headache, and, except for Q fever, by rash. Splenomegaly is variable, and the peripheral white blood cell count is normal or slightly depressed. Pathologically, the chief lesion is a widespread peripheral vasculitis that results from rickettsial multiplication in the endothelial cells of the small blood vessels. In Q fever, however, pneumonia may predominate. The laboratory diagnosis of rickettsial diseases and the distinguishing features of certain of these disorders are described in the following sections.

Typhus Group

Primary Epidemic Typhus (Louse-borne Typhus).
Epidemic typhus is an acute, potentially fatal disease (10 to 40 percent mortality) caused by *Rickettsia prowazekii* and transmitted by the human body louse. The louse becomes infected by sucking blood from febrile patients with the disease and after several days begins to excrete rickettsiae in its feces. Since the louse defecates as it bites, infected feces are deposited on the skin, and rickettsiae are introduced into the new host when the bitten area is scratched. Airborne infection with dried louse feces via the conjunctival or respiratory tract may also occur.

The disease is characterized by an abrupt onset, sustained high fever, severe intractable headache, and generalized aches and pains. By the fourth to seventh day a characteristic maculopapular rash appears, beginning and concentrating on the trunk near the axillae. Occasionally, it is petechial or hemorrhagic; the face, palms, and soles are generally spared. When untreated, the illness lasts for 2 to 3 weeks. Control of this disease is by the use of measures that eliminate lice. An inactivated vaccine is available for prevention.

Murine Typhus (Endemic Typhus). Murine typhus is a natural infection of rodents, caused by *R. mooseri.* It is sporadically spread to man by the rat flea, *Xenopsylla cheopis.* The resulting illness resembles mild epidemic typhus or Brill-Zinsser disease, rarely lasting over 2 weeks; complications are uncommon. There is cross immunity with epidemic typhus. Spread of the disease is controlled by measures to eliminate rodents and their fleas.

Spotted Fever Group

Rocky Mountain Spotted Fever (Tick Typhus).
Rocky Mountain spotted fever is caused by *R. rickettsii* and is representative of a group of related disorders

transmitted by ticks and occurring in various parts of the world (e.g., Siberian tick typhus, Queensland tick typhus). The tick typhus rickettsiae are maintained in nature by transmission to mammals and by trans-ovarial passage in the tick. In the United States the wood tick, *Dermacentor andersoni,* is responsible for most of the western cases of Rocky Mountain spotted fever, and the dog tick, *D. variabilis,* is responsible for most of the eastern cases.

About 7 days after the bite of an infected tick, the patient develops a severe influenzalike illness. Generally, the site of the bite is also evident at this time as a small, dark ulcer. Within 3 to 5 days, a maculopapular rash appears. In contrast to epidemic typhus, the rash begins on the extremities, involves the palms, soles, and occasionally the face, and extends toward the body. In the more severe cases, the rash may become petechial or hemorrhagic or may even progress to necrosis. Fever is usually spiking and may persist 2 weeks or more. Recovery is generally accompanied by a prolonged convalescence. Rocky Mountain spotted fever is a severe disease with a 20 percent mortality rate in untreated cases. A moderately effective killed vaccine is available for persons at high risk. As with other rickettsial infections, this disease responds to specific antibiotic therapy (see under Treatment).

Rickettsialpox. Rickettsialpox is caused by infection with *R. akari.* The reservoir for this agent is the house mouse and possibly other rodents. Infection is transmitted to man by the bite of the mouse mite. Following a 1- to 2-week incubation period, a red papule develops at the site of the bite, progresses to a vesicle, and finally forms an eschar. Within a week after the primary lesion, the patient develops fever and an influenzalike syndrome, followed in several days by a generalized papulovesicular eruption of variable severity. The illness lasts about 2 weeks. The spread of the disease is controlled by measures that are effective against rodents and their mites.

Other Groups of Rickettsial Diseases

Scrub Typhus (Tsutsugamushi Fever; Mite-borne Typhus). Scrub typhus is caused by *R. tsutsugamushi.*

Mites and wild rodents form the reservoirs of the rickettsiae, which are also perpetuated by transovarial passage in the mites. The disorder is found only in a limited area of the Southwest Pacific. It is characterized by an initial lesion at the site of the infection (the mite or chigger bite), a severe influenzalike illness, and a macular or maculopapular rash that appears on the trunk about 1 week after onset and may extend to the arms and legs. The disease is controlled by measures that are effective against mites and rodents.

Q Fever. Q fever, which is primarily a disease of animals, is caused by *Coxiella burnetii.* Cattle, sheep, and other animals, as well as ticks, are natural reservoirs, and the disease is probably spread among animals both by ticks and by contact with infected materials. The agent is resistant to drying, and man is infected chiefly through inhalation of dried dusts or other materials contaminated by products of infected animals, and possibly also by infected milk. Outbreaks of Q fever are most common among people who work with animals or animal products.

The disease is characterized by an influenzalike illness (abrupt onset of fever, chills, headache, myalgia, and weakness) followed after 5 or 6 days by a pneumonitis associated with minimal physical findings in the chest. Recovery generally ensues over the next several weeks. As with the other rickettsial diseases, there is no evidence of direct transmission from man to man. Control measures include the use of inactivated vaccine for workers at high risk and for livestock; pasteurization of milk; and control of infected animals and their products.

Trench Fever. Trench fever is caused by *R. quintana* and is spread by the human body louse. This disease, characterized by fever, headache, myalgia, and a macular rash on the body, has been associated chiefly with armies during war. The etiologic agent differs from the other rickettsiae in that it can apparently multiply extracellularly in vitro.

LABORATORY DIAGNOSIS
The usual technique for the isolation of *Rickettsia* consists in the injection of the patient's blood,

obtained early in the course of the illness, into mice or guinea pigs intraperitoneally, or into the yolk sac of embryonated eggs, which are then observed for signs of infection. The sera of the guinea pigs should be tested serologically for evidence of inapparent infection even if the animals remain clinically well. Smears of the mouse peritoneal exudate or of the egg yolk sac are stained and examined for rickettsiae. Isolates are identified as to species by serologic methods using specific antisera. Epidemiologic considerations, such as geographic location, seasonal occurrence, reservoirs, and vectors in the area, usually provide clues as to the probable species involved.

The technical difficulties of rickettsial isolation make diagnosis by serologic methods simpler, safer, and more satisfactory. Routine serologic procedures for rickettsial infections include complement-fixation and agglutination tests and the Weil-Felix reaction. The Weil-Felix reaction is based on the development during rickettsial infections of antibodies that cross-react with antigens present in *Proteus vulgaris* strains OX-19, OX-K, and OX-2. This reaction is the most commonly employed test for the diagnosis of rickettsial infections and becomes maximally positive 2 to 3 weeks after infection. Sera from patients with epidemic or endemic typhus agglutinate OX-19; those from scrub typhus (tsutsugamushi) react with OX-K; and sera from patients with Rocky Mountain spotted fever may show an increasing titer to all three antigens, although the titer is most often highest against OX-19, and less frequently against OX-2. Patients with rickettsialpox and Q fever fail to react to these antigens.

Treatment

All the rickettsial respond, usually quite promptly, to chloramphenicol or tetracycline in doses of 25 to 50 mg/kg/day. Treatment must be started early to achieve the maximal therapeutic effect. Since the serologic tests are usually not diagnostic until late in the course of the illness, therapy should be initiated on the basis of clinical symptoms, signs, and epidemiologic considerations pending laboratory confirmation.

Exanthematous and Other Common Viral Diseases

MEASLES (RUBEOLA)

An acute, highly contagious disease, *measles* is characterized by fever, a respiratory prodrome, an enanthem (Koplik's spots), and a maculopapular rash. Peak incidence in the temperate zone is in late winter and early spring. Spread is by droplets or by direct or indirect contact with infected persons. The incubation period is 9 to 14 days (usually 10 days). The disease is communicable from about 4 days before to 5 days after onset of the rash.

Signs and Symptoms

Measles is initiated by a 3- to 5-day prodrome consisting of fever, coryza, cough, conjunctivitis (with photophobia), and Koplik's spots (a pathognomonic enanthem on the buccal and labial mucosa). The rash, which is brownish red, appears first on the forehead, face, and neck, and behind the ears. It spreads rapidly downward over the trunk and limbs during the next 2 to 3 days, the temperature reaching its peak at the height of the eruption. The rash then fades in the order of its appearance, leaving a brownish (non-blanching) discoloration that may be followed by a bran-like desquamation. The uncomplicated disease is usually characterized by a granulocytic leukopenia. Measles is more severe in adults.

Complications

The complications of measles are mostly caused either by an extension of the inflammatory reaction in the respiratory tract or by bacterial superinfection. They include otitis media, mastoiditis, laryngotracheitis, and viral (i.e., measles) or bacterial pneumonia. Encephalitis occurs in about 0.1 percent of patients with measles; 15 percent of encephalitic patients die and 25 percent show later brain damage.

Prevention and Treatment

Human immune globulin, given within 5 days after exposure, will protect against measles. The same injection, given after the fifth day but before the prodrome, becomes a moderating, modifying dose. A live, attenuated measles virus vaccine is available and is recommended for immunization of all susceptible individuals during the second year of life; it confers long-lasting immunity. This vaccine also can usually prevent disease if given within 2 days after exposure to natural measles. An inactivated vaccine is no longer recommended because it is less effective and because subsequent exposure to natural measles has resulted in a severe, atypical disease. In such cases, the rash has resembled that of Rocky Mountain spotted fever, both in distribution and appearance.

GERMAN MEASLES (RUBELLA)

German measles is a mild disease characterized by fever, enlargement of the postauricular, suboccipital, or postcervical lymph nodes, and a generalized rash. In the temperate zone, most cases occur in the spring. As with measles, spread is chiefly by droplets or by direct contact with infected persons. The disease may also be transmitted by objects freshly contaminated with the nasopharyngeal secretions, feces, or urine of patients. The incubation period is 14 to 21 days. Patients are infectious from about 7 days before until 4 days after onset of the rash.

Signs and Symptoms

In children the prodrome may be absent. In older persons, it may resemble a mild respiratory illness. Characteristically, the adenopathy precedes the rash and may persist for several weeks. The rash, which is pink and maculopapular, appears first on the face and spreads rapidly downward. It lasts only about 3 days and may be gone from the face by the time it has progressed to the lower extremities. An enanthem consisting of red spots (Forscheimer spots) may be present on the soft palate.

Complications

Complications of German measles are uncommon but may include transitory arthritis, encephalitis, and purpura. Rubella occurring in early pregnancy may result in infection of the fetus (congenital rubella syndrome). This syndrome may be associated with a wide range of dire manifestations including abortion, stillbirth, growth retardation, purpura, and congenital cardiac, ear, eye, and cerebral defects. Infants with congenital rubella may shed virus for many months and are a potential source of infection to susceptible persons.

Prevention

A live, attenuated vaccine is available and is recommended for prevention of the congenital rubella syndrome. The United States Center for Disease Control (CDC) recommends vaccination of all children between the age of one year and puberty, while certain other countries have targeted specific immunization programs at prepubescent females in order to avert subsequent fetal infection. Adolescent and adult females should receive vaccine only if they are shown by serologic testing to be susceptible, and if they agree to avoid pregnancy for 2 months after immunization. Under no circumstances should a pregnant woman be given vaccine. Rash and lymphadenopathy occur occasionally in children after vaccination; however, arthralgia and generally transient arthritis occur more frequently and tend to be more severe in women. Rubella vaccine does not appear to prevent illness if given after exposure.

ENTEROVIRAL EXANTHEMS

Infection with many of the Coxsackie and ECHO virus types may be manifested by febrile illness with rash, either alone or in conjunction with aseptic meningitis. Enteroviral rashes are most commonly maculopapular, but petechial, scarlatiniform, vesicular (such as hand, foot, and mouth disease), and mixed eruptions may also occur. The rashes vary in extent and distribution and, in general, are nonpruritic and do not desquamate. When maculopapular, they have frequently been mistaken for rubella. In the temperate zone, enteroviral infections are most common in the summer and fall. The incubation period for enteroviral disease ranges from 2 to about 7 days.

ROSEOLA INFANTUM (EXANTHEMA SUBITUM)

Roseola infantum is a common benign infectious disease of infants; it is rarely observed after 3 years of age. The illness is characterized by an abrupt onset with high fever that persists for several days and by the appearance of a rubelliform rash as the temperature drops to normal levels. The rash usually begins on the trunk and is generally gone within 1 or 2 days.

ERYTHEMA INFECTIOSUM (FIFTH DISEASE)

Erythema infectiosum is a benign exanthematous infection of childhood, with most cases in the 2- to 12-year-old age group. A low-grade fever may occur, but the predominant feature is a marked erythema of the cheeks, which is followed by maculopapular lesions on the extremities and trunk. The rash may last for 1 to 2 weeks or more and can fade and recur during the illness, particularly in response to changes in temperature, sunlight, and exercise.

DIFFERENTIAL DIAGNOSIS OF MACULOPAPULAR ERUPTIONS

Other disorders characterized by maculopapular eruptions include various rickettsial diseases, infectious hepatitis, infectious mononucleosis, scarlet fever, drug sensitivity, erythema multiforme, meningococcemia, toxoplasmosis, and syphilis.

SMALLPOX (VARIOLA)

An acute, severe, highly contagious disease, *smallpox* is characterized by fever and a vesicular eruption on the skin and mucous membranes. Spread is by direct or indirect contact with respiratory discharges, skin lesions, or crusts of infected persons. The incubation period is commonly 8 to 12 days. Smallpox is communicable from 1 to 2 days before the onset of symptoms, and until all the crusts have disappeared (2 to 3 weeks). The virus resists drying, and it may remain infective for months to years in dried, shed crusts and their dust.

Signs and Symptoms

The disease is initiated by an influenzalike prodrome lasting 3 or 4 days. The rash appears first on the face, neck, and upper extremities and then extends distally; it is heaviest on the exposed surfaces of the body. It begins as macules and papules which progress to vesicles, then to pustules, and finally to crusts over a 1- to 2-week period. Generally, only one crop of lesions is present, and since they evolve slowly, lesions in any one anatomic area are characteristically at the same stage of development.

Prevention

Smallpox vaccine (consisting of vaccinia, an immunologically related virus) is highly effective in pre-venting this disease. Although immunity gradually wanes, it can be renewed or maintained by revaccination. Routine vaccination of children in the United States has been discontinued because the risk of untoward vaccinial side effects from vaccination exceeds the probability of smallpox importation and spread. Exposed susceptible persons should be promptly vaccinated and then given human vaccinia immune globulin. *N*-methylisatin betathiosemicarbazone (Marboran) may also be of short-term value for prevention of smallpox and possibly for treatment of severe vaccinial complications.

CHICKENPOX (VARICELLA)

Chickenpox is caused by the varicella-zoster virus and is one of the most contagious of the exanthemas (see also the section on zoster). It is characterised by a fever and a pruritic papulovesicular rash involving the skin and mucous membranes. Infection is generally transmitted by respiratory tract secretions, less commonly by discharges from the lesions. The incubation period averages 14 to 16 days. It is communicable from 1 day before to about 6 days after onset of the rash.

Signs and Symptoms

The prodrome may be short or even absent. The rash, which spreads centripetally, appears first on the body or head. It begins as macules and papules and quickly progresses (within hours) to vesicles, pustules, and early crusting. The crusting stage may persist for 1 to 2 weeks. In contradistinction to smallpox, the lesions appear in crops so that all the various stages may be found simultaneously in the same anatomic area.

Complications

In adults the disease is generally more severe than in children and may be complicated by a severe varicella pneumonia. Bacterial superinfection of the skin lesions occasionally occurs. Varicella encephalitis occurs in less than 0.1 percent of cases and is frequently associated with a cerebellar ataxia.

Prevention and Treatment

Pooled human gamma globulin may modify (but not prevent) chickenpox if given within 3 days of exposure. Zoster-immune globulin appears to be more effective than pooled globulin for both prevention and modification, but its use is currently restricted by its scarcity to susceptible children with high-risk conditions (e.g., immunodeficiency disorders, leukemia, lymphoma, recipients of immunosuppressive drugs such as steroids). Zoster-immune globulin should be given within 48 to 72 hours after exposure.

ZOSTER (SHINGLES)

Zoster is most common in older persons and involves primarily the posterior (sensory) nerve roots and ganglia. It is characterized by neuralgic pain and crops of clustered vesicles that follow the distribution of the affected sensory nerves. The eruption is usually unilateral and limited to one or two adjacent dermatomes. It can involve the trigeminal ganglion (herpes zoster ophthalmicus), producing pain and a vesicular eruption in the distribution of the ophthalmic division of the fifth nerve, as well as keratitis and uveitis. Corneal scarring can occur. Herpes zoster can also involve the geniculate ganglion (herpes zoster oticus; the Ramsay Hunt syndrome), producing vesicular lesions in the auditory canal with impaired hearing, homolateral facial palsy, and signs of vestibular involvement.

Zoster is caused by the same virus as chickenpox and represents recurrent or reactivated chickenpox in a person whose immunity has waned. Precipitating factors include heavy metals, x-ray, trauma, and certain malignancies, especially lymphomas and leukemias. Although most cases of herpes zoster are not associated with malignancy, if zoster disseminates and becomes generalized, it is frequently found to be associated with lymphomatous malignancy or with immunologic suppression (e.g., use of steroids), in which case it can be particularly severe. Patients with zoster are less infectious than those with chickenpox, but they may transmit chickenpox to susceptible persons.

HERPES SIMPLEX

Acute primary gingivostomatitis is the most common clinical manifestation of the initial or primary infection with herpes simplex virus. Although this disorder is usually encountered in young children, it may also occur in adults. The incubation period is 2 to 7 days. As with other manifestations of primary herpes, the illness is frequently accompanied by the signs and symptoms of a constitutional reaction, including fever and malaise. Characteristic features include a sore mouth; vesicular or ulcerative lesions, or both, in the oral cavity; swollen, reddened, friable gums; and anterior cervical lymphadenopathy. The lesions, which may involve all areas in the mouth including the tongue, are generally located anterior to the tonsillar areas, but may involve the tonsils and occasionally the pharynx (herpetic pharyngitis). Thus, although it is not strictly considered a respiratory virus, herpes simplex can produce tonsillopharyngitis. This illness is self-limited and usually lasts for 1 to 2 weeks. As with most viral diseases, treatment is symptomatic, with emphasis on maintenance of oral hygiene and nutrition. Clinical disease caused by herpes simplex is either primary (occurring in persons without antibodies) or recurrent (occurring in those with antibodies). Herpetic gingivostomatitis is a manifestation of primary, not of recurrent infection; recurrent vesiculoulcerative lesions in the mouth are generally not caused by herpes simplex virus.

Orolabial Herpes

Following primary infection with herpes simplex, the virus is believed to persist at various sites in noninfective form. Activation of this latent virus by a number of nonspecific stimuli — for example, fever, overexposure to sunlight, or local trauma — may result in recurrent herpetic disease. Such localized recurrences are not associated with constitutional symptoms. Herpes labialis is the most common manifestation of recurrent herpetic disease. The lesions are usually located at the mucocutaneous junction of the lips and consist of the characteristic clustered vesicles on an erythematous base. Recurrent herpetic lesions may also involve the skin or mucous membranes. Herpes labialis is common in patients with pneumococcal pneumonia or meningococcemia. Most cases of herpes labialis involving the mouth and lips are caused by herpes simplex virus type 1 strains.

Genital Herpes

Herpes simplex virus type 2 strains commonly produce recurrent episodes of genital infections, which are initially acquired by sexual contact. In women, the cervix is commonly the site for recurrent, asymptomatic vesicular lesions; the vulva and vagina may also be involved, with sometimes painful lesions that can extend to the skin of the perineal area. In men, vesicles and ulcers that are frequently painful occur predominantly on the penis and less commonly on the scrotum and perineal skin. Herpes simplex type 2 infections can also involve the anus or mouth by sexual contact. Primary genital herpes infections are often accompanied by inguinal adenopathy, dysuria, genital soreness, fever, and generalized malaise. Treatment of recurrent genital and orolabial herpes simplex with neutral red and light has been attempted but has been shown to be unsuccessful.

Ocular Herpes

Conjunctivitis and keratoconjunctivitis may each occur as manifestations of either primary or recurrent herpetic infection. Usually only one eye is involved. The conjunctiva is congested, and a slight amount of purulent exudate is present together with edema of the lids. In primary infection, fever and preauricular lymphadenopathy are present. Corneal involvement is manifested by varying types of keratitis and a decrease in corneal sensitivity. Dendritic keratitis is almost pathognomonic of herpes simplex. Ocular herpes usually clears in about 10 days, but it may be associated with residual corneal damage. In patients with primary disease, a history of contact with fever blisters may frequently be elicited. In the recurrent disease the diagnosis can be suspected by the history of previous occurrences or by the presence of herpetic lesions on the lids or adjacent to the eye. Iododeoxyuridine (IDU), a thymidine antagonist applied topically as drops or ointment, is the current treatment of choice for simple herpetic keratitis. Corticosteroids are generally contraindicated since they may lead to perforation of the globe.

Herpetic Meningoencephalitis

Meningoencephalitis is not often produced by herpes simplex virus type 1, but unfortunately when it occurs, it carries a high mortality rate. It appears to be unrelated to either the antibody status or the age of the patient. The disease presents with nondiag-nostic, complex clinical features that can leave surviving patients with severe neurologic deficits. Lesions in the temporal lobes, acute disturbances of consciousness, and epileptiform attacks may occur. Definitive diagnosis requires brain biopsy and demonstration of the virus, since it is not frequently isolated from the spinal fluid. IDU now appears to be ineffective for herpetic encephalitis, but adenine arabinoside (ara-A) and cytosine arabinoside (ara-C) have been used and are awaiting controlled clinical trials to evaluate their efficacy. Recently reported collaborative studies have demonstrated significant enhancement of survival in patients with herpetic encephalitis after treatment with ara-A. Herpes simplex virus type 2 strains can cause aseptic meningitis and ascending myelitis, but they have not been associated with encephalitis.

KAPOSI'S VARICELLIFORM ERUPTION

Infection with either herpes simplex or vaccinia virus in patients with underlying skin disorders may result in a vesicular eruption involving primarily the affected skin areas. Although the underlying disorder is most commonly an atopic dermatitis, a wide variety of other skin conditions may similarly become infected (e.g., seborrheic dermatitis, acne, pyoderma). The resulting disease is known either as eczema herpeticum or eczema vaccinatum, depending on the etiologic agent. It is most severe in patients whose illness represents their primary infection with these viruses. Human vaccinia-immune globulin is useful for prevention or treatment of eczema vaccinatum. Treatment for eczema herpeticum is supportive.

DIFFERENTIAL DIAGNOSIS OF VESICULAR ERUPTIONS

Other disorders characterized by vesicular eruptions include rickettsialpox, impetigo, poison ivy, insect bites, certain enteroviral diseases, and drug eruptions.

INFECTIOUS MONONUCLEOSIS

Infectious mononucleosis is a self-limited viral infection in which both atypical lymphocytes and an absolute lymphocytosis are found in the peripheral blood. Recent persuasive evidence has shown that it is caused by infection with Epstein-Barr virus (EBV). The disease occurs only in persons who lack antibodies to EBV, and following illness a serologic response occurs that is associated with immunity.

Early in mononucleosis, IgM antibodies to EBV develop and then disappear during convalescence. The virus is recoverable from the leukocytes and throat washings of ill patients, and inoculation of nonhuman primates with these materials has reproduced the disease.

Clinical Picture

Mononucleosis, which commonly occurs during the second and third decades of life, has an incubation period of 3 to 7 weeks. The most characteristic findings are severe exudative pharyngitis, generalized lymphadenopathy, and a mild to moderate fever. Palatal petechiae are common, and a transient supraorbital edema may be seen. A variety of organs can be affected; about half of patients have splenomegaly, and 10 percent manifest hepatomegaly. Jaundice is less frequent, but a majority of patients show a mild elevation of liver function tests, particularly transaminase levels. A macular exanthematous rash is occasionally present, and urticarial eruptions occur rarely. A hemolytic anemia, and less commonly an immune-based thrombocytopenia with skin petechiae, are infrequent complications. Minimal neurologic symptoms, notably headache, may be present; however, severe neurologic complications such as meningoencephalitis, transverse myelitis, cranial nerve paresis, or Guillain-Barré syndrome occur in about 1 percent of cases. When neurologic complications appear, mortality increases from the expected less than 1 percent to approximately 10 percent of cases.

Uncomplicated illness can last from several days to several weeks. Rupture of the soft, enlarged spleen is an omnipresent hazard, but occurs rarely; therefore, palpation of the spleen should not be overly vigorous. Additional dangers are respiratory obstruction from massive exudative and edematous tonsillopharyngitis, and neurologic and hematologic complications.

Diagnosis

Diagnosis of mononucleosis is made by the typical clinical findings, an absolute lymphocytosis of 50 percent with at least 20 percent "atypical" lymphocytes, and a positive serum heterophil antibody test. The heterophil antibody is positive in 80 to 90 percent of patients during acute illness; its specificity for infectious mononucleosis is established when it is eliminated by absorption with beef cells but not by absorption with guinea pig kidney. Heterophil-antibody-negative patients with infectious mononucleosis all develop antibodies to EBV. However, since most forms of EBV antibody persist for many years, only the presence of IgM antibody to EBV is diagnostic for the disease. The IgM test for EBV is still experimental and not widely used.

The differential diagnosis of heterophil-negative mononucleosis syndromes includes cytomegalovirus infection, toxoplasmosis, infectious hepatitis, infectious exudative pharyngitis (notably adenoviral, rubella, and streptococcal pharyngitis), infectious lymphocytosis, secondary syphilis, salmonellosis, acute leukemia, and drug reactions (e.g., Dilantin, Mesantoin, para-aminosalicylic acid).

Treatment

Treatment of infectious mononucleosis is symptomatic; no specific therapeutic agent is available. Steroids have no role in therapy, except in the highly unusual patient who experiences respiratory obstruction resulting from massive exudative and edematous tonsillopharyngitis, or the patient who has severe hematologic or possibly neurologic complications.

CYTOMEGALOVIRUS

The clinical manifestations of cytomegalovirus infection are quite varied, and range from common, inapparent infections to severe cytomegalic inclusion disease in newborns and very young infants. The latter disease is characterized by enlarged cells with large intranuclear and occasionally cytoplasmic inclusions in a wide variety of organs, and may resemble erythroblastosis fetalis. Congenital infection can vary from a fatal disease to a severe or a lesser degree of brain damage that may not appear until months after birth. Virus has been recovered from the urine of congenitally infected children for up to several years after birth. Acquired infection in infants and children, while usually asymptomatic, can be accompanied by multisystemic disease, particularly liver disease and bronchopneumonia.

Cytomegalovirus can also produce a mononucleosislike syndrome with fever, atypical lymphocytes, and mild hepatitis. Exudative tonsillitis and lymphadenopathy are usually absent, and the serum heterophil is negative. This form of illness is usually seen in adults, and it can occur naturally or as a complication of multiple blood transfusions received 3 to 6 weeks earlier (postperfusion syndrome). In addition, this illness occurs in disseminated form in patients with malignancies of the hematopoietic-lymphoreticular system and in patients who receive immunosuppressive medications. These patients most commonly have pneumonia, which can be interstitial in character and severe (see the section on viral and *Mycoplasma* pneumonia in Chap. 11). It is not known whether patients who are immunosuppressed or who have malignancy acquire their infection exogenously or by endogenous reactivation of latent infection.

TOXOPLASMOSIS

Toxoplasma gondii is a widespread protozoan parasite that affects man, mammals, and birds (see Chap. 7). Inapparent infections with this agent are common. The disease it causes takes two forms: *congenital* (acquired from the mother), which affects the fetus or newborn infant and is manifested by erythroblastosis fetalis (hepatosplenomegaly, icterus, and rash), and *acquired,* which varies considerably in severity and which may present as (1) a febrile lymphadenopathy resembling infectious mononucleosis, (2) a typhuslike syndrome with rubelliform rash, pneumonitis, or carditis, (3) a meningoencephalitis, (4) an isolated uveitis, or (5) occasionally, pneumonitis as the prominent feature. Diagnosis is usually established by serologic tests. Treatment is supportive except for the more severe cases, in which sulfadiazine and pyrimethamine may be helpful.

Bacterial Infections

STREPTOCOCCAL INFECTIONS
See Chapter 8, Infections of the Upper Respiratory Tract, for a discussion of pharyngitis and other streptococcal infections.

PNEUMOCOCCAL INFECTIONS
See Chapter 11, Bacterial and Viral Infections of the Lower Respiratory Tract, for a discussion of pneumococcal pneumonia.

MENINGOCOCCAL INFECTIONS
Infections produced by *Neisseria meningitidis* may range in severity from completely asymptomatic nasopharyngeal carriage to a rapidly fulminant, lethal bacteremia. Although meningococcal disease is usually considered primarily as a cause of meningitis, as is discussed in Chapter 11, bacteremia is a necessary prerequisite to meningeal localization, whereas nasopharyngeal carriage is the most frequent type of meningococcal infection. The meningococcus may also cause pneumonia.

Meningococci are gram-negative and grow in pairs with their opposing surfaces flattened, giving a microscopic appearance of two closely approximated kidneys. They are relatively fastidious bacteria that prefer special media, such as chocolate agar, enhanced by an atmosphere of 5 to 10% carbon dioxide. Their cultural characteristics and biochemical reactions are similar to those of *N. gonorrhoeae* and almost identical with another species of *Neisseria, N. lactamicus. N. meningitidis,* like the gonococcus, gives a positive oxidase reaction. Meningococci are separated into serotypes on the basis of their capsular polysaccharides. Three major serotypes, A, B, and C, have been known for decades, but recent studies have identified the new serotypes, D, X, Y, Z, 29-E, and 135. Historically, group A strains have been responsible for epidemic outbreaks, but after the 1960s, the frequency of infections caused by groups B and C meningococci has increased until group C currently has become the most prevalent. There has recently been an increase in the number of infections caused by group Y meningococci. For some inexplicable reason, the meningococcus has a peculiar "tropism" for invasion and infection of the meninges.

Asymptomatic colonization of the nasopharynx, which is acquired by inhalation of droplets of respiratory secretions from other carriers, is by far the most frequent type of meningococcal infection. Carriage rates may range from 5 to 70 percent; they rise in winter months, in crowded (e.g., military recruit) populations, and, perhaps, during concomitant viral respiratory infections. The disseminated infection, meningococcemia, occurs within the first few days after acquisition of nasopharyngeal carriage. The onset of meningococcemia may be abrupt, with chills, fever, and myalgias, or the disease may follow a brief prodrome of sore throat and other upper respiratory symptoms. Cutaneous and mucous membrane lesions, which were the basis of the old name "spotted fever," occur in from 50 to 75 percent of patients with meningococcemia. These skin lesions are characteristically hemorrhagic in character and may vary from petechiae, to purpura, to large, cutaneous ecchymoses (suggillations), which are most prevalent on the trunk and upper extremities. Initially, the lesions may be macular or papular before becoming hemorrhagic. Rarely, only macular or papular lesions are seen. The skin lesions may vary in number from one or two to several hundred. Careful search for these skin lesions is extremely important since they can serve to establish the diagnosis.

The course of meningococcemia is quite variable; it may be so mild that the patient may not seek medical attention until meningitis develops, whereas in other instances, it may be so fulminant that death ensues before meningitis is apparent. An unusual form, chronic meningococcemia, also occurs (see below). Reasons for this variation in the severity and course of meningococcemia are unclear but, in the acute fulminant form, few other microorganisms match the ability of the meningococcus to produce overwhelming infection and death within a few hours. This syndrome of fulminant meningococcemia, originally described by Waterhouse and Friderichsen, is associated with profound shock, extensive hemorrhagic lesions of the skin, and hemorrhage into the adrenals and other organs, often found at necropsy. This finding led to the concept that adrenal insufficiency contributes to the circulatory collapse observed, and it influenced the therapy for decades. However, this concept has been definitely disproved by the demonstration that adrenocorticotropic hormone levels are almost uniformly elevated in acute meningococcemia.

A chronic form of meningococcemia may occur, which is characterized by periodic episodes of fever, arthralgias or arthritis, and recurrent skin lesions over several months. Leukocytosis and splenomegaly are common. Patients are usually asymptomatic between episodes, and the diagnosis may be quite difficult to establish. Most patients ultimately become asymptomatic after several weeks or months even without treatment, although a few may develop meningitis or metastatic meningococcal infections.

Pathophysiology

While the exact mechanisms of pathophysiologic changes in meningococcemia and infections caused by other gram-negative bacteria have not been completely defined, several aspects have been clarified in recent years. Measurements of capsular polysaccharide have demonstrated a correlation between the quantity of circulating polysaccharide and the severity of meningococcal disease. Abnormalities of the coagulation system, such as consumption coagulopathy or disseminated intravascular coagulation coupled with bacterial vascular invasion, may account for the hemorrhagic manifestations. In addition, complement activation and bradykinin production have been demonstrated and may contribute to the vascular collapse.

Diagnosis

Absolute confirmation can be made only by isolation of meningococci from blood, skin lesions, or cerebrospinal fluid. Careful incision of a skin lesion followed by Gram's stain of the expressed tissue fluid often allows identification of meningococci within neutrophils. This technique and Gram's stain of buffy coat preparations are two extremely valuable methods for early diagnosis of meningococcemia. In addition, the recent development of countercurrent immunoelectrophoresis has proved to be a most valuable and rapid diagnostic method for the identification of meningococcal capsular antigens in the serum or cerebrospinal fluid.

Treatment

For decades the sulfonamides were the agents of choice for the treatment of meningococcal infections. With the emergence and increasing prevalence of sulfonamide-resistant meningococci in the 1960s, penicillin became the most effective therapeutic agent. The dosage of penicillin for the treatment of meningococcal disease is 12 million to 24 million units per day. Tetracycline and chloramphenicol are satisfactory alternates in patients allergic to penicillin.

STAPHYLOCOCCAL INFECTIONS

Staphylococci are normal inhabitants of the nares, oropharynx, and skin of man and are also important causes of infection. The most frequent type of staphylococcal infection is suppurative disease of the skin and subcutaneous tissues. Clinically inapparent bacteremia may occur with such infections and lead to metastatic infections. Staphylococci also have a propensity to persist within the hospital, to produce infections in debilitated hosts, and to become resistant to antibiotics. These characteristics have made staphylococci an important cause of hospital-acquired infections.

Staphylococci are gram-positive and divide into grapelike clusters of cocci identifiable by Gram's stain. Only two species, *Staphylococcus aureus* and *Staphylococcus epidermidis,* are of medical importance. A number of characteristics may be used to differentiate these two species. The differentiating test used in most laboratories is based on the ability of *S. aureus* to uniformly produce the enzyme coagulase, which causes plasma to clot, whereas *S. epidermidis* lacks this enzyme. *S. aureus* is more pathogenic and may cause skin infections, furuncles, carbuncles, abscesses, wound infections, pneumonia, bacteremia, and acute endocarditis. In contrast, *S. epidermidis* is essentially avirulent and does not cause infections except for an occasional instance of bacterial endocarditis. A large number of toxins and enzymes are produced by *S. aureus,* including hemolysins, leukocidin, coagulase, hyaluronidase, lipase, protease, and DNase, but the role of these toxins in pathogenesis is not well delineated.

Approximately one-third of the population carry *S. aureus* in their anterior nares. Similarly, the skin and gastrointestinal tract may also be sites of carriage. Contact with staphylococci occurs early in life, and many infants become colonized during their stay in newborn nurseries. Transmission of staphylococci occurs primarily by the hands of hospital personnel, with respiratory spread being of minor importance. Autoinfection in nasal carriers is another source of staphylococcal disease.

The most characteristic feature of infection with *S. aureus* is the production of thick, creamy pus in localized abscesses. It has been estimated that as high as 5 percent of the population may have staphylococcal lesions annually, with the vast majority of these involving the skin and subcutaneous tissues (boils, styes, furuncles, carbuncles, and cellulitis). Staphylococci appear to invade the skin through hair follicles and sebaceous glands, whereupon they multiply. Massive leukocytic infiltration then occurs, followed by local tissue necrosis, resulting in the typical lesion with a central core consisting of dead and dying leukocytes and bacteria in the form of creamy pus, surrounded by a fibrous wall. Inflammation of the surrounding tissue is also frequent. Lesions may vary from pustules the size of a pinhead to large carbuncles, deep abscesses that may have several openings to the surface. Extension to the lymphatic or vascular system may also occur, with the development of clinical or subclinical bacteremia and metastatic abscesses in other organs. The factors that predispose to these complications are not well understood, and complications seem to occur as often with minuscule infections as with large abscesses and carbuncles. The most frequent sites of metastatic infection are the kidneys, endocardium, spleen, brain, and the diaphyses of long bones in children (see later in this chapter, under Osteomyelitis). Other staphylococcal infections may develop secondary to bacterial ingress along intravenous catheters, aspiration of oropharyngeal contents containing staphylococci, or introduction of these bacteria into wounds during surgical procedures.

A number of factors may predispose patients to infections with *Staphylococcus.* Any break in the continuity of the skin, as from surgical wounds or dermatitis, may facilitate ingress of staphylococci. Staphylococcal pneumonia, acquired in the community, is rare except following influenza infection. Diabetes mellitus, corticosteroid therapy, antibiotic therapy, and leukopenia also appear to predispose to staphylococcal infection. During the period of time that staphylococcal infections were extremely prevalent in hospitals, the more debilitated patients appeared most susceptible to such infections. It is not clear, however, whether this represented a unique susceptibility of these patients to *Staphylococcus* or whether such patients were more susceptible to all bacterial infections, with *Staphylococcus* being merely the most frequent because it predominates in hospitals. The latter theory appears more likely in view of the increasing frequency of hospital-acquired gram-negative bacillary infections in similar patients, now that these organisms have supplanted *Staphylococcus* as the major component of the flora of hospitals.

The clinical manifestations of staphylococcal infections vary with the site of infection. Local pain and tenderness may be the sole features of boils and small abscesses, whereas chills, fever, and leukocytosis, in addition to local findings, are frequent with more extensive lesions.

Diagnosis

Rapid diagnostic confirmation of the etiology of cutaneous and other accessible lesions may be obtained by Gram's stain of purulent material. Cultures should also be obtained so that antibiotic sensitivity determinations may be performed, since resistance to various antibiotics is frequent among staphylococci. In addition, blood cultures should be obtained from patients with systemic manifestations.

Treatment

Local therapy, especially incision and drainage of purulent accumulations, and administration of appropriate antibiotics are of equal importance in the treatment of staphylococcal infections. Response to antibiotic therapy is usually inadequate in patients with localized collections of pus until adequate drainage has been established. However, incision and drainage of local lesions should be delayed until there is definite purulent accumulation or fluctuation. Frequent application of moist heat helps to accelerate this process.

Penicillin is the antibiotic of choice provided the organism is sensitive. However, penicillin resistance is frequent among "hospital" staphylococci and also occurs in "community" strains, making sensitivity determinations important in delineating therapy. The penicillinase-resistant penicillins — methicillin, oxacillin, nafcillin, cloxacillin, and dicloxacillin — are the agents of choice for the treatment of infections caused by penicillin-resistant *Staphylococcus*. Parenteral therapy is preferable in all but superficial skin

infections. Most penicillinase-resistant penicillins give such low blood levels after oral ingestion that only cloxacillin and dicloxacillin can be relied on for oral use. Optimal parenteral dosage of penicillins for the treatment of staphylococcal infections is somewhat in excess of that recommended in the package inserts, and consists of from 12 to 18 grams per day of methicillin and from 8 to 12 grams daily of nafcillin or oxacillin. Because of the danger of endocarditis and metastatic abscesses, antibiotic treatment of staphylococcal bacteremia should be continued for 4 to 6 weeks. Lack of clinical response, or recurrence of fever and other clinical symptoms in patients with severe staphylococcal infections, should prompt a search for metastatic staphylococcal infections in other sites.

During the past few years, strains of *S. aureus* that are resistant to methicillin have been isolated. These strains, which are also resistant to the other penicillinase-resistant penicillins and the cephalosporins, are a major problem in European hospitals but are rare in the United States. Vancomycin is usually effective against such organisms. Vancomycin and clindamycin, if the *Staphylococcus* is susceptible, are effective alternatives for use in penicillin-allergic patients.

INFECTIONS CAUSED BY GRAM-NEGATIVE BACILLI
Members of the families Enterobacteriaceae and Pseudomonadaceae have become increasingly important causes of infection during the past three decades. In this country, almost all urinary infections are caused by these bacteria, which are also the most frequent cause of hospital-acquired infections and of bacteremias. They are also important causes of intestinal, peritoneal, and burn infections, as well as hospital-acquired pulmonary infections. Except for urinary tract infections, most gram-negative bacillary infections are acquired during hospitalization. *Escherichia coli, Klebsiella pneumoniae, Enterobacter aerogenes, Pseudomonas aeruginosa,* and species of *Proteus* are the most frequent causes of infection among the gram-negative bacilli, but other less prevalent species may produce similar infections.

The relative lack of virulence and the limited invasiveness of gram-negative bacilli in normal hosts would appear to make them unlikely causes of serious infections. There are, however, other factors unique to the practices and the environment of hospitals, to the patients affected, and to the micro-organisms themselves, which more than compensate for the relative avirulence of gram-negative bacilli and explain their paramount importance as causes of hospital-acquired (nosocomial) infections. Among these factors two characteristics of the gram-negative bacilli themselves — their ubiquity and their tendency to develop antibiotic resistance — are important. These organisms constitute a major portion of the bowel flora, are frequent inhabitants of the skin, and may be found in numerous areas within the hospital environment. Since they are often resistant to anti-biotics, the frequent use of antibiotics in hospitals provides a selective reproductive advantage to gram-negative bacilli and results in their becoming the pre-dominant bacterial flora within hospitals. The hos-pital itself provides a population of patients with severe debilitating diseases — individuals who are susceptible to infection with relatively avirulent, noninvasive organisms. Many therapeutic modalities, such as corticosteroids, cytotoxic drugs, and irradi-ation, may further depress host resistance. Finally, many hospital procedures (e.g., indwelling bladder and venous catheters, or the use of ventilatory equip-ment) provide mechanisms for bacteria to circumvent normal host defenses and gain access to the bladder, bloodstream, and lungs. The combination of a very susceptible population, in an environment seeded largely with antibiotic-resistant gram-negative bacilli, together with frequent procedures that enhance the capacity of these organisms to produce nosocomial infections, readily explains the increasing prevalence of gram-negative bacilli as "opportunistic" invaders (see the section later on opportunistic infections). Urinary tract infections, wound infections, bacter-emias, and hospital-acquired pulmonary infections are the most frequent diseases caused by these organisms.

Although there are distinct differences in the epi-demiology and the frequency of infection with the individual species of gram-negative bacilli, once infec-tion is established the clinical manifestations of each type of infection are remarkably similar, irrespective of the etiologic agent. The similarity in the clinical features of infections produced by all these species to the effects observed after the administration of the lipopolysaccharide (endotoxin) component pres-ent in all their cell walls has led to the belief that this material is primarily responsible for the clinical mani-festations. Endotoxin is an extremely active biologic material, capable of producing fever, shock, and leukopenia, followed by leukocytosis, abortion, thrombocytopenia, and death. It also has been shown to activate the coagulation, fibrinolytic, kinin, and complement systems — changes that have been noted in meningococcemia and bacteremia caused by gram-negative bacilli. However, some recent studies have cast doubt on the importance of endotoxin in the pathogenesis of gram-negative infections.

Diagnosis

A number of problems may arise in establishing the role of gram-negative bacilli in individual infections. Since gram-negative bacilli function primarily as opportunistic infectious agents (except in sponta-neous urinary tract infections or Friedländer's pneu-monia) the etiology of a given infection is difficult to predict without bacteriologic cultures. Moreover, interpretation of the etiologic role of gram-negative bacilli isolated from clinical specimens is often diffi-cult. These organisms are extremely hardy and may overgrow fastidious and more pathogenic organisms, such as pneumococci and *Haemophilus,* unless speci-mens are cultured promptly after collection. In addition, gram-negative bacilli frequently colonize various sites without producing infection. The use of methods of bypassing such sites of colonization (e.g., the transtracheal aspiration of uncontaminated sputum) during the collection of diagnostic speci-mens may be of considerable assistance. In addition, Gram's stains of freshly collected specimens are of extreme value for demonstrating the presence of neutrophilic inflammations, as well as leukocytes and various bacteria, in a rough quantitative way.

Treatment

The treatment of gram-negative bacillary infections is complicated by their predilection for patients with severe underlying diseases. In such instances, bacte-riologic cure may be achieved, but death may result

from the underlying disease. The frequency of antibiotic resistance makes selection of an appropriate
antibiotic difficult prior to receipt of antibiotic susceptibility results; thus treatment of mild infections
is often delayed. In more severe infections, early
initial treatment is important, and usually an agent
is selected to which almost all gram-negative bacilli
are susceptible. The species of gram-negative bacilli
most often isolated from such infections and the
antibiotics of choice, with their dosage for *initial*
therapy, are listed below.

Bacterial species	Antibiotic (order of preference)
1. *Escherichia coli*	1. Gentamicin or tobramycin (1.0–1.6 mg/kg q8h) 2. Kanamycin (5 mg/kg q8h)
2. *Klebsiella-Entero-bacteriaceae Serratia species*	1. Gentamicin or tobramycin 2. Kanamycin
3. *Pseudomonas aeruginosa*	1. Tobramycin or amikacin (5 mg/kg q8h) 2. Gentamicin 3. Carbenicillin (4 gm q4h IV; usually in combination with gentamicin)
4. *Proteus mirabilis*	1. Ampicillin (1 gm q4h IV) 2. Kanamycin 3. Gentamicin or tobramycin
5. Indole-positive *Proteus (P. rettgeri, P. morgani, P. vulgaris)*	1. Gentamicin, tobramycin, or amikacin 2. Kanamycin
6. *Acinetobacter (Herellea or Mima)*	1. Kanamycin 2. Gentamicin or tobramycin or amikacin

Since most of these antibiotics possess significant
toxicity, a less toxic agent should be substituted once
sensitivity results have demonstrated the organism to
be sensitive to it. There is little evidence of differences in clinical efficacy of the various systemically
administered antibiotics that are active against gram-
negative bacilli, provided the infecting organism is
susceptible. Ancillary measures such as drainage of
abscesses and correction of obstructing lesions play
an equally important role in the treatment of these
infections.

BACTEREMIA (SEPTICEMIA)
Bacterial invasion of the bloodstream, bacteremia,
occurs during the course of a number of infections.
The term *septicemia* is often used interchangeably
with bacteremia; the former implies ill-defined clinical manifestations (namely, toxemia) in addition to
bacteria circulating in the blood. Since the diagnosis
of septicemia is partially subjective, *bacteremia* seems
a preferable and more exact term. Bacteremia is
almost always secondary to a focal site of infection,
but in rare cases, the original site may not be apparent. Bacteremia may be either transient and asymptomatic (e.g., postdental extraction bacteremia) or
chronic and associated with only mild symptoms
(e.g., subacute bacterial endocarditis); however, in
most instances, patients with bacteremia are acutely
ill.

Bacteria may enter the blood from either intravascular or extravascular foci. Intravascular sources,
such as bacterial endocarditis, bacterial endarteritis,
mycotic aneurysms, septic thrombophlebitis, or
infected vascular grafts, usually result either from
localization from prior bacteremic episodes or from
vascular invasion from an adjacent infection. More
often, bacteria enter the blood from extravascular
septic foci either via the lymphatic system or by
direct involvement of a small blood vessel within a
local area of infection. Rarely, bacteremia may result
from infusion of contaminated fluids.

Isolation of the infecting organism from the blood
is the only means of establishing a diagnosis of bacteremia with certainty. In practice, however, the diagnosis often must be made solely on clinical findings
before culture results are available, to ensure prompt
therapy. Bacteremia occurs with such frequency in
some infections (e.g., meningitis and pneumococcal
pneumonia) that it may be considered an integral
part of the disease process. Although the clinical

manifestations may vary considerably, the occurrence of chills, fever, malaise, and prostration strongly suggests bacteremia. In other instances the onset of bacteremia is less flagrant, and the following clinical situations are often used as indications for taking blood cultures:

1. Fever
2. Prior to antibiotic administration for any reason in hospitalized patients
3. Evidence of meningeal irritation
4. Hypothermia
5. Sudden change in mentation (agitation, stupor, or confusion)
6. Hemorrhagic skin lesions
7. Coma resulting from hepatic insufficiency, diabetic ketoacidosis, cerebrovascular accidents, delirium tremens, or unknown cause
8. Failure of newborn infants to thrive either with excessive bilirubin elevations, or with diarrhea or ileus
9. Granulocytopenia or acute leukemia
10. Hypotension
11. Tachypnea or hyperpnea   } Of unknown or uncertain etiology
12. Oliguria or anuria
13. Thrombocytopenia

The necessity for prompt therapy is never so great that adequate specimens for culture should not be obtained first. These specimens should include two or three aerobic and anaerobic blood cultures, as well as cultures from other appropriate sites such as intravenous catheters, sputum, urine, purulent exudates, and other pathologic body fluids.

It may be difficult to predict accurately the etiologic agent of bacteremia, and whether gram-positive or gram-negative bacteria are involved. Clinical hints may be helpful in other instances; for instance, the appearance of chills, hyperpyrexia ($> 40.5°$C; $105°$F), and tachypnea followed within a few hours by hypotension, occurring after genitourinary manipulation, may strongly suggest bacteremia from gram-negative bacilli. Characteristic black necrotic skin lesions known as ecythyma gangrenosum are indicative of bacteremia from *P. aeruginosa*. Similarly, hemorrhagic skin lesions suggest meningococcemia, gono-

coccemia, or bacterial endocarditis. In general, the diagnosis and selection of therapy are dependent on (1) the most likely clinical diagnosis and primary site of infection, (2) the bacterial species most likely to produce such infections, and (3) selection of the antibiotic or antibiotics known to be most effective against the most likely etiologic agents. Penicillin is the antibiotic of choice for coccal and gram-positive bacterial infections, whereas penicillinase-resistant penicillins are indicated when staphylococcal infections are suspected. The antibiotics of choice for the treatment of gram-negative bacilli have been listed previously.

Bacterial endocarditis and metastatic abscesses may follow bacteremia with cocci, particularly staphylococci, and treatment is often prolonged to prevent these complications. Therapy may then be changed to a more suitable and less toxic agent after receipt of culture and sensitivity results. In contrast, these complications are less frequent with bacteremia caused by gram-negative bacilli; thus shorter courses of treatment are adequate.

Fever of Unknown Origin

Fever of unknown origin (FUO) is a term used to describe febrile illnesses of 3 weeks' duration with daily temperatures exceeding $38°$C ($101°$F) in which the etiology remains obscure after a week of preliminary investigation. There are multiple causes of this perplexing clinical problem; its solution requires repetitive examination of the history and physical findings together with a sequence of laboratory tests, which should be individualized for each patient. Extensive and expensive investigations should be reserved for patients with fever lasting at least 3 weeks, since fevers of shorter duration are usually self-limited. In general, FUOs usually represent atypical presentations of common diseases rather than esoteric illnesses.

The first step in evaluation consists in documenting the occurrence of fever, taking care that the temperature is properly taken per rectum. Although various fever patterns have been described, such as sustained or relapsing fevers, the height or pattern of fever is usually not helpful. An organized search begins with a new, carefully taken history, with particular attention being devoted to the past and present health of family members, exposure to animals or their products, occupation, hobbies, unusual travel, and past surgery. Previous illnesses that are seemingly unrelated may provide important clues. Careful inquiry should be made concerning medications, including nonprescription items that are often not considered medicines by the patient. A history of rigors or shaking chills suggests bacterial infections, but is not specific, since chills also occur with drug reactions, viral infections, lymphomas, and other neoplasms. Physical examination, including the skin, fundi, oral cavity, lymph nodes, diaphragmatic mobility, testes, rectum, prostate, and pelvic organs in the female, should be repeated daily to detect any new signs as the disease evolves. Hastily conceived, blind therapeutic trials are to be avoided.

The diagnostic categories of diseases that cause FUO are listed in the following outline.

I. Infections
  A. Systemic
    1. Tuberculosis
    2. Subacute endocarditis
    3. Mycotic infections
      a. Histoplasmosis
      b. Coccidioidomycosis
      c. Cryptococcosis
      d. Blastomycosis
    4. Less common infections
      a. Infectious mononucleosis
      b. Cytomegalovirus
      c. Toxoplasmosis
      d. Brucellosis
      e. Chronic meningococcemia
      f. Typhoid fever
      g. Malaria
  B. Localized
    1. Liver abscess
    2. Cholangitis
    3. Empyema of gallbladder
    4. Abscesses
      a. Subdiaphragmatic
      b. Tuboovarian
      c. Pelvic
      d. Prostatic
      e. Pancreatic
      f. Perinephric
      g. Appendiceal

II. Neoplasms
  A. Lymphomas
  B. Myeloproliferative disorders
  C. Solid tumors
    1. Kidney
    2. Liver
    3. Pancreas
    4. Stomach
    5. Lung
(Fever is rare in lymphatic leukemia without infection)

III. Collagen and vascular diseases
  A. Systemic lupus erythematosus
  B. Juvenile rheumatoid arthritis
  C. Polyarteritis nodosa
  D. Wegner's granulomatosis
  E. Temporal arteritis

IV. Drug fever
Almost any drug may cause

V. Miscellaneous
  A. Sarcoidosis
  B. Granulomatous hepatitis of unknown origin
  C. Regional enteritis
  D. Ulcerative colitis
  E. Pulmonary emboli
  F. Pelvic thrombophlebitis
  G. Whipple's disease
  H. Familial Mediterranean fever
  I. Thyroiditis

VI. Factitious fever

The majority of patients in whom a diagnosis is finally established have infection (40 percent), neoplasm (20 percent), or collagen vascular disease (15 percent). Extrapulmonary tuberculosis, especially miliary disease, is still common and may occur with a clear chest radiograph and negative tuberculin skin tests. Bone marrow and liver biopsies should be examined for caseating granulomas as well as be stained and cultured for tubercle bacilli. Normal liver function tests do not exclude hepatic granu-lomas. The finding of noncaseating hepatic or bone marrow granulomas is helpful but is not absolutely diagnostic of tuberculosis, and other possibilities should be considered. Subacute endocarditis is also frequent among the infectious causes. Identification of occult abscesses has been enhanced by the devel-opment of hepatic and gallium scans, ultrasound, and arteriography. Inapparent biliary tract infections also may produce protracted fevers. Malaria and other parasitic infections are important causes of fever in endemic areas and should be considered in patients who have traveled in such areas. Acute and convalescent serum should be obtained for detection of diseases such as toxoplasmosis or cytomegalovirus. Lymphomas and tumors of the kidney and liver are common causes of obscure fevers. Any malignant tumor, such as pancreatic or gastric carcinoma, or atrial myxoma, may cause fever. Fever is unusual in patients with uncomplicated multiple myeloma or chronic lymphocytic leukemia, and its occurrence with these diseases suggests bacterial infection.

Drug reactions are an increasingly important cause of a puzzling fever; almost any drug, including those tolerated for years, may induce fever. Patients with drug-related fevers tend to have fewer systemic mani-festations despite high fever, and this may provide a clue to etiology. The presence of inflammatory bowel disease can often pose diagnostic problems since minimal gastrointestinal symptoms may be present.

"Factitious fever" may occur when patients falsify their temperature readings. The methods used are often ingenious, but failure of the pulse rate to increase proportionally to the temperature elevation, lack of diurnal variations in temperature, and lack of sweating with defervescence may provide clues to such manipulation. Other patients may actually inject themselves with bacteria or other foreign materials to produce fevers.

Therapeutic trials are usually of little value in FUO and only delay the establishment of a definitive diag-nosis. Their use may be justified rarely in a rapidly deteriorating patient who is unable to tolerate further diagnostic studies. They also may be helpful when specific drugs, such as antituberculous agents, are

used to help indicate a particular diagnosis. The role of a diagnostic exploratory laparotomy is somewhat controversial, but it should be considered when clues suggest an intraabdominal process. Despite extensive evaluation and even postmortem examination, a definite diagnosis may not be established in a sig-nificant proportion of patients with FUO.

Osteomyelitis

Osteomyelitis, infection of bone, may be either acute or chronic depending on whether it is a first, an acute, or a recurrent, chronic infection. It is the result of hematogenous seeding or extension of adjacent soft tissue infection. Early recognition is dependent on knowledge of the clinical features and settings of the disease, since the characteristic radiographic changes may take 2 to 3 weeks to develop. The long bones are often involved, and in children the femoral and tibial metaphyses are the most frequent sites. In adults, hematogenous osteomyelitis frequently affects the vertebrae, and this diagnosis should be considered in patients with bacteremia, especially staphylococcal, and severe back pain. Osteomyelitis should also be suspected in heroin users who present with bone pain. Bone infections secondary to spread from contiguous foci are common in diabetics with foot infections. Another frequent setting for bone infections is shortly after the reduction of fractures, especially when metallic foreign bodies have been inserted.

Staphylococcus aureus is the most common infec-tive agent in children, but *Haemophilus influenzae* is also quite frequent. Gram-negative bacteria, fungi such as *Candida,* and *Mycobacterium tuberculosis* may also cause osteomyelitis, and a bacteriologic diagnosis is essential for optimal therapy. Several unusual etiologic associations may occur, such as *Salmonella* with sickle cell disease, *Pasteurella multo-cida* with animal bites, and *Pseudomonas aeruginosa* osteomyelitis with puncture wounds of the feet. *Staphylococcus aureus* or enteric gram-negative bacilli are usually responsible for postoperative orthopedic infections as well as for diabetic osteo-myelitis. At times cultures may grow two or three different organisms, but this usually reflects skin contaminants in cultures taken from sinus tracts, whereas cultures of the bone lesion itself usually contain only one organism. Coagulase-negative staphy-lococci *(S. epidermidis)* may cause disease in post-operative patients with foreign bodies such as a hip prosthesis.

Symptoms and signs of acute osteomyelitis include chills, fever, bone pain with localized tenderness and erythema, and limitation of motion. In other instances, acute disease may be present with no fever and only dull bone pain. Chronic osteomyelitis may be less symptomatic, cause only localized pain and tenderness, and produce a recurrent draining sinus, although it may have acute exacerbations. The white blood cell count and the erythrocyte sedimentation rate are usually elevated in acute osteomyelitis; the sedimentation rate usually decreases with adequate treatment and is a useful parameter for following the course of the disease. Radiographic changes consist of soft tissue swelling, periosteal elevation, bone destruction, lytic lesions, and new bone formation or sclerotic lesions. Bone scans may be abnormal before any classic radiographic changes are noted.

Treatment is dependent on the etiologic agent and the stage of the disease. Since a variety of bacteria with markedly different antibiotic susceptibilities may be involved, surgical exploration or needle aspiration is often required to secure a bacteriologic diagnosis. Blood cultures are often positive in acute osteomyelitis. Four to six weeks of high-dose parenteral antibiotics and surgical drainage or removal of sequestra or necrotic bone are usually necessary. Acute osteomyelitis usually responds solely to prolonged high-dose antibiotic therapy (unless an abscess requires drainage), but therapeutic failures are frequent in chronic osteomyelitis. The cure of this disease is dependent on a combination of surgery and prolonged medical treatment with a highly effective antibiotic. Complications may include pathologic fractures, nonunion, bacteremia, and rarely, meningitis or extradural abscess with paraplegia, complicating a vertebral osteomyelitis.

Opportunistic Infections

Certain diseases (e.g., leukemia, Hodgkin's disease) or treatment regimens (e.g., corticosteroids, azathioprine, cytotoxic chemotherapeutic drugs) may lead to alterations in host defense mechanisms. In patients receiving immunosuppressive therapy, certain bacteria, fungi, viruses, and protozoans, ordinarily of low virulence, become invasive and can produce life-threatening disease. Organisms that cause extensive disease in immunosuppressed patients, preferentially if not exclusively, are called opportunistic agents. Infections in such patients are caused most often by opportunistic gram-negative bacilli, which have been discussed previously. A list of the other major opportunistic organisms follows.

Bacteria	*Fungi*
Listeria monocytogenes	Candida
Salmonella species	Cryptococcus
Mycobacterium	Aspergillus
tuberculosis	Mucor
Nocardia	*Torulopsis glabrata*

Viruses	*Protozoa and other parasites*
Cytomegalovirus	*Pneumocystis carinii*
Herpes simplex	*Toxoplasma*
Varicella-zoster	*Strongyloides*

Patients with compromised host defense mechanisms are subject to infection with both these groups of opportunistic organisms as well as with the usual pathogens such as *Streptococcus (Diplococcus) pneumoniae* and *Staphylococcus aureus.*

Depression of cellular immune responses may occur in Hodgkin's disease, or with corticosteroid or cytotoxic drug therapy, as already mentioned; in this setting, one should be alert to the possibility of *Listeria, Cryptococcus,* varicella-zoster, or *Toxoplasma* infections. Defects in humoral immune mechanisms may occur in multiple myeloma, chronic lymphocytic leukemia, and the congenital or acquired gamma globulin disorders. Patients with these diseases have problems with even the common pyogenic organisms such as the pneumococcus or *H. influenzae. Pneumocystis carinii* is an important pathogen in patients with either impaired humoral or depressed cellular immunity. Patients with granulocytopenia frequently become infected with gram-negative bacilli such as *P. aeruginosa* or with fungi such as *Aspergillus* or *Candida.* Splenectomy increases the susceptibility of patients to overwhelming bacteremia and shock from the pneumococcus or *H. influenzae.* Sickle cell disease is associated with an increased incidence of pneumonia, meningitis, and osteomyelitis caused by *S. pneumoniae, H. influenzae,* and *Salmonella.* Rhinocerebral mucormycosis has a predilection for diabetics in ketoacidosis, while *Nocardia* is associated with pulmonary alveolar proteinosis. Narcotic addicts are susceptible to endocarditis and osteomyelitis caused by the usual pathogens as well as by *Candida, Aspergillus,* and the less common gram-negative bacilli such as *Serratia* and *Pseudomonas.* Coagulase-negative staphylococci usually are nonpathogenic; however, these organisms may infect foreign bodies such as hip prostheses, heart valve prostheses, or central nervous system shunts. Defects in granulocyte and complement function have been associated with an increase in pyogenic infections, especially with *S. aureus.*

Immunosuppressed patients are susceptible to a variety of organisms ranging from common gram-positive cocci and gram-negative bacilli to unusual fungi. Recognition of the causative agent requires a thorough history and physical examination along with Gram's stains and cultures of appropriate body fluids. Pulmonary infiltrates, unexplained fever, and central nervous system symptoms and signs are three common presentations of infection in immunosuppressed patients. The symptoms may be subtle when a patient is on high-dose corticosteroid therapy. One should avoid blind therapeutic trials as a substitute for more definitive diagnostic procedures such as an open lung biopsy. The following section describes the clinical features of the different opportunistic organisms.

CANDIDA
The most common fungi infecting leukemic or lymphematous patients belong to the genus *Candida.* The organism is a small, oval, budding yeast that stains gram-positively and forms pseudohyphae which can be cultured from the skin, mouth, vagina, and stool in 10 to 50 percent of normal persons. While colonization with the organism is common, true infection is quite rare. The sputum of patients on antibiotic therapy frequently yields *Candida,* but primary candidal pneumonia occurs rarely if ever.

Disease in the normal host usually consists of oral lesions (thrush) or vaginal infection. The esophagus may be involved, producing pain and dysphagia, with multiple small ulcerations seen on contrast x-ray examination.

Other manifestations of candidal infection seen in the immunosuppressed host are disseminated disease, endocarditis, and focal infection such as arthritis or endophthalmitis. Candidal endocarditis usually involves prosthetic valves. Embolism from the vegetations, occluding medium-sized arteries, is frequent. Whereas disseminated infection primarily involves the kidneys, heart, gastrointestinal tract, and lungs, the symptoms and signs are usually limited to chills, fever, hypotension, and occasionally cutaneous or ocular lesions detectable by fundoscopy. Predisposing factors include the administration of broad-spectrum antibiotics, corticosteroids, and prolonged intravenous infusions, especially with parenteral hyperalimentation fluids, and the occurrence of hyperglycemia. Candidemia occurs most commonly in patients who have recently undergone abdominal surgery and are receiving intravenous hyperalimentation. Such patients may have a transient fungemia that clears promptly when the intravenous catheter is removed. However, persistence of positive blood or urine cultures after an intravenous line or a bladder catheter is changed, or the finding of yeasts in the urine in the absence of a bladder catheter, the presence of predisposing factors, large emboli occluding medium-sized arteries, and clinical deterioration at the time of the candidemia are clues to a deep candidal infection. Blood cultures are positive in only 25 percent of patients with disseminated candidiasis. Serologic tests to date have proved equivocal for diagnosis. If the patient fails to respond to intravenous line removal, amphotericin B, with or without 5-fluorocytosine, may be required. Surgery is essential in candidal endocarditis in addition to treatment with amphotericin B. Oral nystatin is used for esophageal disease. Since this is a hospital-acquired infection, effort should be directed at prevention.

ASPERGILLUS
Fungal infections caused by species of *Aspergillus* are second in frequency to *Candida* in patients receiving immunosuppressive therapy. *Aspergillus*

grows readily in 2 to 5 days on Sabouraud's agar at room temperature. While the fungus occurs widely in nature and is a common laboratory contaminant, hospital outbreaks have been identified and then eradicated after location of the focal source of *Aspergillus* spores.

Aspergillus infection in the normally immune host consists in either an allergic bronchitis with symptoms of asthma, or a colonization of the fungus within a pulmonary cavity to form a fungus ball or aspergilloma. Tissue invasion occurs in the immunosuppressed host, resulting in pulmonary infarction, necrotizing bronchopneumonia, or lung abscesses. The fungus may also disseminate from the lungs to the gastrointestinal tract, brain, or kidney. Endocarditis has also been reported involving prosthetic heart valves.

Diagnosis of invasive disease is difficult because sputum and blood cultures are rarely positive, and serologic and skin tests are not helpful. Biopsy for histologic examination or culture is the best means of diagnosis. Amphotericin B and surgery are employed for the invasive disease. Since this is frequently a hospital-acquired infection, efforts should be directed at identification of environmental sources of exposure.

MUCOR

Mucor, a member of the class Phycomycetes, is a large (5 to 50 microns) fungus; like *Aspergillus*, its hallmark of infection is vascular invasion and tissue infarction. The rhinocerebral form with its characteristic paranasal sinusitis, gangrenous nasal mucosa, ophthalmoplegia, proptosis, and acute cerebral manifestations has a predilection for the diabetic patient in ketoacidosis. Fever and pulmonary infiltrates resembling pulmonary infarction, disseminated respiratory, cerebral, and renal involvement, and gastrointestinal invasion with hemorrhage may occur in the immunosuppressed host. Pulmonary involvement is the principal finding and is limited to the immunosuppressed patient. Sputum and blood cultures are rarely positive, and diagnosis requires biopsy of the involved site with histologic and cultural confirmation. Treatment consists in administration of intravenous amphotericin B, correction of the acidosis, and surgical excision of the infected tissue.

TORULOPSIS GLABRATA

The yeast *Torulopsis glabrata* is an oval-shaped organism 2 to 4 microns in diameter that is slightly smaller than *Candida*. The organism has no capsule and produces no hyphae or pseudohyphae. This yeast should not be confused with *Torula histolytica*, the former name of another fungus, *Cryptococcus neoformans*. The organism occasionally causes a urinary tract infection in patients with diabetes mellitus. In the immunosuppressed host, cases of *T. glabrata* fungemia have been reported. Conditions similar to those that predispose to infection with *Candida* — corticosteroids, broad-spectrum antimicrobials, diabetes mellitus, surgery, parenteral hyperalimentation — are usually present singly or combined. The clinical manifestations of fungemia consist of high fever and hypotension. Diagnosis is dependent on isolation of the yeast from blood or urine. Amphotericin B or 5-fluorocytosine may be effective in treatment.

CRYPTOCOCCUS NEOFORMANS

Cryptococcus neoformans is the most frequent cause of fungal meningitis. The organism, which lacks hyphae, is a budding spherical yeast with a large mucinous capsule. The capsule is usually more than twice the width of the organism. The yeast can be cultured in nature, especially from pigeon droppings, and the infection probably occurs when the organism is inhaled. Infection localized to the lungs resolves without treatment in the majority of cases. The most serious consequence of infection is meningitis. About 50 percent of patients with cryptococcosis have underlying illnesses associated with impaired cellular immunity, and although other hosts may be called normal and lack specific underlying diseases, subtle defects can be detected in their cellular immunity. The most frequently associated conditions are lymphomas and renal transplantation.

Symptoms and signs in patients with meningitis may include headache, nausea and vomiting, alterations in mental status, fever, meningeal signs, and cranial nerve paralysis. The onset is usually gradual, and the clinical manifestations may be quite subtle. The cerebrospinal fluid classically shows an increase in white blood cells, a low sugar level, elevated pressure, and a high protein level. Disease may also be present with atypical cerebrospinal fluid findings.

In about 50 percent of patients the organism can be seen in India ink preparations. Cryptococci may also be identified as gram-positive budding yeasts. A latex agglutination test of the serum and spinal fluid for cryptococcal antigen and antibody is quite useful both in diagnosis and in following the course of treatment. Isolation of the organism by culture from the cerebrospinal fluid is the best diagnostic test; blood, urine, and sputum cultures may also be positive. Intravenous amphotericin B with or without 5-fluorocytosine is the current therapy of choice. Intrathecal administration of amphotericin B is indicated for patients who fail to respond or are unable to tolerate systemic therapy. Cures occur in about 60 percent of treated patients.

TOXOPLASMA GONDII

Toxoplasma gondii has already been discussed earlier in the chapter. This protozoan parasite, like other opportunistic pathogens, may cause fulminant infection in immunosuppressed patients. Neurologic symptoms and signs usually predominate, with findings on examination of a meningoencephalitis or a cerebral mass lesion. Rash, pneumonitis, and myocarditis may also occur. Concomitant infection with cytomegalovirus and herpes virus is common.

LISTERIA MONOCYTOGENES

Listeria monocytogenes is an aerobic, small, motile, gram-positive rod that may be confused with diphtheroids and discarded as a contaminant. Infection in rabbits, unlike man, is associated with a monocytosis. Although the organism can be isolated in nature from plants and animals, its epidemiology in human infections is unknown. A history of animal exposure is rarely obtained. The organism is an intracellular parasite like *Mycobacterium tuberculosis,* *Salmonella,* and *Brucella,* and resistance to it appears to be mediated by the cellular immune system. Infection in adults almost always occurs in patients with impaired cellular immunity as a result of underlying disease or use of corticosteroids or cytotoxic drugs. Meningitis, and less often bacteremia, occurs in the majority of patients with listerial infection. The clinical manifestations of meningitis may be subtle and consist only of fever with minimal head-

ache. High-dose intravenous ampicillin or penicillin is the therapy of choice.

NOCARDIA ASTEROIDES

Nocardia asteroides are aerobic, fine-branching, gram-positive bacteria that fragment into bacillary forms. The organism stains acid fast if decolorized with 3% hydrochloric acid instead of the acid alcohol used for staining mycobacteria. Growth on blood or Sabouraud's agar can occur in 2 to 3 days or may require 2 to 3 weeks. The epidemiology is unknown, and human-to-human transmission has not been documented. The respiratory tract is the usual portal of entry, and infection most commonly involves the lungs, with fever, productive cough, and frequently pleuritic chest pain. The chest radiographic pattern is nonspecific and may show an abscess cavity, or nodular or patchy infiltrates. Sputum smears and cultures may yield the organism, or lung biopsy may be required. Hematogenous dissemination to the brain, skin, or other organs may occur. The organism evokes a suppurative, not a granulomatous, reaction. Prolonged treatment with a sulfonamide such as sulfisoxazole in a dose of 8 to 12 gm per day is indicated.

PNEUMOCYSTIS CARINII

Under the light microscope, *Pneumocystis carinii* appears as a 6-μ cystic structure containing eight oval bodies. The organism is probably a protozoan, although it has never been cultured. Special stains of lung tissue with either silver methenamine or Giemsa's stain are required for identification. Organisms are rarely seen in sputum smears. Lung biopsy, by either bronchial brushing, needle aspiration, bronchoscopy, or thoracotomy, is essential. Infection in adults is limited to immunosuppressed hosts; *Pneumocystis* does not invade even patients with severe alcoholism or diabetes mellitus unless they are also receiving cytotoxic or immunosuppressive therapy. Infection results in a pneumonia with marked dyspnea, a nonproductive cough, and frequently fever. The chest is often clear on examination, although dry rales may be audible. Measurement of arterial blood gases reveals a decreased PO_2 and PCO_2. Characteristic radiographic findings include diffuse bilateral perihilar infiltrates. However, atypical x-ray findings have been reported. Once the diagnosis is established, or pending the pathology report, treatment may be with either pentamidine or trimethoprim and sulfamethoxazole. Response to therapy occurs in about 60 percent of patients.

VIRAL INFECTIONS
Viral infections have been described earlier. However, cytomegalovirus, varicella-zoster virus, and herpes simplex virus deserve emphasis since they may produce disseminated disease in immunosuppressed patients. Generalized cutaneous infection may occur with herpes simplex and varicella-zoster viruses, especially in patients with Hodgkin's disease or leukemia. All three viruses may cause extensive pulmonary involvement.

Sexually Acquired Diseases
Sexually transmitted diseases are increasing in frequency. Whereas such patients often received treatment at public facilities in the past, increasing numbers of patients are currently seeking private medical care. Adequate management of these diseases is dependent on recognition of the symptoms and signs. The usual presenting complaints in patients with sexually acquired diseases, and the other conditions to be considered in the differential diagnosis, are listed below.

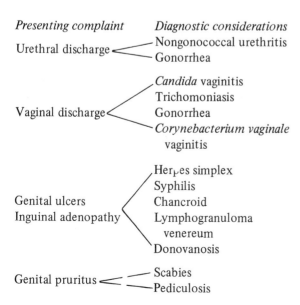

Presenting complaint	Diagnostic considerations
Urethral discharge	Nongonococcal urethritis Gonorrhea
Vaginal discharge	*Candida* vaginitis Trichomoniasis Gonorrhea *Corynebacterium vaginale* vaginitis
Genital ulcers Inguinal adenopathy	Herpes simplex Syphilis Chancroid Lymphogranuloma venereum Donovanosis
Genital pruritus	Scabies Pediculosis

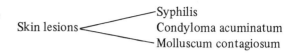

Skin lesions — Syphilis
Condyloma acuminatum
Molluscum contagiosum

URETHRAL DISCHARGE
Urethral discharges are usually infectious in origin and are classified as either gonococcal or nongonococcal. Information should be sought from the patient concerning the temporal relation of sexual exposure previous to the onset of discharge, known diseases in contacts, and the character and duration of the discharge. Gonococcal urethritis usually has an abrupt onset; it follows an incubation period of 1 to 7 days, and the discharge is purulent. In contrast, the onset of nongonococcal urethritis is gradual; it has a longer incubation period of 10 to 14 days, and the discharge is usually mucoid and scanty. Clinical distinction between the two entities is often difficult, however, and Gram's stain and culture are essential for a diagnosis.

Neisseria gonorrhoeae, which are gram-negative, nonmotile diplococci having a coffee-bean appearance, cause gonorrhea. These fastidious organisms grow best on chocolate agar in a 5 to 10% carbon dioxide atmosphere. Thayer-Martin selective agar inhibits the growth of other bacteria and is useful for the direct plating and culturing of clinical specimens. Gram's stain of the urethral discharge will demonstrate gram-negative diplococci within the polymorphonuclear leukocytes in 95 percent of males with gonococcal urethritis. In the remaining 5 percent and in an occasional male with asymptomatic urethral gonorrhea, cultures will be positive for the organism.

A number of organisms, including *Chlamydia, Mycoplasma, Trichomonas,* herpes virus, and cytomegalovirus, have been implicated as causes of nongonococcal urethritis; chlamydiae are responsible for about 50 percent of cases. Gram's stains in nongonococcal urethritis show occasional polymorphonuclear leukocytes and mixed bacteria, but no gram-negative diplococci on smear. Cultures are negative for *Neisseria gonorrhoeae.*

Complications of gonorrhea in men include prostatitis, epididymitis, urethral strictures, and rarely gonococcemia and endocarditis. Anal and pharyngeal infections may occur in homosexual males.

Parenteral aqueous procaine penicillin G given with probenecid is the therapy of choice for gonococcal urethritis. Oral ampicillin is also effective, although oral penicillin is not. Tetracycline and spectinomycin are alternatives in the penicillin-allergic patient. Follow-up cultures should be obtained after treatment to ensure cure. Failure to respond to appropriate therapy is usually a result of reinfection but may be caused by either concomitantly acquired nongonococcal urethritis or antibiotic resistance. Nongonococcal urethritis usually responds to tetracycline.

VAGINAL DISCHARGE

Vaginal discharge is one of the most frequent reasons for which women seek medical care. It may be classified as *physiologic, noninfectious,* or *infectious discharge.* Physiologic discharge often occurs with pregnancy or with the use of oral contraceptives; it contains large numbers of gram-positive rods and sparse polymorphonuclear leukocytes on Gram's stain. Noninfectious causes of vaginal discharge include chemicals (such as feminine hygiene sprays), local foreign bodies, or atrophic vaginitis resulting from estrogen deficiency. Table 6-1 lists the clinical features, diagnosis, and treatment of four diseases responsible for the majority of infectious vaginal discharges.

Trichomonas vaginalis is a pear-shaped, 10-μ, motile, flagellated protozoan which is best seen by microscopic examination of a fresh saline wet mount of vaginal material. Cultures are not necessary for diagnosis.

Candida albicans is a small (2 to 4μ), oval, budding yeast which can be seen by microscopic examination of a potassium hydroxide (KOH) preparation or Gram's stain of vaginal discharge. The organism is gram-positive and may form mycelial-like structures called pseudohyphae. Cultures are not required for diagnosis. Vaginal colonization with *Candida* is extremely common, and only symptomatic patients require treatment.

Gonorrhea causes a spectrum of diseases in women. While asymptomatic vaginal infection is the most frequent, vaginal discharge and pelvic inflammatory disease are also common. Gram's stain and culture of material from the endocervical canal are used to confirm the diagnosis. A Gram's stain showing gram-negative intracellular diplococci will provide a presumptive diagnosis in about 50 percent of patients, but a negative Gram-stained smear does not exclude the diagnosis. Spread of the gonococcus to the uterus, fallopian tubes, and adjacent adnexal structures results in *pelvic inflammatory disease* (PID). The symptoms of PID vary but may include fever, lower abdominal pain, nausea, vomiting, and menstrual irregularities. Gentle cervical motion on pelvic examination usually produces pain. *Neisseria gonorrhoeae* are isolated in from 33 to 50 percent of patients with this syndrome, while mixed anaerobic and aerobic bacteria are cultured from the remainder.

Another complication of gonococcal infection, occurring more frequently in women, is *gonococcal arthritis.* Two clinical forms of gonococcal arthritis have been described. In the *bacteremic syndrome,* clinical features include chills, fever, tenosynovitis, characteristic skin lesions, and polyarthritis with minimal joint effusions. The skin lesions occur predominantly around joints and begin as small red papules or petechiae, which usually evolve to become vesicles or pustules with gray necrotic centers. In the *septic joint syndrome,* features include a monoarticular arthritis with a large effusion and an absence of chills, fever, and skin lesions. However, the clinical features of the two syndromes may overlap, and intermediate forms may occur. Diagnosis is facilitated by obtaining blood cultures, appropriate Gram's stains, and cultures of involved joints, skin lesions, pharynx, rectum, endocervix, and urethra.

Vaginal discharge attributable neither to *Trichomonas, Candida,* nor to *N. gonorrhoeae* has been called *nonspecific vaginitis. Corynebacterium vaginale* (or *Haemophilus vaginalis*) is responsible for a proportion of these cases. The organism is a small, pleomorphic, gram-negative rod. A typical Gram's stain will show few polymorphonuclear leukocytes and sheets of gram-negative rods. Vaginal epithelial cells covered with the organism are also characteristic. Ampicillin, 2 gm per day for 1 week, is the treatment of choice.

GENITAL ULCERS

Table 6-2 lists the clinical features, diagnosis, and treatment of the infectious causes of penile and vul-

Table 6-1. Infectious Vaginal Discharges

Disease & etiology	Epidemiology	Symptoms and signs	Diagnosis	Treatment
Trichomoniasis (*Trichomonas vaginalis*)	60–70% of sexual contacts positive. Usually sexually transmitted	25% asymptomatic, 25% vulvar pruritus, 50% pruritus and discharge. Onset often at menses or immediately after. Creamy, frothy, offensive discharge. Granular vaginitis, punctate hemorrhages of cervix	Wet mount of vaginal secretions. Pap smear unreliable	Symptomatic and, perhaps, asymptomatic females should receive metronidazole (Flagyl) either as a single 2.0 gm p.o. dose or 250 mg p.o., t.i.d. for 7 days. Alcohol should be avoided. Steady male partners of infected females treated as described above. In symptomatic pregnant females, 0.25% acetic acid douches or other local agents should be used and metronidazole avoided.
Candidal (monilial) vaginitis (*Candida albicans*)	Sexual transmission has minor role. Vaginal colonization in 25–50% of asymptomatic sexually active women. Increased prevalence with oral contraceptives, diabetes, late pregnancy, steroids, and antibiotics	Premenstrual onset of marked vulvar pruritus. Discharge odorous, scanty; at times thick, white. Vulva erythematous, edematous, excoriated	KOH preparation or Gram's stain	In symptomatic women only: nystatin vaginal suppositories h.s. for 10 days
Gonorrhea (*Neisseria gonorrhoeae*)	Increase in positive cultures and dissemination during menses	Asymptomatic infection common. Vaginal discharge creamy, thick. Presence of pelvic inflammatory disease	Gram's stain detects 46%; 3% false-positives. Endocervical culture detects 80–90%, rectal culture an additional 6%	Procaine penicillin G, 4.8 million units IM Probenecid 1 gm, p.o.; or Ampicillin, 3.5 gm, p.o. Probenecid, 1 gm, p.o.; or Tetracycline, 500 mg q.i.d. for 5 days; or Spectinomycin, 2 gm IM Ampicillin, 500 mg, p.o., q.i.d. for 1 week
Corynebacterium vaginale or "nonspecific" vaginitis (*Corynebacterium vaginale*)	Sexually active women	Mild to moderate gray-white discharge, mild pruritus. 10–40% asymptomatic	Few PMNs; sheets of small, gram-negative rods. Vaginal epithelial cells covered with cocco-bacilli	

Table 6-2. Diseases with Genital Ulcers or Adenopathy or Both

Disease & etiology	Clinical features	Diagnosis	Treatment
Herpes genitalis (Herpesvirus hominis, type 2)	Itching, burning prodrome Vesicular lesions that evolve to shallow, painful ulcers Recurrence	Tzanck smear from base of intact vesicle shows multinucleated giant cells	Symptomatic
Syphilis (primary) (Treponema pallidum)	Incubation period 10–90 days (3 weeks average) Chancre, usually painless, indurated, solitary Shotty bilateral inguinal adenopathy Extragenital primary lesions (5%) Treated chancre heals in 1 week; untreated chancre heals in 4–8 weeks	Darkfield microscopy Initial serology may be negative (25%)	Benzathine penicillin G, 2.4 million units IM; or Tetracycline, 2 gm p.o. for 15 days or Erythromycin, 2 gm/ day p.o. for 15 days
Chancroid (Haemophilus ducreyi)	Most common in tropical and subtropical areas Incubation period 2–5 days Usually unilateral inguinal adenopathy	Gram's stain of bubo aspirate shows gram-negative coccobacilli Clean ulcer with saline, then do Gram's stain of serous exudate	Sulfisoxazole, 1 gm q.i.d. for 2 weeks
Donovanosis (Granuloma inguinale) (Calymmatobacterium granulomatis)	Incubation period 8–80 days Rare in U.S.A., common in New Guinea & India Beefy, granulomatous ulcers with widespread destruction of tissue Subcutaneous granulomata: pseudobuboes	Wright's stain of tissue smear shows clusters of blue-black organisms in cytoplasm of large mononuclear cells Culture on chick chorioallantoic membrane	Tetracycline, 500 mg p.o., q.i.d. until lesion resolves
Lymphogranuloma venereum (LGV) (Chlamydia trachomatis)	Primary genital lesion usually unnoticed Incubation period 7–12 days Unilateral (70%) inguinal adenopathy usually presenting problem ± fever, abdominal pain, vomiting Rectal stricture, elephantiasis of genitalia	Frei's skin test, 70% positive in 2–6 weeks, but nonspecific LGV-complement fixation test-titer > 1/32	Tetracycline, 500 mg p.o., q.i.d. for 3 weeks

var ulcers. Trauma is the most common noninfectious cause of penile ulceration. Although the genital ulcer may appear insignificant, its location often evokes considerable patient concern.

DISEASES WITH PRURITUS OR ELEVATED SKIN LESIONS

The genitalia, like other skin and hair-bearing areas, may be affected by viruses, lice, and mites, resulting in pruritus or elevated skin lesions. Genital warts or condylomata acuminata are pink papillary growths caused by a papovavirus; the serologic test for syphilis is nonreactive. Treatment consists in application of topical podophyllin or surgery. In contrast, the lesion of condyloma latum is flat and is associated with an abnormal syphilis serology.

Phthirus pubis, or the pubic louse, causes crabs. Patients may be asymptomatic or may note itching in the hair areas. The nits (eggs) or adult lice may be seen attached to hair shafts. Another cause of pruritus (especially at night) and of 1- to 10-mm linear skin lesions is scabies. The mite, *Sarcoptes scabiei,* or its ova may be demonstrated in a wet mount of scraping from an unroofed burrow. Treatment consists in applying 1% gamma benzene hexachloride (Kwell) to the skin from the neck downward after bathing, not to be removed for 24 hours.

SYPHILIS

Syphilis is divided into stages — primary, secondary, latent, and tertiary. The genital or extragenital chancre of primary syphilis is discussed in Table 6-2.

Serologic tests for syphilis are of two types: (1) tests to detect antibody (reagin) directed against the nonspecific cardiolipin antigen, and (2) tests to detect antibody against specific treponemal antigens. Examples of the nontreponemal tests include the Hinton test, the Venereal Disease Research Laboratory (VDRL) test, and the Rapid Plasma Reagin Card (RPRC) test. These tests are useful in screening both asymptomatic and symptomatic patients. Moreover, since the tests can be quantitated, they are helpful in following patients to determine the effectiveness of therapy. If specific therapy is instituted during the primary or secondary states, most patients will show a negative reaction within a year. A small number of patients will fail to convert their tests to negative and

will demonstrate a persistently low antibody titer. An abnormal nontreponemal test suggests four possibilities: a laboratory error, untreated disease, adequate therapy in a "serofast" patient (5 percent), or a false-positive reaction. The fluorescent treponemal antibody absorption (FTA-ABS) test is used to identify false-positive reactions (reactive nontreponemal test but negative FTA-ABS). False-positive nontreponemal reactions may occur with collagen diseases, narcotic addiction, hepatitis, leprosy, or several months after a viral illness or vaccination. The FTA-ABS test is more likely to be reactive in primary and tertiary disease than the nontreponemal tests. The FTA-ABS test, however, is not useful in following the patient's response to therapy since it tends to remain positive indefinitely.

Secondary syphilis must always be considered in a patient with a macular or papulosquamous eruption. The rash is seldom pruritic, and it is usually symmetrical and includes the palms and soles. Other manifestations may be generalized lymphadenopathy, mucous patches, patchy alopecia, annular hyperpigmented lesions, and condylomata lata. The serologic test in secondary syphilis is always positive, with titers of 1/32 being common. Moist lesions reveal spirochetes on dark-field examination and are infective.

The latent stage of syphilis is characterized by an abnormal serologic test in the absence of symptoms and signs of disease.

Tertiary syphilis occurs after a 10- to 30-year delay in about one-third of untreated patients. Patients can present with cardiovascular, neurologic, psychiatric, skeletal, or a variety of other manifestations. The hallmark of cardiovascular involvement is dilatation of the ascending aorta with aortic valvular insufficiency and, rarely, coronary ostial occlusion. Neurologic manifestations are variable and extend from asymptomatic neurosyphilis with only cerebrospinal fluid abnormalities to fulminant sensory, motor, cerebellar, or mental status changes. Nontreponemal serologic tests on the serum are reactive in about 75 percent of patients, while the FTA-ABS test is abnormal in 95 percent. The cerebrospinal fluid shows an increase in cells and protein and a reactive nontreponemal test. Treatment prevents progression of disease but will not repair damage already present.

Bibliography

Bode, F. R., Peter-Pare, J. A., and Fraser, R. G. Pulmonary diseases in the compromised host. A review of clinical and roentgenographic manifestations in patients with impaired host defense mechanisms. *Medicine* 53:255, 1974.

Chervenick, P. A. Infectious mononucleosis. *DM,* December, 1974.

Cluff, L. E., Reynolds, R. C., Page, D. L., and Breckenridge, J. L. Staphylococcal bacteremia and altered host resistance. *Ann. Intern. Med.* 69:859, 1968.

Cohen, J. O. (ed.). *The Staphylococci.* New York: Wiley, 1972.

Gardner, P., and Provine, H. T. *Manual of Acute Bacterial Infections.* Boston: Little, Brown, 1975.

Krugman, S., and Ward, R. *Infectious Diseases of Children and Adults* (5th ed.). St. Louis: Mosby, 1973.

Levine, A. S., Schimpff, S. C., Graw, R. G., Jr., and Young, R. C. Hematologic malignancies and other marrow failure states: Progress on the management of complicating infections. *Semin. Hematol.* 11:141, 1974.

McCabe, W. R. Gram-negative bacteremia. *DM,* December, 1973.

Petersdorf, R. G., and Beeson, P. B. Fever of unexplained origin: Report on 100 cases. *Medicine* 40:1, 1961.

Rein, M. F., and Chapel, T. A. Trichomoniasis, candidiasis, and minor venereal diseases. *Clin. Obstet. Gynecol.* 18:73, 1975.

Ruskin, J., and Remington, J. S. Toxoplasmosis in the compromised host. *Ann. Intern. Med.* 84:193, 1976.

Waldvogel, F. A., Medoff, G., and Swartz, M. N. Osteomyelitis: A review of clinical features, therapeutic considerations and unusual aspects. *N. Engl. J. Med.* 282:198, 260, 316, 1970.

Webster, B. (ed.). Symposium on venereal diseases. *Med. Clin. North Am.* 56:1055, 1972.

Weinstein, L. *The Practice of Infectious Disease.* New York: Landsberger Medical Books, 1958.

Williams, D. M., Krick, J. A., and Remington, J. S. Pulmonary infection in the compromised host. *Am. Rev. Respir. Dis.* 114:359, 1976.

7

Parasitic Diseases

Richard Alan Gleckman

Although it is recognized that parasites infest more than a billion people all over the world, there is a mistaken impression that most parasitic diseases are confined to tropical or underdeveloped countries. However, parasitic infections have received renewed interest recently in the United States as a result of the large-scale immigration of Puerto Ricans, the Vietnamese conflict, the relocation of Vietnamese refugees to America, Peace Corps programs, and the increasing numbers of vacation and business trips by Americans to foreign countries. More than 50 million Americans harbor "worms," and virtually every parasitic disease has been found in the United States. This chapter will attempt to clarify the parasitic diseases, especially those not described elsewhere in the text.

Enterobiasis

Enterobiasis, or pinworm infestation, is the most common parasitic disease in this country. The parasite *Enterobius vermicularis* occurs most frequently in children from 5 to 9 years of age. Man is the only natural host.

Mature eggs that have been ingested develop into adult worms in the cecum and adjacent intestines. The worms do not penetrate tissues but remain free in the intestinal lumen, where they copulate. Gravid female parasites migrate at night to the anus, where they deposit eggs.

Most persons who harbor this parasite are asymptomatic; clinical "disease" is restricted to patients with perianal and perineal pruritus. The development of these symptoms in an individual or in one member of a household or an institution raises the possibility of enterobiasis and requires investigation. Eggs are rarely found in the conventional stool examination; the optimal method for detecting them is to apply a transparent tape swab to the perianal region in the morning, before the patient has bathed or defecated. The tape is then removed and spread on a microscope slide for examination. Repeated examinations on consecutive days may be necessary because of the irregular migrations of the female worms. Infection with pinworms does not elicit a significant blood eosinophilia.

Enterobiasis infection is generally innocuous, and therapy is initiated to eliminate perianal discomfort, insomnia, and mental anguish. All members of a household should be treated simultaneously. Current therapy for pinworm infection is with mebendazole, an oral agent. A single 100-mg tablet, for adults or children, has produced cure rates of more than 90 percent. The drug should not be administered to pregnant women. Pyrvinium pamoate is an effective and safe alternative for nonpregnant women. The latter compound is prescribed as a single oral dose of 5 mg of pyrvinium base per kilogram; a second dose is given in 2 weeks.

Schistosomiasis

Schistosomiasis is a chronic systemic infection caused by trematodes (blood flukes) of three species *(Schistosoma mansoni, S. japonicum, S. haematobium)*, each of which has a distinctive geographic distribution. Man is the exclusive host in the Western Hemisphere. The disease is not transmitted in the United States; *S. mansoni* does, however, constitute a major health problem in this country because of the extensive immigration of persons from areas of the world that are endemic for this schistosome (Puerto Rico, the West Indies).

The life cycle of *S. mansoni* is complex. The eggs, which have been extruded into the feces from mesenteric venules, hatch into miracidia which, in turn, invade specific species of fresh water snails. Within the snail, miracidia develop into cercariae, which subsequently break out and exist as free living organisms. Cercariae eventually penetrate human skin and are transported by the blood through the lungs and into the systemic circulation. The cercariae migrate to the intrahepatic portion of the portal system, where they mature. The adult worms travel to the inferior mesenteric venules to initiate production of eggs. These eggs may remain in the submucosal vessels of the descending colon and rectum, disseminate to the liver, spleen, lungs, and other organs, or reach the intestinal lumen, to be discharged with the feces.

The adult worms do not multiply in the human, but the deposition of eggs continues for the life of the female fluke (which averages 5 to 10 years). The eggs and their secretions (and possibly toxins from the adult worms) are capable of producing endophlebitis of the liver with portal hypertension and esophageal varices.

The severity of the disease is determined by a number of factors: intensity of infection, frequency of infection, and the degree of inflammatory reaction generated by the host. Clinical disease is usually restricted to patients with a heavy infestation, who are only a minority of those infected. Clinical presentations indicative of *S. mansoni* infection in the United States include any or all of the following: unexplained eosinophilia, hepatomegaly or splenomegaly, and hematemesis secondary to ruptured esophageal varices, occurring in patients who have emigrated from or traveled to endemic areas. The disorder simulates blockage of the portal vein (see Chap. 41, Diseases of the Liver).

The definitive diagnosis of schistosomiasis requires the demonstration of the schistosome eggs. Direct examination of a small stool sample is unreliable; concentration techniques are preferable. It is important to quantitate the eggs, both to give an estimate of the severity of the infection and to provide an objective assessment of the therapeutic response. Biopsies of the rectum often demonstrate eggs when examination of the feces has failed to do so. On occasion, the diagnosis is made when a liver biopsy unexpectedly reveals granulomatous reaction and schistosome eggs in a patient being evaluated for hepatomegaly.

The aim of drug therapy is to eliminate the parasites. The inability of patients to be reinfected in the United States and the potential of the treatments to produce severe untoward reactions preclude drug administration to asymptomatic patients with mild infections. Available drugs include niridazole and antimony sodium dimercaptosuccinate; these compounds may be obtained from the Parasitic Disease Drug Service of the Center for Disease Control in Atlanta, Georgia.

Niridazole is administered orally, 25 mg per kilogram for 7 days, but it is contraindicated for patients who have impaired liver function, mental illness, or epilepsy. Patients should be forewarned that their urine will be darker and will have an unpleasant odor. If gastrointestinal intolerance occurs with niridazole, antimony sodium dimercaptosuccinate should be substituted. The latter is injected intramuscularly, 8 mg per kilogram once a week for 5 weeks; it is contraindicated in patients with hepatic, renal, or cardiac insufficiency. Therapeutic efficacy is measured in terms of alleviation of symptoms, reduction of peripheral blood eosinophilia, and disappearance of eggs from the stool.

Trichinosis

Trichinosis is a subacute parasitic disease caused by the nematode *Trichinella spiralis.* It has been estimated that 200,000 Americans harbor this parasite. Trichinosis derives its importance from the fact that either a strategic location or a heavy concentration of organisms may result in a wide range of clinical abnormalities that can resemble other diseases and may even cause death.

Ingested larvae (from pork, beef adulterated by pork, or bear meat) invade the small intestine and develop into adult worms. The adult female releases larvae that are transported through the circulation and disseminated throughout the body. The larvae are capable of encysting only in striated muscle, but they may initiate inflammation in the brain or the myocardium.

Only a small proportion of infected persons have sufficient numbers of parasites to produce clinical disease. Initial symptoms, which occur during the first week after infection, suggest gastroenteritis. From 10 to 21 days after infection, the later clinical manifestations attributable to larval invasion of muscle occur, consisting of fever, periorbital edema, subconjunctival hemorrhage, muscle pain, and headache. Trichinosis is the sole helminthic infection in which a persistent fever may occur. Fatalities result from myocarditis or encephalitis.

Eosinophilia appears on approximately the tenth day of infection in about 90 percent of symptomatic patients. The intradermal test is of limited diagnostic value because it does not differentiate present from past infection. The bentonite flocculation test for antibody will be positive in approximately 90 percent of patients; its major disadvantages are that antibody is not detectable within 2 weeks of infection, and that false-positive reactions may occur in disorders that simulate trichinosis (polyarteritis nodosa, infectious mononucleosis). Biopsy of a tender, swollen muscle performed weeks after the onset of the disease frequently confirms the diagnosis.

Thiabendazole, 25 mg per kilogram administered orally twice daily until symptoms subside, has been recommended as specific therapy, but many experts are skeptical about the ability of this drug to reduce either the symptoms or the number of larvae in muscles. Critically ill patients have been treated with a corticosteroid in order to suppress inflammation, but the efficacy of this form of treatment has not been proved.

Giardiasis

With the recent thaw in the cold war and the larger number of American tourists visiting the Soviet Union, there has been an increased interest in giardiasis, a protozoan infection of the small bowel. This disease occurs worldwide, however. There are both endemic foci and occasional epidemics in the United States.

Infection is initiated by the ingestion of water, vegetables, or fruit contaminated with cysts of *Giardia lamblia*. The organisms excyst in the upper gastrointestinal tract, divide into trophozoites, and mature in the duodenum and upper jejunum. In some patients there is mucosal invasion by the parasite. The time between infection and onset of acute symptoms is 15 days.

Giardiasis has been associated both with achlorhydria and with dysgammaglobulinemia, but the vast majority of patients who develop the disease have no such known defects in host defenses. Infected persons can be asymptomatic, or they may experience either acute enteritis or chronic diarrhea, which can be accompanied by malabsorption. The stools of symptomatic patients are foul smelling but lack blood and pus. Eosinophilia does not occur.

The diagnosis of giardiasis is most readily established by the demonstration of cysts in stools that have been prepared by a concentration technique.

If parasites are not found in a number of stool examinations, an analysis should then be made of duodenal contents, obtained by intubation, Enterotest (a nylon line enclosed in a gelatin capsule), or small intestinal biopsy.

All infected patients require therapy. There are two highly effective oral drug treatments: quinacrine hydrochloride, 100 mg three times per day for a week, and metronidazole, 750 mg three times per day for a week. Quinacrine is contraindicated for patients with a history of psychosis or psoriasis, and for pregnant women. Metronidazole is contraindicated in patients with either an active disease of the central nervous system or a blood dyscrasia; it is currently being investigated as a possible carcinogen.

Malaria

Malaria, a protozoan infection caused by four species of *Plasmodium (P. vivax, P. falciparum, P. ovale, P. malariae)*, is one of the most important parasitic diseases in the world. With the reduction in the number of American troops stationed in Southeast Asia, most cases of malaria in the United States exist in persons who have traveled to endemic areas, particularly Africa. A small number of cases are acquired from infected transfused blood or from the use of contaminated needles by drug addicts.

LIFE CYCLE OF *PLASMODIUM*

The life cycle of *Plasmodium* is highly complex, with an asexual cycle in man and a sexual cycle in the female anopheline mosquito. Man is infected by mosquitoes that have fed on malarious blood about 2 to 4 weeks previously. The biting mosquito injects saliva containing sporozoites which, after a brief period in the circulation, enter the liver, multiply, and become schizonts. Approximately one week later, merozoites are released from the liver to enter circulating red blood cells. In *P. falciparum* malaria the tissue phase ends at the beginning of this erythrocyte phase, but in the other species hepatic forms persist; this explains the propensity of *P. vivax* and *P. ovale* malarias to relapse. The organisms mature in the red blood cells, multiply, and undergo transformation from early trophozoites to schizonts. The erythrocyte cycle is completed as the red blood cells rupture, releasing merozoites, which may either invade additional red blood cells or develop into male and female gametocytes. The discharge of merozoites initiates an episode of shaking chills and fever, and the duration of the erythrocytic cycle is species-specific, resulting in either tertian (*P. vivax* and *P. ovale* paroxysms every second day) or quartan (*P. malariae* paroxysms every third day) episodes. When a mosquito takes a blood meal from an infected person, gametocytes are ingested, undergo a sexual cycle, and become infective sporozoites. Malaria incurred by the parenteral route is not associated with a hepatic phase and thus is not subject to relapse.

Malaria generates a vigorous immune response about one week after parasites are first detected in the blood, and there is a depression of the level of serum complement. Antigen-antibody complexes have been implicated in the nephrotic syndrome caused by *P. malariae.* Virtually all imported cases of *P. falciparum* malaria in the United States develop within 6 months after arrival in this country, whereas only about 25 percent of patients infected with the other three species become ill during this period of time.

SYMPTOMS

The presenting symptoms of malaria, consisting of chills, fever, headache, nausea, vomiting, and diarrhea, often result in an incorrect diagnosis of influenza. Hepatomegaly and splenomegaly occur in about half the patients, more commonly with *P. vivax* than with *P. falciparum.* Anemia may be present; the white blood cell count is usually normal. There is no eosinophilia in protozoan diseases, but thrombocytopenia is frequent. Acute *P. falciparum* malaria has been complicated by renal failure, pulmonary edema, and cerebral hemorrhage. These life-threatening situations are usually associated with high density parasitemia, massive hemolysis, and severe anemia.

DIAGNOSIS

The key to the diagnosis of malaria is to consider it. All patients in whom malaria is suspected should be questioned about their geographic movements and their use of illicit drugs. The diagnosis is confirmed by careful examination of repeated thin and thick

blood smears prepared from drops of fresh blood obtained at different times of the day, particularly after a chill. The smears are stained with Giemsa's stain after the thin smear has been fixed in methyl alcohol. Wright's stain can be substituted, in which case the thin smear is not fixed in methyl alcohol, while the thick smear is dehemoglobinized by immersion in distilled water. It is absolutely vital to identify the exact species of *Plasmodium,* because *P. falciparum,* which requires specific medication, can cause rapid clinical deterioration and death. In fact, *P. falciparum* accounts for all malarial deaths in this country. When the presumptive diagnosis of malaria is not established by blood smears, sera should be mailed to the Parasitic Branch of the Center for Disease Control for antibody determination. Titers of indirect fluorescent antibody greater than 1:16 indicate a recent infection.

TREATMENT

For patients with infections caused by *P. vivax, P. ovale,* or *P. malariae,* chloroquine phosphate should be administered orally as an initial dose of 1 gm followed by 500 mg at 6, 24, and 48 hours to eliminate the erythrocytic stage. Patients with *P. vivax* or *P. ovale* infections that were not acquired through transfusion or contaminated needles require primaquine phosphate in a dose of 26.3 mg daily for 2 weeks to eradicate parasites in the liver. Patients with glucose 6-phosphate dehydrogenase deficiency may experience hemolysis during primaquine therapy.

Chloroquine-sensitive *P. falciparum* malaria infections are treated with chloroquine phosphate in the same dosage as for the other malaria infections. When oral medication cannot be tolerated, parenteral chloroquine hydrochloride (available from the Communicable Disease Center) should be infused, 250 mg every 6 hours. Chloroquine-resistant *P. falciparum* infection is treated with a combination of oral agents: quinine sulfate, 650 mg three times daily for 2 weeks; pyrimethamine, 25 mg twice daily for 3 days; and sulfadiazine, 500 mg four times daily for 5 days. Seriously ill patients who require parenteral treatment should receive intravenous quinine hydrochloride, 600 mg every 8 hours (650 mg every 24 hours by constant infusion if renal failure exists) to eradicate parasitemia. Some experts recommend intravenous dexamethasone, 4 to 6 mg every 4 hours, for adjunctive therapy of cerebral malaria. Renal failure from *P. falciparum* malaria requires careful regulation of fluid and electrolyte balance and control of uremia (dialysis) (see Chap. 53). Surveillance of patients with *P. falciparum* malaria should be continued for 3 months to detect any recurrent symptoms or a parasitemia requiring retreatment.

PREVENTIVE MEASURES
An American traveling to an area of the world where malaria is endemic must be advised to receive chemoprophylaxis. If the person is to reside in a country where chloroquine-sensitive malaria is prevalent, chemoprophylaxis consists of 500 mg of chloroquine weekly (initiated 1 week before departure and continued for 6 weeks after return). Primaquine phosphate, 26.3 mg daily for 2 weeks, is administered in addition when the person leaves the malarious area. A traveler who plans to enter a country where chloroquine-resistant malaria exists (Southeast Asia and parts of South America) should be informed that chloroquine may not be effective against it. The combination therapy of pyrimethamine with sulfadoxine provides complete protection, but this medication is not available in the United States, and sulfadoxine occasionally has produced an agranulocytosis with a 50 percent mortality rate. Additional measures to reduce the risk of malaria include avoiding rural areas at dusk and after dark, and using mosquito repellents, netting, and protective clothing.

Hookworm
Hookworm disease consists in infection of the small intestine by the nematodes *Ancylostoma duodenale* or *Necator americanus.* This parasitic disorder is endemic in some rural Southern states, where it predominates in young white males. Infection is initiated when filariform larvae in the soil are ingested or are permitted to penetrate the skin (by walking barefoot or handling contaminated soil). The larvae, which are transported to the lungs through the vascular system, migrate up the trachea and are swallowed. The larvae mature in the small intestine, where the adult worms will suck blood for years. Hookworms do not multiply in humans. The life cycle is completed when eggs, deposited in the soil by human defecation, hatch into larvae.

Most persons who harbor this parasite have low levels of infestation and are asymptomatic. Hookworm "disease" is manifest when gastrointestinal blood loss caused by the worms exceeds the body's capacity to absorb adequate dietary iron and to sustain optimal erythropoiesis. Patients with chronic hookworm disease develop nonspecific symptoms (weakness, palpitations, headache, dyspnea on exertion), signs (pallor, tachycardia, pale mucous membranes, cardiac murmurs), and laboratory findings (microcytic, hypochromic red blood cells, low hematocrit, low serum iron, elevated iron-binding capacity) that are the hallmarks of prolonged blood loss.

The diagnosis of hookworm infestation is established by the identification of eggs in a direct smear of the patient's feces. Quantitative techniques are utilized to assess the magnitude of the worm burden, since there is a direct relation between the number of parasites in the intestinal tract and the development of anemia. A study performed in Venezuela has demonstrated that anemia is related to fecal egg density (more than 2,000 per milliliter of feces for children and women, more than 5,000 per milliliter of feces for men).

Treatment is restricted to patients with chronic blood loss anemia from heavy infestations; it consists of oral mebendazole (100 mg twice daily for 3 days) and ferrous sulfate (300 mg three times daily). The cure rate exceeds 95 percent, and the egg count decreases significantly in all patients. Infected pregnant females should be treated after delivery, because mebendazole has not been determined to be safe during pregnancy.

Ascariasis
Ascariasis is an intestinal infestation caused by the large roundworm, *Ascaris lumbricoides,* and is the most common helminthic disease of man. It has been estimated that one of every four people in the world harbors this parasite. In the United States ascariasis is endemic in the southeastern parts of the Appalachian range, and in the Southern and Gulf coast states. Man is the only host.

People become infested by ingesting dirt containing the infective eggs. Sources of the contamination include soiled hands and uncooked vegetables that have been fertilized with human excreta. Larvae hatch in the small intestine and migrate through the portal system, lungs, and respiratory passages; they subsequently return to the intestines and develop into adult worms. The adults bridge across the lumen of the jejunum and ileum, where they live from 1 to 2 years, copulate, and discharge eggs into the feces.

During the lung phase of larval migration, respiratory symptoms (cough, wheezing, dyspnea, hemoptysis), signs of pulmonary consolidation, and eosinophilia may develop. Most persons infested with *Ascaris lumbricoides* have few worms and experience either no symptoms or only vague abdominal discomfort. Masses of adult worms, however, may obstruct or perforate the intestine or may migrate into the biliary tract, resulting in suppurative cholangitis or liver abscesses. The eggs, which on occasion are deposited in the liver, gallbladder, or peritoneum, are capable of inciting a granulomatous inflammation, causing cholecystitis or peritonitis.

The diagnosis is established by the detection of ova in direct smear of the feces. Adult worms rarely are passed spontaneously into the feces, and occasionally in the vomitus. All patients should be treated.

The treatment of choice is oral piperazine citrate (3 to 4 gm daily for 2 days), which causes paralysis of the adult worms so that the parasites are no longer able to bridge across the intestinal lumen. Therapy results in transport of the worms into the fecal stream and their passage into the stool. Piperazine does not affect the larvae during their migration. Therapy is repeated if the stools remain positive for ova 2 weeks after treatment.

Strongyloides Hyperinfection Syndrome

Strongyloides stercoralis, a nematode endemic in Kentucky, southern Appalachia, and institutions for the mentally retarded, usually produces an asymptomatic or self-limited pulmonary or small intestinal infection. The parasite is imported to urban areas by immigrants from Puerto Rico and servicemen who were stationed in Southeast Asia. This organism frequently coexists with other enteric helminths (hookworm, *Trichuris trichiuria, Ascaris lumbricoides*). *Strongyloides stercoralis* has recently received considerable attention, however, because it is capable of inducing an overwhelming infection with a fatal outcome, particularly in immunosuppressed patients, and thus it has joined the ranks of the "opportunistic" infections (see Chap. 6).

Although most helminth parasites do not multiply in man, this roundworm undergoes an autoinfectious cycle in which rhabdoid larvae, which are usually passed in the feces, can develop into infective filariform larvae. In immunosuppressed patients who have defects in cell-mediated immunity that are attributable to an underlying disease (lymphoma, leukemia, leprosy) or to therapy, filariform larvae may penetrate the mucosa of the stomach, small intestines, and colon, producing phagedemic ulcers and resulting in an enteritis syndrome that may be associated with bacteremia, fungemia, and shock. There may be additional widespread dissemination of filariform larvae throughout the host. These unfortunate events may suddenly develop in a previously asymptomatic carrier.

The hyperinfection syndrome has to be considered in the differential diagnosis whenever an "enteritis syndrome" develops in an immunosuppressed patient with a past history of possible exposure to *Strongyloides.* The diagnosis must be established as rapidly as possible. Peripheral blood eosinophilia is exceptional in this syndrome, and definitive diagnosis requires demonstration of the larvae in the feces (preferably by a concentration technique), gastric aspirate, or sputum. When these examinations fail to reveal the parasite, duodenal contents should be analyzed.

Therapy consists in supportive measures necessary to maintain the circulation; proper antibiotic and antifungal therapy to meet the challenge of the concomitant bacteremia, fungemia, or both, and thiabendazole, 25 mg per kilogram, given orally twice daily for 2 days. In spite of these maneuvers, the fatality rate remains very high. Undoubtedly, the best therapy is to take preventive measures. Patients with a history of possible exposure to *Strongyloides* should be thoroughly evaluated prior to the onset of immunosuppressive treatment. If an infestation is discovered, it should be eradicated before corticosteroid or cytotoxic drugs are prescribed, and patients receiving these agents should be closely monitored to detect exacerbation of strongyloidiasis.

Bibliography

Brown, H. W. *Basic Clinical Parasitology.* New York: Appleton-Century-Crofts, 1975.

Butler, T., Warren, K. S., and Mahmoud, A. A. F. Algorithms in the diagnosis and management of exotic diseases: XIII. Malaria. *J. Infect. Dis.* 133:721, 1975

Grove, D. I., Warren, K. S., and Mahmoud, A. A. F. Algorithms in the diagnosis and management of exotic diseases: III. Strongyloidiasis. *J. Infect. Dis.* 131:755, 1975.

Grove, D. I., Warren, K. S., and Mahmoud, A. A. F. Algorithms in the diagnosis and management of exotic diseases: VII. Trichinosis. *J. Infect. Dis.* 132:485, 1975.

Lozoff, B., Warren, K. S., and Mahmoud, A. A. F. Algorithms in the diagnosis and management of exotic diseases: VIII. Hookworm. *J. Infect. Dis.* 132:606, 1975.

Mahmoud, A. A. F., and Warren, K. S. Algorithms in the diagnosis and management of exotic diseases: II. Giardiasis. *J. Infect. Dis.* 131:621, 1975.

Warren, K. S., and Mahmoud, A. A. F. Algorithms in the diagnosis and management of exotic diseases: I. Schistosomiasis. *J. Infect. Dis.* 131:614, 1975.

Warren, K. S., and Mahmoud, A. A. F. Algorithms in the diagnosis and management of exotic diseases: V. Enterobiasis. *J. Infect. Dis.* 132:229, 1975.

IV The Lungs and Related Structures

8

Infections of the Upper Respiratory Tract

Neil R. Blacklow, Nelson M. Gantz,
and William R. McCabe

The respiratory tract is the most frequent location of bacterial, fungal, viral, and mycoplasmal infections. Such infections usually involve only a portion of the tract but rarely may involve all of the contiguous system of the nares, oropharynx, trachea, bronchi, bronchioles, and lungs. The contiguity of the various parts of the respiratory tract often results in involvement of more than one site and makes the delineation of the exact anatomic location of infection difficult solely on clinical grounds. As a result there is considerable overlap in the clinical syndromes of respiratory infection that the physician should be able to recognize.

Infections of the Oral Cavity

CANKER SORES
(RECURRENT APHTHOUS STOMATITIS)

Canker sores are self-limited ulcerative oral lesions. They may be single or multiple, tend to recur, and are of uncertain etiology. Initially they appear as vesicles, and then they rapidly progress to ulcers of the mucosal surfaces, particularly in the mucogingival folds. Treatment is symptomatic.

INFECTIOUS AND MEMBRANOUS STOMATITIS

Bacterial infection of the oral mucosa is a rare but serious infection. It may be accompanied by diffuse mucosal inflammation or a false membrane similar to that seen in diphtheria. Group A streptococci are the most frequent cause, but staphylococci have also been implicated. Usually the oral mucosa is diffusely erythematous and so sensitive to irritation that the patient has difficulty with eating and drinking. In the membranous form a grayish white fibrinous exudate surrounded by diffuse erythema covers portions of the oral cavity. Fever, which may reach 102 to 103°F (38.9 to 39.4°C), and regional adenopathy often occur. Frequent rinsing of the mouth with hot water and administration of either penicillin or an antistaphylococcal penicillin parenterally usually result in prompt improvement.

CANDIDIASIS

Infection of the tongue and oropharynx with various species of *Candida,* usually *C. albicans,* occurs primarily in infants (thrush) or in adults with other underlying diseases. Patients with malignant disease or hematologic disorders, or those who have been treated with broad-spectrum antibiotics or corticosteroids, account for almost all cases of oral candidiasis in adults. The typical lesions appear as white patches resembling milk curds on the tongue and buccal mucosa. Removal of the exudate reveals hyperemic shallow ulcers. Occasionally these lesions may extend to involve the tonsils, larynx, esophagus, or respiratory tract; rarely bloodstream invasion and even fungal endocarditis may develop. Diagnostic procedures in candidiasis include staining the scrapings from lesions with either Gram's stain or 20% potassium hydroxide and culture on Sabouraud's agar or blood agar.

Treatment of candidiasis requires improvement of oral hygiene, discontinuation of antibiotics and corticosteroids when feasible, and topical application of 1% gentian violet twice daily. Nystatin or amphotericin B may be used for the treatment of local lesions but is effective only for superficial ones. Amphotericin B given intravenously, 0.5 to 1.0 mg/kg body weight/24 hours, is the only uniformly effective therapeutic agent for systemic infections, but the toxicity of this preparation limits its use to the more severe or systemic infections. A new agent, 5-fluorocytosine, is active against some strains of *Candida.* A search for predisposing causes should be made.

ULCEROMEMBRANOUS STOMATITIS (TRENCH MOUTH, VINCENT'S FUSOSPIROCHETAL DISEASE)

Ulceromembranous stomatitis is caused by synergistic infection with fusobacteria and spirochetes. It ranges in severity from a mild gingivitis with local swelling and bluish reddening to extensive, painful ulceration, marked swelling of the gums, and a gray, foul-smelling membranous exudate. A marked and often characteristic fetor is usually present. Nutritional and vitamin deficiencies, poor oral hygiene, hematologic disorders, and debility are predisposing factors. Diagnostic procedures include a Gram stain for fusiform gram-negative bacilli and spirochetes and anaerobic cultures for isolation of the fusobacterium.

Treatment of trench mouth requires improvement of oral hygiene, removal of calcareous deposits, and local irrigation with dilute sodium perborate or quaternary ammonium compounds. Antibiotic therapy with either procaine penicillin, 600,000 units per day, or tetracycline, 250 mg every 4 hours, is necessary in severe cases and should be continued until the lesions have regressed and the patient has been afebrile for 3 to 5 days.

LUDWIG'S ANGINA

Ludwig's angina disease usually results from entry of bacteria through a mucosal abrasion or through infected tonsils or teeth, and it consists of a submandibular cellulitis followed by a sublingual phlegmon. In the primary form, the lymph nodes are not involved and spread occurs through areolar tissue, while in the secondary form, infection spreads from lymph nodes and through muscular and areolar tissue. Firm, brawny edema of the submaxillary tissue and beneath the tongue produces elevation of the tongue and induration of the floor of the mouth, which is dusky red in appearance. The tongue may be displaced so far upward and anteriorly as to fill the mouth and pharynx. Local swelling, pain, and dysphagia are characteristic, and extensions into the larynx may lead to airway obstruction. Frank suppuration and abscess formation appear late. Fever is often marked, and leukocytosis is regularly observed.

The diagnosis is based on the clinical findings and on cultures of the pharynx or infected teeth. Most such infections are caused by group A hemolytic streptococci, but occasionally staphylococci are responsible. The prognosis is grave. Treatment includes (1) establishment of an airway — a tracheostomy is almost always required; (2) drainage of the space beneath the tongue by external incision — this is of paramount importance; prophylactic tracheostomy is suggested, since otherwise fatal laryngospasm may follow before such a procedure can be done; and (3) administration of penicillin, 600,000 units every 4 hours. Cultures of exudate obtained after drainage may implicate organisms other than streptococci and necessitate the use of other therapeutic agents. The dose of penicillin may be decreased after clinical improvement, but a minimum of 2 weeks of therapy should be given.

MUMPS

Mumps is an acute contagious disease caused by mumps virus, which has an affinity for glandular and central nervous system tissue. Although mumps is most commonly characterized by a nonsuppurative parotitis, other tissues are often involved. In the temperate zones the disease is most prevalent in winter and spring.

The virus is usually spread by direct or indirect contact with saliva or droplets from an infected individual. It probably enters through the nose or mouth, multiplies in the parotid gland or respiratory tract of susceptible persons, and, following a viremia, localizes at various sites. The period of communicability extends from 6 days before onset of parotitis to subsidence of the swelling. The virus has been demonstrated in the blood early in the disease, in the urine as late as 14 days after onset of illness, and in the spinal fluid during "aseptic" meningitis due to this agent. The incubation period ranges from 14 to 21 days.

Signs and Symptoms

Infection is not apparent in 30 to 40 percent of susceptible individuals; the remainder develop a 1- or 2-day prodrome of fever, headache, malaise, or vomiting or combinations of these symptoms. This prodrome is followed by illness of variable severity, the symptoms depending on what bodily sites are involved. The commonest manifestation is a nonsuppurative, painful parotitis that reaches its peak in about 2 days and then slowly subsides. In about 70 percent of cases the parotitis is bilateral, usually with an interval of several days between swellings. Fever generally subsides before the parotitis. The submaxillary and sublingual glands are often also enlarged and rarely may be the only salivary glands involved. The duct openings of the affected glands are frequently reddened and edematous.

Complications

Orchitis occurs in about 20 percent of postpubertal males, beginning 1 to 2 weeks after the salivary gland enlargement. Orchitis is generally preceded by recrudescence of fever and systemic signs, and it usually is unilateral. Although painful and occasionally associated with atrophy, it is rarely followed by sterility. Meningoencephalitis is also common in mumps. About 10 percent of cases show mild encephalitic or meningeal signs, usually within a week after onset of parotitis. In such cases the spinal fluid pressure may be increased with a lymphocytic pleocytosis, a normal glucose, and an elevated total protein. Recovery is usually uneventful; rarely, auditory nerve deafness, facial paralysis, or death results. Pancreatitis occurs in 5 percent of patients and is generally manifested by abdominal pain, subcostal tenderness, nausea, and vomiting. These symptoms usually clear within a week. A wide range of additional manifestations may occur, including thyroiditis, mastitis, oophoritis, prostatitis, lacrimal gland involvement, or, rarely, arthritis or myocarditis. These manifestations may occur either following or preceding the parotitis or even in its absence.

Prevention and Treatment
Normal gamma globulin is ineffective, and even mumps hyperimmune gamma globulin is not proved to be effective. A live attenuated vaccine appears to give long-lasting immunity. It is recommended for children more than 1 year of age and especially for those approaching puberty and for adolescents and adults (especially males) who have not had the disease. Given after exposure, the vaccine gives no protection to mumps contacts.

PURULENT PAROTITIS
A severe pyogenic infection of the parotid gland, purulent parotitis occurs almost exclusively in debilitated or postoperative patients who are dehydrated and who have received anticholinergic agents. The onset may be insidious or abrupt, with chills, fever, and leukocytosis; bacteremia may occur. There is unilateral parotid swelling, and massage of the affected gland leads to expression of pus from Stensen's duct. The usual etiologic agent is *Staphylococcus aureus,* which may be seen on a Gram stain of the pus and may be isolated on culture. Adequate hydration, discontinuation of anticholinergic agents, and vigorous parenteral therapy with penicillinase-resistant penicillins usually control the infection. Incision and drainage are rarely necessary and are indicated only when abscess formation occurs.

SINUSITIS
Acute or chronic infection and inflammation may involve one or more of the paranasal sinuses. Since the sinuses are mucosa-lined cavities that open into the nares or nasopharynx, obstruction of their openings secondary to upper respiratory infection may hamper their drainage and lead to secondary bacterial infection. Nasal polyps, allergic rhinitis, foreign bodies, nasal packing, and forceful nasal injection of water from diving may predispose the sinuses to infection. Occasionally sinusitis may result from a direct extension of infection from the teeth or from a dental extraction.

The patient usually presents with nasal obstruction, purulent drainage, pain over the affected sinus, chills, fever, leukocytosis, and a history of a preceding upper respiratory infection. Examination usually reveals pus in the middle meatus, tenderness over the affected sinuses, fluid levels on transillumination, and fluid levels or opacities on x-ray. Rarely direct extension or spread through venous drainage may lead to osteomyelitis, orbital cellulitis or abscess, cavernous sinus thrombosis, or brain abscess as complications of sinusitis.

Group A beta hemolytic streptococci, *Streptococcus (Diplococcus) pneumoniae, Haemophilus influenzae,* or *S. aureus* are the usual etiologic agents in acute sinusitis. Other bacteria, particularly anaerobes, become more important in chronic sinusitis. *Mucor,* a fungus, is an extremely rare cause of a sinusitis that occurs only in patients with diabetic ketoacidosis or other types of acidosis.

Treatment is directed at (1) promotion of drainage and (2) appropriate antimicrobial therapy. Moist heat over the sinus, humidification of the air, and use of 0.25% phenylephrine (Neo-Synephrine) nose drops promote drainage. Ampicillin or penicillin is the antibiotic of choice unless staphylococcal infection is suspected. Surgical drainage or antral irrigation is occasionally required.

OTITIS MEDIA
Inflammatory disease of the middle ear is frequent in children but is less common in adults. Three different types of otitis media — serous, suppurative, and chronic — may occur. Serous otitis media results from eustachian tube obstruction, which may be

caused by upper respiratory infection, enlarged adenoids, rapid changes in atmospheric pressure, or allergic rhinitis, followed by the absorption of air from the middle ear and its replacement with a serous transudate. The ear drum appears retracted and slightly erythematous, and a fluid level may be seen. Treatment includes symptomatic measures for the relief of pain and the use of nasal vasoconstrictor drops (0.25% phenylephrine). Myringotomy may be required if there is no response to conservative management.

Eustachian tube obstruction also plays a role in the pathogenesis of suppurative otitis media, but the situation is compounded by concomitant infection with pyogenic bacteria. Pneumococci, group A beta hemolytic streptococci, *H. influenzae* (in children), and coagulase-positive staphylococci are the usual etiologic agents. Typically the onset is acute, with fever, occasionally chills, severe pain in the ear, and leukocytosis. On examination the tympanic membrane is fiery red and bulging, with obliteration of the normal landmarks. Rupture of the tympanic membrane may occur, followed by relief of pain and the appearance of a pulsating serosanguineous or purulent discharge.

Treatment consists in promotion of eustachian tube drainage and appropriate antimicrobial therapy. Penicillin is the agent of choice in adults, and ampicillin is used in children except when penicillin-resistant staphylococci are suspected. Myringotomy is indicated if the response to antimicrobial therapy is not prompt.

Chronic otitis media may follow either acute otitis or secondary bacterial infection after tympanic membrane perforation. Granulation tissue forms in response to chronic infection of the tympanic ring and is overgrown by epithelium from the auditory canal. This tissue may extend into the middle ear (cholesteatoma) and serve as a constant nidus of infection. The bacterial flora consist of anaerobic bacteria and aerobic gram-negative bacilli. Hearing loss, chronic malodorous discharge, and recurrent episodes of acute infection are the major manifestations. Management is usually best carried out by specialists in otolaryngology.

Pharyngitis and Other Streptococcal Infections

Pharyngitis is characterized by sore throat that is usually accompanied by infection of the pharynx and red, swollen tonsils. Fever, constitutional symptoms of variable degree, tonsillar exudate, cervical lymphadenopathy, and cough are common. Most cases are caused by viruses (see below), but those caused by bacteria are of greater importance because of their greater severity and the hazards of suppurative and nonsuppurative sequelae. The most important bacterial cause is group A beta hemolytic streptococci, while *Corynebacterium diphtheriae*, *H. influenzae* (in children), and *Neisseria gonorrhoeae* are less frequent causes. Other pathogenic bacteria such as *S. aureus* and *S. (Diplococcus) pneumoniae* may be isolated from the pharynx but do not produce pharyngitis. Since it is not possible to distinguish a viral pharyngitis from one caused by bacteria, a throat culture is essential for etiologic diagnosis.

STREPTOCOCCAL PHARYNGITIS, SCARLET FEVER, AND OTHER STREPTOCOCCAL INFECTIONS

The spectrum of diseases produced by group A streptococci is extensive (Table 8-1). In addition to pharyngitis, skin infections, and infections of the female genital tract, metastatic infections such as purulent arthritis, osteomyelitis, bacteremia, and meningitis can occur. Streptococci are also important in the pathogenesis of acute rheumatic fever and acute glomerulonephritis.

The clinical type of upper respiratory tract illness resulting from a streptococcal infection varies with the age and the immune state of the infected patient. Streptococcal infections in children under 3 years of age are characterized by a mucopurulent nasal discharge with crusting and excoriation around the nares, regional lymphadenopathy, and "streptococcal fever." This syndrome is difficult to distinguish from the common cold, and there is minimal pharyngeal involvement. Children over 3 but less than 10 years of age frequently have pharyngitis with an erythematous skin rash (scarlet fever). Older children and adults with streptococcal pharyngitis usually lack skin manifestations. In addition, as high as 40 percent (10 to 40 percent) of school children may be asymptomatic carriers of beta-hemolytic group A streptococci.

Table 8-1. Streptococcal Infections

Primary sites or complications	Type of disease	Age group primarily affected (yr.)
Upper respiratory system	Streptococcal fever	Under 3
	Scarlet fever (pharyngitis with erythematous skin eruption)	3–10
	Pharyngitis	Under 10
	Asymptomatic carriers	All ages
Skin	Impetigo	All ages
	Cellulitis	All ages
	Pyoderma	Chiefly under 5 and over 40
	Erysipelas	All ages
Genitals	Puerperal sepsis	15–40
	Vaginitis	Under 10
Respiratory	Sinusitis, otitis, cervical adenitis	All ages
Others	Bacteremia, meningitis, pneumonia, purulent arthritis, osteomyelitis, peritonitis, lymphadenitis, wound infections	All ages
Immunologic	Rheumatic fever	All ages
	Glomerulonephritis	Primarily under 25

Microbiology of Streptococci

Streptococci are gram-positive cocci that grow in chains of varying length. Their hemolytic properties on culture with sheep blood agar are useful for their classification. Some organisms produce beta hemolysis, defined as a clear zone of complete lysis of the erythrocytes in the blood agar surrounding the bacterial colony. Others produce hemolysis with only a greening reaction of the blood agar surrounding the colony, called alpha hemolysis. The alpha reaction is characteristic of but not limited to viridans streptococci, which are important causes of subacute bacterial endocarditis but never of respiratory infection. The enzymes produced by the streptococci causing hemolytic reactions include the oxygen-labile streptolysin O and the oxygen-stable streptolysin S. If an organism produces only the oxygen-labile streptolysin O, then subsurface streaking of the blood agar plate is required to demonstrate hemolysis.

Streptococcal cell walls contain three antigens (C, M, and T) that determine their serologic specificity. The C (carbohydrate) substance is used to separate streptococci into serologic groups, of which eighteen have been recognized and designated A through H and K through T. The major human pathogens fit into either group A, group B, or group D. Viridans streptococci are usually nongroupable. Group A streptococci are usually beta hemolytic, and their susceptibility to low concentrations of bacitracin (0.02 unit disk) permits their rapid classification into this group. Group B streptococci are also usually beta hemolytic, but the majority of strains are bacitracin resistant. Neonatal sepsis with meningitis, gynecologic infections, and endocarditis may be caused by group B streptococci. Group D streptococci show either a gamma or an alpha reaction on blood agar and include enterococci; the enterococci may cause urinary tract infections or endocarditis. Rarely group C streptococci may cause respiratory disease, but rheumatic fever and acute glomerulonephritis have been recognized only after group A streptococcal infections.

The M and T antigens are proteins in the group A streptococcal cell wall. M protein is associated with resistance to phagocytosis and hence virulence. Type-specific antibodies usually develop after infection, preventing subsequent attacks by strains of the same M type. There are at least 60 different M types, and prior infection with one type provides no protection against another. Some strains may be M-protein deficient and cannot be typed using the M antigen; the T antigen is useful for subtyping these strains.

A variety of exotoxins and enzymes are produced by streptococci, including streptokinase, streptococcal deoxyribonuclease (streptodornase), hyaluronidase, streptolysin O, streptolysin S, and erythrogenic toxin. Most of these substances are effective antigens, and the antibody responses — in particular antistreptolysin O (ASO titer), antihyaluronidase (AH titer), and antideoxyribonuclease (anti-DNase titer) — are used as serologic evidence of a preceding streptococcal infection. A rise in serum antistreptolysin O (ASO titer) occurs within 2 to 3 weeks following an acute group A streptococcal infection and is considered significant when either a level of more than 250 todd units is found in one sample, or more than a twofold increase occurs between acute and convalescent samples. The majority (85 percent) of patients with acute rheumatic fever will show a significant elevation of the ASO titer. The ASO response is not a satisfactory test in patients with streptococcal skin infections; the anti-DNase, the antihyaluronidase, or the streptozyme tests are more reliable. Antibody formed against the erythrogenic toxin as a result of previous streptococcal infection and the capacity of the infecting strain to produce erythrogenic toxin determine whether a given streptococcal infection will result in an associated skin rash (scarlet fever). Antibodies against erythrogenic toxin protect only against the effects of the toxin and against recurrences of clinical scarlet fever; they do not prevent another streptococcal pharyngeal infection.

Clinical Features

Streptococcal respiratory infections are acquired by contact with the droplets expelled from the throat and nose of infected patients or asymptomatic carriers. Food-borne or milk-borne epidemics have occurred, and one anal carrier has been recognized. If the host does not have antibodies against the infecting serotype, he will contract the infection after an incubation period of 2 to 5 days. The onset of streptococcal sore throat is usually sudden, with frank chills or chilly sensations, headache, malaise, and pharyngeal symptoms that may vary from only slight "scratchiness" to severe pharyngeal pain making swallowing very difficult. Although lesser degrees of fever may occur, temperatures of 102 to 104°F (38.9 to 40°C) are common. Nausea and vomiting may be present. The pharynx is red and swollen; grayish white patches of exudate that can be easily removed without leaving a bleeding surface may appear on the tonsils and posterior pharynx. Tender, enlarged anterior cervical lymph nodes are common. The clinical picture of fever, exudative pharyngitis, and cervical lymphadenopathy is most often observed in streptococcal pharyngitis, but it also may be seen in viral pharyngitis.

Scarlet fever occurs most often in children between 2 and 10 years of age. Although the streptococcal focus of most patients with scarlet fever is in the pharynx, scarlet fever may also occur with streptococcal pharyngitis except that vomiting and general toxicity are somewhat more frequent. The rash is a diffuse erythema that blanches on pressure combined with numerous punctate and papular elevations that give the skin a sandpaper texture; it begins within 2 days after the onset of sore throat. It usually starts on the upper part of the trunk and extends upward onto the neck and down to the extremities. The palms, soles, and area around the mouth (circumoral pallor) are not involved. The rash is a deeper red in color in the inguinal, axillary, and antecubital skinfold areas (Pastia's lines). Small hemorrhagic spots may be noted on the soft palate, and the tongue is coated with a thick, cream-colored fur; whereas the papillae are swollen and bright red (strawberry tongue). The rash begins to fade after the fifth day with peeling of the skin. The white blood cell count is usually in excess of 15,000 cells per cubic millimeter, with a left shift.

Diagnosis

Clinical criteria are inadequate to differentiate streptococcal from nonstreptococcal pharyngitis; a throat culture is essential for diagnostic certainty. The immune response to streptolysin O and other streptococcal exotoxins is useful in diagnosing rheumatic fever. Since about 25 percent of family contacts of patients are infected, family members should be cultured and treated if possible. Usually treatment can be withheld safely until positive bacteriologic identification has been made without appreciably increasing the risk of either acute rheumatic fever or acute glomerulonephritis. Antibiotics are given to prevent the suppurative and nonsuppurative complications and to decrease further spread of the infection. The suppurative complications, less common today than during the preantibiotic era, include peritonsillar or retropharyngeal space abscesses, otitis media, mastoiditis, sinusitis, and cervical lymphadenitis. Other possible complications are meningitis, endocarditis, pneumonia, purulent arthritis, and osteomyelitis. Nonsuppurative complications have also decreased since the widespread use of antibiotics, but cases still occur because of failures to recognize mild streptococcal infections or to treat them adequately.

Treatment

Penicillin is the antimicrobial agent of choice for streptococcal pharyngitis and it is administered in adults as a single intramuscular injection of long-acting benzathine penicillin, 1.2 million units; it can be given orally as phenoxymethyl penicillin, 250 mg (400,000 units) four times per day for 10 days, or as intramuscular procaine penicillin, 600,000 units daily for 10 days. Since clinical recovery occurs in about 5 days with or without antibiotics, it is important to emphasize patient compliance, because a full 10 days of therapy is necessary to eliminate streptococci and prevent sequelae. In patients with penicillin allergy, erythromycin, 250 mg four times per day for 10 days, is adequate. Tetracycline is contraindicated because of the high incidence of resistant streptococci. Careful cardiac auscultation and follow-up urinalysis should be done to ensure that rheumatic fever and glomerulonephritis have not occurred.

PHARYNGITIS AND ACUTE EPIGLOTTIDITIS
DUE TO HAEMOPHILUS INFLUENZAE

Pharyngitis and other respiratory infections in young children are often caused by *H. influenzae,* but this organism rarely causes infections in adults. Clinically an *H. influenzae* pharyngitis cannot be distinguished from streptococcal pharyngitis except that the former is often associated with acute epiglottiditis. The onset is sudden, with high fever and sore throat, but with epiglottic involvement there is often severe inspiratory dyspnea, prostration, and occasionally death. Examination reveals erythema of the pharynx and epiglottis; the latter is often so edematous as to be visible when the tongue is depressed. The vocal cords are not usually involved, but when they are, hoarseness and a barking cough are also present. Epiglottiditis is observed almost exclusively in young children. Gram stains and cultures of the pharynx and epiglottis should be taken and immediate treatment instituted with tetracycline, ampicillin, or chloramphenicol. In patients with severe respiratory obstruction, intubation or tracheostomy may be necessary.

GONOCOCCAL PHARYNGITIS

Gonococcal pharyngeal infection may result from fellatio. Most patients are asymptomatic, but some show symptoms and signs indistinguishable clinically from those of pharyngitis due to other bacteria or to viruses. Throat swabs inoculated onto Thayer-Martin medium are used for isolation of *N. gonorrhoeae.* Gonococcal pharyngitis may be the source of a gonococcal bacteremia, and patients suspected of having disseminated gonococcal infection should have pharyngeal cultures. Treatment with procaine penicillin G or oral tetracycline is usually effective; but treatment failure may occur, and follow-up cultures should be obtained.

DIPHTHERIA

Diphtheria is an acute, contagious infection caused by *Corynebacterium diphtheriae* and characterized by the formation of a fibrinous pseudomembrane involving the respiratory mucous membranes. Contact with early cases and carriers is the principal mode of spread, but both food-borne and milk-borne epidemics have occurred. Diphtheria was once common, but it is observed infrequently in the United States at the present time. With the decreasing incidence of diphtheria, immunity in the general population has decreased; therefore, because of the threat of its dissemination in the nonimmune population, recognition of diphtheria is even more urgent today. It is also important to remember that diphtheria is a completely preventable disease and that physicians should strive to maintain active immunization of their patients with diphtheria toxoid.

Etiology

The causative organism, *C. diphtheriae,* is a pleomorphic, rod-shaped, gram-positive bacillus that appears in slightly curved, clubbed, or branched forms; it tends to stain irregularly and may have granules within its cytoplasm. Löffler's serum medium and potassium tellurite agar are used for its isolation and identification. Three types of strains — gravis, intermedius, and mitis — have been described and have been considered to reflect decreasing virulence in the order listed. Correlation between clinical virulence and the type of strain has not been good, however, especially in the United States.

Clinical Features

Corynebacterium diphtheriae produces a powerful exotoxin that causes the clinical manifestations of the disease both locally and in distant organs. After local invasion, usually in the posterior pharynx, the organism proliferates and produces its toxin. Necrosis of the epithelial cells of the pharynx results from the local effects of the toxin, and a fibrinous exudate then appears. If sufficient antitoxin is present from prior immunization or exposure to diphtheria, the toxin is neutralized and local or systemic manifestations do not occur. In the absence of antitoxin, necrosis continues, polymorphonuclear leukocytes infiltrate into the fibrinous exudate, and additional bacterial multiplication and toxin formation proceed unabated with further exudation or pseudomembrane formation. In the early stage of infection the diphtheritic membrane appears as a patch of soft exudate that can be easily removed. Subsequently a tenacious, sheetlike membrane forms over the tonsils and pharyngeal wall; it peels with difficulty, leaving visible bleeding points. Minimal inflammatory reaction is seen adjacent to the membrane. Relatively few constitutional symptoms occur early in the course, and even the pharyngeal discomfort is often so mild as to be described as only a sense of irritation. Originally the membrane is white, but subsequently it turns gray or black in color.

Nasal involvement may occur either as a primary lesion or secondary to the spread of pharyngeal disease. It is often unilateral and marked by a serosanguineous nasal discharge. Membrane formation may occur on the nasal mucosa. Involvement may also extend to the larynx, trachea, or bronchi and produce fatal respiratory obstruction. Cough, hoarseness, and aphonia are usually observed with laryngeal involvement. In some instances extensive involvement of the pharynx, tonsils, and soft and hard palate may occur, producing the so-called bullneck diphtheria. This form of diphtheria is characterized by marked swelling of the anterior aspect of the neck and submandibular area. Bullneck diphtheria is frequently associated with a concomitant beta-hemolytic streptococcal infection.

Complications

Toxic myocarditis may occur as early as 3 days or as late as 10 weeks after onset of diphtheria. Electrocardiographic evidence of conducting defects indicating myocardial involvement is reported in as many as two-thirds of the patients. In general, the severity of the myocarditis tends to parallel the rapidity with which it appears. The cardiac changes result from the direct effect of the toxin on the myocardium, but on occasion cardiac failure may also be secondary to respiratory obstruction. Clinically the evidences of carditis consist of persistent tachycardia, thready pulse, and indistinct, soft heart sounds. Accentuation of the first sound secondary to prolonged atrioventricular conduction, and fixed splitting of the second pulmonic sound with right bundle branch block may be other clinical indications of myocarditis. A diastolic gallop and various arrhythmias may also occur. Besides conduction defects and arrhythmias, electrocardiographic changes include abnormal T waves and alterations in the ST segment. Mortality in diphtheritic myocarditis tends to vary directly with the intensity of electrocardiographic abnormalities.

Peripheral neuritis may appear at various times during the course of diphtheria. Paralysis of the pharyngeal and palatal muscles tends to occur early and other neural involvement usually later (during the second to sixth week). Cranial nerves, especially those supplying the external ocular muscles, are the most frequently affected, but peripheral neuropathy occurs also. The less severe neural lesions tend to regress early, but more serious involvement recedes more slowly and occasionally may be permanent.

Although quite rare, cutaneous ulcerative diphtheritic infections also occur; these are often incorrectly diagnosed and may be followed by the same complications as respiratory diphtheria. Similarly, involvement of the nasal mucous membrane, the larynx, or rarely the trachea may be observed without pharyngeal involvement.

Diagnosis

All instances of pharyngitis associated with a membrane should be suspected as diphtheritic in origin and proper bacteriologic studies undertaken. With diphtheria, smears reveal the typical organisms arranged in a palisadelike fashion. Similar-appearing nonpathogenic diphtheroids, difficult to distinguish from *C. diphtheriae,* may also be observed in pharyngeal smears; therefore, cultural confirmation should always be obtained. All cases should be reported to local health authorities. Cultures should immediately be inoculated on Löffler serum slants, a tellurite agar plate, and a blood agar plate. Growth may occur within 12 hours. In addition, tests for toxigenicity using intracutaneous injection of the organism into guinea pigs and an agar diffusion precipitation test for toxin production should be made.

Treatment

The primary goals of therapy in diphtheria are neutralization of toxin and maintenance of an adequate airway. Only free toxin can be neutralized by antitoxin; toxin already fixed in the tissues is no longer susceptible to neutralization. Therefore therapy should be instituted as soon as possible. In general, the amount of antitoxin administered should parallel the degree of involvement, as outlined in Table 8-2.

The available antitoxin preparations are produced in horses, and it is essential that antitoxin not be given until tests for host sensitivity to horse serum have been done. One-tenth milliliter of a 1:100 dilution of the antitoxin is injected intradermally in the arm. In the absence of any reaction within 30

Table 8-2. Antitoxin Dosage in Various Forms of Diphtheria

Site	Antitoxin dosage (units)	Route
Nose	5,000	Intramuscular
Tonsils	10,000	Intramuscular
Tonsils and pharynx	30,000–60,000	One-half intramuscular and remainder intravascular in 1 hr
Pharynx, tonsils, soft and hard palate ("bull-neck")	100,000	One half intramuscular and remainder intravascular in 1 hr

minutes, serum therapy may be instituted. Development of a wheal at the site of injection indicates sensitivity to horse serum. Cautious desensitization may be attempted, but extreme care is necessary (see Chap. 45). Injections should be made in an extremity that can be occluded by tourniquet, and epinephrine must be immediately available.

Antibiotics alone cannot be relied on for the treatment of diphtheria, but they may be used as adjuncts to prevent further toxin production by inhibiting bacterial growth. Procaine penicillin, 600,000 units daily, or erythromycin, 250 mg every 6 hours, may be administered. Similar therapy for 12 days is effective in eradicating the carrier state. Obstruction of the larynx or trachea necessitates intubation or tracheostomy. Strict bed rest and mild sedation are indicated in the patient with myocarditis. Some authorities consider that dextrose infusions ranging in concentration from 10 to 50% may be beneficial in the management of diphtheritic myocarditis. Vasopressors may be necessary in patients with severe hypotension.

Viral Respiratory Tract Disease

More than one-half of all acute respiratory tract infections are caused by viral agents, most of which require for identification specialized laboratory techniques not readily available to clinicians. Another third are of unknown etiology and could conceivably

Table 8-3. Viral and Mycoplasmal Infections of the Respiratory Tract

Agent	Ratio of total no. serotypes to no. that produces respiratory illness	Epidemiology	Reinfection	Most important clinical consequences of infection
Myxovirus Influenza	3/2	Epidemic every 8–10 years, usually winter	Common with new variants, less common with same variant	Influenzal disease in all age groups; pneumonia in adults
Parainfluenza	4/4	Endemic, occasionally epidemic	Common; upper respiratory tract disease	Croup in infants, children; also upper and lower tract disease in this age group
Respiratory syncytial	1/1	Epidemic every year; fall, winter, or spring	Common; upper respiratory tract disease	Bronchiolitis, croup, pneumonia in infants; upper and lower tract disease in children
Coronavirus	3/3	Epidemic; winter	Not known	Common colds in children and adults
Picornavirus Coxsackie A and B	29/10	Epidemic; summer, fall	Not known	Febrile pharyngitis in infants, children; colds in military recruits; herpangina (Cox. A); pleurodynia (Cox. B)
Rhinovirus	At least 89/all	Endemic; sporadic flurries of different types	Occurs	Common colds in children and adults
Adenovirus	33/8	Endemic, occasionally epidemic	Uncommon	Upper or lower tract disease in infants, children; same in military recruits
Mycoplasma	9/1	Endemic, occasionally epidemic	Uncommon	Pneumonia in children and adults

be caused by viruses presently unrecognized. Table 8-3 summarizes the many viral and mycoplasmal agents now known to infect the respiratory tract and emphasizes the most important clinical consequences of infection with each agent. It is important to note that a wide variety of clinical syndromes ranging in severity from coryza to pneumonia may be produced by a single species of agent. In addition, it is not possible to recognize a specific etiologic agent as the cause of a respiratory tract illness in any individual on the basis of the clinical picture alone. Because of this fact, viral respiratory disease is described below in reference to the specific clinical infections that are produced.

All the viral agents noted in Table 8-3 are capable of producing disease of both the upper and lower respiratory tracts; some agents, however, have a propensity for one form of disease in certain age groups. Various syndromes affecting the respiratory tract will now be discussed, beginning with upper respiratory tract disease and progressing to lower respiratory tract disease (see Chap. 11).

COMMON COLD (RHINOPHARYNGITIS)
The most common upper respiratory tract infection and also the most frequent illness of man is the common cold (rhinopharyngitis). This familial syndrome, lasting 2 to 7 days, is characterized by sneezing, nasal discharge and obstruction, dry or scratchy throat, and watery eyes and is sometimes accompanied by mild constitutional symptoms and low-grade fever. Secondary acute bacterial infections, particularly sinusitis and otitis media (especially in children), occasionally occur. Rhinoviruses and coronaviruses are important etiologic agents in adults, and parainfluenza and respiratory syncytial viruses are frequent agents in infants and children. Of particular importance are the facts, noted in Table 8-3, that some viruses can reinfect adults many years following a childhood exposure and that reinfection is frequently accompanied by upper respiratory tract disease.

ACUTE PHARYNGITIS
Acute pharyngitis is characterized by a sore throat and is usually accompanied by pharyngeal injection and red, swollen tonsils. Fever, moderate constitutional symptoms, tonsillar exudate, cervical lymph-

adenopathy, and cough are common. Most cases are due to viruses, particularly adenoviruses and parainfluenza viruses. When exudate is present, the etiologic agent is usually either bacterial (beta hemolytic streptococci, C. diphtheriae) or viral (e.g., adenovirus or infectious mononucleosis). An enanthem consisting of vesicles and ulcers suggests either an enterovirus, particularly Coxsackie A, or a primary infection with herpes simplex. Grayish white papulovesicular lesions in the posterior oropharynx that are surrounded by an erythematous zone and that progress to shallow ulcers and clear within a week are findings typical of herpangina produced by Coxsackie A-group viruses. Unilateral or bilateral conjunctivitis and photophobia may be prominent in some patients with pharyngitis. Such illnesses are often caused by adenoviruses, which can also produce epidemic keratoconjunctivitis.

Bibliography

Dowling, H. F. (with the collaboration of L. K. Sweet and H. L. Hirsch). *Acute Bacterial Diseases: Their Diagnosis and Treatment.* Philadelphia: Saunders, 1948.

Evans, A. S., and Dick, E. C. Acute pharyngitis and tonsillitis in University of Wisconsin students. *J.A.M.A.* 190:699, 1964.

Fenner, F. J., and White, D. O. *Medical Virology* (2nd ed.). New York: Academic, 1976.

Howie, V. M., Ploussard, J. H., and Lester, R. L. Otitis media: A clinical and bacteriologic correlation. *Pediatrics* 45:29, 1970.

McCloskey, R. V., Eller, J. J., Green, M. G., Mauney, C. U., and Richards, S. E. M. The 1970 epidemic of diphtheria in San Antonio. *Ann. Intern. Med.* 75:495, 1971.

Wannamaker, L. W., and Ferrieri, P. Streptococcal infections updated. *DM,* October, 1975.

9

Evaluation of Patients with Bronchopulmonary Disease

Gordon L. Snider and Sanford Chodosh[*]

In recent years many older pulmonary diagnostic tools such as the chest roentgenogram have come of age and new ones such as the flexible fiberoptic bronchoscope have become available. The widespread availability of pulmonary function tests, including bedside measurements of arterial blood gases, and the development of sputum cytologic examinations and improved serologic and bacteriologic techniques have not only changed the understanding of pulmonary diseases but have greatly increased the effectiveness of physicians in dealing with them. Despite the expanded use of technology, the physician's role in diagnosis is as great as ever. Laboratory tests are most useful when they are correlated by a thoughtful physician with his own carefully taken history and skillfully done physical examination. In this section various clinical and laboratory techniques for evaluating patients with bronchopulmonary disease will be briefly discussed.

The History

There are only a few strictly pulmonary symptoms: chest pain, hemoptysis, dyspnea, wheezing, cough, and expectoration. The simple presence or absence of any of these is rarely of diagnostic importance; however, the precise manner of their presentation, their sequence, their precipitating and relieving factors, and the context in which they appear often point the way to recognition of the underlying disease.

COUGH

Cough is one of the normal cleansing mechanisms of the lung (see Chap. 10), but persistent cough is never normal. Patients are usually aware of cough of recent origin but may deny chronic cough because they believe that everyone coughs. It is important in sorting out acute infections from exacerbations of chronic

[*]Author of section, Microscopic Examination of the Sputum

bronchitis to determine whether the symptom is really new or is an exacerbation of a chronic complaint. The recent cessation of a long-standing, chronic productive cough may indicate stasis of bronchial secretions in a patient who has impending respiratory failure. A very severe cough may be associated with emesis or syncope.

SPUTUM

A normal person produces up to 100 ml of tracheobronchial secretions per day. This secretion is usually carried to the oropharynx by the mucociliary escalator and is swallowed. Increased amounts of secretion may be expectorated after eating, especially if the food is highly seasoned. The quantity and quality of expectoration are important features in bronchopulmonary disease; the volume is best expressed by some household estimate such as the teaspoonful or tablespoonful. The description of secretions is often valuable; clear and colorless sputum suggests purely mucoid secretion, while a yellow or green color suggests a purulent exudate. Since both neutrophils and eosinophils may be responsible for a purulent appearance, infection cannot be assumed from this gross finding. A fetid odor suggests anaerobic infection. Rusty or brownish red sputum indicates blood cells mixed with mucopus in an acute infection. In coal miners sputum may be black due to large quantities of anthracotic pigment. Three-layered sputum with an uppermost frothy layer, a mucoid layer, and a thick bottom layer is said to be characteristic of bronchiectasis; however, this appearance may also occur with any other extensive bronchitic process. A physician's observation of the patient's sputum often yields information quite different from that obtained from the patient.

HEMOPTYSIS

Hemoptysis is defined as expectoration of blood; the amount of blood may vary from a few streaks mixed with mucus to an exsanguinating hemorrhage. The site of bleeding may be anywhere in the respiratory tract, including the mouth and nose. Bronchial mucosa may bleed because of superficial erosion of passively engorged membranes, such as develop in mitral stenosis, or because of inflamed membranes, such as occur in chronic bronchitis. Bleeding may result from ulceration of a tumor, such as a broncho-genic carcinoma or a bronchial adenoma, or it may occur as the result of penetration of the bronchial wall by an eroding process, such as a calcified lymph node or an aortic aneurysm. Blood may come from the pulmonary parenchyma with the capillary engorgement of pneumonia or with the parenchymal necrosis due to infection or infarction.

The patient may describe expectoration of blood mixed with sputum or the experience of a sudden bubbling sensation in the trachea with expectoration of a mouthful of blood. Bronchopulmonary bleed-ing sometimes is manifested as vomiting of blood. The mechanism here is bleeding during the night with the blood reaching the oropharynx and being swal-lowed. The presence of 300 to 500 ml of blood in the stomach is quite irritating, and several hours later the patient awakens and vomits the blood. Roent-genographic as well as physical examination of the chest is therefore mandatory in the investigation of every patient with hematemesis. A history of epi-staxis must also be sought in evaluating patients with hemoptysis, because blood from the nasopharynx can be aspirated during the night and coughed up in the morning.

WHEEZING

Wheezing is noisy, squeaky, or stertorous breathing that denotes obstruction in the airways. Although common in patients with obstructive airways disease, the presence of wheezing is not very frequently volunteered by the patient but rather is elicited by the physician on direct questioning.

CHEST PAIN

Although there are many causes of chest pain, the physician can gain important insight into the probable cause in a given case from a careful history. Pleuritic chest pain tends to be quite sharply localized, worsens during coughing, deep breathing, or motion, and is relieved by maneuvers that limit the expansion of a particular part of the chest. The pain of a carcinoma invading the spine or ribs tends to be localized, bor-ing, and of a severe, nonremitting character. When nerve roots or brachial plexus trunks are involved, radiation to the affected dermatomes is observed. The pain of vertebral body disease tends to be mid-line, often with girdle radiation, and is associated with tenderness over the affected area. Anginal pain and the pain of myocardial infarction are usually easily identified because of their common midline localization and radiation into the neck or down the left arm (see Chap. 28). Esophageal spasm may pro-duce pain that mimics the pain of myocardial infarc-tion except that it is frequently relieved dramatically by ingestion of an alkali (see Chap. 34). This pain may also be relieved by a change in position from recumbent to upright. The pain of pericarditis is midline, of variable severity, and is often relieved by sitting up and leaning forward. In many instances the history will not identify a probable etiology of chest pain, and appropriate studies must be done to estab-lish a diagnosis.

Precordial catch is a sticking precordial (not mid-line) pain that is variably worsened by deep inspira-tion, is not precipitated by effort, and tends to last only a few minutes. It occurs more often in men than in women and is infrequently observed after the third decade. The pain is not due to heart or lung disease and is probably of chest wall origin. The diag-nosis is made from the history and appropriate clin-ical and laboratory evaluation to exclude visceral disease.

DYSPNEA

Dyspnea is defined as discomfort associated with breathing and is an important symptom of pulmo-nary insufficiency. The character of the dyspnea, such as breathlessness or labored breathing, its dura-tion, its relation to effort and whether it occurs only on exercise or also at rest, should be precisely deter-mined. The evolution of dyspnea on effort can generally be established by asking the patient about his breathlessness during some regular effort such as climbing stairs. Dyspnea at rest in a patient without severe airways obstruction should suggest the possi-bility either of pulmonary emboli or of a diffuse interstitial process. Differentiation of dyspnea of cardiac origin from that of pulmonary origin usually depends on demonstrating the presence of pulmonary or cardiac disease. Paroxysmal nocturnal dyspnea can occur with either left ventricular failure or obstruc-tive airways disease. Left ventricular failure with pulmonary edema rarely occurs without orthopnea, whereas most patients with severe pulmonary insufficiency are able to lie flat.

Eliciting and properly judging historical information in pulmonary disease frequently requires the physician to take the history repeatedly as additional clinical information becomes available. A complete systems review and a review of past illnesses and the family history are valuable, since pulmonary disease is frequently a part of a systemic disorder. A meticulous, chronologically complete history of all occupational exposure should always be recorded, starting with the individual's first job and including all subsequent occupations.

Physical Examination

It is beyond the scope of this section to review all the techniques of physical diagnosis of the chest. Critical analysis of these techniques has resulted in a simplification of both approach and terminology in recent years, and a few key points will be made. Physical examination remains the easiest and certainly the cheapest way of studying the patient, especially on serial examinations. Data gathered from such examinations often increase the accuracy with which chest roentgenograms or pulmonary function studies are interpreted.

Observation of chest expansion yields information on thoracic conformation and on respiratory rate and pattern, and it indicates whether the patient is breathing within the normal range of expansion or near a position of full inspiration, as occurs in high-grade airways obstruction. Percussion of the chest gives information regarding the status of the pleural space, the presence of normal quantities of air in the underlying lung, and the extent of diaphragmatic motion. The normal breath sounds are altered in parenchymal consolidation with patent airways; they assume a character similar to that heard over the trachea. Rales or crackles are discontinuous sounds of very short duration that arise from the parenchyma and indicate the presence of disease, without indicating whether it is acute or chronic. Rhonchi or wheezes are continuous sounds of longer duration than rales, and they arise from the airways and indicate partial obstruction of these structures. Sizable parenchymal lung

abnormalities that are more than 1 to 2 cm beneath the surface of the pleura frequently do not alter the transmission of breath sounds or the spoken or whispered voice, nor do they necessarily produce adventitious sounds.

Auscultation over the larynx permits precise identification of the end of expiration, since sounds are generated there at very low velocities of air flow. A normal person empties his lungs of air during forced expiration in about 4 seconds; a longer forced expiratory time in a cooperating patient indicates airways obstruction.

Needless to say, in many circumstances the remainder of the physical examination may be of as much importance in pulmonary diagnosis as the examination of the chest itself. Such findings as superior vena cava obstruction, digital clubbing, neurologic disease, abdominal organomegaly, and peripheral edema and calf tenderness indicating phlebothrombosis are only a few examples of extrapulmonary physical findings that may be of signal importance.

Pulmonary Function Measurements

In considering tests of pulmonary function, it is helpful to separate arbitrarily the various mechanisms by which the lung carries out gas exchange: (1) the movement of air into and out of the lungs by the action of the thoracic bellows — the chest wall and its musculature, including the diaphragm; (2) the conduction of air to the alveoli in a proper manner through normally patent conducting airways; (3) the appropriately balanced distribution of both inspired air and capillary blood to the alveoli; (4) the diffusion through alveolar membranes of molecular gas; and (5) the proper functioning of the pulmonary circulation. The interpretation of pulmonary function tests requires the coordination of these tests with information obtained from the chest roentgenogram, physical examination, and history.

Derangements of the thoracic bellows can most easily be evaluated by measurements of static lung volumes. The vital capacity measures the "stroke volume" of the respiratory bellows; it may be diminished either as a result of an increased residual volume or because of a decreased total lung capacity. In the absence of airways obstruction, serial measurements of the vital capacity provide useful information regarding changes of bellows function, for example, in rapidly evolving respiratory paralysis. The residual volume increases with age and in emphysema, as a result of loss of elastic recoil of the lung; it also increases in the presence of airways obstruction. The total lung capacity may be decreased by a deformity of the bony thorax, by impairment of neuromuscular function of the bellows, or by loss of lung distensibility due to atelectasis or scarring.

Air conduction into the lungs occurs through a system of branching airways that increase markedly in total cross-sectional area between the level of the trachea and the terminal bronchioles. Consequently an appreciable loss of total cross-sectional area in the upper airway, say to 50 percent of normal, results in an obvious obstructive disturbance of air conduction or flow. On the other hand, a similar reduction of total cross-sectional area at bronchiolar levels has little effect on overall air conduction, since resistance to flow through the small airways makes a relatively small contribution to total airways resistance.

In order to understand the interrelationships between airways driving pressure and total airways flow or conduction during expiration, it is important to recall that the distal airways have thin, collapsible walls and are surrounded by the alveoli. At full inspiration lung recoil pressure is maximal, and the tethering effect of the connective tissue network of the lung holds the small airways widely open. As expiration proceeds, lung recoil pressure diminishes, and the distal, poorly supported airways also diminish in caliber. Since the distal airways are surrounded by alveoli and alveolar pressure must be higher than airway pressure for air to exit from the lungs, an increase in muscular driving pressure during expiration at any given lung volume results in an increase in small airways transmural pressure, tending to collapse the airways. Thus at each lung volume a point is reached at which the increasing muscular driving pressure results in alveolar pressure exceeding airway pressure and collapse of the airway. Further increase in muscular pressure fails to give rise to a further increase in flow through the airways; a flow maximum is reached.

These characteristics determine the shape of the forced expiratory spirogram, which is the volume of air expired plotted against time during a maximal voluntary forced expiration. In the early part of the curve, volume change is determined predominantly by the amount of expiratory muscular effort applied by the patient and the geometry of the large, well-supported airways. In the later part of the curve, volume changes decrease sharply as the small, poorly supported airways diminish in caliber, and flow becomes more independent of driving pressure. Therefore the forced expiratory volume for 1 second, which is measured in the early part of the tracing and reflects predominantly muscular effort and large airway caliber, may be normal in the presence of considerable dysfunction of the small, distal airways. Function of these latter airways is much better reflected in the mean flow rate during the middle half or third quarter of the vital capacity. Values of maximum flow at low lung volume, which also reflect small airways function, are readily obtained from the maximum expiratory flow-volume curve. This curve is made by plotting instantaneous flow against volume during a forced expiration. At present, the expiratory flow-volume curve is more expensive to record than the forced expiratory spirogram and provides little additional information which is useful in clinical practice. However, analysis of the combined inspiratory and expiratory flow-volume record does permit localization of airways obstruction at the level of either the small airways or the large airways within or outside the thorax.

Each inspired breath may be divided into a volume that enters the alveoli and a portion (about one-third of the total) that remains in the conducting airways and does not take part in gas exchange. The latter portion is known as the dead space; the proportion of total ventilation that ventilates the dead space increases when total ventilation is augmented by an increase in rate in preference to an increase in depth.

The adequacy of gas exchange can be determined only by measuring arterial blood gases and interpreting the data in relation to respired gas values. Assuming no change in carbon dioxide production by the tissues, the arterial partial pressure of carbon dioxide (Pa_{CO_2}) varies inversely as the alveolar ventilation. An increase of Pa_{CO_2} above the normal range of 37 to

42 mm Hg denotes alveolar hypoventilation; a decrease in Pa_{CO_2} indicates alveolar hyperventilation.

Hypoxemia is due to one or more of the following causes: (1) a diminution in the inspired partial pressure of oxygen (P_{O_2}); (2) alveolar hypoventilation with a fall in alveolar P_{O_2} (PA_{O_2}); (3) a defect in the mechanism of molecular diffusion of oxygen between alveolus and capillary; (4) the shunting of venous blood into the systemic circulation; or (5) a mismatch between alveolar ventilation and capillary perfusion. Mismatch of alveolar ventilation ($\dot{V}A$) and capillary perfusion ($\dot{Q}c$) is the commonest mechanism of hypoxemia in pulmonary disease. Limited areas of alveolar hypoventilation in relation to perfusion (low $\dot{V}A/\dot{Q}c$ ratios) result in hypoxemia with normal arterial partial pressures of carbon dioxide (Pa_{CO_2}). Increased $\dot{V}A$ in the normal areas of lung readily results in elimination of the excess carbon dioxide contributed by the area of low $\dot{V}A/\dot{Q}c$ ratio, since the carbon dioxide dissociation curve is straight in the physiologic range. Because the upper portion of the oxygen dissociation curve is flat, increased PA_{O_2} in the normal lung resulting from increased $\dot{V}A$ fails to increase the oxygen content in arterial blood, and hypoxemia is not corrected. As the disease becomes more severe and areas of normally ventilated lung diminish, the patient is no longer able to eliminate all excess carbon dioxide from these areas, and hypercapnia and more severe hypoxemia supervene. Portions of lung that are perfused but have no ventilation behave like right-to-left shunts.

Alveoli that have excess ventilation in relation to perfusion may be thought of as behaving like conducting airways or dead space; the dead space or "wasted" ventilation is increased without alteration of blood gases.

Arterial partial pressure of oxygen (Pa_{O_2}) measurements must be interpreted in the light of the inspired partial pressure of oxygen (PI_{O_2}). This is most conveniently done by calculating the difference between alveolar and arterial partial pressure of oxygen ($P[A - a]O_2$). Knowing the PI_{O_2} and the alveolar P_{CO_2} (PA_{CO_2}) and assuming a value of 0.8 for the respiratory ratio (R), one can calculate the alveolar P_{O_2} for bedside use from a simplified version of the alveolar air equation:

$$PA_{O_2} = PI_{O_2} - \frac{PA_{CO_2}}{R}$$

or substituting:

$$PA_{O_2} = PI_{O_2} - (PA_{CO_2} \times 1.25)$$

The PA_{CO_2} is estimated from the Pa_{CO_2}, which serves as a measure of "ideal" or mean PA_{CO_2}. The $P[A - a]O_2$ is then easily determined by subtraction; with the subject breathing room air at sea level, this difference ranges from 5 mm Hg in young normal individuals to 25 mm Hg in elderly, healthy persons. The use of this calculation permits one to determine whether a diminution in the Pa_{O_2} is due to alveolar hypoventilation or to pulmonary disease; in the former instance the $P[A - a]O_2$ is normal, while in the latter the $P[A - a]O_2$ is widened. Note from the alveolar air equation the reciprocal relationship between PA_{CO_2} and PA_{O_2}; as PA_{CO_2} rises, the PA_{O_2} falls and vice versa.

Performance of the diffusing capacity test using carbon monoxide has come into wide use in recent years. The single-breath, bloodless method is the one most widely used. This test is influenced by the intrapulmonary distribution of inspired air, by ventilation-perfusion relationships, by the area of the alveolar capillary surface, and by the character of the alveolar capillary barrier. Although clinically useful in many circumstances, it is not to be construed as an accurate measurement of diffusion function.

Arterial hypoxemia is not regularly observed with decreases of the diffusing capacity until the latter is decreased to as little as 25 percent of the predicted normal. A diminished diffusing capacity measurement in the presence of normal ventilatory function and lung volumes indicates disease in the gas exchange portion of the lung and should lead to a fuller assessment of blood gas exchange by means of respired and arterial blood gas studies at rest and during exercise. Diminution of the diffusing capacity in the presence of airways obstruction and increases in the functional residual capacity and residual volume suggest the presence of emphysema.

Occurrence of occlusive vascular disease of the lung as a result of either multiple pulmonary emboli or pulmonary arteriolosclerosis can be suspected from (1) physical signs of pulmonary hypertension in the absence of valvular or congenital heart disease, (2) hypoxemia in the presence of a normal chest roentgenogram in a patient with normal ventilatory function, and (3) an increase in the ratio of dead space to tidal volume during exercise instead of the usual decrease. Quantitation of pulmonary hypertension requires the performance of right heart catheterization and determination of cardiac output, pulmonary arterial blood pressure, and pulmonary venous-capillary wedge pressure. Regional alterations of the ventilation-perfusion relationships and of the pulmonary capillary circulation can be evaluated in scintigrams made after inhalation of [133]xenon or after the intravenous injection of a solution of [133]xenon or of a macroaggregate of albumin labeled with a radionuclide.

Pulmonary function tests provide information on the nature and severity of pulmonary function abnormalities, but only rarely do they give a diagnosis of the pulmonary disease that has caused them. Different disease entities may produce identical abnormalities of pulmonary function, and any one disease can produce a wide range of pulmonary function abnormalities, depending on the precise anatomic localization and severity of the disease process. On the other hand, results of these tests may be helpful in sorting out a list of differential diagnostic possibilities. These tests also provide valuable information on the progress of disease and the effects of treatment and help in the assessment of pulmonary impairment and claimed disability for specific tasks. They are also of great use in predicting the risks of operative intervention in the presence of lung disease.

The Chest Roentgenogram
X-rays of the chest can detect pulmonary abnormalities that are not evident on either physical examination or pulmonary function measurement, and consequently no examination of the chest is complete without them. On the other hand, a chest roentgenogram, which is almost always taken only in full inspiration, does not reveal the movements of the chest wall and diaphragm, which is information that is easily obtained during physical examination. Par-

tial obstruction of the airways, indicated by rhonchi on auscultation, or lesions in main bronchi easily observed endoscopically, often produce no abnormality in the chest roentgenogram. Rales may be very obvious on physical examination, indicating the presence of parenchymal disease; and abnormalities of pulmonary function may indicate the presence of emphysema or interstitial disease when the chest roentgenogram is quite normal. The conclusion is inescapable that physical examination, pulmonary function measurements, and the chest roentgenogram are complementary and not mutually exclusive methods of investigating the respiratory system.

Microscopic Examination of the Sputum
It is important to select from a specimen aliquots that have come from the lower respiratory tract. This can be determined by picking an opaque fleck or a cloudy area for microscopic examination. When scanned under low power (10X), the presence of macrophages ensures that the origin of the material is the lung; numerous squamous cells indicate an oropharyngeal origin. Staining with an aqueous metachromatic dye simplifies cell identification, but unstained wet preparations examined with the condenser racked down are almost equally useful. Once good material is found, the characterization of the types and numbers of cells should be made using the oil-immersion objective. This information, along with the sputum volume and clinical findings, helps in estimating the nature and severity of the responsible pathology. In addition, such well-identified lower respiratory secretions can be sent with confidence for other indicated studies. A concomitant Gram stain will provide an immediate evaluation of the bacterial flora and a presumptive morphologic identification of the bacterial types and their numbers; this can help in the selection and use of appropriate antimicrobials. While a Gram stain is quicker, cheaper, and more quantitative than culture results, cultures are necessary for precise identification of organisms.

The assessment of a pathologic process requires an understanding of the kinds of bronchial mucosal damage and inflammatory cell response that occur in various diseases. In chronic bronchitis, the bronchial epithelial cells (BEC) are exfoliated as pyknotic, indi-

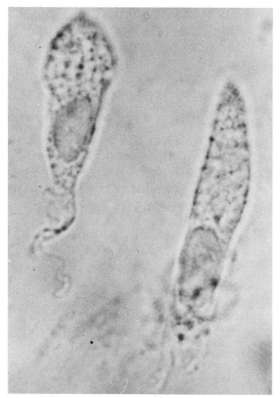

*Figure 9-1.   Degenerated columnar bronchial epi-
thelial cells typical of bronchitis; note loss of cilia
and basal plate and rounding of cell edge.*

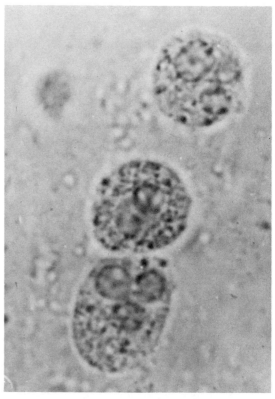

*Figure 9-2. Polymorphonuclear neutrophils with
some toxic granulation in sputum.*

vidual cells that have lost their ciliated borders (Fig.
9-1). Polymorphonuclear neutrophils are the predominant cells (Fig. 9-2) and may represent over 90
percent of all the cells seen. The number of large
round cells (monocytes and macrophages) varies considerably, more being seen in early or mild disease
(Fig. 9-3). A great variety of phagocytized material
can be seen in the cytoplasm of these cells. In allergic
bronchopulmonary conditions, exemplified by
asthma, the exfoliated bronchial epithelial cells are
more numerous, swollen, often occur in clusters, and
tend to retain their cilia; the eosinophil is the characteristic cell, usually representing well over 10 percent
of all cells and often predominating (Fig. 9-4).
Charcot-Leyden crystals, which are elongated rhom-
boids 1 to 40 μ in length, are formed from broken
esosinophils and have the same significance (Fig. 9-5).
Predominance of polymorphonuclear neutrophils sug-

gests the presence of infection even when such a
process is not clinically suspected. Macrophages vary
in numbers. In viral infection the bronchial epithelial
cells look like those in the asthmatic patient, but
eosinophils are seen infrequently; either mononuclear
cells of varying sizes or polymorphonuclear neutrophils may predominate. In bacterial pneumonia, lung
abscess, or bronchiectasis there is a marked predominance of polymorphonuclear neutrophils with a
variable background of granular debris.

Other methods of obtaining secretions should be
used in patients not spontaneously expectorating
sputum. Stimulation with aerosolized hypertonic
sodium chloride, bronchodilator solution, or ultrasonic mist should be tried first. A nasotracheal
catheter and the injection through the catheter of a
bolus of normal saline may induce productive cough.
Transtracheal aspiration by passing a small-gauge

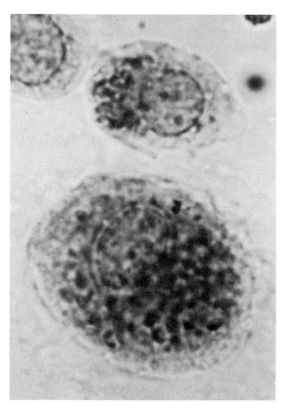

Figure 9-3. Sputum macrophages.

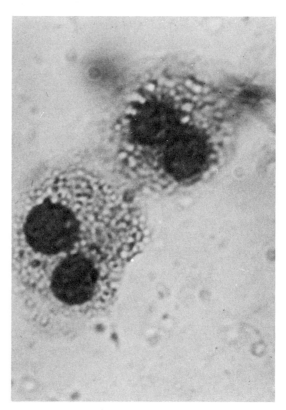

Figure 9-4. Polymorphonuclear eosinophils in sputum with typical bilobed nuclei and large refractile granules.

plastic catheter through a thin-walled needle should be used when other means fail or when material for anaerobic cultures is desired. Where localized disease is suspected, secretions from specific bronchi can be obtained by aspiration under direct visualization through the fiberoptic bronchoscope.

Material for cytologic examination for tumor cells should be prepared as a wet smear, which is immediately fixed with alcohol-ether or an appropriate fixative spray and then is stained by the Papanicolaou method. Cell block examination can be carried out on formalin-fixed sputum aliquots. Cancer of the lung can be detected in 60 to 70 percent of cases if five sputa are examined, and often the specific cell type can be identified.

Cultural discovery of tubercle bacilli and pathogenic fungi provides definitive proof of these infections, but presumptive diagnosis can often be made by microscopic examination of sputum. Acid-fast stains are the standard method for detecting tubercle bacilli. Fungi are classically sought in wet preparations that have been cleared with potassium hydroxide as well as in specially stained preparations. When parasitic infection is suspected, careful examination may detect ova or filaria.

Flexible Fiberoptic Bronchoscopy

The advent of high-quality fiberoptics has made possible a flexible bronchoscope with a 5.0- to 5.2-mm tip and approximately 2-mm aspiration channel. This instrument can readily be passed through the nose or mouth under topical anesthesia.

Flexible fiberoptic bronchoscopy permits inspection of the tracheobronchial tree down to subsegmental bronchi and beyond. Cytologic specimens can be collected on the bronchial brush, and bronchial

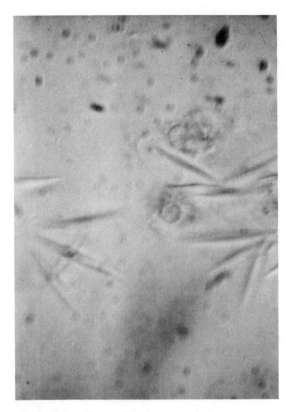

Figure 9-5. Charcot-Leyden crystals in sputum.

brushes or biopsy forceps can be passed directly into solid lesions under fluoroscopic control. Small fragments of diffusely diseased pulmonary parenchyma can be obtained by pushing the bronchoscopic biopsy forceps through the wall of a distal, thin-walled bronchus. Transbronchoscopic lung biopsy has proved useful in the diagnosis of neoplasms, nodular granulomas, and infections in which the organisms can be identified microscopically or by culture.

Biopsy Techniques
Material for cytologic diagnosis can be obtained from solid lung lesions using the method of fine-needle aspiration under fluoroscopic control. When a patient is considered to have an inoperable neoplasm, with the lesion adhering to the pleura, tissue can be obtained by core biopsy with a percutaneous cutting needle. When lesions are diffuse or not suitable for biopsy by one of the above methods, open lung biopsy is performed through a short intercostal incision. This method provides the largest volume of tissue with the least sampling error for histologic examination as well as for culture and biochemistry.

Biopsy of palpable lymph nodes is generally helpful in evaluating inflammatory or neoplastic thoracic disease, especially if the disease is part of a systemic process. When lymph nodes are not palpable, a scalene node situated on the anterior scalene muscle may be biopsied through a small supraclavicular incision. This procedure has a high yield in granulomatous disease, especially if mediastinal nodes are found to be involved on x-ray. There is an even higher yield from mediastinoscopy, which is performed under general anesthesia by making an incision in the suprasternal notch and passing an endoscope into the mediastinum along the tissue planes anterior and lateral to the trachea.

The investigation of pleural disease is discussed elsewhere (see Chap. 21).

Bibliography
Chodosh, S. Examination of sputum cells. *N. Engl. J. Med.* 282:854, 1970.

Felson, B. *Chest Roentgenology.* Philadelphia: Saunders, 1973.

Khan, M. A., Whitcomb, M. E., and Snider, G. L. Flexible fiberoptic bronchoscopy. *Am. J. Med.* 61:151, 1976.

Medici, T. C., and Chodosh, S. Non-malignant Sputum Cytology. In M. J. Dulfano (ed.), *Sputum.* Springfield, Ill.: Thomas, 1973. P. 332.

Snider, G. L. Interpretation of the arterial oxygen and carbon dioxide partial pressures: A simplified approach for bedside use. *Chest* 63:801, 1973.

West, J. B. *Respiratory Physiology.* Baltimore: Williams & Wilkins, 1975.

10

Pulmonary Defense Mechanisms

Wlademir Pereira

In carrying out their primary function of gaseous exchange, the lungs are ventilated with about 10,000 liters of ambient air per day, which exposes them to a wide variety of potentially hazardous substances. These may be gases, liquids, or solid particles suspended in the inhaled air. Microorganisms may be present in droplets or dried particles. The lungs defend themselves by trapping the larger particles in the upper airways, by removing particles of respirable size, and by killing or limiting the growth of potentially pathogenic organisms that reach the lower airways.

Upper Airways

People live in environments widely varying in temperature and humidity. Air that is either frigid or hot (and dry) is "conditioned" by the convoluted, highly vascularized, moist surfaces of the nasal turbinates, so that when it reaches the trachea at the end of an inspiration, it has been warmed (or cooled) to body temperature and is nearly fully saturated with water vapor. Very large particles are trapped in the vibrissae of the nares; most of the remaining particles (greater than 10 μ in diameter) stick to the mucous coating of the nasal turbinates and are moved by the mucociliary system to the pharynx and swallowed. More than 95 percent of the particles greater than 10 μ in diameter never reach the larynx during quiet breathing.

Cough

Cough is a reflex act that may be initiated voluntarily or involuntarily. Sensory points initiating a reflex cough are located in the respiratory tract from the pharynx to about the third- or fourth-order bronchi and are also found in the parietal pleura. The cough sequence consists in a rapid inspiration followed by an expiratory effort against a closed glottis with generation of a high intrabronchial pressure; opening of the glottis is followed by an explosive expiration. High transmural pressure during the expiratory part of the cough results in dynamic compression of intra-

thoracic airways, producing a milking action that tends to move plugs of secretion proximally. Narrowing of the large airways also gives rise to very high linear velocities that cause the secretions to flow upward in a layer on the airway wall and shear off droplets of the secretion, producing a mist. Rapid serial coughs with intermittent opening and closing of the glottis alternately dilate and compress small airways, helping to dislodge tenacious secretions.

Cough effectiveness may be impaired if any phase of this process is abnormal. Asthenia due to age or illness, thoracic or abdominal pain, and neuromuscular disorders that impede an effective inspiratory or expiratory effort may decrease cough efficacy. Glottic closure is helpful but not essential for effective cough; patients with laryngectomy or tracheostomy are able to bring up secretions by a series of rapid forced expirations.

Mucociliary System

The airways are lined from the nose to the terminal bronchioles by ciliated columnar epithelium. Covering the cilia there is a thin layer of secretion, the mucous blanket, which is produced by the submucosal bronchial glands and to a somewhat lesser extent by the goblet cells. The latter can be found in the submucosa of the respiratory tree down to about the fifteenth bronchial generation. The blanket of mucus is continuously propelled toward the pharynx by ciliary motion; the total volume of secretions that reaches the pharynx each day in a normal person is estimated to be about 100 ml.

Vagus nerve stimulation and parasympathomimetic drugs cause an increase in mucous secretions, while atropine blocks the process. Sympathomimetic agents or corticosteroids are unclear in their effect, although there is limited evidence that the former increase secretory activity. Dehydration, cigarette smoke, and other pollutants impair mucociliary performance, and any such impairment contributes to pulmonary dysfunction. An increase in the volume and viscosity of tracheobronchial secretions occurs in association with infection or irritation of the lungs. Qualitative changes in mucus have been shown in chronic bronchitis, asthma, and cystic fibrosis of the pancreas.

Inhaled particles passing below the glottis are mostly under 10 μ in diameter, and almost all particles over 2 μ will be deposited on the sticky mucous layer lining the airways. Particles are propelled upward at a rate of 1 to 3 cm per minute by the beating cilia. Concentrations of particles tend to be gathered at points of branching, but ultimately all particles reach the pharynx. Excessive mucus may overload the system and plug the small bronchi; it should also be remembered that cough is not stimulated unless secretions reach the larger airways.

Alveolar Clearance

The mechanisms involved in the clearance of very small particles (2μ or less in diameter) that reach the alveoli are less clearly understood. The major mechanism appears to be phagocytosis by macrophages. After ingesting particles, macrophages may either move proximally to the terminal bronchioles (and upward by way of the mucociliary system) or directly penetrate the interstitium (and enter the lymphatic or vascular channels). It is known that alveolar clearance is a very slow process, and that although physical removal plays an important role in protection, viable bacteria may be killed within the lung long before they are cleared. In Figure 10-1 the upper dotted line expresses the quantitative contribution of mechanical transport and the solid line represents the phagocytic activity of the lung. The bactericidal activity of the lung is accomplished by both cellular and humoral mechanisms. The alveolar macrophage is a highly phagocytic cell similar to other tissue macrophages that possess the ability to kill organisms after ingesting them. The pulmonary alveolar macrophages are derived from monocytes produced in the bone marrow, and they enter the lung by migration from the vascular bed; however, the factors governing the rate of production, release from the bone marrow, and turnover in the lung of these macrophages are not known.

Numerous influences have been found to impair the efficiency of pulmonary alveolar macrophages, including cigarette smoking, ethanol ingestion, air pollution (ozone, acute hypoxia, hyperoxia), and administration of corticosteroids or immunosuppressive agents. Phagocytosis of noxious particles such as

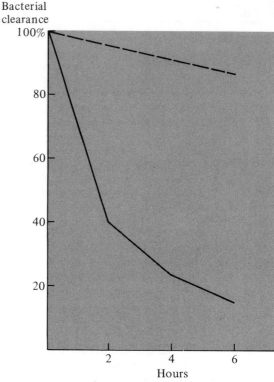

Figure 10-1. *Schema showing clearance of radionuclide-labeled bacteria inhaled by experimental animals. The dotted line represents mechanical removal of bacteria from the lung as determined by diminution of radioactivity in the lung homogenate. The solid line represents bacterial killing as determined by recovery of viable bacteria from culture of the lung homogenate.*

silica may result in rupture of lysosomal membranes and death of the macrophages, with release of their enzymes and possible damage of lung tissues.

Immunoglobulins are the major humoral factors in pulmonary protection against viral and bacterial challenge (see Chap. 44). The predominant immunoglobulin present in the tracheobronchial secretion is IgA produced by plasma cells in the bronchial submucosa. As in other mucous secretions, immunoglobulin A in the tracheobronchial secretions differs from circulating IgA in its sedimentation constant and antigenic properties, and it is called secretory IgA (SIgA). The SIgA molecule consists of two IgA monomers joined by a glycoprotein called the secretory component.

The major defined role of SIgA is its ability to neutralize viruses by preventing their attachment to mucosal cells. Indeed, it has been found that with some respiratory viruses such as influenza, topical immunization (by inhalation) produces more effective immunity than systemic immunization. The protective role of SIgA against bacterial infection is not known; SIgA is not directly bactericidal, does not fix complement, and does not function as an opsonin. However, persons with a SIgA deficiency are abnormally susceptible to bacterial infection.

Whereas the alveolar macrophage and SIgA are the primary defenses against infectious agents in the non-inflamed lung, once inflammation occurs, all the systemic cellular and humoral factors are brought into action. Thus IgG, IgA, polymorphonuclear leukocytes, sensitized T-lymphocytes, and macrophages enter the inflammatory focus, where they function in the inflammatory process as they do in inflammations in all other parts of the body.

Bibliography
Green, G. M. In defense of the lung. *Am. Rev. Respir. Dis.* 102:691, 1970.

11

Bacterial and Viral Infections of the Lower Respiratory Tract

Neil R. Blacklow, Nelson M. Gantz,
and William R. McCabe

Acute Laryngitis and Laryngotracheobronchitis
Acute laryngitis and laryngotracheobronchitis are much more common in children than in adults and usually begin with upper respiratory tract symptoms, although fever, hoarseness, and cough may also occur and be followed by dyspnea, inspiratory stridor (croup) with supraclavicular and infraclavicular retractions, restlessness, and cyanosis. Impaired expiration appears when there is bronchial and bronchiolar involvement with resultant airway obstruction. Parainfluenza and respiratory syncytial viruses are the most common causative agents. Bacterial infections with *Haemophilus influenzae* or diphtheria, although less common, must be considered and evaluated by Gram stains and cultures of the throat, sputum, and epiglottis. Severe cases of acute epiglottiditis with respiratory obstruction and barking cough caused by *H. influenzae* may require emergency tracheostomy. Oxygen and humidified air are helpful in acute laryngotracheobronchitis, regardless of etiology, and maintenance of an adequate airway is always of paramount importance.

Acute Bronchiolitis
Acute bronchiolitis is generally seen only in young infants, and it results from partial obstruction of bronchiolar lumina by exudate and edema. It usually begins as an upper respiratory tract infection that is followed in several days by a dry, persistent cough and increasing dyspnea; it can progress to cyanosis, prostration, and death. In most cases the cause is a virus, particularly respiratory syncytial virus.

Viral and Mycoplasmal Pneumonia
Pneumonia produced by several viral agents is clinically indistinguishable from that caused by a small pleuropneumonialike microorganism, *Mycoplasma pneumoniae* (Table 11-1). The illness tends to have

an insidious onset and is often accompanied by headache, myalgia, malaise, anorexia, nausea, and fever. Usually a dry, nonproductive cough is present. Chest findings on physical examination are often minimal, usually consisting of fine rales or decreased breath sounds. Chest x-rays show more extensive involvement than would be suspected from the physical examination and can consist of localized areas of patchy infiltration or bilateral interstitial lung involvement extending from the hili. A lobar consolidation may rarely be seen in *M. pneumoniae* infection. Leukocyte counts remain normal, and sputum Gram stains are usually devoid of the numerous polymorphonuclear leukocytes seen in bacterial pneumonias; however, mononuclear cells may occasionally be seen. *Mycoplasma pneumoniae* infection, formerly referred to as primary atypical pneumonia, is accompanied in 50 to 70 percent of patients by a rising titer of cold agglutinins in the serum or by a titer of greater than 1:32 that usually appears in the first or second week of illness. Additional serologic and culture studies for viruses and *M. pneumoniae* are not usually readily available to the practicing clinician. Either tetracycline or erythromycin, 500 mg every 6 hours, may be given to adults with severe *M. pneumoniae* infection, although many patients do not require antibiotic therapy.

A variety of viral agents can produce pneumonia. Respiratory syncytial virus is the major cause of severe and sometimes fatal pneumonia in infancy. Parainfluenza viruses, adenoviruses, and influenza viruses are other common causative agents in infants and children. These same viruses also produce pneumonia in adults. Viral pneumonia in adults is also rarely caused by rhinoviruses, Coxsackie viruses, or reoviruses.

Viral pneumonia can also occur as part of a generalized disease. Most notable examples are rubeola, varicella, rubella, herpes simplex, and cytomegalovirus. Patients who are receiving immunosuppressive medications, particularly steroids, are susceptible to cytomegalovirus pneumonia, which can be an extremely severe bilateral interstitial pulmonary infection in these patients. Pneumonia complicating varicella can be especially severe in adults; these patients may have been either previously healthy or have had

Table 11-1. Viral and Mycoplasmal Infections of the Respiratory Tract

Agent	Ratio of total no. serotypes to no. that produces respiratory illness	Epidemiology	Reinfection	Most important clinical consequences of infection
Myxovirus Influenza	3/2	Epidemic every 8–10 years, usually winter	Common with new variants, less common with same variant	Influenzal disease in all age groups; pneumonia in adults
Parainfluenza	4/4	Endemic, occasionally epidemic	Common — upper respiratory tract disease	Croup in infants, children; also upper and lower tract disease in this age group
Respiratory syncytial	1/1	Epidemic every year; fall, winter, or spring	Common — upper respiratory tract disease	Bronchiolitis, croup, pneumonia in infants; upper and lower tract disease in children
Coronavirus	3/3	Epidemic; winter	Not known	Common colds in children and adults
Picornavirus Coxsackie A and B	29/10	Epidemic; summer, fall	Not known	Febrile pharyngitis in infants, children; colds in military recruits; herpangina (Cox. A); pleurodynia (Cox. B)
Rhinovirus	At least 89/all 89	Endemic; sporadic flurries of different types	Occurs	Common colds in children and adults
Adenovirus	33/8	Endemic, occasionally epidemic	Uncommon	Upper or lower tract disease in infants, children; same in military recruits
Mycoplasma	9/1	Endemic, occasionally epidemic	Uncommon	Pneumonia in children and adults

immunosuppressive therapy for malignant processes.

Psittacosis (ornithosis) is produced by small non-viral microorganisms of the *Chlamydia* group. The disease is usually acquired by inhaling dried bird droppings or by handling infected birds, and it can range from inapparent infection or a mild influenza-like illness to a severe viral-like pneumonia. Diagnosis is usually made by serologic techniques. Unlike viral infections, this disease responds to therapy with tetracycline.

Influenza

Influenza virus infection has several unique features that merit discussion apart from the respiratory viruses. Three immunologically distinct groups of human influenza viruses (A, B, and C) exist, of which two (A and B) are known to produce significant respiratory tract disease. Influenza A and B viruses possess the unique capability of undergoing spontaneous genetic mutation that results in the emergence of altered antigenic characteristics in the hemagglutinin (H) and neuraminidase (N) surface coat antigens of the virus. Since immunity is directed against these H and N antigens, major genetic mutations (which occur about every 10 years) result in epidemics of severe influenzal disease among large population groups that then lack immunity to the altered surface-coat antigens. Minor genetic mutations occur every 2 to 3 years with resultant smaller disease outbreaks, and therefore efforts are made to include the latest mutant strains in licensed influenza vaccines.

Influenza occurs in epidemic form primarily during the winter months. The incubation period ranges from 1 to 3 days. Onset can be rapid, frequently with predominance of constitutional over respiratory symptoms. Clinical findings usually include fever, headache, chills, malaise, myalgia, and respiratory symptoms. Rhinitis and pharyngitis, although often present, are not cardinal complaints; a severe tracheitis may occur as well as conjunctivitis. Illness is usually self-limited, lasting 4 to 7 days. Patients are infectious from shortly before until 1 week after the illness.

Although more than 95 percent of influenza cases are benign and self-limited, severe complications can occur; the most common is secondary bacterial pneumonia that follows shortly after recovery from the influenza. Pneumococcal pneumonia is the most frequent type, followed by staphylococcal pneumonia; the latter is almost never found outside the hospital setting except during an influenza outbreak. A less-frequent complication of influenza is primary influenzal pneumonia, which develops shortly after the onset of typical influenza. In this type of pneumonia there is a rapid development of respiratory distress accompanied by profound hypoxia and production of a pinkish, frothy sputum not unlike that found in pulmonary edema. This severe interstitial pneumonia carries a high mortality rate.

The serious complications of influenza can occur in healthy adults but are more likely to develop in certain predisposed individuals. Accordingly, an inactivated polyvalent vaccine consisting of influenza A and B strains identical with or closely related to the strains known to be currently prevalent is commercially available and is recommended for administration to patients who are particularly susceptible to complications of influenza. Such patients include those with the following conditions: congenital and rheumatic heart disease; other cardiovascular disorders, particularly cardiac insufficiency; chronic bronchopulmonary disease; diabetes mellitus and other chronic metabolic disorders; age over 65 years; and pregnancy (only when a major new antigenic strain emerges). The vaccine is not fully protective in all patients, confers only short-term immunity, and therefore must be administered every year. An antiviral drug, amantadine, is available for prophylaxis of infections caused by influenza A H3N2 (Asian) virus strains. This drug must be given before infection has started and should probably be reserved for high-risk patients with chronic debilitating disease in highly specific situations in which they are apt to encounter this specific virus strain.

Pleurodynia

Pleurodynia is a characteristic clinical syndrome caused primarily by Coxsackie B viruses and in which there is a sudden onset of severe, stabbing pain in the muscles of the chest or upper abdomen that is aggravated by movement and respiration. Additional features may include fever, headache, malaise, pharyngitis, and chilliness. The illness usually subsides within 4 days, but it may persist for several weeks. Relapses are frequent. In some cases aseptic meningitis, pleuritis, pericarditis, or orchitis may occur.

Pertussis (Whooping Cough)

Pertussis is an acute, highly communicable infectious disease occurring primarily in younger children. Distinctly uncommon after the age of 17, it is characterized by paroxysmal spasmodic cough that ends with a prolonged, high-pitched, crowing inspiration (whoop). The causative agent is *Bordetella pertussis;* a similar but milder illness is caused by *B. parapertussis.* The incubation period is from 7 to 14 days, and spread is by way of the respiratory route. The infecting organism invades the nasal pharynx, the trachea, and the bronchi. Bacteria localize in large numbers between the cilia, and the resultant inflammatory reaction leads to increased mucus production and decreased ciliary action.

CLINICAL PICTURE

Early in the illness the mucus is normal in consistency, but later it becomes viscid and tenacious. In fatal cases, laryngitis, bronchitis, bronchial pneumonia, and enlargement of the tracheal and bronchial lymph nodes are observed. The illness lasts 6 weeks to 3 months and consists of three stages: catarrhal, paroxysmal, and convalescent. Symptoms during the catarrhal stage, which lasts 7 to 10 days, are nonspecific and include sneezing, lacrimation, coryza, and nocturnal cough. The catarrhal stage is followed by the paroxysmal stage, which lasts from 1 to 6 weeks. Paroxysms of 5 to 15 coughs occur and may be precipitated by the mildest stimuli. After each paroxysm of cough, attempts to inspire are followed by a loud, crowing, inspiratory "whoop." Copious amounts of mucus may be expelled with the paroxysms. These paroxysms are repeated over and over with progressively longer apneic periods. The child's face may become suffused or cyanotic, and often he or she may vomit food or stringy mucus.

Physical findings are usually unremarkable; occasionally crackling inspiratory rales may be heard over the lungs. After prolonged paroxysms, trauma from the lower teeth may cause ulceration of the frenulum of the tongue. Occasionally multiple petechial hemorrhages in the skin and conjunctiva may result from the paroxysms. Complications may appear during the paroxysmal stage and include pneumothorax, subcutaneous emphysema, bronchopneumonia, umbilical hernia, and prolapse of the rectum. Occasionally convulsions may be observed. After a period of a few days to several months, the coughing becomes less frequent and severe and occurs only at night.

DIAGNOSIS

The clinical picture is usually typical, although in early cases and milder forms the diagnosis may be less evident. The leukocyte count may be diagnostic; a white blood cell count of 15,000 or more with approximately 70 percent lymphocytes is usual. Cultures should be obtained early, since the frequency of positive cultures decreases as the illness progresses. Positive cultures are most frequent (90 percent) during the catarrhal stage; they decrease to 75 percent during the early paroxysmal stage and to less than 10 percent by the fifth week. Cultures of either nasopharyngeal swabs or "cough plates" should be made on Bordet-Gengou medium; isolation of *B. pertussis* may be favored by the incorporation of penicillin, 1,000 units per milliliter, in the culture medium.

TREATMENT

Antimicrobial agents have not been demonstrated to affect the course of pertussis materially and are not recommended routinely. Sedation with small amounts of barbiturates at night may be helpful; cough mixtures have little value. It is preferable to maintain a suction apparatus at the bedside. Water, electrolyte, and weight loss from vomiting may be prevented by prompt refeeding; if deficits occur, they should be corrected if possible. The early detection and treatment of complications are among the most important factors in the reduction of mortality. Important complications include bacterial infections of the lung or middle ear and atelectasis of varying degrees that, when severe, may require tracheal suction or bronchoscopy. Immunization against pertussis reduces the risk by more than 90 percent and should be routine for all children.

Pneumonia Caused by Bacteria

Two types of anatomic involvement, lobar and bronchial, may be observed in pneumonia. Involvement of either the major portion of an entire lobe or of several lobes is termed *lobar pneumonia.* Bronchopneumonia involves alveoli adjacent to bronchi in a segmental distribution. Bacterial pneumonias usually have a more acute onset and a greater frequency of chills, high fever, bloody or purulent sputum, pleuritic chest pain, and lobar involvement than observed in viral pneumonia. In addition, a white cell count in excess of 15,000 and a predominance of polymorphonuclear leukocytes in the sputum suggest a bacterial cause. None of these features is absolutely diagnostic, and all may occur occasionally in viral pneumonia. Alcoholism, malnutrition, debility, aspiration, and exposure to inclement weather all predispose to bacterial pneumonia. The relative frequency of bacterial species in the etiology of community-acquired (ambulatory) bacterial pneumonia as observed by Dowling was *Diplococcus pneumoniae,* 98 percent; *Streptococcus pyogenes,* 1.0 percent; *Klebsiella pneumoniae,* 0.6 percent; and *H. influenzae,* 0.3 percent. Pneumonias in hospitalized patients are less often due to these same agents but are more frequently caused by staphylococci or gram-negative bacilli.

PNEUMOCOCCAL (STREPTOCOCCUS PNEUMONIAE) PNEUMONIA

Pneumococci classically produce lobar involvement in adults but are also the most frequent bacterial cause of bronchopneumonia. In children bronchopneumonia is much more frequent than lobar pneumonia. The organism is spread by healthy carriers through the respiratory route.

Pathogenesis

Once pneumococci reach the alveoli, there is an outpouring of serous edema fluid that serves both as a culture medium and as a mechanism to spread the organisms peripherally through the alveolar pores. Dilatation of the alveolar blood vessels occurs and is soon followed by infiltration of leukocytes and dia-

pedesis of a few erythrocytes into the alveolar space. Although some surface phagocytosis occurs, bacterial multiplication proceeds in excess of the ability of the destructive powers of the leukocytes unless the specific antibody against the capsular polysaccharide of the infecting pneumococcus is present. Further leukocytic infiltration occurs until the alveolar spaces are packed with erythrocytes and leukocytes (red hepatization). Subsequently the alveoli become completely filled with leukocytes, and the capillary dilatation disappears (gray hepatization). In areas of advanced consolidation, large quantities of fibrin and debris are present in the alveoli, and macrophages appear to ingest precipitated fibrin and other material as resolution occurs. As the pneumonia spreads, three zones of involvement may be observed: an outer zone consisting of edema fluid and early inflammation, a medial zone of dense consolidation with leukocytes, and an inner zone where some resolution has begun to occur. The histologic pattern of bronchopneumonia is similar except that there is less extensive involvement of the pulmonary parenchyma and proportionally greater bronchial inflammation.

Clinical Picture

Pneumococcal pneumonia tends to occur in persons under 5 or over 40 years of age. Debility and alcoholism are additional predisposing factors, but the disease frequently occurs in otherwise healthy persons. The onset is usually abrupt, but it may be preceded by several days of mild upper respiratory tract symptoms. A single chill, followed by marked temperature elevation ranging from 103 to 105°F (39.4 to 40.6°C), is usual; recurrent chills are infrequent in pneumococcal pneumonia. Sharp, stabbing chest pain accentuated by breathing, coughing, or motion occurs in approximately 80 percent of the patients. Cough is almost universal, but its appearance may be delayed for several hours. The sputum is usually pink or blood streaked but later may become rust colored. The fever tends to persist with only slight fluctuations. Rapid respiration, dilatation of the nares, and grunting expirations are frequent. Physical findings are usually limited to the chest. Splinting or respiratory lag on the involved side is almost uniformly observed. Although physical findings are classically those of consolidation, slight diminution of breath sounds in the area of involvement and fine rales may be the only abnormalities noted early in the illness. Subsequently dullness to percussion, tubular breath sounds, increased fremitus, and medium crepitant rales develop; in more than half the patients a pleural friction rub is present. In bronchopneumonia, similar but less marked findings in several areas may be heard. Leukocytosis in excess of 15,000 cells, with shift to the left, occurs in approximately 75 percent of the patients. Infrequently leukopenia may be observed. X-rays of the chest reveal evidences of lobar involvement, but early in the illness only a portion of the lobe may be affected. Bacteremia occurs in from 15 to 50 percent of the patients.

FRIEDLÄNDER'S PNEUMONIA
Pneumonia caused by *K. pneumoniae* (Friedländer's bacillus) occurs predominantly in alcoholic males in the fourth, fifth, and sixth decades of life. The onset is usually abrupt, and the disease may pursue a rapidly progressive course. Multiple chills are frequent. The sputum tends to be thick and gelatinous and may be brick red or resemble currant jelly. Delirium, prostration, cyanosis, collapse, vomiting, and diarrhea are frequent. The physical findings may be relatively sparse when compared with the extensive consolidation noted on x-ray. The usual findings include dullness to percussion, and often breath sounds are muffled because of the concomitant association of consolidation with extensive atelectasis secondary to bronchial obstruction. On x-ray examination, upper lobe involvement is frequent. The inflammatory enlargement of the lung may be sufficiently great to produce a sagging of the interlobar fissure that is detectable on lateral x-ray views of the chest. Rapid progression leading to early cavitation often occurs. Leukocytosis is usually less marked than in pneumococcal pneumonia; approximately one-third of the patients demonstrate leukopenia. Blood cultures are positive in approximately 50 percent of the patients with Friedländer's pneumonia. Extensive pulmonary destruction and residual cavitation may occur.

STREPTOCOCCAL PNEUMONIA
Streptococcal pneumonia most often appears as a complication of a preceding streptococcal or viral illness, although epidemic outbreaks have been observed in military groups. The onset is abrupt, and the pneumonia tends to be rapidly progressive. Pleuritic chest pain is frequent, and the sputum is usually thin, mucopurulent, and occasionally streaked with blood. Extreme dyspnea and cyanosis are frequent. Empyema occurs in 30 to 60 percent of patients with streptococcal pneumonia and usually appears within 48 to 72 hours after the onset. Physical findings vary, but they usually consist of localized rales and occasional areas of dullness and tubular breathing. The x-ray pattern is that of interstitial bronchopneumonia, frequently with pleural effusion. Bacteremia occurs in only about 10 to 15 percent of the patients.

STAPHYLOCOCCAL PNEUMONIA
Pneumonia caused by *S. aureus* is primarily a disease of infants, hospitalized patients, or patients with altered defense mechanisms. In addition, staphylococcal pneumonia may occur in a community during epidemics of influenza. Careful epidemiologic history frequently can be of great assistance in making the diagnosis. Children with cystic fibrosis are particularly likely to acquire staphylococcal pulmonary infections.

Clinical Picture
The clinical manifestations may vary considerably, and the onset may be either insidious or abrupt. Pleuritic chest pain is relatively infrequent, and the degree of fever may be variable. The sputum is usually thick, purulent, and yellow in color. Lobar involvement may occur, but areas of patchy involvement with central radiolucency are more frequent. Physical findings are usually limited to localized rales and rhonchi, but evidence of consolidation may be found. On the x-ray there are areas of centrally located, patchy infiltrate. Central breakdown and abscess formation are frequent. Thin-walled cysts or pneumatoceles strongly suggest a staphylococcal etiology, and pyopneumothorax is a frequent complication. The leukocyte count generally ranges from 15,000 to 25,000. The frequency of bacteremia varies from 10 to 60 percent.

PNEUMONIA CAUSED BY GRAM-NEGATIVE BACILLI
Pneumonias caused by gram-negative bacilli, except

for those due to *K. pneumoniae* and *H. influenzae,* are almost exclusively hospital acquired. Whereas in Osler's day the pneumococcus was termed the "old man's friend" because of its predilection for producing terminal aspirational pneumonia, gram-negative bacilli have now become frequent causes of terminal pneumonia. Two distinct epidemiologic patterns are important in gram-negative bacillary pneumonias. The first results from aspiration of nasopharyngeal secretions that have become colonized by gram-negative bacilli during hospitalization. Such colonization is enhanced by prior antibiotic therapy. The most frequent bacteria, *Bacteroides, Escherichia coli, Klebsiella,* and species of *Proteus,* are usually those that are also found in the gastrointestinal tract. The second type of gram-negative bacillary pneumonia is usually secondary to the use of ventilatory equipment and is more frequent in patients with tracheotomies. Gram-negative bacilli that are environmental contaminants, such as *Pseudomonas aeruginosa, Serratia marcescens,* and *Enterobacter* species, are the usual causes.

Pneumonias caused by gram-negative bacilli are characterized by the rapid appearance of necrosis of the lung and are associated with high fatality rates. Treatment is similar to that of other infections caused by gram-negative bacilli as described in Chapter 6. When infection has resulted from aspiration secondary to conditions such as coma, repeated infections may occur despite treatment unless the underlying cause is reversed.

HAEMOPHILUS INFLUENZAE PNEUMONIA

Pneumonia due to *H. influenzae* occurs primarily in childhood but may be seen on rare occasions in adults, especially during epidemics of viral influenza. The onset is usually relatively insidious, with cough and variable degrees of fever. Chills and chest pain are not prominent. The sputum tends to be mucopurulent, and the x-ray pattern is that of bronchopneumonia.

DIFFERENTIAL DIAGNOSIS OF THE PNEUMONIAS

Specific, accurate diagnosis is imperative for the proper treatment of pneumonia. Although pneumococci cause the vast majority of bacterial pneumonias, the extremely high fatality rate and the extensive, permanent pulmonary destruction that may result from an incorrectly diagnosed and improperly treated Friedlander's, staphylococcal, or tuberculous pneumonia make their recognition vitally important. No single diagnostic procedure is uniformly successful in establishing the diagnosis; a carefully obtained medical history, physical examination, and laboratory studies must be correlated. Staphylococcal and Friedländer's pneumonia are often suggested by a history of recent illness or hospitalization of the patient or his family. The occurrence of multiple chills tends to lead one away from the diagnosis of pneumococcal pneumonia. Sudden, rapidly fulminating disease associated with cyanosis and extreme prostration tends to suggest staphylococcal or Friedländer's disease, while a state of relative well-being in the face of a high fever and lobar involvement suggests tuberculous disease. Similarly, the absence of chills and a preponderance of generalized symptoms such as malaise, myalgia, headache, and anorexia suggest viral or mycoplasmal pneumonia. Leukopenia favors a viral, mycoplasmal, or tuberculous agent over a bacterial etiology.

Gram stains of the sputum are of inestimable value if their limitations are recognized (see Chap. 9). Sputum often contains bacteria acquired in the oropharynx. Care should be taken to obtain a small fleck of purulent material from the sputum for staining. The presence of large numbers of polymorphonuclear leukocytes in the sputum favors a bacterial etiology. Since pneumococci, streptococci, and influenza bacilli *(H. influenzae)* may be found in healthy carriers, the presence of these organisms in themselves does not ensure a causal relation to the pneumonia. In most bacterial pneumonias, the etiologic agent usually predominates over oral flora in carefully prepared specimens. It is also helpful to search the slide for bacteria that have undergone phagocytosis by polymorphonuclear leukocytes to ensure that the bacteria originated in the bronchi or pulmonary parenchyma. Examination of the sputum is especially valuable for the recognition of pneumonia due to the Friedländer's bacillus *(K. pneumoniae),* since this plump, encapsulated, gram-negative organism is seen infrequently in sputum or flora from the oral cavity except during pneumonia or after antibiotic therapy. Pneumococci appear as lancet-shaped diplococci, but they may occasionally be seen in short chains. *Haemophilus influenzae* is a small, pleomorphic, gram-negative bacillus; and staphylococci appear as grapelike clusters of gram-positive cocci. Sputum smears are relatively valueless in streptococcal pneumonia, since these organisms cannot be distinguished from the streptococci normally inhabiting the mouth and nasal pharynx. Cultures of the sputum should always be obtained from patients with pneumonia, regardless of the suspected clinical diagnosis. Acid-fast stains of the sputum should also be obtained to rule out tuberculous pneumonia. Blood cultures are indicated in all patients. Pleural fluids should be aspirated whenever possible for cell counts, glucose determinations, Gram stains, and cultures. The presence of bacteria within the pleural fluid answers any questions about specific etiology. Viral studies, when available, are of considerable value. Titers of cold agglutinins and determination of specific antibodies against *Mycoplasma* are the only methods available for the diagnosis of mycoplasmal pneumonia during the acute illness.

TREATMENT OF THE PNEUMONIAS

Penicillin is the agent of choice for pneumococcal and streptococcal pneumonias, and a wide range of doses may be used. Parenteral therapy with procaine penicillin, 600,000 units twice daily, or penicillin given by mouth, 2 million units per day, has been demonstrated to be effective, and there is little indication for the use of higher doses. Erythromycin, 500 mg every 6 hours, may be used in patients with a penicillin allergy. Treatment regimens for Friedländer's pneumonia have included chloramphenicol and streptomycin in combination, or kanamycin or gentamicin alone or in combination with cephalothin.

Staphylococcal pneumonia is treated best with either one of the penicillinase-resistant penicillins (methicillin, oxacillin, or nafcillin) or cephalosporin. Benzylpenicillin (G) is still the agent of choice, provided the infecting staphylococcus is sensitive to it. Parenteral rather than oral therapy is always indicated for staphylococcal pneumonia. Twelve to eighteen grams of methicillin, or 6 to 12 gm of oxacillin,

nafcillin, or cephalosporin, should be administered daily in four to six divided doses. Intravenous administration may be used to circumvent the discomfort of the frequent intramuscular injections of large volumes of antibiotic. Probenecid (Benemid), 0.5 gm every 6 hours, decreases renal excretion of the penicillins and doubles their blood levels.

Ampicillin, 100 mg per kilogram of body weight; tetracycline, 50 to 75 mg per kilogram; or chloramphenicol in a similar dose should be given in infections due to *H. influenzae* in children. Tetracycline or erythromycin, 500 mg every 6 hours, are the agents of choice for adults with severe *Mycoplasma* pneumonia, although many such patients do not require any antibiotic therapy. Acute tuberculous pneumonia is treated with a combination of these drugs: isonicotinic acid hydrazide (INH), 5 mg per kilogram in a single dose; ethambutol, 15 mg per kilogram in a single daily dose; and streptomycin, 1 gm per day.

Complete bed rest is preferable for patients with pneumonia. Arterial gases are measured, and oxygen is administered to correct severe hypoxemia. When respiratory failure occurs, as indicated by marked tachypnea and an inability to produce Pa_{O_2} values of 50 mm Hg (except by using inspired oxygen concentrations greater than 75 percent), mechanical assistance to ventilation is used.

Severe pleural pain may be benefited by the judicious use of small amounts of narcotics, but intercostal nerve block may provide a more satisfactory method of managing it. Pleural effusions are tapped, and when secondary to a pneumonia caused by a penicillin-sensitive organism are simultaneously treated by 100,000 units of penicillin bacteria instilled intrapleurally. When empyema is present, daily thoracocentesis with complete removal of the fluid and daily instillation of penicillin are indicated. Failure to respond to such therapy is an indication for surgical drainage.

The overall fatality rate of pneumococcal pneumonia is less than 5 percent. In general, elderly patients and those with involvement of more than one lobe, with complicating diseases, with leukopenia, or in whom treatment has been delayed have a poorer prognosis. The mortality rate in patients with Friedländer's pneumonia has been reduced from 80 percent to approximately 40 percent with adequate antimicrobial therapy, but abscess formation, cavitation, and loss of pulmonary parenchymal tissue are still frequent. Care must be taken to rule out complications that accompany or follow pneumonia — for example, empyema, lung abscess, meningitis, pericarditis, endocarditis, otitis media, and purulent arthritis. These complications are frequently heralded by failure to respond or by a temporary defervescence followed by a secondary temperature elevation. Therefore failure of a temperature response or recurrence of fever in a patient with proved pneumococcal pneumonia should never be considered simply as due to failure of penicillin therapy and as an indication to change to another antibiotic. In such cases a careful search must be made to rule out an incorrect diagnosis, the presence of one of the above complications, or a superinfection with other bacteria.

Lung Abscess

Lung abscesses are areas of tissue necrosis that develop in circumscribed suppurative inflammatory processes of the lung. Aspiration of oropharyngeal secretions is the usual precipitating event, but embolization of infected material to the lung also may lead to abscess formation. Bronchial obstruction such as that caused by bronchogenic carcinoma predisposes to abscess formation. In the past, lung abscess was a frequent complication of surgical procedures such as dental extractions, tonsillectomies, and operations on the paranasal sinuses; but improved surgical and anesthetic techniques have resulted in the virtual disappearance of this complication. Currently, aspiration resulting from alcoholic stupor, grand mal seizures, or diminished consciousness from central nervous system disease, drug overdose, or metabolic abnormalities constitute the most frequent settings leading to a lung abscess.

The usual causative agents of bacterial pneumonia rarely cause lung abscess. Instead, the most frequent agents are mixtures of anaerobic bacteria, *Bacteroides fragilis, B. melaninogenicus, Fusobacterium nucleatum, F. necrophorum,* and microaerophilic streptococci such as the normal constituents of the oral flora. Initially the process begins as a localized pneumonitis; it then rapidly progresses to tissue necrosis and abscess

formation. The posterior segments of the upper lobe and the superior segments of the lower lobe are the most frequent locations, and the right lung is affected more often than the left.

Clinical manifestations consist of progressive fever, malaise, and cough following the initiating event. After 4 to 5 days fever becomes more marked, pleuritic chest pain may appear, and the cough may become productive of copious quantities of purulent sputum that is often foul smelling and may be blood streaked. Physical findings are similar to those observed in bacterial pneumonia. Chest x-rays early in the disease reveal segmental or lobar consolidation in the areas described above. This consolidation subsequently assumes a circular shape with central necrosis and cavitation, often with an air-fluid level. The wall is considerably thicker than that observed with a simple cyst, and there is evidence of inflammatory reaction in the surrounding lung parenchyma. The air-fluid level fluctuates with the adequacy of drainage through the bronchus. Evidence of empyema also may be observed. Leukocytosis is usual. Clubbing of the fingers may be observed, but this is more frequent in chronic lung abscesses. In some instances the disease may pursue a more insidious and chronic course, and underlying bronchogenic carcinoma should then be given even stronger consideration.

DIAGNOSIS

Accurate diagnosis of lung abscess is dependent on a combination of the history and physical findings, chest x-ray, and examination of the sputum. The usual putrid odor of the sputum strongly suggests anaerobic infection. On microscopic examination the sputum is seen to be packed with polymorphonuclear leukocytes and large numbers of bacteria of varying morphology. Chains of small cocci and pleomorphic, slender, gram-negative bacilli are usually present in large numbers. Since the usual etiologic agents are normal constituents of the oral flora, culture of expectorated sputum is of little diagnostic value; specimens obtained by transtracheal aspiration are essential for adequate bacteriologic cultures. These specimens should be immediately placed under anaerobic conditions and promptly transported to the laboratory for anaerobic culture. Such anaerobic cultures are not usually necessary for effective patient management. Bronchoscopy plays an important role in ruling out obstructing lesions. Sputum should also be collected for cytologic studies for malignant cells. The large numbers of inflammatory cells in early sputum specimens often hamper the finding of malignant cells; hence cytologic examination of the sputum should be repeated after subsidence of inflammatory cells in the sputum.

A number of aerobic bacteria and fungi may produce cavitary lesions or multiple small abscesses. These are usually readily distinguishable from aerobic lung abscess on the basis of the clinical course and laboratory findings. Tuberculosis, histoplasmosis, and coccidioidomycosis also cause cavity lesions that may be diagnosed by culture of the etiologic agent or by serologic tests. Staphylococcal pneumonia, Friedländer's *(K. pneumoniae)* pneumonia, and pneumonias caused by *P. aeruginosa* and other gram-negative bacilli are necrotizing in nature and may cause small abscesses. These are often multiple, appear relatively later in the course of disease than in anaerobic lung abscesses, and are readily identifiable by microscopic examination and culture of the sputum. *Actinomyces* and *Nocardia* also may cause chronic necrotizing pneumonia with abscess formation. Bacteremia with *S. aureus* and species of *Bacteroides* may produce embolic pulmonary abscesses. These embolic lesions first appear as 1- to 3-cm pulmonary nodules that progress to central necrosis. Infection in a previously unrecognized lung cyst can pursue a course similar to that of lung abscess and make differentiation difficult.

TREATMENT

Penicillin in doses of 3 million units or greater per day has been a strikingly effective agent for the treatment of anaerobic pneumonia and lung abscess. Clindamycin is an effective alternative in patients allergic to penicillin. Defervescence usually occurs over a period of 3 to 7 days, while diminution of sputum purulence and volume is more prolonged. One of the most impressive indices of the effectiveness of therapy is the rapid disappearance of the foul odor of the sputum, which usually occurs within 12 to 24 hours after the initiation of appropriate antibiotics.

Occasionally fever may recur as a result of inadequate drainage of the lesion, and it is usually associated with a diminution in sputum volume and an increase in the amount of fluid within the abscess. If adequate drainage cannot be reestablished by postural drainage, vigorous suctioning, and physical therapy, bronchoscopy is often effective. Progressive diminution in the surrounding inflammatory response and the size of the cavity occurs within a week, but closure of the cavity may not be complete for several months.

Bibliography

Bartlett, J. G., and Finegold, S. M. Anaerobic pleuropulmonary infections. *Medicine* 51:413, 1972.

Denny, F. W., Clyde, W. A., Jr., and Glezen, W. P. *Mycoplasma pneumoniae* disease: Clinical spectrum, pathophysiology, epidemiology, and control. *J. Infect. Dis.* 123:74, 1971.

Dowling, H. F. (with the collaboration of L. K. Sweet and H. L. Hirsch). *Acute Bacterial Diseases: Their Diagnosis and Treatment.* Philadelphia: Saunders, 1948.

Fenner, F. J., and White, D. O. *Medical Virology* (2nd ed.). New York: Academic, 1976.

12

Tuberculosis and Other Mycobacterial Diseases

Martin L. Spivack

Although tuberculosis has afflicted man since biblical times, many of the current concepts of its epidemiology and pathogenesis have been clarified only in the past few decades, and control of the disease has been possible only since about 1950 with the introduction of effective chemotherapeutic agents.

Pathogenesis

Primary tuberculous infection occurs in the nonimmune host after inhalation of a sufficient number of tubercle bacilli *(Mycobacterium tuberculosis)* suspended in the form of droplet nuclei of respirable size (1 to 5 µm). The initial exudative inflammatory response in the lung is characterized by an outpouring of protein-rich fluid with polymorphonuclear and monocytic phagocytes. Alveolar architecture is preserved. Coincident with the development of hypersensitivity, caseation necrosis and granuloma formation develop. The roentgenographic picture of primary pulmonary tuberculosis is distinctive: a subpleural, midlung zone infiltrate with hilar and mediastinal lymph node enlargement (the primary or Gohn complex). In the majority of infected people, the primary lesions do not cavitate but go on to heal, leaving at most a fleck of calcium in the lungs and regional nodes. In a few cases, particularly in children under age 6, primary infection may evolve directly into progressive primary disease with cavity formation in the lung and widespread organ involvement.

At some point in the primary infection, organisms reach the lymphatics and blood and disseminate throughout the body. Most are killed, but a few organisms may survive in a dormant state for months to years, providing a nidus for later reactivation. The lung itself is seeded with tubercle bacilli during this phase. Most organisms are removed without producing roentgenographically visible lesions; however, those arriving in the apical and posterior segments of the upper lobes commonly produce small caseous foci that either heal without visible scars or leave small residuals (Simon foci). There is substantial evidence that the upper lung zones are more susceptible to tuberculous disease because in upright man in this region there is a higher alveolar oxygen partial pressure resulting from the high ventilation-perfusion relationship. The typical adult type of reactivation or postprimary pulmonary tuberculosis may occur at any time in a patient's life after primary infection. Classically the residual foci in the posterior segments of the upper lobes of the lung become activated, producing the granulomatous lesions with caseation necrosis and cavitary disease that most physicians recognize by x-ray as characteristic of tuberculosis. It should be kept in mind, however, that the deep mycoses (histoplasmosis, coccidioidomycosis, and blastomycosis) as well as the atypical mycobacteria may produce identical roentgenographic lesions. Exogenous reinfection in people previously infected by tubercle bacilli is a rare event. Reactivation of latent foci may occur at any site seeded during the primary spread. It is for this reason that organ tuberculosis (renal, bone, lymph nodes, etc.) frequently occurs in the absence of an active pulmonary lesion. Breakdown of a caseous focus in any organ, but particularly in lymph nodes, may result in spread through the lymphatics into the bloodstream and lead to widespread (miliary) disease.

Pleural effusion develops in about 25 percent of primary infections. It is believed that this is the result of the rupture of a small subpleural focus emptying its contents into the pleural space. Both visceral and parietal pleura become studded with granulomas, and an exudative, lymphocyte-rich effusion evolves. The available evidence suggests that these effusions are manifestations of a hypersensitivity reaction on the pleural surface. The process may be totally silent or may cause pleurisy or dyspnea, bringing the patient to medical attention. Most tuberculous pleural effusions subside spontaneously, but they are of great clinical importance, since 30 percent of patients will develop active pulmonary or extrapulmonary disease within 5 years.

Immunity and Tuberculin Hypersensitivity

When tubercle bacilli are inhaled they undergo phagocytosis by alveolar macrophages, and in the nonimmune host, the bacilli multiply within these cells. Sometime within 3 to 6 weeks after infection cellular immunity develops, so that the macrophages are "activated" and are capable of not only phagocytizing but also of killing the organisms. Coincident with the development of cellular immunity, the delayed type of skin hypersensitivity to tuberculoprotein can be demonstrated. There is good reason to doubt whether allergy to tuberculoprotein can be equated with immunity, but there is little question that both phenomena most often coexist and are manifestations of an activated T-lymphocyte system.

Purified protein derivative (PPD) of tuberculin, a crude culture filtrate of *M. tuberculosis,* is now the standard substance used in intradermal testing. The classic (Mantoux) test is carried out by the intradermal injection of 0.1 ml of PPD containing 5 tuberculin units (TU) (intermediate strength) and then measuring the diameter of induration produced 48 to 72 hours later. A reaction of less than 5 mm is considered negative, 5 to 10 mm doubtful, and more than 10 mm positive. A positive tuberculin skin test indicates tuberculous infection, with or without disease (Table 12-1). First-strength PPD (1 TU) was developed to avoid severe reactions to the 5-TU test in very sensitive patients. Since a severe reaction rarely happens and the number of false-negative tests is high, this material should not be used. Second-strength PPD (250 TU) is of limited usefulness, since nonspecific cross reactions to the atypical mycobacteria are common.

For undefined reasons, 10 to 25 percent of patients with active tuberculosis will have negative intermediate-strength skin tests when first seen. False-negative reactions may also be caused by inability of the patient to react due to an abnormality in his T-lymphocyte system. Such anergy is seen in miliary or overwhelming tuberculosis, sarcoidosis, Hodgkin's disease, advanced age, malnutrition, recent viral infection, or in patients under treatment with immunosuppressive drugs (see Chap. 44).

Atypical Mycobacterial Infection

Before proceeding, it is necessary to describe the current understanding of atypical mycobacterial disease and its epidemiologic interrelationships with

Table 12-1. The Classification of Tuberculosis[*]

Class	Definition
0	No tuberculous exposure, not infected
I	Tuberculous exposure, no evidence of infection
II	Tuberculous infection, without disease (positive tuberculin test, no evidence of disease; treated or untreated)
III	Tuberculous infection with disease (described by organ location, bacteriologic status, roentgenographic findings, and tuberculin skin test; treated or untreated)
Tuberculosis suspect	A temporary classification while evaluation is underway

[*] Adapted from Diagnostic Standards and Classification of Tuberculosis and Other Mycobacterial Diseases, American Lung Association, 1974.

typical tuberculosis. The existence of atypical mycobacteria had been known for many years, but their etiologic role in human disease was not appreciated until 1951. In 1959 Runyon published the scheme of classification (Table 12-2) in use today. The prevalence of skin hypersensitivity to these organisms was revealed by large-scale tuberculin testing, using antigens prepared from each group. Fifty to seventy percent of young adults from the southeastern United States reacted to PPD-B; and while hypersensitivity to PPD-Y was widespread, it was most frequent in Illinois, Kansas, and Texas. Cross reactions occurred between the skin test antigens made from atypical mycobacteria and antigens derived from *M. tuberculosis* (PPD-S). Thus in areas of the country in which hypersensitivity to atypical mycobacteria is frequent, reactions to PPD-S of less than 10 mm usually represent cross hypersensitivity to atypical organisms. The epidemiology of atypical mycobacterial infections is not clear. Case-to-case spread of disease has never been proved; hence it is assumed that infection is acquired from the environment, most likely the soil. Because of this, isolation of hospitalized patients is not necessary.

Disease due to *M. kansasii* and *M. intracellularis* can mimic in every way that due to *M. tuberculosis.*

Table 12-2. Atypical Mycobacteria Classification[*]

Runyon group	Skin test antigen	Proper name	Associated disease states
Group I (photochromogens)	PPD-Y	M. kansasii	Cavity pulmonary and disseminated disease
		M. marinum (balnei)	Skin infection (swimming pool granuloma)
Group II (scotochromogens)	PPD-G	M. scrofulaceum	Cervical adenitis
		Tap water organisms, no proper name	
Group III (nonphoto chromogens)	PPD-B	M. intracellularis (Battey bacillus)	Cavity pulmonary and disseminated disease
		M. avium	Cervical adenitis
		M. xenopi	Rare pulmonary disease
Group IV (rapid growers)	–	M. fortuitum	Skin lesions; rare pulmonary disease
		M. chelonei (abscessus)	Rare pulmonary disease
Bovine tuberculosis	–	M. bovis	Uncommon; adenitis and systemic disease

[*]Adapted from E. H. Runyon, Anonymous mycobacteria in pulmonary disease. *Med. Clin. North Am.* 43:273, 1959.

In addition to pulmonary disease, disseminated disease, particularly of bone, has been described. The atypical mycobacteria tend to be resistant to the usual antituberculosis drugs, although *M. kansasii* is strikingly sensitive to rifampin. Treatment frequently requires combinations of four to five drugs, but it must be individualized based on the results of sensitivity testing. Surgical resection of involved lung may be necessary when effective chemotherapy is unavailable.

Epidemiology
In the United States tuberculosis has become a disease of the middle and later years of life, occurring for the most part in people from the urban centers of the country. In 1973 the U.S. Public Health Service estimated that 7 percent of the population had been infected with the tubercle bacillus as indicated by a positive tuberculin test. Seventy percent of these 15 million people were over age 35, with the peak prevalence being in the 55- to 59-year age group. Only 5 percent were under age 25. This was a complete reversal of the situation that existed from 1900 to the 1930s, when tuberculous infection was common early in life, with positive skin reactivity by age 20 present in more than 80 percent of the population. At that time, active disease and death occurred most frequently in children under age 5, during adolescence, and in early adulthood. Presently only 0.2 percent of first graders and 0.7 percent of high school students are tuberculin positive. The slow decline in the prevalence of tuberculosis prior to the advent of chemotherapy was attributed to improved standards of living and the removal of active cases from the community through sanatorium care. The pace of this decline quickened markedly after the introduction of effective chemotherapeutic agents.

Where are the new cases of tuberculosis coming from now? Figure 12-1 graphically depicts the situation as it existed in 1971. A number of facts become obvious from these data:

1. Among 190 million Americans, 70,000 previously uninfected (tuberculin negative) became infected, that is, converted their skin tests to positive; and of these, 3,000 developed active disease. Thus the

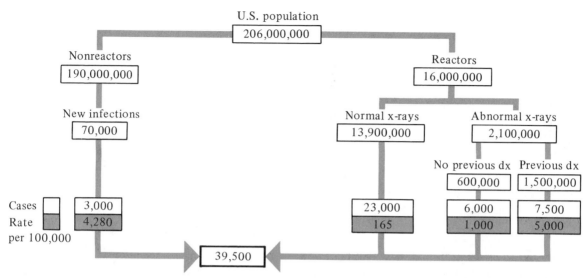

Figure 12-1. Schema of tuberculosis epidemiology in the United States of America in 1971. [Reprinted with permission from Tuberculosis Programs 1972, *DHEW Publication No. (CDC) 74-8189. See text for discussion.]*

risk of becoming infected if an individual is previously uninfected is low (1 in 2,850), *but* the risk of developing active disease within a few years after tuberculin conversion is high (1 in 25).

2. The bulk of tuberculosis cases arises in the population with positive skin tests and normal chest x-rays, even though the attack rate of active disease in this group is low (1 in 600).

3. A positive skin test in association with an abnormal chest x-ray carries a much greater risk of reactivation (1 in 100 to 200).

Further attempts to reduce the number of new active cases of tuberculosis must take these facts into account.

Diagnosis of Tuberculosis

The new classification of tuberculosis developed by the American Lung Association in 1974 (see Table 12-1) makes a clear distinction between tuberculous exposure, tuberculous infection, and the disease tuberculosis. *Infection* means that at some time in the past the tubercle bacillus became established in the body (a tuberculin skin test is positive). A defi-

nite diagnosis of tuberculous disease due to *M. tuberculosis* depends on the isolation of this bacillus from secretions or tissues in association with a compatible roentgenographic, clinical, or pathologic picture. Since culture takes 3 to 12 weeks, the presence of acid-fast bacilli in the sputum and a suggestive roentgenogram are considered sufficient evidence on which to institute therapy. In tissue specimens, the finding of caseating granuloma with demonstrable acid-fast bacilli is also acceptable for diagnosis; the finding of caseating granuloma without acid-fast bacilli is less certain.

A patient with tuberculous pulmonary disease will come to the physician for one of three reasons: (1) suggestive symptoms; (2) a positive finding on routine tuberculin testing; or (3) a suspicious routine chest roentgenogram. In each situation it is the x-ray that alerts the physician to proceed in obtaining further studies. However, about a third of the cases will be radiologically atypical, showing midzone, lower lobe, or diffuse pulmonary infiltrates rather than typical upper lobe cavitary disease. Therefore the physician's index of suspicion with regard to tuberculosis should remain high in evaluating any pulmonary process of undefined etiology.

Symptoms of tuberculous disease are variable. Primary infection often either is asymptomatic or causes such mild constitutional symptoms that the patient does not seek attention. The typical adult type of reactivation tuberculosis starts insidiously over weeks to months with anorexia, weight loss, fevers, night sweats, and increasing cough and sputum production. Hemoptysis and pleurisy are less frequent. In older patients the physician may interpret these symptoms as suggestive of malignancy. Laboratory findings are nonspecific, with anemia, elevated sedimentation rate, leukocytosis, and monocytosis being variably present.

ORGAN TUBERCULOSIS

A brief overview of the diagnosis of tuberculous disease in extrapulmonary sites is presented below. The student is referred to specialized texts for more detailed descriptions.

Tuberculous pleural effusion is seen both in children and adults; any exudative pleural effusion with lymphocyte predominance is suspect. Smears are positive in less than 20 percent, and cultures are positive in less than 50 percent. A needle biopsy of the pleura should be done; it will demonstrate a granuloma or positive culture in 75 percent of cases. By combining histology and culture, diagnostic yields as high as 93 percent have been reported.

Peritoneal tuberculosis, particularly in alcoholic patients with ascites, may present in an insidious manner. Most of these patients have peritoneal fluid protein contents greater than 2.5 gm per 100 ml and cell counts greater than 250 per cubic millimeter with lymphocyte predominance; acid-fast bacilli are rarely seen, and cultures are positive in only about 50 percent. Needle biopsy of the peritoneum may reveal granuloma; and peritoneoscopy, when available, is usually diagnostic.

Meningeal tuberculosis in adults is only rarely associated with active pulmonary disease, but even in children as many as 50 percent may have normal x-rays. The disease starts insidiously with headache and low-grade fever. After 1 or 2 weeks, mental status may alter and ocular palsies, particularly of the sixth nerve, are common. Diagnosis before the onset of coma is essential, as a successful outcome depends primarily on early treatment. Evaluation of the cerebrospinal fluid should be carried out at the earliest possible time; elevated protein (100 to 300 mg per 100 ml) with lymphocytes predominating and a

low cerebrospinal fluid glucose are sufficient evidence to start the patient on antituberculosis therapy while a vigorous search for fungi (cryptococci particularly) and other causative agents is continued. Acid-fast bacilli are visualized microscopically in only 10 percent, but cultures should be positive in 60 to 80 percent of cases.

Renal tuberculosis is perhaps the most insidious form of tuberculosis. Organisms seeded to the kidney during the primary lymphohematogenous dissemination form small cortical abscesses that may heal; but some settle in the medulla, where large, caseous excavations develop. Spread down the ureters may infect the ureters, prostate, testes, and epididymis. The process of renal destruction usually proceeds silently for years, until the patient presents with a totally destroyed kidney. Ureteral fibrosis with stricture and secondary hydronephrosis may predominate. Silent "sterile" pyuria and hematuria remain the key to alerting the physician to the diagnosis. Cultures of early morning urine for *M. tuberculosis* are usually positive, and intravenous pyelography showing medullary necrosis and ureteral strictures is highly suggestive. Acid-fast stains of urine may be falsely positive, but in the appropriate setting they should not be ignored.

Vertebral tuberculosis is frequently misdiagnosed during the early months of the disease. Systemic manifestations of infection can be minimal, and x-rays may demonstrate only rarification of the superior or inferior margins of the vertebral body with slight narrowing of the disk space. Eventually the disk space is destroyed, and one or more vertebral bodies collapse. Disk involvement is an important clue differentiating tuberculosis from neoplasm. Spinal cord involvement and a cold abscess in the paraspinal region are possible complications. In the absence of associated pulmonary tuberculosis, bone biopsy or aspiration of the abscess is necessary for definitive diagnosis.

Tuberculous pericarditis begins slowly with mild anterior chest pain, low-grade fever and sweats, and eventually dyspnea on exertion as the pericardial effusion begins to interfere with cardiac output (see Chap. 33). This insidious presentation contrasts with the more dramatic and sudden onset of severe pain found in viral pericarditis. The pericardial fluid is a lymphocyte-rich exudate in which acid-fast bacilli are rarely seen. These clinical findings in association with a positive tuberculin skin test provide adequate presumptive evidence on which to start treatment. A definitive diagnosis may require pericardial biopsy.

Miliary tuberculosis has changed strikingly since the introduction of chemotherapy. It was once chiefly a complication of progressive primary disease in children, but it has now become a disease of middle and late life. The diagnosis may be unsuspected if miliary shadows are not present on the roentgenogram. Other indications of miliary spread include choroidal tubercles, which have been uncommon in recent series, and hepatosplenomegaly, adenopathy, and skin lesions, which are only variably present in adults. Headache is an ominous sign suggesting tuberculous meningitis. Anemia is common, and pancytopenia or a leukemoid reaction may be present if the bone marrow is involved. Sputum smears are positive in only 25 percent of patients, and cultures are positive in 50 to 60 percent. Liver, bone marrow, and transbronchoscopic lung biopsy are excellent techniques to establish the diagnosis.

Principles of Chemotherapy

The institution of a good drug regimen followed for a significant period of time is the dominant factor in curing tuberculous disease. Failure of chemotherapy is due either to the emergence of resistant organisms or to failure of the patient to take the drugs. When drugs are taken faithfully, a successful outcome can be anticipated in 95 percent of patients with a very low relapse rate.

Isoniazid (INH) is a highly effective chemotherapeutic agent against *M. tuberculosis.* Isoniazid-resistant mutants occur spontaneously about once in every 10^6 organisms, and since bacterial populations in cavitary disease may reach 10^8 or 10^9 organisms per gram of tissue, the likelihood of their presence is great. Use of INH alone would suppress the INH-sensitive bacilli, while allowing resistant organisms to flourish. This concept has led to the use of *two-phase chemotherapy,* which begins with an early intensive phase using three drugs for 60 to 90 days to prevent the emergence of INH-resistant bacilli and is followed

by a regimen of two drugs for 18 to 24 months to eradicate the persisting drug-sensitive organisms.

Currently the standard initial treatment program in adults consists of INH, 300 mg, and ethambutol, 15 mg per kilogram of body weight, given as a single dose once daily. In patients with cavitary disease, streptomycin, 1 gm daily, is added for the first 60 to 90 days. All forms of tuberculosis including meningitis can be effectively treated with this standard regimen. Rifampin is a highly effective antituberculosis drug that is used by some groups in combinations with INH in initial treatment regimens. The second-line drugs, pyrazinamide, para-aminosalicylic acid (PAS), ethionamide, cycloserine, viomycin, and kanamycin, are used in special circumstances based on resistance studies. Since the major problem in treating tuberculosis is poor compliance with the drug regimen on the part of the patients, attempts to find alternative treatment programs continue. Twice-weekly monitored chemotherapy and short-course chemotherapy regimens are currently in use or are under study.

DRUG TOXICITY

Since the inception of chemotherapy for tuberculosis, drug reactions due to hypersensitivity and direct toxicity have been a problem. Streptomycin carries a risk of ototoxicity involving the vestibular mechanism, may produce nephrotoxicity, and can cause eosinophilia, with or without drug fever and rash. Two second-line drugs, pyrazinamide and ethionamide, were placed in that category because of their risk of hepatotoxicity, and cycloserine may produce serious psychosis and seizures. Ethambutol in doses greater than 15 mg per kilogram can lead to optic atrophy that may be irreversible.

It is clear that INH is a direct hepatotoxin; in the first 90 days of treatment, 10 to 15 percent of patients have rises in serum glutamic oxaloacetic transaminase (SGOT). The vast majority of these will be asymptomatic, and their liver function tests will return to normal despite continued therapy; a small percentage become jaundiced with symptoms suggesting hepatitis. If the drug is continued in the face of clinical hepatitis, fatal hepatic damage may ensue. Serious hepatotoxicity is rare in children but is a problem in persons over 35, particularly if alcohol is used excessively.

Rifampin also appears to possess hepatotoxicity, and its combination with INH has raised concern. However, the administration of these two drugs together does not seem to cause abnormal liver function tests more frequently than either one alone, even in patients with abnormal tests at the beginning of therapy. Acute allergic reactions to rifampin may also occur, particularly when the drug is used in intermittent chemotherapy regimens.

ISONIAZID PREVENTIVE THERAPY VERSUS BCG IMMUNIZATION

Loud and sometimes bitter arguments rage among public health authorities on the relative merits of preventive chemotherapy versus immunization. The BCG (bacille Calmette-Guerin) vaccine contains viable attenuated bacilli. When inoculated into tuberculin-negative individuals, a self-limited infection occurs resulting in tuberculin conversion. Some studies have demonstrated protection in the range of 80 percent, while others, most notably those conducted under the auspices of the U.S. Public Health Service, have shown little protection. A glance at Figure 12-1 suggests to the unbiased observer that if less than 10 percent of all active cases of tuberculosis arise in the United States among tuberculin-negative people, it makes no sense to immunize 95 percent of the population to prevent this small risk. However, in areas in which tuberculous infection remains in the 70- to 90-percent range by age 20, widespread use of an effective vaccine in children might have a dramatic impact.

Isoniazid preventive therapy (chemoprophylaxis) has been widely used in the United States. If the drug were totally without toxicity, it would be a simple matter to treat the 16 million tuberculin-positive people in this country in an attempt to eradicate the disease. However, since hepatotoxicity is major, one must select for treatment only those individuals at highest risk. Table 12-3 lists the groups currently recommended by the U.S. Public Health Service and the American Thoracic Society to receive preventive therapy.

It should be understood that this form of treatment is in fact full and effective therapy for minimal

Table 12-3. Isoniazid Preventive Therapy[*]

Candidates for chemoprophylaxis	Risk of developing tuberculous disease
1. Household contacts	2.5 percent in first year; 5.0 percent if tuberculin positive
2. Tuberculin converters	5 percent in first year after conversion
3. Positive tuberculin test, abnormal chest x-ray — previously untreated	1.0—2.0 percent per year
4. Positive tuberculin test in children under age 6	5—10 percent
5. Positive reactors, age 6—35 (relative indication), but normal chest x-ray	Variable
6. Special circumstances — positive tuberculin test in patients on adrenal corticoids or immunosuppressive therapy, with hematologic malignancy, diabetes mellitus, silicosis, or gastrectomy	Unknown but increased

[*]Current recommendations of the U.S. Public Health Service and the American Thoracic Society.

noncavitary tuberculous disease where bacterial populations are small and the presence of resistant organisms unlikely. A large amount of data has been accumulated to show that INH chemoprophylaxis will produce a decrease in active cases by some 75 to 90 percent; the major effect is noted within the first 2 years of treatment, and some protection extends to at least 10 years.

Prolonged rest is unimportant as treatment for tuberculosis, provided the patient follows an effective chemotherapeutic regimen for a sufficient period of time. Patients are hospitalized in a general hospital to carry out diagnostic studies, to treat symptoms due to the disease or complicating illnesses, and to start appropriate therapy; the only isolation required is a private room with an appropriate air flow system. The patient should be counseled on the communicable nature of his disease and its mechanism of spread.

A simple mask is adequate for the patient to travel within the hospital. Once chemotherapy is instituted, the number of viable bacilli in the sputum falls off rapidly and contagiousness decreases. After 2 to 3 weeks the patient may return home, even if his sputum continues to show acid-fast bacilli. His family is not at risk, because heavy, prolonged exposure has already occurred prior to the detection of the patient's disease. All exposed family members should have tuberculin tests and chest x-rays and those at greatest risk should be placed on INH preventive therapy. There is no evidence that prolonged hospital care leads to better adherence to a drug regimen by the recalcitrant patient. Early hospital discharge, however, does not obviate the need for an effective ambulatory care program to monitor the patient's clinical progress and chemotherapy regimen. Once treatment has been completed, lifelong follow-up in tuberculosis clinics as formerly practiced is unnecessary. Patients should be discharged from care and told to return promptly if any pulmonary or systemic symptoms of recurrent disease are noted.

Bibliography

Fraser, R. G., and Pare, J. A. P. *Diagnosis of Diseases of the Chest.* Philadelphia: Saunders, 1970.

Johnston, R. F., and Wildrick, K. H. The impact of chemotherapy on the care of patients with tuberculosis. *Am. Rev. Respir Dis.* 109:636, 1974.

Wolinsky, E. Non-tuberculous mycobacterial infections of man. *Med. Clin. North Am.* 58:639, 1974.

13

The Mycoses

M. Anees Khan and Gordon L. Snider

Advances in epidemiology over the past 30 years, improvement in histopathologic and immunodiagnostic techniques, and the emergence of amphotericin B and other potent antifungal agents have greatly increased medical awareness of systemic fungal infections. On the other hand, the widespread use of corticosteroids, ionizing irradiation, and immunosuppressive and cytotoxic agents has greatly increased the invasiveness of fungi, which are ubiquitous in nature. For these reasons, fungal infections are likely to continue to be of great medical concern.

It is clinically helpful to separate the fungi that produce human disease into two groups. (1) The opportunistic fungi, such as *Aspergillus* and *Candida* species, are widespread in nature and are usual inhabitants of the mouth or other body cavities. These organisms invade and produce disease only in compromised hosts. (2) Primary pathogenic fungi, such as *Histoplasma capsulatum, Coccidioides immitis, Blastomyces dermatiditis,* and *Nocardia asteroides,* on the other hand, are comparatively restricted in their distribution and are never found in man as opportunistic invaders; their presence indicates infection or disease.

Most of the primary pathogenic fungi have a number of other features in common. The usual reservoirs for these organisms are the soil, decaying vegetable material, or bird excreta. They are usually not transmitted from man to man or animal to man; the portal of entry is usually the respiratory tract, and the tissue response is usually granulomatous. Finally, delayed cutaneous hypersensitivity as well as circulating antibodies are demonstrable in many of these infections.

HISTOPLASMOSIS

Histoplasmosis is a systemic fungal disease caused by *H. capsulatum.* The process may be asymptomatic; it may be acute, self-limited, and benign; or it may be chronic, progressive, disseminated, and fatal. *Histoplasma capsulatum* is a dimorphic fungus found in filamentous form in soil, especially that contaminated with bird or bat excreta; conversion into the yeast form occurs after entry into animal tissues. The infection is acquired in both animals and man by inhalation of spores that multiply within the mononuclear cells of the reticulendothelial system and spread through the lymphatics and the bloodstream to mediastinal lymph nodes, spleen, liver, adrenal glands, gastrointestinal tract, kidneys, skin and mucous membranes, heart, and other organs. The disease is not transmissible from man to man.

Histoplasmosis is a widely disseminated disease in North America and has been reported in many other countries in South and Central America, India, and the Far East. It is rare in Europe, Australia, England, and Japan. The highest endemicity in North America is in the Ohio, Mississippi, and St. Lawrence river valleys, where as high as 80 percent of the population may be infected. Localized epidemics of acute histoplasmosis have occurred in persons exposed to infectious soil from areas of bird or bat roosting or from buildings heavily contaminated with pigeon or chicken excreta.

The organism produces a granulomatous reaction, sometimes with caseation necrosis, and healing is by fibrosis or resolution. Calcification is very frequent, especially in lesions in lungs, lymph nodes, and spleen.

Clinical Manifestations

The clinical and roentgenographic manifestations are related to the size of the infecting dose. However, infants, the elderly, patients with lymphoma, or patients receiving corticosteroids are more likely to have a virulent form of the disease.

In low-dose infections, the primary focus in the lungs may be either not demonstrable or evident as a single parenchymal focus, with or without a nodal component. This resembles the primary tuberculous focus and goes on to either resolution or calcification in a high proportion of cases. Symptoms are mild or absent. Residual solitary, or rarely, multiple circumscribed granulomas (histoplasmomas) may mimic neoplasms.

High-dose infections, on the other hand, are characterized by varying degrees of fever, prostration, cough, dyspnea, pleuritic chest pain, and weight loss. Bilateral diffuse nodular infiltration may be noted in the chest roentgenogram, or there may be homogeneous parenchymal consolidation of a nonsegmental distribution. Hilar adenopathy is often present. The multinodular lesions either regress slowly or calcify. Disseminated, severe disease occurs in a small minority of those infected by *H. capsulatum*. All the organs of the body may become involved; adrenal gland involvement leading to hypoadrenalism is well known, and there is a high incidence of splenic calcification.

Histoplasmosis also may present as chronic cavitary disease of the lungs, probably as a result of postprimary endogenous reactivation or progression. Fibrosing and cavitary lesions occur predominantly in the posterior segments of the upper lobes and are roentgenographically indistinguishable from tuberculosis; in fact, the two infections may coexist. This form of the disease is particularly apt to occur in men over age 40.

Calcified or fibrocaseous lymph nodes infected with *H. capsulatum* may compress or erode into bronchi or compress mediastinal structures. They may cause dysphagia as a result of esophageal involvement, and rarely, they may produce superior vena caval obstruction.

Diagnosis
The presence of hilar or parenchymal calcification in an individual who has lived in an endemic area and who is tuberculin negative suggests a past *Histoplasma* infection. This may be confirmed by a positive histoplasmin skin test in which 0.1 ml of 1 : 100 histoplasmin solution is injected intradermally; a positive reaction is indicated by a local induration of 5 mm or more after 48 hours. In some patients in whom active histoplasmosis is a diagnostic possibility, the histoplasmin skin test may only confuse the issue because the skin test may be negative in disseminated disease. Furthermore, the skin test may increase the level of complement-fixing antibodies to *Histoplasma* antigen in the serum, even when active disease is not present. Finally, the skin reaction to histoplasmin is not a highly specific one, as cross reactivity with coccidioidin and blastomycin are well known.

For these reasons, serologic tests must be used for confirmation and many clinics have stopped using the histoplasmin skin test in routine diagnostic work. Precipitin tests are positive after a recent infection but become negative within a few weeks. Comple-

ment-fixing antibodies to both yeast- and mycelial-phase antigens become positive about 1 month after infection. Values of 1 : 8 for mycelial and 1 : 32 for yeast antigens are suggestive; a rising titer is stronger evidence of disease. A latex fixation test is also in use. Serologic tests are negative with most histoplasmomas; they are also negative in 25 percent of patients with chronic active pulmonary disease and 40 percent of patients with disseminated disease.

In disseminated and chronic cavitary forms of histoplasmosis, cultures of the sputum, urine, and bone marrow are helpful. The fungus may be identified in tissue biopsies with the periodic acid–Schiff (PAS) stain or with a silver impregnation method.

Treatment
Most infections are benign and self-limited. Chemotherapy with amphotericin B is indicated in severely ill patients, in patients with disseminated disease, or in patients before and after surgery for cavitary disease.

COCCIDIOIDOMYCOSIS
Coccidioidomycosis is a systemic fungus infection caused by the dimorphic organism *C. immitis,* which exists only in the mycelial phase in nature; infection is caused by inhalation of the airborne arthrospores. The organism then reproduces itself in tissues by endosporulation into spherules, which rupture and spread the infection either locally to adjacent structures or hematogenously to distant tissues. The disease is not transmissible from man to man; it is endemic in desert regions of the United States Southwest (California, Arizona, New Mexico, southern Utah, Nevada, and Texas) and also occurs in northern Mexico, Argentina, and Paraguay.

The lung is the primary site of infection. The initial polymorphonuclear response may arrest the infection completely, resulting in a small, inconsequential lesion. A granulomatous response may ensue, with giant cells, caseation, and cavitation and then spread to regional lymph nodes and the pleura. Among distant tissues, the skin, bone, and meninges are especially liable to involvement; the lesions may be both granulomatous and suppurative; spherules may be observed in the tissues. The lesions may ultimately heal by fibrosis or residual granulomatous nodules may mimic carcinoma.

Clinical Manifestations

Fifty percent of infections are asymptomatic. The majority of symptomatic infections present as an influenzalike illness with fever, backache, severe arthralgias, headache, and nondescript respiratory symptoms. Erythema nodosum is seen in 10 percent of patients. Roentgenographic abnormalities, which consist of focal infiltrates, hilar or mediastinal lymphadenopathy, nodules or cavities, and occasionally pleural effusion, usually resolve within several weeks. In some cases, however, a cavitary or nodular pulmonary lesion persists. A coccidioidal cavity is characteristically thin-walled and situated peripherally; such lesions are usually asymptomatic but occasionally may cause recurrent hemoptysis or may rupture into the pleural space and produce coccidioidal empyema.

Primary infection goes on to complete recovery in more than 50 percent of patients, continues as a chronic cavitary or nodular disease in 40 percent, and may progress to a disseminated form in a few patients. The risk of dissemination is said to be greater among blacks, American Indians, and Filipinos. The clinical picture then consists in fever, generalized weakness, and weight loss, accompanied by skin ulcerations as well as bone and meningeal involvement. Such a clinical course, if unattended, often culminates in death in less than a year.

Diagnosis

Roentgenographic evidence of hilar lymphadenopathy accompanied by multiple foci of infiltration or the presence of a thin-walled cavity without surrounding parenchymal disease in a patient who lives in or has visited an endemic area is highly suggestive of the diagnosis. An intradermal test with coccidioidin (1:100) is positive within several weeks of primary infection. In disseminated disease, however, the coccidioidin intradermal test may be negative.

Serologic tests are also helpful in establishing the diagnosis. The precipitin reaction becomes positive by the third week of primary infection and fades after several weeks. A titer of 1:16 or above is diagnostic of recent infection. Complement-fixing anti-bodies appear later and last longer; a titer of 1:32 suggests active disease, and a rising titer, especially above 1:64, suggests dissemination. *Coccidioides immitis* is easily recovered from the lesions by direct examination and cultures of exudates or biopsy materials. However, culture should be attempted only by experienced microbiologists because of the risk of laboratory dissemination.

Therapy

The disease is self-limited in most cases and does not require specific treatment. Intensive therapy with amphotericin B intravenously is indicated in severe infections with threatened or proved disseminated disease. Pulmonary resection is used for enlarging subpleural cavities and for recurrent hemoptysis. Appropriate tube drainage is helpful in treating empyema.

BLASTOMYCOSIS

Blastomycosis, a chronic systemic fungal infection caused by *B. dermatiditis,* is commonest by far in North, Central, and South America; it affects men much more often than women and is most frequent in the third and fourth decades of life. The infection is acquired by inhalation of the spherical forms (conidia) of the fungus, but the reservoir in nature, although thought to be the soil, is not certain.

The infection may be localized to the lung, or it may spread to the skin, bones, lymph nodes, liver, spleen, and central nervous and genitourinary systems. The characteristic histopathology seen in the lungs and other tissues is a combination of epithelioid and giant cell granulomatous inflammatory reaction and pyogenic abscess formation. Pulmonary lesions may vary in size from small nodules to diffuse pneumonitis; cavitation and calcification are distinctly uncommon. Marked epithelial cell hyperplasia is seen in skin lesions that simulate squamous cell carcinomas. The causative agent may be found in tissues as a budding yeast cell with a double-contoured, thick refractile wall. In culture the organism grows as a white mycelium producing smooth, spherical forms or conidia which, in contradistinction to the yeast phase, are infectious.

Clinical Manifestations

Benign subclinical cases are not well documented. However, in a recent outbreak of blastomycosis presumed due to a common source, 18 of 21 persons with repeated exposure developed evidence of infection by the fungus. Of the seven with symptoms, three were severely ill and four had a mild illness of short duration. An additional eleven asymptomatic persons were believed to have been infected on the basis of abnormalities in the chest roentgenogram or a positive blastomycin skin test or both. All the patients recovered without specific antifungal therapy. Thus it appears that human infection with *B. dermatiditis* is clinically similar in all aspects to histoplasmosis and coccidioidomycosis; "primary" pulmonary blastomycosis is an acute disease with a benign outcome.

The infection is usually insidious in onset, producing symptoms of low-grade fever, persistent cough, and weight loss. Chest roentgenograms may show evidence of pneumonitis. Single or widely disseminated nodular densities, usually without cavitation, are quite nonspecific. Bone lesions occur in 25 percent of patients, and skin ulcerations are as common as pulmonary disease. Most skin lesions probably represent dissemination from a pulmonary infection rather than direct cutaneous inoculation.

Diagnosis

No clinical or radiologic features are characteristic. In suspected cases, microscopic examination of the sputum or pus and histologic examination of biopsy material for the characteristic budding yeast with a double refractile wall should be made. *Blastomyces dermatiditis* can be isolated by culturing pus or sputum on Sabouraud agar at room temperature. Skin and serologic tests are of no value in the disseminated disease.

Treatment

A course of amphotericin B is the treatment of choice; 2-hydroxystilbamadine is less effective. Surgical resection of localized disease may sometimes be necessary.

CRYPTOCOCCOSIS

Cryptococcosis is a systemic fungus infection caused by *Cryptococcus neoformans,* a saprophytic spherical yeast with a thick mucopolysaccharide capsule that is found in the soil and bird droppings; the organism reproduces entirely by budding. In most cases the portal of entry is considered to be the respiratory tract, where the fungus characteristically disseminates to the central nervous system and occasionally to other viscera, skin, and bones. Pulmonary foci are often minor and produce no symptoms. Individuals with diabetes mellitus, lymphoma, and leukemia are particularly vulnerable to disease from *C. neoformans.* However, the disease is not transmissible from man to man. The inflammatory response to *C. neoformans* is characteristically scanty. Early lesions are rather gelatinous, owing to the presence of large masses of organisms. Older lesions show a granulomatous reaction with histiocytes, giant cells, and mononuclear cells. Necrosis is unusual.

Clinical Manifestations

Although the lungs are considered to be the portal of entry in most cases, clinical pulmonary disease is rarely seen. Most patients present only after the onset of neurologic manifestations, which consist of signs and symptoms of meningitis, meningoencephalitis, or a space-occupying intracranial lesion. Headaches are generally followed by slowly progressive malaise and fever with eventual appearance of vomiting, nuchal rigidity, and other manifestations of elevated intracranial tension; the course is rarely fulminant. Untreated cryptococcal meningitis usually terminates fatally within several months, although chronic infection lasting many years has been described. In chronic disease the neurologic manifestations are those of an intracranial lesion in about 25 percent of the patients.

Roentgenographic examination of the chest may reveal a localized, dense infiltrate in the lower lobes. Miliary infiltrates or solitary coin lesions may also occur, especially in the compromised host. Calcification or hilar lymphadenopathy is extremely rare. Because of its tendency to involve compromised hosts, cryptococcal disease should alert one to the possibility of underlying Hodgkin's disease, lymphoma, leukemia, or diabetes mellitus.

Diagnosis

The sediment from the centrifuged cerebrospinal fluid should be stained with india ink to help identify the encapsulated budding yeast. Diagnosis is confirmed by culturing the spinal fluid on Sabouraud agar at room temperature; sputum, blood, urine, pleural fluid, skin, or bone marrow may also yield the organism on culture. In lung disease without meningitis, the diagnosis is often not possible except from biopsy.

Circulating antigen in blood or especially in spinal fluid indicates continuing active disease, and the tests are highly specific and helpful in both diagnosis and treatment. Antibodies are found only after treatment has been given and antigen levels have decreased.

Treatment

Intensive therapy with amphotericin B given intravenously is the treatment of choice. Intrathecal administration of amphotericin B is helpful in patients with severe, life-threatening meningitis or in those who have relapsed after intravenous therapy; 5-fluorocytosine has shown some promise, but its role is not yet clear.

NOCARDIOSIS

Nocardiosis is a systemic fungus infection caused by *N. asteroides,* an aerobic actinomycete found in infected tissue and exudates as branching mycelial as well as fragmented bacillary forms. The gram-positive and partially acid-fast organism has a worldwide distribution in the soil, but transmission from man to man does not occur. The lung is the usual portal of entry and is the most commonly involved organ; acute suppuration and abscess formation are more prominent tissue responses than granulomas. Hematogenous dissemination occurs; and brain abscess, usually without meningitis, is an important clinical feature. Spread to liver, kidney, spleen, and subcutaneous tissues may also be observed.

Clinical Manifestations

The majority of patients with nocardiosis present with an acute pneumonic illness with fever and cough productive of purulent or blood-streaked sputum. The

chest roentgenogram usually shows patchy or confluent widespread infiltration that may be bilateral. Pleural involvement, often with effusion, is seen in 25 percent of cases. Unequivocal cavitation is uncommon, and miliary lesions are rare. Patients with lymphoma, leukemia, and alveolar proteinosis are particularly susceptible to this infection. Brain abscess occurs in about one-third of the patients. Systemic dissemination is usually fatal.

Diagnosis

In the chronic pulmonary form, nocardiosis may be confused with tuberculosis. The confusion is compounded because *N. asteroides* is weakly acid fast and may mimic *M. tuberculosis* in preparations stained by the Ziehl-Neelsen method. The diagnosis is confirmed by aerobic cultivation on Sabouraud or blood agar; the organism is rarely saprophytic in man.

Treatment

Sulfonamides are the drugs of choice, and treatment must be prolonged. A therapeutic blood level of sulfonamide should be maintained for 3 or more months.

Opportunistic Fungal Diseases

ACTINOMYCOSIS

Actinomycosis, a chronic suppurative infection that may involve the jaw, the ileocecal area, or the thorax, is caused by *Actinomyces israelii,* a branching, gram-positive, filamentous anaerobic organism normally present in the oral cavity and the bowel. The reasons for tissue invasion are unclear, but when such invasion occurs, the inflammatory response is characteristically suppurative, with a chronic granulomatous reaction, few giant cells, and extensive scarring. Formation of sinus tracts that do not respect tissue planes is characteristic. The pus may contain white to yellow conglomerates, 1 to 2 mm in diameter, of mycelial filaments; these mycelial masses, known as sulfur granules, are also found in tissue sections.

Clinical Manifestations

The cervicofacial form of the disease makes up 50 percent of all cases of actinomycosis. The disease is more common in men than in women. A painful, indurated swelling appears at the angle of the mandible as a complication of periodontal sepsis, an infected tonsillar crypt, or a tooth extraction. The swelling increases in size and soon presents one or several draining sinuses in reddened skin with a characteristic woody induration. Pain is seldom prominent, even with bony involvement.

The thoracic form of the disease occurs in about 15 percent of collected series. Pulmonary lesions usually appear to be due to aspiration and tend to involve the lower lobes. The pneumonic phase is accompanied by low-grade fever and mild, productive cough. Pleural involvement with empyema, which is usually localized, is frequent; and the infection tends to burrow through the chest wall to the skin surface. Extensive generalized empyema is infrequent. Systemic symptoms of chronic infection are often prominent, but the course varies from subacute to one of great chronicity.

Abdominal actinomycosis is most frequent in the ileocecal region and generally follows appendicitis or an appendiceal abscess. The abdominal mass is usually large, and extensive burrowing sinus tracts are often present.

Hematogenous dissemination occurs in about 10 percent of the patients. Any organ of the body, including the central nervous system, heart valves, anorectal area, and subcutaneous tissue, may become involved.

Diagnosis

Acthinomyces israelii can be easily demonstrated by microscopic examination of sulfur granules in pus obtained from sinuses, empyema fluid, or abscess cavities. These appear as gram-positive, branching hyphae that often have a beaded appearance. The organism may not be found in cerebrospinal fluid. The diagnosis is confirmed by isolation of the organism in anaerobic culture. Roentgenographic findings of pneumonic consolidation accompanied by periosteal proliferation in the adjacent ribs are suggestive of actinomycosis.

Treatment

Penicillin in large doses for several weeks is curative; tetracycline and streptomycin are also effective.

Surgical drainage of pus or resection of chronically infected tissues are adjunctive modes of therapy.

ASPERGILLOSIS

Aspergillosis may be either a bronchopulmonary or a disseminated systemic disease; it is caused by dimorphic, usually saprophytic fungi of the genus *Aspergillus*. Several species can cause disease, but *A. fumigatus* is the most frequently implicated, followed by *A. niger*. All the *Aspergillus* species are widely distributed in nature. The mycelia grow on damp soil or grain and bear masses of tiny spores that may become readily suspended in the air and be inhaled. The concentration of spores in ambient air varies geographically and seasonally and likely accounts for the differences in incidence of the disease in different parts of the world.

Four main types of human disease have been recognized: (1) Primary pneumonic infection with *Aspergillus* is a rare occurrence in previously well people; there is usually no history of significant occupational exposure. (2) Allergic bronchopulmonary aspergillosis is characterized by the development of focal plugs of mucus, eosinophils, and mycelia of *Aspergillus* in the bronchi, usually in known asthmatics but occasionally in normal persons. Subsegmental, segmental, or, uncommonly, more extensive atelectasis and consolidation may develop. Focal bronchial damage with residual ectasia may result. (3) A third type of pulmonary involvement, mycetoma, occurs as a super-infection in residual cavitary air spaces in the lung, primarily caused by other diseases such as histoplasmosis, sarcoidosis, tuberculosis, bronchiectasis, giant bullae, or neoplasms. The fungus produces a mycelial mass or fungus ball that usually only partly fills the cavity. In most cases tissue invasion is minimal. (4) A more destructive lesion may occur as a bronchopneumonia with lung abscesses in a host whose resistance has been compromised by an underlying disease such as lymphoma, leukemia, or Hodgkin's disease. Such aspergillosis is usually a sequel to therapy with corticosteroids, ionizing irradiation, or antineoplastic drugs and may cause invasion of the pulmonary vessels with thrombosis, necrosis, and hemorrhage; hematogenous dissemination may be observed.

Clinical Manifestations

Primary aspergillosis presents with a very nonspecific picture of cough, chest pain, low-grade fever, and expectoration that may be purulent and bloody. The roentgenographic features are those of nonsegmental homogeneous consolidation, often with cavity formation. In the allergic variety, the patient presents with recurrent episodes of asthma, migrating pulmonary infiltrates, and peripheral eosinophilia accompanied by expectoration of brown plugs of mucus containing *Aspergillus* mycelia. This syndrome, though frequently seen in Great Britain, is rare in the United States. Hemoptysis is the most frequent symptom in patients with aspergilloma. In the invasive form of the disease, pulmonary symptoms may be overshadowed by constitutional and neurologic symptoms.

Diagnosis

A positive sputum culture must be interpreted cautiously because of the ubiquitous nature of the fungus. Repeated positive sputum cultures in the presence of rising serum precipitins against *Aspergillus* antigen are very suggestive. In invasive aspergillosis in the compromised host, mycelia may be seen in bronchial secretions but may not grow on culture.

Mycetoma of the lung presents with a unique roentgenographic picture of a crescentic radiolucency surrounding a circular mass; the mass often shifts in films made in different positions. The presence of precipitins is also a constant feature of aspergilloma, but the highest levels of precipitins against *Aspergillus* antigen are found in the allergic variety, in which the sputum may also contain mycelial plugs.

Treatment

Surgical resection of a fungus ball is indicated when hemoptysis occurs. Ten percent of aspergillomas resolve spontaneously. Invasive aspergillosis and disseminated forms warrant treatment with amphotericin B. Hypersensitivity aspergillosis usually responds to treatment with corticosteroids.

CANDIDIASIS

Candidiasis (moniliasis, thrush) is an infection usually caused by *C. albicans* and, less commonly, by other *Candida* species. The organism usually causes a mild mucocutaneous infection, although widespread visceral infection occasionally occurs in susceptible hosts.

Pathogenesis

Candida albicans is a budding yeast that also forms false or true hyphae in infected body fluids or tissue. The organism is commonly present in the mouth, gastrointestinal tract, and vagina. In infants, in debilitated, diabetic, or pregnant individuals, and in persons treated with antibiotics or corticosteroids, an increased number of organisms is usually found, and the proportion of such individuals with clinical candidiasis is increased. Hematogenous dissemination is particularly likely to develop in susceptible patients who have indwelling intravenous plastic catheters. With active infection, a delayed cutaneous hypersensitivity as well as an increased titer of circulating antibodies may be found; the latter are currently under investigation as a means of differentiating a carrier state from active disease.

Clinical Manifestations

Mucocutaneous candidiasis, or thrush, presents as white patches of exudate appearing on reddened and painful mucosa of the mouth and tongue; the process may spread to the pharynx and esophagus, producing dysphagia. A similar process may involve the rectovaginal area. Cutaneous infection takes the form of reddened, weeping lesions that commonly involve the intertriginous areas; the nails and paronychial tissues may also be involved. The budding yeast form and mycelia are easily observed microscopically, and the organism is readily grown in scrapings from superficial infections.

Pulmonary candidiasis is a rare occurrence even in the compromised host. The clinical and roentgenographic pictures are quite nonspecific; the diagnosis is difficult because the organism is frequently recovered on culture in patients receiving antibiotics; and even the microscopic observation of large numbers of yeast and mycelial forms in sputum does not prove that the fungi have caused parenchymal pulmonary invasion. Pulmonary candidiasis can be diagnosed with certainty only by demonstration of the organism in tissues.

Table 13-1. Characteristics of Phycomycosis, Paracoccidioidomycosis, Maduromycosis, Sporotrichosis, Geotrichosis, and Torulopsosis

Name and geographic distribution	Organism and portal of entry	Host factors	Pathology	Diagnosis	Clinical features	Treatment
Phycomycosis (mucormycosis); worldwide	*Absidia, Rhizopus,* and *Mucor* species (bread molds); respiratory and GI tracts	Diabetes in 40%; leukemia; lymphoma; burns; corticosteroid, antibiotic treatment	Necrosis, suppuration; blood vessel invasion with thrombosis and infarction	Nonseptate hyphae in tissues; culture	Rhinoophthalmic: necrotizing disease nose and paranasal sinuses with extension to orbit and cranium; pneumonic: consolidation, infarction, cavitation; intestinal ulcers; septicemia	Amphotericin B
Paracoccidioidomycosis (South American blastomycosis); Central and South America	*Paracoccidioides brasiliensis;* oral or nasal mucosa	Males predominate; manual laborers and farmers	Granulomatous reaction with suppuration in GI mucosa, lymph nodes, spleen, lungs, and liver	Skin test; complement-fixing antibodies are supporting; culture of organism	Widespread benign, asymptomatic infection; primary ulcer in oral or nasal mucosa with regional suppurative lymphadenopathy; spread to adrenals, lungs, liver via bloodstream	Amphotericin B
Maduromycosis (Madura foot, allescheriasis); tropical regions of the world	Many species of ten genera — *Madurella mycetomi, Nocardia brasiliensis, Allescheria boydii;* skin of bare feet	Adult males predominate	Granulomatous reaction with fibrosis and suppuration; fungal cells in pus or epithelioid cells	Fungal cells in tissue or pus; culture	Progressive, relatively painless swelling of foot with induration and multiple sinus tracts; opportunistic pulmonary infection may occur	Sulfonamides, amphotericin B tetracycline — depending on infecting organism
Sporotrichosis; worldwide	*Sporothrix schenckii;* skin and respiratory tract	Males; laborers, farmers, florists	Varied; acute or chronic suppurative or granulomatous process	Culture; skin tests and serologic tests helpful but not usually available	Papules or pustules in skin and along draining lymphatics. Less common systemic forms: bones and joints, eye, lung, GI tract, or central nervous system	Iodides, amphotericin B
Geotrichosis; worldwide	*Geotrichum candidum* and other species; ~spiratory tract	Saprophyte in mouth, sputum in chronic pulmonary disease	Tissue invasion is rare	Culture; skin test and agglutination test not generally available	Superficial bronchial infection with asthma and eosinophilia in some cases; pneumonic form is rare	—
Torulopsosis; worldwide	*Torulopsis glabrata;* opportunistic in urinary or respiratory tract	Debilitation, immunosuppression	Ovoid yeast forms	Culture	Mycetoma, urinary tract infections	—

Candidemia may represent only transient blood-stream invasion, but when it is associated with demonstration of the fungus in the urine in a patient with the clinical picture of septicemia, there is strong evidence for disseminated candidiasis. Candidal meningitis is usually less acute than bacterial meningitis and is manifested by headache, stiff neck, and delirium. Endocarditis due to this fungus is particularly likely to occur after cardiovascular surgery and in addicts using drugs intravenously.

Treatment
Mucocutaneous candidiasis responds to improved hygiene and to nystatin given as a cream, mouthwash, or vaginal suppository. Gastrointestinal or vulvovaginal thrush can also be treated with oral nystatin tablets; this agent is not absorbed from the gastrointestinal tract and is not available for parenteral use. Candidemia and heavy sputum infection may subside rapidly on stopping antibiotics and removing intravenous catheters. Therapy with amphotericin B or 5-fluorocytosine is indicated for established disseminated infections.

Less Common Mycoses
The characteristics of a number of the less common mycoses are summarized in Table 13-1.

Bibliography
Buechner, A. H., Seabury, H. J., Campbell, C. C., et al. The current status of serologic, immunologic and skin tests in the diagnosis of pulmonary mycoses. *Chest* 63:259, 1973.

Hammerman, J. K., Powell, E. K., Christianson, S. C., et al. Pulmonary cryptococcosis: Clinical forms and treatment. *Am. Rev. Respir. Dis.* 108:1116, 1973.

Lewis, L. J., and Rabinovich, S. The wide spectrum of cryptococcal infections. *Am. J. Med.* 53:315, 1972.

Louria, D. B., Deep-seated mycotic infections, allergy to fungi and mycotoxins. *N. Engl. J. Med.* 277:1065, 1126, 1967.

Louria, D. B., Stiff, D. P., and Bennell, B. Disseminated moniliasis in the adult. *Medicine* 41:307, 1962.

Sarosi, A. G., Hammerman, J. K., Tosh, F. E., and Kronenberg, R. S. Clinical features of acute blastomycosis. *N. Engl. J. Med.* 290:540, 1974.

Sarosi, A. G., Parker, D. J., Doto, L. I., et al. Chronic pulmonary coccidioidomycosis. *N. Engl. J. Med.* 283:325, 1970.

Smith, W. J., and Utz, P. J. Progressive disseminated histoplasmosis. *Ann. Intern. Med.* 76:557, 1972.

Weese, W. C. A study of 57 cases of actinomycosis over a 36 year period. *Arch. Intern. Med.* 135:1562, 1975.

Young, C. R., Bennett, E. J., Vogel, L. C., et al. Aspergillosis: The spectrum of the disease in 98 patients. *Medicine* 49:147, 1970.

Young, L. S., Armstrong, D., Blevins, A., and Lieberman, P. *Nocardia asteroides* infection complicating neoplasmic disease. *Am. J. Med.* 50:356, 1971.

14

Bronchiectasis

Bruce F. Bachus and Gordon L. Snider

Bronchiectasis is a disease characterized by permanent, abnormal dilatation of one or more bronchi, often with an associated destruction of the bronchial wall. The disease process may be either localized or diffuse; women are as commonly affected as men, and more than one-half of the cases occur in children. The true incidence of the disease is unknown, although it is reported to be present in 4 percent of random autopsies. Bronchial dilatation that may accompany an acute pulmonary infection but then resolves upon recovery from the infection is termed *pseudobronchiectasis.*

Bronchiectasis may be classified on anatomic or bronchographic grounds into three groups: (1) Cylindrical bronchiectasis involves dilatation of the bronchi in a uniform manner, with preservation of the full number of generations of the bronchial tree. (2) Varicose bronchiectasis is the most common form of the disease and is characterized by irregular dilatation of the bronchi with areas of focal constriction. (3) Saccular or cystic bronchiectasis is the most severe, advanced form and is characterized by marked bronchial dilatation with preservation of only four to six generations of the bronchial tree.

Bronchiectasis usually affects the lower lobes bilaterally, occurring less commonly in a unilateral or segmental distribution. The right middle lobe and the lingular division of the left upper lobe are next in frequency of involvement. The upper lobes are rarely involved alone, except secondarily to a fibrosing process such as tuberculosis. The first- and second-order bronchi are usually spared, while the disease process is concentrated in the third- and fourth-order bronchi. These bronchi are markedly dilated, can be traced out to the pleural surface, and are often filled with a suppurative exudate. Enlargement of and an increase in the number of bronchial arteries and anastomosis of the bronchial to the pulmonary arteries are frequent findings. Areas of adjacent atelectasis may be seen.

The histologic findings depend on the severity and duration of the disease in the areas sampled. Destruc-

tion of the elastic and muscular tissues of the bronchial wall is often prominent. Mucous gland enlargement is common. The mucosa is congested with many engorged, thin-walled capillaries just beneath the epithelium, which may be ulcerated or show foci of squamous metaplasia. The bronchial wall may be intensely infiltrated with polymorphonuclear leukocytes, and the inflammation may extend through the bronchial wall into an adjacent area of pneumonia; necrosis may be present with formation of a bronchiectatic lung abscess. In areas of more chronic disease, fibrosis of the bronchial wall may develop along with an infiltration of plasma cells and lymphocytes, at times with the formation of geminal centers in dense lymphoid accumulations.

Two mechanisms are generally accepted as being of major importance in the pathogenesis: (1) infection and (2) obstruction with associated collapse. The initiating roles and the relative contribution of each of these mechanisms are not completely settled and indeed are probably different from patient to patient. In the early stages of bronchiectasis, if infection has caused little or no necrosis of bronchial wall tissues, the dilatation associated with collapse due to retained secretions may be readily reversible on relief of the obstruction. If, on the other hand, infection with its destructive changes has been the predominant feature, the ectasia that results when the damaged bronchi are subjected to the recoil forces of normal lung, or to the much greater retractile forces generated by the atelectatic lung, will be permanent. Bronchi that are not yet ectatic but are damaged by the same infectious process may be prone to dilate later if they are subjected to increased distending forces. This may occur after a surgical resection of more severely diseased portions of the lung, when the residual lung expands to fill the hemithorax. Recurrent suppurative infections may aggravate the disease process long after the initiating infection has subsided. Bronchiectasis tends to be localized when it is secondary to obstruction from a tumor, a lymph node, or a foreign body, whereas it is usually more generalized when caused by a viral or bacterial infection. With obstruction the bronchi may be distended with glairy, opalescent, uninfected mucus, while the adjacent lung may show consolidation with lipid-laden macrophages.

Infection and collapse can lead to the development of bronchiectasis in a normal person, but the process develops more readily in individuals with underlying congenital abnormalities. Cystic fibrosis, which will be discussed more fully below, is almost always complicated by bronchiectasis. In Kartagener's syndrome, bronchiectasis is associated with situs inversus and paranasal sinusitis. Agammaglobulinemia and dys-gammaglobulinemia are also frequently associated with bronchiectasis and paranasal sinusitis (see Chap. 44).

Clinically the typical patient with bronchiectasis presents with a cough productive of copious amounts of sputum, which in untreated cases may be foul smelling. Hemoptysis occurs at some time in about 50 percent of cases; it may be recurrent, commonly in association with exacerbations of infection. Occasionally the hemoptysis may be massive, but it is rarely life-threatening. Patients with bronchiectasis frequently present with recurring pneumonia in the same segments of the lung. Episodes of unexplained fever may result from retention of secretions in the involved areas. Physical examination may reveal evidence of weight loss, malnutrition, and cyanosis. Clubbing of the digits is common. Examination of the chest may show localized rales due to parenchymal disease and rhonchi indicating airways obstruction; evidence of cor pulmonale and right-sided heart failure may be present in advanced cases, but the physical examination may be entirely normal.

The chest x-rays may appear normal, but atelectasis or nonspecific accentuation of linear markings may be present. Cystic spaces with air-fluid levels are pathognomonic, but these are observed only in severe, cystic bronchiectasis. The appearance of the bronchogram, a study necessary to confirm the diagnosis, is characteristic for each type of bronchiectasis. In cylindrical bronchiectasis the bronchi are of regular outline and do not increase greatly in diameter distally. Their lumina end squarely and abruptly due to plugs of mucus that block further passage of contrast media peripherally. In varicose bronchiectasis there is greater dilatation of the bronchi with areas of local constriction and irregular, bulbous terminations; on the average only four bronchial subdivisions may be seen. In saccular bronchiectasis bronchial dilatation

increases progressively toward the periphery, and usually no more than five bronchial subdivisions are seen.

Bacteriologic analysis of the sputum commonly shows mouth flora, *Streptococcus pneumoniae, Haemophilus influenzae,* or anaerobic organisms. Staphylococci and gram-negative organisms appear in patients previously treated with antibiotic therapy. Untreated bronchiectasis may be complicated by lung abscess, brain abscess, empyema, cor pulmonale, and amyloidosis, but these sequelae have become rare since the advent of antibiotic therapy.

The effect of bronchiectasis upon pulmonary function depends on the type of bronchiectasis and the extent and distribution of the disease. Obviously the more localized the disease, the less impairment of overall pulmonary function. In moderate disease, atelectasis and fibrosis may contribute to modest losses of both total lung capacity and vital capacity; but airways obstruction is a regular feature of severe disease, in which marked increases of residual volume may contribute to losses of vital capacity. Hypoxemia tends to be more severe than expected from the degree of airways obstruction because of shuntlike effects in the lung. When ventilation-perfusion mismatch and airways obstruction are severe, hypercapnia is present. Hypoxemia as well as bronchial-to-pulmonary arterial anastomoses may result in pulmonary hypertension and cor pulmonale. Studies have documented deterioration of pulmonary function following each exacerbation of the disease, especially when the disease becomes more extensive.

The diagnosis of bronchiectasis is based on the history, physical examination, and x-ray studies. Bronchography is essential. The procedure should not be carried out for 3 or more months after a slowly resolving pneumonia in order to avoid confusion with pseudobronchiectasis. Underlying predisposing conditions should also be ruled out. In young patients a sweat test should be done to rule out cystic fibrosis, and an immunoglobulin electrophoresis study should also be performed.

In the therapy of bronchiectasis, vigorous medical efforts are made to improve drainage from the bronchi, to decrease the quantity of sputum, and to change the quality of the sputum from purulent to mucoid. The goals are to minimize exacerbations of infection and to prevent complications of the disease. Medical measures include inhalation therapy and postural drainage designed, respectively, to thin and to mobilize secretions; cessation of smoking; and the use of appropriate antibiotics to control infection. Surgical intervention is usually successful but is indicated only in patients with bronchographically documented localized disease who remain significantly symptomatic in spite of a prolonged trial of vigorous medical therapy. Surgery is generally contraindicated in patients whose bronchiectasis, even though localized, is a part of a more generalized underlying disorder. Treated early and appropriately, mild or moderate bronchiectasis usually does not significantly decrease longevity.

Cystic Fibrosis

Cystic fibrosis is a disease involving widespread dysfunction of the exocrine glands, predominantly in the skin, pancreas, lungs, and liver. The disorder is inherited as an autosomal recessive trait, occurs in about 1 in 2,000 live births, and affects primarily members of the Caucasian race. Cystic fibrosis is not often seen in black Americans and is rare in black Africans and Orientals.

The major clinical manifestations of the disease stem from involvement of the gastrointestinal and respiratory systems. Gastrointestinal manifestations include meconium ileus, pancreatic insufficiency with malabsorption, volvulus, diabetes mellitus, and biliary cirrhosis. Over 95 percent of adult males with cystic fibrosis have azoospermia and sterility.

Involvement of the lungs begins with bronchiolar obstruction by the abnormally viscous, tenacious secretions characteristic of the disease. The bronchiolar obstruction is complicated by a spectrum of pathologic changes, including focal atelectasis with resultant pneumonitis, multiple abscess formation, bronchiectasis, and areas of hyperinflation. *Staphylococcus aureus* and *Pseudomonas aeruginosa* are the most common organisms cultured from the sputum of these patients. The clinical manifestations of pulmonary involvement include chronic sputum production, dyspnea, wheezing, hemoptysis, digital clubbing, and eventually signs of cor pulmonale. Diagnostic

criteria include a sweat chloride of greater than 60 mEq per liter, chronic suppurative bronchopulmonary disease, and evidence of pancreatic insufficiency. Apart from cystic fibrosis, an elevated level of sweat chloride is seen only in patients with either renal diabetes insipidus or adrenal insufficiency.

The main thrust of treatment of cystic fibrosis should be against the pulmonary involvement, which has a crucial effect on the prognosis. The goals of pulmonary therapy are to clear the copious secretions through physical and aerosol therapy and to prevent further loss of function by therapy with adequate antibiotics during acute infections. With early diagnosis and treatment, more affected individuals are surviving into adulthood; the mean survival is now about 20 years.

Bibliography

Cherniack, N. S., and Carton, R. W. Factors associated with respiratory insufficiency in bronchiectasis. *Am. J. Med.* 41:562, 1966.

Cherniack, N. S., et al. The role of acute lower respiratory infection in causing pulmonary insufficiency in bronchiectasis. *Ann. Intern. Med.* 66:489, 1967.

Crozier, D. N. Cystic fibrosis, a not-so-fatal disease. *Med. Clin. North Am.* 21:935, 1974.

DiSant'Agnese, P. A., and Talamo, R. C. Pathogenesis and physiopathology of cystic fibrosis of the pancreas. *N. Engl. J. Med.* 277:1287, 1344, 1399, 1967.

Konietzko, N., et al. Causes of death in patients with bronchiectasis. *Am. Rev. Respir. Dis.* 100:852, 1969.

Ogilvie, A. G. The natural history of bronchiectasis: A clinical, roentgenographic and pathologic study. *Arch. Intern. Med.* 68:395, 1941.

Perry, K. M. A., and King, S. Bronchiectasis: A study of prognosis based on a follow-up of 400 patients. *Am. Rev. Tuberc.* 41:531, 1940.

Reid, L. M. Reduction in bronchial subdivision in bronchiectasis. *Thorax* 5:223, 1950.

Shwachman, H. Changing concepts of cystic fibrosis. *Hosp. Pract.* 9:143, 1974.

Whitwell, F. A study of the pathology and pathogenesis of bronchiectasis. *Thorax* 7:213, 1952.

15

Asthma

Michael E. Whitcomb

Bronchial asthma is a complex clinical disorder characterized by acute airways obstruction that is reversible, either spontaneously or after appropriate drug therapy. Although such obstruction may occur in a variety of diseases, the diagnosis of asthma should be reserved for patients whose primary difficulty is reversible airways obstruction. Although the incidence of asthma in the United States cannot be determined accurately, between 5 and 10 percent of people may be affected with it during their lives. The disease may have its onset at any time from infancy through adulthood; complete remissions of childhood asthma are common during puberty.

Pathogenesis

In considering the pathogenesis of acute airways obstruction, it is important to review the idea that a partial blockade of the beta-adrenergic sympathetic nervous system exists in patients with asthma. Bronchial tone is thought to be controlled by the level of cyclic adenosine monophosphate (cyclic AMP) within the bronchial smooth muscle cells. Intracellular cyclic AMP, a bronchodilator, can be generated by stimulation of beta-adrenergic receptors on the cell surface and is degraded within the cell by the action of the enzyme phosphodiesterase. Under normal circumstances, a balance seems to exist between the mechanisms that stimulate bronchial smooth muscle contraction and the generation of bronchodilating cyclic AMP; thus normal airway dimensions are maintained. It is hypothesized, however, that in individuals with asthma, beta-adrenergic stimulation results in subnormal levels of intracellular cyclic AMP. Thus these individuals have an innate tendency to develop bronchial smooth muscle contraction under circumstances that would not affect a normal individual. Although this theory has not been completely proved, it provides a basis for understanding both the potential mechanisms involved in the development of acute airways obstruction and the rationale for the various pharmacologic agents used in its treatment.

Although the pathogenesis of acute bronchospasm has not been completely elucidated, two major mechanisms have been postulated to be of importance — intrapulmonary mast-cell mediator release and bronchial parasympathetic nerve stimulation. Each of these mechanisms can be demonstrated to cause bronchial smooth muscle contraction under experimental conditions. The mechanism of immune-mediated, mast-cell mediator release has received considerable attention in recent years and is thought to be the mechanism of airways obstruction in extrinsic allergic asthma. It is currently believed that patients with this form of asthma become sensitized to specific allergens against which they develop IgE antibodies on the surface of the mast cells. When the offending allergen combines with the surface-bound antibody, mast cell degranulation is in some way triggered; and histamine, slow-reacting substance of anaphylaxis, and eosinophilic chemotactic factor are released. These humoral mediators appear to cause bronchial smooth muscle contraction, bronchial wall inflammation, and mucosal edema.

Bronchial smooth muscle contraction can also be mediated by stimulation of the parasympathetic nervous system supplying the bronchi. It has been proposed that the bronchial mucosa contains irritant receptors, which may, on contact with a number of nonspecific irritants, result in vagally mediated bronchial smooth muscle contraction, mucosal edema, and increased bronchial secretions; these in combination lead to obstruction of air flow within both large and small bronchi and result in the physiologic and clinical abnormalities of asthma.

Etiology and Precipitating Factors

In the majority of adult asthmatics it is impossible to identify specific factors that precipitate acute airways obstruction. This condition is often referred to as intrinsic asthma. It is presumed that the inhalation of nonspecific bronchial irritants may be important in precipitating an asthmatic attack in such patients. Respiratory tract infection may also play a role, although the mechanism by which infection causes airways obstruction has not been elucidated. Most such patients have perennial symptoms.

In certain patients specific precipitating factors can be identified by taking a careful history or by obtaining selected laboratory studies. The majority

170

of these patients have immune-mediated asthma caused by extrinsic allergens; therefore the condition is usually referred to as extrinsic asthma. The most commonly implicated environmental allergens are grass, tree, or plant pollens, although animal proteins, fungal spores, and a variety of industrial allergens may be of importance in selected patients. Patients with extrinsic asthma frequently have a past or a family history of childhood eczema or allergic rhinitis. Symptoms tend to be seasonal in patients with extrinsic asthma caused by pollens. However, patients with allergic asthma may also develop airways obstruction on exposure to nonspecific bronchial irritants such as dust, smoke, or changes in environmental temperature, and thus, like intrinsic asthmatics, they may have perennial symptoms.

Pathophysiology

The major pathophysiologic effect of smooth muscle contraction, mucosal edema, and increased bronchial secretions is obstruction to air flow. Therefore tests of lung function that measure flow rates are abnormal during an acute asthmatic attack. In the majority of patients the forced expired volume in 1 second ($FEV_{1.0}$) will be decreased. In patients with minimal bronchospasm or in those in whom the predominant site of response is in the terminal airways (bronchioles), the $FEV_{1.0}$ may be normal. In such patients, tests that measure flow in the terminal bronchioles such as the forced expiratory flow for the middle half of the forced vital capacity will generally be abnormal (see Chap. 9). The distribution of gas within the lung also becomes abnormal during an asthma attack. The residual volume is usually increased, and the vital capacity may be decreased. The degree to which these abnormalities occur is dependent on the site and severity of airways obstruction.

Blood gas abnormalities are usually observed in patients with acute airways obstruction. Hypoxemia is almost uniformly present as the result of ventilation-perfusion mismatching within the lung. During mild to moderate asthmatic attacks the arterial P_{CO_2} is decreased; however, as the severity of airways obstruction increases, the arterial carbon dioxide tension tends to normalize, and in severe status asthmaticus, hypercapnia may occur. It is important to appreciate that, with the institution of therapy, patients may show marked symptomatic improvement and still have little change in flow rates. In this situation a marked reduction in the residual volume usually accompanies the symptomatic improvement. As progressive clinical improvement occurs, flow rates also begin to return toward normal. Patients in remission may retain certain physiologic abnormalities. Although the routine tests of lung function are usually normal, mild hypoxemia may persist. In addition, persistent obstruction in the small airways can also be detected in certain patients by employing sophisticated physiologic studies.

Pathology

In uncomplicated asthma, pathologic changes are restricted to the airways. Diffuse mucous plugging of both small and large airways may be present in patients who die of status asthmaticus. In addition, an increase in the number of mucosal goblet cells, hyperplasia of submucosal glands, and infiltration of the submucosa with neutrophils and eosinophils may be present. Hypertrophy of the bronchial smooth muscle and thickening of the bronchial basement membrane may be prominent. In selected patients, immunoglobulin deposits can be identified in the bronchial basement membrane.

Clinical Manifestations

With the development of acute airways obstruction, patients may note the onset of audible wheezing, cough, chest tightness, dyspnea, or any combination of these symptoms. In most episodes symptoms begin gradually and progress in severity over a period of days. On physical examination patients usually appear quite anxious. Diffuse musical wheezes may be audible over all lung fields. As obstruction becomes more severe, breath sounds may be markedly diminished in intensity and the wheezes may develop a high-pitched quality. With severe obstruction, retraction of the intercostal muscles may be noted and a pulsus paradoxus may develop. During prolonged episodes patients may become extremely fatigued, confused, and disoriented.

With successful therapy the clinical manifestations of asthma resolve in an orderly fashion. Intercostal retraction and pulsus paradoxus are the first signs to disappear. With further improvement in airways obstruction, symptoms disappear; and finally auscultatory findings resolve. As a general rule, patients become asymptomatic when pulmonary function has returned to 60 to 70 percent of normal, that is, while subclinical airways obstruction is still present. Therefore symptoms may recur if therapy is abruptly discontinued. Subclinical airways obstruction may persist for weeks following an acute episode. As a result, exertional dyspnea may be a persistent complaint of patients after an acute episode has apparently resolved. As has been mentioned previously, many patients in complete remission will have normal routine pulmonary function studies, but on special testing will manifest physiologic abnormalities indicative of obstruction in the small airways.

Laboratory Data

There are only a few helpful laboratory studies for evaluating a patient with asthma. In selected patients in whom the history or physical findings are not classic, demonstration that the patient has irritable airways is of some value in suggesting the diagnosis of asthma. Patients with asthma usually develop acute bronchospasm on inhalation challenges with histamine or methacholine in concentrations that do not affect normal individuals. If obstruction to air flow is demonstrated in the laboratory after inhalation of an appropriate concentration of these drugs, it is highly likely that the patient has asthma.

Patients with extrinsic asthma have IgE antibodies against a variety of allergens. The amount of circulating IgE antibody is characteristically elevated in these patients. In addition, specific IgE antibodies against a variety of potential allergens can be demonstrated by cutaneous scratch testing. Although the development of the classic wheal and flare reaction within 15 to 30 minutes after the intradermal application of the test antigen is evidence that the patient has IgE antibody against that antigen, it does not necessarily implicate it as the precipitating factor in the development of airways obstruction. This association may be made either on the basis of a highly reliable history of the development of bronchospasm on repeated exposure to the allergen, or by producing bronchospasm in the laboratory after inhalation challenge with the allergen in question.

During an episode of asthma, peripheral blood eosinophilia and sputum eosinophilia characteristically occur in patients with asthma. Curschmann's spirals and Charcot-Leyden crystals may less frequently be observed in the sputum of patients during an acute asthma attack. All other routine laboratory studies may be normal both during acute airways obstruction and when the patient is in remission.

The chest roentgenogram may be abnormal during an acute episode of asthma, revealing evidence of pulmonary hyperinflation. An increase in the retrosternal air space and flattening of the diaphragm in the lateral view are the most commonly observed abnormalities. Although hyperlucency of the lung fields may also be present, this is often difficult to distinguish in young individuals.

Treatment

The treatment of asthma should be divided into prophylactic therapy and therapy of the acute attack of bronchospasm. Clearly, prevention would be the ideal approach to the management of asthma. Hyposensitization therapy has long been used as a form of preventive therapy. However, despite the theoretical basis of hyposensitization therapy (see Chap. 44), its value in asthma has yet to be convincingly demonstrated. Many allergists believe that this form of therapy may be beneficial in children but has little value in adults.

It has been documented that cromolyn sodium prevents acute bronchospasm in certain patients. This drug has been demonstrated to prevent the degranulation of mast cells despite the surface interaction of antigen with IgE. Currently the therapy is of limited use for two reasons: (1) The drug is of value only in patients with extrinsic asthma, which is relatively uncommon in adults, and (2) the drug has to be administered by inhalation at frequent intervals, which is not feasible in patients who have only sporadic episodes. Despite these limitations, cromolyn sodium is effective in preventing asthmatic episodes in true extrinsic asthma and may be of great benefit in some patients.

The treatment of acute bronchospasm often requires a combination of several drugs: the beta-adrenergic stimulants, the methyl xanthines, and the corticosteroids. A large number of beta-adrenergic stimulants are available; epinephrine subcutaneously and isoproterenol by inhalation are the agents most commonly used in acute asthma. As already mentioned, these drugs stimulate the generation of cyclic AMP, producing bronchodilation. Since the beta-adrenergic stimulants also affect the cardiovascular system, they may cause tachycardia and hypertension. Therefore other drugs have been developed selectively to stimulate only the beta-2 receptors of the bronchi. Although in theory these drugs should be advantageous, they have not completely eliminated the troublesome cardiovascular side effects observed with the nonspecific beta-adrenergic stimulants.

The xanthine derivatives are the next most commonly used drugs in the treatment of acute asthma. The xanthines may be administered in a variety of ways, but during acute airways obstruction intravenous administration is the most efficacious. The xanthines also produce bronchodilation by increasing intracellular cyclic AMP in bronchial smooth muscle cells. In contrast to the beta-adrenergic stimulants, however, the xanthines decrease the intracellular metabolism of cyclic AMP by interfering with the action of phosphodiesterase, the major enzyme responsible for breaking down cyclic AMP. Gastrointestinal disturbances, arrhythmias, and hypotension are commonly observed side effects of parenteral aminophylline.

In recent years it has been demonstrated that the bronchodilating effect of aminophylline is directly related to its blood level. In general, the higher the blood level, the greater the bronchodilation. The dosage is limited, however, by the development of toxicity in a predictable fashion with levels higher than 20 mg per liter. Therapeutic blood levels can be achieved most rapidly by administering an intravenous loading dose of aminophylline, followed by a constant infusion of the drug. The amount of loading dose is based on body weight; infusion rate should be based on blood levels (page 205).

The corticosteroids are also of great benefit in the treatment of acute asthma. The exact mechanism by which the corticosteroids act to abort episodes of acute airways obstruction has not been clearly defined. Although bronchial secretions may decrease and inflammation may be reversed, it is apparent that steroids have a direct effect on bronchial muscle tone also.

When severe or persistent airways obstruction leads to the development of respiratory failure, endotracheal intubation and mechanical ventilation may be required as an integral part of the total management of the patient. In general, patients with asthma should be considered candidates for mechanical ventilation at a PCO_2 level far less than that which would be considered an indication for similar therapy in patients with the chronic bronchitis-emphysema syndrome. Since hypocapnia is usually present during acute bronchospasm, any degree of hypercapnia represents a significant deterioration in total alveolar ventilation. The development of a PCO_2 in excess of 50 mm Hg should be considered a grave prognostic sign, and intubation and mechanical ventilation must be considered.

Other general measures are usually included in the management of acute asthma. Hydration may be of importance in these patients, although its value as an integral part of therapy has not been clearly demonstrated. Nonetheless, the presence of inspissated bronchial secretions suggests that hydration may be valuable. In some patients, airways infection is an important contributing factor in the pathogenesis of the disease; therefore broad-spectrum antibiotic therapy may be beneficial in selected patients. As a general rule, sedatives or other drugs that suppress central ventilatory drive should not be administered to patients during an acute asthmatic episode. Suppression of ventilatory drive in such patients may lead to progressive respiratory failure and complicate the management of the patient profoundly.

Bibliography

Austen, K. F., and Lichtenstein, L. M. (eds.). *Asthma: Physiology, Immunopharmacology, and Treatment.* New York: Academic, 1973.

McFadden, E. R., Kiser, R., and DeGroot, W. J.
      Acute bronchial asthma: Relations between
      clinical and physiologic manifestations. *N. Engl.
      J. Med.* 288:221, 1973.
McFadden, E. R., and Lyons, H. A. Arterial blood
      gas tension in asthma. *N. Engl. J. Med.* 278:
      1027, 1968.

16

Interstitial Lung Disease

Jerome S. Brody

Although acute interstitial reactions in the lung occur in a variety of diseases and with a variety of distinctive clinical and pathologic pictures, chronic, end-stage interstitial lung disease presents with common clinical and pathologic patterns, the original causes of which frequently are no longer distinguishable. Interstitial lung disease involves damage and repair of the alveolar wall, the surface of which is lined by a continuous, thin epithelial layer of two types of cells. The first are the highly differentiated, platelike alveolar epithelial cells (type 1 pneumonocytes, Fig. 16-1); these cells have long, thin cytoplasmic extensions that make up the major gas-exchange surface of the alveolus. The second are the rounded granular cells (type 2 pneumonocytes), the functions of which appear to be (1) the production of surfactant coating of the alveolar surface and (2) the repair of lung damage. Both types of alveolar epithelial cells rest on a common basement membrane that frequently fuses with the basement membrane of the alveolar capillaries, thus minimizing the thickness of the alveolar wall and providing an extremely thin gas exchange surface. The capillary endothelium not only provides for gas exchange but also serves an important metabolic function. The endothelial surface consists of small caveolli that appear to be intimately involved in the inactivation or metabolism of a variety of substances that pass through the lung.

Where the basement membranes of epithelium and endothelium are separated, the interstitial space contains a network of collagen and elastin fibers, fibroblasts, and macrophages. There are also rare mast cells, nerve fibers, and lymphocytes within this interstitial space. The tissue plane of this interstitium broadens and becomes continuous with the perivascular and peribronchial connective tissue, providing an avenue of escape for fluids that exude from the pulmonary capillaries.

Injury to the lung parenchyma and interstitium may occur either through the airways and air spaces or through the capillaries. The initial insult may

result in cellular necrosis, with the endothelial and the type 1 alveolar cells being the most susceptible to injury. Upon injury of endothelial cells, leakage of protein-rich fluid into the interstitium and the alveolar space occurs; inflammatory cells then appear, and organization of the edema fluid begins. The capillary endothelial cells are capable of undergoing mitosis and repair, but type 1 alveolar cells do not appear to do this. Instead, the epithelial repair process is initiated by a proliferation of type 2 alveolar cells, which gradually assume the shape and functions of type 1 cells. This alveolar type 2 proliferative response has been shown to occur in situations as diverse as oxygen or ozone toxicity, nitrogen dioxide inhalation, and damage from experimental pneumonia. The repair process may or may not be associated with pulmonary fibrosis, and what determines this is not known. It appears that the immunologic status of the host plays a role in the process, in view of the high incidence of nonspecific immunologic factors found in interstitial lung disease. In addition, the nature and chronicity of an exposure to injurious agents may play important roles.

Because of the great physiologic reserves of the lung, symptoms and pulmonary function abnormalities tend to occur only with extensive interstitial lung disease. Early symptoms usually include dyspnea on exertion and nonproductive cough. Late symptoms are related primarily to dyspnea and to the sequelae of chronic pulmonary hypertension and cor pulmonale, which result from hypoxia and obliteration of the pulmonary vasculature. Physiologic changes are directly related to the amount of lung tissue involved. Local pathology that leaves normal lung tissue intervening may have little effect on pulmonary function, while diffuse involvement may have dramatic effects.

The characteristic changes in respiratory mechanics associated with diffuse interstitial lung disease relate to altered distensibility of the lung. As the interstitium becomes more involved, the lung volumes begin to diminish. This diminution is manifested by a proportional decrease in the total lung capacity, the functional residual capacity, and the vital capacity and a somewhat smaller diminution in the residual volume. Thus the residual volume—total lung capac-

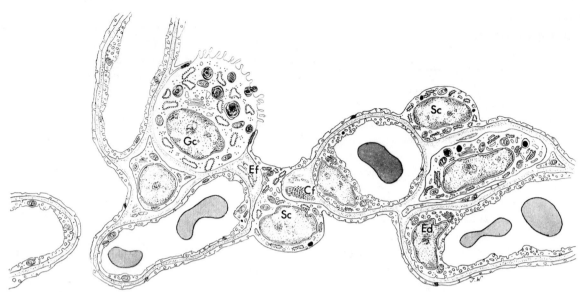

*Figure 16-1. The alveolar wall. Cf = collagenous
fiber; Ed = endothelial cell of the blood capillary;
Ef = elastic fiber; Gc = great alveolar epithelial cell;
Sc = squamous alveolar epithelial cell. (From T. Ebe
and S. Kobayashi,* Fine Structure of Human Cells
and Tissue, *New York: Wiley and Sons, Inc., 1972.
P. 170. Reproduced by permission.)*

ity ratio may increase slightly, even though obstructive lung disease is not present. Air-flow rates are
usually well preserved, because the stiffening lung
tends to hold airways open (see Chap. 9).

The pulmonary diffusing capacity characteristically decreases in interstitial lung disease, although
arterial oxygen transport at rest tends to be maintained until the disease is far advanced. Patients with
interstitial disease may, however, develop significant
hypoxemia during moderate degrees of exercise.
Hyperventilation with lowered arterial carbon
dioxide tension and respiratory alkalosis is a frequent
occurrence, although the mechanism responsible for
the hyperventilation is uncertain. Because of the
wide variability of normal values, it is frequently
difficult to determine whether any one patient with
interstitial lung disease has a significant impairment
of pulmonary function. However, changes in pulmonary function tests are extremely useful in following
the course of a patient's disease and his response to
therapy. In far-advanced interstitial lung disease with
severe fibrosis and formation of bullae, pulmonary

function abnormalities begin to show the features of
air trapping and airways obstruction seen in pulmonary emphysema.

Since there are no therapeutic agents that produce
regression of chronic pulmonary fibrosis, therapy at
this stage of the disease is limited to supportive
measures such as oxygen inhalation. Therapy is more
effective in the early stages of disease, prior to the
development of chronic fibrosis. In many circumstances, definition of the cause and elimination of
the sources of injury are more important than any
specific drug therapy. Figure 16-2 illustrates the four
main categories of disease that are associated with
lung injury leading to pulmonary fibrosis.

Pulmonary Granulomas

Although most chronic inflammatory diseases produce nonspecific morphologic changes in the lung,
a few are characterized by a distinctive histologic
feature — the granuloma. Histologically, a pulmonary
granuloma consists of a central aggregation of macrophages and epithelioid cells surrounded by fibroblasts,
lymphocytes, and plasma cells. Multinucleated giant
cells, which are of macrophage origin, are frequently
found in the center of a granuloma.

Classically, granulomas have been divided into
epithelioid and nonepithelioid granulomas; the epithelioid are believed to be immunologic or hypersensitive in origin, while the nonepithelioid are thought

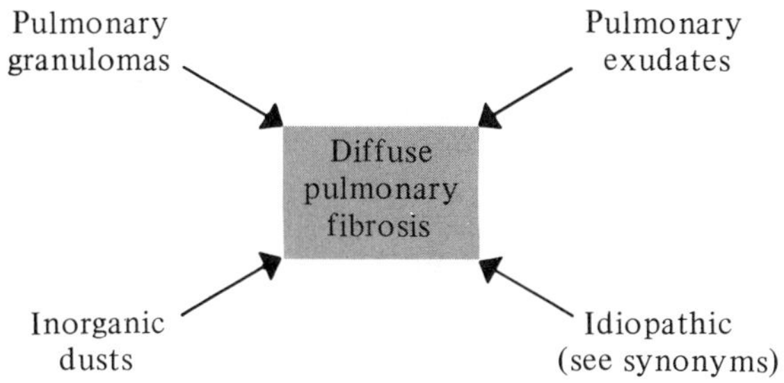

Figure 16-2. The major causes of diffuse pulmonary fibrosis.

to be foreign body reactions. The exact nature of the immunologic process and the contributions of cell-mediated immunity or of serum antibodies in the genesis of the granulomas are not clear; initial exposure to an antigen will not result in granuloma formation, provided the antigen does not persist, whereas reexposure will result in a rapid granulomatous response. In nonimmunologic granulomas, the histologic response is induced by a chemical mediator of inflammation and begins rapidly.

During the repair process, the granulomatous reaction may either resolve completely, leaving no residual morphologic changes, or be replaced by a fibroblastic proliferation and scarring. It is unclear what determines whether a granuloma resolves or progresses toward fibrosis and what factors determine the rate of fibrosis when it occurs. The most important noninfectious chronic granulomatous reactions involving the lung are those due to sarcoidosis, eosinophilic granuloma, and allergic alveolitis. Sarcoidosis will be discussed in Chapter 24.

EOSINOPHILIC GRANULOMA
A disease of unknown etiology, eosinophilic granuloma is characterized pathologically by pulmonary granulomas; these may be focal but are usually diffuse, and they are comprised chiefly of histiocytes and eosinophils, though at times they contain neutrophils and lymphocytes. The histiocytes are often filled with lipid. The process may either resolve or undergo progressive fibrosis with the formation within the pulmonary parenchyma of characteristic multiple, air-filled cysts of varying size (honeycombing). The cysts usually are most evident in the upper lung fields. Lung and bone are the organs most fre-

quently involved, but lymph nodes, skin, central nervous system, liver, spleen, and kidneys may also be affected. Letterer-Siwe disease is a widespread, fulminant form of eosinophilic granuloma seen in infants and children. The characteristic triad of Hand-Schüller-Christian disease — exophthalmos, diabetes insipidus, and osteolytic lesions of the skull — is rare. In adults, eosinophilic granuloma is usually confined to the lungs, occurs in the 20- to 50-year age group, is relatively indolent or only slowly progressive, and occasionally regresses spontaneously. Pneumothorax may occur as a result of rupture of subpleural cystic spaces. It appears that corticosteroids are of therapeutic benefit.

EXTRINSIC ALLERGIC ALVEOLITIS
A wide variety of antigens are now recognized to produce an acute Arthus, or type III, reaction in the lung upon inhalation (Table 16-1). Four to six hours after a reexposure to the antigen, the patient will develop fever, cough, dyspnea, and bilateral, diffuse nodular infiltrates in the lung. Pathologically there is evidence of bronchiolitis and diffuse, nodular granulomatous pneumonitis. The nodules represent the proliferation of type 2 alveolar cells and the accumulation of lymphocytes, mononuclear cells, and foreign-body giant cells. Prolonged or repeated exposures lead to a picture of diffuse interstitial fibrosis that is often indistinguishable from the fibrotic stage of sarcoidosis. Diagnosis of allergic alveolitis is made by careful history, positive skin test (a delayed Arthus reaction), and positive precipitin reactions to the specific antigen. Therapy in early stages involves the removal of the offending agent, and when disease is severe, the use of corticosteroids.

Pulmonary Exudates
Pulmonary exudates arise from the leakage of edema fluid, first into the interstitium and ultimately into the alveoli. The edema results either from damage to the capillary endothelial cells, making them more permeable, or from excessive intravascular pressures causing the capillaries to leak (see Chap. 30). Endothelial damage may be due to inhalation of the offending or initiating agent, but most such substances

Table 16-1. Antigens Producing Extrinsic Allergic Alveolitis[*]

Disease	Exposure	Antigen
Farmer's lung	Moldy hay	*Micropolyspora faeni, Thermoactinomyces vulgaris*
Bagassosis	Moldy sugar cane	*T. vulgaris*
Mushroom picker's lung	Mushroom dust	*M. faeni* and *T. vulgaris*
Maple bark disease	Moldy maple bark	Fungal spores of *Coniosporium corticale*
Bird breeder's lung	Pigeon, parakeet, etc., droppings	Serum proteins
Pituitary snuff lung	Porcine or bovine posterior pituitary powder	Serum proteins
Sequoiosis	Moldy redwood dust	Graphium and *Aureobasidium pullulans*
Cheese washer's lung	Moldy cheese	*Penicillium casei*
Malt worker's lung	Moldy barley and malt dust	*Aspergillus*

[*]Partial listing.

reach the lung through the pulmonary circulation. In general, the resulting process tends to predominate at the lung bases because blood flow is greater in those areas. The outline below lists the general categories of agents that can produce pulmonary exudates and gives examples in each category.

Altered permeability
  Drugs
    Cytotoxic: oxygen, busulfan, bleomycin, oxides of nitrogen
    Hypersensitivity: nitrofurantoin, ? heroin, methadone
  Chemicals
    HCl (aspiration pneumonia), ozone, phosgene, NO_2
    Smoke inhalation
  Infection
    Viral pneumonia
  Connective tissue diseases
    Systemic lupus erythematosus, rheumatoid arthritis, scleroderma
  Miscellaneous or unknown mechanisms
    Fat embolus, uremia, radiation pneumonitis
    Idiopathic pulmonary fibrosis
Increased capillary pressure
  Mitral stenosis, myocarditis, pulmonary veno-occlusive disease

Both the alveolar and the interstitial reactions may resolve, or they may go on to fibrosis. It appears that in each case the ultimate development of fibrosis depends on (1) the amount of tissue necrosis produced by the initial inflammation, and (2) the persistence of the active injuring agent. It is clear from the outline at left that the patient's history will often depend on the inciting agent, as will his physical examination and laboratory manifestations. Indeed, a careful history is often of great help in defining the causative agent. In some instances, removal of the inciting agent by eliminating the source of injury may reverse the disease, while in other instances, the initial insult may be so severe that fibrosis ensues despite all therapy. Therapy for exudates due to altered permeability has been limited to supportive measures during the acute phase (see Chap. 23) and to the use of corticosteroids. It is generally believed that the antiinflammatory action of corticosteroids is of value in preventing fibrosis subsequent to injury, although there are few controlled data to substantiate this.

The collagen (connective tissue) diseases comprise a widely divergent group of disorders with fibrinoid necrosis as a common denominator (see Chap. 46). Three entities characteristically produce diffuse pulmonary fibrosis: (1) Scleroderma is the one most frequently (over 90 percent) associated with diffuse pulmonary fibrosis; (2) rheumatoid arthritis may be associated with a variety of pulmonary changes ranging from nonspecific exudative pleural effusions and nonspecific pulmonary fibrosis to relatively specific necrobiotic nodules in the lung; (3) systemic lupus erythematosus is often associated with pleural effusions and fleeting pulmonary infiltrates and on occasion with diffuse pulmonary fibrosis.

Idiopathic Pulmonary Fibrosis

Idiopathic pulmonary fibrosis is a catchall category that undoubtedly will include fewer disorders as more and more specific inciting agents are identified. A wide variety of synonyms have been applied to idiopathic pulmonary fibrosis, including Hamman-Rich syndrome, cryptogenic fibrosing alveolitis, usual interstitial pneumonitis, and idiopathic pulmonary fibrosis. In general, the disease runs a variable course from acute, rapidly progressive, fatal pulmonary infiltrates to chronic, indolent, nonprogressive disease. The age spectrum is wide, including infants and individuals in the eighth decade of life. There are instances of familial idiopathic pulmonary fibrosis and suggestions that at least in some patients hypersensitivities or autoimmune phenomena are of importance, as illustrated by the associated occurrence of hyperglobulinemia, positive rheumatoid factor, and nonspecific antilung antibodies.

The pathologic picture ranges from an acellular, dense connective tissue with considerable destruction of lung to an extremely cellular pulmonary infiltrate, often with massive proliferation and desquamation of large alveolar cells into the alveolar lumina. The latter form, in which there usually is minimal fibrotic disease, has been labeled *desquamative interstitial pneumonitis*. The roentgenogram is variable, depending on the stage and severity of the disease. With desquamative interstitial pneumonitis the chest x-ray frequently has a diffuse, ground-glass appearance with little evidence of scarring and retraction. With acellular, end-stage fibrotic disease there may be widespread scarring and retraction of the lung with formation of bullae and extensive loss of lung volume.

Currently, therapy of these entities is limited. Corticosteroids have been used with variable success, beginning with relatively high doses of 60 to 80 mg of prednisone daily or its equivalent and tapering down to maintenance doses of between 10 and 40 mg given every other day. In general, there seems to be a rough correlation between the cellularity of the lung on biopsy and the response to therapy: Patients with desquamative interstitial pneumonitis tend to have a fairly favorable response, while patients with severe fibrotic scarring and few cellular infiltrates have a poor response. Immunosuppressive agents may be used in patients who have major medical indications against corticosteroid therapy; unfortunately, only patients who respond to corticosteroids appear to respond to the immunosuppressive agents.

Bibliography

Spencer, H. Interstitial pneumonia. *Annu. Rev. Intern. Med.* 18:423, 1967.

Turner-Warwick, M. A perspective view on widespread pulmonary fibrosis. *Br. Med. J.* 2:371, 1974.

17

Environmental Lung Disease

Edward A. Gaensler

The respiratory system differs in three important related aspects from other organ systems discussed in this book. First, both mortality and morbidity from chronic lung disease, with the exception of tuberculosis, have increased constantly during the last 50 years, whereas death rates and disability from chronic disease of other organs have remained stable or declined. Second, the lungs, except for the skin, are the only organs constantly exposed to the atmosphere: They have a total surface area about the same as a tennis court and during a lifetime are exposed to approximately 30 million liters of air. Third, unlike disorders of many other organs, most diseases of the lungs have a known cause, namely the inhalation of noxious substances that are either mined, manufactured, grown, or burned by man. Clearly the removal of such noxious materials from the environment would immediately halt the increase in prevalence of most chronic lung disorders and eventually might lead to their virtual disappearance.

Cigarette smoking without a doubt is the most common, the most prolonged, and the most concentrated form of air pollution. The role of smoking in the gamut of environmental lung disease is difficult to quantitate but, with respect to the most disabling of the pulmonary disorders — chronic bronchitis, emphysema, and bronchogenic carcinoma — the only question is whether smoking is the chief, or the sole, pathogenic environmental factor. Furthermore it is now established that other important environmental pulmonary diseases, such as those of coal miners and asbestos workers, are greatly increased in cigarette smokers.

Industry produces a huge quantity of chemical substances, many of which are distributed to the public before their effects on health are fully known and some of which eventually prove to be harmful. One example is the tragic introduction of beryllium in the coating of fluorescent light bulbs, x-ray tubes, and other electronic devices three decades ago. More recent examples include the use of toluene diisocya-

nate in urea foam, which was developed as a replacement for natural foam rubber, and the introduction of enzyme detergents and certain aerosol sprays. Even in certain well-recognized hazardous occupations, where there is already great awareness of the dangers, disturbing new information has emerged. Thus the dust control measures for asbestosis, long considered adequate, have now been shown to be clearly ineffective; preventive measures in coal workers' pneumoconiosis are being questioned; and byssinosis of cotton workers has reemerged as an underestimated health hazard.

The principal role of the practicing physician is to maintain a high index of suspicion of the possible occupational hazards whenever he is confronted with a patient with a respiratory problem. A close working relationship with local public health officers and agencies responsible for industrial hygiene is of inestimable value. Inasmuch as there is no specific treatment for most of these disorders, the best contribution the physician can make is to the understanding of their epidemiology and to their prevention.

Classification

Occupational lung disease refers to disorders caused by the inhalation of inorganic or organic dusts, gases, fumes, or infectious agents at a place of work. The term *environmental lung disease* is preferable, because the same disorders have also been found to occur in individuals whose exposure did not occur in a work area. The following is a working outline of the environmental noxious agents of chief concern:

I. Inorganic dusts
   A. Free silica
      1. Crystalline: quartz, flint, tridymite, cristobolite
      2. Amorphous: diatomaceous earth [Submicron: Hi-Sil, etc.] *
   B. Silicates
      1. Asbestos
         a. Serpentine: chrysotile (90% of all)
         b. Amphiboles: crocidolite (blue), amosite, anthophyllite, tremolite

*Substances in brackets are most likely not pathogenic.

2. "Talc": magnesium silicate (also asbestos amphiboles, silica)
3. [Kaolin, fuller's earth, bentonite, vermiculite, sillimanite]

C. Coal and graphite: ? anthracosilicosis
D. Inert dusts
   1. Low radiodensity: [carbon, limestone, gypsum, cement, silicon carbide]
   2. High radiodensity: [iron, tin, barium, chromium, rare earths]

II. Toxic metals and compounds
Beryllium, cadmium, zirconium

III. Noxious gases
Oxides of nitrogen, sulfur dioxide, ozone, chlorine, phosgene, ammonia

IV. Biologic dusts causing allergic alveolitis
Moldy hay, bagasse, moldy malt and barley, cork, infected bark, cheese, redwood dust, pigeons, parrots, budgerigars, green coffee, weevil-infested flour, air conditioners, humidifiers

V. Dusts that may cause asthma
A. Animal: silk hair and butterfly squamae; feathers and moths; sheep, cattle, horse dander epidermis; chitin, screwworm fly
B. Vegetable: cotton, flax, hemp, sisal; castor bean meal, linseed; cedar and boxwood; *Penicillium casei*
C. Organic chemicals: heated polyvinyl film, penicillin, toluene diisocyanate, formaldehyde, proteolytic enzymes
D. Inorganic chemicals: thallic anhydride, platinum salts, chromates

VI. Infections related to occupation
A. Bacterial: tuberculosis, anthrax, glanders, Q fever
B. Rickettsial: ornithosis-psittacosis
C. Fungal: coccidioidomycosis, histoplasmosis, North American blastomycosis

VII. Pulmonary carcinogens
A. Asbestos, especially crocidolite and chrysotile (both mesothelioma and, in smokers, bronchogenic carcinoma)
B. Nickel and nickel carbonyl
C. Chromium, as in monochromate dusts, fumes, mists
D. Coal tar, pitch, soot, and smoke
E. Ionizing radiation: pitchblende, carnotite (yellow cake), hematite, and fluorite
F. Arsenic: trioxide, sheep-dip, vineyards
G. Isopropyl oil
H. Mustard gas
I. Bis (chloromethyl) ether

Silica Dust Exposure

Pneumoconiosis is the term applied to lung disease resulting from inhalation of dust, usually inorganic, and capable of being demonstrated in the lung tissue. *Silicosis* is pneumoconiosis due to the inhalation of silica dust, which constitutes a major problem, probably because of its fibrogenicity and ubiquity. Silica may be inhaled in pure form but more often is a contaminant of other mined materials or is carried into a mine shaft to provide traction on the rails. Disease appears to be dose-related: Inhalation of only small quantities, as in a well-supervised operation, may not result in significant disease for 20 to 40 years, whereas inhalation of high concentrations, as can occur during tunnel drilling, the handling of silica flour, or the cleaning of boilers, may result in fatal disease within a few months. In regions without heavy industry or mining such as New England, pure silicosis is seen most commonly in granite cutters, foundry workers, and in the abrasive industry.

Coal Dust Exposure

Coal workers' pneumoconiosis, allegedly the most common form of pneumoconiosis, is still a poorly defined disorder. The problem is that while coal mining is always associated with some degree of silica exposure, reliable data concerning pulmonary disease in American coal miners are lacking. It is believed that miners have a higher prevalence of lung diseases than the general male population. However, emphysema and chronic bronchitis seem to account for most of the higher prevalence; hence, the problem of cigarette smoking further confounds the picture.

Simple coal workers' pneumoconiosis (black lung) results largely from the inhalation of pure coal dust and usually causes no symptoms and only slight or equivocal changes in lung function. The major importance of the syndrome is that it may be a precursor of a more complicated disease, progressive massive fibrosis.

Progressive massive fibrosis, or complicated pneumoconiosis, is defined as any radiographic opacity greater than 1 cm in diameter in an exposed worker who has no evidence of other disease. Unlike simple pneumoconiosis, progressive massive fibrosis statistically is associated with severe, progressive respiratory impairment and premature death, although spontaneous arrests in the disease do occur. Here again the pathogenesis is obscure; the belief is still widely held that progressive massive fibrosis is usually the result of an infection with *Mycobacterium tuberculosis* or atypical acid-fast bacilli.

Asbestos Exposure

Asbestos, in contrast to coal dust, is one of the most dangerous substances encountered in industry. This mineral has an infinite half-life and is constantly present — in houses with asbestos siding, roofing, or vinyl asbestos floors; in cars with asbestos undercoating, brake linings, and clutch facings; in asbestos paper filters, and in industrial plants with fireproof ceiling tiles or steel girders coated with asbestos. Although the dangers of asbestos have been appreciated for 50 years, asbestos-related diseases presently appear to be entirely out of control. This is probably related to two peculiarities of this material. First, inhalation of a quantity of asbestos fibers sufficient to cause fatal disease generally does not lead to signs or symptoms until 8 to 15 years later. As a result, the effects of attempts to improve industrial hygiene do not become evident until many years later, making an evaluation of such efforts exceedingly difficult. Second, asbestos is mined, cleaned, and processed by a few large companies that are well acquainted with the health hazards. The products, however, are then dispersed to industries and individuals who are often unconcerned with asbestos. As a result, most asbestos-related disease is seen in these secondary users.

Asbestos causes three distinct types of problems. The first is *asbestosis* (white lung), an interstitial pneumonia indistinguishable from the usual or idiopathic type except for the presence in the former of asbestos bodies (see Table 17-1). Asbestosis appears to be dose-related, but regardless of dosage, it develops slowly over a period of years. However, it appears to progress relentlessly even after cessation of exposure. The second problem is *bronchogenic carcinoma,* which is 5 to 10 times more common in cigarette-smoking asbestos workers than in other cigarette smokers. In nonsmoking asbestos workers, however, bronchogenic carcinoma is as rare as it is in other nonsmokers.

The third problem caused by asbestos is a *pleural complication* of four types, all of which appear to be unique in persons exposed to the fibrous silicates, mainly asbestos and talc: (1) peculiar pleural plaques that often calcify after 20 to 40 years, generally are benign, cause no functional impairment, are merely a marker of exposure, are only slightly dose-related, and are seen in individuals living at some distance from mines and asbestos plants; (2) diffuse pleural thickening that may be associated with restrictive functional impairment; (3) asbestos pleural effusion that is usually bloody, often bilateral, and, lacking distinctive features, is usually not recognized; and finally, (4) pleural or peritoneal *mesothelioma,* a rare tumor that now can be shown to be related to asbestos in more than 80 percent of cases. Though still relatively rare, this last problem is the most worrisome of the pleural complications, both because it is apparently only weakly dose-related (it is found also in so-called neighborhood cases) and because it is invariably fatal.

Talc Exposure

Talc is closely related to asbestos, both in that it contains asbestos amphiboles and in that all the asbestos-related disorders, with the exception of mesothelioma, have been demonstrated also to be caused by talc, albeit after much longer and more intense exposure. Talc is also important because talc consumption in the United States exceeds even that of asbestos. Most patients come from the rubber industry, but talc miners, ceramic and cosmetic workers, and even parachute packers have all developed the disease.

Table 17-1. Pathologic Reactions of Lung

Lung reaction	Occupational example	Nonoccupational example
Phagocyte and dust macule with relatively little scarring	Coal workers' pneumoconiosis with minimal silica	City dwellers
Phagocyte and dust nodule with relatively marked scarring	Silicosis of sandblasters, foundry workers	None
Progressive massive fibrosis	Silicosis of sandblasters, foundry workers	None
Acute interstitial pneumonia or acute alveolar injury	NO_2 from welding in confined space	Viral pneumonia
Chronic interstitial pneumonia		
1. Usual type	Asbestosis of insulation workers	Idiopathic, collagen disease
2. Desquamative type	? Talc, e.g., rubber industry workers	Idiopathic
Sarcoid reaction	Berylliosis, allergic alveolitis	Sarcoidosis
Infection		
1. Viral	Ornithosis of turkey dressers	Any
2. Bacterial	Tuberculosis of pathology residents	Any
3. Fungal	Coccidioidomycosis of agricultural workers	Any
Acute bronchiolitis and bronchiolitis obliterans	SO_2 inhalation — Maraschino cherry processers	? Viral, ? bacterial
Acute and chronic bronchitis	Chemical workers	Cigarette smokers
Bronchial asthma	Toluene diisocyanate — "atopic"	—
Malignant tumors	Mesothelioma of shipyard workers	Any

Exposure to Inert Dusts

Inert dusts by definition are not fibrogenic and generally do not cause disease unless exposure to them is so massive and prolonged that lung clearance mechanisms are overwhelmed, resulting in an increased susceptibility to infection. Dusts with high radiodensity cause a benign pneumoconiosis associated with well-defined opacities throughout the lung fields, while dusts of low radiodensity lead to no evident radiographic abnormalities. The high-radiodensity dusts include iron (siderosis, which occurs mainly in steel grinders and welders); tin (stannosis); barium; antimony; and some of the rare earths. The principal inert dust of low radiodensity is carbon, which in the absence of silica causes a benign pneumoconiosis (page 181). Exposure to carbon uncontaminated by silica may occur in carbon black and soot workers or in those producing channel coal or charcoal, while graphite miners are exposed also to variable amounts of silica. It is well to remember that widely used materials such as limestone, cement, gypsum, and Carborundum belong in this inert class.

Biologic Dust Disease

The biologic dust diseases (allergic alveolitis) are discussed in Chapter 16. Suffice it to say here that, with the exception of byssinosis and farmer's lung, the magnitude of the problem has become apparent only recently, and the lists of organic substances capable of causing allergic alveolitis are growing monthly.

Noxious Gas Exposure

This is easy to define in the context of industrial accidents when workers, trapped in confined spaces, sustain acute chemical pneumonitis from chlorine, phosgene, sulfur dioxide, ozone, or ammonia. All but the last of these may be involved in smoke inhalation, a problem that is much more difficult to evaluate and one that is usually compounded by the inhalation of carbon monoxide and burns of the upper respiratory tract. Other difficult examples include oxyacetylene or electric arc welding in confined spaces, where oxides of nitrogen are formed and might cause acute alveolar injury; this should not be confused either with welder's lung due to inhalation of vaporized iron oxide fumes, which causes a harmless siderosis, or with a brief metal-fume fever resulting from inhalation of vaporized zinc or copper. Silo filler's disease is also the result of acute exposure to oxides of nitrogen; its characteristic clinical features consist of a period of acute edema followed by apparent recovery and then usually a relapse, with a second acute illness a few weeks later. Whether chronic exposure to acid-forming radicals causes disease is still more difficult to establish. Threshold values for sulfur dioxide may be exceeded in certain industrial processes such as are used in the bleaching of paper or in the production of maraschino cherries or dried fruit. Much lower concentrations are found in polluted air.

Toxic Metal Exposure
Among the toxic metals, beryllium has received the most attention. It may cause an acute pneumonitis or a chronic, insidious, multisystemic granulomatosis that was thought originally to be a variant of sarcoidosis (Salem sarcoid). Because chronic berylliosis sometimes becomes manifest only after a latent period of up to 20 years, the importance of a detailed occupational history is apparent. Cadmium oxide fumes are so toxic that they have been considered for chemical warfare. Oxyacetylene welding of cadmium-plated metal is especially hazardous. Cadmium has produced emphysema in experimental animals in some studies but is not well established as a cause of chronic obstructive lung disease in cadmium workers.

Organic Chemicals
The role of a variety of organic chemicals in relation to lung disease often is very difficult to define, both because of the multiplicity of such compounds in modern chemical plants and because the pulmonary reaction to them consists of acute or chronic bronchitis, bronchospasm, and asthma, disorders that have a very high prevalence in the population at large.

Both immediate and late types of asthmatic reactions may be provoked by a large number of substances, including some of the organic dusts referred to under Biologic Dust Disease, as well as by complex platinum salts, aluminum soldering flux, piperazine, and a number of proteolytic enzymes, especially those derived from *Bacillus subtilis* and used in "biological" washing powders. The most interesting are the isocyanates used in the manufacture of polyurethane fibers, plastics, elastomers, adhesives, surface coatings, and a variety of flexible and rigid foams. The most common of these is toluene diisocyanate, which may cause a chemical bronchitis in high doses but may provoke asthmatic reactions in concentrations as low as 0.003 parts per million. In most cases the almost infinite number of possible organic compounds makes evaluation difficult. Personal hypersensitivity or idiosyncrasy is often the major factor when patients have severe respiratory symptoms when at work or on inhalation challenge while their fellow workers remain unaffected despite similar exposures.

Occupational Respiratory Infections
The diseases listed on page 181 generally are acquired in unusual circumstances and are caused by unusual organisms. Only a detailed occupational history can distinguish a causal relationship from a similar disease contracted in a nonoccupational context.

Environmental Respiratory Carcinogens
A number of occupations clearly are associated with an increased prevalence of bronchogenic carcinoma. This was first demonstrated in pitchblende miners in Joachimsthal, Czechoslovakia, at the beginning of this century. With the greatly increased demand for uranium during the past 30 years, much greater prevalence of bronchogenic carcinoma has been demonstrated among so-called yellow cake miners in Utah and Colorado. It is now well established that the ionizing radiation of uranium dust stored in the lung and lymphatics is carcinogenic. Other materials that have been incriminated are listed on page 181. Currently of most serious concern is the increased prevalence of bronchogenic carcinoma among asbestos workers alluded to previously. Approximately 15 percent of all cigarette-smoking insulation workers are likely to die of bronchogenic carcinoma. It is thought that the effects of tar and nicotine are potentiated by the irritating effect of the asbestos fibers. Chromium, tar, soot, and smoke as well as nickel and arsenic have been definitely incriminated. Indeed, some studies show that bronchogenic carcinoma is

slightly more prevalent in nonsmoking city dwellers than it is in nonsmokers who live in the country.

Diagnosis

The lung can react to insult in only a limited number of ways. These reactions are discussed in Chapter 16 and are listed for environmental diseases in Table 17-1. Most of these reactions, be they interstitial or granulomatous, pneumonic or bronchiolitic, may result from environmental or nonenvironmental injury or both. It is therefore not surprising that the symptoms, signs, laboratory data, roentgenographic findings, and even pathologic pictures may fail to establish that an occupational hazard has caused a disease. Therefore the occupational history not only gives the initial clue but is indispensable in relation to all other findings.

THE OCCUPATIONAL HISTORY

An exhaustive occupational history should be obtained from every patient with signs or symptoms of lung disease. One must list in chronologic order every single job, including part-time work, as well as recreational activities. In discussing these it is necessary to determine what materials were worked upon; whether any intermediary compounds were used to facilitate the job, such as graphite, talc, or oils; the composition of tools such as grinding wheels; the raw materials that were supplied to the plant; and the nature of the finished products.

Also of interest are preventive measures at the plant, such as special ventilation, the availability of masks, and the extent and frequency of industrial hygiene inspections either by the company or by outside state or federal inspectors. Finally, simple epidemiologic information concerning respiratory disease or deaths among fellow workers may be of interest. Information relating to well-publicized hazards such as mining, sandblasting, or asbestos manufacture is generally uninformative because it is now volunteered by well-educated workers. Thus answers to questions relating to dust at work usually are slanted, because most patients with respiratory complaints and knowledge of abnormal roentgenograms are likely to answer in the affirmative. Respiratory disease in some circumstances may be the result of the patient's

exposure to nearby workers who use dangerous materials. Contact or neighborhood cases probably were first described in relation to chronic beryllium disease, in which persons living at some distance from the plant were affected.

Symptomatic items of special interest are those concerning the duration, precise time relationship to the patient's work, and periodicity. Dyspnea, with or without cough, is by far the most common complaint. An insidious onset is usual with pneumoconiosis, while paroxysmal or recurrent dyspnea may be the result of a bronchospasm from inhaled agents, a chemical pneumonitis, or an allergic alveolitis. An interval of several hours between exposure and dyspnea, fever, and chills is common in farmer's lung. By contrast, attacks indistinguishable from allergic asthma occur immediately after contact with toluene diisocyanate. With byssinosis, dyspnea and wheezing are most marked on resuming work after the weekend (Monday blues).

THE CHEST ROENTGENOGRAM

The chest film is indispensable for screening and not uncommonly brings the patient to the physician. Unfortunately it also is often used to adjudicate disability, either because of ignorance or sometimes because it is prescribed by law. Therefore certain principles in the interpretation of chest films may be helpful. The classification of the International Labor Office simply describes pulmonary densities as rounded or irregular (linear) and grades them on the basis of size, configuration, degree of profusion, and location. Pleural thickening and calcification as well as an indistinct cardiac contour, so important in asbestosis, are also to be documented. This classification avoids expressions that imply a pathologic process, such as "interstitial disease," "granulomatous foci," or "fibrotic nodule."

In general, the pneumoconioses lead to generalized or diffuse x-ray opacities. In silicosis, coal workers' pneumoconiosis, and benign pneumoconioses these shadows usually have a rounded contour and vary from 1 to 10 mm in diameter. Larger shadows are equated with massive fibrosis. Rounded opacities are recognized at a relatively early stage, because the normal roentgenogram does not contain such shadows.

By contrast, in the interstitial pneumonias caused by asbestos or other fibrous silicates, the opacities tend to be irregular or linear. These are not recognized until a late stage of the disease, because the normal roentgenogram does contain the normal irregular lines of vascular shadows. As a corollary, the functional impairment in silicosis and coal workers' pneumoconiosis tends to be overestimated from the appearance of the roentgenogram, whereas the opposite is true in asbestosis. The chest roentgenogram is unsuitable for evaluation of functional impairment, especially in disorders associated with airways obstruction. Following exposure to inert heavy metals, even quite astonishing diffuse opacities may not be associated with any functional abnormality or symptom, whereas in allergic alveolitis the chest roentgenogram may appear quite normal, even when there are profound disturbances of respiratory gas exchange and severe exertional dyspnea. From the diagnostic standpoint the chest roentgenogram is most helpful when abnormalities are characteristic, as with the progressive massive fibrosis and the so-called eggshell calcifications seen in silicosis, or as with the basal irregular opacities associated with pleural thickening and the plaques or pleural calcifications seen in asbestosis.

SPECIAL DIAGNOSTIC PROCEDURES

The pneumoconioses are not associated with known systemic, hematologic, or biochemical manifestations. Generally they can be recognized only on epidemiologic grounds or by direct examination of lung tissue. Lung biopsy is necessary in about one-quarter of the patients; its usual indication is a pulmonary infiltration of unknown etiology. However, other patients with a suspicious occupational history may prove to have a treatable though totally nonoccupational lung disease. Infections and tumors are recognized by conventional tests, and any association with occupation is derived from the history. The cause of biologic dust diseases may be clarified by immunoserological reactions or by bronchial provocation tests described elsewhere in this text.

Pathology

The pathogenesis of some of the pulmonary lesions is relatively obvious. For example, gases of acid radicals combine with lung water to form the corresponding acids and cause direct injury to the bronchiolar and alveolar walls. In other occupational disorders, much less is known about the mechanisms. The fibrogenic activity of silica has been investigated for many years without clear-cut answers. Also, the various reactions that are outlined in Table 17-1 most often occur in various combinations. For example, acute interstitial pneumonia is often associated with acute bronchiolitis that progresses to distortion and even obliteration of the bronchioles (bronchiolitis obliterans). When the lesions are typical and are associated with dust particles, a suggestive diagnosis is possible. However, if no dust is seen with either transmitted or polarized light and if the lesion does not belong among the first three reactions of Table 17-1, then a diagnosis of environmental lung disease is not possible without a history.

Pathophysiology

Environmental lung disease may be associated with the entire spectrum of lung pathology, and therefore any of the patterns of physiologic deficit may result (see Chap. 9). In recent years it has been recognized that occupational lung diseases may cause significant impairment of respiratory gas exchange with little or no mechanical abnormalities. Hypoxemia may result from ventilation-perfusion discrepancies and perhaps also from interference with membrane diffusion. Early stages of asbestosis exemplify this situation, and impaired gas exchange with elevated alveolar-arterial oxygen differences and reduced diffusing capacity predominate in the toxic or allergic granulomatoses. Uneven perfusion may result from irregular obliteration of the pulmonary vascular bed, as may occur with perivascular cuffing by silicotic nodules; from a hypersensitivity type of arteriolitis; or from vasoconstriction resulting from local underventilation.

For purposes of this discussion, correlation of physiologic abnormalities with clinical and radiologic findings might be summarized as follows:

1. Physiologic studies are most useful in delineating the type of pathophysiology and, by inference, the general nature of the structural alterations; they are also useful in estimating the severity of the func-

tional impairment and in following the course of the disease. Lung function studies have no diagnostic value, because occupational and nonoccupational disorders may cause the same types of lesions and therefore may be responsible for a similar range of functional disorders (see Table 17-1).

2. Correlations of functional and structural changes suggest that the important functional determinant is not the number or size of obvious nodules, but rather the severity and distribution of cellular and acellular infiltration of the intervening alveolar spaces and interstitial tissue.

3. The severity of roentgenographic abnormalities correlates poorly with both functional and histologic changes, and by inference the roentgenograph is of limited value as a screening device, especially in lesions primarily associated with interstitial pneumonia.

4. Concerning disability, the obstructive syndromes lead to a marked increase in the work of breathing and therefore quickly lead to dyspnea; in these cases subjective complaints usually correlate well with objective measurements of functional abnormality. Restriction without marked impairment of gas exchange is well tolerated, and sometimes there are no complaints until the vital capacity is reduced to less than one-half its normal value; right heart failure then appears to be the principal risk. Primary impairment of gas exchange has variable subjective consequences. Arterial oxygen tension and diffusing capacity correlate poorly with dyspnea. Usually shortness of breath is most closely related to the degree of hyperventilation, probably resulting from hypoxemia and abnormal lung and chest wall reflexes.

Disability Evaluation

Physicians should be qualified to judge impairment either of organ systems or of the whole man. Impairment exists when the individual's performance is less than that of a group of normal individuals of the same sex, age, and stature. Generally physicians are not trained nor do they have the necessary information to adjudicate disability, which concerns judgment of the worker's capacity for gainful employment. It is an administrative decision and must take into account not only the functional impairment but

also the patient's age, education, social milieu, rehabilitation potential, as well as the local employment situation and related factors. Indeed, disability is much more closely related to these other factors than to the degree of pulmonary impairment. The pulmonary reserve is so great, there may be marked impairment of lung function without serious disability, particularly today in an era of extensive mechanization with heavy manual labor largely a thing of the past. Conversely, a worker may be totally disabled without significant functional impairment because of excessive cough, generalized toxicity, recurrent pulmonary infection, or because of his physician's advice to take an extended rest.

Bibliography

American Lung Association. *Air Pollution Primer* (3rd ed.). New York, 1974.

Biological effects of asbestos. *Ann. N.Y. Acad. Sci.* 132:138, 1965.

Brodeur, P. The magic mineral. *The New Yorker Magazine,* Oct. 12, 1968. P. 117.

Coal workers' pneumoconiosis. *Ann. N.Y. Acad. Sci.* Vol. 200, 1972.

Dinman, B. D. *Nature of Occupational Cancer.* Springfield, Ill.: Thomas, 1974.

Gaensler, E. A., and Wright, G. W. Evaluation of respiratory impairment. *Arch. Environ. Health* 12:146, 1966.

Goldsmith, J. R. Health effects of air pollution. Basics of RD. *Am. Thorac. Soc.* 4:1, 1975.

The Health Consequences of Smoking. Washington, D.C.: U.S. Department of Health, Education and Welfare, U.S. Public Health Service, 1973.

Higgins, I. T. T. Trends in respiratory cancer mortality. *Arch. Environ. Health* 28:121, 1974.

Hunter, D. *The Diseases of Occupations* (5th ed.). London: The English Universities Press, 1975.

Morgan, W. K. C., and Seaton, A. *Occupational Lung Diseases.* Philadelphia: Saunders, 1975.

Parkes, W. R. *Occupational Lung Disorders.* London: Butterworth, 1974.

18

Neoplasms of the Respiratory Tract

Michael E. Whitcomb

Bronchogenic Carcinoma

Bronchogenic carcinoma is the most common form of adult cancer; approximately 30 percent of all men and 7 percent of all women who die from cancer in the United States have lung cancer. More deaths occur in men from lung cancer than from the next five most common forms of cancer combined. The number of deaths caused by lung cancer in women is currently exceeded only by those caused individually by breast, colon, and rectal cancers. It is estimated that about 75,000 persons die in this country each year from lung cancer.

EPIDEMIOLOGY

The incidence of bronchogenic carcinoma in any population is determined to a great extent by exposure to carcinogens, the most important of which is cigarette smoke. Although still somewhat controversial, epidemiologic data strongly implicate cigarette smoking in lung cancer. Not only do nonsmokers comprise a very small percentage of patients with lung cancer, but analysis of the histologic types of cancers in nonsmokers reveals that squamous cell carcinoma and small cell carcinoma, the most common types in smokers, occur only rarely in nonsmokers. Adenocarcinoma accounts for more than 50 percent of all lung tumors in nonsmokers, with bronchial adenoma being the second most common.

Since cigarette smoking is ubiquitous, other possible environmental carcinogens are difficult to identify in the development of lung cancer. Certain industrial exposures seem to be hazardous: Arsenic, nickel, chromium, hematite, asbestos, mustard gas, and radioactive minerals have been shown to be associated with an increased risk of developing lung cancer (see Chap. 17). With the exception of small cell carcinomas associated with exposure to radioactive minerals, squamous cell carcinoma has been the most common form of lung cancer identified in patients exposed to environmental carcinogens.

Recent evidence suggests that the risk of developing lung cancer associated with cigarette smoking is related to the breakdown of hydrocarbons to highly carcinogenic metabolites, a function of the enzyme aryl hydrocarbon decarboxylase. Individuals who develop bronchogenic carcinoma generally have higher levels of this enzyme than individuals with similar smoking habits who do not have lung cancer. Another factor that may play a role is the presence of certain types of lung disease; for example, there is an increased frequency of bronchogenic carcinoma, usually adenocarcinoma, in patients with interstitial pulmonary fibrosis of the idiopathic variety or associated with scleroderma. There may also be an increased incidence of lung cancer in patients with bullous lung disease. The apparent association of bronchogenic carcinoma with chronic bronchitis or with emphysema is probably simply related to the fact that cigarette smoking is a common factor associated with both of those diseases.

PATHOLOGY

Bronchogenic carcinoma has been classified into four major pathologic categories: (1) epidermoid or squamous cell carcinoma; (2) small cell carcinoma; (3) adenocarcinoma; and (4) large cell carcinoma. The histopathologic features of each are beyond the scope of this discussion; however, it is important to know that significant variability exists even among experienced pathologists in classifying lung tumors. In addition, variability in the histologic pattern may be observed within a single tumor. Despite these limitations, the histologic tumor type has definite prognostic significance, and it influences the therapeutic approach to the patient.

Squamous cell carcinoma accounts for 40 to 50 percent of all lung cancers. These tumors appear most commonly as hilar or perihilar masses and are the most frequent form of lung cancer to undergo cavitation. Because of their central location, a high percentage of cases can be diagnosed by either bronchoscopy or sputum cytologic examination. Although these tumors grow rapidly, they tend to stay localized in the thorax and thus have higher resectability and survival rates than the other cell types.

Twenty to thirty percent of all lung cancers are small cell carcinomas, the most malignant form of bronchogenic carcinoma. These tumors generally present as hilar lesions and are frequently associated with massive mediastinal adenopathy. Systemic metastases are almost invariably present at the time of initial diagnosis, and therefore these tumors are not usually amenable to surgical resection. In most centers the diagnosis of small cell carcinoma is considered evidence of inoperability even if distant metastases cannot be documented. Of all the forms of lung cancer, small cell carcinoma is the most responsive to radiotherapy and chemotherapy. Despite favorable response rates, however, mean survival time seems little affected by these forms of therapy.

Adenocarcinomas account for 20 to 30 percent of bronchogenic carcinomas. These tumors most commonly present as masses in the periphery of the lung. Because of their peripheral location, they are uncommonly diagnosed by bronchoscopy or by sputum cytologic examination. The degree of histologic differentiation of these tumors is of prognostic significance. Well-differentiated peripheral adenocarcinomas less than 4 cm in diameter have the highest 5-year survival rates of all forms of lung cancer. Poorly differentiated or undifferentiated adenocarcinomas tend to metastasize early, giving them a poorer prognosis. Pleural effusions occur most commonly in this form of lung cancer.

Large cell carcinomas occurring with a frequency of about 20 percent tend to mimic undifferentiated adenocarcinomas in clinical and roentgenologic presentation and biologic activity. There are no other distinctive features of these tumors.

CLINICAL MANIFESTATIONS

The clinical manifestations of lung cancer are related to their local effects within the thorax, the effects of disseminated metastases, and the systemic biologic effects of the tumor. Symptoms caused by tumors within the thorax may be predominantly either pulmonary or extrapulmonary. The most common pulmonary symptoms are those caused by irritation of the bronchial mucosa — cough, sputum production, or hemoptysis. In addition, obstruction of a major bronchus may result either in atelectasis or in a distal obstructive pneumonitis with symptoms indistinguishable from those of a primary pneumonia. The extra-

pulmonary manifestations of lung cancer result from direct extension or from metastasis to vital structures. Involvement of the pleural space with development of significant pleural effusion may cause progressive dyspnea. The syndromes of superior vena cava obstruction, left recurrent laryngeal nerve paralysis, and phrenic nerve paralysis may be caused either by direct extension of the tumor or by encroachment upon these structures by mediastinal lymph node metastases. Involvement of the pericardium and heart may result in pericardial effusion or arrhythmias. Chest wall involvement may result in pain simulating parietal pleurisy, intercostal neuritis, or bone erosion. Horner's syndrome and muscle atrophy may occur when superior sulcus tumors extend into the sympathetic ganglion and brachial plexus.

A variety of symptoms may occur as a result of systemic metastases. The most common symptoms are due to metastases to the brain, bones, and liver. Central nervous system involvement may be manifested by headaches, personality changes, seizures, or focal neurologic deficits. Bone involvement is almost always manifested by pain. Liver involvement may occasionally cause jaundice. Although adrenal gland metastases are present in a high percentage of cases at postmortem examination, clinical manifestations of adrenal involvement are hardly ever recognized.

A number of systemic manifestations of lung cancer cannot be attributed to the local effects of systemic metastases. Although the pathogenesis of some of these systemic manifestations is known, it remains obscure in many cases. The varied manifestations include weight loss, anorexia, fatigability, hypertrophic pulmonary osteoarthropathy, and paraneoplastic endocrine and neurologic syndromes. The pathogenesis of hypertrophic pulmonary osteoarthropathy and of the neurologic syndromes is unknown. The paraneoplastic endocrine syndromes are caused by the synthesis and secretion by bronchogenic carcinomas of a variety of polypeptides that are identical or similar to normally produced hormones. Although these syndromes may be associated with all forms of bronchogenic carcinoma, the majority occur in patients with small cell carcinoma. The major exception is hypercalcemia due to ectopic parathormone secretion by squamous cell carcinoma. Adrenocorticotropic (ACTH) secretion is probably the most common form of ectopic hormone production associated with bronchogenic carcinoma. In contrast to the hyperadrenocorticism that may occur in patients without bronchogenic carcinoma, the excess ACTH secretion in patients with bronchogenic carcinoma is manifested chiefly by severe hypokalemic and hypochloremic alkalosis.

At the time of diagnosis, patients with bronchogenic carcinoma may be asymptomatic or may have any combination of local, systemic, or metastatic symptoms. Approximately 10 percent of patients are asymptomatic; 30 percent have only pulmonary symptoms, and another 30 percent have either systemic symptoms or symptoms attributable to metastatic disease. Within any group of patients with nearly identical lesions and similar cell types, those who are asymptomatic have a more favorable prognosis than those who have symptoms. Patients with pulmonary symptoms alone have a better prognosis than those with systemic symptoms, while patients with metastatic symptoms at the time of diagnosis have the worst prognosis.

DIAGNOSIS

Although a presumptive diagnosis of lung cancer can usually be made on the basis of the roentgenogram, cytologic or histologic proof of neoplasm is necessary for choosing between surgery and alternate treatments and for planning irradiation or chemotherapy. Cytologic examination of the sputum (see Chap. 9) is a technique that can confirm the presence of tumor, often with effective diagnosis of the histologic type. The technique can establish the diagnosis in a very high percentage of centrally located tumors, especially if multiple specimens and methods of sputum induction are used; sputum cytology is less helpful in midzonal tumors and is of little value for peripheral lesions.

Use of the flexible fiberoptic bronchoscope coupled with the bronchial brush and biopsy forceps has increased the percentage of cases of bronchogenic carcinoma that can be directly visualized and sampled; diagnostic accuracy when the lesion is endoscopically visualized is 80 to 85 percent. When the lesion cannot be directly visualized, diagnostic accuracy is 50 to 60 percent. Other procedures may be required or preferable in selected patients; an obvious and accessible metastasis, such as to skin or lymph node, should be biopsied. Bone marrow biopsy is diagnostic in about 50 percent of patients with small cell carcinoma and 10 percent of patients with adenocarcinoma; the yield is negligible in squamous cell carcinoma. Mediastinoscopy is positive in approximately 40 percent of patients considered potentially resectable who undergo this procedure prior to thoracotomy and may at times be a worthwhile diagnostic procedure; bilateral scalene lymph node biopsy (in the absence of palpable nodes) is positive in 15 to 20 percent of patients.

STAGING EVALUATION

It is important that a thorough staging evaluation be performed before lung cancer patients are selected for surgery, so that those who have unresectable lesions will not have to undergo a thoracotomy unnecessarily. From a practical standpoint, the important thing to determine is whether lung cancer is localized to the lung parenchyma or whether mediastinal lymph node or extrathoracic metastases have occurred. Thirty to forty percent of patients otherwise considered potential candidates for resectional surgery have mediastinal lymph node metastases demonstrated by mediastinoscopy. In general, the yield of metastases to lymph nodes discovered by mediastinoscopy is higher in patients with lesions in the hilum or perihilar region and in patients with undifferentiated tumors. It is also important to recognize that false-negative mediastinoscopies occur in 10 to 15 percent of patients who in fact do have mediastinal metastases; in the majority of these patients the tumor is located in the left upper lobe or left hilum, has metastasized to mediastinal lymph nodes in the aortic window area, and is thus inaccessible to the mediastinoscope. Mediastinal lymph node metastases should be considered a contraindication to surgery except in unusual circumstances.

In the absence of symptoms attributable to any specific metastatic site, diagnostic techniques to detect extrathoracic metastases are, for the most part, grossly inadequate. The most common sites of metastases of bronchogenic carcinoma are brain, bone, liver, and adrenal glands. Brain scans are positive in approximately 5 percent of patients with no central nervous symptoms and in 50 to 60 percent of patients with such symptoms. Neither an electroen-cephalogram nor a lumbar puncture increases the sensitivity of detecting central nervous system metastases. Liver scan has likewise been demonstrated to be of little value in diagnosing patients with bronchogenic carcinoma because it gives a large percentage of false-positive and false-negative results. Peritoneoscopy with direct needle biopsy of the liver is the most specific and most sensitive technique for detecting liver metastases. Bone marrow biopsy is the most sensitive technique for detecting bone metastases. Bone scans are positive in 15 percent of patients with a negative biopsy and in only 5 percent of patients with a positive biopsy. At present there are no satisfactory diagnostic techniques to detect adrenal gland metastases.

TREATMENT
The overall 5-year survival rate for patients with bronchogenic carcinoma is between 5 and 10 percent. It is clear, therefore, that no single form of therapy has had great success. The approach to therapy must be based on knowledge of the extent of the disease and, if possible, of the histologic tumor type. In general, surgical resection of a tumor localized to the lung parenchyma is the only form of curative therapy and should be done in patients who do not have demonstrable intrathoracic or systemic metastases. The inadequacy of staging procedures in identifying patients with truly localized disease is illustrated by the fact that less than 50 percent of patients with apparently localized peripheral nodules survive 5 years.

Mediastinal lymph node metastases are as unfavorable for prognosis as systemic metastases; patients with mediastinal metastases who have undergone resectional surgery have 5-year survival rates of less than 10 percent. Neither adjuvant chemotherapy nor radiotherapy in patients with mediastinal lymph node metastases has had a significant effect on mean survival or long-term survival rates, except possibly in patients with squamous cell carcinoma. Recent studies suggest that the combination of resectional surgery and radiation results in a 5-year survival rate of between 20 and 30 percent in patients with squamous cell carcinoma, even when they are known to have

mediastinal lymph node involvement. Otherwise, radiotherapy should be considered palliative therapy and should be reserved for patients with symptoms directly related to local tumor growth (bronchial obstruction, hemotysis, bone pain, and central nervous system involvement). Systemic chemotherapy has been disappointing for the most part; multiple chemotherapeutic regimens are currently undergoing intensive investigation, with the greatest success to date being in the treatment of small cell carcinoma. Another palliative measure that should be mentioned is corticosteroid therapy (either alone or with local radiotherapy) in patients with symptomatic brain metastases. Recent studies demonstrate that steroids have a favorable effect on local cerebral blood supply and the control of edema in the region of brain metastases.

In patients with hypercalcemia, appropriate therapy to lower the serum calcium may also relieve disturbing symptoms and improve the patient's well-being. Acute therapy usually consists in maintaining a forced diuresis, either alone or in conjunction with oral phosphates, while long-term therapy depends on the pathogenesis of the hypercalcemia; steroids, mithramycin, or indomethacin may be beneficial in certain patients. The newest form of therapy being investigated in bronchogenic carcinoma is immunotherapy; most studies in this area are evaluating the effect of systemic administration of bacille Calmette Guérin (BCG) vaccine or other nonspecific adjuvants on tumor rejection.

Solitary Pulmonary Nodule
The evaluation and management of patients with a solitary pulmonary nodule will be considered in this chapter, since the principles involved are governed by the fact that a high percentage of such lesions are bronchogenic carcinomas. For the purpose of this discussion a solitary pulmonary nodule will be defined as a circumscribed lesion, 3 cm or less in cross-sectional diameter, located in the periphery of the lung.

The approach to the evaluation and management of such lesions is limited by the fact that the list of conditions that can give rise to a solitary pulmonary nodule is quite long; due to the size and location of these lesions, it is extremely unusual to make a specific etiologic diagnosis without resorting to an exploratory thoracotomy. Since it is usually impossible to make a specific diagnosis, the major goal of the preoperative evaluation is simply to differentiate benign from malignant lesions. Unfortunately very little information can be obtained preoperatively to differentiate malignancy from benignity. Routine laboratory studies and skin tests do not allow one to make this distinction. Furthermore, bacteriologic and cytologic examination of expectorated sputum specimens is rarely diagnostic. Although fluoroscopically controlled brushing of such lesions may be diagnostic in an occasional patient with a malignant lesion, this procedure is rarely diagnostic in benign disease. Thus negative results cannot be used to differentiate benign and malignant lesions.

As a general rule, indirect evidence of benignity is used to select those patients who need not undergo an exploratory thoracotomy. Since bronchogenic carcinomas are extremely rare in patients less than 35 years of age, lesions that occur in patients in this age group may be presumed to be benign and only those lesions that grow during subsequent observation need be surgically removed. In patients over 35, roentgenographic criteria are employed to distinguish between benign and malignant lesions. Although a number of roentgenographic signs suggest benignity, there are only two criteria that can be confidently employed. The presence of earlier central or diffuse calcification within the lesion strongly suggests that the lesion is benign. However, the best criterion for benignity is the demonstration that the lesion has been stable on serial chest roentgenograms for a 24-month period. This criterion implies that an old chest roentgenogram is available for comparison purposes and does not mean that the lesion should be observed for growth before decisions regarding surgical intervention are made.

If indirect evidence of benignity is not present, then the lesion should be surgically resected. Clinical experience has demonstrated that extensive roentgenologic and laboratory evaluation to detect either metastases from a primary lung cancer or an extrathoracic primary tumor is unnecessary when the patient is asymptomatic and has a normal physical examination. Thus patients in the cancer age group

with a solitary pulmonary nodule should undergo an exploratory thoracotomy without extensive laboratory evaluation unless the lesion meets acceptable criteria for benignity.

This approach necessarily results in removal of a number of benign lesions. However, since the highest survival rates for patients with bronchogenic carcinoma occur in patients with solitary pulmonary nodules, such an approach is considered acceptable. The dilemma of managing patients with bronchogenic carcinoma is exemplified by this group of patients, since the 5-year survival rate for patients with malignant solitary nodules is still less than 50 percent.

Bronchial Adenoma

Bronchial adenomas are histologically distinct tumors that usually arise from the proximal bronchi. Approximately 90 percent of these tumors are bronchial carcinoids, while the remainder are cylindromas and mucoepidermoid tumors.

The most common presenting complaints of patients with bronchial adenomas are cough and hemoptysis. Because of their central location, these tumors may also cause bronchial obstruction resulting in atelectasis or postobstructive pneumonitis. In many cases the lesion is detected on a routine chest roentgenogram in an asymptomatic individual. Since more than 80 percent of these tumors are centrally located, a specific diagnosis can usually be made by biopsy of the lesion at the time of bronchoscopic examination.

Although these tumors were originally thought to be benign lesions, they have clearly been demonstrated to have a malignant potential. Metastases, however, are usually confined to local or regional lymph nodes and rarely occur outside the thorax. The treatment is surgical, usually lobectomy or pneumonectomy; occasionally the latter operation can be avoided by excising a segment of main bronchus bearing the tumor and performing a plastic reconstruction of the airway. The 5-year survival rate of patients with these tumors exceeds 80 percent.

Bibliography
Feinstein, A. R., Gelfman, N. A., and Yesner, R.
    Observer variability in the histopathologic

diagnosis of lung cancer. *Am. Rev. Respir. Dis.* 100:671, 1970.

Lillington, C. A. The solitary pulmonary nodule — 1974. *Am. Rev. Respir. Dis.* 110:699, 1974.

Mathews, M. J. Morphologic classification of bronchogenic carcinoma. *Cancer Chemother. Rep.* 4:299, 1973.

Muggia, F. M., and Chervo, L. R. Lung cancer: Diagnosis in metastatic sites. *Semin. Oncol.* 1:217, 1974.

Paulson, D. L., and Urschel, H. C. Selectivity in the surgical treatment of bronchogenic carcinoma. *J. Thorac. Cardiovasc. Surg.* 62:544, 1971.

Senior, R. M., and Adamson, J. S. Survival in patients with lung cancer. *Arch. Intern. Med.* 125:975, 1970.

19

Pulmonary Embolism and Infarction

Frank F. Davidson

Pulmonary embolic disease is encountered in every branch of clinical medicine. Feared by all clinicians, it is the cause of 15 percent of the deaths in hospital patients and may be found in more than 50 percent of patients at autopsy. This common disorder is often extremely difficult to diagnose. Small emboli may produce only minor symptoms, and the clinical picture of overt pulmonary embolic disease is often indistinguishable from the very conditions predisposing to it, such as prolonged hypotension or myocardial infarction.

The immediate cause of pulmonary embolism is a thrombus that forms in the veins, presumably due either to venous stasis or to a hypercoagulable state, or both. The clot or a portion of it becomes dislodged, thus becoming an embolus, and passes with the venous blood into the right atrium and ventricle and finally into a pulmonary artery. *Pulmonary embolism* refers to the occlusion of a pulmonary artery by such a clot; *pulmonary infarction* refers to the lung necrosis that may result hours after the embolism. Catastrophic sudden death occasionally occurs from acute pulmonary embolism, but in such cases there is usually evidence of prior pulmonary emboli that, had the emboli been detected clinically, might have led to prevention. An understanding of blood clotting and of venous thrombosis is central to an understanding of thromboembolic disease; these subjects are covered in Chapters 27 and 52.

Pathology

Since pulmonary embolism is so commonly associated with severe disease and death, postmortem studies and clinicopathologic correlations have been available since the time of Virchow in the early nineteenth century. The usual source of the embolus is a thrombus in the deep veins of the legs or thighs. The clinical conditions predisposing to thromboembolic disease are prolonged bed rest or immobility of any sort, congestive heart failure, myocardial infarction, malignancy (especially of the pancreas, stomach, and lung),

polycythemia, and posttraumatic and postsurgical states. Elderly patients with recent hip fractures have a particularly high risk of developing thromboembolic disease. The disease occurs only rarely in children or in normal, healthy individuals, although there is a slightly increased incidence of venous thrombosis and pulmonary embolism during pregnancy and in women taking birth control pills.

Occasionally the source of the thrombus is in the pelvic or periprostatic veins, especially when there is adjacent infection or malignancy, or in the right atrium in patients with atrial fibrillation. Often no source can be found. Carried by the flow of blood, a large clot may lodge in the heart or at the main pulmonary artery bifurcation (saddle embolus). Most clots, however, are smaller or at least are broken up in passage through the heart, and these smaller clots lodge in the segmental or smaller arteries of the lung, particularly in the lower lobes where blood flow is normally greatest. Clinical experience and experimental studies indicate that infarction occurs only when there is underlying pulmonary disease, pulmonary congestion due to heart failure, or a compromised bronchial circulation. Rarely does infarction occur in individuals who are otherwise apparently well.

Often no lung tissue damage occurs with pulmonary embolism, and there may be few if any clinical clues that such a potentially dangerous condition exists. The area fed by the plugged artery may become hemorrhagic and atelectatic and may resolve without actual necrosis; this has been termed *incomplete infarct*. With true infarction, the initially hemorrhagic area develops coagulation necrosis and inflammation over several days. This process accounts for the clinical signs of hemoptysis, low-grade fever, neutrophil count elevation, pleuritic pain, and pleural effusion. The hemorrhagic infarcted area is, as one would expect, bounded by costal or diaphragmatic pleura or interlobar fissures and is usually either segmental or subsegmental in size. Infection with cavity formation is rare unless the embolus is infected, as can be the case if the source of the embolus is pelvic or abdominal sepsis or right-sided bacterial endocarditis. Microscopically the area simply shows alveolar hemorrhage and death of the various cellular components of the lung, followed by inflammation and subsequently by organization and repair. Small scars may remain visible in the lung parenchyma. The emboli in the pulmonary arteries may resolve by lysis, which may be evident within 48 hours, although the process usually takes several weeks or longer. Alternatively the thrombi may undergo organization and recanalization; webs will then remain in the pulmonary arteries as anatomic remnants of the embolus.

Pathophysiology

Some aspects of the clinical presentation of pulmonary embolism are puzzling in view of the observed pathology. The area of hemorrhagic edema or infarction often correlates poorly with the size of the clot, because either the thrombus only partially occludes an artery, thus allowing some blood to pass, or there is a double circulation of the lung. Although simple mechanical blockage of the pulmonary circulation best explains the hemodynamic changes (chiefly, a fall in cardiac output with hypotension and tachycardia due to diminished filling of the left heart), some patients exhibit a much greater degree of hemodynamic instability than that expected from the size of the recent embolus. This hemodynamic instability may be due either to an already compromised pulmonary vascular bed from antecedent emboli or other lung disease or, conceivably, to the release of vasoactive substances (similar to serotonin) from platelets in the impacted clot, although the latter phenomenon has not been demonstrated in man.

Arterial hypoxemia, although characteristic of pulmonary embolus, is difficult to explain. Physiologically it appears to result from venous admixture or shunting due to a decrease or complete absence of ventilation in the area of the lung that is still being perfused with pulmonary arterial blood. Pulmonary embolism pathologically represents predominantly a decrease in perfusion with little obvious cause for a decrease in ventilation. Thus occlusion of a pulmonary artery would be expected to cause an increase in physiologic dead space rather than hypoxemia, since presumably the affected area could be ventilated though not perfused. Nevertheless, as just stated, hypoxemia that is often severe and not easily correctable with oxygen is the predominant clinical abnormality in pulmonary embolism. One explanation is that the ventilation-perfusion mismatch of pulmonary embolism is caused by atelectasis in areas that are still perfused with pulmonary arterial blood from adjacent nonoccluded vessels. Another is that decreased surfactant production may result in impaired alveolar stability and may be a factor contributing to microatelectasis. Although the atelectasis is often not evident on chest x-ray, the hypoxemia may improve transiently with deep inspirations, supporting the concept that the atelectasis exists. Acute hypocapnia is also characteristic of acute pulmonary embolism and is probably caused by a combination of anxiety, hypoxemia, and reflexes from the lungs, all of which could cause alveolar hyperventilation.

Diagnosis

Clinical manifestations of pulmonary embolism range widely from none at all to the serious hemodynamic changes alluded to above. Typically an individual at high risk may either suddenly or over a period of several hours develop mild to severe substernal or pleuritic chest pain, tachycardia, slight fever, and tachypnea. Hemoptysis occurs in about one-third of the patients. In postsurgical patients the clinical picture usually occurs in 7 to 10 days rather than immediately after an operation, whereas in medical patients it may occur at any time. Frequently there is no evidence of deep vein thrombosis, although occasionally leg or thigh swelling or palpable cords in the popliteal area or thigh indicate the presence of clots and make a clinical diagnosis of pulmonary embolus much more obvious. The patient is often anxious and sweating. Fever may or may not occur but is rarely over 103°F (39.4°C), even with infarction. Auscultatory findings may be normal or subtle, such as diminished breath sounds, faint rales, or dullness over the affected area, and they reflect atelectasis, effusion, or an elevated hemidiaphragm. Wheezing may occur but usually indicates other lung disease. A pleural friction rub may be present. With extensive embolization, signs of pulmonary hypertension may develop, such as a right ventricular lift felt in the left lower parasternal area and a palpable valve closure noted in the second or third intercostal space; an increased pulmonic component of the second sound and a pulmonary systolic murmur may be heard. Postural or persistent hypotension may develop, and prominent a waves and engorgement of the neck veins may be observed, indicating failure of the right ventricle.

The chest x-ray may be perfectly normal, particularly at first. Frequent but nonspecific findings on a plain chest film after the initial event include elevation of one hemidiaphragm, pleural effusion, and horizontal or wedge-shaped infiltrates suggestive of atelectasis. Only occasionally are shadows due to the infarct actually observed; these are wedge-shaped segmental densities with their bases on the pleural surface and their more central parts slightly rounded and convex toward the hilum. Oligemia may be noted in the lung distal to the embolus, and the affected pulmonary artery shadow may be enlarged proximally but not evident distally.

The electrocardiogram, in addition to tachycardia (rarely bradycardia), may show signs of sudden right ventricular dilation and strain or a right ventricular conduction defect, although the supposedly classic transient deep S waves in lead I and Q waves in lead III are more often absent (see Chap. 32). Inversion of the T wave may occur in the anterior precordial leads, and atrial fibrillation may be present either as a result of the embolism or as a cause of the emboli (there may be clots in the right atrium). Unfortunately the electrocardiogram is frequently normal or, if there is underlying heart or lung disease, the electrocardiogram may already have been so abnormal that it is of little diagnostic value.

The routine blood count is of little value early, except to document occasional preexisting polycythemia. With subsequent infarction an elevation of the neutrophil count, serum lactic acid dehydrogenase, bilirubin, and even transaminase may occur, but these are nonspecific changes that may occur under many circumstances and are usually of no help in establishing a diagnosis. Pleural fluid, if present, is a clear or bloody exudate, the cytologic study of which often reveals numerous shed mesothelial cells.

The peripheral arterial blood characteristically shows a reduced PO_2 on room air breathing. The PCO_2 is also usually reduced, indicating an acute respiratory alkalosis. The finding of normal arterial PO_2 and PCO_2 on room air usually excludes acute pulmonary embolus as a diagnostic possibility, but the converse is not true, since a reduction in Pa_{O_2} is totally nonspecific, occurring in many types of lung disease as well as in congestive heart failure. However, if no other cause is evident clinically, a reduced arterial PO_2 with decreased PCO_2 should always raise the possibility of pulmonary embolus. Thus it is unusual to have an arterial PO_2 of greater than 80 mm Hg with this disease. It occasionally does occur, particularly if the arterial PCO_2 is also markedly reduced, indicating a high alveolar PO_2 and an increased alveolar-to-arterial oxygen tension difference. Pulmonary function tests are not helpful in the acute phase; however, in chronic occlusive pulmonary vascular disease with or without emboli the pulmonary diffusing capacity is usually reduced and the physiologic dead space is elevated, particularly during exercise. There may or may not be hypoxemia and respiratory alkalosis.

The best noninvasive diagnostic test for pulmonary emboli is the lung scintiscan, which is performed after intravenous administration of albumin macroaggregates labeled with radioactive technetium. These aggregates lodge in a small percentage of the pulmonary arterioles and follow the pattern of blood flow through the lungs. The scintiscan pattern thus demonstrates the vascular perfusion of each lung. The proportion of small vessels embolized is so small that they induce no detectable change in the circulation and there is virtually no morbidity from the procedure. The intravenous perfusion scan, which must be performed using anterior, posterior, and both lateral views, is so sensitive that with very rare exceptions no pulmonary emboli are ever demonstrated subsequent to a normal lung scan. The typical lung scan defects seen in pulmonary embolism are lobar or segmental wedge-shaped defects at the periphery of the lungs. The defects are often multiple or bilateral and may change from day to day. When this type of abnormality is present, provided the chest x-ray is otherwise normal and the clinical setting is appropriate, a diagnosis of pulmonary embolism can be made with reasonable certainty without proceeding to a pulmonary arteriogram.

Unfortunately the x-ray often is not normal. Furthermore, intravenous perfusion lung scans, like peripheral arterial oxygen measurements, do not give specific information; many common lung diseases may distort them. Pneumonia or atelectasis, for example, may cause segmental consolidation on x-ray and a corresponding perfusion defect on the lung scan. Even with emboli, the intravenous perfusion scan may not show typical defects but rather smaller peripheral, ill-defined ones; such changes are nonspecific and are frequent in asthma and chronic obstructive pulmonary disease, especially with severe airways obstruction or bullae. This finding can be clarified somewhat by combining the intravenous perfusion scan with a ventilation scan using radioactive xenon gas. If the ventilation scan is normal but the perfusion lung scan is abnormal, the implication is that there must be pulmonary vascular occlusive disease rather than primary air space disease. However, if atelectasis, alveolar hemorrhage, or infarction has occurred in the area of the embolus, both the ventilation and the perfusion scan will be abnormal, and the combination will not help differentiate emboli from other pulmonary parenchymal disease. A ventilation scan thus occasionally makes a diagnosis more secure, although it more often adds little to careful clinical examination plus a review of the chest x-rays and a perfusion scan. A ventilation scan rarely obviates a pulmonary arteriogram in a doubtful case. Finally, if an infiltrate is present on chest x-ray and the lung scan shows defects not only in that area, but also in other radiographically clear areas of the lung, pulmonary emboli should be strongly suspected, provided there is not an alternate explanation such as severe obstructive lung disease.

The pulmonary arteriogram is the most definitive diagnostic test for pulmonary embolism. It should be performed whenever doubt exists after the studies outlined above, since treatment with anticoagulants or vena cava interruption carries risk. Morbidity due to arteriography is acceptable, and the mortality is very low. Serious arrhythmias or even death is rare but may occur during the procedure in severely ill patients or in those with severe pulmonary hypertension; these conditions, therefore, are relative contraindications to the test. Selective pulmonary arterial catheterization and injection of contrast material may

be required to demonstrate the occluded sites. The clot may actually be outlined as a filling defect in the pulmonary artery, or there may be an abrupt cutoff of the vascular shadows. It is preferable to perform arteriography within 48 hours of initial symptoms, since some clots may be dissolved by this time and hence will not be seen on the arteriogram. Finally, a measurement of pulmonary artery pressure can be made simultaneously to aid in subsequent management. The pulmonary artery pressure and central venous pressure measurements are frequently normal unless the embolic occlusion is massive or there has been antecedent pulmonary hypertension. The pulmonary capillary wedge pressure is normal in the absence of left ventricular failure. The cardiac output, if measured, is found to be reduced in severe pulmonary arterial occlusion.

The selection of appropriate diagnostic tests obviously depends on the particular situation. In patients with vague chest pain or dyspnea, but in whom the index of suspicion is relatively low, an arterial PO_2 of greater than 80 mm Hg may be adequate to exclude the diagnosis. However, if the Pa_{O_2} is reduced and the suspicion is high, a lung scan should be done; if this is normal the diagnosis again can be excluded. If typical segmental or lobar defects are present on scan (particularly in an area where the routine chest x-ray is clear) and if the individual is known to be at high risk for pulmonary embolism, the diagnosis can be made with reasonable certainty and without arteriography. When the scan is abnormal but not typical for embolism, or if doubt exists about the scan interpretation because of coexisting lung disease, arteriography should be done before committing the patient to more than a brief period of anticoagulation therapy. In very seriously ill patients a scan may not be practical and the diagnosis must be made clinically, or, if vena cava interruption or pulmonary embolectomy is being considered, an inferior vena cavogram and pulmonary arteriogram can be done directly without a scan.

Unfortunately many other common and uncommon conditions cause chest pain, dyspnea, hypoxemia, tachycardia, fever, or pulmonary hypertension, and hence they must be included in the differential diagnosis. These include pneumonia or atelectasis, coronary artery disease, left-sided congestive heart failure, dissecting aneurysm, tuberculosis, pleural effusion, pericarditis, systemic lupus erythematosus with pleurisy, rib fracture, costochondritis, and other musculoskeletal chest pain.

Treatment

Preventive measures are obligatory once the diagnosis of pulmonary embolism is made, because other clots may be either present or forming in the leg veins and another embolus could be catastrophic. Administration of heparin intravenously is indicated and usually should be continued for 7 to 10 days, at which time the patient should be changed to an oral anticoagulant for varying time periods (3 months to 1 year). Hemoptysis due to lung infarction is not a contraindication to anticoagulation therapy. If immediate angiography is not available and the suspicion of embolism is high, the heparin should be started and the angiogram done later. Proper anticoagulation therapy is discussed in Chapter 52. If anticoagulant therapy is contraindicated because of remote bleeding, or if embolism recurs despite adequate anticoagulation, interruption of the inferior vena cava by surgical plication is preferred or, in patients too ill for such surgery, an umbrella type of filter may be passed by the transvenous route under fluoroscopy to partially occlude the vena cava. These procedures must be done only after angiography has been done to define preexisting clots. Vena cava interruption with plication is also frequently carried out after pulmonary embolism in patients in whom long-term anticoagulant therapy might be difficult, such as paraplegics who remain immobilized for long periods. Because of the risk and inconvenience of prolonged anticoagulation, when the diagnosis of pulmonary emboli is not obvious on clinical examination and lung scan, the diagnosis should be confirmed by angiography, before making a commitment to carrying on long-term anticoagulation therapy. After anticoagulation is begun, the initial clots in the lungs may resolve within several weeks; the diagnosis is then impossible and the patient could be committed to long-term anticoagulation unnecessarily.

Direct treatment of the embolus is usually neither possible nor necessary. Pulmonary embolectomy is indicated rarely, and only if large clots are demonstrated by angiography and systemic hypotension is present. The mortality of massive pulmonary embolism is high, even with surgery. Fibrinolytic enzymes such as urokinase have been given in attempts to hasten dissolution of the embolus once it has occurred; however, this form of therapy has not yet appeared to alter mortality.

In certain high-risk patients, anticoagulation appears to be beneficial and preventive when it is initiated before there is evidence of pulmonary emboli. In addition to patients with deep vein thrombosis, such treatment should be considered in those with recent hip fracture (in whom prophylactic anticoagulation has been conclusively shown to reduce thromboembolic complications), myocardial infarction, and those with congestive heart failure confined to bed. The best choice and dose of anticoagulant agent is controversial; recommendations include low-dose subcutaneous heparin, sodium warfarin (Coumadin), aspirin, and low-molecular-weight dextran (see Chap. 52). Other preventive measures include early mobilization of surgical patients and (possibly) properly fitted elastic stockings in all patients on bed rest.

Other types of pulmonary embolic disease do occur. Multiple small pulmonary emboli (or in situ thrombi) may cause some otherwise unexplained cases of pulmonary hypertension; a few of these may benefit from anticoagulants. Thrombosis of large pulmonary arteries occurs rarely from trauma or other injury to a main pulmonary artery. Fat emboli occur after fractures, amniotic fluid embolism occurs in obstetric patients, and foreign body emboli occur in intravenous drug users. Patients with right-sided bacterial endocarditis or others with sources of septic pulmonary emboli may present with single or scattered pulmonary infiltrates that often cavitate. These types of embolic disease are treated differently, but usually they can be recognized by the clinical setting in which they occur. The ultimate prognosis in patients with pulmonary embolism depends on the underlying disease and on whether recurrent embolism can be prevented. Chronic cor pulmonale is rarely a result of recurrent pulmonary embolism.

Bibliography

Cook, D. J., and Lauder, H. The diagnosis of pulmonary embolism: A review with particular reference to the use of radionuclides. *Postgrad. Med. J.* 47:214, 1971.

Dalen, J. E. Pulmonary angiography in acute pulmonary embolus: Indications, techniques, and results in 367 patients. *Am. Heart J.* 81:175, 1971.

Hampton, A. D., and Castleman, B. Correlation of post-mortem chest teleroentgenograms with autopsy findings with special reference to pulmonary embolism and infarction. *Am. J. Roentgenol.* 43:305, 1940.

Sasahara, A. A. Therapy for pulmonary embolism. *J.A.M.A.* 220, 1795, 1974.

Spencer, H. *Pathology of the Lung.* New York: Pergamon, 1968.

Szucs, M. M., Brooks, H. L., Grossman, W., Banas, J. S., Jr., Meister, S. G., Dexter, L., and Dalen, J. E. Diagnostic sensitivity of laboratory findings in acute pulmonary embolism. *Ann. Intern. Med.* 74:161, 1971.

Wilson, J. E., III, Pierce, A. K., Johnson, R. L., Jr., Winga, E. R., Harrell, W. R., Curry, G. C., and Mullins, C. B. Hypoxemia in pulmonary embolism, a clinical study. *J. Clin. Invest.* 50:481, 1970.

20

Chronic Bronchitis and Emphysema

Sanford Chodosh and Gordon L. Snider

Although pulmonary disorders associated with chronic cough, expectoration, wheezing, and dyspnea have been of interest to physicians for thousands of years, the first descriptions of pulmonary emphysema in autopsy specimens were published in the late eighteenth century. Laennec in the early nineteenth century made the first clear-cut distinction between emphysema proper and interstitial emphysema and correlated the anatomic and clinical findings in these two entities. Modern knowledge of the anatomy of emphysema began with the classic papers of Gough and Leopold in the 1950s and subsequent meetings of experts to develop precise definitions of chronic bronchitis, emphysema, and asthma.

Epidemiologic studies have shown that in the decade between 1960 and 1970, chronic bronchitis increased by tenfold in the industrialized areas of the United States. These disorders have now replaced tuberculosis as the pulmonary entity most often treated by physicians.

Definitions and Pathology

Chronic bronchitis is defined clinically as the presence of chronic productive cough for 3 months in each of 2 successive years when other causes of cough such as tuberculosis, carcinoma of the lung, mycosis, and chronic congestive heart failure have been excluded.

Morphologic evidence of hypersecretion in chronic bronchitis consists in hypertrophy and hyperplasia of the tracheobronchial seromucous glands. The mucous gland ducts are usually dilated. Plugging of small bronchi with mucus is not unusual, and patchy areas of squamous metaplasia replacing the normal ciliated epithelium are often observed. Polymorphonuclear neutrophils and lymphocytes may infiltrate the mucosal layers. The epithelial and glandular changes lead to decreased mucociliary clearance and relative stasis of secretions; these in turn lead to bacterial infection and airways obstruction.

Emphysema is defined as dilatation of the respiratory air spaces beyond the terminal bronchioles asso-

ciated with irreversible destructive changes of the alveolar walls. Localization of the early lesions serves as a basis for classification of the various types of emphysema. In centrilobular emphysema the initial lesion is in the respiratory bronchioles, with scarring, irregularity, and focal dilatation of the airways and adjacent alveoli resulting in localized emphysema in the central zone of the secondary lung lobule. Centrilobular emphysema is irregular in distribution, tending to involve the upper and posterior portions of the lungs more than the lower portions. Centrilobular emphysema is the form of emphysema most frequently associated with chronic bronchitis and is more commonly seen in men.

In panlobular emphysema all air spaces of the secondary lung lobule are involved. Panlobular emphysema may be either focal or diffuse; if focal, the lesions are more frequent at the lung bases. Focal panlobular emphysema has a predilection for older persons and women; diffuse panlobular emphysema is the lesion most often associated with alpha$_1$-antitrypsin deficiency.

In paraseptal or subpleural emphysema the respiratory air spaces next to the fibrous septa are involved, often sparing most of the rest of the lung. Irregular or paracicatricial emphysema, a process associated with scarring, is commonly observed by the pathologist but is only rarely extensive or symptomatic. This form of emphysema is characterized by a nonuniform pattern of involvement of the lung and by proximity to foci of scarring.

Bullae, which are areas of marked focal dilatation of air spaces, may result from the coalescence of adjacent areas of emphysema, from locally severe panlobular emphysema, or from a ball-valve effect in the bronchi supplying an emphysematous area. Giant bullae are particularly likely to complicate subpleural or panlobular emphysema.

The different anatomic patterns, age and sex distributions, and associated diseases suggest differing etiology and pathogenesis for the various types of emphysema. However, disruption of the elastic tissue network of the lung is the common pathologic feature in all forms of emphysema. The resultant loss of elastic recoil gives rise to an impaired tethering of the small bronchi. Consequently the small airways collapse at much higher lung volumes than normal, accounting for the irreversible airways obstruction in emphysema.

Chronic Obstructive Pulmonary Disease (COPD)

Chronic bronchitis and emphysema can both occur without airways obstruction as determined either clinically or by standard spirometric tests; asthma, by definition (see Chap. 15), is always associated with airways obstruction. However, if airways obstruction supervenes in chronic bronchitis or emphysema, their differentiation from one another or from asthma may become difficult. Furthermore, chronic bronchitis often occurs together with emphysema or with asthma; indeed, some patients have all three disorders. Bronchiectasis, diagnosable with certainty only by bronchography, may be associated with a diffuse bronchiolitis that causes airways obstruction. Although for prognostic and therapeutic reasons it is always desirable to identify precisely the entities present in any patient, this may at times be difficult; consequently the terms *chronic obstructive airways disease, chronic obstructive lung disease,* and *chronic obstructive pulmonary disease* have come into widespread usage to denote a syndrome of chronic airways obstruction associated with productive cough and dyspnea.

Pathogenetic Relations

Chronic bronchitis and emphysema most often co-exist: About two-thirds of bronchitic patients have emphysema, and about 80 percent of severely emphysematous patients have bronchitis. Fibrosis, distortion, and cellular infiltration of the terminal and adjacent respiratory bronchioles are regularly noted in centrilobular emphysema, suggesting that the inflammatory response of chronic bronchitis precedes the development of this type of emphysema. In panlobular emphysema, chronic bronchitis appears as a consequence of the altered structure and function of the diseased lung. The features characterizing the relatively infrequently observed patients with either pure emphysema or pure chronic bronchitis are summarized in Table 20-1 and are discussed later.

Epidemiology and Etiologic Factors

Prevalence figures from the 1970 National Health Survey and other epidemiologic studies estimate about 8 million cases of chronic bronchitis and emphysema in the United States; 20 to 30 percent of adult men and 10 to 15 percent of adult women have the chronic productive cough of chronic bronchitis. The 1971 figures for Social Security Disability Benefits indicate that 4.8 percent were awarded because of chronic bronchitis and emphysema. In the United Kingdom, respiratory ailments are the most common cause of loss of time from work, and the mortality rates for chronic bronchitis and emphysema in 1974 were 2.2 and 9.3 per 100,000, respectively.

Although full understanding of the causes of these diseases is uncertain, a number of relationships are apparent. The patient's current cigarette-smoking status and lifetime smoking history are the most important correlates of chronic productive cough and airways obstruction in epidemiologic surveys and of pulmonary emphysema in autopsy studies. Chronic bronchitis and emphysema are more common in men than women, and mortality is greater in men than women by threefold to fourfold. Although smoking habits may account for much of this difference, other factors may well be operative. There is evidence that frequent respiratory infections in childhood predispose to chronic obstructive lung disease in adults, and chronic bronchitis often appears to begin in the late teens. The slightly increased prevalence in urban as compared to rural areas is usually attributed to differences in air pollution, and occupations with high dust exposure appear to contribute to increased mortality (although these factors are small as compared with cigarette usage; see Chap. 17).

A role for genetic factors has been confirmed by the discovery of the relation between homozygous alpha$_1$-antitrypsin deficiency and emphysema beginning in the second and third decade of life (see later). A family history of chronic airways obstruction is commoner in women than in men, and occasional instances of familial emphysema without alpha$_1$-antitrypsin deficiency have been observed. Genetic factors may determine why some heavy smokers develop progressive, disabling disease while others do not.

Table 20-1. Characteristics of Patients with Predominant Emphysema or Chronic Bronchitis

Characteristic	Predominant emphysema	Predominant chronic bronchitis
Weight	Thin — frequent history of major weight loss	No marked weight loss
Sputum	Usually scanty, mucoid	Usually over 10 ml/24 hr, often purulent
Cardiovascular system	Narrow cardiac shadow PA film; chronic cor pulmonale rare	History of heart failure due to chronic cor pulmonale frequent
Roentgenogram	Overdistention marked; attenuation of vascular markings; bullae	Accentuated markings frequent; overdistention mild
Lung volumes	VC usually only slightly reduced RV markedly increased TLC increased	VC often very low RV usually only moderately increased TLC usually within normal limits, occasionally low
Arterial PCO_2	Usually normal or low except during acute exacerbations or terminally	Usually persistently elevated when $FEV_1 < 1.0$ liter
Arterial PO_2	Hypoxemia usually mild except during exacerbations	Hypoxemia usually severe
Diffusing capacity (breath holding)	Usually less than 70% of predicted	Often normal or only slightly low
Polycythemia	Rare	Occasional
Cardiac output	Relatively low	Relatively high
Ventilation	Relatively high	Relatively low
Exercise tolerance	Relatively low	Relatively high

Note: PA = posteroanterior; VC = vital capacity; RV = residual volume; TLC = total lung capacity; PCO_2 = partial pressure, carbon dioxide; FEV_1 = forced expiratory volume in 1 sec; PO_2 = partial pressure, oxygen.

Even among those who have chronic bronchitis, it is not possible to predict who will go on to disabling disease, with or without emphysema.

Alpha$_1$-antitrypsin is the glycoprotein comprising the majority of the alpha$_1$ globulin in serum electrophoresis; it inhibits several proteases. Its concentration is 180 to 280 mg per 100 ml in normal serum, and the concentration increases with inflammation or pregnancy. More than 20 phenotypes of this polymorphic protein have been identified; the principal normal gene is termed *PiZ*. The homozygous ZZ phenotype is manifested by low levels of serum alpha$_1$ antitrypsin (about 20 mg per 100 ml). This homozygous phenotype also carries with it a 20 to 30 percent risk of neonatal hepatitis and cirrhosis and a 70 to 80 percent risk of chronic bronchitis and emphysema. The emphysema characteristic of the ZZ group often begins before the fourth decade, occurs more frequently than expected in women, need not be preceded by chronic bronchitis, and is accelerated by cigarette smoking.

In patients with alpha$_1$-antitrypsin deficiency, the basis for destruction of tissue is hypothesized to be the release of protease with elastolytic activity from inflammatory cells; the enzyme is not appropriately inhibited because of the lack of antiprotease activity. The physiologic consequence of a loss of elastic tissue is the development of emphysema, as has been recently demonstrated in elastase-induced emphysema in hamsters. A similar hypothesis has been put forward for the patient with chronic bronchitis and emphysema but without alpha$_1$-antitrypsin deficiency. In this instance it is suggested that the chronic inflammatory process releases concentrations of protease in localized areas that overwhelm the host's normal antiprotease mechanism. Controversy still surrounds the question of whether heterozygous alpha$_1$-antitrypsin deficiency predisposes to the development of chronic bronchitis and emphysema, although most evidence indicates that it does not.

Clinical Features

The first symptom in patients with predominant emphysema is usually the insidious development of dyspnea on exertion; wheeze and cough are minimal until late in the course of the disease. Weight loss is frequent, and because hypoxemia is usually moderate and hypercapnia is often not present until the final stages of the disease, chronic cor pulmonale is less frequent than it is in chronic bronchitis.

Physical examination of the chest in emphysema reflects the hyperinflation of the lungs. The thorax is held near the position of full inspiration; the diaphragms are low and do not move appreciably with a maximum inspiratory effort. The use of accessory muscles of respiration to achieve movement of the chest cage, paradoxical retraction of the lower rib interspaces, and a depressed zone of liver dullness and a palpable liver edge without actual hepatic enlargement are also often noted. Breath sounds and heart sounds are generally diminished, the forced expiratory time is prolonged, and rhonchi are heard on auscultation, especially during forced expiration.

The patient with advanced, predominant emphysema has been referred to as the "pink puffer."

Patients with chronic bronchitis usually present with the complaint of dyspnea on exertion beginning in the fifth decade, but there is generally a history of many years of chronic productive cough. The volume of sputum varies considerably but it is rarely more than 60 ml per day and is usually between 5 and 15 ml per day. Because of the much larger cross-sectional area of the small airways than of the trachea, involvement of small airways must be widespread before obvious global airways obstruction (and dyspnea) occurs due to small airways dysfunction. A history of frequent chest colds characterized by increased cough, purulent sputum, wheezing, and dyspnea is common; as the disease progresses, the symptom-free periods between acute exacerbations tend to become shorter. The presence of wheezing with exacerbations may lead to the erroneous diagnosis of asthma. Late in the course of the disease, hypoxemia, often associated with chronic hypercapnia and polycythemia, may result in cyanosis. Personality change, either insomnia or somnolence, and headache are indications of severe disruption of blood gas exchange and acid-base balance. Swelling of the legs may be a symptom of cor pulmonale with heart failure. Weight loss is not usually observed.

In chronic bronchitis, hyperinflation of the lungs and thorax is not very prominent. Rhonchi tend to be lower pitched and more numerous than in emphysema and to vary more between examinations. Because of pulmonary overdistention, evidence of pulmonary hypertension and right ventricular hypertrophy is usually not detectable on physical examination. An enlarged, tender liver indicates heart failure. Asterixis, typical of many metabolic disorders, is evidence of severe hypercapnia.

The combination of plethora, cyanosis, and edema has led to the term *blue bloater* being used to characterize the late stages of chronic bronchitis.

Laboratory Findings

CHEST ROENTGENOGRAPHY

Since the definition of emphysema is based on a distinctive pathologic change, the most conclusive antemortem evidence for the diagnosis is obtained from the chest roentgenogram. The presence of bullae and excessively rapid tapering of the vascular shadows are the specific roentgenographic findings in emphysema, but these are not detectable before the disease is severe, at least locally. Bullae are radiolucent areas larger than a centimeter in diameter that are completely or partially outlined by arcuate hairline shadows. Evidence of persistent overdistention of the lungs is strongly suggestive of emphysema; the findings include low, flat diaphragms and, on lateral projection, increased retrosternal air space and loss of the acute angle formed by the diaphragm and anterior chest wall. The heart shadow tends to be long and narrow.

In chronic bronchitis, evidence of marked overdistention of the lungs in the chest roentgenogram is unusual, even when airways obstruction is severe. The vascular pattern is characteristically accentuated as opposed to the attenuation noted in emphysema. In a bronchogram, filling of the dilated ducts of enlarged submucosal mucous glands is often observed. With complicating cor pulmonale, serial films may reveal the transverse cardiac diameter to be slightly increased with prominent hilar vascular shadows; enlargement of the heart anteriorly indicates right ventricular hypertrophy.

PULMONARY FUNCTION TESTING

The physiologic status of the lungs may help in differentiating chronic bronchitis from emphysema as well as in detecting asthma, but the results are not pathognomonic. These measurements are helpful in assessing severity, following progress, and making a prognosis.

As noted above, airways obstruction may be absent in both chronic bronchitis and emphysema or may be detectable only with very sensitive tests. The forced expiratory spirogram is the most widely available and useful test of airways dynamics. The forced expiratory flow for the middle half of the vital capacity is often abnormal with mild airways obstruction, while measurements of forced expiratory volume for 1 second and of airways resistance, both of which reflect large airways dynamics, tend to remain normal until late in the course of the disease. Patients with chronic bronchitis or emphysema usually have little or no improvement in spirometric indices when studied in the laboratory before and after bronchodilator treatment, whereas asthmatics may have a dramatic response (more than 25 percent increase). However, the absence of response to bronchodilators on a single study in the laboratory should never be used as a reason to withhold bronchodilator drug therapy or to exclude the diagnosis of asthma; serial studies of a patient treated for weeks or months may demonstrate unexpected reversal of airways obstruction.

The predominantly emphysematous patient tends to have a total lung capacity above normal, a modest decrease in vital capacity, and a marked increase in residual volume. In chronic bronchitis, the total lung capacity is often normal or only slightly low, with a relatively marked decrease of vital capacity and a modest increase of residual volume. Measurement of static volume-pressure relationships is the most specific means of identifying emphysema, but this is a research procedure. Compliance of the lungs is increased and transpulmonary pressure at total lung capacity is decreased, reflecting disruption of the elastic tissue framework of the lungs. The single-breath diffusing capacity is decreased in emphysema (but not in bronchitis) because of destruction of the capillary bed.

Arterial blood gases measured during stable clinical conditions in emphysematous patients reveal a modest hypoxemia without hypercapnia. Only terminally, or with superimposed bronchitis, does the hypoxemia become severe and hypercapnia become evident. The patient with severe, chronic bronchitis tends to have severe hypoxemia associated with chronic hypercapnia and increased serum bicarbonate levels. Secondary polycythemia is seen much more often in chronic bronchitis than in emphysema. The more severe hypoxemia and hypercapnia of chronic bronchitis is due to widespread hypoventilation in relation to perfusion; in emphysema the destructive process tends to impair capillary perfusion as well as alveolar ventilation, and the blood gas abnormality is therefore less.

Forced expiratory spirometry and arterial blood gas measurements are the pulmonary function tests most useful in following these patients.

SPUTUM EXAMINATION

The sputum characteristics are the most important features of an exacerbation of bronchitis, since in most instances neither fever nor leukocytosis is present. In stable bronchitis the sputum is mucoid, and microscopic examination reveals predominance of macrophages and few organisms. During an exacerbation, sputum becomes purulent due to an influx of polymorphonuclear neutrophils, while the number of organisms seen on the Gram stain characteristically increases.

The pathogens most often cultured from the sputum are *Streptococcus pneumoniae* and *Haemophilus influenzae*. Cultures provide only qualitative data; the numbers of organisms observed in the Gram stain provide quantitative information that is important in deciding whether bacterial infection is playing an important pathogenic role and if antibiotic therapy should be started.

Diagnosis

The diagnosis is made from the history, physical examination, and chest roentgenographic studies, with appropriate laboratory data to exclude other pulmonary diseases such as tuberculosis, carcinoma, or cystic fibrosis, which may produce the same symptom complex. The physiologic diagnosis is made from pulmonary function studies. Asthma causes the greatest confusion in differential diagnosis, since it can clinically mimic both chronic bronchitis and emphysema.

Treatment

The ambulatory management of patients with chronic bronchitis and emphysema may be considered under three categories — specific, symptomatic, and secondary. There is little specific therapy to offer; cessation of cigarette smoking should be urged and supported; occupational and other environmental inhalants should be evaluated and dealt with as well as possible. Influenza vaccine should be given annually.

Symptomatic therapy should be directed against the reversible elements of airways obstruction, namely mucosal congestion and edema, increased secretion, bronchial muscle spasm, and cellular infiltration and inflammation. A trial of bronchodilator therapy should be undertaken in all patients. These drugs are generally helpful in patients with bronchitis, but they offer little to patients with predominant emphysema. Methyl xanthines and sympathomimetic amines have different modes of action at the cellular level (see Chap. 15), and both drugs should be given to more severely ill patients; the dosage of each drug is individualized rather than given in fixed combinations. Recent studies have shown that gastrointestinal toxicity generally is not noted at theophylline blood levels below 10 mg per liter, and more serious toxicity such as tachycardia and central nervous system stimulation is not usually observed until theophylline levels rise above 20 mg per liter. Optimal bronchodilator efficacy also lies in the range of 10 to 20 mg theophylline per liter, so gastrointestinal toxicity may be used as a rough guide to the level of medication in the blood. Recent studies suggest that an effective theophylline blood level can be attained in most patients with oral administration, but individuals vary greatly in the rate of metabolism of these drugs, and caution must therefore be used with fixed dosage

regimens. Hepatic disease particularly interferes with theophylline excretion.

The value of sympathomimetic amines in these patients has not been established by controlled clinical trials, but there is a widespread clinical impression that these drugs are efficacious in chronic bronchitis. Ephedrine is a weak bronchodilator agent. A number of orally effective long-acting beta-2 agonists, such as terbutaline and metaproterenol, have recently become available and may be tried. One of these newer drugs or even the older beta agonist, isoproterenol, is often helpful when given by inhalation.

Thinning and mobilization of intrabronchial secretions is one of the most important goals in decreasing airways obstruction. Dehydration increases sputum viscosity, and patients should be instructed to drink enough fluids to keep their urine pale in color except for the initial voiding after sleep. The value of expectorants is questioned because most studies have failed to document objective changes. Glyceryl guaiacolate in doses of 200 to 600 mg four times daily may be tried.

The administration of an aqueous aerosol or mist therapy using a simple nebulizer powered by compressed air for 15 minutes several times daily is often helpful. Saline, alone or with a beta-adrenergic drug, may be given two to four times daily in the nebulizer. Intermittent positive-pressure breathing devices do not deliver these agents any more effectively than simpler nebulization systems and have little value except in patients who cannot carry out simple breathing maneuvers. Acetylcysteine and pancreatic deoxyribonuclease solutions are not effective thinners of bronchial secretions when given by aerosol.

Physical methods of clearing secretions are helpful in many patients. Postural drainage uses gravity to help patients with impaired cough efficacy to expectorate their secretions. Shock waves set up by cupped hand percussion may help move secretions from smaller to larger airways, where they are more easily mobilized. A member of the family can generally be trained to carry out these procedures.

Although long-term prophylactic antibiotic therapy has been shown to shorten exacerbations of bronchitis, the discrete treatment of individual exacerbations is the preferred method. Ampicillin is then the drug of choice and should be given for 10 to 14 days; the tetracyclines offer comparable efficacy. Treatment to effect sputum thinning and mobilization is equally as important as the administration of antibiotics in the management of exacerbations of bronchitis.

Corticosteroids are not indicated in clear-cut chronic bronchitis and emphysema. However, if there is reason to suspect an important asthmatic component, as indicated by a family history of atopy, by a history of dramatic responsiveness of episodes of airways obstruction to bronchodilator drugs, or by the presence of peripheral blood and sputum eosinophilia, then a trial of corticosteroid therapy should be undertaken. Drugs should be given in a defined course of 2 to 3 weeks while objective evidence of improvement is sought if the nonspecific tonic effects of corticosteroids are not to confuse the issue.

Treatment designed to improve the functioning of the whole person is important, even when it has little effect on the diseased respiratory system. Patients living a sedentary life or confined to bed for a long period of time develop skeletal muscle deconditioning, and as a result they have an increased ventilatory and cardiovascular requirement during exercise. These effects can be reversed by a program of graded exercise. Chronic obstructive lung disease with severe hypoxemia during exercise may limit one's ability to undertake any effort. Oxygen supplementation may then improve the patient's comfort during exercise so that the skeletal muscles can be reconditioned. In patients who are chronically hypoxemic at rest with worsening during exercise, exercise tolerance may be improved by the administration of oxygen with an ambulatory liquid oxygen system. Because of its considerable expense, such therapy should be prescribed only after very careful evaluation of arterial blood gases in the laboratory.

In patients with cor pulmonale and recurrent bouts of right heart failure, the major approach is the treatment of the lung disease. Hypoxemia and acidemia are the chief causes of pulmonary hypertension in chronic bronchitis and emphysema, and measures designed to improve alveolar ventilation are therefore a central part of the treatment of cor pulmonale. The administration of controlled low-dose oxygen therapy,

particularly at night, helps in selected patients, although its precise mechanism has not been finally established. Diuretic therapy should be used to control edema, but digitalis should be given with the greatest caution because of the frequency of hypokalemia and hypoxemia in these patients. Although it has been shown that digitalis will increase cardiac output in certain patients with chronic bronchitis and emphysema and a high pulmonary resistance, the effect is often a slight increase in pulmonary arterial pressure; hence, the overall improvement in the function of the stressed heart is dubious.

Prognosis and Course

The prognosis in patients who have chronic bronchitis with mild or no airways obstruction is generally favorable. Most chronic bronchitics show improvement in cough and expectoration with treatment, especially if they stop smoking. The outlook for patients with moderate or severe airways obstruction is less favorable. These patients tend to present during an exacerbation of their disease. Even though there is improvement with initial treatment, ventilatory function generally declines with age at a rate greater than that observed in normal individuals. The FEV_1 falls inexorably at an average rate of 50 to 75 ml per year, and the prognosis is closely related to the severity of airways obstruction. Over a 5-year period mortality rates are slightly greater than normal in patients who have values of FEV_1 greater than 1.35 liters, but there is more definite excess mortality by 10 years. The prognosis is generally poor in patients with severe obstruction, especially if this is accompanied by hypercapnia or cor pulmonale; in patients presenting with values of FEV_1 of less than 0.75 liters, the approximate mortality at 1 year is 30 percent and by 10 years is 95 percent. Death generally occurs from some accident such as an overwhelming infection, retained secretions with atelectasis and pneumonia, pneumothorax, a cardiac arrhythmia, or pulmonary embolism.

Bibliography

Burrows, B., Fletcher, C. M., Heard, B. E., et al. The emphysematous and bronchial types of chronic airways obstruction: A clinicopathological study of patients in London and Chicago. *Lancet* 1:830, 1966.

Ferris, B., Jr. Chronic bronchitis and emphysema: Classification and terminology. *Med. Clin. North Am.* 57:637, 1973.

Kueppers, F., and Black, L. Alpha$_1$-antitrypsin and its deficiency. *Am. Rev. Respir. Dis.* 110:176, 1974.

Macklem, P. T. The pathophysiology of chronic bronchitis and emphysema. *Med. Clin. North Am.* 57:669, 1973.

Petty, T. L. Ambulatory care for emphysema and chronic bronchitis. *Chest* 58:441, 1970.

Thurlbeck, W. M. Chronic bronchitis and emphysema. *Med. Clin. North Am.* 57:651, 1973.

21

Diseases of the Pleura

Gordon L. Snider

The *pleura* is a thin membrane composed of a layer of mesothelial cells supported by vascular connective tissue. It invests the lungs (the visceral pleura) and lines the cavities of the hemithoraces (the parietal pleura). The parietal pleura is subdivided into costal, diaphragmatic, and mediastinal pleurae. The spaces between the visceral and parietal pleural surfaces normally contain a total of no more than 30 ml of serous fluid, which serves to lubricate the surfaces, facilitating the gliding movements of chest wall and lungs. The lungs within the chest cavity are inflated or stretched, tending always to recoil toward the hili. This recoil force normally results in subatmospheric pressures within the pleural space.

Pleural Transudates

In systemic disorders associated with extracellular accumulation of fluid in such conditions as congestive heart failure, edematous renal disease, and cirrhosis of the liver, serous fluid containing little protein and few cells may collect in one or both pleural spaces because the fluid is transuded into the pleural spaces faster than it is absorbed. Pleural transudate may also occur in myxedema and rarely as part of a triad along with ascites and benign tumor of the ovary (Meigs syndrome). In heart failure, fluid accumulates predominantly on the right side; unilateral left-sided effusion should raise the suspicion of a complicating process such as pulmonary embolism. Predominantly right-sided pleural effusion may also complicate cirrhosis with ascites in the absence of general anasarca, because ascitic fluid enters the pleural space through the lymphatic channels perforating the diaphragm. The differentiation of pleural transudates from exudates is discussed below. Treatment of pleural transudates is that of the underlying disease; aspiration of fluid is usually indicated only to establish the diagnosis and is therapeutically unnecessary except to relieve dyspnea from a large effusion.

Pleurisy

Pleurisy is inflammation of the pleura due to either an infectious or noninfectious cause, and it may occur

with or without pleural effusion. The process may be part of disease in the underlying lung, such as a mycoplasmal or bacterial pneumonia or a pulmonary infarction; alternatively the pleura may be injured by a toxic or infectious agent that enters the pleural space directly, as in pleurisy complicating pancreatitis or in an empyema complicating a subphrenic abscess. Infectious or noxious agents may be transported directly to the pleura through either the lymphatics or the vascular system, as occurs in neoplastic pleural disease or uremic pleurisy. Direct trauma to the pleura due to penetrating chest wounds or to blunt trauma with rib fractures may cause a local inflammatory reaction; irritation due to blood, air, or other contaminating substances may cause widespread pleurisy.

In the early stages of inflammation, the pleura becomes congested and edematous. Cellular infiltration ensues and with an increase in vascular permeability, a fibrinous, cellular exudate covers the pleural surfaces. The pleuritic process may run its course without a significant accumulation of fluid, a process known as dry or fibrinous pleurisy. More often, however, a pleural exudate rich in plasma protein collects and contains cells that reflect the nature of the pleuritic process. Healing of the pleura may be either by resolution or by organization of the exudate, with fibrous scarring and often the formation of adhesions between the visceral and parietal pleurae.

Clinical Presentation

The onset of acute fibrinous pleurisy is usually dramatic, with severe, localized pain that is aggravated by deep breathing and coughing. Less frequently the pain is mild and is felt only during deep inspiration. Pain arises only from inflammation of the parietal pleura; the visceral pleura does not contain pain-sensitive nerve fibers. Because the parietal nerve fibers are derived from the intercostal nerves, the pain may be referred to relatively distant sites. For example, irritation of the lower parietal pleura and the peripheral portions of the diaphragm may cause pain referred to the abdomen, simulating intraabdominal disease. The phrenic nerves innervate the central tendon of the diaphragm; involvement of this area often produces pain in the neck and shoulder. When pleural effusion develops, pleural pain generally subsides as a result of chest wall splinting. Pleural effu·

sion may develop with no pleuritic pain but rather with dyspnea as the presenting symptom.

Physical examination in pleurisy varies considerably, depending on the nature of the accompanying lung or systemic disease; it usually discloses rapid, shallow respirations, impaired chest wall motion, intercostal tenderness, and decreased breath sounds over the affected area. A pleural friction rub is the characteristic physical sign, but it is often entirely absent or only audible for 24 to 48 hours after the onset of the pain. Impaired percussion note, absent tactile fremitus, decreased or absent breath sounds, and E to A change of the spoken voice (egobronchophony) at the upper border of the fluid are frequent signs of pleural effusion.

Diagnosis

Acute fibrinous pleurisy is readily diagnosed when there is characteristic pain; a pleural friction rub is pathognomonic. Diaphragmatic pleurisy masquerading as abdominal disease should be suspected from the presence of respiratory symptoms; careful physical examination of the lungs and a chest roentgenogram may reveal an otherwise occult intrathoracic process. In intercostal neuritis the pain is rarely aggravated by respiration and the signs of pleuritic involvement are absent. A characteristic eruption will establish the diagnosis of herpes zoster, in which pain may precede the vesicles by several days. A pericardial friction rub is usually easily distinguished from a pleural friction rub by its synchrony with the heartbeat.

An area of fibrinous pleurisy casts no roentgenographic shadow, but an associated pulmonary or chest wall lesion may. Except for thoracentesis, the chest roentgenogram is the most precise method of detecting pleural fluid. When adhesions between visceral and parietal pleura are absent, the fluid seeks the most dependent portion of the thorax; the upper border of the resultant dense shadow is concave upwards because of the recoil force generated by the lung. Adhesions between the visceral and parietal pleura or within the interlobar fissures may result in atypical localization (loculation) of pleural fluid. The minimal amount of free fluid that is detectable with a patient in the upright position ranges between 300 and 500 ml. However, when frontal chest films are taken by a horizontal x-ray beam with the patient

lying on the affected side (decubitus views), less than 100 ml of fluid is easily detectable.

Ultrasonography may be helpful in localizing a small pleural effusion that is in contact with the chest wall; the technique is often useful in determining the correct site for performance of a thoracentesis.

When pleural fluid is thought to be present, thoracentesis should be done to establish its presence and characteristics. Clear yellow fluid is called serous; bloody or blood-tinged fluid is sanguineous or serosanguineous; while thick, opaque fluid is called purulent. Milky white fluid is referred to as chylous, and rarely cholesterol crystals give fluid a shimmering quality. Specimens should be taken for chemical, bacteriologic, and cytologic examination, and tubes for the cytologic specimen should contain an anticoagulant.

Pleural fluid transudates generally have a specific gravity of less than 1.015, total protein of less than 2.5 gm per 100 ml, lactic dehydrogenase of less than 200 IU, pleural fluid—serum lactic dehydrogenase ratios of less than 0.6, and very low cell counts. Pleural exudates have a specific gravity greater than 1.018, total protein greater than 3 gm per 100 ml, and pleural fluid—serum lactic dehydrogenase ratios of greater than 0.6. In infectious effusions the glucose may be moderately decreased, say to half the serum values, but in rheumatoid effusions the glucose is characteristically less than 10 mg per 100 ml. Total and differential cell counts are indicated except for grossly purulent pleural fluids.

A predominance of polymorphonuclear leukocytes suggests that bacterial infection is the cause. The etiology may be a bacterial pneumonia with synpneumonic effusion; the effusion itself is usually sterile. When bacterial contamination of the pleural fluid has occurred, the fluid may or may not be visibly purulent. Any such bacteria may be seen in a Gram stain, often within polymorphonuclear leukocytes, which are the predominant cells. A predominance of small lymphocytes, particularly with a few mesothelial cells, and a total cell count above 1,000 per cubic millimeter strongly suggest tuberculosis; however, tubercle bacilli are rarely observed in acid-fast stains and are not common on culture (less than 50 percent).

Pleural fluid is usually blood stained in pleural carcinomatosis and in pulmonary infarction. The presence of cancer cells in appropriately fixed and stained cytologic preparations is diagnostic of neoplastic pleural involvement; but lymphoma of the pleura cannot be reliably diagnosed by cytology. In pulmonary infarction a mixture of polymorphonuclear leukocytes, lymphocytes, and numerous mesothelial cells is usual. Lupus erythematosus cells may be seen in the pleural fluid in systemic lupus erythematosus. Eosinophils may constitute 30 percent or more of all cells in the pleural fluid, but they have no diagnostic significance except to indicate the chronicity of the process. The pleural fluid complicating pancreatitis usually demonstrates an amylase concentration several times higher than that in serum. The causes of pleural effusion are summarized in the following list:

Hydrothorax
  Congestive heart failure
  Edematous renal disease
  Hypoalbuminemia
  Hepatic cirrhosis
  Myxedema
  Fibroma of ovary (Meigs syndrome)
Infections
  Tuberculous
  Bacterial
  Mycotic
  Viral
  Mycoplasma
Pulmonary infarction
Connective tissue or autoimmune disorders
  Systemic lupus erythematosus
  Rheumatoid disease
  Acute rheumatic fever
  Following myocardial infarction or cardiotomy
Neoplasms
  Bronchogenic carcinoma
  Metastatic carcinoma
  Pleural mesothelioma
  Lymphoma
Subdiaphragmatic lesions
  Acute pancreatitis
  Subphrenic abscess
  Hepatic abscess
Trauma
  Blunt to thorax

With rib fracture
Ruptured esophagus
Ruptured mediastinal vessel (including thoracic duct)
Pneumoconiosis
  Asbestosis

Needle biopsy of the pleura carried out with either a Cope or an Abrams pleural biopsy needle should be considered whenever the diagnosis is not readily made by the clinical findings and pleural fluid analysis. Histologic examination of the tissue obtained may yield a diagnosis of neoplasm or suggest a specific infectious etiology; tissue sections should be examined for microorganisms using appropriate stains. Culture of parietal pleural tissue may yield mycobacteria when the pleural fluid culture is negative.

Pleural fluid analyses and pleural biopsies provide specific diagnoses only for diseases of neoplastic or infectious etiology, but these methods can also be of great value in other diseases when integrated with the total clinical presentation. Thus tuberculous pleural effusion generally presents with variable systemic and respiratory symptoms but no underlying pulmonary disease. A positive tuberculin test should then immediately raise the possibility of tuberculosis; a pleural exudate with lymphocyte predominance would be supportive evidence sufficient to begin antituberculosis drug treatment. The finding of caseating epithelioid cell granulomas on pleural biopsy would provide an additional assurance of tuberculosis, while culture of fluid and tissue should give absolute confirmation in more than 80 percent of cases. On the other hand, with a similar clinical presentation but an exudate revealing a predominance of polymorphonuclear leukocytes, alternative diagnoses such as pulmonary infarction or synpneumonic effusion with an occult pneumonia should be vigorously explored.

Treatment
Treatment for many pleural effusions, whether transudates or exudates, is primarily for the underlying pulmonary or systemic disease. Indolent infections of the pleural space such as tuberculosis should be treated by long courses of appropriate chemotherapy (see Chaps. 8 through 24). Dyspnea produced by a

large effusion is readily relieved by thoracentesis. Because cardiovascular collapse very occasionally complicates the removal of large amounts of pleural fluid (pleural shock), more than 1,200 to 1,500 ml should not be removed at a single thoracentesis. Pneumothorax may complicate thoracentesis if the visceral pleura is punctured or if air is allowed to enter the pleural space.

Empyema of the thorax is treated with high doses of parenteral antibiotics and drainage of the pleural space. One or two needle aspirations may be used to drain small collections of thin pus, but water-sealed tube thoracostomy is usually preferable (see later). Antibiotic choices depend upon identification of the organism microscopically, upon cultures, and upon results of antibiotic sensitivity tests; however, while awaiting cultural identification, drugs may often have to be chosen on the basis of the probable causes as predicated on Gram stains and clinical circumstances. When the exudate becomes very thick, open drainage for weeks or months through an intercostal tube or rib resection may be necessary to permit the space to obliterate by granulation from below. If the lung is trapped in a collapsed position with a thick cortex lining a large empyema space, thoracotomy and surgical decortication is the best way to expand the lung and obliterate the space. Surgical treatment, at times with lung resection, may be necessary when a bronchopleural fistula complicates the empyema.

Therapy of pleural effusion due to malignant involvement of the pleural surfaces is difficult. Occasionally fluid does not reaccumulate after a needle aspiration, especially if systemic antitumor therapy is begun. When fluid does reaccumulate, it generally responds to obliteration of the pleural space by instillation of a pleural irritant such as tetracycline or quinacrine; the process of adherence of visceral and parietal pleura may be aided by keeping the pleural space empty for a few days with water-sealed tube thoracostomy after instillation of the mild pleural irritant.

HEMOTHORAX
Hemothorax, or blood in the pleural space, may be a sequel of trauma or of the rupture of an aneurysm; rarely it occurs spontaneously from a coagulation defect or from the tearing of a small vessel in a parietopleural adhesion with spontaneous pneumothorax. Pleural blood often does not clot and can be readily removed by needle aspiration or by tube drainage. Streptokinase-streptodornase may be instilled once or twice to dissolve clots and to lyse adhesions, but if this is not promptly successful in dealing with clotted hemothorax, surgical decortication is the treatment of choice.

CHYLOTHORAX
Injury to the thoracic duct from trauma or neoplasm (most often lymphoma) may produce chylous pleural effusion. The lipid content of the fluid is high, as manifested microscopically by sudanophilic fat droplets and a high concentration of neutral fat and fatty acids. Cholesterol content is low. Treatment is surgical for traumatic rupture; antineoplastic therapy is used for underlying tumor.

CHOLESTEROL EFFUSION
Also known as pseudochylous effusion, cholesterol effusion is characterized by pleural fluid that is golden greenish and iridescent due to the presence of cholesterol crystals. Cholesterol concentration is high, up to 1,000 mg per 100 ml, but neutral and fatty acid concentrations are low. The effusion is usually small and is a result of long-standing chronic pleural disease, most commonly either tuberculosis or rheumatoid disease, both of which must be carefully sought.

FIBROSIS OF THE PLEURA
Inflammation of the pleura has great potential for healing by resolution rather than by fibrosis, but slight residual scarring, often manifested only as blunting of the costophrenic angle, is common. Occasionally the lung becomes encased in a thick layer of fibrous tissue that limits chest wall motion and retracts the mediastinum toward the side of disease. Blood flow to the affected lung is usually decreased as much as or even more than ventilation, so the mixed arterial blood gases are not disturbed. Thoracentesis or ultrasonography may be necessary to distinguish an area of localized pleural thickening from a loculated pleural effusion.

Extensive pleural fibrosis, also known as fibro-thorax, should be minimized by appropriate early therapy of the pleural disease. Surgical decortication of pleural fibrous tissues does not usually improve lung function unless a sizable collection of fluid or air is also removed.

CALCIFICATION OF THE PLEURA
Calcification of the pleura presents as focal (but some-times widespread) fenestrated plaques on the costal surfaces as a sequel of hemorrhage or empyema. However, a history of the antecedent illness is often not obtainable. Many years following inhalation of asbestos, focal plaquelike pleural fibrosis may be observed, at times with calcification. Calcific plaques involving the diaphragmatic pleura are almost invari-ably related to asbestos exposure (see Chap. 17).

Pneumothorax
Pneumothorax is the presence of air in the pleural space. As noted earlier, the pleural space normally contains only a few milliliters of fluid under sub-atmospheric pressure. If a manometer is connected through a needle and tubing to a localized pneumo-thorax, the pressure within the pleural space during quiet breathing will be observed to be about -8 cm H_2O at end-inspiration and about -4 cm H_2O at end-expiration. Pressures in the range of -30 to -40 cm H_2O may be produced during deep inspiration and may rise to $+100$ to $+200$ cm H_2O during cough or straining against a closed glottis.

Pneumothorax may be produced as a result of rupture of a localized bulla, a process called simple pneumothorax. Pneumothorax may also occur as a result of bullous disease in generalized emphysema, or it may accompany serious infection in the lung. When associated with severe underlying lung disease it is referred to as complicated pneumothorax. A pene-trating wound of the chest or a rib fracture with puncture of the lung may give rise to a traumatic pneumothorax. The deliberate introduction of air into the pleural space through a needle is known as artificial pneumothorax. Air may also enter the pleural space from the mediastinum; pneumomedi-astinum may be either spontaneous (see later) or secondary to traumatic rupture of the esophagus or a bronchus.

SPONTANEOUS PNEUMOTHORAX
Spontaneous pneumothorax is the common form of pneumothorax seen in clinical practice. Simple spon-taneous pneumothorax occurs as a result of rupture of a localized bulla. The underlying bullous disease is rarely severe or widespread enough to impair pul-monary function. Complicated spontaneous pneumo-thorax occurs in association with severe obstructive pulmonary diseases such as chronic bronchitis, emphysema, and asthma, or with other processes such as widespread interstitial lung disease, pneumonia and lung abscess, and diseases of the mediastinum.

Simple Spontaneous Pneumothorax
Simple spontaneous pneumothorax occurs about five times more commonly in men than in women, usually during the third decade of life, and is due to rupture of a small subpleural bulla, almost always in the apex of a lung. The genesis of these bullae is not under-stood. The right side is involved more commonly than the left, but simultaneous bilateral involvement is rare. However, recurrence on the side of the orig-inal pneumothorax is high (about 30 percent), whereas recurrent pneumothorax on the contralateral side is low (10 percent).

The precipitating cause of the rupture of bullae is obscure; only a very small percentage occur with active effort. Rupture seems likely to be due to a check-valve mechanism in the draining bronchus of a bulla, resulting either from retained secretions or from anatomic distortion of the bronchus. A simple spon-taneous pneumothorax may occur with rapid vari-ations in intrathoracic pressure such as occur during ascent to high altitudes in an airplane or during rapid decompression after diving. Pilots who have to eject at high altitude have an increased risk of developing a pneumothorax, as do skin divers who surface with the glottis closed.

Clinical Presentation. Simple spontaneous pneumo-thorax is usually signaled by chest pain and dyspnea. The functional abnormalities of small pneumotho-races are not striking; since pulmonary ventilation and perfusion tend to diminish in parallel, most patients have little respiratory distress. Such is not the case when a tension pneumothorax develops as a result of persistence of a bronchopleural fistula; in this type of pneumothorax a valvelike mechanism develops and allows air to continue to enter the pleural space during each inspiration, but not to leave during the succeeding expiration. The lung may then become completely collapsed, with shift of the mediastinum to the contralateral side and distortion of the great veins giving rise to striking respiratory embarrassment as the entire cardiac output is shifted to the contralateral lung.

The dyspnea tends to subside within about 24 hours even if the pneumothorax remains the same in size, since the patient accommodates to the altered mechanical state of the lung and hemithorax. Increased resonance on percussion, decreased motion of the hemithorax, and shift of the mediastinum to the contralateral side may be observed in tension pneumothorax. However, with small-sized and intermediate-sized pneumothoraces, percussion changes are usually not helpful, and the most impressive finding of pneumothorax is depression of breath sounds on the ipsilateral side.

Diagnosis. The diagnosis is confirmed by a chest roentgenogram, which reveals a sharply defined pleural margin of lung separated from the shadow of the chest wall by a clear zone devoid of vascular markings. If the pneumothorax is very small, it may be difficult to detect unless a chest film is taken in full expiration. During such expiration air leaves the lung, so the lung becomes denser while the pneumothorax alters in size but not in volume or density. This increases the contrast between the pneumothorax space and the adjacent lung, rendering the sharp pleural margin more visible. Pleural effusion, which presents as a horizontal air-fluid level immediately above the diaphragm, is detectable in fewer than 25 percent of patients with pneumothorax. It is usually not possible to detect the bulla that causes a pneumothorax; occasionally, however, the bulla stands out as a cystic air-filled space because the lesion retains its volume while the surrounding lung collapses. The margins of the lung may sometimes be irregular and distorted as a result of adhesions between visceral and parietal pleura. In tension pneumothorax the lung collapses toward the hilus and presents as an irregular, ovoid,

or globular density.

Treatment. Treatment is selective; when the pneumothorax is small (perhaps less than 20 percent of the lung being collapsed), when the patient's physiologic status has become stabilized, and when two films done at intervals of several hours have shown no increase in the size of the pneumothorax, management may be ambulatory and the lung allowed to reexpand spontaneously. As long as the lung remains partially collapsed, there is danger that the pleural space will become filled with fluid, with added risks of secondary infection and of trapping of the lung by an organizing fibrinous epipleural membrane. Small pneumothoraces can be expected to reexpand promptly, and the risk of these complications is low. However, large pneumothoraces usually require some means to reexpand the lung promptly; the most effective way is by the insertion of a chest tube with its distal end in a water bottle approximately 1 cm beneath the surface of the water (water-sealed tube thoracostomy). Reexpansion will occur promptly, since every time the patient coughs, strains, or turns over in bed, pleural pressures will rise above atmospheric levels and air will bubble out beneath the surface of the water. If the fistulous communication between the bronchus and pleural space persists, reexpansion of the lung can be hastened by application of up to 20 cm H_2O subatmospheric pressure above the surface of the water. Negative pressure should not be applied to the water-seal system unless a fistulous communication is present, since too rapid a reexpansion of the lung may result in the development of unilateral pulmonary edema. The tube should be left in place for 2 or 3 days after the lung is completely reexpanded. Prognosis is uniformly excellent.

Surgical therapy with excision of the bulla should be considered for all patients who have a third recurrence of spontaneous pneumothorax on the ipsilateral side. When a simple spontaneous pneumothorax is complicated by severe bleeding into the pleural space as a result of partial or complete rupture of a pleural adhesion, thoracotomy may be needed to control the bleeding. Atelectasis may complicate a spontaneous pneumothorax, and while it usually responds to respiratory and physical therapy, it may at times require bronchoscopy for reexpansion. Empyemas complicating pneumothorax should be treated as described earlier, with immediate water-sealed drainage and appropriate, vigorous antibiotic therapy.

Complicated Spontaneous Pneumothorax

A spontaneous complicated pneumothorax occurs as a result of a rupture of the visceral pleura in a patient with important underlying lung disease. Widespread emphysema is the commonest pulmonary process underlying a complicated pneumothorax. Less common pulmonary diseases are bronchial asthma, rupture of a pneumatocele in staphylococcal pneumonia, and rupture of subpleural cavities in necrotizing lung disease due to tuberculosis, deep mycotic infections, or anaerobic suppuration. Rupture of bullae may occur in diffuse interstitial fibrosing processes in the lung, but eosinophilic granuloma perhaps more frequently complicates a pneumothorax than any other interstitial lung disease.

In patients over age 40, complicated pneumothorax is much commoner than simple pneumothorax. In contradistinction to the excellent prognosis in simple pneumothorax, complicated pneumothorax is difficult to treat and is associated with significant mortality. Whereas pulmonary insufficiency is mild with simple pneumothorax, in the complicated variety there is often already serious underlying lung disease; when this disease is combined with a pneumothorax, the symptoms and clinical findings of pulmonary insufficiency may become striking. Persistent bronchopleural fistulas are common, and recurrence of pneumothorax is frequent. The severe impairment in pulmonary function due to the underlying lung disease often greatly increases the risk of therapeutic thoracotomy. All these factors lead to increased morbidity and mortality.

Treatment. This is much the same as for simple spontaneous pneumothorax, with early, vigorous application of water-sealed tube thoracostomy. In a patient who is not a suitable candidate for more vigorous surgery, the application of up to 20 cm H_2O negative pressure will often be necessary to overcome the effect of a persistent bronchopleural fistula and to obtain reexpansion of the lung with obliteration of the pleural space.

TRAUMATIC PNEUMOTHORAX

Accidental puncture of the lung during thoracentesis is probably the commonest cause of traumatic pneumothorax. Injury of the pleura due to penetrating wounds of the chest or to rib fractures is a more important cause. When there is a persistent opening between the pleural space and the skin, the patient has an open pneumothorax, and complete collapse of the lung will result as pressure within the pleural space reaches atmospheric levels. An open pneumothorax should be promptly converted to a closed pneumothorax by closing the skin and starting water-seal drainage. Any complicating hemothorax or infection should be sought out and treated promptly.

SPONTANEOUS PNEUMOMEDIASTINUM

Air may enter the mediastinum either as a result of a break in the esophagus or tracheobronchial tree, or because of dissection of air from ruptured alveoli along the perivascular sheath into the mediastinum. Rupture of the esophagus may occur from instrumentation, as a result of penetration by a foreign body, or spontaneously. Pneumomediastinum resulting from alveolar rupture may occur in individuals with no known underlying lung disease; it may also be a complication of severe diffuse lung disease or of its treatment by intermittent positive-pressure mechanical ventilation. Alveolar rupture occurs because of a bronchiolar check-valve mechanism or because of great variability in the compliance of the alveoli. If air can get into the alveoli but cannot readily escape, or if the lung must be exposed to a very high transpulmonary pressure in order to ventilate it, resulting in overdistention of the most compliant alveoli, these air spaces may rupture into the perivascular sheath and air will be pumped through the rupture into the mediastinum.

In adults, pneumomediastinum ordinarily gives rise to no significant physiologic abnormality. In about two-thirds of the cases air will rupture through the mediastinal pleura and produce a complicating pneumothorax, which rarely may be bilateral. The air may dissect into the subcutaneous tissues of the neck and produce generalized subcutaneous emphysema. In children the air may collect within the mediastinum, giving rise to obstruction of venous return and requiring subxyphoid insertion of a needle for aspiration of the air as an emergency measure.

Patients with pneumomediastinum may be asymptomatic or at times may develop midline substernal pain indistinguishable from that of myocardial infarction. When pneumothorax occurs, lateralizing pleuritic pain may be observed. On physical examination, in addition to detection of subcutaneous emphysema in the neck, auscultation often reveals so-called mediastinal crunch, a crackling sound best heard over the left sternal border from the third to the sixth intercostal spaces when the patient is sitting up or is in the left lateral recumbent position. The crackling sounds are strikingly synchronous with cardiac systole. Although this sound is generally pathognomonic, it may occasionally be present in left-sided pneumothorax without demonstrable mediastinal emphysema. The chest roentgenogram may show air in the fibrous pericardium, but air in the soft tissues of the neck is a more obvious and easily detectable roentgenographic sign.

Rupture of the esophagus gives rise within a few hours to pleural effusion, almost always left sided, and the development of empyema and very frequently a complicating pneumothorax. If this condition is suspected, the pH of the aspirated fluid should be checked, since it is often heavily contaminated by gastric contents and therefore reveals an acid pH.

A simple spontaneous pneumomediastinum usually subsides without treatment. When pneumomediastinum complicates either bronchial or tracheal rupture, esophageal disease, or severe lung disease, the underlying disease must be vigorously treated.

Bibliography

Carr, D. T., and Mayne, J. G. Pleurisy with effusion in rheumatoid arthritis with reference to the low concentration of glucose in pleural fluid. *Am. Rev. Respir. Dis.* 85:345, 1962.

Hammarsten, J. F., Honska, W. L., Jr., and Limes, B. J. Pleural fluid amylase in pancreatitis and other diseases. *Am. Rev. Respir. Dis.* 79:606, 1959.

Hyde, L. Benign spontaneous pneumothorax. *Ann. Intern. Med.* 56:746, 1962.

Macklin, M. T., and Macklin, C. C. Malignant interstitial emphysema of the lungs and mediastinum as an important occult complication in many respiratory diseases and other conditions: An interpretation of the clinical literature in the light of laboratory experiment. *Medicine* 23:281, 1944.

Reynolds, J., and Davis, J. T. Injuries of the chest wall, pleura, pericardium, lungs, bronchi and esophagus. *Radiol. Clin. North Am.* 4:383, 1966.

Snider, G. L., and Saleh, S. S. Empyema of the thorax in adults: Review of 105 cases. *Dis. Chest* 54:12, 1968.

Sulavik, S., and Katz, S. *Pleural Effusion.* Springfield, Ill.: Thomas, 1963.

22

Disorders of the Diaphragm and Mediastinum

Gordon L. Snider

The Diaphragm

The *diaphragm* is a sheet of muscle and tendon lined on its superior surface by diaphragmatic pleura and on its inferior surface by peritoneal membrane. The muscle fibers arise from the lower six ribs, the lateral margins of the first, second, and third lumbar vertebrae on the right side, and the lateral margins of the first and second lumbar vertebrae on the left. These fibers converge and insert into the margins of the crescentic central tendon of the diaphragm. The aorta, inferior vena cava, and the esophagus normally perforate the diaphragm. The muscle fibers arising anteriorly from the xyphoid process and from the seventh ribs are separated bilaterally by triangular spaces filled with areolar tissue that is poor in both muscle and tendinous fibers. These triangular weak points in the diaphragm are known as the parasternal spaces, or foramina of Morgagni. Potentially weak areas called the foramina of Bochdalek may form because of deficiencies in the origin of the muscle slips arising from the posterolateral rib cage.

DISORDERS OF MOTION

Hiccough (singultus) is caused by spasm of the diaphragm followed by sudden closure of the glottis during an inspiratory effort. A characteristic sound is produced as the glottis closes, and discomfort is often experienced as thoracic pressure is sharply lowered because of the continued contraction of the diaphragm. Repeated contractions occur with more or less regularity. Although hiccough is usually limited to a few minutes, occasionally it is prolonged. Causes of hiccough are numerous and include central nervous system disorders, irritation of the phrenic nerve, direct irritation of the diaphragm, and irritation of the diaphragmatic pleura or peritoneum.

Diaphragmatic "Stitch." This is a pain that occurs in normal persons after an effort; the pain may be on one side or the other, always is related to exertion, and tends to occur more readily after eating. The process subsides in a few minutes, and its only importance is that it may be considered by patients to be an indication of disease.

Diaphragmatic Flutter. This is a rare disturbance in which there are rapid, rhythmic contractions of the diaphragm at a rate of 70 to 200 times per minute occurring either unilaterally or bilaterally and tending to be episodic; associated symptoms are pain and breathlessness. The etiology is poorly understood; it has been described as following encephalitis lethargica or as a complication of drug abuse.

Paralysis of the Diaphragm. This occurs as a result of interruption of the phrenic nerve anywhere from its origin in the C3 to C5 (cervical) nerve roots to the entry into the diaphragm. The commonest cause is invasion of the nerve by tumor, usually a bronchogenic carcinoma. Idiopathic cases comprise the second commonest category; phrenic paralysis occurs more frequently on the right and more often in males.

Paralysis of the diaphragm usually produces few symptoms. On the left side, elevation of the diaphragm may alter the relations of the viscera in the left upper quadrant of the abdomen. Left upper quadrant discomfort may occur due to retention of gas in the stomach or in the splenic flexure of the colon. Elevation of the diaphragm is usually detectable on physical examination, while roentgenographically the three major findings are elevation of the hemidiaphragm above the normal position in full inspiration; diminished, absent, or paradoxical diaphragmatic motion during respiration; and paradoxical motion during conditions of increased load such as sniffing or coughing. Dynamic studies of the diaphragm by fluoroscopy should always be used to augment chest x-rays in establishing this diagnosis.

Eventration. This is a localized ballooning of the diaphragm due to impairment of muscle structure or function. It is believed to be due either to failure of muscular development of part of the hemidiaphragm or to local impairment of neural function with subsequent atrophy of muscle fibers. The resultant elevation of the diaphragm often involves the right side and the anteromedial portion of the diaphragm. The process is usually manifested in the middle years of life in company with the development of severe obesity, which tends to raise intraabdominal pressure. The process is rarely symptomatic, is usually recognized roentgenographically, and requires differentiation from neoplasms or hernias through the diaphragm.

DIAPHRAGMATIC HERNIAS
Herniation of abdominal or retroperitoneal structures may occur through congenitally weak areas of the diaphragm, may result from traumatic diaphragmatic rupture, or may occur through the esophageal hiatus. The last is the commonest hernia through the diaphragm and is discussed in Chapter 34.

Hernia through the foramen of Bochdalek (pleuroperitoneal hiatus) is the commonest form of hernia in infancy, and it occurs much more often on the left side than on the right. The hernial opening may be large because of an almost complete absence of the diaphragm due to failure of its posterolateral portion to close, a process that normally occurs at about the eighth week of gestation. When the defect is small, the peritoneum and pleura usually fuse, producing a sac that contains the herniated contents. However, when the opening is large, the abdominal viscera may herniate freely into the left pleural space, producing striking respiratory embarrassment and requiring immediate surgical therapy for survival.

In adults when the diaphragmatic defect is small, the patient is usually asymptomatic; the lesion is discovered accidentally on chest roentgenogram. These defects are almost always situated posterolaterally, and the hernial contents are usually retroperitoneal fat, or occasionally the upper pole of the kidney, or rarely the spleen.

Hernias of the foramina of Morgagni (parasternal hernias) are comparatively rare and tend to occur in adults who have become obese, with a resultant increase in intraabdominal pressure. The hernial sac commonly presents as a round density anteriorly in the region of the right cardiophrenic angle. The herniated organ is usually omentum, but in a very small percentage of cases in which the opening is larger, the stomach or bowel may herniate, with strangulation or obstruction. In these larger hernias auscultation of borborygmi over the chest is an important sign and

should make the physician consider whether a stomach tube should be passed or contrast studies carried out before he does a thoracentesis. The induction of pneumoperitoneum followed by an upright roentgenogram of the abdomen may sometimes help in making the diagnosis.

Therapy is usually not needed, especially when old films demonstrate that the mass has been present a long time. Occasionally surgical exploration is required to differentiate the hernia from other mediastinal masses and to establish the diagnosis.

Traumatic rupture of the diaphragm is usually a consequence of severe blunt trauma as in an automobile accident or a serious fall. Symptoms and signs may occur immediately after the injury due to entry of abdominal viscera into the pleural space with resultant obstruction or strangulation. A latent period, which may extend for many years, often intervenes between the time of injury and the development of symptoms. The diagnosis is established with plain and contrast roentgenography and the treatment is surgical.

SUBPHRENIC ABSCESS
Subphrenic abscess is a collection of pus beneath the diaphragm. The infection may be a complication of a ruptured abdominal viscus or of abdominal surgery. The process occurs with equal frequency on the two sides and in the anterior and posterior subphrenic spaces. Antibiotic therapy may suppress the infection postoperatively and delay the onset of low-grade fever, vague upper abdominal pain, weight loss, and other signs of chronic infection for a long period of time. Physical examination shows evidence of an elevated hemidiaphragm and perhaps of a pleural effusion on the affected side. These findings are confirmed by chest roentgenogram. The pleural fluid is usually a sterile exudate containing a predominance of polymorphonuclear leukocytes. The diagnosis is suspected by taking a careful history and carrying out appropriate roentgenographic studies to demonstrate displacement of abdominal viscera by the subphrenic mass. Ultrasound studies of the abdomen may disclose the abnormal collection of fluid. Treatment consists in surgical drainage and appropriate antibiotic therapy.

The Mediastinum

The *mediastinum* is the compartment bound laterally by the parietal pleura adjacent to the medial aspects of both lungs, superiorly by the thoracic inlet, inferiorly by the diaphragm, anteriorly by the sternum, and posteriorly by the anterior surfaces of the thoracic vertebral bodies. It is convenient for clinical purposes to divide the mediastinum into three compartments: anterior, middle, and posterior. The *anterior mediastinal compartment* is bound posteriorly by the pericardium, ascending aorta, and the brachiocephalic vessels; it is bound anteriorly by the sternum. This compartment contains the thymus gland and the anterior mediastinal lymph nodes, and it is much narrower inferiorly than superiorly. The *middle mediastinal compartment* is bound anteriorly and posteriorly by vertical planes extending upward from the pericardium below. It contains the pericardium and heart, the ascending and transverse arch of the aorta, the superior and inferior venae cavae, the brachiocephalic vessels, the phrenic nerves, the upper portions of the vagus nerves, the trachea, the main bronchi and contiguous lymph nodes, and the main pulmonary vessels. The *posterior mediastinal compartment* contains the descending thoracic aorta, the esophagus, the thoracic duct, the azygos and hemiazygos veins, the sympathetic chains, the lower portions of the vagus nerves, and the posterior group of mediastinal lymph nodes.

MEDIASTINAL MASSES

A variety of mediastinal masses of neoplastic, inflammatory, or vascular origin may present in the chest roentgenogram. It is useful for differential diagnosis to know that many processes tend to occur more often in one of the three mediastinal compartments than in the others (Table 22-1). While some lesions such as aortic aneurysms can occur in any compartment (see Chap. 27), lymphomatous lymph nodes occur with equal frequency in the anterior and middle mediastinal compartments but rarely in the posterior compartment.

Half of all patients with mediastinal masses have no symptoms, and their masses are discovered by shadows in their chest roentgenograms. Symptoms that may bring the patient to the physician include

Table 22-1. Predominant Localization of Mediastinal Masses in the Three Mediastinal Compartments

Process	Mediastinal compartment		
	Anterior	Middle	Posterior
Thymoma	++	0	+
Germinal cell tumors	++	0	+
Thyroid masses	++	0	+
Parathyroid masses	++	0	0
Lipoma	++	+	+
Mesenchymal tumors	++	+	+
Neoplastic lymphadenopathy	+	++	+
Granulomatous lymphadenopathy	+	++	+
Bronchogenic cyst	0	++	+
Hernia of foramen of Morgagni	0	++	0
Pleuropericardial cyst	+	++	0
Dilatation of pulmonary artery	0	++	0
Dilatation of superior vena cava	0	++	0
Dilatation of azygos vein	0	++	0
Dilatation of aorta (aneurysm)	++	++	++
Neurogenic tumors	+	+	++
Meningocele	0	0	++
Gastroenteric cysts	0	0	++
Esophageal lesions	0	0	++
Hernia of foramen of Bochdalek	0	0	++

Note: 0 = almost never; + = rare; ++ = common predilection.

a sense of fullness or pain substernally, breathlessness or cough because of compression of the tracheobronchial tree, hoarseness because of recurrent laryngeal nerve paralysis, and edema of the face and upper extremities because of compression of the superior vena cava. A broad range of techniques is often required to establish the diagnosis of mediastinal mass. A careful history and physical examination may provide evidence of an unusual infection or may indicate that the process is part of a more widespread systemic disease. A scintiscan made after administration of radioactive iodine is useful in identifying

intrathoracic goiter. Bronchoscopy may prove that
an upper mediastinal mass is due to metastatic involvement from bronchogenic carcinoma. A barium esoph-
agram often provides very useful information on the
anatomic relationships of a mass lesion. Contrast
studies of the great vessels may confirm the presence
of obstruction of the superior vena cava or may indicate an aneurysm of one of the great arteries in the
thorax. Mediastinoscopy often provides histologic
material permitting precise diagnosis of neoplasm or
infection. However, in many instances thoracotomy
with exploration or biopsy is the only successful
diagnostic approach.

Bibliography

Fraser, R. G., and Paré, J. A. P. *Diagnosis of Diseases
    of the Chest.* Philadelphia: Saunders, 1970.

Leigh, T. F., and Weens, H. S. *The Mediastinum.*
    Springfield, Ill.: Thomas, 1959.

Lyons, H. A., Calvy, G. L., and Simmons, B. P. The
    diagnosis and classification of mediastinal
    masses: I. A study of 782 cases. *Ann. Intern.
    Med.* 51:897, 1959.

23

Acute Respiratory Failure

Frank F. Davidson and Jerome S. Brody

Acute respiratory failure may be defined as a decrease in arterial partial pressure of oxygen (Pa_{O_2}) below 50 mm Hg or an increase in arterial partial pressure of carbon dioxide (Pa_{CO_2}) above 50 mm Hg that is of recent origin (30 days or less) or is accompanied by recent clinical deterioration. Recognition of respiratory failure depends on measurements of arterial blood gases, since clinical signs of hypoxemia and hypercapnia are notoriously imprecise and misleading. Sudden carbon dioxide elevations may be associated first with vasodilatation (warm, flushed skin; tachycardia) followed by neurologic signs (mental depression, increased tendon reflexes, tremulousness, and asterixis) and ultimately by cardiovascular and central nervous system depression (hypotension and coma). However, absence of these signs does not rule out hypercapnia; patients with chronic hypercapnia frequently have no symptoms at all, suggesting that many of the clinical findings related to acute hypercapnia are due to changes in pH. Signs and symptoms of hypoxemia may be equally vague and nonspecific, including restlessness, personality change, confusion, and ultimately coma. Cyanosis is not consistently recognized until arterial saturation is less than 85 percent. Thus arterial blood gases should be measured in patients with severe respiratory system disease and, in addition, in patients who are in shock or who are severely and acutely ill from any cause.

Classification of Respiratory Failure

The causes of respiratory failure may be classified into three broad groups on the basis of the localization of the deranged portion of the respiratory system: (1) disease of the respiratory bellows with normal lungs; (2) diseases affecting the airways and pulmonary system; and (3) mixed disorders. Another classification groups diseases into those producing hypoxemia without hypercapnia and those producing hypoxemia with hypercapnia. In the following list, all thoracic bellows defects (category I), disorders of the conducting airways (category IIA), and mixed disorders (category III) fall into the latter group of diseases that

produce hypoxemia with hypercapnia. Diseases affecting the lung parenchyma (category IIB) are characterized by hypoxemia without hypercapnia.

I. Thoracic bellows disease — normal lungs
   A. Impaired respiratory control
      1. Neurologic disease* (encephalitis, bulbar poliomyelitis, trauma, idiopathic)
      2. Metabolic abnormalities (alkalosis, myxedema)
      3. Drug intoxication (barbiturates, opiates)
   B. Impaired neural transmission
      1. Spinal cord (anterior poliomyelitis, trauma, amyotrophic lateral sclerosis)
      2. Peripheral nerves (Guillain-Barré syndrome)
      3. Neuromuscular junction (myasthenia gravis, curare intoxication, botulism, tick paralysis)
   C. Myopathies (muscular dystrophies, polymyositis, dermatomyositis)
   D. Rib cage defects
      1. Trauma (flail chest)
      2. Kyphoscoliosis
      3. Thoracoplasty
      4. Bilateral fibrothorax
II. Airways and pulmonary disease
   A. Airways disease
      1. Upper airways disease (tonsillar hypertrophy, tumors)
      2. Lower airways disease (asthma, chronic bronchitis, emphysema)
   B. Alveolar disease
      1. Bilateral severe pneumonia
      2. Adult respiratory distress syndrome
III. Mixed problems (obesity-hypoventilation syndrome, postoperative respiratory failure in patients with obstructive airways disease)

A combination of both classifications — localization and respiratory result — provides the most useful operational approach to management. Hypercapnia denotes the presence of alveolar hypoventilation

---

*Examples are given in parentheses. Categories I, IIA, and III present with hypoxemia and hypercapnia; category IIB presents with hypoxemia without hypercapnia.

(ventilatory failure) but does not indicate the mechanism. In bellows defects, overall or global hypoventilation can be alleviated only by mechanical assistance to ventilation; in chronic airways obstruction, ventilation-perfusion mismatch has become so severe that the patient can no longer do the work to eliminate carbon dioxide through the portions of the lungs that are the best ventilated. In the latter group, medical measures may relieve obstruction of the small airways and simple measures such as tonsillectomy, tracheal intubation, or tracheostomy may relieve upper airways obstruction.

RESPIRATORY BELLOWS DYSFUNCTION
Patients with respiratory bellows dysfunction (see list preceding) develop respiratory failure because they fail to ventilate their lungs adequately; and with this global hypoventilation, they develop hypercapnia and hypoxemia. The process may develop rapidly (e.g., following barbiturate overdose or trauma) or more slowly over days, weeks, or months (e.g., with neuromuscular disease). An alert patient who is not severely dyspneic and who has normal arterial blood gases does not require mechanical ventilation. Patients with neuromuscular disease should be followed with tests of muscle strength and measurements of the vital capacity. When the vital capacity decreases to below 10 ml per kilogram of body weight, particularly if the change occurs over a period of hours, the patient should be intubated and placed on mechanical ventilation. The basic cause of depressed respiratory drive should be treated (e.g., treat metabolic alkalosis with potassium chloride or acidifying agents or a drug overdose with specific antagonists and diuresis), and the patient should be followed closely with aggressive chest physiotherapy and measurements of ventilation and blood gases. Patients comatose from drug overdosage are intubated to prevent aspiration and are mechanically ventilated until oxygen exchange is adequate and they are alert enough to perform adequate vital capacity maneuvers (at least 10 ml per kilogram). These patients frequently develop hypoxemia without carbon dioxide retention because their low vital capacity prevents effective coughing and deep breathing, which in turn leads to pooling of tracheobronchial secretions, atelec-

tasis, and often pneumonia. In any paralyzed or unconscious patient, whether on or off the ventilator, careful and frequent turning onto each side along with physical therapy permits optimal drainage of secretions from the tracheobronchial tree. Occasionally fiberoptic bronchoscopy with aspiration of secretions in atelectatic segments appears to be beneficial. Carbon dioxide retention develops late in the course of neuromuscular disease, and patients should be intubated and ventilated prior to this time.

THE ADULT RESPIRATORY DISTRESS SYNDROME
Patients seriously ill from trauma, shock, and severe infection develop a type of severe lung injury that takes the form of damage to the alveolar epithelium and the development of markedly increased capillary permeability. The injury presents as a state of acute interstitial and alveolar pulmonary edema that is not due to left ventricular failure. Although many names have been applied to this state, such as shock lung and stiff lung syndrome, the term *adult respiratory distress syndrome* (ARDS) will be used here. The etiology of the syndrome is unknown, but a wide variety of diseases have been shown to produce it, as listed below.

Pneumonia: viral, mycoplasmal, or bacterial
Chemical pneumonia (e.g., smoke inhalation, gastric acid aspiration)
  Fat embolization
  Hemorrhagic pancreatitis
  Postextracorporeal perfusion lung injury
  Hypotensive lung injury
  Gram-negative sepsis
  Drug induced (e.g., heroin, methadone)
  O_2 toxicity

The pulmonary pathology is often complicated by additional lung damage due to infection or oxygen toxicity. At postmortem examination the lungs have the appearance of liver, being heavy and congested, and the pathologic picture is nonspecific. The interstitium of the lung is edematous, often with cellular infiltrates and fibroblastic proliferation; edema fluid and hyaline membranes may be seen in the alveoli.

The distinguishing clinical feature of the syndrome is refractory hypoxemia without hypercapnia (except terminally) associated with the roentgenographic features of pulmonary edema but no evidence of left ventricular failure. The early manifestations of this condition are an increased respiratory rate with respiratory alkalosis and arterial hypoxemia but with few other clinical or x-ray abnormalities. Eventually the x-ray shows a progressive, usually symmetrical, fluffy alveolar infiltrate that progresses to involve all portions of the lung. Breath sounds are normal, and rales and rhonchi are not prominent. Pulmonary secretions are not increased, and cough and nasotracheal suction are unproductive unless there is coincident infection.

At this point, every possible effort should be made to identify and treat the underlying condition and to rule out local or systemic infection as a precipitating event. Pulmonary edema of cardiac origin must be excluded; this is best done by measurement of pulmonary capillary wedge pressure. The balloon-tipped pulmonary artery catheter necessary for these measurements can also be used for cardiac output measurements by the thermodilution technique or for measurement of mixed venous oxygen saturation which, if decreased below 75 percent, indicates that the cardiac output is inappropriately low for metabolic demands. Serial measurements may be used as a guide to fluid therapy, but the catheters increase susceptibility to infection and if at all possible should not be left in place more than 48 hours after the initial wedge pressure measurement has been made.

Treatment

Most experienced physicians believe that relatively early intubation and mechanical ventilation are beneficial in the treatment of adult respiratory distress syndrome. This practice improves oxygen exchange and permits management with a lower concentration of inspired oxygen. The patient is ventilated at high tidal volumes (15 ml per kilogram), and if oxygen concentrations higher than 50 percent are required to procure a safe arterial PO_2, positive end-expiratory pressure (PEEP) is used to increase functional residual capacity and decrease airway or alveolar collapse. Positive end-expiratory pressure may produce a decrease in cardiac output with resultant hypotension because of diminished venous return to the thorax.

Fluid therapy usually counteracts this effect. It should be remembered that the arterial PO_2 does not reflect tissue oxygenation and that oxygen delivery is better related to the product of cardiac output and blood oxygen content. It is important to transfuse anemic patients to provide more circulating hemoglobin.

Albumin may be given if serum oncotic pressure is low; however, large amounts must be given to achieve a measurable rise in serum albumin concentration and may cause an increase in blood volume and pulmonary capillary pressure as well as further transudation of fluid into the lungs. Provided the cardiac output is adequate (as judged by direct measurement or estimation from the mixed venous oxygen saturation), the pulmonary capillary wedge pressure should be kept low (less than 10 mm Hg) to prevent additional lung edema from developing on a hydrostatic basis. Steroids are occasionally given empirically. As peak and end-expiratory pressures are raised to improve oxygen exchange, pneumomediastinum or pneumothorax may occur, requiring placement of a chest tube. Finally, if progressive hypoxemia persists, sedation, muscle paralysis, or hypothermia may be used to decrease the metabolic rate. Although hypoxemia can be overcome by these means in most patients, the mortality rate is very high, usually because of the underlying disease and other complications such as sepsis, gastrointestinal bleeding, infection, and pulmonary embolism. A membrane oxygenator has been used as an artificial lung in some patients, but results to date have been disappointing.

CHRONIC OBSTRUCTIVE AIRWAYS DISEASE

Respiratory failure in chronic obstructive airways disease is characterized by carbon dioxide retention and hypoxemia. Although the hypoxemia is usually easily corrected with oxygen administration, the accompanying removal of hypoxemic ventilatory drive may cause further respiratory depression and carbon dioxide retention to the point of frank narcosis. Every attempt should be made to avoid intubation and mechanical ventilation, since results are comparable, if not better, with more conservative therapy. Although respiratory failure may represent the end-stage of a terminal disease, many episodes are reversible and are brought on by exacerbations of bronchitis, pneumonia, inappropriate sedation, or pneumothorax. It is in such patients that an aggressive approach with artificial ventilation may be required. The clinical features of an exacerbation of chronic bronchitis are discussed in depth in Chapter 20.

Treatment

Most patients with acute respiratory failure due to chronic obstructive airways disease arrive at the hospital awake and with a Pa_{CO_2} of less than 75 mm Hg provided they have not received supplemental oxygen. Approximately one-third of these patients (especially those with chronic elevation of Pa_{CO_2}) will hypoventilate to the point of coma when given uncontrolled amounts of oxygen. Hypoventilation results because these patients depend primarily on hypoxic peripheral chemoreceptor ventilatory drive, since central carbon dioxide and pH-related respiratory drive is in large part buffered by high levels of bicarbonate in the central nervous system. If the patient does develop marked elevations in Pa_{CO_2} with acidemia and resultant carbon dioxide narcosis, then immediate intubation and mechanical ventilation are mandatory. Special care is then required to avoid excessively rapid lowering of the Pa_{CO_2} with resultant alkalosis in patients who have chronically elevated serum bicarbonate levels.

If the patient has not received excessive oxygen and is alert, controlled 24 or 28% oxygen therapy should relieve dangerous hypoxemia but preserve some hypoxic drive to ventilation. Usual modes of oxygen administration (Table 23-1) such as the traditional face mask or nasal prongs providing a flow of 5 to 6 liters per minute may increase the Pa_{O_2} too much and suppress respiration. Specially designed Venturi masks that entrain air are uncomfortable but deliver quite precise percentages of oxygen that usually suffice to raise the Pa_{O_2} from very dangerous levels (below 40 mm Hg) to the shoulder of the dissociation curve (50 to 60 mm Hg), where oxygen content is much greater but some hypoxemic drive is retained. Individual variability makes a Pa_{O_2} of 50 mm Hg a rough guideline, although some patients will be alert at lower levels of oxygen tension and retain

carbon dioxide excessively even at a Pa_{O_2} of 50. While Pa_{O_2} values below 50 mm Hg are hardly desirable, patients rarely develop severe tissue hypoxia with lactic acidosis, particularly if the hypoxemia is of long duration, the hematocrit is normal or above normal, and the cardiac output is adequate.

In addition to controlled oxygen therapy, bronchodilator drugs are given. Sympathomimetic aerosol solutions may be inhaled with or without positive pressure as often as every 2 to 4 hours. Aminophylline is usually given intravenously and acts as a bronchodilator and central respiratory stimulant. In the occasional patient, corticosteroid administration relieves airways obstruction, although objective assessment of benefit is needed to avoid unnecessary complications with prolonged therapy. Antibiotics such as tetracycline or ampicillin are beneficial only in patients with evidence of infection on Gram stain of sputum. Physical therapeutic measures as tolerated, such as vigorous encouragement of cough and deep breathing, chest percussion, nasotracheal suction, and postural drainage, all improve gas exchange. Such aggressive physical measures with the controlled use of oxygen are the key features of conservative management. Phlebotomy is rarely indicated in hypoxic polycythemia, since this would decrease blood oxygen-carrying capacity; however, patients with very high hematocrit readings (over 60 percent) may benefit from the removal of 300-ml amounts of blood to reduce the hematocrit below 60 percent.

In some patients conservative management fails and the Pa_{CO_2} remains high; intubation and mechanical ventilation are then required. Many patients at this stage have little reversible disease, and weaning from artificial respiration may be prolonged or unsuccessful. Tracheostomy is performed for comfort and convenience if prolonged endotracheal intubation is required. Patients derive long-term benefit from tracheostomy after recovery from the acute episode only if management of secretions is otherwise impossible or if mechanical ventilation is to be used for a long period of time.

The syndrome of obesity hypoventilation and sleep apnea is the combination of periodic respiration during sleep, somnolence, and alveolar hypoventilation occurring occasionally in grossly obese persons.

Table 23-1. Forms of Oxygen Therapy

Equipment	Flow (L/min)	Approximate O_2 concentration (%)
Nasal cannula	1–6	24–40
Face mask	6–8	30–45
	10–12	45–65
Partial rebreathing mask	6–8	40–80
Nonrebreathing mask	6–8[*]	80–100
Venturi masks		
24 or 28% O_2	4	24 or 28
35 or 40% O_2	8	35 or 40
T-tube adapter for use with endotracheal or tracheostomy tubes (with or without reservoir tube)	Use with Venturi nebulizer with appropriate O_2 flow; reservoir tube prevents entrance of ambient air and increases concentration of O_2	

[*]Oxygen flow should be high enough to prevent emptying of reservoir bag during inspiration.

There may be associated heart failure due to hypoxia, polycythemia, and the resultant increase in pulmonary arterial pressure. The mechanism is decreased chest wall compliance and increased work of breathing in obese individuals, coupled with altered respiratory center sensitivity. Some patients also develop periodic upper airway obstruction. Relief occurs with weight loss and, if oropharyngeal obstruction is a feature, with tracheostomy. Controlled oxygen therapy and physical measures are the initial forms of treatment, although artificial ventilation is often required.

Bibliography

Bendixen, H., Egbert, L., Hedley-Whyte, J., Laver, M., and Pontoppidan, H. *Respiratory Care.* St. Louis: Mosby, 1965.

Campbell, E. The management of acute respiratory failure in chronic bronchitis and emphysema. *Am. Rev. Respir. Dis.* 96:626, 1967.

Pontoppidan, H., Geffin, B., and Lowenstein, E. Acute respiratory failure in the adult. *N. Engl. J. Med.* 287:690, 1972.

24

Sarcoidosis

Jerome S. Brody and Wlademir Pereira

Sarcoidosis is a multisystemic disease of unknown etiology and variable clinical manifestations characterized by noncaseating epithelioid cell granulomas in all affected organs and tissues. Because the histologic appearance is not pathognomonic, the pathologist can only describe the findings and indicate whether they are compatible with sarcoidosis. Special stains to exclude infectious agents and an appropriate clinical picture are essential to confirm the diagnosis.

Sarcoidosis is worldwide in distribution. Although it can occur at any age, it is most frequent between 20 and 40 years; the racial predominance in the United States is 10 to 17 times greater in blacks than in Caucasians. Women have a slightly greater incidence than men.

Sarcoidosis most frequently affects the hilar lymph nodes and lung. About one-third of the patients are totally asymptomatic, and their disease is first recognized on routine chest roentgenogram. Respiratory symptoms such as cough and dyspnea occur in one-third to one-half of the patients. The remaining patients also have extrathoracic manifestations of sarcoidosis such as enlarged peripheral lymph nodes and eye and skin abnormalities.

The roentgenographic manifestations of intrathoracic sarcoidosis are conveniently divided into four groups:

Group 0:   Normal
Group I: Hilar adenopathy
Groups II: Bilateral hilar adenopathy associated
             with pulmonary infiltration
Groups III: Pulmonary infiltration without hilar
             adenopathy

The pulmonary infiltrates seen in stages II and III may be disseminated miliary or nodular lesions resembling miliary tuberculosis, diffuse or confluent patchy shadows, bilateral massive opacities, or diffuse fibrosis. Long-standing fibrosis often leads to distortion of lung tissue with formation of cystic spaces and cavitation. On occasion, fungus balls (most often

aspergillomas) form within these cavities. Roentgenographic abnormalities involving the pleura are rare in sarcoidosis, although pleural lesions are not infrequent at autopsy. Sarcoidosis does not necessarily progress chronologically from group 0 through group III, nor is there a clear relation between the roentgenographic stage and symptoms.

Pulmonary function tests tend to correlate more closely with symptoms than with chest roentgenograms. However, functional abnormalities and histologic evidence of pulmonary granulomas have been found in group 0 and group I patients. In general, when granulomas are diffuse but circumscribed with normal lung tissue intervening, pulmonary function tests tend to be normal. When interstitial granulomatous infiltration is widespread, often with fibrosis, pulmonary function tests tend to reveal loss of total lung and vital capacity, diminished diffusing capacity, good preservation of airways patency, and hypoxemia without hypercapnia. Recent studies have revealed a high incidence of small airways disease in sarcoidosis.

Extrapulmonary Lesions

While intrathoracic manifestations of sarcoidosis predominate, the diversity of clinical manifestations is such that a patient may present with symptoms relating to virtually any organ system. Pulmonary lesions are almost always present in patients who have extrathoracic sarcoidosis.

Hilar and paratracheal lymph glands are most frequently involved in sarcoidosis. Enlargement of any of the superficial lymph glands may occur, and these nodes provide readily accessible tissue for biopsy. The parotid glands may be enlarged, and when this enlargement is associated with fever, uveitus, and facial palsy (due to involvement of the seventh cranial nerve), the illness is called uveoparotid fever.

Ocular involvement occurs in 20 to 25 percent of patients with sarcoidosis. The eyes should be examined routinely with a slit lamp, since lesions may not produce symptoms. Uveitis is the most frequent manifestation, often producing pain and clouded vision. Conjunctivitis and keratoconjunctivitis sicca, retinal lesions, and lacrimal gland enlargement are also seen. These lesions may lead to blindness in a small number of patients.

The skin may be involved in several fashions. The commonest lesion in Caucasian populations, particularly in Europe, is erythema nodosum. This lesion appears to be an early manifestation of sarcoidosis and is associated with hilar adenopathy and frequently with polyarthralgia; it carries a very good prognosis. Maculopapular eruptions, subcutaneous nodules, plaques, and purple raised nodular lesions known as lupus pernio are also seen. The last frequently involve the face and may produce disfiguration. Skin lesions other than erythema nodosum tend to be associated with a poor prognosis.

The musculoskeletal system is frequently involved in extrathoracic sarcoidosis. Sarcoid granulomas are found in 40 to 60 percent of random muscle biopsies. Muscle symptoms, when present, may range from mild pain to severe weakness, wasting, and incapacitation. Sarcoid foci have been reported in almost every bone, although the incidence is less than 5 percent. Cystic lesions in the phalanges of hands and feet are most characteristic, but diffuse infiltration and cortical thinning may also occur. Sarcoid arthritis has been reported in 10 to 20 percent of patients. It is frequently associated with erythema nodosum and is mild in nature.

Next to the lung and lymph nodes, the liver is most frequently involved in sarcoidosis. Despite the 60 to 80 percent incidence of positive liver biopsies, clinically significant liver disease rarely occurs, although a few cases of jaundice and portal hypertension have been reported. Sarcoidosis rarely involves other portions of the gastrointestinal tract.

Sarcoidosis may affect the kidneys in two ways, both of which can lead to functional impairment. The kidneys may be infiltrated with sarcoid granulomas, but the most common development is nephrocalcinosis. Hypercalcemia, apparently due to an unexplained increase in sensitivity to vitamin D, occurs in 2 to 4 percent of patients. Excess calcium may be deposited in the cornea and subcutaneous tissues, but nephrocalcinosis is the major consequence of hypercalcemia.

Sarcoidosis may produce cardiac disease as a result of extensive pulmonary fibrosis (cor pulmonale) or because of sarcoid involvement of the myocardium. Conduction disturbances and paroxysmal arrhyth-

mias are the most common manifestations of primary cardiac disease, with sudden death occurring in two-thirds of patients with myocardial sarcoidosis. Electrocardiographic abnormalities usually appear in the absence of cardiac symptoms. Granulomatous involvement of vessels other than the pulmonary arteries is rare.

Sarcoid involvement of the nervous system may result in a variety of clinical pictures. Peripheral neuropathy, meningitis, space-occupying lesions, and involvement of the posterior pituitary gland have been reported. The diagnosis is often difficult to establish, and the disease frequently has a chronic course with a poor prognosis.

Diagnosis

The diagnosis of sarcoidosis needs maximum precision when corticosteroid treatment is contemplated. In patients with few or no symptoms who are only to be observed, the diagnosis may be based on a chest roentgenogram showing group I or II changes and careful studies to exclude infectious causes.

The most accessible lesions, such as cutaneous lesions, conjunctival or subcutaneous nodules, or enlarged lymph nodes, should be biopsied first because of the high yield, ease of performance, and safety of such biopsies. When the predominant lesions are in the lung with no specific peripheral manifestations, lung biopsy is the best approach. Flexible fiberoptic transbronchial lung biopsy offers a high yield with very low morbidity. Scalene lymph node biopsy yields granulomatous changes in about 80 percent of patients with sarcoidosis, but it should be remembered that drainage through these nodes may produce noncaseating granulomas in other diseases as diverse as carcinoma, Hodgkin's disease, and tuberculosis. Lymph node tissue obtained at mediastinoscopy has an even higher yield of granulomatous tissue but still is not 100 percent specific. The differential diagnosis should include infectious granulomatous diseases such as tuberculosis, coccidioidomycosis, histoplasmosis, cryptococcosis, and brucellosis, all of which may present pathologic and clinical pictures similar to those in sarcoidosis. Special stains of granulomatous tissue are necessary to rule out the above infectious diseases. Occasionally the granulomas may contain extensive areas of central eosino-philic necrosis, making histologic differentiation from tuberculosis difficult.

The Kveim test is an intradermal injection of a suspension of sarcoid tissue. When positive, a biopsy of the site of the injection 2 to 3 weeks later will show a noncaseating granuloma. The test gives a positive yield in up to 80 percent of active cases. There is continuing controversy about the specificity of the different antigen suspensions, with some anti-gens giving a high incidence of false-positive results. This test remains largely a research tool.

The most common biochemical abnormalities are elevated levels of serum globulins (30 to 50 percent of patients) and of serum calcium (5 to 10 percent of patients). Eosinophilia and anemia as well as throm-bocytopenia may be seen in sarcoidosis. The level of angiotensin-converting enzyme in the serum has been recently shown to be elevated in half the patients with sarcoidosis, although the ultimate value of this test remains to be determined.

The depression of delayed-type hypersensitivity is a characteristic immunologic phenomenon in sarcoi-dosis. Skin tests (mumps, *Candida,* trichophytin, etc.) that evaluate delayed-type hypersensitivity (cell-mediated immunity) are characteristically depressed, while circulating antibody responses are normal. The depression is variable and correlates roughly with the extent and activity of disease. The specific immuno-logic reason for depressed and delayed hypersensitiv-ity is unclear.

Treatment

There is no known cure for sarcoidosis, although corticosteroids can usually suppress the manifesta-tions of disease activity. In general, corticosteroids should be used if vital organs (e.g., heart, eye, or brain) are involved or if there is evidence of func-tional compromise of the lung.

The asymptomatic patient with pulmonary disease should not be treated but instead should be followed closely with serial chest roentgenograms and vital capacity measurements. The decision to use cortico-steroids in pulmonary sarcoidosis should be based on the presence of troublesome respiratory or systemic symptoms or on the progressive loss of lung function

rather than on the roentgenographic appearance. Patients usually respond in early disease to 40 to 50 mg of prednisone per day, tapered down to 20 mg every other day. If the patient demonstrates no objective response in 4 to 6 weeks, the drug is dis-continued. If the patient responds, steroids are con-tinued for at least 6 months and are tapered cautiously with close attention given to possible rebound of the disease. Some patients may be committed to steroids for life because their disease rebounds whenever steroids are discontinued. Local corticosteroids should be used in all patients with ocular sarcoidosis. It is generally agreed that hypercalcemia and central nervous system and myocardial involvement require systemic corticosteroid therapy, although the results in the last two have not been dramatic.

The prognosis of sarcoidosis depends in part on the stage at which it is diagnosed, in part on how long it has been present, and in part on the extent of sys-temic involvement. Asymptomatic patients with group I x-rays (hilar adenopathy) and disease of recent onset have an extremely good prognosis, with 70 to 90 percent spontaneous cure rates. Patients with group II or group III chest x-rays and disease of several years' duration who also have skin or myo-cardial disease have a poor prognosis, with little chance of spontaneous cure. The overall 5-year mortality as determined from large series (that were weighted somewhat with poor prognosis cases) is 6 percent.

Bibliography

Cummings, M. M., and Hammarsten, J. F. Sarcoi-dosis. *Annu. Rev. Med.* 13:19, 1962.

Mayock, R. L., Bertrand, P., Morrison, C. E., and Scott, J. H. Manifestations of sarcoidosis. *Am. J. Med.* 35:67, 1963.

Mitchell, D. H., and Scadding, J. G. Sarcoidosis. *Am. Rev. Respir. Dis.* 110:774, 1974.

V The Heart and Blood Vessels

25

Hypertensive Diseases

William Hollander

Hypertension is one of the most important risk factors for cardiovascular morbidity and mortality as well as for death from all causes. It is a leading factor in stroke, kidney failure, and congestive heart failure and is frequently implicated in ischemic heart disease and sudden death. Hypertension is believed to be the cause of at least one-fourth and perhaps as many as one-half of all cardiovascular deaths. Although a systolic blood pressure greater than 150 mm Hg or a diastolic blood pressure greater than 90 mm Hg is usually regarded as abnormal, epidemiologic studies have shown that there is a progressive increase in cardiovascular disease with any increase of blood pressure, even within the range generally regarded as normal.

It is estimated that about 15 percent of American adults have definite hypertension, while another 15 percent have borderline hypertension. The frequency of hypertension increases with advancing age, and more than 25 percent of individuals over the age of 55 have definite hypertension. Elevation of blood pressure also is more common in men than in women up to the age of 50. After this age, the reverse is true.

In studies of hypertension among children, a major problem has been that of establishing normal values for blood pressure. Blood pressure levels regarded as normal in adults may be abnormally high for children. Blood pressure in normal infants averages about 80/45 mm Hg; it then rises in childhood to an average of about 95/65 mm Hg and in adolescence it reaches levels of 110 mm Hg systolic and 70 mm Hg diastolic. Thereafter the blood pressure rises gradually and attains an average level of 150 to 160 mm Hg systolic and 85 to 90 mm Hg diastolic by age 65.

CLASSIFICATION

There are two general types of arterial hypertension — systolic hypertension and diastolic hypertension. Systolic hypertension is characterized by an elevation of the systolic blood pressure, with diastolic pressure normal, decreased, or mildly elevated. Disproportion-ate rises in systolic as compared with diastolic pressure result in an increase of pulse pressure. In "pure" systolic hypertension the diastolic pressure is either normal or decreased.

Systolic hypertension is caused hemodynamically by an increase in stroke output of the left ventricle or by a decrease in the distensibility of the great vessels or both. It is found commonly in elderly persons, in whom it is mainly a manifestation of increased rigidity of an arteriosclerotic aorta. Diastolic hypertension is characterized by an elevation of diastolic blood pressure and usually (but not always) of systolic pressure. The hypertension appears to result from an increase in the absolute level of the peripheral vascular resistance relative to the cardiac output.

A clinical classification of arterial (systolic and diastolic) hypertension based on its etiology, course, and complications is shown below.

I. A. Diastolic hypertension
    1. Essential hypertension
       a. Labile (intermittent)
       b. Established (fixed)
    2. Renal hypertension
       a. Parenchymal kidney disease
         (1) Pyelonephritis
         (2) Glomerulonephritis
         (3) Diabetic nephropathy
         (4) Polycystic kidneys
         (5) Collagen diseases
         (6) Gouty nephritis
         (7) Renal tumors (juxtaglomerular cell tumor, hypernephroma, Wilms' tumor)
         (8) Renal hematoma
         (9) Other (tuberculosis, amyloidosis, radiation nephritis)
       b. Obstructive vascular kidney disease
         (1) Atherosclerotic obstruction of renal artery
         (2) Fibromuscular diseases of renal artery
         (3) Thrombotic obstruction of renal artery
         (4) Embolic obstruction of renal artery

(5) Other diseases of the renal artery: hypoplasia, aneurysm, inflammation, pseudoxanthoma elasticum
c. Obstructive uropathy — hydronephrosis
d. Renoprival hypertension
  (1) Renal failure
  (2) Anephric state
3. Adrenal hypertension
  a. Mineralocorticoid hypertension
    (1) Primary aldosteronism (adrenal adenoma)
    (2) Idiopathic aldosteronism (adrenal hyperplasia)
    (3) Deoxycorticosterone (DOC) hypertension
    (4) 18-hydroxy-DOC hypertension
    (5) Hydroxylase-deficiency hypertension
  b. Pheochromocytoma
  c. Cushing's syndrome
  d. Adrenogenital syndrome
4. Diabetic hypertension
5. Neurogenic hypertension
  a. Brain tumors
  b. Epilepsy
  c. Diencephalic syndrome
  d. Lead encephalopathy
  e. Bulbar poliomyelitis
  f. Encephalitis
  g. Ganglioneuroma
  h. Tabes dorsalis
  i. Neuroblastoma
  j. Spinal cord transection
  k. Polyneuritis
  l. Porphyria
6. Hypertension of coarctation of the aorta
7. Hypertension of toxemia of pregnancy
  a. Preeclampsia
  b. Eclampsia
8. Drug-induced hypertension
  a. Oral contraceptives
  b. Steroids
  c. Sympathomimetic drugs (amphetamines, phenylephrine)
  d. Monoamine oxidase inhibitors with tyramine
  e. Tricyclic antidepressants (antagonize, guanethidine, and clonidine)
9. Other causes of hypertension
  a. Smoking
  b. Licorice ingestion
  c. Hypercalcemia
  d. Myxedema
  e. Polycythemia
B. Systolic hypertension
  1. Caused mainly by an increased output of the left ventricle
    a. "Hyperkinetic" systolic hypertension
    b. Thyrotoxicosis
    c. Aortic regurgitation
    d. Complete heart block
    e. Anemia
    f. Arteriovenous fistula
    g. Patent ductus arteriosus
    h. Paget's disease of bone
    i. Beriberi

II. Course
A. Gradual phase (benign or nonmalignant hypertension)
  1. Course — long duration (usually more than 10 years)
  2. Onset — gradual and frequently asymptomatic
  3. Encephalopathy — rarely complicates course
  4. Diastolic blood pressure — usually below 130 mm Hg
  5. Fundi — usually grade 0 to 2 retinopathy (no papilledema)
  6. Blood urea nitrogen — usually normal
  7. Urine — normal or slight albuminuria
B. Accelerated phase ("malignant" hypertension)
  1. Course — short duration (usually less than 2 years)
  2. Onset — usually sudden and symptomatic
  3. Encephalopathy — often complicates course
  4. Diastolic blood pressure — usually above 120 mm Hg
  5. Fundi — grade 3 to 4 retinopathy (papilledema usually present)

6. Blood urea nitrogen — may be elevated
7. Urine — albuminuria, hematuria, and casts frequently present

III. Severity and extent of cardiovascular complications
   A. Uncomplicated
   B. Complicated
      1. Fundi
         a. Grade 1 (vascular spasm)
         b. Grade 2 (vascular sclerosis)
         c. Grade 3 (hemorrhage or exudates or both)
         d. Grade 4 (papilledema)
      2. Heart
         a. Left ventricular hypertrophy
         b. Congestive heart failure
         c. Coronary heart disease
         d. Myocardial infarction
      3. Aorta and main branches
         a. Atherosclerotic and/or thrombotic narrowing or occlusion
         b. Aortic (atherosclerotic) aneurysm (with or without rupture)
         c. Dissecting aneurysm
      4. Brain
         a. Cerebrovascular insufficiency
         b. Encephalopathy
         c. Cerebral thrombosis
         d. Intracerebral hemorrhage
         e. Subarachnoid hemorrhage
      5. Kidneys
         a. Benign nephrosclerosis
         b. Malignant nephrosclerosis
         c. Impaired renal function — proteinuria, hematuria, reduced creatinine clearance, low urinary specific gravity
         d. Renal insufficiency — blood urea nitrogen 25 mg per 100 ml; serum creatinine 1.2 mg per 100 ml

COURSE OF HYPERTENSION

The course of arterial hypertension may be divided into two phases: a gradual (benign) one and an accelerated (malignant) one. In the benign phase of hypertension the course is relatively slow but progressive, and lasts about 10 to 20 years in the average patient. In the malignant phase of hypertension the course is short and predictable. Malignant hypertension if left untreated runs a rapid, downhill course and terminates in uremia as a result of complicating renal necrotizing arteriolitis. The average survival time in malignant hypertension without treatment is about 8 months and the mortality is close to 100 percent in 2 years.

The malignant phase may complicate any form of hypertension, but it appears to be commoner in renal than in other forms. It occurs at least ten times more frequently in chronic glomerulonephritis than in essential hypertension. The cause of malignant hypertension is not known, but it is currently viewed as being due to, or at least associated with, injury of arterioles caused by high levels of arterial pressure and intense vasoconstriction.

The renin-angiotensin-aldosterone system also may play a role, since the activity of this system is often increased in malignant hypertension. Hypersecretion of aldosterone appears to be caused by adrenocortical stimulation by angiotensin resulting from the renin release attributable to renal involvement. Such secondary hyperaldosteronism in malignant hypertension may produce biochemical findings in the blood and urine similar to those found in primary aldosteronism (see later). Papilledema, low serum sodium, increased plasma-renin activity, and absence of a blood pressure lowering response to the aldosterone antagonist spironolactone favor the diagnosis of malignant hypertension over primary aldosteronism.

The diastolic blood pressure in accelerated (malignant) hypertension is usually over 120 mm Hg and is accompanied by blurring of the optic disc margins (papilledema). Papilledema is an early sign of malignant hypertension and usually precedes the development of renal insufficiency. Although some patients with accelerated hypertension may not have papilledema, almost all do have retinal hemorrhages and exudates. In such patients, the diagnosis and treatment of malignant hypertension should not be deferred until papilledema, signs of hematuria, or renal insufficiency occurs. At the onset or early in the course of the accelerated phase, urinalysis, standard renal function tests, and renal biopsy may be essentially normal. The findings of competent renal function without elevation of the blood urea nitrogen in accelerated as well as in gradual hypertension are favorable prognostically and increase the likelihood of effective antihypertensive treatment. A rise in the blood urea nitrogen and creatinine signals the onset of necrotizing renal arteriolitis (malignant nephrosclerosis) and has a much graver prognosis.

COMPLICATIONS OF HYPERTENSION

The adverse effects of hypertension on the cardiovascular system appear mainly due to the mechanical effects of the elevated blood pressure on the heart and arterial system. By increasing the work load and oxygen requirements of the myocardium, hypertension not only may cause cardiac hypertrophy and congestive heart failure but also may precipitate or aggravate coronary insufficiency (Fig. 25-1). A high level of arterial pressure with resulting increase in tangential stress on the arterial wall also can cause structural changes in the arterial wall that may result in hypertensive vascular disease, aggravation of atherosclerosis, aneurysmal dilatation of arteries, and rupture of diseased vessels. Although vasoactive hormones such as angiotensin, catecholamines, and prostaglandins may influence the metabolism and function of the arterial wall, their role in vascular disease has not been established.

The sequelae of hypertension may be classified into hypertensive or atherosclerotic complications. Those directly due to the hypertension are commonly referred to as hypertensive complications. They appear to be caused by the direct mechanical effects of the hypertension on the heart and blood vessels and are preventable by effective antihypertensive treatment. These complications include (1) left ventricular hypertrophy, (2) congestive heart failure, (3) dissecting aneurysms, (4) hypertensive retinopathy, (5) malignant hypertension, (6) hypertensive crises or encephalopathy, (7) cerebral hemorrhage, and (8) renal failure. The atherosclerotic complications of hypertension are manifestations of advanced atherosclerosis and include (1) coronary heart disease, and its sequelae of angina pectoris, myocardial infarction, and sudden death; (2) atherothrombotic strokes; (3) aortic aneurysm; (4) peripheral vascular disease; and (5) renal artery stenosis. There is substantial evidence

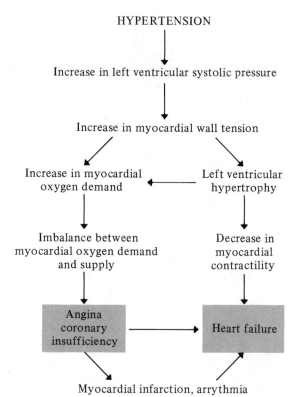

Figure 25-1. *Mechanisms by which hypertension may aggravate coronary heart disease.*

in man and experimental animals that a sustained elevation of arterial blood pressure regardless of its cause aggravates and accelerates atherosclerosis. However, it has not been demonstrated that hypertension per se, in the absence of other atherogenic factors, can cause atherosclerosis. The atherosclerotic complications of hypertension are much more difficult to control than the hypertensive complications and are largely responsible for the current morbidity and mortality in hypertension.

Although hypertension per se does not appear to cause atherosclerosis, it does produce structural changes in the large and small arteries and in the arterioles. These vascular changes resulting in hypertensive vascular disease are characterized by fibromuscular thickening of the intima and media with marked deposition of acid mucopolysaccharides. Involvement of the small vessels may cause luminal narrowing and result in an increase in peripheral vascular resistance and reduction of blood flow, particularly to the brain, kidney, and heart.

Hypertensive encephalopathy, or acute hypertensive crisis, is not uncommon in accelerated or malignant hypertension. The syndrome may complicate any form of hypertension and is usually signaled by a sudden, marked rise in blood pressure to levels greater than 220/120 mm Hg. In children, however, lower levels of hypertension may accompany this medical emergency. Hypertensive encephalopathy is manifested initially by severe headache, nausea, or vomiting; later by convulsions; and finally by coma. The early manifestations may resemble those of brain tumor and include a change in personality with mental confusion and disorientation. Papilledema and an elevated cerebrospinal fluid pressure commonly occur, but these findings are not necessary for the diagnosis. Cerebrovascular accidents and congestive heart failure are frequent complications of hypertensive encephalopathy that has not been treated early and effectively with antihypertensive drugs. Uremic encephalopathy in a patient with hypertension may be difficult to differentiate from hypertensive encephalopathy. A blood urea nitrogen over 75 mg per 100 ml and a failure of the symptoms to respond to a lowering of the blood pressure favor the diagnosis of uremic over hypertensive encephalopathy. The differential diagnosis of hypertensive encephalopathy, brain tumor, and other intracranial diseases is discussed in the section on neurogenic hypertension later in this chapter.

The view that hypertensive encephalopathy is due to cerebral ischemia caused by intense vasoconstriction of the cerebral arteries has been challenged by recent studies. These studies suggest that an acute rise in blood pressure causes a breakdown of the normal autoregulation of cerebral blood flow and thereby results in hyperperfusion of the cerebral blood vessels and an increase in capillary hydrostatic pressure, which is followed by brain edema.

Cerebrovascular disease and resulting stroke are major complications of hypertension. These complications are generally due to (1) atherosclerotic narrowing of the cerebral vessels, (2) cerebral thrombosis associated with atherosclerosis, (3) small vessel disease due to hypertension, or (4) intracerebral hemorrhage.

The most common cause of intracerebral hemorrhage in hypertensive patients over the age of 40 appears to be the rupture of intracerebral microaneurysms of the Charcot-Bouchard type. These aneurysms appear to result from the destruction of the arterial media by the hypertension. Rupture of a berry aneurysm with bleeding into the subarachnoid space also is an important cause of cerebrovascular accidents. These aneurysms involve the extracerebral arteries and occur with increased frequency in hypertensive patients with coarctation of the aorta or with polycystic kidney disease.

LABORATORY FINDINGS

The laboratory studies employed in the diagnosis and evaluation of hypertension are outlined below.

1. Routine studies
   a. Blood pressure (both arms, lower extremities, lying, standing)
   b. Optic fundi — grade of retinopathy (0 to 4)
   c. Peripheral arterial pulses and bruits
   d. Blood studies — complete blood count, serology, creatinine, blood urea nitrogen, glucose, sodium, potassium, cholesterol, triglycerides, and uric acid
   e. Urinalysis and urine culture
   f. Chest x-ray
   g. Electrocardiogram
   h. Excretory pyelogram
2. Special tests
   a. Radioisotope renogram
   b. Arteriogram
   c. Renin assay — peripheral and renal veins
   d. Urine catecholamines and metabolite excretion
   e. Urinary and plasma steroid levels
   f. Differential renal function studies
   g. Retrograde pyelogram
   h. Renal biopsy
   i. Others as indicated

The routine studies in conjunction with the history and physical examination will lead to an accurate diagnosis in the vast majority of cases. The special tests listed above, however, may be required to confirm the diagnosis and establish the site of origin of hypertension.

Arterial (Diastolic) Hypertension

CLINICAL FEATURES

Symptoms are often absent in the early stages of hypertension, which is usually diagnosed during a routine physical examination. Among the early complaints of patients with hypertension, the most frequent include headache, palpitations, nervousness, dizziness, light-headedness, and fatigability. For the most part these early symptoms appear to be functional and not the result of vascular complications of hypertension. The typical hypertensive headache is throbbing, occipital in location, and occurs early in the morning. It is usually relieved by a cup of coffee or a caffeine-containing drug and generally disappears completely after effective control of the blood pressure. Tension headaches characterized by stiffness and tenderness of the posterior cervical and occipital muscles also are common and frequently respond to tranquilizers, aspirin, or antihypertensive treatment. As the hypertension progresses, more serious symptoms may develop due to complicating cardiovascular disease.

Early symptoms of malignant hypertension may be similar to those of benign hypertension but in addition may include blurring of vision (due to the retinopathy), weight loss, and hematuria. The headache is usually severe and may be accompanied by nausea and vomiting. Weight loss may occur without a noticeable change in appetite. Hand tremors, prominent eyeballs, and emotional lability may also be present, even though thyroid function tests are normal.

PHYSIOLOGIC CHARACTERISTICS

The major physiologic function of the arterial pressure is to perfuse the tissues with blood. The mean arterial pressure is determined by the cardiac output and peripheral vascular resistance and is approximately equal to the diastolic blood pressure plus one-third of the pulse pressure. The primary determinants of pulse pressure are the velocity and volume of left ventricular ejection in relation to the arterial distensibility. In general, the pulse pressure (and systolic pressure) rises both with increases in ventricular ejection rate and volume and with decreases in aortic distensibility. The diastolic pressure is determined

primarily by the peripheral vascular resistance and is affected by heart rate, as this changes the duration of diastole. Usually the higher the peripheral vascular resistance, the higher the diastolic blood pressure. Systolic pressure generally rises with increasing levels of diastolic pressure, because the systolic blood pressure is equal to the diastolic pressure plus the pulse pressure.

Increased peripheral resistance is no longer considered the only hemodynamic abnormality of diastolic hypertension. In addition to the resistance vessels (arterioles), the heart, arteries, veins, and capillaries also appear to participate in the hemodynamic and fluid volume changes that occur in hypertension. The contribution of peripheral vascular resistance and cardiac output to the level of blood pressure appears to vary in different stages and forms of hypertension. However, peripheral resistance usually is inappropriately high for the level of cardiac output in this disease.

A number of systems operating in an integrated manner play an important role in controlling the cardiac output and peripheral resistance and hence the arterial pressure. These systems include (1) autonomic nervous system (sympathetic and parasympathetic), (2) baroreceptors, (3) catecholamines, (4) renin-angiotensin-aldosterone system, (5) blood volume and extracellular fluid volume, and (6) resistance vessels. Different forms of hypertension, as discussed below, may arise from different abnormalities in these blood pressure controlling mechanisms. There also is some evidence that the mechanisms which initiate certain forms of hypertension may not necessarily be the same ones that sustain it.

ESSENTIAL HYPERTENSION

Essential hypertension is a disease (or diseases) of unknown cause and accounts for the vast majority of patients with diastolic hypertension. As more is learned about various types of high blood pressure and better methods of diagnosis are developed, the percentage of cases in which essential hypertension is diagnosed appears to be slowly decreasing. There is growing evidence from endocrinologic and hemodynamic investigations that essential hypertension is a heterogeneous disorder that can be separated into several subgroups. Essential hypertension occurs frequently as a familial disease, with about 75 percent of the patients having a family history of high blood pressure or of its sequelae. The familial tendency to hypertension may begin in childhood or even earlier. The children of hypertensive parents have been found to have higher levels of blood pressure than the children of normotensive parents. It appears that the higher the pressure of the parents, the higher the pressures of their offspring at any given age. Studies in man and animal indicate that hypertension or the predisposition to hypertension can be transmitted genetically. There also is strong experimental evidence that the interaction of genetic factors with environmental factors operates to cause hypertension. Some of the environmental factors implicated in the pathogenesis of essential hypertension include behavioral stress and a high dietary intake of salt (NaCl).

While behavioral stress is difficult to quantify, it appears to be an important factor in hypertension. It is well recognized that emotional stress may elevate the blood pressure and aggravate hypertension, whereas rest and relaxation often lower the arterial pressure, particularly in the early stages of hypertensive disease. Recent studies suggest that psychotherapy may lower arterial pressure in mild or labile hypertension as a result of reducing sympathetic neural activity. Evidence is accumulating that a high dietary salt intake may be a major etiologic factor in hypertension. Diets high in sodium often increase blood pressure and aggravate hypertension, while diets low in sodium may lower pressure and ameliorate hypertension. There is some experimental and clinical evidence that excessive sodium intake may increase arterial pressure and vascular resistance as a result of stimulating sympathetic nerve function. The importance of dietary salt in the pathogenesis of essential hypertension is supported by epidemiologic studies in acculturated and unacculturated societies. These studies have shown that populations with high salt intake have a high incidence of hypertension, whereas populations with low salt intake (less than 4 gm of NaCl daily) have a low incidence of hypertension and a blood pressure that does not rise with advancing years. Studies in inbred rats suggest that genetic factors may exert a powerful

influence on the response of the blood pressure to dietary salt. These experiments also suggest that hypertension induced by a high-salt diet may persist indefinitely, even after a normal diet is resumed.

Pathologic Physiology

There is a growing body of evidence that there is some abnormality in the autonomic control of the blood pressure in patients with essential hypertension. In addition to overactivity of the sympathetic nervous system, a decrease in parasympathetic and baroreceptor neural function has been described. There also is some evidence that these changes of autonomic function may originate in the hypothalamus and medulla and result from disturbed activity of the alpha- and beta-adrenergic receptors located in these centers. The hemodynamic responses to experimental hypothalamic stimulation are not unlike those seen in early labile hypertension or in emotional stress and appear to be mediated by the central beta-adrenergic receptors. In contrast, activation of the alpha-adrenergic receptors in the brainstem appears to cause lowering of blood pressure and reflex withdrawal of sympathetic drive. Recent studies suggest that a decrease in the activity of these alpha-adrenergic receptors may be responsible for the hypertension induced in animals by a high-salt diet and mineralocorticoids.

The cardiac output, stroke volume, and heart rate are frequently elevated in labile or borderline hypertension. Total peripheral resistance may be either reduced or within normal limits but is inappropriately high for the level of cardiac output. In established hypertension, the cardiac output is normal and peripheral resistance is elevated. It is likely that the increased peripheral resistance in the early stages of "fixed" hypertension is due mainly to functional arteriolar vasoconstriction, whereas in the later stages of the disease structural changes in the arterioles also contribute to the abnormally high peripheral resistance. Several investigators have proposed that labile hypertension leads to established hypertension by causing autoregulatory adjustments in the circulation. According to this concept, the rise in blood pressure is initiated by an increase in cardiac output in the early stages of hypertension and leads in turn to either myogenic vasoconstriction or structural change in the arterial wall, which results in an increase in peripheral vascular resistance. The increased resistance acts at first to restrict cardiac output, but finally a new balance is established with a normal cardiac output and an elevated peripheral resistance. Thus established arterial hypertension, a vascular disease in its later phases, may be cardiogenic in its inception.

The vasomotor tone of the veins as well as of the arteries may be altered in hypertension. Forearm venous distensibility has been reported to be lower in patients with essential hypertension than in normal subjects and to be increased toward normal by drugs that suppress sympathetic neural activity.

Reports of urinary and plasma catecholamine levels in essential hypertension are conflicting. The overall evidence indicates that urinary and plasma norepinephrine levels are elevated in a significant proportion of patients with essential hypertension. Excessive catecholamine responsiveness to mental stress and to postural stimulation also has been reported in some hypertensive patients. There is some evidence that plasma levels of dopamine beta-hydroxylase may be elevated in a number of patients with borderline or established hypertension. The plasma concentration of this enzyme could reflect sympathetic nervous activity, since the enzyme is stored in the vesicles of the sympathetic nerve terminals and is released (with norepinephrine) by exocytosis upon nerve stimulation. Urinary excretion of cyclic AMP has been used as an index of overall beta-adrenergic receptor stimulation and has been reported to be normal at rest in borderline hypertension but to show an excessive response to postural stimulation.

The activity of the renin-angiotensin system is generally normal in essential hypertension. However, plasma renin is reported to be low in about 25 percent of the patients and high in about 10 percent of the patients. Low-renin hypertension is more common in blacks than in whites and occurs with increased frequency after the age of 30. Although plasma renin activity appears to decrease with age and duration of hypertension, a number of patients with low-renin hypertension have been reported to have a disturbance in mineralocorticoid metabolism. Some of the mineralocorticoids suspected of playing

an etiologic role in this form of hypertension include aldosterone, DOC, 18-hydroxy-DOC, and 16-oxygenated steroids (16-beta-hydroxy-dehydroepiandrosterone). Among the high-renin forms of hypertension, two types can be identified. One type represents borderline and mild hypertension of early onset and is believed to be due to overactivity of the sympathetic nervous system. In the second type the hypertension is more severe and is associated with complicating renal disease.

A deficiency of vasodilator or antihypertensive hormones such as the prostaglandins (PGA, PGE), bradykinin, and kallikrein has been postulated as a cause of hypertension. Plasma PGA has been reported to be reduced in a significant number of patients with essential hypertension. In addition, urinary kallikrein excretion also may be reduced. At present the role of these agents in essential hypertension is uncertain.

Total body sodium, potassium, and extracellular fluid volume are normal in uncomplicated hypertension. However, plasma volume is reported to be reduced and to be inversely related to the degree of diastolic hypertension. When the hypertension progresses to a malignant phase, extracellular fluid volume generally increases in association with an increased activity of the renin-angiotensin-aldosterone system. Abnormalities in the renal excretion of sodium have been observed in hypertension with hyperexcretion of sodium in response to saline loads and a paradoxical natriuresis with angiotensin administration. These changes appear to be due to the elevated blood pressure, since they are corrected by effective antihypertensive treatment.

Increased sodium, calcium, and water content in arteries from animals with experimental hypertension has been demonstrated by a number of studies. It is uncertain whether these changes are causally related or are a consequence of the hypertension. It has been suggested that an increase in the water content of arteries thickens the vessel wall and causes narrowing of the arteriolar lumen, which in turn results in an increase in peripheral vascular resistance and hypertension. It also has been proposed that increases in arteriolar calcium and sodium might influence the contractility of smooth muscle and lead to hypertension.

I. Brachial artery pressure responses to straining (Valsalva maneuver)

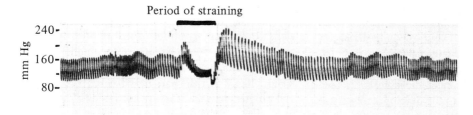

II. Brachial artery pressure responses to cold (ice water test)

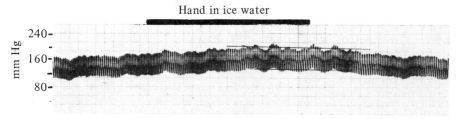

Figure 25-2. Hyperreactivity of the blood pressure to pressor stimuli in a 30-year-old woman with essential hypertension. In the upper tracing the overshoot in the blood pressure following the straining period of the Valsalva maneuver is unusually marked, being 80/65 mm Hg higher than the control blood pressure. In the lower tracing the blood pressure response to cold is similarly exaggerated, the increase in blood pressure being 40/25 mm Hg.

Patients with essential hypertension, especially those with borderline or labile hypertension, frequently have exaggerated blood pressure and vasoconstrictor responses to a number of pressor stimuli both before and after the development of hypertension (Fig. 25-2). Increased vascular reactivity has been demonstrated in the prehypertensive offspring of patients with essential hypertension (that is, before hypertension develops in the offspring). Why hypertensive and prehypertensive persons hyperreact to vasopressor agents (e.g., norepinephrine, angiotensin, serotonin); to procedures such as cold exposure or straining (Valsalva maneuver); and to emotional stimulation is not known. It has been postulated that such hyperreactivity is related to an increase in sympathetic neural activity or to functional or structural changes in the arterial wall. Experimental studies in rats with genetic hypertension suggest that the vascular hyperreactivity that occurs in these animals may be due mainly to inherited disturbances in the excitation and contraction of the arterial smooth muscle cells. There also is some evidence that this disorder might involve changes in membrane permeability and contractile protein function as well as an altered metabolism of intracellular calcium, adenosine triphosphate, and cyclic AMP.

Clinical Course

In the early or prehypertensive phase of essential hypertension, which may last a number of years, the blood pressure is characteristically labile and rises above the normal levels only intermittently. After this initial phase and usually between the ages of 25 and 30 years, the blood pressure gradually becomes continuously elevated but may show wide fluctuations above the normal level. In both the early and late phases of hypertension a rapid pulse rate is a characteristic finding. The course of mild and labile forms of hypertension is often one of gradual progress to higher and more sustained levels. However, in many of these patients the blood pressure may remain the same or even revert to normal.

Symptoms are often absent in the early stages of essential hypertension, but they appear with increasing frequency as the disease persists. Hyperglycemia, hyperlipidemia, and hyperuricemia are common findings in these disorders and are associated with the subsequent development of cardiovascular disease. The average case of essential hypertension without treatment runs a gradual course for 10 to 20 years and terminates in death from cardiovascular disease in the fifth decade. Prior to the development of antihypertensive drug treatment, congestive heart failure and coronary heart disease accounted equally for a total of about 80 percent of the cardiovascular deaths, whereas cerebrovascular and renovascular disease accounted for about 15 and 5 percent of the deaths, respectively. A small percentage of patients, probably less than 5 percent, progressed to a malignant phase.

Diagnosis

Although essential hypertension has certain characteristic clinical features, the diagnosis of this condition is usually firmly established only after all other known causes of hypertension have been excluded. This is because other forms of hypertension may have similar clinical features. The typical findings in a patient with essential hypertension are family history of either hypertension, coronary disease, or both; a gradual onset of hypertension between the ages of 25 and 35 years; a long history of hypertension before the appearance of cardiovascular complications; a normal urinalysis, blood urea nitrogen, and creatinine; and an absence of orthostatic hypotension (instead, the blood pressure often rises in the upright posture). Proteinuria and reductions of creatinine clearance are late findings that correlate with the degree of nephrosclerosis. An early appearance of more than slight proteinuria and impaired renal function frequently indicates either an accelerated phase of hypertension or primary or complicating renal disease (see Chap. 53).

Prognosis

Considerable evidence exists that the prognosis in hypertension is closely related to the height of the blood pressure itself and to the extent and severity of cardiovascular disease at the initial examination. Patients with labile or borderline hypertension also have been shown to have an increased risk of developing premature cardiovascular disease, although the

risk is less than that of patients with established or "fixed" hypertension. A family history of hypertension also has important adverse prognostic implications. In a parent or sibling, a history of early disability or death from a hypertensive complication such as stroke, heart failure, and heart attack makes it more likely that the patient with mild hypertension will progress to a more severe and complicated form of hypertension. Prognosis is less favorable when hypertension develops in the earlier decades of life. The prognosis in men, especially young men, is worse than in women, and it is worse in black patients than in white. Hypertension also develops earlier and in a higher percentage of blacks than whites. The risk of developing coronary artery disease is significantly higher in the hypertensive patient who has an elevated blood cholesterol or sugar than in the patient who does not. Cigarette smoking and obesity also increase the risk of ischemic heart disease. In addition, cardiomegaly or electrocardiographic signs of left ventricular hypertrophy are associated with an unusually high risk of cardiovascular complications. Nitrogen retention indicates a very grave prognosis. Changes in the optic fundi appear to be one of the more accurate guides to prognosis in essential hypertension, with or without complications. When complications are absent, the survival rates appear to be closely related to the level of the diastolic blood pressure and the appearance of the optic fundi. Also, with any given complication of hypertension, the prognosis becomes increasingly grave as the grade of retinopathy increases in severity (see III.B.1. in the outline at the beginning of this chapter).

Principles of Therapy

Before antihypertensive treatment is instituted, it is of paramount importance that the patient be carefully evaluated, since the choice and urgency of treatment depend on the pathogenesis, severity, and complications of the hypertension. The initiation of therapy without adequate diagnostic workup may obscure the cause of the hypertension or aggravate other associated diseases. However, when the hypertension is in the malignant or accelerated phase, antihypertensive treatment is instituted promptly and not delayed until the patient has had a full workup, since severe renal insufficiency (malignant nephrosclerosis) may complicate this condition within a period of days.

The major goals of treatment of hypertension are to relieve symptoms and to prevent, to arrest, or if possible, to reverse the cardiovascular complications of the disease. Therefore management is directed not only at the elevated blood pressure but also at other risk factors that may have an adverse effect on the cardiovascular system such as obesity, smoking, hyperlipidemia, and diabetes. These factors appear to interact with hypertension to multiply the risk of cardiovascular complications.

One of the most important factors in the successful management of hypertension is good rapport between a cooperative patient and a sympathetic, reassuring doctor. Reassuring the patient frequently leads to a lessening of his anxiety, headache, and other functional symptoms. Sedatives and tranquilizers may help to relax the patient and to relieve his headache. In the obese patient, a diet low in calories plus appropriate exercise may not only induce weight loss and reduce serum lipids but also lower blood pressure. Restriction of saturated fat and cholesterol in the diet also is useful in lowering serum cholesterol and low-density lipoproteins. A diet restricted in sodium chloride may exert an antihypertensive effect and potentiate the effects of antihypertensive drugs. However, many patients will not adhere to this diet, which should contain less than 2 gm of sodium chloride per day to be effective. Reduction of salt intake in adults and children alike, especially in those with a family history of hypertension, could prove to be of great value in the prevention of the disease. Although the general measures of reassurance, sedation, weight reduction, salt restriction, and elimination of smoking are often effective in patients with mild elevation in blood pressure, many of these patients require additional antihypertensive therapy.

Antihypertensive Drugs. A number of different types of drugs are available for the treatment of hypertension. They may be classified into the three broad groups listed below.

1. Diuretics — for example, the thiazides, spironolactone, and furosemide

2. Sympathetic nervous system antagonists
   a. Adrenergic blocking agents such as reserpine, alpha-methyldopa, and guanethidine
   b. Propranolol, a beta-adrenergic blocking agent
   c. Clonidine, a central alpha-adrenergic receptor stimulator
3. Vasodilators, including hydralazine, minoxidil, diazoxide, and nitroprusside

When used in combination, the different types of antihypertensive drugs have been shown to have additive or potentiating effects in lowering the blood pressure. These effects are likely due to the different modes and sites of action of the drugs on the mechanisms that control the blood pressure.

In all patients without clinically significant cardiovascular disease, treatment should be directed toward reducing the blood pressure to normal. In patients with advanced vascular disease, moderate and gradual lowering of the blood pressure is indicated, at least initially, because sudden and excessive reduction of blood pressure may aggravate instead of relieve symptoms of vascular insufficiency. An initial reduction of blood pressure to about 160/100 mm Hg appears to be tolerated by most patients with vascular complications. In some patients, maintenance of relative hypertension may be necessary to sustain adequate blood flow through the diseased arteries.

The response to a particular drug or to a given dosage of that drug may vary considerably from patient to patient. Therefore in benign hypertension therapy is instituted in small doses and increased gradually toward an optimal range in order to minimize the development of side effects. Little is to be gained by using maximally effective doses in a patient who as a result may have disturbing or intolerable side effects. Combinations of drugs are usually more effective and sometimes are less likely to produce symptoms than one drug pushed to its maximal effectiveness.

In addition to drug dosage, other factors may augment the hypotensive action of drugs. Such hypotensive factors include rest, sleep, upright position, exercise, fever, hot weather, eating, alcohol ingestion, salt-restricted diet and salt depletion, dehydration, blood loss or anemia, sedatives, vasodilators, and anesthesia. These factors themselves often operate to lower blood pressure, but their hypotensive effects may not be obvious because they are counteracted by other mechanisms that control the blood pressure, especially the sympathetic nervous system. However, after these other mechanisms are blocked or depressed pharmacologically, these hypotensive factors may produce strong hypotensive effects (and increase the antihypertensive action of the blocking drugs used). When these factors are present or are to be anticipated, it may be wise to reduce or omit drug dosages in order to avoid excessive falls in blood pressure. Drug and dose requirements in individual patients on continued treatment may also increase or decrease without apparent cause. Therefore it is necessary to maintain frequent, continued supervision and to adjust dosages as necessary. When drugs are withdrawn or dosages are reduced, it is important to observe the patient closely, since excessive rises in blood pressure may occur and lead to a complicating vascular accident, particularly in the brain.

It should be recognized that the blood pressure generally is lower and more responsive to hypotensive drugs in the morning after awakening than later on in the day, in the home than in the clinic or office, and during bed rest in the hospital than when ambulatory. In individuals who sleep during the day and work at night, the diurnal variations of the blood pressure are reversed. Such variations probably are related to a number of physiologic and psychological factors and likely account for the greater frequency of postural dizziness and hypotension soon after awakening in the morning than later on in the day, particularly if the patient is on therapy with sympathetic blocking agents or has had a splanchnicectomy.

All the antihypertensive drugs are capable of producing serious side effects that may appear either abruptly or insidiously days or years after the initiation of treatment. The major side effects of the various drugs are listed in Tables 25-1 and 25-2. It is extremely important that patients treated with these drugs be followed carefully and at frequent intervals with history, physical examination, and laboratory tests for early detection of untoward reactions. In general, drugs should be withdrawn when any potentially serious side effect occurs or when the etiologic

relationship between symptoms and drug administration is not clear. Drug dosages should be reduced or antidotes employed to manage mild side effects.

Antihypertensive Treatment. The drugs most commonly used in the treatment of mild hypertension are the diuretics, *Rauwolfia* derivatives, and propranolol. *Rauwolfia* derivatives and propranolol are generally preferred to the thiazides and related diuretics in the treatment of young individuals with uncomplicated mild hypertension, because the diuretics, when given over a prolonged period, may lead to an impaired glucose tolerance. Propranolol is particularly useful in younger patients with labile or borderline hypertension who have signs of a hyperkinetic circulation such as an increased cardiac output, pulse rate, and systolic blood pressure. A *Rauwolfia* compound or alpha-methyldopa is generally used as the initial agent in patients who are anxious or have symptoms or signs suggesting overactivity of the sympathetic nervous system, such as increased sweating, nervousness, or tachycardia. The vast majority of patients with moderate hypertension will respond to a diuretic in combination with propranolol, alpha-methyldopa, or a *Rauwolfia* derivative. Stronger drug regimens may be required for the control of severe or malignant hypertension. These regimens generally include a diuretic and a vasodilator (hydralazine) in combination with propranolol or alpha-methyldopa. Guanethidine also may be needed to control the hypertension. Refractory cases of accelerated or malignant hypertension often require intravenous therapy with powerful vasodilator drugs such as diazoxide or nitroprusside. In addition, furosemide is generally given to augment the hypotensive action of the vasodilators and to prevent the salt and water retention caused by these drugs. Following prolonged control of the blood pressure with drug therapy, the severe arteriolar damage caused by the elevated blood pressure appears to regress; and as a result of this regression, the hypertension becomes easier to manage.

Results of Antihypertensive Treatment. Effective antihypertensive treatment has caused a significant increase in the life span of patients with malignant hypertension. Survival is closely related to the con-

Table 25-1. Oral Drugs Commonly Employed in the Treatment of Hypertension

Drug	Type of drug	Average total daily dose	Antihypertensive action	Major side effects
Chlorothiazide (and related diuretics)	Diuretic	250–500 mg, in 1–3 doses	Moderate	Hypokalemia, digitalis intoxication, gout, hyperglycemia
Spironolactone	Diuretic, aldosterone antagonist	25 mg, in 2–4 doses	Moderate	Hyperkalemia, acidosis, gynecomastia, menstrual irregularity
Triamterene	Diuretic	50–100 mg, in 2–3 doses	Mild	Nausea, diarrhea, vomiting, weakness, headache
Propranolol	Beta-adrenergic blocking agent	20–80 mg, in 2–4 doses	Moderate	Heart failure, bronchial asthma, Raynaud's disease
Reserpine (and other *Rauwolfia* derivatives)	Adrenergic neuron blocker	0.1–0.25 mg, in 1–2 doses	Mild	Sedation, mental depression, loss of libido, parkinsonianlike syndrome
Methyldopa	Adrenergic neuron blocker	250–500 mg, in 2–4 doses	Moderate	Sedation, drowsiness, fever, hemolytic anemia, liver disorder
Guanethidine	Adrenergic neuron blocker	25–50 mg, in 2–4 doses	Strong	Postural dizziness and faintness, diarrhea, impaired ejaculation
Hydralazine	Vasodilator	25–50 mg, in 2–4 doses	Moderate	Lupus-like syndrome, headache, palpitation, aggravation of angina pectoris
Clonidine	Alpha-adrenergic receptor stimulator	0.1–0.2 mg, in 1–3 doses	Moderate	Sedation, drowsiness, dry mouth, marked rise of blood pressure following drug withdrawal
Phenoxybenzamine	Alpha-adrenergic blocking agent	10–20 mg, in 3–4 doses	Moderate	Tachycardia, postural hypotension, impotence, nasal congestion

Table 25-2. Parenteral Drugs Employed in the Treatment of Hypertensive Emergencies

Drug	Type of drug	Indications	Usual dosage	Route of administration	Onset of action	Maximum action	Duration of action	Major side effects
Nitroprusside	Vasodilator	Hypertensive crises, encephalopathy, cerebral hemorrhage, acute pulmonary edema	0.05–0.20 mg/min	IV infusion	½–1 min	1–2 min	3–5 min	Hypotension, thiocyanate toxicity, restlessness, nausea, muscular twitching, cramps
Diazoxide	Vasodilator	Hypertensive crises, encephalopathy	300 mg	IV injection	1–2 min	5–15 min	3–12 hr	Hypotension, angina, fluid retention, hyperglycemia, hyperuricemia
Trimethaphan	Ganglionic blocker	Hypertension complicated by dissecting aneurysm or acute pulmonary edema	1–10 mg/min	IV infusion	1–2 min	2–5 min	10 min	Hypotension, adynamic ileus, urinary retention
Reserpine	Adrenergic neuron blocker	Hypertensive crises, encephalopathy	1–2.5 mg	IM injection	1½–3 hr	…	6–12 hr	Drowsiness, somnolence, parkinsonian-like syndrome
Methyldopa	Adrenergic neuron blocker	Hypertensive crises, encephalopathy	250–500 mg	IM injection	2–3 hr	3–5 hr	6–12 hr	Drowsiness, parkinsonianlike syndrome
Furosemide	Diuretic	Acute pulmonary edema, also used to prevent salt and water retention of other drugs and to augment their antihypertensive effects	40–120 mg	IM injection	5–10 min (diuretic effect)	60 min	2–4 hr	Electrolyte imbalance, hypokalemia, transient nerve deafness
Hydralazine	Vasodilator	Sometimes used as additive drug in treatment of acute hypertensive crises	10–40 mg	IV injection	5–20 min	20–60 min	3–6 min	Angina pectoris, headache, palpitation, flushing
Phentolamine	Alpha-adrenergic blocking agent	Hypertensive crises caused by pheochromocytoma, monoamine oxidase inhibitors, or clonidine withdrawal	2.5–10 mg	IV injection	1 min	1–2 min	5–60 min	Hypotension, palpitation

trol of blood pressure with therapy as well as to the extent of renal impairment before the institution of therapy. Effective lowering of the blood pressure increases life expectancy in part by preventing rapid deterioration of renal function. In less severe forms of hypertension, a Veterans Administration study has presented convincing evidence that antihypertensive drug treatment is capable of preventing serious cardio-vascular complications (see Bibliography). Life table analysis of the results in patients with an initial dia-stolic blood pressure of 90 through 114 mm Hg indi-cated that the risk of a fatal or nonfatal complication over a 5-year period was reduced from 55 to 18 per-cent by combination drug treatment with hydrochlo-rothiazide, reserpine, and hydralazine. Congestive heart failure, stroke, and progressive renal damage were sharply reduced or eliminated in the treated patients. However, the incidence of myocardial in-farction and sudden death was essentially the same in the control and the treated groups. These and other studies indicate that coronary heart disease remains a major problem in the hypertensive patient.

The failure of the Veterans Administration study to demonstrate a significant benefit from effective antihypertensive treatment on complicating ischemic heart disease does not necessarily contradict the clin-ical and experimental evidence that elevated blood pressure accelerates and aggravates atherosclerosis. It is possible that if treatment had been started at an earlier age, before the development of advanced coro-nary atherosclerosis, the results might have indicated a protective effect of antihypertensive treatment against ischemic heart disease. Recent population studies suggest that antihypertensive treatment may be beneficial in hypertensive individuals with clinical manifestations of ischemic heart disease. In these studies the patients with ischemic heart disease and borderline or established hypertension had a higher mortality rate than normotensive patients with similar heart disease. Antihypertensive treatment appeared to improve survivorship and was associated with a decrease in the incidence of congestive heart failure, myocardial infarction, and cardiac (including sudden) death. Since there is no evidence that antihyperten-sive treatment alone can cause atherosclerosis to regress, the reported beneficial effects were likely due,

at least in part, to an improvement in cardiac perfor-mance as well as in supply-demand ratio of the coro-nary circulation as a consequence of reducing the mechanical load of hypertension on the heart.

RENAL HYPERTENSION
Of the recognizable causes of secondary hypertension, renal disease is the most common, accounting for probably 5 to 10 percent of all cases of hypertension; parenchymal disease of the kidney appears clinically to be a commoner cause than renovascular disease (see Chap. 53). Renal hypertension is often preceded by a history of renal disease or by abnormal urinary findings. It occurs more frequently in the advanced stages of kidney disease, but it may occur early, when no signs of renal insufficiency are present. In the latter instance hypertension is often associated with complicating renovascular disease or some alteration in renal hemodynamic function. Severe accelerated or malignant hypertension occurs with greater fre-quency in renal hypertension than in essential hyper-tension. The onset of hypertension before age 25 or the early onset of albuminuria, especially with impair-ment of renal function, should make one suspect underlying kidney disease as a possible cause. A fam-ily history of hypertension is of limited value in the differential diagnosis, since it is frequently positive in patients with renal hypertension. When the diag-nosis of renal hypertension is made, it is important to determine whether it is due to unilateral or to bilat-eral kidney disease, since treatment and prognosis depend on this finding. An elevated blood urea nitro-gen in the absence of either dehydration or heart failure often indicates the presence of bilateral kidney disease with a loss of at least two-thirds of the func-tioning renal mass.

Pathogenesis
The exact manner in which the kidney gives rise to hypertension has not been fully established. How-ever, there is growing evidence that the renin-angio-tensin system plays a major role in the pathogenesis of a number of forms of renal hypertension. In these forms of hypertension the activity of the renin-angio-tensin system is generally increased and the hyperten-sion responds readily to treatment with angiotensin

antagonists. Renin is made in the juxtaglomerular cells of the renal arterioles, and it acts as a proteolytic enzyme on a serum polypeptide substrate (renin substrate) to form the decapeptide angiotensin I, which in turn is hydrolyzed to the octapeptide angiotensin II by a converting enzyme (peptidase) located primarily in the pulmonary circulation. Angiotensin II can in turn be converted to angiotensin III, a heptapeptide that appears to be more potent than angiotensin II in stimulating aldosterone secretion. A number of factors operate to stimulate renin secretion and hence increase the formation of angiotensin. These stimulants include a reduction in systemic arterial pressure; a decrease in blood and extracellular fluid volume; sodium depletion; and reduction in intravascular pressure (or tension) within the afferent juxtaglomerular arterioles. Changes in the sodium load or concentration within the renal tubules (macula densa) also may influence renin secretion. Increases in sympathetic neural activity and catecholamines appear to enhance renin secretion through the renal beta-adrenergic receptors. Beta-adrenergic blockage results in a decrease in plasma renin activity, and angiotensin itself exerts a negative feedback control over renin release.

Angiotensin II is the most powerful pressor agent yet discovered. Its pressor effect is due largely to direct vasoconstriction of the arterioles. The hormone also has stimulant effects on the peripheral and central sympathetic nervous systems that could contribute to its pressor activity. These sympathetic effects of angiotensin similarly may play a role in the high cardiac output and peripheral vascular resistance reported in renovascular hypertension. In addition to its potent vasoconstrictor and hypertensive effects, the other major actions of angiotensin II include both the direct stimulation of the adrenal cortex to secrete aldosterone and the reduction of renal blood flow, glomerular filtration rate, and electrolyte and water excretion. Competitive antagonists of angiotensin II, such as 1-sarcosine-8-alanine-angiotensin II (Saralasin), have been shown to reduce blood pressure in many conditions in which plasma renin activity is elevated, that is, hypertension due to high renin levels and states associated with sodium depletion, low cardiac output, and shock. Studies using angiotensin antag-

onists in experimental hypertension suggest that some forms of renal hypertension are initiated by the renin-angiotensin system but then are sustained by other mechanisms. In these forms of hypertension plasma renin activity is elevated in the early stages of the disease but is normal in the later stages.

In addition to having a vasopressor or hypertensive function, the kidney may have a vasodepressor or antihypertensive function. Some of the renal substances currently being investigated as responsible for antihypertensive functions include (1) prostaglandins, especially PGA_2 and PGE_2; (2) kallikreins; (3) renin inhibitors such as phosphatidylserine; and (4) antihypertensive neutral lipid from the adrenal medulla. In animals the removal of both kidneys may result in hypertension, especially in the presence of an expanded extracellular fluid volume; it has not been demonstrated that true renoprival hypertension can be produced in man. Recent reports indicate that patients with end-stage kidney disease and normal blood pressure do not develop hypertension following bilateral nephrectomy. Furthermore, the failure of transplanted kidneys to normalize the blood pressure in hypertensive patients with end-stage diseased kidneys suggests that lack of an antihypertensive function of the kidney does not play a major role in the pathophysiology of their hypertension.

The hypertension of chronic renal failure is frequently associated with expanded extracellular fluid volume and increased body sodium. Plasma renin, which might be expected to be reduced, is usually normal or only slightly elevated in these patients. This form of hypertension appears to be *sodium dependent,* since it can be controlled by reducing extracellular fluid volume by dialysis. In other patients the hypertension is associated with high levels of renin and is not lowered by dialysis treatment; this hypertension appears to be *renin dependent,* since the blood pressure decreases following bilateral nephrectomy while plasma renin falls. It has been postulated that both the sodium-dependent and the renin-dependent hypertension in chronic renal failure are due to inappropriately high circulating levels of renin and angiotensin in proportion to extracellular fluid volume and body sodium.

The cardiac output and peripheral vascular resistance are often increased in hypertensive patients with chronic renal failure. Following dialysis or nephrectomy, the fall in blood pressure is associated with a decrease in peripheral resistance.

In the anephric state there appears to be a striking difference in the blood pressure response to salt and water loading between previously normotensive and previously hypertensive patients. Previously hypertensive patients have been reported to respond to a high dietary sodium intake with a progressive increase in blood pressure and peripheral resistance, whereas previously normotensive patients fail to elevate their blood pressure and peripheral resistance significantly. The reasons for these different responses are not clear from the available human studies, but they might be related to changes in autonomic nervous system function, structural and functional changes in the blood vessels caused by previous long-standing hypertension, or to the genetic predisposition to hypertension. It has been demonstrated in inbred animals that genetic factors critically control the response of the blood pressure to high salt intake.

Renovascular Hypertension
The prevalence of renal arterial stenosis as a cause of hypertension is higher than previously recognized. However, renovascular hypertension probably accounts for less than 1 percent of all cases of hypertension. The commonest cause of renal arterial stenosis appears to be atherosclerosis, which accounts for about 75 percent of the cases. This lesion occurs more often in older individuals, particularly males. When arteriosclerotic plaques involve the main renal artery, they usually are located at or near the orifice of the renal artery, involving both renal arteries in about 30 percent of the cases. Selective renal arteriography indicates that lesions of the main renal artery are usually accompanied by lesions in the primary branches, which occur more frequently than lesions of the main arterial trunk alone. Stenosing fibromuscular hyperplasia of the renal artery is the next most common cause of renal arterial occlusive disease, occurring in about 15 percent of the cases. This lesion is most frequently encountered in relatively young women and characteristically involves the distal two-thirds of one or both renal arteries. Other

medium-sized vessels also may be affected. Fibromuscular disease of the renal artery can be of many types, but the most common form is associated with marked intimal or medial fibrosis, elastic tissue degeneration, and aneurysmal dilatation. Fibromuscular disease appears on the arteriogram as multiple discrete areas of narrowing with poststenotic dilatation beyond each constricting point. Other less common stenosing diseases of the renal artery include aneurysm, thrombosis, embolism, and coarctation (of the abdominal aorta in the region of the origin of the renal arteries). Renal artery hypoplasia also appears to be a cause of renal hypertension.

Clinical Features. The clinical manifestations of renovascular hypertension may be indistinguishable from those of essential hypertension, but the following findings favor a diagnosis of renal hypertension: (1) the onset of hypertension before 25 or after 50 years of age; (2) the absence of a family history of hypertension; (3) unexplained, severe hypertension, especially hypertension unresponsive to antihypertensive therapy; (4) sudden onset of severe or malignant hypertension; (5) preexistence or early appearance of diffuse vascular disease; (6) abnormal renal findings or early impairment of renal function; (7) systolic bruit heard in the epigastrium or on either side of the midline of the upper abdomen; (8) flank pain presumably due to renal infarction; (9) hypokalemia and other biochemical findings of secondary aldosteronism; and (10) postural hypotension. It is noteworthy that one-third of the patients with arterial occlusive disease have a family history of hypertension that may be mild or paroxysmal and may respond to drugs and bed rest.

Laboratory Findings. The characteristic urologic findings in hypertension due to renal arterial stenosis include an abnormal excretory pyelogram — that is, a disparity in the size of the two kidneys of at least 1 cm, and a difference in the concentration of the injected contrast materials. The involved kidney early in the disease shows an increase in concentration of the radiopaque dye, whereas later on this concentration decreases as ischemic atrophy of the kidney progresses. A delayed appearance of the injected dye in the renal pelvis, especially within the first 3 minutes after the dye injection, is another early sign of renal ischemia. Retrograde pyelography frequently shows the involved kidney to have a small pelvis but normal calyces. Intravenous pyelography is the most useful screening procedure for renovascular hypertension, and it indicates an abnormality in approximately 85 percent of patients with this disease. The radioisotope renogram (usually performed with intravenous ^{131}I-labeled iodohippurate sodium [Hippuran]) may also have some value as a screening test for renal hypertension. The test is based on the external detection of the injected radioactive iodohippurate in the kidney, as the iodohippurate is transported from blood to urine through the renal parenchyma. In renal arterial occlusive disease the radioactive iodohippurate is retained for a longer time in the involved than in the uninvolved kidney. The difference in the excretion of the Hippuran is likely related to the increased water reabsorption in the affected kidney. A scintiscan or echogram of the kidneys may be useful in the differentiation and localization of certain types of unilateral renal disease such as tumor, cyst, infarct, and ischemia.

Renal arteriography is the most accurate way of demonstrating occlusive disease of the renal arteries. However, demonstration of a renal arterial lesion does not establish that the lesion is the cause of the hypertension, since such stenosis may be a result and not the cause of the hypertension. Also, it is well known that occlusive disease of the renal arteries can occur in normotensive persons without causing hypertension.

The measurement of renin activity in the renal venous blood is the most specific and sensitive method for determining the functional significance of renal artery stenosis. It has been shown that a significant correlation exists between curability of renovascular hypertension and the demonstration of increased renin activity in the venous blood of the involved kidney. When renin activity in the renal venous blood from an ischemic kidney is elevated and more than 50 percent greater than the renin values from the normal contralateral kidney, surgery will cure or greatly improve the hypertension in approximately 80 percent of the cases. Factors that stimulate renin release such as low sodium diet, diuretics, and hydralazine may enhance the diagnostic sensitivity of the renin assays, since they widen the resting differences in renin activity between the involved and uninvolved kidney. Drugs that inhibit renin secretion such as propranolol, methyldopa, and guanethidine may narrow differences in renin in the two renal veins and reduce the sensitivity of the test.

The differential split renal function studies introduced by Howard and Stamey have been used widely in the diagnosis of renovascular hypertension. However, the tests do not appear to be as sensitive or as specific as the renin assay test, particularly in patients with lesions in the arterial branches. In addition, infections of the genitourinary system and, occasionally, attacks of pulmonary edema or hypertensive crisis have been precipitated by these tests. The distinguishing features of an ischemic kidney as shown by split renal function studies are a decreased urinary volume and sodium concentration on the affected side in association with an increased concentration of nonreabsorbable, nonelectrolyte solute such as para-aminophipuric acid (PAH), inulin, or creatinine when these values are compared to the contralateral normal kidney. These changes in renal function are usually associated with a reduction in the glomerular filtration rate. When an ischemic lesion involves both renal arteries or branches of both renal arteries, such split renal function studies may not reveal the ischemic lesion and so may be falsely negative. Split renal function studies do provide valuable information concerning differential renal function and renal blood flow, and they may be performed in certain patients with impaired renal function, equivocal renin assays, or demonstrated bilateral arterial stenosis.

Other Diagnostic Procedures. There are strong correlations between the renal venous renin activity, the pressure gradient measured across the stenosis, and the juxtaglomerular cell counts on the involved side. As a rule, patients with a gradient of less than 35 mm Hg do not benefit from surgery. These measurements are not performed routinely, since they do not add significantly to the diagnosis and treatment of renovascular hypertension.

The use of the angiotensin antagonist 1-sarcosine-8-alanine-angiotensin II appears to have considerable value in the diagnosis of renin-dependent hypertension. This agent could prove useful in the diagnosis of surgically curable renovascular hypertension.

Treatment of Renovascular Hypertension. In general, the treatment of hypertension due to renal arteriostenosis is surgical, with the stenotic portion of the renal artery being either resected or bypassed with a graft. Surgery is generally advisable in patients with severe hypertension who have marked renal arteriostenosis and hypersecretion of renin from the ischemic kidney. Surgical therapy also is usually indicated in young patients with functionally significant unilateral arterial stenosis. The hypertension will be cured or improved after surgical repair in approximately 80 to 90 percent of such patients. These patients may also be managed medically with antihypertensive drugs, but this requires life-long treatment with drugs that may produce disturbing side effects. In older patients with apparent atherosclerotic lesions of the renal artery, a conservative approach using medical therapy is recommended. Many such patients have complicating coronary, cerebral, or peripheral atherosclerotic vascular disease and represent a significant surgical risk. In addition, the possibility of cure or improvement of their hypertension is only 60 to 70 percent. The long-term results of medical as compared with surgical therapy in patients with atherosclerosis of the renal artery appears to be related primarily to the degree of success of controlling the hypertension. Beta-adrenergic blockade with propranolol reduces renin activity and may be particularly useful in the medical management of renovascular hypertension.

Other Causes of Renal Hypertension
Some of the less common causes of renal hypertension are listed in the outline at the beginning of this chapter. Myeloma of the kidney, with or without advanced renal insufficiency, is not included, since hypertension rarely occurs in this condition. Tuberculosis, hypernephroma, Wilms' tumor, perinephritis, and renal trauma are other causes of unilateral kidney disease that may give rise to hypertension which is surgically curable.

Renal juxtaglomerular cell tumors that produce large amounts of renin have recently been described.

The tumors tend to be small and difficult to visualize radiographically. However, they can produce very severe hypertension, hyperreninemia, and other findings of secondary aldosteronism. Wilms' tumors may also produce renin on rare occasions and therefore may induce a similar syndrome. The diagnosis of primary reninism should be suspected when renal arteriostenosis is not demonstrable by renal arteriography and one kidney secretes a good deal more renin than the opposite one. The hypertension is curable after the renin-secreting tumor has been removed.

OTHER CONDITIONS CAUSING HYPERTENSION

Diabetic Hypertension
The incidence of hypertension in patients with diabetes mellitus is greater than in the nondiabetic population and increases with both the age of the patient and the duration of the diabetes. In many reports, elevated blood pressures have been recorded in from 40 to 80 percent of the diabetic populations studied. The hypertension associated with diabetes may be of three types: (1) essential hypertension, usually occurring with maturity-onset diabetes; (2) systolic hypertension secondary to arteriosclerosis (arteriosclerotic hypertension); and (3) diabetic hypertension, which appears to be a form of renal hypertension accompanying the clinical syndrome of diabetic nephropathy most commonly observed in juvenile-onset diabetes. The renin-angiotensin system is suppressed in patients with long-standing diabetes and evidence of diabetic complications such as renal disease and retinopathy. The low plasma renin activity may explain the rarity of malignant hypertension in this condition. Some studies suggest that either a decrease in the activity of the sympathetic nervous system and in the levels of circulating catecholamines or destruction of the juxtaglomerular cells by the diabetic glomerulosclerosis is responsible for the suppression of the renin-angiotensin system in diabetic hypertension. Microvascular and macrovascular diseases are major complications of both hypertension and diabetes and are likely responsible for the unusually high incidence of coronary heart disease and stroke in patients who have both diseases.

Cushing's syndrome, primary aldosteronism, and

pheochromocytoma can be associated with a mild to moderate impairment of glucose tolerance, or so-called secondary diabetes, which is frequently revers-ible with correction of the metabolic defect of the primary disease. Thiazide diuretics are another important cause of hyperglycemia. These agents may precipitate or aggravate diabetes, especially in patients with a family history of hypertension and diabetes. Long-term treatment with thiazide diuretics also may lead to impairment in glucose tolerance, even in patients with an initially normal glucose metabolism. The relationship of these effects to the risk of devel-oping cardiovascular disease is not known.

Coarctation of the Aorta

Coarctation of the aorta is a congenital vascular abnor-mality in which the aorta is greatly narrowed or com-pletely occluded (Fig. 25-3; see Chap. 29). Coarcta-tion of the aorta causes a type of hypertension that can be reduced by surgical repair of the stricture. The hypertension appears due to increased resistance to flow through the narrowed aorta and collateral vessels. In cases in which the hypertension is severe, renal ischemia may also be a contributory factor (see earlier in this chapter under Renovascular Hypertension). The hypertension in the upper extremities is mainly systolic. It is rarely severe or of the accelerated type unless it is complicated by renovascular disease. In coarctation of the aorta the systolic blood pressure is lower in the legs than in the arms. In addition, the femoral pulse is weaker and arrives later than the radial. In some patients in whom the coarctation is proximal to the left subclavian artery, the blood pressure in the left arm is less than that in the right.

Surgical treatment of coarctation includes the removal of the obstruction and reconstruction of the aortic pathway, usually by anastomosis. Whenever possible, an excision of the coarctation and union of the remaining aortic ends is the operation of choice. In the vast majority of patients the hypertension will respond to surgical correction of the coarctation, although many months may be required after surgery for the blood pressure to return to satisfactory levels.

Neurogenic Hypertension

Disease or functional disturbances of the central and

autonomic nervous systems may either cause or aggra-vate preexisting hypertension. Neurogenic hyperten-sion is especially prone to result from lesions involving the vasomotor centers in the medulla, pons, or dien-cephalon or from those producing an increase in cerebrospinal fluid pressure. The prompt, striking response of neurogenic hypertension to sympatho-lytic drugs as well as the finding of elevated urinary and blood catecholamines in some cases suggests that neurogenic hypertension may be mediated through the sympathetic adrenal system.

Neurogenic hypertension may be either paroxys-mal or sustained. The paroxysmal form is usually accompanied by other signs suggestive of sympathetic overactivity such as tachycardia, sweating, and flush-ing and also by signs suggestive of pheochromocytoma. It also may be accompanied by paroxysmal abdominal pain. Some of the neurologic conditions that cause this type of hypertension are tabes dorsalis, transverse myelopathy, diencephalic syndrome, postinfectious encephalitis, and acute porphyria. Neurogenic hyper-tension may be complicated by malignant hyperten-sion or by hypertensive encephalopathy.

Encephalopathy caused by preexisting disease in the brain itself, especially a brain tumor, may be con-fused with encephalopathy caused by hypertension. The findings that favor a primary hypertensive rather than a primary cerebral cause for the encephalopathy are diastolic blood pressure over 120 mm Hg; a clear, normal cerebrospinal fluid having a pressure less than 400 mm H_2O; and striking improvement of the encephalopathy following effective antihypertensive drug treatment. Additional studies that may be neces-sary in differentiating the cause of the encephalopathy are x-ray studies of the skull, scintiscan of the brain, electroencephalography, cerebral angiography, and ventriculography. Whenever possible, the cause of neurogenic hypertension should be removed. In non-curable forms of neurogenic hypertension, the alpha-adrenergic blocking agent phenoxybenzamine may prove useful in addition to the other antihypertensive drugs.

Oral Contraceptive Hypertension

It is estimated that about 7 to 15 percent of women taking oral contraceptives have a rise in blood pres-

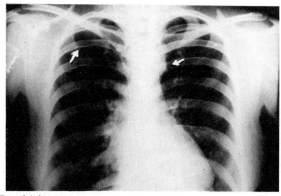

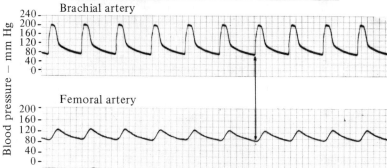

Figure 25-3. Typical findings of coarctation of the aorta. In addition to an enlarged left ventricle, the chest film shows a small aortic knob and notching of the inferior margins of the upper ribs (arrow at left). The arterial pressure tracings reveal that the systolic pressure is considerably higher in the upper than in the lower extremities. They also show an arrival of the brachial pulse before the femoral pulse. The patient was 45 years old.

sure that is usually mild and can be reversed by withdrawing the drugs. Many patients who develop hypertension have a positive family history of the disease, suggesting that a genetic predisposition to hypertension may influence this response to the drugs. The mechanism for the hypertension has not been clearly established, but it may involve abnormalities in the renin-angiotensin-aldosterone system. Increases in plasma renin activity and aldosterone secretion have been noted in about one-half of the patients and an increase in renin substrate in almost all.

Systolic Hypertension

Elevation of systolic blood pressure independent of diastolic blood pressure is associated with increased morbidity and mortality from cardiovascular disease. There also is some evidence that increased systolic arterial pressure may have even a stronger association with ischemic heart disease, congestive heart failure, and stroke than increased diastolic pressure.

There are two common forms of systolic hypertension. One form, designated as hyperkinetic systolic hypertension, occurs in young adults before the age of 35 and is a frequent manifestation of labile or borderline hypertension. Patients with this form of hypertension have a hyperkinetic circulation as manifested by elevations in the heart rate, cardiac output, and left ventricular ejection rate. An overactive sympathetic nervous system probably plays a role in this disorder, since the hypertension generally responds to treatment with beta-adrenergic blocking agents. The second common form of systolic hypertension, referred to as arteriosclerotic hypertension, occurs in the elderly and is mainly due to arteriosclerotic changes in the aorta. Hemodynamic studies suggest that many of these individuals have a reduced cardiac output and an increased peripheral vascular resistance.

ARTERIOSCLEROTIC HYPERTENSION

Arteriosclerotic hypertension is commonly observed in persons past the fifth decade. It appears to be one of the chief manifestations of aging and results from arteriosclerotic involvement of the aorta and major arteries. The systolic blood pressure is usually over 175 mm Hg, whereas the diastolic blood pressure may be normal or only slightly elevated (less than 110 mm Hg). Many of the patients with elevation of diastolic pressure give a history of antecedent essential hypertension.

Pathogenesis

With aging there is an increase in blood pressure that is associated with a progressive loss of the elasticity of the aorta and other peripheral arteries. The increased rigidity of the aorta does not appear to be due to a decrease in the medial elastin content but to changes in the physiochemical nature of the elastic tissue of the aorta. It has been shown that uncoiling and fracture of the helical elastic lamellae of the aortic wall occur as collagen increases between the elastic fibers. In addition, increased amounts of calcium ions are laid down in the medial elastic tissue. The changes in the media are usually accompanied by atherosclerotic involvement of the intima, which accounts for much of the morbidity and mortality in arteriosclerotic hypertension. The increased rigidity of the aorta seems to be responsible for the elevated systolic and pulse pressures observed in this form of hypertension, while sclerosis of the arterioles caused by aging and hypertension may explain the increased peripheral vascular resistance.

Clinical Features

One of the most frequent symptoms of patients with systolic arteriosclerotic hypertension is persistent dizziness or light-headedness that often responds to mild lowering of the blood pressure. Many of the patients also experience postural dizziness, which may be due to an inability of the cerebral circulation to adjust rapidly to changes in posture or to orthostatic falls in blood pressure. A high (as well as a sudden relatively low) blood pressure may lead to a stroke in such patients or to other manifestations of circulatory insufficiency. The marked fluctuations of blood pressure in arteriosclerosis may be due to hypoactive pressor and depressor reflexes caused by an impairment in autonomic and baroreceptor functions. The diabetes commonly seen in arteriosclerotic hypertension may play a role in both the autonomic and the vascular disorders.

The serious complications of arteriosclerotic hypertension are often due to occlusive disease of the cerebral, coronary, and peripheral arteries. Aneurysm formation and rupture of diseased arteries, particularly in the brain or abdomen, also contribute to morbidity and mortality. When the blood pressure suddenly increases in severity, atherosclerotic occlusion of the renal artery should be suspected as a complication.

Although many of the sequelae of systolic hypertension in the elderly are due primarily to atherosclerotic disease, many of the complications appear to be precipitated and aggravated by the systolic hypertension itself. These complications include cerebral hemorrhage and stroke due to rupture of a Charcot-Bouchard aneurysm and congestive heart failure associated with an increase in the left ventricular systolic blood pressure and a resulting increase in myocardial wall tension.

A systolic murmur, due either to a tortuous ascending aorta or to calcification of the aortic valve, is often heard over the base of the heart, which may be normal in size. The electrocardiogram also may be normal, but it frequently shows nonspecific T-wave changes and signs of left ventricular hypertrophy or of an old myocardial infarction. Roentgenographically, arteriosclerosis of the aorta is recognized by the tortuosity and calcification of the vessel.

Treatment

Although the increased morbidity and mortality rates associated with systolic hypertension have been well substantiated, no long-term controlled study has been carried out to assess the efficacy of therapy of arteriosclerotic hypertension. However, gradual, cautious moderation of the blood pressure with mild antihypertensive drugs in small dosages may be attempted, particularly when diastolic pressure is elevated, since such treatment may relieve symptoms and protect against heart failure, cerebral hemorrhage, and stroke. Excessive reduction of blood pressure should be avoided, because it can precipitate a cerebrovascular accident and other forms of circulatory insufficiency. A systolic blood pressure reduced slowly to a level of 170 mm Hg is usually well tolerated. If symptoms or signs of inadequate circulation appear, antihypertensive drug treatment should be reduced or withdrawn. Strong antihypertensive drugs such as guanethidine are contraindicated.

Bibliography

Blood Pressure: Insurance Experience and Its Implications. New York: Metropolitan Life Insurance Co., 1961.

Dustan, H. P., Tarazi, R. C., Bravo, E. L., and Dart, R. A. Plasma and extracellular fluid volume in hypertension. *Circ. Res.* 32:I, 1973.

Genest, J., and Koiw, E. *Hypertension '72.* Berlin: Springer, 1972.

Hollander, W. Hypertension, antihypertensive drugs and atherosclerosis. *Circulation* 48:1112, 1973.

Kannel, W. B., and Sorlie, P. Hypertension in Framingham. In O. Paul (ed.), *Epidemiology and Control of Hypertension.* New York: Stratton Intercontinental Medical Book Corp., 1975.

Laragh, J. H. *Hypertension Manual.* New York: Yorke Medical Books, 1974.

Page, I. H., and McCubbin, J. W. *Renal Hypertension.* Chicago: Year Book, 1968.

Veterans Administration Cooperative Study Group on Anti-hypertensive Agents. Results in patients with diastolic blood pressure averaging 90 through 114 mm Hg. *J.A.M.A.* 213:1143, 1970.

26

Atherosclerosis and Hyperlipoproteinemia

Aram V. Chobanian

Atherosclerosis and its clinical sequelae represent the major cause of death in western society. Most myocardial infarctions as well as cerebral thromboses, peripheral vascular diseases, and aortic aneurysms can be attributed to the complications of atherosclerosis. This disease appears to be a continuous process, beginning in infancy or childhood and increasing in severity with advancing age. It is widespread and eventually afflicts most adults.

The intimal lesions in atherosclerosis may vary from localized, superficial plaques to areas of extensive thickening and ulceration, with elastic tissue degeneration and marked accumulation of lipids, mucopolysaccharides, and collagen. The intimal thickening may produce narrowing or complete obstruction of the arterial lumen. Arterial occlusion may also occur from a thrombus forming at the site of an intimal ulceration or from a hematoma due to rupture of intimal vasa vasorum. Clinical manifestations result from interference with blood flow to tissues.

Etiologic Factors

It is now accepted that multiple factors are involved in the causes of atherosclerosis and its major complication, ischemic heart disease. The simplistic view that atherosclerosis is an inevitable process of aging no longer appears tenable. *Endothelial cell injury* and increased vascular permeability to plasma lipoproteins and other substances appear to be important factors in the development of atherosclerosis. Lesions can be induced by almost any experimental approach involving endothelial damage. The response to the injury depends in part on the level of serum lipoproteins. In general, lipid-rich lesions develop in the presence of hyperlipoproteinemia, whereas only fibrous plaques or intimal scars result when serum lipoproteins are normal.

Smooth muscle cell proliferation is a characteristic and very important feature of the developing atherosclerotic lesion. Vascular injury leads to the migration of smooth muscle cells from the media into the intima and to the proliferation of these cells. Low-density lipoproteins and a factor released from platelets may induce the proliferative response. The smooth muscle cell is the major cell type in the plaque and is the primary source of connective tissue components in the vessel wall. Benditt recently has suggested that the smooth muscle cells in a plaque may be derived from a single cell, and the plaque could be looked at as a smooth muscle cell tumor. This intriguing monoclonal cell hypothesis is currently under intense investigation.

Abnormal lipid metabolism almost certainly plays a role. The induction of hypercholesterolemia or of hyperlipoproteinemia has been a necessary component of almost all experimental atherosclerosis, and the most significant chemical abnormality in the atherosclerotic lesion is a marked intimal accumulation of cholesterol and other lipids. The source of most of the lipids in the lesion appears to be plasma lipoproteins. Epidemiologic studies indicate that the risk of developing a clinical episode of coronary heart disease is directly related to the plasma level of cholesterol. Significant coronary heart disease is rare in areas where the average plasma cholesterol ranges between 100 and 170 mg per 100 ml; whereas in the United States, where the mean plasma cholesterol in the adult population is approximately 245 mg, the incidence of atherosclerotic disease is high. Within our population, the average risk of significant ischemic heart disease is four to five times greater in subjects with plasma cholesterols over 250 mg than it is in those with cholesterol below that level. Elevations in plasma triglycerides, low-density lipoproteins (beta), and very low density lipoproteins (prebeta) also are associated with an increased incidence of vascular disease, although the relative risks may vary with the different types of hyperlipoproteinemia (see below). On the other hand, high-density lipoproteins may have an opposite protective role, and recent epidemiologic studies have pointed to an inverse relationship between the level of plasma high density lipoproteins and risk for coronary disease.

Arterial lipid metabolism also appears to contribute to the atherogenic process. The intimal smooth muscle cells may be stimulated to synthesize markedly increased amounts of cholesteryl esters, and this increased local synthesis, as well as an increased delivery of lipid from plasma, probably contributes to the lipid accumulation. Impaired mechanisms for the transport and removal of lipid may also be involved. The hydrolysis of cholesteryl esters carried on in lysosomes may not keep pace with the delivery of cholesteryl esters to the vessel wall. It is of interest that two congenital disorders involving a defect in the hydrolysis of cholesteryl esters, namely, cholesteryl ester storage disease and Wolman's disease, are both associated with an exaggerated tendency to develop atherosclerotic disease. In addition, lipids bind to arterial elastin and collagen, and such binding could contribute to the accumulation of lipids in the arterial wall. High-density lipoproteins may facilitate the removal of cholesterol from cells, and a deficiency of high-density lipoproteins could also lead to arterial lipid accumulation.

Arterial hypertension is a major accelerator of atherogenesis. The number and extent of atherosclerotic lesions, both fatty streaks and fibrous plaques, are increased in hypertensive patients, particularly if other abnormal risk factors are present. A progressive increase in risk of developing various cardiovascular complications has been observed as systolic blood pressure rises above 120 mm Hg and diastolic above 80 mm Hg (Fig. 26-1). If hypertension is combined with other positive risk factors such as hypercholesterolemia, glucose intolerance, or cigarette smoking, the adverse effects on vascular complications are multiplied (Fig. 26-2).

The mechanism by which hypertension influences atherogenesis is unclear, but endothelial cell injury, increased vascular permeability, smooth muscle cell proliferation, and increased deposition of connective tissue components all appear to be involved. With hypertension, the vessel wall first becomes thickened; then degenerative changes can occur that damage the elastin fibers and weaken the vessel wall, particularly if there are marked rises in blood pressure.

Factors that facilitate *thrombus formation* or fibrin deposition also contribute to the atherosclerotic process. Endothelial damage may cause blood platelets to adhere to the intima, subsequently leading to thrombus formation. Complete occlusion of the vessel may result if the thrombus is large, as in areas of fibrous plaques. However, it is also conceivable that smaller thrombi or platelet aggregates could gradually result in the buildup of a plaque. In addition, recent studies have suggested that a factor present in platelets with a molecular weight of approximately 13,000 may stimulate the proliferation of arterial smooth muscle cells.

Marked increases in *arterial lysosomal activity* have been demonstrated in experimental atherosclerosis and hypertension. The lipid accumulating in the early stages of a lesion appears to be associated with lysosomes that may be involved in lipid degradation as well as in the degradation of other cellular constituents. The release of lysosomes from cells could have an injurious effect on arterial tissue.

Immunologic injury to the artery may also play a role. For example, recent studies have demonstrated severe atherosclerosis developing in the coronary arteries of transplanted hearts.

Hormonal influences appear to be related to atherogenesis. Men have a marked *sex predisposition* for coronary atherosclerosis and myocardial infarction as compared with premenopausal women; after the menopause, however, the incidence of atherosclerotic complications in women gradually approaches the incidence in men. The serum levels of cholesterol, triglycerides, and low-density lipoprotein are somewhat lower and high-density lipoproteins somewhat higher in premenopausal women than in men of corresponding age, but these differences probably do not account entirely for the major sex differences in coronary atherosclerosis.

Diabetes also markedly accelerates the atherosclerotic process. Most patients with long-standing diabetes show evidence of advanced vascular disease, and approximately 70 percent of diabetic deaths can be attributed to vascular complications. The hyperlipoproteinemia found in many diabetic patients must be an important factor contributing to the acceleration of atherosclerosis. In addition, primary vascular changes in diabetic patients such as basement membrane thickening and mucopolysaccharide deposition may also be important. Hyperglycemia itself is an independent risk factor and is associated with approx-

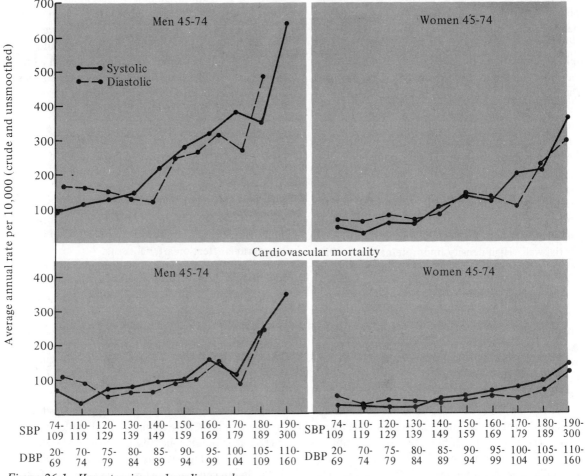

Figure 26-1. Hypertension and cardiovascular morbidity and mortality according to systolic (SBP) *versus diastolic* (DBP) *blood pressure in an 18-year follow-up in the Framingham population. (Reproduced by permission from O. Paul (ed.),* Epidemiology and Control of Hypertension. *New York: Stratton Intercontinental Medical Book Corp., 1975. P. 555.)*

imately a twofold increase for coronary heart disease.

Heavy *cigarette smoking* is a major risk factor and is associated with an increased incidence of atherosclerotic disease as well as a twofold to threefold increase in frequency of sudden death from myocardial infarction. The mechanism of this effect has not been delineated, although the increased levels of carbon monoxide in the blood that occur with smoking have been postulated to be important.

The observed *familial predisposition* for atherosclerosis suggests that genetic as well as environmental influences are also involved. Many of the hyperlipidemias associated with increased risks of atherosclerotic disease are genetically determined (see below). Hypertension and diabetes also frequently represent inherited traits. In addition, genetic factors may help to determine the structure and function of the intima and its inherent susceptibility to atherosclerosis.

An increased incidence of clinically significant coronary disease may occur during periods of severe *emotional stress.* The high frequency of coronary atherosclerosis in this country as compared with underdeveloped areas has been attributed to the greater anxieties and tensions of our civilization.

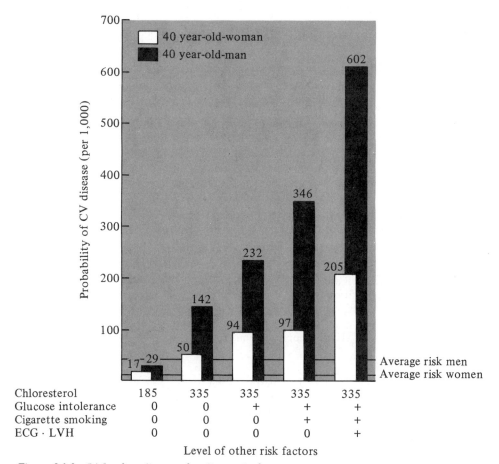

Chloresterol	185	335	335	335	335
Glucose intolerance	0	0	+	+	+
Cigarette smoking	0	0	0	+	+
ECG · LVH	0	0	0	0	+

Level of other risk factors

Figure 26-2. Risk of cardiovascular disease in 8 years at a systolic blood pressure of 165 mm Hg according to other risk factors during an 18-year follow-up in the Framingham population. ECG = electrocardiogram; LVH = left ventricular hypertrophy. (Reproduced by permission from O. Paul (ed.), Epidemiology and Control of Hypertension. *New York: Stratton Intercontinental Medical Book Corp., 1975. P. 560.)*

There is little evidence, however, that changing to a tranquil life-style will retard the development of atherosclerosis.

Clinical observations indicate that a number of other poorly understood factors may influence atherosclerosis. *Obesity, hyperuricemia,* and *elevated blood hematocrit* are associated with an increased frequency of atherosclerotic complications. A positive correlation between *physical inactivity* and increased atherogenesis has also been reported, but there is considerable controversy about this.

Recently it has been observed that patients with elevated levels of blood and urinary *homocysteine* develop a markedly increased predisposition to atherosclerotic disease. Experimental studies have suggested that homocysteine may damage the arterial endothelium, thereby producing platelet adherence, smooth muscle cell proliferation, and eventual plaque formation.

A summary of the proposed sequence of events involved in atherogenesis is illustrated in Figure 26-3.

Classification of Hyperlipoproteinemias

Characterization of hyperlipoproteinemias according to serum lipoprotein patterns has been considered to be of value in identifying individuals susceptible to atherosclerotic disease, in differentiating between the primary and the secondary lipid disorders, and in planning appropriate therapy. Five major patterns

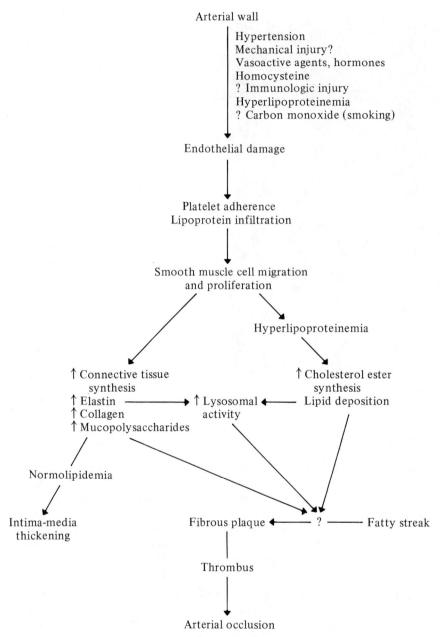

Figure 26-3. Proposed sequence of events in atherogenesis.

have been described (Fredrickson et al.). These types and their principal characteristics are summarized in Table 26-1. Types II and IV are the most common forms in the general population and account for more than 95 percent of all hyperlipoproteinemias and both types II and IV are associated with a markedly increased incidence of atherosclerotic disease. The rare type III disease is also associated with a greater risk of vascular disease, particularly of the peripheral type.

These patterns of hyperlipoproteinemia can generally be distinguished by means of serum lipoprotein electrophoresis, although ultracentrifugal analysis is needed to prove the presence of the type III variety. A fairly accurate estimation of the lipoprotein pattern can also be made from the appearance of the serum combined with its concentrations of cholesterol and triglycerides. In type I the serum, upon standing, has a creamy upper layer and a clear infranate, and its triglyceride level is markedly elevated. In type II the serum is generally clear, its cholesterol is increased, and its triglycerides are either normal (type II-A) or somewhat elevated (II-B). Types III and IV have turbid serum and are associated with higher concentrations of triglycerides than cholesterol. Type V serum has a creamy upper pellet and a cloudy infranate along with elevated cholesterol and triglycerides.

There has been a recent trend away from lipoprotein phenotyping and measurement of only serum cholesterol and triglyceride. The lipoprotein phenotype may not be constant in some of the individual patients or families with genetically determined hyperlipoproteinemia. Separate genetic inheritances appear to exist for familial hypercholesterolemia, familial hypertriglyceridemia, or combined hyperlipidemia. The latter appears to be the commonest genetic type. Familial hypercholesterolemia and the combined form are associated with an increased risk for atherosclerotic disease although familial hypertriglyceridemia may not be. Whenever a genetic form of hyperlipoproteinemia is apparent, it is important to examine other members of the family so that therapy can be instituted in them at an early age.

Cellular Metabolism of Cholesterol and Lipoproteins
Recent in vitro studies of cultured fibroblasts have

indicated that both low-density lipoproteins and very low density lipoproteins normally bind to receptors on the surface of the cell. The level of cellular cholesterol may regulate the number of these surface receptors. The lipoprotein bound to the receptor is taken up into the cell by pinocytosis and is incorporated into lysosomes. Lysosomal degradation of the apoprotein and of the cholesteryl ester of the lipoprotein appears to occur, and the lipoprotein cholesterol may then inhibit the cellular synthesis of cholesterol by a negative feedback effect on the rate-limiting enzyme 3-hydroxy-3-methylglutaryl coenzyme A reductase. In patients with familial hypercholesterolemia, a genetic deficiency in the number of specific cell receptors for low-density lipoproteins appears to be present. The problem is most severe in the homozygous form of the disease, where receptor binding may be almost totally absent. In heterozygous individuals, the binding defect appears to be less severe. A deficiency in binding of low-density lipoproteins is associated with a failure to inhibit cholesterol synthesis in the cell. As a result, an elevated cellular synthesis of cholesterol may occur in familial hypercholesterolemia.

Treatment of Atherosclerosis
Numerous forms of therapy have been advocated to prevent or retard the development of atherosclerosis. None of these measures has as yet been clearly demonstrated to be effective, but available evidence suggests that the following may have merit.

Therapy of Hyperlipoproteinemia
The therapy of specific forms of hyperlipoproteinemia is summarized in Table 26-2.

Dietary Management. Weight reduction appears desirable for all obese patients. In some obese individuals, particularly those with a predominant increase in serum low-density lipoproteins and triglycerides, weight reduction alone may be associated with a decrease in serum lipids and may constitute the most important aspect of the therapeutic regimen.

Moderate reduction in total dietary fat is justified for the general population, whose average consumption of fat is 40 to 45 percent of their total calories. A change in the quality of the fat to favor polyun-

Table 26-1. Characteristic Features of the Hyperlipoproteinemias

Characteristic	Type I	Type II II-A	Type II II-B	Type III	Type IV	Type V
Lipoprotein type	Chylomicron	LDL	LDL and VLDL	Abnormal LDL	VLDL	VLDL and chylomicron
Plasma cholesterol level	↑	↑	↑	↑	Normal or ↑	↑
Plasma triglyceride level	↑	Normal	↑	↑	↑	↑
Plasma appearance	Creamy top layer, clear infranate	Clear	Clear to turbid	Turbid	Turbid	Creamy top layer, turbid infranate
Electrophoretic pattern	↑ Chylomicron band	↑ beta bands	↑ beta and prebeta bands	↑ broad beta band	↑ prebeta band	↑ chylomicron and prebeta bands
Atherosclerosis risk	Normal	↑	↑	↑	↑	Normal or ↑
Xanthomas	Eruptive	Xanthelasma, tendinous corneal arcus	Xanthelasma, corneal arcus	Palmar, tuberous, eruptive	Tuberous, eruptive	Eruptive
Carbohydrate tolerance	Normal	Normal	Normal	Normal	Normal or ↓	↓
Postheparin lipolytic activity	↓	Normal	Normal	Normal	Normal or ↓	Normal or ↓
Mechanism	↓ Clearance of chylomicra	? ↓ clearance or ? ↑ synthesis of LDL	LDL and VLDL abnormality	↓ conversion VLDL to LDL	? ↓ clearance or ↑ synthesis of VLDL	Insulin deficiency, decreased chylomicron clearance, VLDL abnormality
Associated clinical abnormalities	Hepatosplenomegaly	...	...	Diabetes mellitus	Diabetes mellitus, gout	Abdominal pain, diabetes mellitus, gout
Secondary causes	High fat meal, ? leukemia	High saturated fat and cholesterol diet, nephrotic syndrome, hypothyroidism, multiple myeloma, obstructive liver disease		...	High carbohydrate diet, diabetes mellitus, alcoholism, pancreatitis, hypothyroidism, myeloma, nephrotic syndrome, glycogen storage disease, Gaucher's disease, pregnancy, gestational hormones	Diabetes mellitus (with ketoacidosis), pancreatitis, alcoholism, hypothyroidism

Note: LDL = low-density lipoproteins; VLDL = very low density lipoproteins.

Table 26-2. Summary of the Treatment of Hyperlipoproteinemias

Abnormality		Treatment		
Lipoprotein type	Class of hyperlipo-proteinemia	Diet	Major drugs	Other
Chylomicron	I	Decrease in total fat and medium-chain triglyc-erides	None	. . .
LDL (beta-lipoproteins)	II	Decrease in saturated fats and cholesterol; ? decrease in sucrose	Cholestyramine or colestipol, neomycin, clofibrate, nicotinic acid, beta-sitosterol	Ileal bypass surgery, ? portacaval shunting
Broad-band beta-lipoproteins	III	Weight reduction, decrease in saturated fats and cholesterol	Clofibrate	. . .
VLDL (prebeta-lipoproteins)	IV	Weight reduction, decrease in carbo-hydrates	Clofibrate	. . .
VLDL and chylomicron	V	Weight reduction, decrease in total fat and/or carbohydrates	Clofibrate	Insulin (uncon-trolled diabetes), alcohol withdrawal, ? progestins

Note: LDL = low-density lipoproteins; VLDL = very low density lipoproteins.

saturated varieties also seems of value. Metabolic studies indicate that the ingestion of highly saturated fats tends to increase serum cholesterol, whereas either reduction of saturated fats or substitution of polyunsaturated for saturated fats produces moderate reductions in serum cholesterol, triglycerides, and low-density lipoproteins. From the practical standpoint, it is appropriate to increase the intake of foods rich in polyunsaturated fats, such as vegetable oils, fish, and poultry, and decrease the consumption of meats and dairy products, in which the fat is predominantly of the saturated type. Restriction of dietary choles-terol itself also has value in lowering serum choles-terol, particularly in patients with type II and type III hyperlipoproteinemias. While much of the cholesterol that is metabolized is derived from endogenous syn-thesis rather than from dietary sources, severe restric-tion of dietary cholesterol to 250 mg or less per day will produce a moderate reduction in serum choles-terol. Most diets low in both total and saturated fat are also restricted in cholesterol content. Obese

patients with type IV hyperlipoproteinemia (very low density lipoprotein excess) should reduce their body weight. In addition, a decreased consumption of simple sugars such as sucrose has been advocated for lowering serum cholesterol, but the benefits of this appear to be minimal.

The influence of dietary changes on the athero-sclerotic process in man has not been clearly defined, but circumstantial evidence suggests that maintenance of low lipid levels may retard the development of atherosclerosis. In addition, it appears reasonable that the general population should moderately restrict their total dietary fat and cholesterol, increase their consumption of polyunsaturated in preference to saturated fats, and limit their total calories so as to maintain an optimum weight.

Hypolipoproteinemic Drugs. Drugs presently avail-able to lower serum lipids are limited, and none is entirely satisfactory for widespread use. The effects of the most important of these compounds are summarized in Table 26-3. Combinations of dietary man-agement, drug therapy, and the use of drugs with different sites of action are frequently necessary to substantially moderate severe forms of hyperlipidemia.

Ileal Bypass Surgery. This surgery, which interferes with bile acid reabsorption in the intestine, may be effective in lowering serum lipids, particularly in the patient with type II hyperlipoproteinemia. In selected patients with severe type II disease, ileal bypass surgery may be the treatment of choice, since it may be more effective in these individuals than any available pharmacologic approach. Portacaval venous shunting has also been used recently to lower serum lipids in patients with familial hypercholesterolemia, but the long-term safety of this procedure remains to be determined.

Other Therapeutic Measures. The use of drugs that inhibit platelet aggregation, such as aspirin and dipyrimidazole, has recently been advocated in the treatment of atherosclerosis. Preliminary reports have been promising, but the ultimate value of this approach must await the results of large-scale clinical trials now in progress. Long-term anticoagulant therapy has also been recommended but appears to be of questionable value (see Chap. 28).

Antihypertensive therapy should be employed in all patients with persistent diastolic hypertension unless it is specifically contraindicated. Marked reduction in morbidity and mortality can be expected with effective control of hypertension (see Chap. 25), although it is uncertain whether the atherosclerotic process itself is influenced by blood pressure lowering.

Cessation of cigarette smoking is strongly recommended, and educational programs to deter individuals from smoking appear to be of crucial importance. The cultivation of physical fitness in adults should also be encouraged, even though the effects of physical activity on the atherosclerotic process have not yet been fully defined.

Proper management of diabetes may be of value in decreasing serum lipids and in reducing the incidence of atherosclerotic complications. Unfortunately, the clinical manifestations of atherosclerosis continue to be frequent, even in patients whose dia-betes is well controlled. In fact, treatment with oral hypoglycemic drugs may be associated with an increased incidence of coronary disease. Earlier recognition and more vigorous treatment of mild or latent diabetes may prove important.

Surgical treatment of atherosclerosis may be of value if the disease is localized to a relatively small area. Thromboendarterectomy and arterial reconstructive surgery with vascular prostheses have been performed with gratifying results, particularly in patients with aortic aneurysms (see Chap. 27). Unfortunately, the atherosclerotic process is usually generalized, and not all patients benefit from such surgery.

Rationale of Therapy

There is little information concerning the prevention or reversal of atherosclerosis in man. In the experimental animal model such as the cholesterol-fed monkey or rabbit, both prevention and regression of atherosclerotic lesions have been demonstrated. Fatty streak lesions can be made to disappear almost completely, although fibrous fatty plaques regress only in part. During regression, atherosclerotic lesions have shown marked decreases in cholesterol content, and some increases have been observed in the lumen of the involved arteries as well. The collagen concentration of arteries may actually increase during regression of atherosclerotic lesions, but it is uncertain whether this change may later lead to arterial narrowing or to thrombotic complications. If prophylactic measures are to have maximum effects in man, they probably have to be instituted long before any clinical manifestations of atherosclerosis develop. There is no evidence as yet to indicate that advanced atheromatous plaques which are severely fibrotic, calcified, or necrotic can be resorbed.

Clinically, the beneficial effects of cholesterol-lowering procedures in patients with known vascular disease appear to be doubtful. No significant improvement in mortality or in the incidence of coronary events was observed in the Coronary Drug Study following treatment with clofibrate or nicotinic acid (see Bibliography). Dietary therapy also appears to have inconsistent benefits once clinically significant vascular disease is already present.

Table 26-3. Summary of the Action of the Major Hypolipoproteinemic Drugs

Drug	Usual daily dose	Mechanism of action	Predominant hypolipidemic effect	Side effects
Cholestyramine and colestipol	12–24 gm	Bile acid sequestration to decrease GI absorption of cholesterol	LDL cholesterol	Constipation, steatorrhea, fat-soluble vitamin deficiency, reduced effect of digitalis glycosides
Clofibrate	1.5–2.0 gm	Increased cholesterol excretion, decreased cholesterol and cholesteryl ester synthesis, decreased VLDL release into plasma	VLDL triglycerides, and cholesterol; also occasionally LDL cholesterol	Myositis, abnormal liver function tests, potentiation of coumarin anticoagulants
D-thyroxine	4.0–8.0 mg	Increased cholesterol excretion and degradation	LDL cholesterol	Angina pectoris
Nicotinic acid	1.5–5.0 gm	? decreased lipolysis, decreased conversion of VLDL to LDL, increased cholesterol oxidation	LDL cholesterol	Flushing, rash, nausea and vomiting, abnormal liver function, hyperuricemia
Neomycin	0.5–2.0 gm	Inhibit cholesterol absorption, ? increased bile acid deconjugation	LDL cholesterol	Decreased renal function, nausea, diarrhea
Beta-sitosterol	12.0–24.0 gm	Decreased intestinal cholesterol absorption	LDL cholesterol	Nausea, diarrhea

Note: GI = gastrointestinal; LDL = low-density lipoproteins; VLDL = very low density lipoproteins.

Early detection of positive risk factors is important for the control of atherosclerosis. Such approaches as the measurement of blood pressure, blood sugar, and serum lipids in children and young adults should prove to be of value in any major prevention program.

Bibliography

Armstrong, M. L., Warner, E. D., and Connor, W. E. Regression of coronary atheromatosis in rhesus monkeys. *Circ. Res.* 27:59, 1970.

Brecher, P. I., and Chobanian, A. V. Cholesteryl ester synthesis in normal and atherosclerotic aortas of rabbits and rhesus monkeys. *Circ. Res.* 35:692, 1974.

Brown, M. S., Dana, S. E., and Goldstein, J. C. Regulation of 3-hydroxy-3-methylgluteryl coenzyme: A reductase activity in cultured human fibroblasts. *J. Biol. Chem.* 249:789, 1974.

Coronary Drug Project Research Group. Clofibrate and niacin in coronary heart disease. *J.A.M.A.* 231:360, 1975.

Dayton, S., Pearce, M. L., Hashimoto, S., Dixon, W. J., and Tomiyasu, U. A controlled clinical trial of a diet high in unsaturated fat in preventing complications of atherosclerosis. *Circulation* 40(Suppl. II):1, 1969.

Fredrickson, D. S., Levy, R. I., and Lees, R. S. Fat transport in lipoproteins — an integrated approach to mechanisms and disorders. *N. Engl. J. Med.* 276:33, 94, 148, 215, 273, 1967.

Geer, J. C., McGill, H. C., and Strong, J. P. The fine structure of human atherosclerotic lesions. *Am. J. Pathol.* 38:263, 1961.

Goldstein, J. L., Hazzard, W. R., Schrott, H. G., Bierman, E. L., and Motulsky, A. G. Hyperlipidemia in coronary heart disease. *J. Clin. Invest.* 52:1133, 1544, 1569, 1973.

Jones, R. J. *Atherosclerosis: Proceedings of the Second International Symposium.* New York: Springer, 1969.

Kannell, W. B., Dawber, T. R., Kagan, A., Revotskie, N., and Stokes, J., III. Factors of risk in the development of coronary heart disease — six year followup experience. The Framingham Study. *Ann. Intern. Med.* 55:33, 1961.

Kannel, W. B., and Sorlie, P. Hypertension in Framingham. In O. Paul (ed.), *Epidemiology and Control of Hypertension.* New York: Stratton Intercontinental Medical Book Corp., 1975.

Page, I. H. National diet-heart study final report. *Circulation* 37(Suppl. I):1, 1968.

Peters, T. J., and deDuve, C. Lysosomes of the arterial wall: II. Subcellular fractionation of aortic cells from rabbits with experimental atheroma. *Exp. Mol. Pathol.* 20:228, 1974.

Ross, R., and Glomset, J. A. Atherosclerosis and the arterial smooth muscle cell. *Science* 180:1332, 1973.

Schettler, F. G., and Wissler, R. W. *Third International Symposium on Atherosclerosis.* Berlin: Springer, 1974.

Sloan, H. R., and Fredrickson, D. S. Enzyme deficiency in cholesteryl ester storage disease. *J. Clin. Invest.* 51:1929, 1972.

Stemerman, M., and Ross, R. Experimental atherosclerosis: I. Fibrous plaque formation in primates: An electron microscopic study. *J. Exp. Med.* 136:769, 1972.

U.S. Department of Health, Education and Welfare, Public Health Service. *The Dietary Management of Hyperlipoproteinemia: A Handbook for Physicians.* Washington, D.C.: U.S. Government Printing Office, 1970.

27

Diseases of the Aorta and Peripheral Blood Vessels

Jay D. Coffman

Diseases of the Aorta

ANEURYSMS

Clinical Picture. Aneurysms of the aorta produce signs and symptoms by progressively dilating the aortic wall and exerting pressure on surrounding structures. In their early stages, aneurysms are asymptomatic, and their first presenting symptom may be the steady, severe pain due to rupture; the patient will usually then be in shock. In the aortic arch, aneurysms may cause venous distention and edema of the head and neck (compression of great veins); dysphagia (pressure on esophagus); dyspnea, stridor, and a brassy cough (compression of air passages); hoarseness (pressure on the recurrent laryngeal nerve); or pain in the substernal region and left scapular area (erosion of ribs and sternum). Angina may develop if coronary ostia are involved, or cardiac failure may result if aortic valvular insufficiency is produced by the aneurysm.

The physical signs of aortic aneurysm may include a systolic murmur, widened area of mediastinal dullness, diastolic heave of the thorax, displacement of the trachea, or a tracheal tug. Aneurysms of the descending thoracic aorta may cause excruciating pain by erosion of ribs and vertebrae, but abdominal aortic aneurysms produce symptoms in less than half the cases, the pain being located in the middle or lower abdomen most often and in the back less frequently. An abdominal mass (tender or not) with expansile pulsation is a frequent finding, and a systolic bruit over the aneurysm is also very common. Abdominal aneurysms may present with symptoms of small intestinal obstruction or even renal colic with hydronephrosis due to ureteral obstruction.

Etiology. Atherosclerosis is the leading cause of aneurysms; usually the descending aorta, particularly the abdominal aorta, is involved in a fusiform enlargement. Syphilitic aortitis, the second leading cause of aneurysms, usually affects the thoracic segment,

especially the arch of the aorta, in a sacciform enlargement. Rarer etiologic factors include trauma and infection. Atherosclerotic aneurysms usually occur in the sixth and seventh decades, with a male-to-female ratio of 10:1; syphilitic aneurysms are most frequent in the fifth and sixth decades, with an M/F ratio of 5:1. The latent period between the primary syphilitic infection and the onset of symptoms and signs is usually more than 10 years, and the serologic tests for syphilis are usually positive.

Diagnosis. X-ray examination, echography (ultrasound), and angiography are helpful in the diagnosis of aneurysms; but angiograms may fail to delineate the lesion due to thrombus formation within the aneurysm. A curvilinear calcification in a soft tissue mass is often seen in lateral or oblique x-ray films of an abdominal aneurysm. A dilated ascending arch of the aorta with a convex prominence extending outward beyond the right atrial shadow and increased pulsations may be seen by fluoroscopy of aneurysms of the aortic arch.

Prognosis and Treatment. The average life span after symptoms of a thoracic aneurysm appear is less than 1 year; 50 percent of patients live 5 years and 30 percent, 10 years; only about one-third die from rupture of the aneurysm. For abdominal aneurysms, the 5-year survival is less than 20 percent. The larger the aneurysm, the shorter the life expectancy. For sacciform aneurysms treatment consists in excision and lateral aortorrhaphy. Fusiform aneurysms are excised with graft replacement. Antisyphilitic treatment may prolong life in patients with syphilitic aneurysms.

DISSECTING ANEURYSMS

The usual pathologic change of dissecting aneurysm is cystic necrosis, which is characterized by focal accumulation of mucoid material in the media. Although the cause is unknown in most cases, dissecting aneurysm may occur in the Marfan syndrome, hypertension, coarctation, syphilitic aortitis, arteriosclerosis, pregnancy, trauma, and kyphoscoliosis. Rupture of the vasa vasorum in the degenerated areas causes an intramural hematoma and an intimal tear that dissects proximally, distally, or both. Aortic branches may be dissected or may shut off. Reentry tears may occur into the aortic lumen, producing a double channel; or external rupture of the dissection may occur into the pericardial, pleural, or peritoneal cavities or into the mediastinum or gastrointestinal tract. Men are affected two to three times more frequently than women, with the greatest incidence being in the sixth and seventh decades. More than one-half of dissecting aortic aneurysms begin in the ascending portion, and about one-third are distal to the subclavian artery. The aorta is most frequently affected by dissection, but rare cases have been reported of isolated dissection of almost all other vessels in the body.

Clinical Picture. Dissecting aneurysms of the aorta are characterized by the sudden onset of excruciating, persistent, tearing pain in the anterior thorax or epigastrium, sometimes radiating through to the intrascapular area. The pain follows the route of dissection; it may involve the legs and then subside in a few days. The patient is sweaty, pale, and shocklike, but the blood pressure is elevated in about 80 percent of the patients. Neurologic findings occur in 42 percent of the patients, and the symptoms comprise a spectrum ranging from paralyses to coma. The characteristic sign is absent pulses in one or both carotid arteries or in the arms or legs, depending on which vessels are occluded. Other symptoms and signs are extremely variable. Anginal pain with or without myocardial infarction may occur from involvement of the coronary ostia. If the aortic valve is deformed, an aortic diastolic murmur may appear. Bleeding into the pericardium may produce a pericardial friction rub or tamponade. Congestive heart failure often follows the acute onset. Rarely, the disease causes no symptoms at all, or at least none recognizable during life. This is especially true of dissections distal to the left subclavian artery.

Diagnosis. Dissecting aneurysm is often difficult to differentiate from myocardial infarction, which may also be present. An x-ray film of the chest may reveal an increase in the diameter of the aortic shadow. An angiogram may be helpful in the diagnosis by demonstrating a double lumen in the aorta. Anemia and

leukocytosis are common; hematuria and a rising blood urea nitrogen may occur with renal involvement.

Prognosis and Treatment. The survival in dissecting aneurysm is greatest if the ascending aorta is spared. Currently the initial treatment is medical and is designed to reduce the systolic ejection force of the heart and the blood pressure. Medications usually include sodium nitroprusside or trimethaphan, reserpine or guanethidine, and propranolol (if hypertension is not present). Early surgery is necessary if large vital vessels are occluded, if severe aortic insufficiency occurs, or if dissection progresses despite medical treatment. Medical treatment has reduced the mortality from approximately 70 to 14 percent. In the period following medical treatment, about 25 percent of patients will require surgery for aortic insufficiency or enlarging saccular aneurysms.

Diseases of the Peripheral Blood Vessels

OBSTRUCTIVE ARTERIAL DISEASES

Arteriosclerosis Obliterans

Clinical Picture. Arteriosclerosis obliterans is the leading cause of occlusive arterial disease of the extremities in patients over 40. The obstructing lesions are very often localized and segmental, although other parts of the same vessel are also atherosclerotic (the etiology and pathology are discussed in Chap. 26). Below the obstruction there is a decreased blood pressure, and there may be a decreased blood flow. The clinical picture is a result of inadequate oxygenation of the tissues during exercise or even at rest. Men are affected more frequently than women; the highest incidence occurs in the sixth and seventh decades. The commonest lesion occurs in the superficial femoral artery in the adductor canal; the deep femoral artery is infrequently obstructed and its collaterals may be adequate to supply the limb. Aortoiliac and popliteal arteriosclerosis obliterans are next in incidence. Patients with diabetes mellitus develop arteriosclerosis at an earlier age and have an increased involvement of the vessels between the knee and the ankle, though less in the aortoiliac area, than do nondiabetics. Diabetics do not have small vessel (arteriolar) disease but do have an increased capillary basement membrane thickness with increased permeability. Diabetics may have foot ulcers with good pulses; such ulcers are evidently due to trauma undetected because of neuropathy.

Pain is the commonest occlusive symptom and presents early as intermittent claudication — usually a gripping pain and tightness but sometimes only aching, cramping, or fatigue on exercise of the affected muscle group. The amount of exercise producing the pain is relatively constant in each patient, and the pain is relieved promptly by rest. The lower extremities are involved most frequently. Other symptoms and signs include unilateral extremity coldness and paresthesias. Pain at rest is a late and grave occurrence due to tissue anoxia or ischemic neuritis. Such pain is worse at night, is aggravated by heat, and is relieved by dependency of the affected part. Examination may reveal deformed toenails; hair loss; atrophic, thin skin; pallor; cyanosis; or rubor. Ulcers and gangrene are late occurrences. Arterial pulsations are diminished or absent; if pulses are present, they may disappear for up to 5 minutes after exercise of the limb. Systolic or continuous bruits may be heard over the artery below an obstruction; continuous bruits denote an inadequate collateral blood flow.

To test the presence and degree of ischemia, the limb is raised to a 45° angle with the patient supine. Pallor of the plantar surface indicates a deficient blood supply; if pallor of the foot in this position occurs only after ankle exercise, the disease is less severe. The patient is then asked to sit up with the extremities dependent. Flushing of the foot should occur immediately, and the veins should fill in about 10 seconds. Flushing and venous filling times of greater than 30 seconds denote a severely ischemic limb with inadequate collateral circulation. These tests should be performed in a warm room to rule out vasospasm; varicosities invalidate the measurement of the venous filling time. The use of a Doppler systolic blood pressure measurement over the pedal arteries before and after exercise (for comparison with brachial arterial pressure) has proved to be a very useful diagnostic test. (Pedal systolic pressure should equal or exceed arm pressure.) Arteriography will reveal the location and extent of both the obstructive lesion and the collateral circulation.

Prognosis and Treatment. Intermittent claudication secondary to femoral arteriosclerosis obliterans remains stable or improves over a period of years in more than 90 percent of the patients. The prognosis is worse if diabetes mellitus is present, because progression of the disease is then usually unrelenting.

Treatment of intermittent claudication consists in having the patient walk more slowly, cease smoking, and do graded exercises, and in controlling hyperlipoproteinemias, hypertension, or diabetes mellitus when present. Vasodilator drugs are ineffective. Careful attention to cleanliness and dryness of the feet is emphasized. If the claudication is progressive or interferes with employment and the obstructing lesion is segmental with good arterial runoff below the lesion, vein graft bypass or surgical endarterectomy is recommended. If pain at rest is present and the lesion is not segmental, a period of strict bed rest with the affected limb in a dependent position is imperative; narcotics and even crushing the sensory nerve supplying the ischemic area may be necessary to control the pain. Ulcers should be kept moist and clean, and appropriate antibiotics should be used. Lumbar sympathectomy will often increase the cutaneous blood flow enough to relieve pain at rest or to heal small areas of ulceration or gangrene. If there is unrelenting pain at rest or if there is ulceration or gangrene, amputation is indicated when bypass surgery cannot be performed.

Aortoiliac Occlusive Disease

Aortoiliac occlusive disease (Leriche syndrome) is due overwhelmingly to arteriosclerosis. As an isolated lesion it occurs a decade earlier than more peripheral disease and is usually not associated with diabetes. Rarer causes are thromboangiitis obliterans, syphilis, and trauma. Men are affected eight times more frequently than women. The arteriosclerotic process gradually narrows the aortoiliac lumina until a thrombus forms to cause complete or partial obstruction. Both legs are usually involved. Since the whole process is a gradual one, a large collateral circulation usually develops.

Clinical Picture. Aortoiliac occlusive disease is usually characterized by intermittent claudication (in the low back, buttock, thigh, calf, or foot) and by leg weakness. Other symptoms and signs include impotence, pallor, and muscle atrophy. Trophic changes are not frequent; if they appear, concomitant disease of more peripheral vessels should be suspected. Femoral pulses are usually absent but may be felt if collateral circulation is well developed. Systolic bruits over the abdomen and over the femoral arteries are very common. The arms often have an elevated blood pressure. The diagnosis is confirmed by aortography, and treatment (surgical endarterectomy, graft replacement, or bypass) is very successful because the involved vessels are large. In elderly, high-risk patients, axillofemoral and femorofemoral grafts have been extremely effective.

Thromboangiitis Obliterans

The cause of thromboangiitis obliterans (Buerger's disease) is unknown; tobacco sensitivity, infectious agents, metabolic abnormalities, exposure to dampness and cold, and trauma have all been incriminated. Lately the incidence of the disease has decreased markedly, and there has been controversy as to whether it is a disease entity distinct from arteriosclerosis. It is generally agreed now that it is a syndrome that can have several causes.

The pathologic changes in thromboangiitis obliterans relate to a chronic inflammatory infiltrate of small- and medium-sized arteries and veins of the extremities, although rarely the mesenteric, coronary, cerebral, or renal vessels are involved. Lesions are focal in nature and are interspersed with areas of normal vessels. Characteristically, red thrombi form containing multiple sterile microabscesses and multinucleated cells; gradually these organize and become fibrotic.

Clinical Picture. Thromboangiitis obliterans is characterized by symptoms and signs of ischemia occurring in a relapsing course with quiescent periods of varying duration. It may be differentiated from arteriosclerosis obliterans by the following points: occurrence almost exclusively in men 20 to 40 years of age who smoke cigarettes; migratory thrombophlebitis in 30 to 40 percent of cases; frequent involvement of the upper extremities; and vasospasm (often with Raynaud's phenomenon) as a prominent early feature. No association with diabetes mellitus or hypercholesterolemia is apparent, and cardiac involvement is rare. Arteriograms may be helpful in diagnosis by demonstrating absence of atheroma, normality of vessels between lesions, corkscrew tortuosity of affected arteries, and involvement of the vessels of the upper extremities.

Treatment. The treatment of thromboangiitis obliterans is the same as in arteriosclerosis obliterans. It is imperative that tobacco never be used; the disease may be arrested by stopping smoking.

Arterial Embolism and Acute Arterial Thrombosis

Clinical Picture. Arterial embolism and acute arterial thrombosis are characterized by symptoms and signs of ischemia below the site of obstruction. About one-half the patients have a sudden onset of pain; in the remainder the symptoms begin insidiously. Pain is present in 80 percent of cases, paresthesias in about 60 percent, and weakness or paralysis in 20 percent. Nausea, vomiting, and shock are common in a so-called saddle embolus at the aortic bifurcation. The involved extremity shows sharply demarcated color changes (pallor that may later change to cyanosis) and coolness below the obstruction site, collapsed veins, absent arterial pulses, and decreased to absent reflexes and sensation. Massive gangrene may develop later.

Acute arterial thrombosis occurs in obstructive vascular disease, polycythemia, or following trauma, and it can be distinguished from an embolus only by the absence of the underlying causes of emboli. Most arterial emboli occur in patients afflicted with myocardial infarction, atrial fibrillation with mitral valvular disease, chronic congestive heart failure, or endocarditis.

Emboli usually lodge at the bifurcations of the larger arteries; the commonest site is the junction of the superficial femoral and the deep femoral arteries. The pathophysiology relates to the cessation of blood flow in the vessel and secondary extension of the thrombus above and below the obstruction site.

Vasospasm may contribute to the ischemia, but experimental evidence is not conclusive on this point.

Prognosis and Treatment. Important factors in the prognosis of arterial embolism and acute arterial thrombosis are the size of the artery involved, the presence of patent companion vessels and collateral circulation, and the speed of treatment. Gangrene is much commoner after age 60. Except for embolus to the aortic bifurcation, where surgery is the best treatment, conservative care often gives equally good results. Pain should be relieved and the limb positioned in 15° dependency; anticoagulation therapy is necessary to prevent further emboli and extension of the thrombus. Measures to increase blood flow include body warming (except for the involved limb) and sympathetic blockade. If conservative treatment is not effective in greatly improving the circulation of the extremity within 2 to 4 hours, embolectomy is indicated. Fibrinolytic agents (streptokinase and urokinase) have been used with success in about a third of patients with embolism or acute thrombosis.

Pulseless Disease
Pulseless disease (Takayashu syndrome; aortic arch syndrome) results from a diminishing blood supply to the upper half of the body. The pathologic changes relate to a chronic, slowly progressive, obliterative panarteritis of the large vessels arising from the arch of the aorta; the abdominal aorta and branches are seldom affected. The cause is unknown.

Clinical Picture. Ocular symptoms are very common, varying from transitory visual disturbances to blindness; headache, vertigo, mental confusion, and hemiplegia may occur in pulseless disease. The classic sign is an asymmetrical absence or diminution of pulses in the neck or arms; blood pressure is low in the affected arm. Murmurs may be heard over the stenosed vessels. The blood pressure is often elevated in the lower extremities. Pulseless disease cannot be diagnosed until arteriosclerosis, syphilitic aortitis, dissecting aneurysm, congenital malformations, emboli, thrombi, and neoplasms have been ruled out. Since only women are affected, usually in the second to fifth decades, age and sex are helpful clues; the erythrocyte sedimentation rate is elevated, and a nonspecific hyperglobulinemia is often found.

Treatment. The treatment of pulseless disease has been unsatisfactory. Continuous anticoagulation and steroid therapy are said to be of benefit on the basis of a small experience. Endarterectomy is helpful in some cases. The life expectancy of patients with this disease is usually 5 to 10 years.

VASOSPASTIC DISEASES

Raynaud's Disease and Phenomenon
The cause of Raynaud's disease is unknown. Experimental evidence supports the theory that there is an abnormal susceptibility of the small arteries or arterioles to vasoconstrictive stimuli, but the nature of this local abnormality is unknown. Other factors that have been implicated are overactivity of the sympathetic nervous system and excess production or interference with the metabolism of catecholamines or serotonin. Women are affected more frequently than men (5:1), and the disease is most common between puberty and age 40.

Raynaud's phenomenon (as distinct from the disease) is secondary to some underlying cause such as connective tissue disease (especially scleroderma), rheumatoid arthritis, neurogenic vasoconstriction (cervical rib, scalenus anticus, costoclavicular, and hyperabduction syndromes), occlusive arterial disease, posttraumatic states (pneumatic hammer, piano player diseases), intoxications (ergot, methysergide), cryoglobulinemia, macroglobulinemia, or cold hemagglutinins. An association with primary pulmonary hypertension has been reported.

Clinical Picture. Raynaud's disease and phenomenon are characterized by attacks of digital pallor or cyanosis, or both. As the attack passes off, the digits may become red. The first attacks appear on exposure to cold and may involve only one digit, but later the attacks become bilateral and symmetrical and may be induced by emotional stimuli. Attacks may last from a few minutes to hours. The fingers alone are involved in about half the cases; the fingers and toes in the remainder. The blush areas of the head may be affected in rare patients. Other symptoms and signs include numbness and excess perspiration during attacks and burning, throbbing pain and swelling after attacks. Large vessel pulsations are usually normal. In severe, progressive cases, the fingers become thin, tapering, smooth, and shiny with tight skin (sclerodactyly); small, painful areas of cutaneous gangrene may occur on the fingertips.

Pathophysiology. The pathophysiology of Raynaud's disease and phenomenon relates to vasoconstriction of the digital arteries, leading to pallor, and then cyanosis secondary to stasis of blood. When the arteries reopen, the red (hyperemic) phase occurs. In the early stages the digital arteries are histologically normal. In advanced cases there is presumably secondary arterial intimal thickening; muscular hypertrophy and small arterial thromboses may also be present.

Prognosis. Raynaud's disease usually improves slowly or remains stationary for years. Approximately one-third of cases are progressive, but amputation of terminal phalanges has been necessary in less than 1 percent of cases. The prognosis of Raynaud's phenomenon depends on the underlying condition. Since scleroderma may be manifested only by Raynaud's attacks for several years, differentiation from Raynaud's disease is important but often difficult.

Treatment. Mild cases of Raynaud's disease without trophic changes may be treated by protection from cold exposure, abstinence from smoking, and mild sedation. Reserpine has proved remarkably effective in some cases; tolazoline may also be added if necessary. Regional sympathectomy has been used in patients with progressive disease and trophic changes and, although it does not cure the disease, may provide relief for 6 months to 2 years. The treatment of Raynaud's phenomenon consists in control of the underlying condition; sympathectomy is not used.

Acrocyanosis
Acrocyanosis is characterized by persistent, symmetrical, painless cyanosis and coldness of the hands, and, less commonly, of the feet. The cyanosis is accentuated by cold and diminished by warmth. Other signs and symptoms include swelling and profuse sweating, but trophic changes do not occur.

Although acrocyanosis is often associated with endocrine disorders (e.g., pituitary insufficiency) or with asthenia, the cause is unknown. As in Raynaud's disease, local abnormality of the arterioles with heightened sensitivity to cold has been blamed; the sympathetic nervous system has also been implicated. The pathophysiology relates to arteriolar constriction associated with dilatation of the capillaries and venules. Acrocyanosis must be differentiated from Raynaud's disease (which is judged by the persistence of color change) and from chronic cyanosis of the extremities secondary to obstructive vascular disease, cardiac or pulmonary disease, and polycythemia.

Reassurance is often the only treatment necessary, as the prognosis is good. For cosmetic reasons, protection from cold is advised and vasodilator drugs may be administered. Sympathectomy, though helpful, is seldom warranted.

Ergot and Methysergide Toxicity
Ergot or methysergide toxicity can cause ischemic symptoms and signs, including intermittent claudication, coldness and pallor of the extremities, pain at rest, absence of pulses of small and large arteries, loss of sensation in the limbs, typical Raynaud's phenomenon, ulceration, and gangrene.

Excessive use of ergot can induce intense vasospasm of large and small arteries and veins, while small doses (1 mg) of methysergide can have the same effect in sensitive persons. Ergot toxicity may cause vasospasm (slowing the blood flow) and intimal hyperplasia and thromboses of arteries and capillaries; the last may lead to gangrene, especially of the digits, nose, and ears. The pathology has not yet been studied in methysergide toxicity.

Treatment and Prognosis. The treatment of ergot and methysergide toxicity consists in stopping the medication; symptoms will usually subside and vessels reopen within 3 days. Ancillary treatment consists in therapy with vasodilators (which are usually ineffective) and anticoagulants. The prognosis depends on the extent of irreversible changes induced by thrombosis. Syndromes similar to Raynaud's phenomenon or erythromelalgia may follow the acute episode.

Erythromelalgia

Erythromelalgia is considered here, although it is not a vasospastic disease. It is a rare condition characterized by attacks of burning pain and redness of both feet and, less often, of both hands. At first only small, circumscribed areas may be involved, but later an entire sole, palm, or even a whole extremity may be affected. Other symptoms and signs include warm or hot skin and swelling. Arterial pulsations are normal in the extremities. Attacks are induced by warming, exercising, or dependency of the affected limb and usually last 2 to 3 hours.

The cause of idiopathic cases of erythromelalgia, which occur in healthy middle-aged men and women, is unknown. Secondary cases occur in polycythemia vera, arterial hypertension, or arteriosclerosis obliterans. No uniform vascular pathologic changes have been found. Symptoms are probably due to a hypersensitivity of the cutaneous pain fibers to heat or tension; the pain is not due to an increase in blood flow.

Prognosis and Treatment. The prognosis in idiopathic erythromelalgia is guarded, since the severe pain may become disabling; in secondary cases the outcome depends on the underlying disease process and its treatment. Treatment consists in therapy with aspirin, vasoconstrictor agents, or sedatives and avoidance of attack-producing stimuli. During attacks the extremity should be elevated, rested, and cooled. In severer cases, nerve block or section is occasionally necessary.

Peripheral Vascular Disease due to Exposure to Cold

Chilblain (pernio, erythrocyanosis), immersion (trench) foot, and frostbite are diseases involving a reaction of the peripheral blood vessels to cold exposure, with or without dampness.

Clinical Picture. Symptoms and signs of chilblain may occur yearly with the onset of cold weather and include bluish red swelling with pruritus and burning on exposed areas of the body (hands, feet, lower legs). The lesions may go on to bleb formation and hemor-

rhagic ulceration, which can leave residual scarring and pigmentation. The etiology is unknown, but it occurs only in cold, damp climates.

Immersion foot is produced by prolonged exposure to low, not necessarily freezing, temperatures plus dampness. An ischemic vasospastic phase consisting of cold, swollen, white or blue pulseless extremities with decreased to absent sensation is followed by a hyperemic (warming) phase, during which the skin is dry, hot, and red and there are bounding pulses; swollen tissues; blisters; throbbing, lancinating pain; and paresthesias. Extensive exfoliation and gangrene may follow. After healing occurs, the feet may remain pale and cold and exhibit hypersensitivity to cold. Warm-water immersion foot occurs in southeastern Asia; in this type of disease the plantar surfaces are painful, wrinkled, white, and convoluted, and sometimes there is maceration. There are usually no residua.

Frostbite causes numb, yellowish white patches; if severe, the involved part may be white in appearance and feel cold and solid to touch. Depending on the depth of tissue freezing, there may be only erythema and transient anesthesia or superficial bullae; deeper freezing may cause secondary thromboses, livid cyanosis, deep-tissue destruction, and even gangrene. In the healing phase a black eschar usually covers the area.

Pathologic Changes. The pathologic findings in chilblain consist of subcutaneous tissue inflammation, angiitis, and tissue necrosis. The anoxia from vasoconstriction in cold immersion foot leads to tissue necrosis, increased capillary permeability with a protein-rich edema, and nerve degeneration. Warm immersion foot is evidently due to swelling of the stratum corneum and to abrasion from footwear. Frostbite, besides causing damage by vasoconstriction, involves actual freezing of tissue; ice crystal formation occurs in extracellular fluid, damaging cells by dehydration.

Treatment. Chilblain is treated by protection from cold; reserpine may be helpful. The treatment of immersion foot is supportive: bed rest, cleaning, and moderate elevation of the extremities. Cooling during the hyperemic phase may help relieve the pain. Frostbite is treated by rapid thawing in warm water (40 to 42°C; 104 to 105.8°F) and meticulous care to prevent trauma (no rubbing) or infection of the involved areas. Early sympathectomy may lead to a better outcome. Anticoagulants and analgesics should also be used. In both immersion foot and frostbite, extensive gangrene may necessitate amputation.

ARTERIOVENOUS FISTULAS

Arteriovenous fistulas are direct communications between arteries and veins. Since arterial blood follows the path of least resistance into the venous system, there is increased blood flow in the fistular area but decreased arterial pressure distally. The venous pressure locally in the extremity is increased.

Clinical Picture. Symptoms and signs of arteriovenous fistula include aching pain and increased skin temperature locally; a continuous murmur and thrill over the fistula; swollen, reddened, or cyanotic tissue in the area of the fistula; and venous tortuosities and varicosities (often with venous pulsations) of the limb. There are decreased diastolic and increased systolic and pulse pressures secondary to the lowered peripheral resistance. About 50 percent of patients have a fistula large enough to cause an increased cardiac output and blood volume; even congestive heart failure may occur. Compression of the artery feeding a large fistula may cause a decrease in heart rate (Branham's sign). Distal to the fistula there may be decreased skin temperature, edema, stasis pigmentation, ulcers, gangrene, and rarefaction of bone. Higher venous blood oxygen saturation in the involved extremity as compared to that in the opposite extremity and visible arteriovenous communications on arteriography are helpful diagnostic aids.

Congenital fistulas are present from birth, are often multiple, and occur most frequently in the lower extremities. Acquired fistulas are usually single and follow penetrating wounds or intervertebral disk surgery. Treatment includes arterial repair, grafting, mass ligation, or amputation. Sympathectomy will increase blood flow to the limb distal to the fistula.

DISEASES OF PERIPHERAL VEINS

Varicose Veins

Dilated, elongated, tortuous varicose veins with a loss of elasticity and incompetent valves lead to an increased local venous pressure and formation of edema in the involved extremity.

Clinical Picture. Symptoms may be absent, even with large varicosities. Some patients experience aching pain, fatigue, congested feelings, paresthesias, or soreness of the limb after ordinary activities. Symptoms are usually relieved by rest with the limbs elevated. In severe cases the edema and local pressure lead to petechiae, stasis dermatitis with brownish pigmentation, subcutaneous fibrosis, and ulcers (postphlebitic syndrome). Generally the varicosities are easily seen and traced if the patient is in the standing position. Retrograde blood flow and incompetent perforating veins may be demonstrated by elevating the limb to empty the varicosities, applying tourniquets or pressure at appropriate levels, and then observing the veins with the patient in the standing position before and after release of the tourniquets.

Etiologic Factors. Varicose veins are caused by defective valves (due to hereditary or familial weakness of the vein wall or to a previous thrombophlebitis), obstructed venous blood flow (due to pressure, e.g., from a pregnant uterus, neoplasm, scar tissue), or a combination of these factors. Chronic constipation from the low-residue diet of Western civilization has been implicated as a cause of varicosities, hemorrhoids, and diverticula of the colon. About one-sixth of the adult population is affected with varicosities, with women predominating. The veins of the lower extremities are involved most frequently.

Treatment. The treatment of uncomplicated varicosities involves frequent periods of rest with leg elevation above heart level, elastic support, and ligation or vein stripping. When ulcers are present, pressure dressings, gelatin boots, or excision and skin grafting may be necessary.

Thrombophlebitis (and Phlebothrombosis)

Thrombophlebitis is usually due to thrombus formation in a vein. Without local reaction or symptoms, the term *phlebothrombosis* is applied; in thrombophlebitis there is, in addition, a local inflammatory reaction.

Clinical Picture. Symptoms and signs of thrombophlebitis are produced by the local elevation of venous pressure and inflammatory reaction, if present. Venous thrombosis may involve either the superficial or the deep veins. Since local symptoms are usually absent in phlebothrombosis, it is usually suspected only after a pulmonary embolism occurs; however, local pressure may cause pain at a much lower level (160 mm Hg) than in normal extremities when a blood pressure cuff is inflated around the involved segment of the extremity.

Deep phlebitis may be gradual or sudden in onset, usually with continuous throbbing pain; some patients only experience aching during the night. Swelling of the limb may be noticed. Malaise, anorexia, and fever can occur if large veins are affected. Examination reveals tenderness or pain over the thrombosed vein, which is sometimes felt as a cord. Resistance to dorsiflexion of the foot (Homans' sign) may be found. Edema, increased circumference, and cyanosis of the limb may be present if collateral venous flow is inadequate. The muscles are often tense and firm, even when edema is not obvious. A local increase in temperature may occur.

Arterial pulses may be decreased secondary to vasospasm; in acute iliofemoral venous thrombosis the vasospasm may be severe enough to lead to gangrene. Detection of a feeble pulsation by an oscillometer helps to differentiate vasospasm from arterial embolism, in which no pulsation can be found. An increased erythrocyte sedimentation rate and leukocytosis are usually not present unless large veins are involved. In superficial phlebitis there are elevated warm, red, tender, indurated areas; other signs are absent. In migratory phlebitis, veins in different areas are affected in succession.

Etiologic Factors. Predisposing factors in thrombophlebitis frequently involve venous stasis secondary to prolonged immobility (particularly postpartum, after operations, in heart disease, or general debility) or external pressure (long periods of sitting), although local injury to the vein from trauma, chemicals, or infectious agents and blood alterations favoring coagulation (polycythemia, birth control pills) are not uncommon factors. Phlebitis also may be idiopathic and recurrent. A significant correlation has been found between the use of oral contraceptive hormones and thrombophlebitis. The cause of the high incidence of thrombophlebitis in patients with ulcerative colitis (30 percent) or with carcinoma is unknown. Venous thrombosis and phlebitis are commonest with carcinomas of the lung but have been reported with tumors of many other organs, particularly the stomach and the body and tail of the pancreas. The phlebitis associated with carcinoma is often superficial and migratory, but deep veins may also be involved. A migratory type of phlebitis is also seen in thromboangiitis obliterans (page 268).

Pathologic Changes and Complications. It is commonly believed that phlebothrombosis precedes thrombophlebitis, although thrombophlebitis can be produced by direct infection or irritation of veins (i.e., from indwelling catheters or intravenous drugs). The venous thrombus is usually red (contains red cells) and has a propagating tail proximally, and it causes an inflammatory reaction involving various layers of the venous wall.

Pulmonary embolism is the most serious complication of deep phlebitis; it does not occur in superficial phlebitis (see Chap. 31). After several years, recurrent episodes of deep phlebitis may cause varicosities or even the postphlebitic limb (swollen, pigmented, fibrosed limb with a tendency to ulcerate).

Diagnosis. Thrombophlebitis is often a very difficult clinical diagnosis to make from symptoms and signs. Phlebography is the most helpful test available. Peripheral venous scanning with radioisotope-tagged fibrinogen may become of great use as more experience with it is acquired. Examination with the Doppler or impedance plethysmograph yields many false-negative results except when large veins such as the iliac or popliteal veins are totally occluded.

Treatment. The treatment of superficial phlebitis consists in application of moist heat locally, elevation of the limb several times a day, restricted use of the limb, and elastic support. The medical treatment of deep phlebitis is complete bed rest, elevation of the limb above heart level, and continuous application of hot packs. Anticoagulation therapy is used to prevent propagation of the thrombus and consequent pulmonary emboli. Sympathetic ganglionic blockade or even epidural anesthesia may be necessary to relieve vasospasm. Intensive medical treatment is continued until local tenderness and edema totally subside. Then gradual ambulation with elastic support is allowed. Fibrinolytic agents are being evaluated in the treatment of thrombophlebitis, but more extensive experience is needed. When severe vasospasm accompanies iliofemoral thrombophlebitis, early surgical removal of the thrombus may prevent gangrene.

Proximal venous ligation is recommended by some authorities in the treatment of thrombophlebitis, especially after a pulmonary embolus has occurred. Since some emboli originate in the thigh and pelvic veins, ligation of the superficial or common femoral veins has declined in popularity, while inferior vena cava plication or ligation is more favored. Venous ligation should be performed for pulmonary embolus if there is a contraindication to anticoagulant therapy, if complications from anticoagulant therapy develop, or if pulmonary embolism recurs despite adequate anticoagulation. In patients too ill for surgery, an umbrella filter may be inserted in the inferior vena cava through a subclavian vein.

Prophylaxis against phlebitis in bedridden or surgical patients can be practiced by frequent exercise of the extremities, the use of mildly compressive elastic stockings, and the administration of anticoagulants. Anticoagulation therapy is the only treatment that has been shown to be of definite value. Recent studies tagging clots with radioisotope-labeled fibrinogen indicate that there is a reduced incidence of postoperative thrombi if low-dose (clotting time not affected) subcutaneous heparin prophylaxis is started before surgery.

DISEASES OF THE PERIPHERAL LYMPHATIC VESSELS

Lymphangiitis
Lymphangiitis is an acute or chronic infection of the lymphatic vessels. A small reddened patch appears at the source of infection and spreads upward toward regional lymph nodes as red, warm, firm, tender streaks. The lymph nodes become swollen and tender. Other symptoms and signs may include severe chills, fever, and malaise. The commonest cause is strepto-coccal infection; skin ulcers and areas of trichophytosis are common portals of entry. An idiopathic variety of lymphangiitis occurs in which organisms cannot be cultured. Treatment consists in rest, local applications of moist heat, specific chemotherapy or antibiotics, and drainage of the infected foci.

Lymphedema
Lymphedema is characterized by a slowly progressive enlargement of a limb with soft edema that later becomes fixed due to fibrosis. The skin becomes thick, coarse, folded, and hard; in the late stages the descriptive term *elephantiasis* is used. Recurrent episodes of lymphangiitis are often present. Primary (idiopathic) lymphedema is classified into three types: (1) congenital or familial (Milroy's disease), (2) praecox, affecting girls, usually at puberty, or (3) tarda (occurring after the second decade). The pathologic changes relate to aplasia, hypoplasia, or varicose dilatation of the lymph vessels. Secondary lymphedemas may be either noninflammatory (e.g., due to invasion of lymphatics by malignancy or surgical removal of nodes) or inflammatory (e.g., due to infections or thrombophlebitis). Diagnosis may be confirmed by lymphangiography.

Treatment of lymphedema consists in elevation of the extremity, use of elastic compression, administration of diuretics, and a low-salt diet. Eradication of infection in recurrent lymphangiitis is important. Advanced cases may require radical surgical removal of tissue (modified Kondoleon operations).

Bibliography

Aneurysms and Dissecting Aneurysms
Anagnostopoulos, C. E., Prabhaker, M. J. S., and Kittle, C. F. Aortic dissections and dissecting aneurysms. *Am. J. Cardiol.* 30:263, 1972.
Crane, C. Arteriosclerotic aneurysm of the abdominal aorta. *N. Engl. J. Med.* 253:954, 1955.
Joyce, J. W., Fairbairn, J. F., II, Kincaid, O. W., and Juergens, J. L. Aneurysms of the thoracic aorta: A clinical study with special reference to prognosis. *Circulation* 29:176, 1964.

Diseases of the Peripheral Blood Vessels
Amery, A., Deloof, W., Vermylen, J., and Verstraete,

M. Outcome of recent thromboembolic occlusions of limb arteries treated with streptokinase. *Br. Med. J.* 4:639, 1970.

Askey, J. M. Embolism and atrial fibrillation. *Am. J. Cardiol.* 9:491, 1962.

Atkins, P., and Hawkins, L. A. Detection of venous thrombosis in the legs. *Lancet* 2:1217, 1965.

Babb, R. R., Alarcon-Segovia, D., and Fairbairn, J. F., II. Erythermalgia: Review of 51 cases. *Circulation* 29:136, 1964.

Barritt, D. W., and Jordan, S. C. Anticoagulant drugs in treatment of pulmonary embolism: Controlled trial. *Lancet* 1:1309, 1960.

Byrd, R. B., Divertie, M. B., and Spittell, J. A. Bronchogenic carcinoma and thromboembolic disease. *J.A.M.A.* 202:1019, 1967.

Coffman, J. D., and Cohen, A. S. Total and capillary fingertip blood flow in Raynaud's phenomenon. *N. Engl. J. Med.* 285:259, 1971.

Coffman, J. D., and Mannick, J. A. Failure of vasodilator drugs in arteriosclerosis obliterans. *Ann. Intern. Med.* 76:35, 1972.

Edwards, E. A. Recurrent febrile episodes and lymphedema. *J.A.M.A.* 184:858, 1963.

Gifford, R. W., Jr., and Hines, E. A., Jr. Raynaud's disease among women and girls. *Circulation* 16:1012, 1957.

Jacobs, A. L. *Arterial Embolism in the Limbs.* Edinburgh: Livingstone, 1959.

Kinmonth, J. B. *The Lymphatics: Diseases, Lymphography and Surgery.* Baltimore: Williams & Wilkins, 1972.

McKusick, V. A., Harris, W. S., Ottesen, O. E., Goodman, R. M., Shelley, W. M., and Bloodwell, R. D. Buerger's disease: A distinct clinical and pathological entity. *J.A.M.A.* 181:5, 1962.

Mannick, J. A., and Coffman, J. D. *Ischemic Limbs.* New York: Grune & Stratton, 1973.

Meryman, H. T. Tissue freezing and local cold injury. *Physiol. Rev.* 37:233, 1957.

Mobin-Uddin, K., Collard, G. M., Bolooki, H., Rubinson, R., Michie, D., and Jude, J. R. Transvenous caval interruption with umbrella filter. *N. Engl. J. Med.* 286:55, 1972.

Schirger, A., Harrison, E. G., Jr., and Janes, J. M. Idiopathic lymphedema: Review of 131 cases. *J.A.M.A.* 182:14, 1962.

Washburn, B. Frostbite. *N. Engl. J. Med.* 266:974, 1962.

Wessler, S., and Yin, E. T. Theory and practice of minidose heparin in surgical patients. *Circulation* 47:671, 1973.

28

Coronary Artery Disease

Athanasios P. Flessas and Thomas J. Ryan

Coronary artery disease may cause no symptoms at all, or, conversely, it may produce myocardial ischemia that is clinically expressed as angina pectoris, arrhythmias, myocardial infarction, congestive heart failure, or sudden death. Ischemic coronary artery disease may be referred to as either ischemic heart disease or coronary heart disease. In this presentation, the term *coronary artery disease* will denote both asymptomatic and symptomatic conditions.

Pathology

In almost all cases, coronary artery disease is due to intimal atherosclerosis (see Chap. 26). Nonatheromatous lesions include various arteritides; embolism; coronary ostial stenosis due to syphilitic aortitis, aortic atherosclerosis, or calcification; dissecting aneurysms; and congenital anomalies of the coronary arteries. Thickening of the coronary arteries has also been observed in gargoylism (Hurler syndrome), the Marfan syndrome, and in homocystinuria.

In patients with clinical manifestations of coronary artery disease (angina pectoris, myocardial infarction, or sudden death), significant atherosclerotic lesions obstructing more than 70 percent of the lumen may be present in only one artery (20 to 30 percent of cases), or such lesions may be found in two (40 percent of cases) or three arteries (30 percent of cases). In patients with angina pectoris uncomplicated by myocardial infarction there is usually more than 50 percent, but not total, obstruction. Even total obstruction may occur without producing a myocardial infarction, especially when there are well-developed collaterals. In the majority of transmural myocardial infarctions the underlying pathology is the total obstruction of an artery by a thrombus formed when a significantly obstructing atheromatous plaque ruptures on its endothelial surface. Nontransmural myocardial infarctions are uncommon after such total obstruction; they usually follow a subtotal obstruction of the vessel. Sudden coronary death is usually the result of electrical instability resulting from ischemia. In about 60 percent of cases of sudden death and in about 35 percent of acute myocardial infarctions, acute coronary changes (plaque, rupture, thrombus formation or, rarely, hemorrhage inside the plaque) are seen.

The ultimate effect of any coronary artery obstructive lesion is to compromise coronary blood flow and myocardial oxygen supply. Whereas the oxygen requirements of skeletal muscle are met both by an increase in arterial inflow and by a greater extraction of oxygen from each unit of blood passing through the capillaries (venous oxygen content decreasing from 12 to 5 volumes per 100 ml or less on exercise), the venous blood of the heart, even under normal "resting" (working) conditions, contains only 2 to 5 volumes of oxygen per 100 ml. Therefore, when oxygen demands increase in the heart, they must be met mainly by augmented coronary flow. In addition, the myocardium is especially vulnerable to oxygen lack because of its very limited (up to 1 minute) supplies of phosphate anhydrite energy bonds, which make it unable to generate sufficient anaerobic glycolysis. Finally, in a physiologic or functional sense the coronary arteries are end arteries, and while they do have fine communications of an arteriolar nature, these are of limited value and cannot prevent an infarction when a large coronary artery is suddenly occluded.

Normal coronaries can increase their flow five times above resting values, but manifestations of myocardial hypoxia will appear whenever the increase cannot meet the myocardial demands. There is a dynamic interplay between oxygen supply and demand in which a number of factors should be considered. Oxygen supply depends on (1) the patency of coronary vessels, (2) the diastolic aortic pressure, (3) the oxygen-carrying capacity of blood, and (4) the collateral circulation. As already stated, the patency of the coronaries is affected primarily by atherosclerotic obstructive lesions. Arterial spasm superimposed on asymptomatic stenosis may precipitate acute anoxia in a few patients; however, in the vast majority its role has not been elucidated. As an obstruction becomes more critical, the flow depends more on the aortic diastolic pressure; and the flow will fall critically if the diastolic pressure drops below 60 mm Hg.

This explains why hypotension, sometimes precipitated by an arrhythmia, may aggravate symptoms of ischemia. A decrease in the oxygen-carrying capacity of the blood, such as occurs in anemia, also may aggravate or even precipitate symptoms in otherwise asymptomatic coronary obstructions. The development of collateral vessels distal to an obstructive lesion may compensate to a limited extent for an obstruction. Through a mechanism not well understood but possibly related to recurrent ischemia, the collaterals enlarge until they can fill the stenotic or occluded vessel retrogradely. Such compensation by collaterals is highly variable, depending on a number of factors, including the rate of progression of the obstructive lesions, the development of obstruction in the collateral vessels, the location of the original obstruction, and whether there is disease in the vessel distal to the original obstruction. Many patients do not have time to develop collaterals, while in others an existing compensation may become disturbed by further progression of disease.

Myocardial oxygen demands vary considerably and are determined grossly by the mass of the myocardial tissue and the work of the heart. In some forms of myopathy, aortic stenosis, and aortic regurgitation, the myocardial mass is great and the oxygen demands are high even at rest. Exercise increases the demands until even fully patent coronary arteries may not meet them, with the result that typical angina pectoris may occur. For a given myocardium, oxygen consumption varies with heart rate, contractility, and wall tension (a function of heart size and systolic intracardiac pressure). Thus tachycardia, thyrotoxicosis, anxiety, or hypertension all may precipitate or exaggerate anoxia.

Clinical Manifestations

ANGINA PECTORIS

Angina pectoris (AP) is a clinical symptom indicative of myocardial ischemia. It may be the first clinical manifestation of coronary disease. Indeed 38 percent of the new coronary events in men and 62 percent of new coronary events in women are AP attacks unassociated with myocardial infarction (uncomplicated AP). Angina pectoris may also appear shortly before or sometimes after a myocardial infarction (complicated AP). Half the men and 15 percent of the women with AP have had a myocardial infarction in the past. The overall incidence both of complicated and uncomplicated AP is twice as high in men as in women, with women lagging behind by 10 years; but after age 60 there is little difference between the sexes in incidence of AP.

Typical Angina Pectoris

Typical AP was described by Heberden as follows: "They who are afflicted with it, are seized, while they are walking (more especially if it be uphill and soon after eating) with a painful and most disagreeable sensation in the breast, which seems as if it would extinguish life, if it were to increase or continue, but the moment they stand still, all this uneasiness vanishes." Thus effort or an equivalent of effort such as anger precipitates AP, while rest relieves it. Walking in cold weather, particularly against a cold wind or after eating, or effort that involves the use of the arms above the head, is especially liable to precipitate AP. Angina pectoris may occur on relatively light effort early in the day and yet not be evoked by more strenuous effort later on. Chest discomfort that appears sometime after rather than during the physical effort is unlikely to be due to AP. The location of the discomfort, though generally in the anterior or posterior chest, is not crucial for the diagnosis, provided it is not confined to the lower extremities or head. Thus pain may represent AP even if it is confined to or located predominantly in the upper extremities or the abdomen, provided it is induced by effort or emotion and is relieved by rest. Pain limited to the left axilla or beneath the left breast is seldom caused by coronary artery disease.

The character of the discomfort in AP may be described in different ways, for example, as dull pain, pressure, tightness, heaviness, or burning. Sometimes it is described as shortness of breath with a sense of constriction around the larynx or upper trachea. A characteristic feature is the build up or gradual increase in the intensity of the anginal pain, which is followed by a gradual fading away of the sensation. Certain features of a chest discomfort weigh heavily against the diagnosis of AP. Angina is seldom described as "catching" or "stabbing" and is seldom affected by changes in posture or by deep breathing. In describing the discomfort, the patient with AP tends to indicate a sizable area of discomfort with his whole hand or his clenched fist. The designation with a single finger is unusual with true AP. Anginal pain is usually a few minutes in duration, with extremes lying between 30 seconds and 30 minutes. Shorter or longer durations argue against the diagnosis. Radiation of the pain is not essential for a diagnosis, but radiation to the upper extremities, predominantly to the inner aspect of the left arm, is helpful in excluding certain other possible causes. However, left arm radiation is not specific for AP, since this may also be due to cervical radiculitis or to injury or strain of the pectoral muscle. With AP, radiation to the jaws, teeth, or face is more specific but is relatively infrequent. The relieving effect of sublingual nitroglycerin is often helpful in the diagnosis and is a positive sign of AP, but it may require numerous trials to be sure, with careful timing of the duration of pain. The effect of nitroglycerin is apparent within 1 to 2 minutes and should come at the time the patient feels fullness or aching in the head. One should recognize that even severe attacks of AP may not respond even to several sublingual nitroglycerin tablets and that atypical forms of angina may appear to respond to a placebo.

Atypical Angina Pectoris
Atypical AP is a poorly defined syndrome with some or all the characteristics of true AP except for the clear relation to effort. In addition, chest pains similar to AP may arise from diseases of the pericardium, pleura, lungs, esophagus, abdominal organs, muscles, joints, spine, and nerve roots. Atypical AP also usually differs from typical angina in its quality, duration, location, radiation, and its lack of response to nitroglycerin.

Pathogenosis
Typical Angina Pectoris. Myocardial ischemia perceived as angina may be due to lesions in the coronary arteries, to functional causes (when no significant lesions are present), or to a combination of both. In a very small percentage of patients, no obvious cause

is ever found (angina pectoris with normal coronary arteries). The anatomic lesions have already been discussed (see earlier in this chapter, under Pathology).

Functional causes include aortic insufficiency, aortic stenosis, myopathies, or asymmetric septal hypertrophy with or without obstruction, all of which increase oxygen demand because of excessive hypertrophy of the myocardium. In pulmonary hypertension, a discomfort similar to angina pectoris is frequently observed; however, systemic hypertension in the absence of coronary artery disease is a very uncommon cause of AP. In cases of AP without myocardial infarction, there are usually no large fibrous scars in the myocardium, but small scars or increased areas of fibrosis are not uncommon.

Atypical Angina Pectoris. A small percentage of patients with atypical angina will show evidence during coronary angiography or at autopsy of obstructive lesions of their coronary arteries. Another few patients may have myopathy of any variety. It is also becoming increasingly evident that patients, mainly women, with prolapse of mitral valve leaflets may present with atypical AP. In the majority of patients with atypical AP, however, no underlying pathogenic mechanism can be found.

Left Ventricular Function
Left ventricular function as studied at cardiac catheterization is usually normal in AP without myocardial infarction, in spite of extensive coronary disease. The size and wall thickness of the left ventricle and the diastolic filling pressure are all normal. During systole, the wall contracts symmetrically and adequately, effecting a normal systolic emptying and a normal cardiac output. In about 20 to 30 percent of patients, a segment of the wall corresponding to the area of a critically narrowed artery does not move vigorously during systole. Such segmental abnormalities usually disappear after nitroglycerin therapy or following successful bypass surgery, indicating that the abnormalities were ischemic, not fibrotic. During either spontaneous or stress-induced AP, a number of other abnormalities may be seen; segments of the left ventricular wall that contract normally at rest fail to contract during the AP, and the stroke volume falls

significantly. There is also a sharp elevation of the diastolic filling pressure of the ventricle, probably due to incomplete relaxation of the myocardium. Such reversible left ventricular dysfunction helps explain the transient shortness of breath, gallop rhythms, and occasional systolic apical murmurs often found during attacks of AP. Another interesting and diagnostically helpful phenomenon found during AP is an increase in heart rate and blood pressure, which may appear even before the pain; the cause is unknown.

Natural History
Following the initial occurrence of AP, one of the following courses may develop:

1. Stable angina precipitated by essentially the same factors day after day.
2. Spontaneous disappearance of AP. Some patients with AP (30 percent in some reports) will spontaneously stop having symptoms. Various reasons are given for this; for example, elimination of contributing factors, development of collaterals, and unrecognized myocardial infarctions that replace the ischemic myocardial segment by a scar. Fifteen percent of patients who have a myocardial infarction lose their anginal symptoms; patients who develop congestive failure generally do not continue to have AP.
3. Myocardial infarction. It is difficult to predict which anginal patient will develop a myocardial infarction. Almost all anginal patients who do develop myocardial infarction do so after a period of acceleration of symptoms; silent myocardial infarction is extremely rare in these patients.
4. Sudden death. Almost half the deaths occurring in patients with AP are sudden and unexpected, and such deaths are threefold to fivefold higher in anginal patients than in the asymptomatic population.

Prognosis
The average annual mortality of patients with AP is 4 percent; women below the age of 60 have a slightly lower mortality. The prognosis in a given patient can be approximated best by studying the coronary anatomy and left ventricular function with coronary angi-

ography and left ventriculography. Patients with obstructive lesions in only one coronary artery have a low annual mortality (1 percent if the occlusion is subtotal; 2 percent if it is total). However, even minimal disease in a second vessel doubles the mortality. Total occlusion of one vessel with good distal collaterals has an annual mortality of 1.5 percent, but without collaterals it may have as high as an 8 percent mortality in older men. Single-vessel disease has a higher mortality when it involves the left anterior descending coronary artery than when it involves the right coronary artery. Significant obstructive lesions of two main vessels carry an annual mortality of 7 percent, and of three vessels, 11 percent. Any degree of left ventricular dysfunction increases the mortality; severe left ventricular dysfunction with congestive heart failure has a 1-year mortality of 50 percent and a 5-year mortality of 85 percent.

Diagnosis
Patients with typical AP usually have a vivid recollection of their first attack, whereas patients with atypical symptomatology are vague about it. One should remember that patients with typical angina may also have chest pains due to other causes (musculoskeletal, etc.) and that during the course of the disease the angina may change its characteristics. The differentiation of typical AP from noncoronary causes and from atypical angina is based in part on observations by the physician of changes in heart rate, blood pressure, and the ST and T waves of the ECG during an attack. Even when typical angina is clearly present, one must still rule out noncoronary conditions that may produce it: aortic stenosis; asymmetric septal hypertrophy, with or without obstruction; aortic regurgitation; some forms of myopathy; and pulmonary hypertension. The diagnosis of all these is usually easy, although echocardiography is required to diagnose asymmetric septal hypertrophy. When one of the above conditions is present with AP, there may also be coexistent coronary artery disease. For example, as many as 50 percent of patients with aortic stenosis and AP have coexistent coronary artery disease. Only coronary angiography can differentiate between coronary and noncoronary causes of AP. When a patient has typical AP and all the above con-

ditions have been ruled out, coronary atherosclerosis may be diagnosed with exceptionally high accuracy.

A positive exercise ECG response adds some certainty to the diagnosis of AP (95 percent of patients with a typical history and a positive exercise response do have significant obstructive coronary lesions). However, a few patients with normal coronaries and the typical AP history may have a positive exercise response (see Chap. 32). When AP is atypical, one must rule out possible diseases of chest and abdominal organs that may be responsible for the pain (chest pain syndromes), including

1. Hiatal hernia, which may produce a burning or compression over the lower sternum, often at night in the recumbent position or on bending over. As a rule, the symptoms have no relation to effort, but when there is a serious doubt, exercise electrocardiography or even coronary arteriography may be needed to settle the issue.
2. The Tietze syndrome (costochondral inflammation), which is recognized by swollen, tender costochondral junctions.
3. Posthepatic neuralgias.
4. Injury or strain of the pectoral muscle.
5. Pleurodynia caused by viruses; pleurisy; diseases of the lungs, spine, or nerve roots; or pericarditis.
6. Pulmonary embolism.
7. Aneurysms of the thoracic aorta.

If all the above conditions can be ruled out, one must consider the possible cardiac disorders that can present as atypical AP. These include the myopathies and prolapse of the mitral valve leaflet. A negative exercise ECG lessens the probability that coronary disease is the cause of angina to only about 10 percent and justifies the physician in not proceeding with coronary angiography. A positive exercise test indicates a 30 per cent probability of coronary disease and may justify coronary angiography in order to make the final diagnosis.

Management

Asymptomatic patients who have either multiple risk factors for coronary disease or a positive exercise ECG response must be considered to have asymptomatic coronary artery disease, because they are very likely to develop clear-cut clinical manifestations in the future. It should be obvious, however, that not all these individuals inevitably develop clinical manifestations. Therefore, a tight control of the risk factors may be helpful in these patients. The onset of symptoms of AP in a previously asymptomatic patient is a critical matter for two reasons: First, some patients will rapidly accelerate their symptoms and develop myocardial infarction or sudden death. When chest pains become frequent, appear with minimal effort, or occur at rest, the patient should be hospitalized. The second reason is that a definitive diagnosis is required because of its crucial importance to the patient. The physician should take the time to make such a diagnosis, and the patient should keep a detailed diary of his activities and episodes of discomfort. A clear-cut relation between activity and discomfort establishes the diagnosis. Once the diagnosis of AP has been established and the pattern is relatively stable, the following therapeutic approach is indicated:

1. Elimination or moderation of aggravating factors: anemia, hyperthyroidism, hypertension, excessive weight, and physical and emotional stress.
2. Control of risk factors: cigarette smoking, hypercholesterolemia, diabetes mellitus (see Chap. 26).
3. Drug therapy.

Nitrates. Sublingual nitroglycerin (glyceryl trinitrate) is the most commonly used preparation for the relief of angina, and there is no convincing evidence that any other nitrate offers additional benefits. Its overall effects include arterial dilatation, relaxation of the capacitance vessels, decrease in the venous return, decrease in the filling pressure of the ventricles, and decrease of the diastolic size of the heart. The cardiac output falls, as does the systolic arterial pressure, and there is a decrease in heart wall tension. As a result, both cardiac work and oxygen requirement decrease; and these decreases are considered to be the main benefits of nitrates.

Although nitrates dilate the coronary arteries, they do not increase the coronary blood flow. However, they do redistribute blood flow through collaterals to ischemic areas and improve the perfusion of the subendocardium. They also improve the exercise capacity of patients with AP before they experience angina. Furthermore, nitrates diminish the ST segment depression seen in the ECG during exercise. The effects of nitroglycerin should begin within 1 to 2 minutes and last 30 to 60 minutes except for the improvement in exercise capacity, which does not last longer than 20 minutes. However, nitroglycerin may be given cutaneously as a 2% ointment in a dose of about 5 mg, thus providing much longer hemodynamic effects and an improvement in the exercise capacity for up to 3 hours. Patients also learn to use nitroglycerin not only for relief of pain but also prophylactically, *before* undertaking physical effort that might precipitate angina.

Nitroglycerin is volatile and deteriorates unless kept tightly sealed. Isorbide dinitrate and erythrityl tetranitrate may also be given sublingually, but there is no convincing evidence that they are of any additional benefit over nitroglycerin. Isorbide dinitrate and erythrityl tetranitrate are also available for oral use, but because nitrates given orally are degraded in the liver and their effective levels cannot be predicted, their overall hemodynamic effects are less reliable than those produced by sublingual preparations, although occasionally their actions may be longer.

Beta-adrenergic Receptor Blocking Drugs. As a group, these agents decrease resting heart rate, cardiac output, and myocardial oxygen consumption. These effects give them a prophylactic action against AP and increase exercise tolerance. Propranolol is the drug used almost exclusively in this country; its therapeutic action is determined mainly by its plasma level, which can vary widely among individuals treated with the same dose orally. Therefore the effective dose of propranolol has to be determined in each patient by starting with 10 mg four times per day and increasing the dose as necessary up to 100 mg four times per day. Rarely will larger doses be needed, and some therapeutic effect should be seen with smaller doses such as 40 to 80 mg four times per day. Though propranolol is effective prophylactically against AP, there is no evidence that it alters the overall prognosis of patients with coronary disease.

Side effects are observed in about 9 percent of patients on oral propranolol; these include precipitation of congestive heart failure, hypotension, shock, and various degrees of atrioventricular block. Deaths reported soon after its intravenous use in critically ill patients have been attributed to either complete heart block or shock. It is interesting that most of the cardiovascular complications during oral administration occur with very small doses and during the first days of treatment in patients with already compromised left ventricular function. Treating these patients first with digitalis and diuretics corrects the failure and allows propranolol to be used with relative safety. Asthma is another contraindication for propranolol, which aggravates it. Rare side effects include fatigue, decrease of libido, nightmares, depression, and gastrointestinal irritability.

Surgical Treatment
Aortocoronary bypass operations using saphenous veins (and less often internal mammary arteries) are now being performed with increasing frequency and less than a 5 percent mortality. The rationale for bypass operations is that atherosclerotic lesions are usually focal and involve (at least in the left anterior descending coronary artery) mainly the proximal parts of the vessel. This, of course, is not always the case, especially in the right coronary artery, and therefore widespread disease imposes limitations on surgery in some patients. Another limitation is imposed by large myocardial scars, which cannot be revitalized after revascularization. The main indication for bypass operation is AP, especially accelerated AP that is not controlled by medical treatment and which interferes with the capacity of a patient to work and enjoy life. With improvement in surgical techniques and experience, about 80 percent of the grafts remain patent indefinitely. Symptomatic improvement is evident in about the same percentage of patients, because there is a good correlation between graft patency and symptomatic improvement. Improvements in exercise capacity, exercise response, coronary flow response to exercise, and abnormalities of contraction have also been demonstrated postoperatively. However, a high incidence (up to 15 percent) of intraoperative myocardial infarction has been reported, and there is a high mortality in patients

with severely compromised left ventricular function. Also it is not clear as yet whether surgery actually improves long-term survival.

MYOCARDIAL INFARCTION

Myocardial infarction (MI), or ischemic necrosis of the myocardium, is due to interruption or severe compromise of the myocardial blood supply. A severe manifestation of coronary artery disease, it is not only associated with high mortality but also almost invariably compromises left ventricular function, and frequently it results in intractable congestive heart failure with a poor prognosis. Almost all instances of MI are atherosclerotic in nature. Myocardial infarctions do occur rarely in very young persons (usually below the age of 20) in whom subsequent coronary angiography fails to demonstrate coronary artery pathology.

Pathologic Changes

As MI develops, the involved muscle becomes pale gray while the surrounding tissue becomes hyperemic. The muscle cells degenerate and are infiltrated with polymorphonuclear leukocytes and red blood cells. Organization and gradual resorption of the necrotic material and its replacement with fibrous tissue ensue, and when healing is complete, a dense scar is the end result. In the first 2 weeks, when the infarcted myocardium is soft and weak, cardiac rupture may occur. If the resultant scar tissue does not give sufficient strength to the infarcted zone, a myocardial aneurysm may develop. Mural thrombi are often formed over the damaged endocardium and may lead to embolism.

Clinical Features

The characteristic feature generally dominating the clinical picture in MI is severe, prolonged chest pain, which is associated with restlessness, anxiety, and a fear of impending death. The pain may have the same distribution and radiation as AP, but generally it is more severe and prolonged, usually persisting for more than 30 minutes. The initial pain of myocardial infarction then usually subsides within a few hours and, except for some residual soreness, is gone almost always within 24 hours. When chest pain persists

longer or recurs after the first day, a diagnosis of extending myocardial infarction is made unless pericarditis is present or pulmonary emboli have occurred. Unlike angina pectoris, MI as a rule is not precipitated by effort. Instead, more than half the cases occur during sleep or rest and only 2 percent during unusual effort. Myocardial infarction may develop either as a new event in otherwise asymptomatic patients (in men, 50 percent of the new coronary events are MIs) or in patients with previous symptoms of angina. Prodromal signs in the form of accelerating angina, marked fatigue, and shortness of breath are the rule in patients with preexistent AP, especially in those developing anterior infarctions. A significant number of patients develop so-called silent or symptomless infarctions as revealed by routine repeated electrocardiograms. Also, a significant number of MIs are dominated by symptoms of congestive heart failure, shock, and cerebrovascular accidents, with pain being minimal or absent.

On physical examination, there are no specific findings in uncomplicated MI. A low-grade fever and mild tachycardia are common during the first 24 to 72 hours. Paradoxical pulsations between the left sternal border and the apex may be felt in some patients, usually those with large infarctions complicated by heart failure. The first sound is faint, the second sound may be paradoxically split, and a fourth sound may be heard. In a number of cases a pericardial friction rub develops, becoming audible on the second or third day after the attack and persisting for a few minutes up to a number of days. Hemodynamic measurements during acute infarction have shown that the filling pressure of the left ventricle may be elevated in many patients who are not clinically in congestive heart failure and in whom cardiac output may be normal. Patients with symptoms of left ventricular failure have higher filling pressures and lower cardiac outputs.

Laboratory Studies

An increase in the white blood count to the range of 10,000 to 20,000 cells per cubic millimeter is observed during the first 24 to 48 hours of MI. Almost all patients have an increase in the erythrocyte sedimentation rate during the first 72 hours; this may persist for a number of weeks. Increase in the blood levels of various enzymes may also occur: serum glutamic oxaloacetic transaminase rises within 8 to 12 hours, reaches a peak in 18 to 36 hours, and declines to normal within 3 to 4 days; creatinine phosphokinase increases within 3 to 6 hours, reaches a peak in 12 to 24 hours, and declines to normal in 3 days; while lactic dehydrogenase rises in 24 to 48 hours, reaches a peak in 3 to 6 days, and declines to normal within 8 to 14 days.

Lipid Changes. Soon after the onset of infarction, free fatty acids increase considerably. An increase in triglycerides and a decrease in cholesterol follow. Therefore determinations of the lipids during the course of acute infarction may not give an accurate picture of the baseline lipid profile.

Electrocardiograms (see Chap. 32). The cardinal ECG sign of an acute MI is the development within the first 2 or 3 days of an abnormal Q wave (> 0.04 second) not present before the onset of the infarction. The ST segments are elevated immediately and return to baseline gradually in the next few days, usually within the first week. Persistence of ST elevation after the second week is suggestive of an aneurysm. The T wave may become very high in the first hours after infarction but soon becomes inverted and remains symmetrically inverted for a variable time, sometimes permanently.

Diagnosis
Diagnosis of acute MI is based on at least two of the three following criteria: (1) a history of chest pain consistent with myocardial ischemia; (2) an initially normal or abnormal ECG evolving over a period of 48 to 72 hours in a specific sequence that includes development of new Q waves in appropriate leads; (3) a characteristic rise and fall in the serum enzyme activities with no other obvious cause.

Completed Myocardial Infarction. The disappearance of cardiac pain (excluding pleural and pericardial pain) without pain-relieving drugs and associated with a decline in serum enzymes and a gradual fall in the elevated ST segments is suggestive that the infarc-

tion is essentially completed and that tissue repair is proceeding.

Complicated Acute Myocardial Infarction. Myocardial infarction is said to be complicated when one or more of the following is present on the fourth or fifth day:

1. Repeated attacks of typical ischemic pain; this increases the risk of extension of the infarction
2. Recurrence of pain with a second rise in enzymes and reelevation of the ST segments
3. Evidence of left ventricular failure after the first 48 hours
4. Cardiogenic shock
5. Significant mitral regurgitation or rupture of the intraventricular septum (usually associated with left ventricular failure)
6. Important disturbances of the cardiac rhythm (frequent ventricular ectopic beats; atrial, junctional, or ventricular tachycardia; atrial flutter or fibrillation; unexplained sinus tachycardia)
7. Second- and third-degree atrioventricular block and the new development of right or left bundle branch block
8. Severe ongoing pericarditis or pleurisy
9. Serious diseases of the lungs, kidney, gastrointestinal tract, impaired circulation to the brain or limbs, and peripheral venous thrombosis

Nontransmural Myocardial Infarction. When a typical clinical presentation and elevation of enzymes is not followed by abnormal Q waves in the ECG, the infarction is characterized as nontransmural. The T waves may become symmetrically inverted for a prolonged time, or the ST segments may be depressed. Pathologically, the whole thickness of the wall is not involved, only the inner and middle layers; thus the outer layer is left intact. Abnormalities of contraction are limited, and often left ventricular contraction is normal; arrhythmias occur as with transmural infarcts, but heart failure and shock are less frequent.

Right Ventricular Infarction. Right ventricular infarction is relatively rare (14 percent of all infarcts), in spite of the common involvement of the right coronary artery. In most instances an associated infarct of the left ventricle is present, and left ventricular dysfunction dominates the clinical picture. Rarely, the right ventricle only or predominantly is affected, and right ventricular dysfunction and failure are the dominant signs.

Atrial Infarction. Atrial infarction is rarely diagnosed but may be suspected from shifts in the P-Q interval in the ECG and frequent supraventricular arrhythmias.

Complications

Mild to Moderate Congestive Heart Failure. Congestive heart failure (CHF) is seen in about 40 percent of acute MIs, and severe failure (Class III — pulmonary edema) occurs in about 10 percent of cases; chest roentgenograms are helpful in evaluating the severity of CHF (see Chap. 31). Congestive heart failure is treated with diuretics and digitalis; nitrates and sodium nitroprusside may be helpful in reducing the pulmonary congestion. The overall prognosis of CHF with MI is grim, as compared with a mortality of about 5 percent when there is no CHF; Class II CHF has a mortality around 20 percent and Class III CHF, about 40 percent.

Cardiogenic Shock. Cardiogenic shock is similar clinically to shock from other causes (see Chap. 31). As a complication, it occurs in only 12 percent of acute MIs, but it has a mortality approaching 90 percent. Some patients develop shock at the onset of MI and may die within minutes or a few hours. A second group of patients develop shock in the hospital, secondary to a cardiac arrest with an extension of the infarction; or their shock may arise through relatively slow deterioration and progressive hypotension, oliguria, and central nervous system depression. Shock may be precipitated by other factors such as abnormalities of heart rate or rhythm, hypovolemia due to low intake or excessive loss of fluids, hypoxemia, or acidosis. If these are corrected and the patient continues to exhibit the shock syndrome, then and only then is a diagnosis of cardiogenic shock appropriate.

Treatment of shock involves careful monitoring of the filling pressures of the left ventricle and cardiac output while all contributing factors, especially hypovolemia, are corrected. Although widely used, catecholamine therapy does not improve the prognosis. Circulatory assist using the intraaortic balloon pump may be helpful in temporarily improving the hemodynamic abnormalities and allowing time for emergency coronary angiography and bypass surgery.

Rupture of the Intraventricular Septum. This rupture accounts for 2 percent of infarction-related deaths (see Chap. 30). It is usually associated with an anteroseptal MI, and it occurs near the apex of the septum, primarily within the first week. The patient's condition suddenly deteriorates, and a loud pansystolic murmur and associated thrill appear along the lower left sternal border. Clinically, rupture of the intraventricular septum is difficult to distinguish from mitral incompetence complicating acute MI, and in fact the two conditions sometimes coexist. Surgical closure of the defect may be attempted after 6 weeks; the mortality of early operation has been reported to be as high as 56 percent.

Mitral Regurgitation. This finding displays varying severity and is common during the course of an MI (see Chap. 30). It may be due to transient ischemia of a (usually posterior) papillary muscle; or it may be caused by permanent necrotic or fibrotic changes in one or two papillary muscles. Mitral regurgitation may also occur with left ventricular aneurysms or extreme dilatation of the left ventricle. Complete rupture of a papillary muscle is very rare (1 percent of fatal infarctions) and results in sudden deterioration with pulmonary edema and shock. Rupture of chordae tendineae causes less deterioration and may allow time for surgical repair.

Rupture of the Heart. This has been reported to be the cause of death in 4 to 13 percent of fatal cases of acute MI and is a less frequent cause of death than cardiogenic shock or arrhythmias. It occurs within 2 weeks of onset (50 percent within the first 3 days), and the anterior wall is usually involved. Hemopericardium, cardiac tamponade, and death follow within a short time.

Ventricular Aneurysm. This event complicates MI in 20 to 25 percent of cases, and four out of five of these aneurysms occur in the anterior wall and apex. Ventricular aneurysm may become apparent in the acute phase but usually is not evident for weeks, months, or years. Chest x-rays may show a distinct bulge of the left ventricle, or, more frequently, non-specific cardiomegaly. Paradoxical pulsations may be seen on fluoroscopy and felt in palpation of the precordium. Congestive heart failure, persistent ventricular arrhythmias, and arterial embolism are the main clinical manifestations. Aneurysmectomy may be performed, preferably 3 or more months following the MI. Untreated aneurysms have a 3-year mortality of more than 70 percent.

Thromboembolic Complications. These complications include pulmonary and systemic emboli and deep vein thromboses, which have been reported as occurring in 11 percent of MI cases in older studies. The incidence is probably lower at present due to early ambulation, the use of elastic stockings, and proper attention to hydration.

Postmyocardial Infarction Syndrome. This rare complication of MI includes unexplained fever, pleurisy, and pericarditis developing during the convalescent period. Another unusual complication is the development of pain and limitation of motion in the shoulder, arm, or hand (see Chap. 27).

Arrhythmias in Myocardial Infarction
Arrhythmias are common in MI and are almost invariably present in one form or another (see Chap. 32).

Atrial Tachyarrhythmias. Atrial tachyarrhythmias are estimated to occur in approximately one-fourth of patients with acute MI. Compromise of the circulation to the sinus node and heart failure are considered to be the main mechanisms.

Sinus tachycardia, seen in one-third of acute cases of MI, is mainly a reflection of heart failure, although fever, anxiety, pericarditis, and cardioaccelerator drugs may contribute. Sinus tachycardia is associated with a higher mortality, basically because it usually reflects failure. Treatment is of the underlying heart failure.

Atrial premature beats have been detected in 15 to 30 percent of myocardial infarctions, and they are frequently the harbinger of atrial tachyarrhythmias. No treatment is indicated.

Paroxysmal atrial tachycardia is seen in 1 to 2 percent of infarctions. If prolonged, it may induce hypotension or heart failure. Carotid sinus pressure, induced gagging, or the Valsalva maneuver may terminate the attack. Short-acting digitalis preparations (ouabain, 0.25 to 0.5 mg, or digoxin, 0.5 to 0.75 mg, given in divided doses of 0.1 and 0.25, respectively, over a 24-hour period) may be effective. Cardioversion may be necessary.

Atrial flutter is encountered in less than 5 percent of patients with acute infarction, and it frequently appears in the form of a 2 : 1 block with an effective ventricular rate of 150 beats per minute. Atrial flutter is usually resistant to digitalis, but it corrects easily with small shocks of 25 to 50 joules using synchronized DC cardioversion. However, digitalis in half its loading dose should be administered before cardioversion is attempted.

Atrial fibrillation occurs in 7 to 10 percent of acute infarctions (usually extensive). Digitalis is the treatment of choice, and if that fails, cardioversion should be tried. This arrhythmia may be intermittent, and if it recurs, the patient should have anticoagulation medication. Quinidine, 0.8 to 1.6 gm daily, and procainamide, 250 to 300 mg every 3 to 4 hours, may be used for control of arrhythmia along with digitalis. The first two medications are discontinued after discharge, but digitalis should be continued for several weeks.

Junctional (nodal) tachycardias in acute myocardial infarction are of two types, accelerated junctional rhythm and paroxysmal junctional tachycardia. The first type is an acceleration of a junctional pacemaker focus to rates of between 60 and 100 beats per minute. Paroxysmal junctional tachycardia, usually at rates of between 120 and 180 beats per minute, is seen rarely in infarction. Its significance is analogous to that of atrial arrhythmias in that it may occur spontaneously as a consequence of pump failure or (rarely) from digitalis intoxicity. The consequences of this arrhythmia are analogous to those of paroxysmal atrial tachycardia, and therapy is similar.

Ventricular Premature Beats (VPBs). In at least 80 percent of monitored patients, VPBs occur during acute MI. The hazards of VPBs, particularly when they occur in the vulnerable phase of the cardiac cycle, have been carefully investigated. Attention has been called to the importance of the ratio of the time interval between the Q waves of normally conducted beats and the R wave of the VPB compared to the Q-T interval of the normally conducted beat (Q-R$'$/Q-t ratio). It has been found that VPBs which occur with a Q-R$'$/Q-T ratio of 0.60 to 0.85 second are likely to precipitate ventricular tachycardia or fibrillation. The criteria for attempting supression of VPBs in the setting of MI are as follows:

1. When they occur with a frequency of more than five per minute
2. When they fall in the vulnerable phase of the cardiac cycle
3. When they are multifocal in origin
4. When they are coupled or occur in salvos

However, recent experience points out that ventricular fibrillation often occurs even in the absence of these criteria.

Ventricular Tachycardia. The incidence of ventricular tachycardia in acute infarctions is approximately 10 percent. Physical examination reveals intermittent cannon waves in the jugular venous pulse, varying intensity of the first sound, variation in the systemic peak blood pressure, and extra heart sounds consisting of atrial, ventricular, and summation gallop sounds. Ventricular tachycardia usually results in significant hemodynamic embarrassment with hypotension and heart failure, though a few patients with good left ventricular function are able to sustain fair vital signs for long periods. Lidocaine is the therapy of choice if the hemodynamic embarrassment is not serious. If ventricular tachycardia results in significant clinical deterioration, cardioversion with synchronized DC shock should be undertaken.

Ventricular Fibrillation (VF). Ventricular fibrillation is regarded as primary when it occurs suddenly and unexpectedly in patients with little or no ventricular failure. Secondary VF represents the end stage of progressive left ventricular failure or shock. Primary VF may occur in as many as 18 percent of acute infarctions, usually within the first 2 hours; its incidence declines exponentially with time subsequent to the onset of symptoms. Premonitory VPBs or other ventricular arrhythmias are not seen in many instances of VF, and it is recommended that all acute infarcts be treated with lidocaine in their early stages for prevention of VF. Though the prophylactic value of lidocaine has been demonstrated in some studies, different reports have indicated that VF may occur even during treatment with lidocaine. Primary VF may respond to DC shock, but the results of treatment are poor in secondary VF.

Sinus Bradycardia. The incidence of sinus bradycardia in monitored patients with acute MI ranges from 10 to 30 percent and is substantially higher in the early hours (40 percent). Inferior MIs are three times more frequently associated with sinus bradycardia than anterior. Pain and fear have been shown to be factors in producing reflex sinus slowing. Many drugs used for the treatment of the patient with acute MI also have the potential for slowing of impulse formation. Morphine with its vagomimetic action, tranquilizers with their central nervous system depression, and antiarrhythmics with their local anesthetic effects may all exert a negative chronotropic influence on the sinus node. However, this arrhythmia is not associated with a bad overall prognosis. Treatment consists first in alleviating the pain. In the majority of cases under observation in the coronary care unit, no other treatment is necessary. When hypotension, ventricular irritability, or heart rates below 40 beats per minute occur, atropine, 0.6 to 0.8 mg, may be given.

Sinus Pause. This arrhythmia includes the sinus arrest and sinus exit block, in which a sinus impulse does not reach the atrium. This arrhythmia is seen in 4 percent of acute infarctions and if persistent may require insertion of a temporary pacemaker.

Atrioventricular Block. Atrioventricular block in the setting of an acute myocardial infarction is highly influenced by the relationship of the conduction system to the obstructed coronary circulation and the resultant muscle necrosis. Pathologic studies of patients with inferior infarction and atrioventricular block have revealed necrosis either within or adjacent to the proximal conduction system. The extent of neither the infarction nor the necrosis of the conduction system need be great. In the setting of anterior infarction, however, pathologic studies of atrioventricular block have shown a pronounced extent of infarction and prominent necrosis of the distal conduction system.

In anterior infarction, progression to high degrees of block is usually sudden, resulting in the 2:1 or 3:1 pattern of second-degree type II block but often producing many consecutive nonconducted P waves. The idioventricular escape rhythm is slow, often with a bizarre morphology of wide QRS patterns. Syncope is much more likely than it is with inferior infarction and type I block. The development of atrioventricular conduction disturbances is two to three times more frequent in patients with inferior than in those with anterior MI. In the majority of patients, atrioventricular block lasts from a few hours to several days, with an average of 2 or 3 days. Complete block is associated with relatively low mortality in the absence of failure (20 percent), but there is a very high mortality when failure is present (80 percent). Currently the routine treatment of atrioventricular block is temporary pacing.

Prognosis
Half of the deaths in acute MI occur before the patient reaches the hospital; the in-hospital mortality of 10 to 20 percent is basically determined by the extent of the myocardial damage, both present and past. Older patients, those with previous infarctions, and those with anterior infarctions have a worse prognosis. The mortality of the uncomplicated MI is about 5 percent; complications such as those discussed above increase the mortality.

The long-term prognosis after an MI heals depends on both the extent of residual myocardial damage and the remaining coronary anatomy.

Treatment of Acute Myocardial Infarction
The benefits of coronary care units in preventing arrhythmia deaths in MI have been well established. Patients with clinical symptomatology suggestive of infarction should therefore be admitted to the coronary care unit within the shortest possible time. General measurements include relief of pain with morphine, administration of oxygen, mild sedation, adequate hydration, application of elastic stockings, prevention of constipation, and a bland, low-sodium, 1200-calorie diet.

Uncomplicated Myocardial Infarction. Starting 24 hours after the relief of pain, the patient is allowed to use a bedside commode, to dangle his feet by the side of the bed, and to sit in a chair for 15 minutes twice per day. He is encouraged to do mild exercises involving his ankles, knees, and abdominal and respiratory muscles. In 3 to 4 days he may be transferred to the general ward, and he is allowed to start gradual ambulation between the seventh and tenth days. After 2 to 3 weeks of total hospitalization, he may go home and gradually increase activity and resume work, at first on a part-time basis and then, after 1 or 2 months, full time.

Complicated Myocardial Infarction. The treatment of arrhythmias is based on the use of digitalis for supraventricular tachyarrhythmias; lidocaine is used to control ventricular tachyarrhythmias. When tachyarrhythmias cause hemodynamic embarrassment, DC cardioversion is used; and for atrioventricular blocks temporary pacing is employed. Atropine is used for severe sinus bradycardia. Because infarcted myocardium is sensitive to the arrhythmogenic complications of digitalis, digitalis preparations are given initially in only 50 to 70 percent of the recommended digitalizing dose. In using lidocaine, a loading dose as a bolus of 1 to 2 mg per kilogram of body weight is administered for quick therapeutic effect and is followed by an infusion of 2 to 3 mg per minute continuously for at least 24 hours after the last episode of arrhythmia. In rare cases in which lidocaine fails to suppress arrhythmias, procainamide, quinidine, or a combination of different antiarrhythmic drugs may be used. Persistent ventricular irritability requires continuous treatment with procainamide or quinidine during hospitalization and after discharge. In intractable ventricular tachyarrhythmias, rapid cardiac pacing either in the right atrium or right ventricle may suppress the irritability. Propranolol is rarely needed, and it is contraindicated in the presence of severe left ventricular failure.

Congestive heart failure may be treated with digitalis and diuretics. In addition, agents that decrease pulmonary congestion and left ventricular work may be used, such as nitroglycerin and sodium nitroprusside, especially if hypertension is present. Circulatory assist devices (diastolic counterpulsation using an intraaortic balloon pump) are used in cardiogenic shock, rupture of the interventricular septum, and severe mitral regurgitation. Emergency cardiac surgery may be necessary in cardiogenic shock, interventricular septal rupture, and mitral regurgitation not responding to medical treatment. Cardiac catheterization is necessary in these cases to determine whether there is enough viable myocardium left and to outline the coronary lesions, which will be bypassed during corrective surgery. Severe left ventricular dysfunction demonstrated during cardiac catheterization is a contraindication to surgery. In general, emergency surgery during acute myocardial infarction has a high mortality.

The controversy over the value of anticoagulant therapy has raged for the last 25 years. It is agreed that anticoagulants reduce the incidence of thromboembolic episodes during the acute phase. However, with the current tendency for early ambulation, most physicians omit anticoagulation. In complicated cases with prolonged confinement to bed, especially when congestive failure is present, anticoagulation has a place during the period of hospitalization.

SUDDEN CORONARY DEATH

Fifty to sixty percent of all deaths attributed to coronary artery disease are unexpected and occur suddenly. Of course, these do not include deaths clearly due to myocardial infarction. Among persons dying suddenly with severe coronary artery disease but no other cause to explain the death, 60 percent have no prior coronary symptoms. Forty percent of all deaths in symptomatic coronary patients are sudden. The cholesterol level is not clearly associated with sudden death, but cigarette smoking is strongly related; hypertension, ECG evidence of left ventricular hypertrophy, and excessive weight are also significant contributors. A small percentage of the victims — about 25 percent — have some warning symptoms on the day of death (angina, fatigue, or shortness of breath).

The mechanism of sudden death is arrhythmia. Ventricular fibrillation occurs in more than 70 percent of cases, and there are other serious arrhythmias in the remainder (asystole, complete atrioventricular block, ventricular tachycardia). New arterial lesions superimposed on chronic obstructive lesions have been demonstrated in about 60 percent of cases, and 60 percent of these are ruptures of a plaque. A fresh myocardial infarction may be found in about one-third of the cases.

CONGESTIVE FAILURE

Although multiple vessel involvement with repeated infarcts is usual in patients with coronary heart failure, very often a single infarct due to obstruction of only one vessel — commonly the left anterior descending coronary artery — may result in severe congestive failure. There is a direct relation between the extent of abnormal segmental contraction seen on ventriculography and the degree of left ventricular dysfunction. In the chronic state, the left ventricle first dilates and then hypertrophies to compensate for the segmental failure. If the segmental abnormalities are large, so that the ejection fraction falls below 40 percent (normal 65 percent), there is not enough healthy muscle left to hypertrophy and compensate. Mitral regurgitation, seen in almost 40 percent of cases after an infarct, and ventricular aneurysms may contribute further to a decreased cardiac output.

Congestive heart failure is seen clinically in about one-third of patients surviving an MI. Tachycardia, a third heart sound, basilar rales, venous hypertension, and cardiomegaly may be present. Very often, however, many of these signs are missing. It is also surprising that some patients with severe left ventricular dysfunction demonstrated by catheterization deny all symptoms of congestive heart failure. Pulmonary hypertension and right ventricular failure usually develop when the ejection fraction falls below 30 percent. The prognosis in sustained congestive heart failure is poor, with a 5-year survival of no more than 15 to 20 percent. Surgical treatment is indicated when an isolated, well-circumscribed aneurysm is present and the remaining myocardium contracts well. A mitral valve prosthesis may be inserted in patients with severe mitral regurgitation, provided overall left ventricular function is not significantly depressed.

Bibliography

Brutsaert, D. L., and Sonnenblick, E. H. Cardiac muscle mechanics in the evaluation of myocardial contractility and pump function: Problems, concepts and directions. *Progr. Cardiovasc. Dis.* 16:337, 1973.

Dunkman, W. B., Perloff, J. K., Kastor, J. A., and Shelburne, J. C. Medical perspectives in coronary artery surgery ... a caveat. *Ann. Intern. Med.* 81:817, 1974.

Flessas, A. P., Connelly, G. P., Handa, S., Tilney, C., Kloster, C. K., Rimmer, R. H., Keefe, J. F., Klein, M. D., and Ryan, T. J. Effects of isometric exercise on the end diastolic pressure, volumes and function of the left ventricle in man. *Circulation* 53:839, 1976.

Heberden, W. Some account of a disorder of the breast. *Med. Trans. R. Coll. Physicians* 2:59, 1772.

Kannel, W. B., and Feinleib, M. Natural history of angina pectoris in the Framingham study: Prognosis and survival. *Am. J. Cardiol.* 39:154, 1972.

Kuller, L., Lilienfeld, A., and Fisher, R. An epidemiological study of sudden and unexpected deaths due to arteriosclerotic heart disease. *Circulation* 34:1056, 1966.

Master, A. M., Dack, S., and Jaffe, H. L. Activities associated with the onset of acute coronary occlusion. *Am. Heart J.* 18:434, 1939.

Reeves, T. J., Oberman, A., Jones, W. B., and Sheffield, L. T. Natural history of angina pectoris. *Am. J. Cardiol.* 33:423, 1974.

Robinson, B. F. Relation of heart rate and systolic blood pressure to the onset of pain in angina pectoris. *Circulation* 35:1073, 1967.

Wolfson, S., and Gorlin, R. Cardiovascular pharmacology of propranolol in man. *Circulation* 40:501, 1969.

29

Congenital Diseases

Burton J. Polansky

The rapid advances in cardiac surgery within the last decade have radically altered the viewpoint of physicians toward the problems of congenital heart disease. Previous to the modern era of cardiac surgery, all that was required was a general diagnosis of congenital heart disease. Now, almost of necessity, both an accurate localization and a specific type of cardiac lesion must be defined. In the past, the great majority of patients with congenital cardiac lesions who reached adulthood either had mild abnormalities or had undergone simple surgical repairs that were almost completely curative for the uncomplicated, relatively minor defects then operated upon. Technical advances now enable the surgeon to attempt the correction of even the most complicated major defects. Thus many of the present generation of patients with congenital cardiac disease enter adulthood with complex corrected or palliated lesions. Such patients will present adult cardiologists and primary care physicians with new therapeutic challenges. These considerations demand a basic understanding of the anatomy, physiology, and natural history of congenital heart disease as well as a knowledge of the natural history of the postoperative problems that will now be encountered in ever-increasing numbers.

Incidence and Etiology

Congenital heart disease occurs in approximately 0.5 percent of all live births and constitutes 2 to 5 percent of heart diseases recognized after infancy. The etiology of the specific congenital heart lesions is unknown. Various environmental factors have been implicated, such as viruses that affect the mother during early pregnancy, and recently some drugs have been shown to cause a variety of congenital malformations. It is important to attempt a careful elucidation of all possible etiologic influences occurring during the first trimester, although this effort will often prove fruitless. Avoidance of both unnecessary medication and exposure to viral illness should be encouraged in early pregnancy. Certain lesions seem to be sex-related, such as patent ductus arteriosus and

atrial septal defects in girls or pulmonary stenosis and ventricular septal defects in boys. Other lesions are commonly seen in association with congenital syndromes such as Down's syndrome (ostium primum) and the Turner syndrome (coarctation of aorta or atrial septal defect). The familial recurrence rate of a congenital heart defect is estimated to be between 1 and 5 percent for the first offspring. This may be higher for some specific defects, particularly ventricular septal and atrial septal defects. Since in the past only patients with mild forms of congenital heart disease survived long enough to procreate, the longer life span now available to those with more severe defects may increase the familial incidence above that previously encountered. The clarification of genetic influences merits further study.

Diagnostic Techniques

A detailed history is vital in the diagnosis of congenital heart disease. The history-taking often serves to educate parents concerning important observations they can make but may easily overlook. Common occurrences such as cyanosis when crying, anoxic spells, squatting, excessive perspiration, recurrent respiratory infections, difficult feeding, and failure to thrive must be clearly documented. A prenatal history and a knowledge of earlier examinations (e.g., the time of the first appearance of a murmur) should be obtained along with a careful chronologic charting of the patient's growth and development.

PHYSICAL EXAMINATION
Examination should include close attention to the following points: blood pressure in both arms and legs; the presence of cyanosis, digital clubbing, arterial and venous pulsations in the neck, or thrills; the prominence of the chest wall (a left parasternal heave indicates right ventricular hypertrophy); and the position of the ventricular impulses. One should note the character and intensity of the heart sounds and the position, timing, intensity, and quality of any murmurs. Whenever possible, such murmurs should be identified completely — that is, not as "diastolic murmur" but as "a long decrescendo diastolic blowing murmur of grade 2/6 intensity, heard best at the left sternal border." Such descriptions denote careful,

thoughtful auscultation and leave little doubt that the examiner is describing aortic or pulmonary insufficiency and not a diastolic rumbling murmur of mitral or tricuspid stenosis. Particular emphasis should be placed on abdominal examination, since an enlarged liver may be due to congestive heart failure. If the femoral pulses are examined and compared to the radial pulses, the diagnosis of coarctation of the aorta will seldom be missed.

FUNCTIONAL OR NONSIGNIFICANT MURMURS

An important problem in the evaluation of patients in the pediatric age group is the evaluation of murmurs that may be of no significance. This problem is often magnified because the evaluation of the murmur is often made out of context, without any attention to the electrocardiogram or chest x-ray. Several points need to be emphasized in this brief discussion, and the interested reader is referred to the excellent discussions of this problem in the standard textbooks of pediatric cardiology (see Bibliography).

Murmurs in newborns are relatively rare and are more common in premature infants and in those with respiratory distress syndrome. At the age of 1 year the incidence of murmurs rises to approximately 7 percent, and in normal children and adolescents murmurs may be heard in anywhere from 30 to 50 percent. The classic concept has been to separate murmurs into two categories, functional versus organic, and to suggest further that systolic murmurs grade 3 or higher in intensity are often related to organic lesions, while diastolic murmurs of whatever intensity, either rumbling or blowing, have all been considered to be organic in nature. However, many loud systolic murmurs disappear with normal growth and development, and soft systolic murmurs, which indicate pulmonary stenosis, have a remarkably benign prognosis but should be appropriately considered organic. Furthermore, diastolic murmurs are heard in patients with idiopathic pulmonary regurgitation who have anatomically normal hearts. Probably the wisest course to follow in evaluation of murmurs in the pediatric group would be to properly describe the murmur in terms of its characteristics, make use of the electrocardiogram and the chest x-ray, and then designate the murmur as being either

significant or not significant at the time of a given evaluation. Certainly murmurs associated with cardiac symptoms, x-ray evidence of cardiac enlargement, pulmonary plethora, pulmonary overcirculation, or an abnormal electrocardiogram should be considered significant; and the statement previously made concerning the loudness of systolic murmurs and the significance of any murmur in diastole should be followed as a general rule.

The problem, then, basically relates to the analysis of murmurs of systole. Grade 1 murmurs are considered to be the faintest murmurs that can be heard and are usually heard only after a rather prolonged period of auscultation. Grade 2 murmurs are slightly louder than grade 1 murmurs and are usually heard immediately on auscultation. Grade 3 murmurs are those that are of moderate intensity. Grade 4 are loud murmurs often accompanied by a palpable thrill, and grade 5 are the loudest murmurs that can be imagined with the stethoscope on the chest. Grade 6 are murmurs that are heard with the stethoscope slightly off the chest wall.

The typical systolic murmur is then one of low intensity and of short duration, usually occupying midsystole, and it is most often best heard maximally along the left sternal border or at the apex and transmits poorly. These murmurs may show considerable variation from cycle to cycle, with respiration or changes in position, or on repeated examination. One murmur that has been characterized as insignificant is one that has a musical component to it or sounds like the plucking of a string.

The major problem that occurs is in the evaluation of a systolic murmur. The differential diagnosis, as mentioned elsewhere, usually rests between (1) a nonsignificant murmur that usually is generated in the pulmonary artery; (2) the murmur of mild pulmonary stenosis that occurs, of course, in the same area; and (3) the murmur of atrial septal defect, one of the more common types of congenital lesions that also is generated in the pulmonary artery. Helpful clues to the differentiation come from the chest x-ray, which may show pulmonary stenosis with poststenotic dilatation of the pulmonary artery, mild right ventricular hypertrophy, and evidence of reduced circulation to the lungs. Observations that would suggest that the murmur is related to atrial septal defect include pulmonary overcirculation, right ventricular dilatation, and wide fixed splitting of the second sound with incomplete right bundle branch block noted on the electrocardiogram.

Since mild pulmonary stenosis and atrial septal defect have very benign natural histories, there is usually no urgent need to seek full cardiac evaluation, and a period of follow-up is certainly indicated to decide whether or not the murmur is significant. This may even extend to a matter of years before an appropriate decision need be made to establish an exact etiologic diagnosis.

Finally, mention should be made of the murmur that is referred to as a venous hum, which is best heard just above the clavicle and is often continuous, occurring in both systole and diastole. This murmur is loudest with the patient sitting, is decreased by lying down, and is obliterated by compressing the cervical veins or by turning the head away from the side of the murmur. This murmur is often mistaken for patent ductus arteriosus. Bruits are often heard in the supraclavicular area, usually on the right side, and they may be transmitted toward the first and second interspace. These occasionally may be mistaken for the murmurs of aortic or pulmonic stenosis, but an important differential point is that they are always loudest in the neck. It should also be kept in mind that systolic murmurs, particularly those that sound like pulmonary ejection systolic murmurs, are common in pediatric patients, in whom there is a thin chest wall. These systolic murmurs are the same type that occur when extracardiac causes produce increased flow. Such causes include exercise, sinus tachycardia, hyperthyroidism, fever, anemia, and peripheral arteriovenous fistulas.

ELECTROCARDIOGRAPHY

The electrocardiogram is of great aid in the diagnosis of congenital heart disease. In children the electrocardiogram is not usually deranged by the changes of coronary heart disease, chronic lung disease, or rheumatic involvement. Thus the type and location of any overloading (right or left sided, systolic or diastolic) may be diagnosed in each case and fitted to the physiology of the lesion. The high voltages in the electrocardiograms of children often cause confusion between normal and abnormal tracings. Vectorcardiograms correlate well with the type of lesion and serve to clarify many of the electrocardiographic patterns. The electrocardiographic findings and their significance are briefly discussed below within the framework of each specific lesion.

X-RAY EXAMINATIONS

Special x-ray and fluoroscopic examinations are a necessary part of any complete cardiac evaluation. Specific information can be gained as to the size of the various chambers and the position and status of the great vessels. Of great importance is the analysis of the pulmonary vasculature. Left-to-right shunting lesions (atrial septal defect or ventricular septal defect) produce increased pulmonary arterial markings, while obstructive lesions at the level of the pulmonary valve (stenosis, tetralogy of Fallot) are associated with a marked reduction of the pulmonary vasculature. It should be constantly borne in mind that an enlarged chamber may be either dilated or both dilated and hypertrophied; hypertrophy alone will usually not be revealed either by an x-ray plate or by fluoroscopy. The anatomy of the congenital cardiac lesion often fits very well with the findings seen by x-ray.

CARDIAC CATHETERIZATION

Cardiac catheterization is invaluable in indicating the status and needs of a given patient with congenital heart disease, particularly when catheterization is combined with angiography, intracavitary phonocardiography, and electrocardiography. The risk of catheterization in careful hands is small, whereas the information gained from it permits the clinician to assess both the physiologic and the anatomic status of the patient and to determine the need and risks of surgery. The technique for catheterization is outlined in many texts, and it is sufficient to note here that all the chambers of the heart may be entered so that pressure tracings and blood samples for gas analysis can be obtained. The pressure tracings give important information as to the presence and severity of obstructive lesions. The measurement of cardiac output may be made either by the Fick principle or by the use of dye-dilution curves, and the size of each valvular orifice may then be calculated. Levels of oxygen saturation that change suddenly, for example, a sudden increase from right atrium to right ventricle, indicate that oxygenated blood is shunting from left to right. In a similar fashion, desaturation appearing suddenly on the systemic side indicates that there could be a shunt from right to left. By the application of appropriate hemodynamic formulas, the degree of shunting can be grossly estimated.

Dye-dilution techniques using a variety of different substances have become useful in the demonstration of shunts that might otherwise be missed. The basic principle involved is the selective injection of a foreign substance at one site and sampling at a site downstream for spectrophotometric analysis of any change in the concentration of the substance. The graph obtained is in essence a time-concentration curve from the distal sampling site. Shunting toward the downstream site produces a curve that rises earlier than normal. Conversely, shunting away from the downstream site produces a curve that is lower and more prolonged than normal. Dye-dilution techniques may also be used to evaluate valvular insufficiency, although angiography is more useful in this situation.

CINEANGIOGRAPHY
Cineangiography has proved to be an invaluable diagnostic tool in the clarification of both simple and complicated congenital heart defects. By means of selective catheterization of the cardiac chambers and great vessels, radiopaque dye can be injected at one or several sites, and the course of the flow of the dye can be followed by recording it on moving x-ray film. This permits a later, more leisurely study and analysis. Information can be obtained relative to shunting lesions (atrial septal defect, ventricular septal defect, or patent ductus arteriosus), obstructive lesions (pulmonary stenosis, aortic stenosis, coarctation), the size of individual chambers or vessels, and the relationship of the great vessels (tetralogy of Fallot, transpositions, and anomalous pulmonary venous drainage). Though small, the risk of both catheterization and cineangiography is real, and it is greatest in patients with pulmonary vascular obstruction.

ECHOCARDIOGRAPHY
Echocardiography, which is discussed elsewhere

(Chap. 30), has become an important adjunct to the analysis of congenital heart lesions. Although initial interest in this technique centered mainly on acquired heart disease, echocardiography is now becoming quite useful in congenital heart lesions because of its noninvasive nature and safety. It should be kept in mind that important differences exist between echocardiography in adult and in pediatric patients, such as the occasional necessity for sedation in order to obtain better cooperation in children and the ability to use a higher frequency transducer in infants, giving better resolution and less distortion of the ultrasonic beam. Since many congenital heart lesions sometimes involve malposition of cardiac structures, it is essential that the interpreter of an echocardiogram know the position of the transducer and the direction of the beam in every instance. Reference to the more common and accepted echocardiographic findings using the conventional single-crystal method will be made below, under the specific lesions.

Problems Peculiar to Congenital Heart Disease

CONGESTIVE HEART FAILURE
In the first year of life, congestive heart failure occurs commonly in patients with congenital heart disease. Frequent causative lesions are large ventricular septal defects, transposition of the great vessels, large patent ductus arteriosus, and coarctation of the aorta. Myocarditis and endocardial fibroelastosis must also be considered.

The recognition of congestive heart failure in an infant may be difficult, since the clinical picture differs from that in the adult. Fatigue when feeding is an early sign, from which follows a failure to gain weight. Tachypnea, tachycardia, and increasing cardiac size are important findings. Respiration is difficult, with marked use of accessory muscles and retraction of the ribs. Cough is common, as is diaphoresis. On physical examination, rales may or may not be heard in the lungs, and evidence of elevated venous pressure is lacking. One of the most reliable signs of congestive heart failure is an enlarged liver, which is often tender. Peripheral edema is uncommon. Repeated pulmonary infections are often seen in infants with congestive heart failure, making the diagnosis more difficult. Occasionally prophylactic administration of antibiotics will be found useful in such patients.

Therapy for congestive heart failure in children is essentially the same as for adults. Sedation, oxygen, proper positioning of the patient, digitalis and diuretics, as well as low-salt diets are all useful. The doses of the drugs vary according to the age and body weight of the patient. Adequate medical management of severely ill patients often gives gratifying results and permits the infant to develop so that further study and consideration of surgery may be postponed until the size of the child represents a more favorable risk.

FAILURE TO THRIVE

This is a common problem in many patients with congenital heart disease. In certain lesions, such as patent ductus arteriosus or ventricular septal defect with a large shunt, closure of the defect may result in the attainment of normal growth and development. Growth retardation is generally dependent on the anatomic lesion and its functional effects. Most children with mild defects grow normally, while those with more severe defects are retarded in their growth and may also exhibit deficiencies in motor skills and intellectual development. There is often an accelerated period of growth immediately after surgery, and this growth is more notable in patients who display congestive heart failure prior to operation. A persistent retardation in growth pattern in patients whose congenital lesions have been repaired is often the result of other associated congenital abnormalities. It should be noted that an increased incidence of scoliosis has been reported in young adults with congenital heart disease. It is therefore important that patients with a history of congenital heart disease be observed carefully before the eventual development of scoliosis, and this is particularly true of patients with cyanotic heart disease, coarctation of the aorta, or cardiomegaly, or of patients who have had previous open heart surgery.

PULMONARY VASCULAR OBSTRUCTION SYNDROME

This syndrome may occur as an isolated finding, but more commonly pulmonary vascular obstruction is seen in patients who have defects that cause left-to-right shunting. The incidence of this syndrome in all patients with congenital heart disease is probably 8 to 10 percent. The cause of the syndrome is unclear, and explanations of its pathogenesis have involved mechanisms that relate to the degree and duration of the shunting into the pulmonary vascular tree, to the height above sea level at which the patients live, or to the persistence of a fetal type of pulmonary arterial musculature. The major physiologic deficit is a greatly increased pulmonary resistance, usually at the arteriolar level. This increased pulmonary resistance in turn causes pulmonary hypertension and right ventricular hypertrophy. The pressure in the right ventricle ultimately approaches systemic levels, and cyanosis is quite common. These patients are referred to as having the Eisenmenger syndrome, which is discussed later in this chapter and at greater length. It should be noted that the findings of pulmonary hypertension and elevated pulmonary vascular resistance increase the risk of cardiac catheterization and may preclude the possibility of surgical correction in a given patient, because the mortality in such operations is greatly increased.

ELECTROCARDIOGRAM

A right bundle branch block pattern is commonly seen following corrective surgery that has involved a right ventriculotomy. Complete heart block may occur in some patients because of damage to the conducting system, and such block may require the insertion of an artificial pacemaker. Injury to the sinus node may result in postoperative arrhythmias, and this is most commonly seen in patients who have had total correction of transposition of the great arteries. In some instances, episodes of supraventricular tachycardia or ventricular ectopic beats will require long-term antiarrhythmic therapy, although this is unusual.

PROPHYLAXIS AGAINST SUBACUTE
BACTERIAL ENDOCARDITIS

It is well recognized that prophylactic administration of antibiotics is necessary in patients with various forms of uncorrected congenital heart disease in order to avoid the development of bacterial endocarditis (see Chap. 33). Bacterial endocarditis can occur following procedures that produce bacteremia, such as various types of surgery, dental manipulations, skin infections, and labor. Palliative cardiac surgery does not appear to decrease the incidence of bacterial endocarditis, and although there is not a large body of data available, it would seem worthwhile to seriously consider administering prophylactic antibiotics during risk periods to most patients with surgically corrected congenital heart disease. This would not be necessary in patients who have had repairs of patent ductus arteriosus or atrial septal defects without mitral valve abnormalities, since the incidence of bacterial endocarditis following these types of complete correction is almost nonexistent.

CEREBROVASCULAR ACCIDENTS AND THROMBOEMBOLISM

Cerebrovascular accidents and thromboembolism occur for the most part in patients with lesions that cause markedly reduced arterial oxygen tensions and severe cyanosis. Early repair of cyanotic heart disease therefore may contribute to a reduced incidence of these complications. Postoperative thromboembolism is unusual in patients with congenital heart disease, with the exception of those who have had mitral valve replacement (who should be on long-term anticoagulant therapy). The added risk of thromboembolism in patients with pulmonary vascular obstruction is great. Because of this risk, the use of oral contraceptives should be discouraged in any female patient with congenital heart disease and pulmonary vascular obstruction.

PHYSICAL ACTIVITIES

If surgery is primarily corrective and not palliative, there are often no postoperative deficits in cardiovascular function, particularly at rest, although some patients may exhibit an abnormal response to exercise. In general, hemodynamic abnormalities usually revert to normal following successful correction. Particular attention must be paid to patients who have residual aortic stenosis, since these patients, even after successful surgery, risk sudden death by engaging in rough competitive sports. An excellent summary regarding physical, recreational, and occupational guidelines for patients with congenital heart disease has been made available by the congenital

heart disease study group of the American Heart Association (see Bibliography).

Types of Congenital Lesions

ATRIAL SEPTAL DEFECTS

Interatrial communications usually have as their basic physiologic defect the shunting of blood from left to right.

Embryology and Anatomy. Early in intrauterine life the septum primum develops high in the roof of the common atrium and grows caudally, partitioning the common atrial chamber into right and left sides. This septum is incomplete caudally, leaving an opening (ostium primum) just above the atrioventricular valves that permits blood to flow from right to left, bypassing the lungs. As the process of atrial partition continues, another septum develops to the right of the septum primum (septum secundum) and grows in a crescent-shaped fashion leaving a large central opening (foramen ovale). The ostium primum of the septum primum then closes, while reabsorption occurs higher in the septum primum (ostium secundum). The right-to-left extrapulmonary flow of fetal blood thus proceeds through the foramen ovale and ostium secundum. Closure of the foramen ovale takes place toward the end of the first year of life but does not occur at all in 25 percent of normal hearts. If the foramen ovale is probe-patent, right-to-left shunting may occur, but only when pressure in the right atrium exceeds that in the left atrium. Usually the higher left atrial pressure serves to keep the valve of the foramen ovale functionally closed. The lower portions of the interatrial septum are believed to contribute some components to the upper portions of the interventricular septum, which may explain the common association of interatrial and interventricular septal defects in the so-called endocardial cushion defects.

Defects of the atrial septum allow shunting of blood from the left to the right atrium, thus overloading the right ventricle and the pulmonary vasculature. The major types of defects seen in the interatrial septum are those within the area of the foramen ovale; defects at the site of the ostium primum are less common, as are high defects in the area of the ostium secundum. Ostium primum defects are discussed in the section on endocardial cushion defects.

Physical Findings. Patients with atrial septal defects are usually asymptomatic and acyanotic. The male-female ratio is 1:2. On physical examination these patients are slender in build. The major auscultatory finding is a systolic murmur of the ejection type, grade 2/6 or 3/6, heard best along the left sternal border. This murmur is produced by the increased flow of blood across the pulmonary valve. There is delay of the pulmonary component of the second sound that is unchanged by inspiration. Thus a fixed split second sound is found in almost three-fourths of the cases. Thrills are rarely noted in atrial septal defect. There may be a middiastolic rumble heard close to the sternum, which is ascribed to a relative tricuspid stenosis due to the excess flow across the tricuspid valve.

Laboratory Studies. Electrocardiography reveals almost all patients with interatrial septal defect to have incomplete right bundle branch block and slight prolongation of the P-R interval (see Chap. 32). The finding of incomplete right bundle branch block is a common normal variation in children, but if congenital heart disease is believed to be present, this finding is of considerable aid in the differential diagnosis. Incomplete right bundle branch block is also seen in some patients with ventricular septal defect and in some patients with pulmonary stenosis.

X-ray examination usually reveals slight cardiac enlargement, often to the right, with prominence of the pulmonary artery along the left border of the heart and marked increase in the pulmonary vasculature. On fluoroscopy, these patients show bounding pulmonary arteries (referred to as hilar dance) because of the increased flow.

Cardiac catheterization reveals an increase in oxygen saturation in the atrium as compared to the venae cavae, with either normal ventricular pressures or slight elevations due to the increased flow. The presence of pulmonary hypertension is a late finding in atrial septal defect. The catheter may often be passed through the septal defect. If a left atrial injec-tion of radiopaque dye can be made, angiography will be of great aid in the diagnosis. Anomalous pulmonary venous drainage to the right atrium is not uncommon in atrial septal defect.

Echocardiographic Findings. The echocardiogram in atrial septal defect shows evidence of paradoxical septal motion and right ventricular enlargement, but these are nonspecific findings also seen in other conditions producing right ventricular overload.

Treatment. The natural history of atrial septal defects is more benign than that of many other congenital lesions. Because of this, atrial septal defect may be regarded as one of the commonest previously undiagnosed congenital lesions to be discovered in adult life. Pulmonary hypertension is a late finding. Early operation is not urgent. At present, patients with pulmonary flow twice that of systemic flow due to the left-to-right shunt should be operated on at an optimum time. As the mortality of the procedure continues to lessen, the number of smaller defects considered for operation will probably grow larger. Following surgery, most patients with atrial septal defect could be considered for all practical purposes to have normal hearts.

VENTRICULAR SEPTAL DEFECTS

Embryology and Anatomy. The ventricular portion of the embryonic heart quickly becomes separated into a right and left ventricular chamber by the development of the primitive septum, which in adult life becomes the muscular portion of the interventricular septum. Somewhat later the truncoconal complex shifts toward the midline and comes to lie above the muscular interventricular septum. Then components from the endocardial cushions, which are forming the mitral and tricuspid anuli, and components from the cristae, which separate the truncus into pulmonary artery and aorta, combine with a component from the atrial septum to close the muscular interventricular septum at its base. This is the so-called membranous septum, and it completes the separation of the right from the left ventricle. It should be noted that the aorta and pulmonary artery are in close relation to the interventricular septum in its anterior portion (outflow tract), while the mitral and tricuspid valves are in close relation to the septum in its posterior portion (inflow tract).

A convenient anatomic classification of ventricular septal defect (VSD) divides it into (1) defects that occur as isolated lesions and (2) defects related to a primary disturbance in some other structure. An example of the latter would be a VSD associated with a common truncus arteriosus. In this situation, the septum that separates the truncus into the pulmonary artery and aorta has not developed, hence there is an absence of the components of the membranous interventricular septum normally derived from the truncal septum. Therefore *every* case of common truncus arteriosus is associated with a large anterior, high interventricular septal defect.

Isolated interventricular defects may occur either in the muscular portion of the septum (rare) or in the membrane portion of the septum at its base (most common). The crista supraventricularis of the right ventricle is a convenient landmark. Anterior defects lie in front of the crista, medial defects just behind, and posterior defects farther behind this structure. Pulmonary stenosis commonly occurs in association with, but is not an intrinsic embryologic component of, isolated VSD. The major physiologic abnormality is a shunting of blood from the left (high pressure) to the right (low pressure) ventricle during both phases of the cardiac cycle.

Physical Findings. Cyanosis is unusual in VSD. There is slight prominence of the left sternal border, and commonly a systolic thrill is felt at the lower left sternal border. There may be a slight increase in pulse pressure. The first heart sound is normal; the second heart sound is accentuated and may be slightly split. As pulmonary vascular resistance rises, the split becomes narrower and pulmonary closure becomes even more accentuated. The characteristic finding in VSD is a loud, rather harsh systolic murmur heard best at the lower left sternal border but transmitted well to the right sternal border. This murmur is often pansystolic and may be difficult to distinguish from that of pulmonary stenosis, which is commonly present as an associated defect.

Small interventricular defects with no evidence of overloading are believed to be benign lesions. Children with large VSDs usually are symptomatic and have dyspnea and fatigue. Common to the symptomatic group is the presence of repeated attacks of pneumonia and early congestive heart failure with cyanosis. Often these patients do very well if they can be supported over the first 2 years of life with medical management. Careful evaluation is needed in terms of the problem of severe pulmonary hypertension, which greatly magnifies the risk of catheterization and of surgery.

Laboratory Studies. At catheterization, one finds in the simplest VSD lesions an increasing oxygen saturation as the catheter is moved from the right atrium to the right ventricle or pulmonary artery. Pressure in the right ventricle and pulmonary artery may be elevated, depending on the amount of shunting and the degree of pulmonary vascular resistance. In the smallest lesions (maladie de Roger) the shunt may be very minor with no x-ray or electrocardiographic abnormality and only auscultatory phenomena. In general terms, therefore, the findings in VSD are related to the amount of shunting and the degree of pulmonary vascular resistance.

X-ray and fluoroscopy in VSD may reveal either a normal-sized heart or one with marked biventricular enlargement. The pulmonary vasculature is engorged; the aorta is usually small or hypoplastic.

The electrocardiogram may be normal in VSD, or it may only reveal evidence of left ventricular diastolic overloading. In many cases the electrocardiogram shows biventricular hypertrophy characterized by incomplete right bundle branch block, with deep Q waves in V_5 and V_6 and high voltage in the left precordial leads. A small number of patients show predominantly right ventricular hypertrophy.

Echocardiography reveals no characteristic features in VSD. With very large defects, a portion of the septum may be recognized as being absent with appropriate technique. Right ventricular, left atrial, and left ventricular dimensions may all be increased as a result of the left to right shunt.

Differential Diagnosis. In patients with small VSDs, differential diagnosis includes atrial septal defect, pulmonary stenosis, mitral regurgitation, and aortic stenosis, or simply functional murmurs (page 291). Endocardial cushion defects or a single common ventricle must be differentiated from larger ventricular septal defects. It may be necessary to perform repeated catheterizations to determine the degree of progression of pulmonary vascular resistance and the optimal timing of surgery. Some patients show evidence of pulmonary hypertension from the time of birth.

Treatment. Most patients who have had a successful repair of VSD can be expected to live a normal life following surgery. Postoperatively the electrocardiogram may show right bundle branch block, and auscultation may reveal a soft left sternal border systolic murmur with mild cardiac enlargement on x-ray. In some patients small residual shunts remain, but such shunts may not require further intervention. Patients with severe pulmonary vascular obstruction and little or no left-to-right shunt may improve after surgery, but they should be encouraged to avoid vigorous physical activity, since acute changes in the pulmonary or systemic hemodynamics carry a risk of sudden death. Travel to high altitudes should be avoided, since this has been found to increase acutely the degree of pulmonary vascular resistance.

COMMON ATRIOVENTRICULAR CANAL
OR ENDOCARDIAL CUSHION DEFECT
In a general sense, endocardial cushion defect lesions may be considered as varying combinations of atrial septal defect and ventricular septal defect but with a much poorer prognosis than either one of these alone. The incidence is low — approximately 2 percent of patients with congenital heart disease.

Embryology and Anatomy. The endocardial cushions arise from the ventral and dorsal aspects of the common atrioventricular canal. These grow and fuse in the midline, thus dividing the atrioventricular canal into a right (tricuspid) and a left (mitral) valve orifice. Complete separation of the atrioventricular canal into a right and left side is accomplished by a contribution from the septal primum of the atrial septum. Also the endocardial cushions supply components to the

posterior portions of the interventricular septum. These last two facts explain why both ostium primum defects of the atrial septum and interventricular septal defects are intimately related to endocardial cushion defects. As mentioned earlier, a wide variety of combinations is possible, and many workers have referred to these defects as partial or complete forms of a common atrioventricular canal. Of great importance is the common anatomic finding of cleft mitral and tricuspid valves with these defects.

Physical Findings. In patients with endocardial cushion defect the findings include evidences of right and left ventricular hypertrophy. The characteristic murmur is a long, blowing systolic murmur heard at the apex and transmitted well to the axilla. This arises from mitral insufficiency due to the valvular defect. Third heart sounds are commonly present in the apical area. A frequent finding is that of a rumbling middiastolic murmur heard best just within the apex.

Laboratory Studies. X-rays in endocardial cushion defect reveal left and right ventricular enlargement as well as left and right atrial enlargement. The pulmonary vascular markings are usually increased because of the increased pulmonary blood flow.

The electrocardiographic findings are reasonably typical in that they reveal the uncommon association of right bundle branch block with left axis deviation. Cardiac catheterization shows evidence of a large left-to-right shunt, usually at both the atrial and the ventricular level. The course of the catheter as it moves from the right to the left atrium and on into the left ventricle is very characteristic in ostium primum defects and is helpful in differentiating these from atrial septal defects. In the former, the catheter crosses from right to left at a *low* level, while in atrial septal defect the catheter passes to the left much *higher*. Finally, bidirectional shunting is often found because of the free and intimate relationship of the four cardiac chambers that is usual in endocardial cushion defects.

Echocardiographic features include abnormal septal motion, narrowing of the left ventricular outflow tract, prolonged approximation of the anterior mitral leaflet to the ventricular septum during dias-

tole, and a double echo from the cleft anterior leaflet of the mitral valve.

Treatment. The mortality with medical management is high in patients with endocardial cushion defect, and at least 50 percent of the patients die within the first year of life. Attempts at early surgery are mandatory in patients who respond poorly to medical management. Because of the complex nature of the anatomic defect in endocardial cushion lesions, complete closure and correction may be technically difficult. Residual mitral insufficiency is encountered, and residual shunts may be common.

TRUNCOCONAL MALFORMATIONS

Embryology and Anatomy. The common truncus of the embryonic heart is joined originally to a primitive right ventricle, but it migrates toward the midline as the torsion of the straight cardiac tube occurs and the ventricular portion of the heart becomes separated into a right and left side. Division of the common truncus into pulmonary artery and aorta takes place by the development of a septum which, as it arises, makes a 180-degree rotation from above downward. The lower portions of this septum give rise to structures that close the upper anterior and medial portions of the interventricular septum, as mentioned previously.

The various possibilities of maldevelopment of the truncoconal structures are given in the following listing. (Note that almost all are associated with interventricular septal defects as an obligatory part of the lesion.)

1. Lateral displacement of the entire structure, with pulmonary artery and aorta arising from the right ventricle (Eisenmenger complex)
2. Unequal partitioning of the truncus at the expense of either the aorta or the pulmonary artery (tetralogy of Fallot)
3. Failure of any septation at all to develop (common truncus)
4. Failure of the septum to achieve rotation (transposition of the great vessels)

The embryologic evolution of transposition of the great vessels has received considerable attention in the recent literature, which indicates that the embryologic explanation given above may not be entirely accurate. However, it does serve to separate the major entities in this group, which are tetralogy of Fallot, common truncus, and transposition of the great vessels.

TETRALOGY OF FALLOT

Tetralogy of Fallot consists of (1) pulmonary stenosis, either valvular or infundibular, (2) a high medial interventricular septal defect just behind the crista supraventricularis, (3) overriding of the aorta toward the right ventricle (this is more apparent than real), and (4) right ventricular hypertrophy that is secondary to the pulmonary stenosis. There is often an underdeveloped pulmonary artery, while in one-third of the cases the aortic arch is right-sided. This entity is probably the commonest form of cyanotic congenital heart disease.

Physical Findings. Tetralogy patients may be cyanotic at birth or may develop cyanosis up to the age of 1. Anoxic spells are common and, as the child grows, squatting is often present. There is also clubbing of the fingers. Examination of the chest reveals a left parasternal bulge indicating right ventricular hypertrophy. A normal first sound is heard; the pulmonic second sound is decreased or absent. The aortic closure is well heard along the lower left sternal border. A loud systolic ejection-type murmur is present along the left sternal border. Congestive failure does not occur in uncomplicated tetralogy of Fallot; however, patients may die during an anoxic spell. Brain abscess is frequent, particularly in patients who are severely polycythemic. The polycythemia may be difficult to manage.

Laboratory Studies. Catheterization of tetralogy patients reveals evidence of increased pressure in the right ventricle, with normal pressures in the pulmonary artery. There is a right-to-left shunt and often a small left-to-right shunt at the ventricular level. Angiography clarifies the type of pulmonary stenosis present as well as the size of the pulmonary artery, thus providing information essential to the surgical approach. X-rays show a small right heart (hypertrophied but not dilated), a large aorta, absence of the main pulmonary artery segment, and reduced pulmonary vasculature.

In the electrocardiogram there is evidence of marked right ventricular hypertrophy with tall, slurred R waves in the right precordial leads and with small R and deep S waves in leads V_5 and V_6, indicating right ventricular overloading. The T wave is negative in lead V_1 but becomes positive in V_2 to V_6.

Echocardiographic features include evidence of discontinuity of the ventricular septum with the anterior wall of the aorta, which suggests overriding of the aorta on the septum.

Differential Diagnosis. Major problems of differential diagnosis in tetralogy of Fallot center on transposition of the great vessels. Many patients with pulmonary stenosis and ventricular septal defects will gradually develop right-to-left shunts. These cases are referred to in their early stages as "pink" or "rosy" tetralogies.

Treatment. Surgical approach is directed toward complete correction of the tetralogy defects under cardiac bypass techniques. However, this may not be technically feasible, and some surgeons still rely on either the Blalock-Taussig procedure (anastomosis of subclavian artery to pulmonary artery) or the Potts-Smith-Gibson procedure, which joins the aorta to the pulmonary artery. Both are designed to deliver more blood to the lungs, thus reducing the degree of cyanosis and disability. In patients in whom full correction has been attempted, late follow-up may show a residual right ventricular-to-pulmonary artery pressure gradient, a persistent VSD, and pulmonary insufficiency.

TRUNCUS ARTERIOSUS

Embryology and Anatomy. Truncus arteriosus is a rather rare lesion that is due to a failure of normal partitioning of the common truncus into the pulmonary artery and aorta, and it is always associated with a large defect of the interventricular septum. Both the systemic and pulmonary circulations are supplied completely from this common outflow canal. A variety of anatomic types of persistent truncus arteriosus have been described, based primarily on the relationship of the pulmonary arteries to the common

truncus. The physiologic defect relates to the fact that the common canal produces a rather complete mixture of oxygenated and unsaturated blood, but the degree of cyanosis is determined by the status of the pulmonary arteries. Thus patients with normal pulmonary arteries and no pulmonary hypertension have little cyanosis, whereas those with small pulmonary arteries or pulmonary hypertension will exhibit marked cyanosis.

Physical Findings. Truncus arteriosus patients are usually underdeveloped and cyanotic. There is a loud pansystolic murmur at the lower left sternal border and a loud, accentuated single second sound. Many patients also have a diastolic blowing murmur.

Laboratory Studies. At catheterization in truncus arteriosus patients, an increase in oxygen content is found inside the right ventricle, but there is a variable degree of unsaturation of arterial blood. A common finding is the presence of a similar degree of saturation in both the systemic and the pulmonary arteries. Right ventricular and pulmonary artery pressures are close to systemic levels.

The x-rays show cardiac enlargement with pulmonary vascular engorgement and a large aorta that often has its arch on the right side. It may be possible to recognize the absence of the main pulmonary artery. Cineangiography is of great value in determining the exact anatomic defect. The electrocardiogram is consistent with combined hypertrophy.

Echocardiographic studies may be confused with those of tetralogy of Fallot, since in both there is a large overriding vessel with interruption of the ventricular septum.

Diagnosis and Treatment. Differential diagnosis in truncus arteriosus includes a large VSD, patent ductus arteriosus, aorticopulmonary window, and tricuspid atresia. With medical treatment alone, this defect has previously been universally fatal. However, complete correction is now being accomplished by closure of the ventricular septal defect and insertion of a conduit from the right ventricle to the pulmonary artery.

TRANSPOSITION OF THE GREAT VESSELS

Transposition of the great vessels is an entity not commonly seen in the previous everyday practice of pediatrics or cardiology, because the vast majority of these patients died at a very early age. This condition was formerly the commonest cause of death from congenital heart disease in the first month of life.

Embryology and Anatomy. The embryologic defect in transposition is a failure of rotational septation of the common truncus. As stated above, the septum, which eventually separates the pulmonary artery and the aorta, normally undergoes a 180° rotation from above downward. Therefore the normal pulmonary artery is posterior above but anterior below. This accounts for the fact that the aorta and pulmonary artery cross one another in an oblique fashion in the normal heart. In transposition of the great vessels, the aorta and pulmonary artery are completely parallel because the dividing septum has developed in a straight (nonrotated) line. The pulmonary artery is posterior throughout its course, while the aorta lies anteriorly. Thus the great vessels are transposed and the pulmonary artery now arises from the left (posterior) ventricle. This situation in its pure form is incompatible with life, and these patients survive only because of the presence of large septal defects that permit some form of mixing. A patent ductus would serve the purpose.

As previously noted, there have been renewed attempts to explain the complicated anatomic disturbances in these entities, and more complicated classifications than those given above are now available. Also, recent surgical advances have improved the previously grave prognosis for patients with transposition of the great vessels. These facts have increased the attention given to this disease.

Physical and Laboratory Findings. The physical findings in transposition of the great vessels are cyanosis from the time of birth and early congestive heart failure. At the time of cardiac catheterization, there is evidence of shunting at the atrial or ventricular level. X-ray findings are usually those of a heart that has a narrow aortic waist in the presence of pulmonary plethora. The electrocardiographic findings are not characteristic and consist of various combinations of right ventricular hypertrophy and combined hypertrophy. The echocardiogram can be diagnostic by demonstrating continuity of the mitral and pulmonic valves, separation of the aortic valve from the right ventricle by an outflow tract, and abnormal positioning of the aortic valve anterior and superior to the pulmonic valve.

Diagnosis and Treatment. Differential diagnosis of transposition of the great vessels includes severe tetralogy of Fallot, truncus arteriosus, hypoplastic left heart syndrome, and complete transposition of the pulmonary veins. The poor prognosis that previously obtained, with death occurring in the early neonatal period, has now been improved with the introduction of balloon atrial septostomy, which can be performed at the time of the initial cardiac catheterization. It is relatively easy during an early diagnostic catheterization to pass a catheter from the right atrium to the left atrium, since the foramen ovale is patent to probes during the first year of life. A small balloon on the end of the catheter can then be inflated and the catheter rapidly withdrawn from the left atrium to the right atrium with the balloon inflated, thereby rupturing the intraatrial septum and permitting a greater mixture of blood between the venous and arterial systems. This procedure allows for survival until the patient has grown sufficiently to survive a second-stage corrective operation, which in essence rechannels atrial blood flow to the opposite ventricle (Mustard procedure). This operation is usually carried out between 1 and 2 years of age.

Since many patients with transposition of the great arteries have additional cardiac lesions, other forms of palliative surgery may also be necessary. Persistent abnormalities are often seen postoperatively in patients with transposition of the great vessels. These abnormalities consist of residual intraatrial shunts, superior or inferior vena caval obstruction, pulmonary venous obstruction, tricuspid regurgitation, cardiac dysrhythmias, and pulmonary vascular obstructive disease. As previously mentioned, the rhythm disturbances are often supraventricular tachycardias due to injury to the sinus node and perhaps also due to interruption of the atrial conducting tracts.

CORRECTED TRANSPOSITION OF THE GREAT VESSELS
Brief mention should be made of the entity known as
corrected transposition of the great vessels. This
lesion has a complicated embryologic derivation, the
essential features of which are (1) transposition of
the great vessels and (2) inversion of the ventricles so
that the right atrium delivers blood to the aorta in
spite of the transposition of the great vessels. This
situation alone is completely compatible with a
normal life. Unfortunately there is also a common
association of pulmonary stenosis and ventricular
septal defect, the physiologic deficits and clinical
symptoms of which are essentially the same as when
these lesions occur without transposition; however,
the electrocardiographic, x-ray, and angiographic
findings are different. It is important to define the
anatomy before undertaking surgery to ensure a
proper approach and correction. Complete atrioventricular block may be seen in patients with corrected
transposition of the great vessels.

EISENMENGER SYNDROME
A great deal of confusion exists concerning the exact
definition of the Eisenmenger syndrome. The confusion seems to have arisen because the term has both
anatomic and physiologic connotations. The *anatomic*
Eisenmenger anomaly consists in a lateral positioning
of both the pulmonary artery and aorta toward the
right ventricle, with an associated large ventricular
septal defect. The *physiologic* Eisenmenger syndrome
is caused by a severe degree of pulmonary vascular
obstruction in conjunction with either a shunting
lesion (i.e., atrial septal defect, ventricular septal
defect, or patent ductus arteriosus) or an obstructive
lesion on the left side of the heart (e.g., mitral stenosis, aortic stenosis, or coarctation of the aorta).
The physiologic variety is the more common of the
two types of Eisenmenger syndrome. The anatomic
basis of the pulmonary obstruction is usually marked
hypertrophy of the muscular layer of the medium-
sized pulmonary arteries.

Physical Findings. The clinical picture in the common physiologic type of the Eisenmenger syndrome
is usually the same regardless of the basic underlying
defect. The patients have exertional dyspnea and

transient or permanent cyanosis, and they often present themselves to the physician complaining of chest
pain, syncope, or hemoptysis. On auscultation, the
most striking finding is the markedly accentuated
second sound. This sound is heard best in the pulmonic area and is the hallmark of pulmonary hypertension. There is usually a grade 2 to 3/6 systolic
murmur along the left sternal border. The murmur
of pulmonary insufficiency may also be heard.

Laboratory Studies. Cardiac catheterization in the
Eisenmenger syndrome may reveal arterial oxygen
unsaturation, right ventricular and pulmonary arterial
pressure elevations to systemic levels, and a varying
degree of right-to-left shunting. The risks of catheterization are increased in patients with pulmonary
hypertension.

   The x-ray shows right ventricular enlargement,
a very prominent pulmonary artery, prominence of
the pulmonary vasculature at the hilus, but a markedly diminished peripheral pulmonary vasculature
referred to as the so-called cutoff sign. The electrocardiogram reveals severe right ventricular hypertrophy with an increase in the height of the R waves
in the right precordial leads.

Treatment. Medical therapy has little to offer in the
treatment of the Eisenmenger syndrome, and surgical
mortality is greatly increased by the presence of pulmonary hypertension. The decision as to whether to
operate, therefore, is difficult. Surgery is usually
decided against if there is evidence of only right-to-
left shunting.

PULMONARY STENOSIS
Pulmonary valvular stenosis is among the more common congenital heart lesions, and it occurs either
alone or in combination with various types of VSD.
Although secondary infundibular stenosis is often
seen, the incidence of true primary infundibular
stenosis is probably quite low.

   The physiologic defect that must be overcome is
obstruction at the pulmonary valve. This demands
greater work from the right ventricle, particularly if
the septum is intact; thus right ventricular hypertrophy supervenes.

Physical Findings. Patients with pulmonary valvular stenosis are usually asymptomatic or complain only of mild dyspnea and exertional fatigue. Cyanosis, if it is ever present, is a late finding. The patients are well developed with no general evidence of illness. Examination reveals a loud, harsh, diamond-shaped systolic murmur at the second to fourth left intercostal space, with good transmission to the neck. There is usually a thrill in the same area that may be felt in the suprasternal notch. Other findings include a systolic ejection click, a decreased pulmonic heart sound, and late pulmonic closure compared to aortic closure.

Laboratory Studies. Cardiac catheterization in pulmonary valvular stenosis is not essential to the diagnosis of pure pulmonary stenosis. It does, however, reveal an increase in right ventricular pressure and affords some estimation of the severity of the lesion.

On x-ray there is little enlargement of the heart, since the major anatomic lesion in pulmonary valvular stenosis consists only of thickening of the right ventricular myocardium without dilatation. The main pulmonary artery may be dilated; however, peripherally the pulmonary vasculature appears to be diminished. This is a point of great diagnostic significance in relation to atrial septal defects or ventricular septal defects, in both of which the peripheral pulmonary vasculature is increased in the absence of pulmonary hypertension.

The electrocardiogram in pulmonary valvular stenosis reveals evidence of both right ventricular and right atrial hypertrophy. This consists in an increase in the R waves in the right precordial leads and right axis deviation in the standard leads. The P waves are high and peaked in leads II and III. Incomplete right bundle branch block is also seen, particularly in milder cases.

Treatment. Although the murmur of pulmonary valvular stenosis is often noted at birth, symptoms do not develop until later in life, with the exception of a small group of infants who have critically narrowed valves. A large proportion of the patients have no symptoms and little progression of their findings, which suggests that they have a mild nonprogressive pulmonic stenosis not requiring surgical intervention.

Critically ill infants must have early surgical intervention. Patients with the clinical picture of severe right ventricular overloading should probably have surgery after the age of 5. Patients with mild symptoms need only to be followed. Cardiac catheterization often helps to classify patients with pulmonary valvular stenosis properly. Differential diagnosis includes tetralogy of Fallot and, in patients with severe right ventricular overloading, the pulmonary vascular obstruction syndrome. However, the differential diagnosis of the murmur of mild pulmonic stenosis includes such entities as atrial septal defect, anomalous pulmonary venous drainage, and innocent systolic murmurs. Critical examination of the electrocardiogram and particularly of the chest x-ray serves to differentiate these more benign entities from each other. Happily, for the most part mild pulmonic stenosis does not require urgent intervention and may be followed leisurely in order to arrive eventually at an appropriate diagnosis and choice of therapy.

AORTIC STENOSIS

Aortic stenosis is a common congenital anomaly. The lesion may be divided anatomically into valvular, subvalvular, and supravalvular types. The valvular type is the commonest, occurring in approximately three-fourths of all cases. The major physiologic defect is overloading of the left ventricle. In order to maintain an adequate cardiac output through the reduced valvular orifice, high pressures that subsequently lead to marked left ventricular hypertrophy must be developed. There are two major clinical groups: (1) those that do not survive the first year of life and (2) those whose disease is discovered on routine examination during early childhood.

Physical Findings. The commonest auscultatory finding in aortic stenosis is that of a diamond-shaped systolic murmur that is loud, best heard at the base, and transmitted toward the neck vessels. Another common finding is an early systolic click heard at the lower left sternal border. A systolic thrill is present in most patients. The expected reduction of pulse pressure is often not present in children.

Laboratory Studies. The x-ray shadow of the heart is often within normal limits in aortic stenosis, and a useful sign is poststenotic dilatation of the ascending arch of the aorta. In the majority of patients with aortic stenosis the electrocardiogram reveals left ventricular hypertrophy, with tall R waves and flat or inverted T waves in the left precordial leads. The vectorcardiogram is believed to show left ventricular hypertrophy before characteristic changes are seen in the scalar electrocardiogram. Somewhat disturbing is a small group of patients who have severe aortic stenosis without any abnormality in the electrocardiogram.

The echocardiogram is less useful in pediatric aortic stenosis than it is in adult forms.

Differential Diagnosis and Treatment. Aortic stenosis may be a lethal lesion in the first few weeks or months of life, and the early diagnosis may be quite difficult. The major finding pointing to the diagnosis is left ventricular hypertrophy in the electrocardiogram. Patients with mild to moderate aortic stenosis have few symptoms, and many lead normal lives. A disturbing feature is the high incidence of sudden death in this group, apparently associated with excessive physical exertion. Careful continuing observation is important. Patients with progressive symptoms should be considered for left-sided heart catheterization, since this is the only objective way of measuring the degree of difficulty prior to surgery. Differential diagnosis depends mainly on distinguishing mild aortic from mild pulmonic stenosis. Aortic stenosis may also be seen in association with coarctation of the aorta, patent ductus arteriosus, and more rarely, subaortic stenosis.

Aortic valvulotomy for aortic valvular stenosis during infancy and childhood is a palliative procedure. The gradient between the left ventricle and the aorta is usually not completely abolished, since efforts must be made to avoid causing significant aortic insufficiency. However, the palliative procedure is useful in that it serves to protect the left ventricular myocardium until total valve replacement can be carried out at a later age, and it may lessen the possibility of sudden death.

HYPERTROPHIC SUBAORTIC STENOSIS
There has been much recent interest in patients with the entity hypertrophic (muscular) subaortic stenosis. In this situation the obstruction is not at the valve area but in the outflow tract of the left ventricle. During systole, hypertrophied muscle obstructs the flow of blood from the left ventricle. Cardiac catheterization and angiography serve to identify this lesion. Other helpful points are the systolic murmur, heard best at the apex; the absence of poststenotic dilatation of the aorta; and a positive family history (see Chap. 30).

MITRAL OR TRICUSPID LESIONS
Congenital lesions of the mitral valve are rare. Mitral stenosis may occur either as part of the hypoplastic left heart syndrome or as a solitary lesion. Congenital mitral insufficiency is commonly seen as part of an endocardial cushion defect and more rarely as an isolated defect.

Defects of the tricuspid valve are also uncommon. Tricuspid atresia or stenosis will usually be associated with an atrial septal defect, which permits the maintenance of life. Because of the atrial septal defect these patients show considerable cyanosis, and there is marked left ventricular preponderance since the right ventricle receives no blood and is underloaded. The Ebstein anomaly of the tricuspid valve is related to a malpositioning of the tricuspid valve leaflets, which extend down into the right ventricle. There may also be a defect in the right ventricular musculature. Thus the right side of the heart may be primarily atrial from the functional viewpoint. This lesion may be compatible with a relatively symptom-free life. The x-ray will be abnormal, and the electrocardiogram characteristically shows complete right bundle branch block with very large, peaked P waves. The Wolff-Parkinson-White syndrome is also seen with increased frequency in the Ebstein anomaly.

Tricuspid atresia may be relieved by creating an anastomosis between the superior vena cava and the pulmonary artery; such surgery (Glenn procedure) is only palliative.

PATENT DUCTUS ARTERIOSUS
Patent ductus arteriosus is a common congenital defect. In most large series it is second or third in frequency; it is more common in girls. The ductus arteriosus in fetal life is the channel through which the

oxygenated maternal blood bypasses the pulmonary system and reaches the aorta for peripheral distribution. In most instances the ductus closes a few days to a few weeks after birth. The physiologic defect consists in shunting of blood from the high-pressure system of the aorta to the lower-pressure system of the pulmonary artery. This shunting occurs both in systole and in diastole. The overloading involves primarily the left ventricle; the right ventricle is enlarged only when there is pulmonary hypertension.

Physical Findings. The physical findings in patent ductus arteriosus are usually those of an asymptomatic child with a prominent left ventricular impulse. The diagnosis may be established by careful auscultation of the typical murmur, which is a continuous so-called machinery murmur occupying both systole and diastole and heard best at the upper left sternal border and beneath the left clavicle. The second sound is loud and often single; a third sound is common at the apex.

Laboratory Studies. At catheterization in patent ductus arteriosus a step-up of oxygenation is found at the level of the pulmonary artery. The presence of a patent ductus may be demonstrated by selective angiography with the injection of contrast material into the aorta near the mouth of the ductus.

X-ray findings range from normal-sized hearts in patients with small shunts to left ventricular and left atrial enlargement, a prominent pulmonary artery, a dilated ascending aorta, and pulmonary vascular engorgement in patients with larger shunts.

The electrocardiogram is often within normal limits, or it may show left ventricular overloading of the diastolic type, with a deep Q wave and high-peaked T waves in the left ventricular leads.

Differential Diagnosis and Treatment. The differential diagnosis for patent ductus arteriosus includes aortico-pulmonary window, pulmonary arteriovenous fistulas, aneurysm of the sinus of Valsalva, or venous hum. The last entity is simply an auscultatory phenomenon arising in the great veins of the neck or mediastinum, and it can often be obliterated by extension of the neck or pressure on the jugular veins.

The indications for operative intervention in all patients who have patent ductus arteriosus are related to the dangers of bacterial endocarditis, pulmonary hypertension, or congestive failure (in patients with very large shunts). The major problem is the proper timing of the operation. Optimal age for surgery lies between 3 and 10 to 15 years.

COARCTATION OF THE AORTA
Aortic coarctation is a rather common congenital anomaly that consists of a narrowing of the lumen of the aorta at the level of the insertion of the ligamentum arteriosum. A commonly used classification has been a division into preductal and postductal coarctation. The former is also referred to as the infantile type, the latter as the adult type. The major physiologic difficulty in coarctation of the aorta centers around the maintenance of adequate flow and pressure to the lower half of the body and obstruction to outflow from left ventricle. The classic terminology should probably be disregarded in favor of the more physiologic terminology proposed by Nadas and Fyler (see Bibliography) — namely, coarctation with systemic left ventricle and coarctation with systemic left and right ventricles. The latter is accomplished by means of a persistent patent ductus arteriosus (page 306). Coarctation may often be associated with one or more other anomalies, including a defect of the subclavian arteries, bicuspid aortic valve, patent ductus arteriosus, ventricular septal defect, and mitral insufficiency. A small group of patients with coarctation and systemic left ventricle present very early with marked congestive heart failure, which is a common cause of death in the first month of life. These patients may respond well to medical measures, but early operation is indicated in the face of continued heart failure.

Physical Findings. The majority of children with coarctation of the aorta and systemic left ventricle are asymptomatic. The diagnosis is made at the time of routine physical examination. Auscultatory findings include normal heart sounds and a systolic murmur that is quite loud and rough. The murmur is heard best at the base of the heart and is transmitted very well to the back. Diastolic rumbles at the mitral area have been described. Hypertension in the upper extremities is a common finding, while the femoral pulses are either absent or weak and delayed when compared to the radial pulses. The blood pressure in the arms is higher than the blood pressure in the legs (see Chap. 25).

Laboratory Studies. Catheterization is of little aid in coarctation of the aorta unless there is an associated lesion. On x-ray, the heart shadow may be within normal limits, but the aorta may show a characteristic indentation described as the "E" sign. The presence of collateral circulation with erosion of the inferior aspect of the ribs by the dilated intercostal arteries does not usually occur until the age of 6 or 7. The diagnosis can be proved by angiography, but this usually is not necessary. The electrocardiogram may be within normal limits or may show only varying degrees of incomplete right bundle branch block during the first few years of life. Ultimately left ventricular hypertrophy will appear.

In terms of therapy, it is believed that elective surgery should be undertaken during the optimal age range of 7 to 20 years. The more severe the abnormalities in the electrocardiogram and x-rays, the more urgent the indications for earlier operation.

Coarctation of the aorta with systemic right and left ventricles is a rare condition in which the association of a patent ductus arteriosus with coarctation causes marked overloading of both the right and the left ventricles. Accordingly these patients may have differential cyanosis, with the upper half of the body pink and the lower half blue. Usually there are associated complicated cardiac defects. The mortality in this group is high during the first few months of life. A few patients survive, and the diagnosis in these survivors may be suspected by the finding of right ventricular hypertrophy in the electrocardiogram in the presence of physical findings suggesting coarctation.

Arterial hypertension may persist postoperatively, and because of the presence of bicuspid aortic valves, the late development of aortic stenosis is not uncommon. Late narrowing of the surgical anastomosis with recurrence of differential pressures in the arms and legs may develop.

HYPOPLASTIC LEFT HEART SYNDROME
Hypoplastic left heart syndrome has as its common denominator an obstructive lesion on the left side of the heart with a hypoplastic left ventricle and a large, dilated, hypertrophied right ventricle. The possible obstructive lesions include hypoplasia of the aortic arch, mitral atresia or stenosis, and aortic valve atresia. Hypoplastic left heart syndrome may be the second leading cause of death in infants with congenital heart disease.

The embryologic defect is not clear. The recognition of the syndrome in general is not difficult; usually the infants appear normal at birth, do well for a short time, but within a matter of a few hours to days develop both right-sided and left-sided congestive heart failure with a mild degree of cyanosis.

Physical findings are not striking and include a nonspecific soft systolic murmur, which generally is heard to the left of the sternum, and weak pulses in all extremities. X-ray reveals moderate cardiac enlargement; pulmonary markings may be increased or normal. The electrocardiogram shows right axis deviation with right ventricular hypertrophy and P pulmonale.

Surgical alleviation of hypoplastic left heart syndrome is quite difficult, particularly because there are often multiple congenital cardiac defects in association with the basic lesion.

Bibliography
American Heart Association Ad Hoc Committee on Rehabilitation of the Young Cardiac (W. H. Weidman, Chairman). Recreational activity and career choice recommendations for use by physicians counseling physical education directors, vocational counselors, parents and young patients with heart disease (committee report). *Circulation* 43:459, 1971.

De La Cruz, M., Polansky, B. J., and Navarro-Lopez, F. The diagnosis of corrected transposition of the great vessels. *Br. Heart J.* 24:483, 1962.

Gould, S. E. *Pathology of the Heart* (2nd ed.). Springfield, Ill.: Thomas, 1960.

Keith, J. D., Rowe, R. D., and Vlad, P. *Heart Disease in Infancy and Childhood.* New York: Macmillan, 1958.

Nadas, A. S., and Fyler, D. C. *Pediatric Cardiology*
    (3rd ed.). Philadelphia: Saunders, 1972.
Sonnenblick, E. H., and Lesch, M. Symposium:
    Postoperative congenital heart disease. I. *Progr.*
    Cardiovasc. Dis. 27:401, 1975.
Sonnenblick, E. H., and Lesch, M. Symposium:
    Postoperative congenital heart disease. I. *Progr.*
    Cardiovasc. Dis. 28:1, 1975.
Zimmerman, H. A. (ed.). *Intravascular Catheteriza-*
    tion (2nd ed.). Springfield, Ill.: Thomas, 1966.

30

Valvular Heart Disease

Thomas J. Ryan

Traditionally the term *valvular heart disease* has been applied to disorders of the heart resulting either from rheumatic carditis or from some other inflammatory condition that causes deformity of one or more of the heart's valves. These *acquired* lesions were formerly distinguished from *congenital* valvular disorders because the latter became clinically manifest in a separate pediatric population, had a far different natural history, and appeared to have little relevance to adult heart disease. Studies in the past decade, however, have suggested that a significant proportion of adult valvular disease is related to congenital abnormalities of the valves. For example, both bicuspid aortic valve and redundant mitral valve with myxomatous degeneration are congenital abnormalities that can lead to heart disease that only appears to be acquired later in life. Whether acquired or congenital, each specific valvular disorder is discussed here in the light of the altered physiology it produces. This altered physiology fundamentally determines the natural history as well as the symptoms, physical findings, and hemodynamic abnormalities characteristic of each lesion.

Pathogenesis

A specific causative relationship between streptococcal infections and rheumatic fever has been well established, with evidence that group A streptococcal antigens cross-react with the structural glycoprotein of heart valves. With the initial episode of rheumatic fever, acute inflammation is usually seen on the endothelial lining of the heart valves, often associated with acute inflammatory changes of both the myocardium and pericardium. During the initial endocarditis there is a temporary malfunction of the heart valves, frequently resulting in clinical signs of mitral regurgitation but not necessarily indicating permanent damage. Often the initial inflammatory process may be so mild as to pass unnoticed; a clinical history of acute rheumatic fever is obtainable in approximately one-half of all patients with rheumatic valvular disease. Damage

to valvular structures does not end with the subsidence of the acute inflammation; rather, the damage seems to continue chronically, producing further scarring or fibrosis that ultimately interferes with valve function. This long-term process accounts for the latent period between the initial episode of acute rheumatic fever and the appearance of signs and symptoms of permanent valve damage. In a study of 1,000 patients followed for 20 years, Bland and Jones found that more than a decade was required to develop definite clinical evidence of mitral stenosis. The pathogenesis for the later development of valvular disease was originally thought to relate to smoldering chronic rheumatic activity. This is now disclaimed, and the current belief is that the early scars of rheumatic valvulitis are perpetuated in a nonspecific manner. Abnormal flow patterns are thought to traumatize the valve, leading to thickening, fibrosis, and calcification of the cusps. It can be appreciated that adhesions of the valve commissures, either from acute carditis or from congenital fusion, as in bicuspid aortic valve, can also alter flow patterns through the valve orifice and set up progressive valvular damage on a traumatic basis.

Natural History

These considerations of pathogenesis are fundamental to the understanding of valvular heart disease, since they determine the life history of the patient. Knowledge of the natural history of each specific disorder also is important, because this is the yardstick by which one must judge the efficacy of therapy. The four valves of the heart are not affected with equal frequency either by the rheumatic process or by congenital abnormalities. From large autopsy series of rheumatic heart disease it is widely accepted that the mitral valve is involved in 80 to 90 percent, the aortic valve in 40 to 60 percent, the tricuspid valve in 5 to 20 percent, and the pulmonary valve in 1 to 2 percent of the cases. These represent maximal figures and include lesions so mild as to escape clinical recognition. It is also evident that many patients have more than one valve involved and that disorders of the aortic and mitral valves are far more common than those of the pulmonary and tricuspid valves. Table 30-1 presents the salient features of the natural

Table 30-1. Natural History of Valvular Disease

Lesion	% Survival		Latent period (yr)	Duration of symptoms (yr)
	5 Yr	10 Yr		
MS	80	60	20	8
Class III*	60	40		
Class IV*	15	0		
MR	80	60	0–5	Variable: 5–25
AR	75	50	10	2
AS	40	10	38	3
MS + MR	66	33		

*New York Heart Association functional classification.
Note: MS = mitral stenosis; MR = mitral regurgitation; AS = aortic stenosis; AR = aortic regurgitation.

history of the various valvular lesions, both alone and in combination. The *latent* period is the time from the acute rheumatic infection to the point of earliest symptoms, while the *duration* of symptoms refers to the period from the earliest symptoms to the point of total disability. It can be seen that while aortic stenosis requires the longest time to cause symptoms, it is associated with a rather rapid course once symptoms do appear. Survival rates are timed from the patient's coming to the attention of a medical center until the patient's death and presumably include his receiving the benefits of modern care.

Pathophysiology

In the simplest terms, the function of normal valves may be defined as the maintenance of an unimpeded, one-way (forward) flow of blood through the heart. Expressed hemodynamically, each valve should allow the entire stroke output of the heart to pass freely during one phase of the cardiac cycle (diastole in the case of the atrioventricular valves, systole in the case of the semilunar valves) with no measurable pressure gradient between the two chambers separated by the valve, and no backflow occurring during the alternate phase of the cycle despite the considerable pressure gradient then existing.

It follows that damage to a valve may interfere with its function in either or both of two ways: (1) by narrowing *(stenosis)* of the valve, creating an obstacle to the free forward flow of blood and (2) by

impaired closure, allowing backward leakage of blood (*regurgitation,* insufficiency, or incompetence). Valvular stenosis exists when the cardiac output can pass through the valve only as a result of a measurable pressure gradient (during diastole between atrium and ventricle or during systole between ventricle and great vessels). Stenosis and regurgitation in the same valve are by no means mutually exclusive; in many cases they coexist, even though one or the other may predominate.

Mitral Valve Disease

The mitral valve, so named because of its resemblance to a bishop's miter, is more than an orifice between the left atrium and ventricle. It is a complex apparatus comprised of the anulus fibrosis; the anterior (medial, aortic, or septal) and posterior (lateral or mural) leaflets; the first-, second-, and third-order chordae tendineae, numbering 120 to 124 in all; and the two papillary muscles that are specialized portions of the left ventricular myocardium. During ventricular systole, contraction of the papillary muscles produces tension in the chordae tendineae, pulling the leaflets together along their free margins and sealing the valve orifice. During diastole the papillary muscles relax, the chordae tendineae fan out, and the leaflets separate widely from one another as blood flows freely from the left atrium into the left ventricle.

The two major functional types of disturbances that can occur at the mitral valve, stenosis and regurgitation, cause sharply different circulatory abnormalities. Mitral stenosis causes a systolic overload on the left atrium and ultimately creates pressure work for the right side of the heart, while mitral regurgitation, on the other hand, represents a diastolic overload on the left ventricle and creates increased flow work for that chamber. Thus it is understandable that mitral stenosis and mitral regurgitation differ in natural history, clinical symptoms, physical findings, and hemodynamic measurements.

MITRAL STENOSIS

Incidence. Mitral stenosis, as either the sole or the dominant lesion, is encountered in about two-thirds of all cases of mitral valvular involvement. The predilection for women to develop pure mitral stenosis is well established (the M/F sex ratio is 1:4), though it is poorly understood. In pure mitral regurgitation the M/F ratio is 1:1.

Pathophysiology. Three distinct components of mitral stenosis may be seen pathologically: (1) commissural (fusion of commissures), (2) cuspal (thickened, fibrous leaflets that eventually calcify), and (3) chordal (chordae are fused, thickened, and shortened and principally interfere with valve mobility). The clinical course and natural history are basically determined by which of these three pathologic components predominates. In certain instances the acute rheumatic process results in commissural fusion only, causing minimal trauma and no significant blockade to flow from atrium to ventricle. Such mild mitral stenosis may persist for life. In other instances more severe involvement of the commissures occurs, with both cuspal and chordal involvement and alteration of flow patterns through the mitral orifice. This sets up progressive valvular deformity on a traumatic basis, and there is a slow progression of symptoms. Accordingly, symptoms are usually delayed until the fourth and fifth decades, although there is evidence that in poorer economic areas the course of mitral stenosis is considerably accelerated, progressing rapidly

atic, since the rise of left atrial pressure is accompanied by a similar rise of the blood pressure in the lungs and in the right ventricle. The increased transudation of fluid from the pulmonary capillaries under high hydrostatic pressure is partially offset by an increase in the capacity of the lymphatics to drain away the excess fluid. The pulmonary capillaries are the locus minoris resistentiae, and when their pressure rises above the osmotic pressure of plasma (25 mm Hg), they transude fluid freely into the alveoli. As the resultant pulmonary edema becomes chronic in mitral stenosis, pulmonary vascular changes cause further obstruction to blood flow and a reduction in cardiac output. Thus there are two kinds of stenosis — the primary structural blockade at the mitral valve and the secondary functional blockade at the pulmonary arterioles. It has been reasoned that the secondary arteriolar obstruction, by reducing blood flow, allows the pressure in the left atrium to remain at or near 25 mm Hg, even though the valve becomes smaller. At the same time, pressure in the pulmonary artery rises inordinately as blood is forced through to the left side of the heart.

Pulmonary hypertension is the important factor in the altered hemodynamics of mitral stenosis. An adaptation of the Poiseuille equation is used to quantify pulmonary vascular resistance:

$$\text{Resistance (R)} = \frac{\text{mean PA pressure} - \text{mean LA pressure (mm Hg)}}{\text{Pulmonary blood flow (CO, L/min)}} \quad \text{(Wood units)}$$

to serious disability early in life.

Mechanical obstruction of blood flow arising from mitral stenosis results in a rise in pressure proximal to the mitral valve, and this accounts for the primary hemodynamic abnormalities measured at cardiac catheterization. The orifice size of the normal adult mitral valve is approximately 5 sq cm. A normal cardiac output of 5.0 to 6.0 liters per minute is associated with a normal left atrial pressure that ranges from 6 to 10 mm Hg. When orifice size is reduced to approximately 1.5 sq cm, left atrial pressure rises above these normal values; and when the narrowing reaches the critical level of 1.0 sq cm, left atrial pressure rises to 20 to 25 mm Hg. All patients with this degree of valve narrowing are thoroughly symptom-

where PA = pulmonary artery
  LA = left atrium
  CO = cardiac output

While pulmonary hypertension and elevated pulmonary vascular resistance are common findings in mitral stenosis, neither value ordinarily reaches the extremes often seen in congenital heart disease with pulmonary vascular obstruction. Thus only in an unusual case of mitral stenosis is pulmonary artery pressure equal to the systemic pressure, as is often found in congenital heart disease. Similarly, the pulmonary hypertension associated with mitral stenosis is reversible, suggesting that it must be due in part to a vasoconstrictor response to left atrial hypertension. This suggestion is supported by the observation that either the infusion of hexamethonium or successful valve surgery markedly decreases the pulmonary hypertension.

Early in the course of mitral stenosis the cardiac output is lowered, often before the advent of symptoms. This lowering seems to relate primarily to the degree of mitral valve narrowing, and it may be effected by baroreceptors (stretch receptors) located in the left atrium or pulmonary veins. The lowered cardiac output should be considered one of the hallmarks of mitral stenosis. The salient features of the pathophysiology of mitral stenosis appear in Table 30-2.

Clinical Profile. The classic description of mitral stenosis continues to be Wood's treatise based on his personal experience with more than 350 cases up until 1954. Although considerable sophistication has been added to hemodynamic studies over the past two decades, Wood's clinical picture and general hemodynamic profile have been substantiated in most other large series reported (see Bibliography).

Dyspnea is the cardinal symptom of mitral stenosis and, as explained above, it can be attributed to the increased rigidity of the lungs caused by interstitial changes. Since mitral stenosis develops gradually over a period of time, the pressure increments in the pulmonary capillaries are small and permit adaptive processes to take place. Translated into a patient's history, it is important to appreciate both the gradual onset and gradual adaptation that occur. Often the subjective awareness of shortness of breath is obscure and may even be denied by the patient, so the physician must probe beyond the traditional query of how many stairs can be climbed. Today the climbing of stairs can often be totally avoided, and the doctor frequently gets the first clue to dyspnea by asking about a once pleasurable activity such as bike riding or swimming. Frank pulmonary edema occurs much less frequently in mitral stenosis than in other forms of heart failure, in which sudden elevations of left ventricular end-diastolic pressure result in equally elevated levels of left atrial pressure. In these other forms of heart failure there is insufficient time for the secondary adaptive mechanisms to develop and prevent the transudation of fluid from the pulmonary

Table 30-2. Pathophysiology of Mitral Stenosis

Systolic overload of LA; increased pressure work for right heart.

Increased rigidity of lungs due to interstitial tissue changes (engorgement of lymphatics, perivascular cuffing).

Decrease in cardiac output.

Pulmonary arteriolar constriction (secondary, reversible).

Resultant pulmonary hypertension; rarely equals systemic BP (8 percent).

Atrial fibrillation frequent — relates to patient's age and disintegration of atrial muscle.

Myocardial factor.

Note: LA = left atrium; BP = blood pressure.

capillaries into the alveoli. In mitral stenosis the chronic elevation of intravascular pressure results in perivascular cuffing, creating a capillary-alveolar interstitial barrier that retards transudation of fluid. Since pressure is a function of flow × resistance, it is apparent that the level of cardiac output is another major determinant in the production of pulmonary edema. This is suggested in Wood's finding that among patients who gave a history of acute pulmonary edema, normal sinus rhythm was twice as frequent as atrial fibrillation. The average age of Wood's patients with pulmonary edema was 32 as compared with 37 in his series as a whole, suggesting that in time protective mechanisms developed against pulmonary edema.

Hemoptysis occurs in approximately 35 percent of patients with mitral stenosis and is an important early symptom. Since the bronchial veins drain into the pulmonary veins, edema and bleeding of the bronchial mucosa can occur secondary to elevated pulmonary venous pressure. This and a susceptibility to infection are believed to be mainly responsible for the severity of pulmonary symptoms.

Systemic embolism ranges in incidence from 9 to 21 percent in patients suffering from rheumatic mitral valve disease, and in 60 percent of instances the embolism is cerebral. For patients in atrial fibrillation, the incidence has been approximated at 5 percent per patient-year as compared with 0.7 percent per patient-year in patients with sinus rhythm. There is also evidence that systemic embolism is as common with mitral regurgitation as it is with mitral stenosis, and hence the size of the atrial appendage has no influence on the occurrence of embolic phenomena.

Other less common symptoms of mitral stenosis include anginal chest pain, dry cough, and hoarseness. In his series that was dominantly female with an average age of 36, Wood found a 10 percent incidence of chest pain indistinguishable from that encountered in occlusive coronary disease. He attributed this pain to functional impairment of coronary blood flow rather than to occlusive coronary disease, and he found it twice as often in patients with extreme stenosis and high pulmonary vascular resistance than in patients without these symptoms. In contrast, experience derived from selective coronary cineangiography performed at the time of cardiac catheterization indicates that when anginal chest pain occurs in a patient with mitral stenosis, it is associated with demonstrable coronary disease.

Physical Signs. Physical findings in mitral stenosis are extensively covered in standard textbooks of cardiology, and the emphasis here will be placed on features that are of most benefit in diagnosis.

Inspection. The malar flush ascribed to mitral stenosis is found in many patients with rheumatic valvular disease, but certainly it is not specific for mitral stenosis. Patients with mitral stenosis are usually slender and only rarely obese. The jugular venous pulse is helpful in assessing the degree of congestive failure, but it is nonspecific in mitral stenosis. It is well to remember that the negative shadow of the skin deflection coincides with the y trough and calls attention to the next rising v wave. A striking venous pulsation should not be ignored or erroneously attributed to a carotid pulsation. It is therefore important to palpate as well as to inspect pulsations, since an arterial pulsation is readily palpable. A striking v wave bespeaks associated tricuspid regurgitation, whereas an absent or delayed y trough strongly suggests tricuspid stenosis or at least an elevated right ventricular end-diastolic pressure. The precordium is usually quiet in patients with mitral stenosis, but a gentle heave along the left

sternal border is frequently visible when there is significant pulmonary hypertension.

Palpation. The carotid pulse is never bounding in patients with pure mitral stenosis, and if it is present, it indicates some associated problem such as aortic regurgitation, anemia, or thyrotoxicosis. The carotid upstroke in mitral stenosis is normal, although the amplitude characteristically is small. The precordium is nonheaving. The point of maximal impulse is located in the fifth intercostal space, although frequently the point of maximal impulse is displaced laterally as far as the anterior axillary line due to right ventricular enlargement. The point of maximal impulse should not be displaced downward to the sixth intercostal space unless there is associated left ventricular enlargement caused by other conditions. A right ventricular heave may be appreciated as a significant lift across the palm of the hand when the heel of the hand is placed along the manubrium with the fingers extended horizontally toward the anterior axillary line. The heave may extend to, but not beyond, the metacarpophalangeal joints; any lift of the distal phalanges of the hand in this position is strongly suggestive of associated left ventricular enlargement. A diastolic thrill at the apex is virtually pathognomonic of mitral stenosis.

Auscultation. The first heart sound (S_1) is generated primarily by the closure of the atrioventricular valves, as ventricular pressure exceeds atrial at the beginning of systole. Mitral valve closure usually precedes tricuspid valve closure, and the resultant S_1 is often normally reduplicated, or split. Because of the stiffening of the valve leaflets in mitral stenosis, mitral valve closure is delayed and coincides with closure of the tricuspid valve, resulting in the characteristically loud and somewhat snapping first heart sound. The second heart sound (S_2) is increased in intensity due to accentuated pulmonic closure, and there is persistence of physiologic splitting. Normally aortic valve closure precedes pulmonary valve closure, resulting in asynchrony or splitting of the second heart sound. This asynchronous closure is further accentuated by respiration. During inspiration and increased negative intrathoracic pressure there is increased venous return to the right heart, and this in turn prolongs right ventricular ejection time. The result is a split second heart sound, the first component of which is due to aortic valve closure and the second to pulmonic valve closure. When searching for this normal sequence it is important to remember that the inspiratory and expiratory changes should be elicited with the patient breathing continuously. If the examiner asks the patient to take a deep breath so that he can focus his attention at the end of inspiration, the patient will often hold his breath at the end of inspiration or perform a Valsalva maneuver. This will completely obliterate physiologic splitting.

As left ventricular pressure falls below atrial pressure after the end of systole, the mitral valve opens. Normally this opening is inaudible, but due to the pathologic changes in the valve in mitral stenosis, opening of the valve produces a characteristic third heart sound referred to as the opening snap. It occurs 0.06 to 0.12 second after the second sound at the left sternal edge or at the apex. While there is nothing *snapping* about the sound, it does differ considerably from the other third heart sounds. Instead of a dull *thud* typical of the ventricular diastolic gallop, or S_3, this sound, although quite faint, is sharp in quality and seems close to the ear. It is occasionally extremely loud, and then it can be heard even in the aortic area. The higher the left atrial pressure, the sooner the mitral valve opens and thus the earlier the opening snap. The more severe the stenosis, the shorter the S_2-opening snap interval. When the mitral valve is very heavily calcified, it becomes rigid and totally immobile. In this situation the sounds produced by its closure and opening may become almost inaudible. Therefore in the presence of well-established mitral stenosis, a diminished S_1 and an absent opening snap are indications of a heavily calcified valve. Following the opening snap, the flow starts from atrium to ventricle. Passage of blood across the narrowed orifice causes turbulent flow, which results in the typical diastolic murmur of mitral stenosis. It is appreciated as a low-pitched rumble following the opening sound and, with rare exceptions, extends to S_1 if mitral stenosis is significant. It usually requires an extremely light pressure on the bell to hear this murmur, and it is often well localized to a small point

at the apex. It should never be judged absent until several provocative maneuvers have been carried out, such as having the patient turn to the left lateral decubitus position, cough, or perform several sit-ups. Anything that increases heart rate will shorten diastole, augment the pressure gradient, and in turn accentuate the auscultatory findings.

In addition to these specific auscultatory events, there is a characteristic overall cadence in mitral stenosis. In patients with normal sinus rhythm the dominant beat of this cadence is a presystolic accentuation of the diastolic rumble that leads to the characteristically loud first sound. With atrial fibrillation the presystolic accentuation lessens, but it does not totally disappear. There is a striking accentuation of some of the irregularly occurring first heart sounds, that is, the ones occurring after the shorter R-R intervals (two preceding beats that are close together). This specific cadence is particularly helpful in differentiating mitral stenosis from other conditions that mimic it, as when there is an accentuated pulmonic second sound, a loud first sound associated with an early third sound, or a diastolic rumble. Conditions commonly confused with mitral stenosis on auscultation include thyrotoxicosis, atrial septal defect with a large left-to-right shunt, and occasionally a cardiomyopathy. None of these conditions has the cadence of mitral stenosis. A reduplicated first sound virtually excludes significant mitral stenosis, but before relying on this, one must be careful not to confuse it with an early ejection click.

Concomitant findings of congestive heart failure indicate that the mitral stenosis is hemodynamically significant. The absence of failure or even of symptoms, on the other hand, does not mean that significant stenosis is excluded. The presence of a right ventricular heave is perhaps the most reliable sign of pulmonary hypertension; it never occurs in mild stenosis. It is well to remember that the loudness of the murmur of mitral stenosis relates more to the level of cardiac output than it does to the degree of mitral stenosis. A high-pitched diastolic blowing murmur can occasionally be heard at the base of the heart, and when it is clearly located in the pulmonic valve area, it can represent insufficiency of the pulmonary valve. This situation is referred to as the Graham

Steell murmur. In most instances, however, a high-pitched diastolic blowing murmur along the left sternal edge relates to associated aortic regurgitation.

Electrocardiographic Findings. A broad-notched P wave, often most visible in lead II, has been labeled P mitrale because of its frequent association with mitral stenosis and sinus rhythm. Strict criteria for left atrial enlargement, which is a frequent accompaniment of mitral stenosis, have been established and are determined from an analysis of the P terminal force in lead V_1. The algebraic product of the duration (seconds) and the amplitude (millimeters) of the V_1 terminal force ranges from +0.01 to −0.03 in normal people and from −0.03 to −0.30 in subjects with left-sided heart disease. The most helpful electrocardiographic finding in assessing the severity of mitral stenosis is the mean QRS axis in the frontal plane. Rightward displacement of +60 degrees or greater correlates well (90 percent) with a mitral valve area of 1.3 sq cm or less, provided the patient does not have either another valvular disease or significant hypertension.

X-ray. A mitral configuration of the cardiac silhouette may be defined as a wide-waisted heart with a diminutive aortic knob and a distinct pulmonary vascular pattern. The legendary "straight left heart border" is nonspecific and is found in many normal subjects. An enlarged left atrium first appears in the posteroanterior projection of the chest x-ray as a convex bulge immediately below the main pulmonary artery trunk (pulmonary conus). As left atrial hypertrophy ensues, there is an increased density of the left atrial shadow that is recognizable as a double density within the center of the cardiac silhouette, immediately below the bifurcation of the trachea. Continued enlargement results in a convex bulge along the right heart border. In the lateral projection, left atrial enlargement is seen as a discrete bulge fairly high on the posterior margin of the cardiac silhouette. A more gentle bulge lower down on the posterior margin is indicative of left ventricular enlargement and is not apparent in pure mitral stenosis. Thus the typical heart x-ray in severe mitral stenosis may show five separate convex bulges along the left sternal border,

from above downward being (1) a small aortic knob, (2) a prominent pulmonary conus, (3) an enlarged atrium, (4) a dilated right ventricle, and (5) a normal-sized left ventricle. In addition to the dilated main pulmonary artery segments, the vascular pattern in mitral stenosis shows increased blood flow to the upper lung fields.

Echocardiogram. Echocardiography has become a well-established, noninvasive means of studying cardiac motion and has been particularly helpful in the study of the mitral valve with its demonstration that a distinctive mitral echo originates from the anterior mitral leaflet. The reader is referred to the bibliography for articles on this waveform and its correlation to the various phases of the cardiac cycle.

Complications. Congestive heart failure, hemoptysis, and systemic embolism have already been mentioned. Atrial fibrillation deserves further comment, as it can cause serious circulatory embarrassment and in addition can give rise to thromboembolic complications. Atrial systole, appearing at the very end of ventricular diastole, normally plays only a minor role in ventricular filling, which is accomplished passively, for the most part, during early diastole. In mitral stenosis, however, in which left atrial emptying is impeded, the active contraction of the atrium functions more significantly to increase the filling (and output) of the left ventricle. In atrial fibrillation this function is lost. Even more deleterious is the rapid ventricular rate that accompanies atrial fibrillation when conduction in the atrioventricular node is intact. Because the duration of systole is relatively constant, any increase in heart rate takes place at the expense of diastole. Normally the shortening of diastole that accompanies rapid heart rates has little effect on atrial emptying and ventricular filling, but in mitral stenosis it results in further blockage of blood within the left atrium and pulmonary veins, increasing the pulmonary congestion and at the same time reducing left ventricular output. Measurements of cardiac output, ventricular volume, and ejection fraction are reduced below normal in patients with mitral stenosis, with or without atrial fibrillation. Atrial fibrillation exaggerates these abnormalities and requires that the heart rate be controlled by the use of digitalis, which, through its blocking effect on the atrioventricular node, reduces the ventricular rate and hence is very effective therapeutically. The incidence of atrial fibrillation is related more to the patient's age (fibrillation increases with age) than to any other factor. It is precipitated by left atrial enlargement and eventually is perpetuated by disintegration of the atrial muscle.

Differential Diagnosis. Other conditions resulting in blockade to the inflow of the left ventricle include left atrial tumors, extreme calcification of the mitral anulus, and cor triatriatum. These conditions are all exceedingly rare, and one should consider first the more common entities that are often confused with mitral stenosis: atrial septal defect with partial anomalous pulmonary venous drainage, thyrotoxicosis, and cardiomyopathy.

Treatment. Medical therapy for mitral stenosis cannot correct the basic pathologic defect, but it is effective in relieving some of the circulatory consequences. The efficacy of digitalis for congestion, particularly when due to atrial fibrillation with rapid ventricular response, has already been discussed. In the presence of sinus rhythm, digitalis is of less value. Pulmonary hemorrhage is rarely severe in mitral stenosis and usually responds to bed rest and codeine. Anticoagulants are useful in preventing recurrence of systemic emboli, and all patients with atrial fibrillation and mitral stenosis who are essentially asymptomatic should receive anticoagulants unless they are to be considered for surgery. Any patient having a systemic embolus in association with mitral stenosis is promptly placed on anticoagulants, and early cardiac catheterization study is planned unless a severe neurologic deficit persists. If the valve area is found to be 1.5 sq cm or less, the patient is recommended for surgery since only in the presence of a significantly stenotic valve is the number of emboli reduced by surgery. Atrial appendagectomy has no influence on postoperative emboli. Prophylactic penicillin therapy reduces the incidence of both beta-hemolytic streptococcal infections and recurrences of rheumatic carditis. Large doses must be employed to prevent infective endocarditis and should be given

to all patients who are at risk of bacteremia, such as those facing dental procedures, urologic studies, or the incision and drainage of abscesses.

The role of surgery has been clarified over the past 25 years; today it offers the only possibility of "cure" by relieving the mitral obstruction. The relatively low, though definite, postoperative mortality and morbidity and the distinct possibility of recurrence of stenosis following mitral valvuloplasty makes surgery unwarranted in an asymptomatic patient. On the other hand, the operative results in general are so satisfactory that no patient should be allowed to reach serious incapacity without being offered surgery. The selection of patients will be influenced by such factors as age, occupation, and the presence or absence of associated mitral regurgitation and other valvular lesions. The choice of operation, of prosthetic valve replacement, or of mitral valvuloplasty is determined by the age of the patient and by the presence of severe calcification and other variables such as the degree of subchordal fusion. Prosthetic replacement of the mitral valve commits the patient to lifelong anticoagulant therapy.

MITRAL REGURGITATION

In mitral regurgitation of rheumatic origin, fibrosis and scarring produce retraction of the mitral valve leaflets so that the free margins no longer come into apposition during systole. Consequently, during ventricular systole the mitral orifice is not sealed, and backflow of blood into the left atrium results. Unlike mitral stenosis, in which the cardinal circulatory abnormality is a delayed inflow into the left ventricle, mitral regurgitation is best characterized as an abnormality of unloading of the left ventricle during systole.

Incidence. Mitral regurgitation is the dominant or sole lesion in about one-third of all cases of mitral valve involvement. The sex ratio is nearly equal, with a slight preponderance in men.

Pathophysiology. Systolic regurgitation of blood into the left atrium places a volume load on the left ventricle. The primary adaptive mechanism of the left ventricle in this situation is a decline in tension during systole. This allows the contractile energy of the

Table 30-3. Pathophysiology of Mitral Regurgitation

Abnormal unloading of LV: Low impedance to outflow allows peak velocity of ejection to occur early
and rapidly.

Rapid reduction in wall tension allows contractile
energy to be expended in shortening, not in developing tension.

Twenty percent of total SV ejects backward into LA
prior to aortic opening.

Diastolic inflow is augmented (increased EDV), but
flow work is accomplished with reduced afterload.

Myocardial VO_2 not substantially increased.

Progressive dilatation and thinning of LA wall.

Myocardial contractility is depressed (? mechanism).

Note: LV = left ventricle; SV = stroke volume; LA = left
atrium; EDV = end-diastolic volume; VO_2 = oxygen consumption.

heart to be expended in shortening rather than in
developing tension, without a significant increase in
myocardial oxygen consumption. To maintain normal forward flow, the left ventricular stroke output
must be increased by an amount that approximates
the volume of regurgitation. One of the compensatory mechanisms that permits the stroke output to
increase is elongation of the diastolic myocardial
fiber length; this is achieved by ventricular dilatation
(Starling's law). Left ventricular enlargement is
therefore a prominent feature of mitral regurgitation.
When the left ventricle is no longer able to sustain the
added work load, it fails, causing the characteristic
symptoms and signs of left ventricular decompensation.

Following systolic regurgitation of blood into the
left atrium as the result of mitral incompetence, there
is prompt and massive early ventricular filling in diastole. There is no impairment to decompression of the
atrium during diastole; therefore pulmonary congestion and pulmonary hypertension are less liable to
occur. Even a short diastole does not prevent proper
ventricular filling, and hence atrial fibrillation and
tachycardia are relatively better tolerated. These considerations contribute significantly to the natural history and clinical findings of patients with pure mitral
regurgitation (Table 30-3).

Natural History. It is generally believed that patients
with mitral regurgitation have had a more severe form

of acute rheumatic fever and that the condition has
existed unchanged from the time of active carditis,
that is, with virtually no latent interval. The early
and easy recognition of the systolic murmur of mitral
insufficiency, in contrast to the easily missed and
later developing diastolic murmur of stenosis, may be
responsible for the large number of patients with
regurgitation being diagnosed as having rheumatic
fever during the acute stage. Since flow work is
better tolerated than pressure work by the myocardium, these patients also are symptom-free longer
than patients with mitral stenosis. However, there is
considerable disagreement about the clinical course
once symptoms have developed. Wood observed a
more progressive downhill course that averaged 5.3
years, but recent series suggest that many patients
with severe mitral regurgitation have a prolonged and
often benign course.

There are multiple etiologies of organic mitral
regurgitation in addition to acute rheumatic fever and
bacterial endocarditis. These include rupture of the
chordae tendineae, rupture of papillary muscles
secondary to trauma or infarction, calcification of
the anulus fibrosis, and congenital malformations that
include ostium primum defects and myxomatous
degeneration of the mitral valve leaflets. A clinical
spectrum of severe mitral regurgitation includes at
one end, patients with acute mitral regurgitation
resulting from spontaneous rupture of chordae
tendineae, and, at the other end, patients with long-
standing mitral regurgitation due to rheumatic heart
disease. Patients with acute mitral regurgitation have
thick-walled small left atria with marked left atrial
hypertension, while patients with chronic mitral
regurgitation have markedly dilated left atria and
low atrial pressures. Although these two groups of
patients may be equally disabled, their clinical
examinations may differ significantly.

Clinical Profile. The symptoms of mitral regurgitation
are predominantly those due to a low cardiac output,
and the primary complaint is often fatigue. In comparison to mitral stenosis, there is less exertional dyspnea and only half the incidence of pulmonary edema,
hemoptysis, and angina. The physical signs include a
characteristic peripheral pulse that rises rapidly and

sharply but is poorly sustained. This is the result of a high peak velocity of left ventricular ejection, which is more rapid and occurs earlier than normal. The precordium reveals a hyperdynamic apex with the point of maximal impulse displaced downward and to the left. There is often a visible but false right ventricular heave; it is seen as a sustained lift of the precordium just to the left of the sternal edge and is the result of anterior displacement of the heart due to atrial expansion during ventricular systole.

Auscultation. The most striking finding in mitral regurgitation is a holosystolic murmur that is well heard along the left sternal border but is usually maximal at the apex and frequently radiates to the axilla. The murmur begins with the first sound and extends to or through the second sound, since, with an incompetent mitral valve, left ventricular pressure exceeds left atrial pressure from the onset of isometric contraction to isometric relaxation. The murmur has several features that distinguish it from the murmur of aortic stenosis, which may be equally intense at the apex. The murmur of aortic stenosis invariably begins after the first sound and ends before the second. A very helpful clue to the origin of a systolic murmur is its character after a compensatory pause due to a premature ventricular beat. During the compensatory pause there is greater filling of the left ventricle, and the next beat ejects a greater stroke volume. In the case of aortic stenosis this results in an intensification of the systolic murmur, whereas in mitral regurgitation there is no such intensification. The administration of a peripheral vasodilator such as amyl nitrite results in a diminution of intensity of the regurgitant murmur, since it lowers the impedance to left ventricular outflow and temporarily lessens the degree of mitral regurgitation. It is well to remember that the murmur of mitral regurgitation can radiate anteriorly to the base of the heart and simulate aortic stenosis. This radiation results from incompetence of the posterior mitral leaflet, which directs the regurgitant stream forward and immediately against the atrial septum. The holosystolic murmur of mitral regurgitation is often followed by an early diastolic to mid-diastolic rumble, and in severe cases this may suggest a to-and-fro murmur at the apex.

The first heart sound in mitral regurgitation is usually quite soft and single. The second heart sound at the base is almost invariably split to some degree. Due to the regurgitation, the left ventricle is unable to sustain intraventricular pressure, which falls off abruptly as systole proceeds. Therefore aortic valve closure occurs prematurely, and the first component of the second heart sound occurs earlier than normal. This explains the splitting of the second heart sound with maintenance of normal respiratory variations. Following the systolic regurgitation of blood into the left atrium, there is prompt and massive ventricular filling in diastole. This gives rise to a prominent ventricular diastolic gallop heard as a third heart sound following the second sound in early diastole. Fourth heart sounds or atrial gallops are extremely uncommon in established mitral regurgitation. An atrial gallop is considered the hallmark of a recent onset of mitral regurgitation, and it persists until the left atrium finally loses normal compliance. In the average case this takes 9 to 18 months after, for example, the sudden onset of mitral regurgitation due to ruptured chordae.

X-ray. Mitral regurgitation is characterized by left atrial enlargement, and its x-ray appearance is frequently difficult to distinguish from that of mitral stenosis. However, the largest atria result from mitral regurgitation. Frequently there is left ventricular enlargement, and the aortic knob tends to be larger than in patients with pure mitral stenosis. Calcification of the mitral valve is rarely seen in pure mitral regurgitation.

Electrocardiographic Findings. As compared to pure mitral stenosis, in which left ventricular hypertrophy (LVH) is rarely present, the ECG in mitral regurgitation frequently indicates LVH. The frontal plane axis is usually less rightward in mitral regurgitation than in stenosis, but atrial fibrillation is more common and occurs earlier. It is also well to remember that in one-third of the cases LVH is not present and, when present, is rarely as striking as with the concentric hypertrophy of aortic valvular disease.

Echocardiogram. This is less helpful in mitral regurgitation than in stenosis.

Complications. The principal complication in mitral regurgitation is left ventricular failure, which occurs when progressive dilatation of the heart can no longer accommodate the volume overload. In only a third of the cases does extreme pulmonary hypertension develop. Originally it was thought that the regurgitant stream and the rapid diastolic emptying of the left atrium would tend to prevent stagnation of blood and, as a result, the occurrence of atrial thrombosis and arterial embolization. However, in one large series of patients embolism was as common in mitral regurgitation as it was in mitral stenosis. Infective endocarditis is a constant hazard, and it occurs more frequently in mitral regurgitation than in mitral stenosis.

Differential Diagnosis. An apical systolic murmur developing after an episode of rheumatic carditis, along with the physical, radiologic, and electrocardiographic signs discussed above, poses no great problem; the diagnosis is mitral regurgitation. Often, however, the situation is less clear, and a knowledge of the differential diagnosis of apical systolic murmurs and the use of special diagnostic methods (cardiac catheterization and angiocardiography) may be required for proper evaluation.

Other causes of organic mitral regurgitation have been mentioned earlier. Rupture of chordae tendineae may occur (1) spontaneously without known cause, (2) as a result of sudden extreme effort, (3) following trauma, or (4) due to infective endocarditis. Following such rupture, even though the valve leaflets themselves are normal, they cannot seal the valve orifice during systole because they have lost their anchorage. The condition is often associated with a rapid downhill course requiring surgical intervention with valve replacement. Papillary muscle rupture usually results from acute myocardial infarction and leads to fulminating mitral regurgitation and left ventricular failure. It should always be suspected when a loud apical systolic murmur occurs suddenly in the early stages of an acute myocardial infarction. Papillary muscle dysfunction can occur without rupture, and then it is the result of fibrosis and scarring associated with coronary artery disease. It results in faulty mitral valve closure and is manifested by an apical systolic murmur; however, hemodynamically the regurgitation is usually not severe. Calcification of the anulus fibrosis of the mitral valve, commonly found in older people, often produces a holosystolic apical murmur consistent with mitral regurgitation. It rarely produces hemodynamically significant regurgitation, and the murmur is attributed to turbulent blood flow over the jutting margins of the calcified anulus. The loss of sphincteric action by the calcified anulus results in an orifice too large to be bridged by the leaflets.

The entities difficult to distinguish from mitral regurgitation are (1) ventricular septal defect, (2) tricuspid regurgitation, and (3) idiopathic hypertrophic subaortic stenosis. All three are associated with holosystolic precordial murmurs. Tricuspid regurgitation almost invariably causes prominent systolic venous pulsations in the neck, and its murmur is often augmented with inspiration. Since tricuspid regurgitation usually occurs in association with mitral stenosis, a careful search for the characteristic opening snap and diastolic rumble of mitral stenosis in the lateral precordium is required. The murmur of ventricular septal defect is usually located closer to the sternum than it is in mitral regurgitation, and the murmur extends to the right sternal border. Most often the ventricular septal defect murmur is associated with a palpable systolic thrill, and the chest x-ray presents the characteristic congested appearance of the pulmonary vasculature consistent with the left-to-right shunt. Idiopathic hypertrophic subaortic stenosis is usually associated with some degree of mitral regurgitation. The Valsalva maneuver is most helpful in identifying idiopathic hypertrophic subaortic stenosis; it is the only condition in which a systolic murmur intensifies during the strain phase of the Valsalva maneuver, whereas in other primary valvular disorders the systolic murmur will diminish as the stroke volume is reduced.

Treatment. Medical treatment of mitral regurgitation is the same as for left ventricular failure due to any cause, with the addition of antibiotic therapy to prevent rheumatic fever and endocarditis. It is well to remember that many patients with congestive heart failure from other causes such as cardiomyopathy, aortic stenosis, or coronary artery disease will manifest an apical systolic murmur indicative of cardiac dilatation and secondary (functional) mitral regurgitation. As their congestive failure responds to therapy, the systolic murmur will diminish and usually will disappear. Conversely, when there is congestive heart failure due to organic mitral regurgitation, the apical systolic murmur is less intense; and as the cardiac output improves on treatment, the apical systolic murmur will become louder.

Reconstruction of the incompetent mitral valve by surgery has not proved successful. Surgical therapy therefore consists in prosthetic valve replacement. The accepted surgical mortality ranges from 5 to 10 percent for this procedure, and the operation generally results in improved cardiac function. Emboli from the prosthesis are a continued hazard and require lifelong anticoagulation therapy. The operation is therefore reserved for patients who have had at least one episode of congestive heart failure and are beyond New York Heart Association Functional Class II in disability.

MITRAL VALVE PROLAPSE: THE BARLOW SYNDROME
In recent years a syndrome has been described in patients with clinical findings of a nonejection click and a late systolic murmur ascribed to the mitral valve. Barlow demonstrated that the late systolic murmur behaved like the murmur of mitral regurgitation and showed that it was associated with protrusion of the mitral valve leaflets into the left atrium during the middle third of systole. These findings, coupled with a distinctive electrocardiographic pattern, now constitute the syndrome that appropriately bears Barlow's name. Anatomic features have been documented both at the time of surgery and at postmortem examination. These features include voluminous, scalloped leaflets of the mitral valve as well as myxomatous degeneration of the valve substance without any inflammatory changes. Barlow's syndrome is often referred to as the "floppy mitral valve syndrome."

Incidence. As the Barlow syndrome is a newly emerging entity, there is much yet to be learned about its natural history. It has a striking predilection for women, and since it also has a characteristic echocardiographic pattern, there is opportunity to study normal populations to determine its exact incidence. Presently it is estimated to occur in 6 to 18 percent of young healthy women.

Clinical Profile. The syndrome occurs most frequently in young or middle-aged women who present with a variety of symptoms that include chest pain, lightheadedness, dyspnea, fatigue, and palpitations. Chest pain has been found in 60 percent of patients with symptoms, and it has been attributed to ischemia of the posterior papillary muscle due to excessive stretching of the chordae tendineae that are attached to the billowing mitral leaflet.

Auscultation. This reveals a snapping extra sound in middle to late systole. The extra sound is heard loudest at the apex or just inside the apex, and it is considered to be the auscultatory hallmark of the Barlow syndrome. In some patients the sound has a scratchy quality or makes multiple clicks that may create the erroneous impression of a friction rub. The click is often followed by a late systolic murmur, but not invariably so. In other patients, only a pansystolic murmur is audible. It is important to realize that the midsystolic click may not be present in the supine position, but it may emerge as the patient assumes the left lateral decubitus or upright position. The click occurs earlier during inspiration, in the straining phase of the Valsalva maneuver, and following inhalation of amyl nitrite.

Electrocardiographic Findings. The ECG in the Barlow syndrome often shows inversion of the T waves in leads II, III, and aVF, with or without minimal ST depression. Similar changes may appear in the left precordial leads as well. Ventricular irritability is considered a frequent accompaniment of this syndrome and is estimated to occur in 25 percent of the cases. Often an exercise stress test is required to unmask the ventricular irritability. No associated abnormalities of the coronary arteries have been found to account for the electrocardiographic changes.

X-ray. This demonstrates no distinct features; however, the left cineventriculogram obtained at cardiac catheterization is diagnostic of the Barlow syndrome.

It shows a billowing posterior and oftentimes anterior leaflet protruding into the left atrium during systole.

Echocardiogram. This has proved helpful in diagnosing the Barlow syndrome by demonstrating abnormal waveforms of the mitral valve echo in systole. There is separation of the posterior leaflet in systole in most cases. In addition, there is usually exaggerated excursion of the anterior mitral leaflet in diastole.

Complications. While ruptured chordae tendineae have been found in association with myxomatous degeneration of mitral valve leaflets, this is probably rare in the Barlow syndrome. The most disturbing feature is the occurrence of palpitations and, in certain instances, marked ventricular irritability. Originally it was thought that sudden death might be more common in patients with this syndrome, but as larger population studies are being reported, this has not become statistically significant. Infective endocarditis is a known risk and a recognized complication.

Treatment. Only in rare instances is the degree of associated mitral regurgitation severe enough in the Barlow syndrome to warrant mitral valve replacement. Medical therapy is directed toward control of bothersome arrhythmias. Propranolol therapy has been suggested to reduce the tension on stretched chordae tendineae, and this beta-adrenergic blocking agent is occasionally effective in reducing the frequency of arrhythmias as well. Prophylaxis against subacute bacterial endocarditis is recommended for all patients.

Aortic Valve Disease

AORTIC STENOSIS

Valvular aortic stenosis may be congenital, rheumatic, or purely sclerotic in origin. The pathogenesis of traumatic changes leading to progressive deformity with fibrous thickening and heavy calcification of the aortic cusps has already been discussed. The normal orifice of the aortic valve measures approximately 3 sq cm, and physiologic stenosis is considered to be present when the orifice is less than 0.8 sq cm. The three semilunar leaflets of the aortic valve have neither chordae tendineae nor papillary muscles, and their opening and closing is determined solely by the relative pressures in the left ventricle and aorta. Each cusp is attached to the fibrous ring of the aortic base, and each encloses a localized dilatation of the aortic wall known as the sinus of Valsalva. Two of these contain the ostia of the right and left coronary arteries. It is estimated that 25 percent of all cases of chronic rheumatic heart disease involve stenosis of the aortic valve.

Natural History. Aortic stenosis has the longest latent period of all the rheumatic lesions, averaging 38 years from the acute rheumatic process to the onset of symptoms. However, it is rapidly fatal once symptoms begin, with an average duration of 3 years after symptoms begin. The age at onset of symptoms, however, does not influence the rapidly downhill course. In the United States the average age at death from aortic stenosis is 63 years. Compared to other valvular lesions, there is a higher incidence of sudden death from aortic stenosis, estimated to be 15 to 20 percent. In children with significant aortic stenosis from birth, the incidence of sudden death is estimated to be 7.5 percent during the first decade. If a child with aortic stenosis reaches age 10 without any clinical symptoms or any ECG abnormalities, sudden death rarely occurs. When the stenosis is severe enough to lead to congestive failure during infancy, mortality approaches 30 percent.

Pathophysiology. Impedance to left ventricular outflow results in increased pressure work for the left ventricle. Pressure work is one of the primary determinants of myocardial oxygen consumption and of demand for coronary blood flow. In response to the stenosis, the myocardial fibers hypertrophy, resulting in marked thickening of the chamber walls. There is a raised initial tension and an elevated maximum pressure within the left ventricular chamber, while the pressure in the aorta is significantly lower than normal and reaches a maximum later in systole; consequently, left ventricular ejection is prolonged and aortic valve closure is delayed. The narrowed aortic orifice often results in a jetlike expulsion of blood into the aorta, resulting in increased turbulence of blood flow and secondary changes in the aortic wall.

Occasionally these changes compromise the coronary ostia located distal to the valvular narrowing.

Clinical Profile. The symptoms most commonly associated with significant aortic stenosis are effort syncope, angina pectoris, and complaints referable to left ventricular failure. Exertional light-headedness or frank syncope is thought to be the result of abnormal vasodilatation that prevents an adequate maintenance of blood pressure. The angina pectoris is indistinguishable from that associated with occlusive coronary disease, and indeed many patients in their sixth decade do have associated coronary lesions. An equal number, however, have no significant coronary disease but complain of angina presumably because coronary blood flow cannot keep pace with the demand of the hypertrophied muscle fibers working under an extreme load. Coronary filling is also diminished by the low mean blood pressure in the aorta. Dyspnea heralds the onset of left ventricular failure and this, the gravest of the clinical symptoms, indicates a survival of rarely more than 6 to 18 months.

Physical Findings. The classic physical findings of aortic stenosis are those of a small carotid pulse with a delayed upstroke, a palpable thrill over the aortic area, a late-peaking ejection-type systolic murmur, and a markedly reduced or absent aortic second sound. The parvus et tardus carotid pulse may not be evident in the elderly patient, whose sclerotic vessels may actually present a full and rather rapidly rising carotid upstroke. A systolic thrill over the base of the heart is an important finding, because it correlates well with the severity of stenosis. The ventricle-to-aorta systolic gradient is usually 50 mm Hg or greater when a thrill is palpable and less than this when a thrill is absent.

Auscultation. Many features can alter the intensity of the aortic stenotic murmur, such as concomitant pulmonary disease with an increased anteroposterior diameter of the chest, and therefore the intensity is a poor index of the degree of stenosis. The murmur is characteristically ejection in type, beginning after the first sound and ending before the second sound, and its crescendo-decrescendo characteristic is an impor-

tant clue to the severity of stenosis. The more severe the stenosis, the more time required to overcome the obstruction and, consequently, the later the peaking of the murmur. Since aortic ejection is prolonged, aortic closure is delayed, often until well after pulmonic valve closure. In this case the normal physiologic splitting will be reversed. A single second sound is heard at the end of inspiration, and a split sound is heard during expiration. This is referred to as paradoxical splitting. The thickened, fibrosed aortic valve produces a sound on opening much like that produced by a diseased mitral valve. This opening sound is heard in early systole just after S_1 and is referred to as an ejection click. Following the loud ejection systolic murmur, it is often possible to hear a faint diastolic blowing murmur indicating a mild degree of aortic regurgitation. When significant aortic incompetence is associated with aortic stenosis, the peripheral manifestations of aortic regurgitation will be present. These are discussed below.

The systolic murmur of aortic stenosis may actually be loudest at the apex, and the uninitiated may misinterpret this to represent mitral regurgitation. However, at the apex the murmur maintains its ejection form and should be readily distinguishable from the holosystolic murmur of mitral regurgitation. As one inches the stethoscope from the aortic area to the apex, the harsh systolic murmur of aortic stenosis can often be noted to become higher pitched and even musical. This change, known as the Gallavardin phenomenon, should not make the observer postulate an additional cardiac lesion. It is also well to remember that the aortic stenotic murmur is louder after the compensatory pause following a premature ventricular beat.

Palpation. Since the left ventricle undergoes marked concentric hypertrophy in response to aortic stenosis, the point of maximal impulse is often located in the normal position in the fifth intercostal space within the midclavicular line. There is, however, a sustained systolic lift to this impulse that occupies more than half of systole. There is often also a palpable atrial systole that is felt as a double apical impulse.

Electrocardiographic Findings. The ECG will invariably show marked LVH in adults with severe aortic stenosis who do not have a conduction abnormality. In children, hemodynamically significant aortic stenosis can be present without the ECG showing extremes of LVH.

X-ray. The appearance of significant aortic stenosis can frequently be quite subtle. Since initially there is no dilatation, overall cardiac size is often within normal limits. As dilatation occurs, there is progressive prominence of the left ventricular chamber. The ascending aorta almost invariably shows poststenotic dilatation, and this can be appreciated by seeing the ascending aorta projecting beyond the right cardiac border in the posteroanterior projection. In the lateral projection, calcification can often be seen in the region of the aortic valve. The calcification is frequently dense and has a mulberrylike appearance.

Echocardiogram. This can provide helpful information, although it is not useful in quantifying the aortic stenosis. In addition to the enlarged dimensions of the dilated aorta, it shows the waveform characteristic of a calcified, thickened aortic valve. The echocardiogram is particularly helpful in identifying a congenital bicuspid aortic valve by indicating eccentricity of the valve opening.

Diagnosis. Perhaps more important and challenging than the differential diagnosis of aortic stenosis itself is the assessment of the degree of outflow obstruction and a determination of the status of ventricular function. These evaluations invariably require cardiac catheterization and the measurement of the pressure gradient and flow across the aortic valve. In addition, by performing coronary cineangiography at the same time it is possible to determine whether there is associated obstructive coronary disease.

The most important entities to be distinguished from aortic valvular stenosis are subvalvular (idiopathic hypertrophic subaortic stenosis) and supravalvular stenosis. Coarctation of the aorta and pulmonic stenosis are also associated with an ejection type of systolic murmur but are usually quite readily distinguishable on clinical grounds. In rare instances, very severe aortic stenosis can be clinically silent; this occurs when severe left ventricular failure results in

marked reduction of the cardiac output and a diminished intensity of the systolic murmur to the point at which it is virtually inaudible.

Treatment. Medical treatment is directed at left ventricular failure, while surgical treatment consists in aortic valve correction with a prosthetic device, an aortic valve allograft, or a porcine valve. The allografts and xenografts, being natural tissue valves, do not require long-term anticoagulation therapy, but they do have a higher incidence of postoperative aortic regurgitation. Hence the prosthetic valve continues to be the most commonly used, both because surgical mortality has been reduced to 3 to 8 percent and because the course of aortic stenosis is so malignant, once symptoms develop, that enthusiasm for its surgical correction may be expected to continue.

AORTIC REGURGITATION

The most common cause of aortic regurgitation (aortic insufficiency, aortic incompetence) continues to be rheumatic valvulitis, with 20 percent of the cases of valvulitis occurring during the initial attack. It is estimated that the aortic valve is involved in 45 percent of all cases of chronic rheumatic heart disease; half of these have clinical manifestations within 5 years and 90 percent within 15 years. Scarring, distortion, and retraction of the valve cusps prevent their apposition during diastole and permit backflow into the left ventricle. A congenital bicuspid aortic valve usually presents with mild incompetence before it progresses to significant stenosis. Syphilitic aortitis produces dilatation of the ascending aorta by destruction of the elastic and muscular fibers and ultimately allows free regurgitation. Infective endocarditis can result in the perforation or the destruction of one or more valve cusps; other causes of aortic regurgitation include dissecting aneurysm, chest wall trauma, ankylosing spondylitis, Reiter's disease, severe hypertension, and atherosclerosis.

Pathophysiology. The main features of the pathophysiology of aortic regurgitation are listed in Table 30-4. Aortic regurgitation creates a volume overload for the left ventricle by virtue of the blood that leaks back during diastole. The ventricle initially adapts

Table 30-4. Pathophysiology of Aortic Regurgitation

Volume overload, LV dilatation, increased T ($\frac{P \times r}{h}$); LVH develops to normalize wall stress.

Ventricular shape, V_{cf}, wall thickening, fiber orientation remain intact (in contrast to dilatation 2° to myocardial injury).

Preserved D/L results in increased equatorial stress.

Aortic regurgitation present at end of index rheumatic attack in 20 percent; will appear in 45 percent at 5 yr and 90 percent in 15 yr.

Combination of LVH, BP 140/40, cardiomegaly identifies high-risk group (25 percent mortality in 3 yr, CHF or angina in 88 percent within 6 yr).

Low-risk patients have only 7 percent chance of developing symptoms and 4.4 percent chance of sudden death.

Note: T = wall tension; P = intracavitary pressure; r = radius; h = wall thickness; V_{cf} = rate of circumferential fiber shortening; D/L = ratio of short axis to long axis; LV = left ventricular; LVH = left ventricular hypertrophy.

by dilating, with the stretched myocardial fibers augmenting the force of contraction according to the Starling mechanism. The stroke volume is consequently increased, as is the initial tension. According to the Laplace relationship, increased left ventricular wall tension results because of the higher pressure and the increased radius of curvature. This tension later becomes normalized by an increasing wall thickness as left ventricular hypertrophy ensues. Since maximum pressure is attained earlier in systole, the ejection phase is shortened and the pressure falls away rapidly in late systole. In this regard the ejection phase is similar to mitral regurgitation, with the pressure curve so altered that early systole is loaded and late systole unloaded. This type of left ventricular ejection results in a rapidly rising percussion wave followed by a late systolic collapse. Since part of the blood leaks rapidly out of the aorta, back through the incompetent valve, diastolic pressure is lower than normal. The primary determinant of the diastolic blood pressure, however, continues to be the resistance vessels — the peripheral arterioles — which dilate and increase the rate at which blood leaves the central aorta. Both regurgitation and vasodilatation contribute to the bounding arterial pulse that is the hallmark of aortic regurgitation. Left ventricular dilata-

tion and hypertrophy progress inexorably to produce some of the largest hearts seen in clinical medicine.

Clinical Profile. The symptoms of aortic regurgitation are basically those of left ventricular failure. Many individuals with severe disease are aware of vigorous heart action prior to the onset of failure, and often they observe their neck vessels pulsating and their beds rocking. A small percentage of patients have angina pectoris because of poor coronary perfusion secondary to a lowered diastolic pressure. This is considered an ominous symptom of severe aortic incompetence; it can occur without coronary obstructive disease and results in part from an excessive myocardial demand.

The diagnosis of significant aortic regurgitation is usually made on the basis of a water-hammer (Corrigan) pulse, a wide arterial pulse pressure, and abnormalities relating to vasodilatation and pulse wave transmission. The abnormal pulse wave transmission accounts for the higher systolic blood pressure found in the lower as compared to the upper extremities, known as Hill's sign. When present, this sign indicates severe aortic regurgitation, but it can be unreliable in the presence of congestive heart failure. Another indication of aortic regurgitation is capillary pulsation that is visible (and often palpable) when the nailbeds are lightly compressed (Quincke's sign). In aortic regurgitation the Korotkoff sounds normally elicited during the recording of blood pressure have a characteristic "pistol shot" quality, even without the cuff fully inflated. The Duroziez sign refers to a to-and-fro bruit heard over a large artery when it is compressed with a bell stethoscope.

Inspection, Palpation, and Auscultation. The precordium invariably reveals hyperdynamic pulsations, with the point of maximal impulse displaced downward to the sixth left interspace and extended laterally beyond the midclavicular line. Often a systolic thrill can be felt in the aortic area; if so, it does not necessarily mean that there is a critical aortic stenosis. It is the rule rather than the exception to hear a prominent ejection-type systolic murmur in association with the diastolic blow of aortic regurgitation. This systolic murmur is created by a *relative* aortic stenosis resulting from the augmented stroke volume. The diastolic blow of aortic regurgitation is frequently heard in the aortic area but often radiates to a midposition along the left sternal edge. It is comprised of high-frequency vibrations and is therefore best appreciated with the diaphragm stethoscope firmly applied against the chest. In severe aortic regurgitation the diastolic vibrations are also well heard at the apex, where they often assume a lower frequency and may be confused with a diastolic rumble. The regurgitant jet from the aortic valve can interfere with complete opening of the aortic leaflet of the mitral valve and can produce a distant diastolic rumble identical to that of mitral stenosis (Austin Flint murmur). Radiation of the diastolic blow along the sternal edge is often a clue to the etiology: When the aorta is markedly dilated, as in syphilitic aortitis or dissecting aneurysm, radiation is more prominent along the right sternal border. By contrast, rheumatic valvulitis usually results in radiation of the murmur along the left sternal border, where it is heard best.

X-ray and Electrocardiographic Findings. The cardiac silhouette in patients with chronic aortic regurgitation has a characteristic appearance: The left ventricle predominates, it has an elongated and somewhat globular appearance, and its apex often disappears behind the diaphragm. The aortic knob is prominent and, in regurgitation due to syphilis, there is frequently linear calcification in the aortic wall. Under fluoroscopy a characteristic vigorous pulsation of the aorta can be seen. Extreme calcification of the valve is never seen in pure aortic regurgitation. The ECG shows the characteristic pattern of LVH. Very young patients (less than 16) often show excess voltage in the precordial leads, even with a normal chest wall configuration.

Natural History. In general, the clinical course will depend on the etiology of the regurgitation; when aortic regurgitation accompanies dissection of the aorta, the prognosis is grave and even immediate surgical intervention is accompanied by a high mortality. On the other hand, individuals with mild aortic regurgitation in association with ankylosing spondy-

litis often show no ill effects during a normal life span. In patients with rheumatic heart disease with aortic regurgitation, the prognosis relates to the degree of incompetence. A high-risk group of individuals may be identified by the triad of a wide pulse pressure (systolic in excess of 140 mm Hg or diastolic below 40 mm Hg), pronounced LVH by ECG, and significant cardiomegaly by x-ray. Any two of these findings, even in an individual who may be asymptomatic, indicate a 25 percent mortality within 3 years and an 88 percent chance of congestive heart failure or angina within 6 years. Individuals without this triad are considered to be at low risk and have only a 7 percent likelihood of ever developing symptoms; their greatest risk is from infective endocarditis.

Differential Diagnosis. Because of the striking peripheral manifestations of significant aortic regurgitation, there is rarely any difficulty in diagnosing it. To-and-fro murmurs at the base of the heart can be heard in other conditions; most of these arise from some kind of arteriovenous fistula such as patent ductus arteriosus, pulmonary arteriovenous fistula, rupture of an aortic sinus into the right atrium, or right ventricle and coronary arteriovenous fistula. While these conditions are associated with a rapidly rising and collapsing peripheral pulse, they rarely produce the striking peripheral findings seen in aortic regurgitation. The location of the to-and-fro murmur near an arteriovenous communication is also frequently an important clue.

Treatment. Medical therapy is directed at relief of left ventricular failure and prophylaxis against infective endocarditis. Surgical valve replacement using a prosthetic device or allograft valve constitutes the only definitive therapy; the overall operative mortality is 6 percent. Individuals in frank congestive heart failure at the time of surgery have a higher risk (15 percent), whereas those with minimal or early symptoms have an operative risk of only 2 to 4 percent. The late mortality following surgery (20 to 25 percent) appears to be closely related to the size of the left ventricle at the time of operation.

Tricuspid Valve Disease

TRICUSPID STENOSIS

Organic involvement of the tricuspid valve is found at autopsy in 10 to 20 percent of patients with chronic rheumatic heart disease. It rarely occurs as an isolated valvular lesion but is nearly always accompanied by mitral stenosis and often by aortic valve disease as well. For this reason, it is frequently overlooked at the time of clinical evaluation. In Wood's carefully studied group of rheumatic patients the incidence was 4 percent. Disseminated lupus erythematosus, argentaffinoma, and the metastatic carcinoid have each been incriminated as rare causes for lesions involving the right side of the heart, including both the tricuspid and the pulmonic valves.

Pathophysiology. Tricuspid stenosis prevents proper filling of the right ventricle and therefore results in a lowered cardiac output. When it is associated with mitral stenosis, as it usually is, it tends to lessen pulmonary venous congestion. The elevation of right atrial pressure is transmitted directly backward to the systemic venous circuit and produces marked distention of the neck veins with characteristic waveforms, engorgement of the liver, and the development of ascites and dependent peripheral edema.

Clinical Profile. The symptoms associated with tricuspid stenosis may relate merely to an awareness of the venous pulsations in the neck, which may become quite distracting and noticeable. More commonly, however, the patient becomes symptomatic from associated mitral or aortic valve disease. Whenever a patient is found to have the murmur of mitral stenosis and an inordinate amount of peripheral edema with comparatively little pulmonary vascular congestion, one should think of tricuspid stenosis.

The physical signs of tricuspid stenosis are actually plentiful, and it is surprising that the diagnosis is frequently overlooked. Murmurs emanating from the tricuspid valve characteristically intensify during inspiration. This is due to the increased venous filling of the right heart when intrathoracic pressure becomes more negative. The murmur of tricuspid stenosis is often indistinguishable from that of mitral

stenosis except that it is located in the third and fourth left intercostal spaces adjacent to the sternal edge in comparison to mitral stenosis, which is heard more laterally. The opening snap tends to be closer to the second sound, and the rumble is usually louder than a mitral rumble because of the more superficial location of the tricuspid valve. When the rumble intensifies during inspiration, the observer can be quite certain of its tricuspid origin. The diastolic murmur of tricuspid stenosis tends to be higher pitched than a mitral rumble, and it may be confused with a diastolic murmur thought to emanate from the aortic or pulmonic valve.

The principal clue to tricuspid valve disease is the jugular venous pulse. Normally the jugular waveform is triphasic, consisting of three positive waves separated by two negative troughs or descents for each cardiac cycle. The first of the positive waves is the presystolic a wave caused by contraction of the right atrium, and it is followed by the x descent as the atrium relaxes during ventricular systole. The x descent is interrupted by the c wave, which represents an artifact thought to be due to transmitted carotid pulsations. The eye rarely appreciates this small notch in the waveform as a positive deflection. The c wave is followed by the most prominent positive wave, the v wave, which is produced during late systole by the rising pressure in the right atrium due to venous inflow against the closed tricuspid valve. The v wave is followed by the most prominent negative deflection, the y descent, which develops as the valve opens and atrial pressure falls. In tricuspid stenosis there is an overall distention of the jugular venous column and a striking intensification of the atrial systolic (a) wave when sinus rhythm is present. In patients with atrial fibrillation this "giant a wave" is absent, of course, while the v descent is noticeably delayed or absent. Hepatomegaly, ascites, and pronounced peripheral edema are also usually present.

X-ray and Electrocardiographic Findings. Right atrial enlargement is pronounced, with the cardiac silhouette extending well to the right of the spine. The overall configuration of the heart shadow is determined largely by any associated valvular lesions present in the aortic or mitral area. Pulmonary venous congestion often is noticeably absent. In patients with normal sinus rhythm, the ECG shows a combination of an unusually tall and widened P wave that is actually a combination of P pulmonale and P mitrale. Right ventricular hypertrophy is usually absent.

Diagnosis. Other conditions associated with prominent *a* waves in the jugular venous pulse include pulmonary hypertension, pulmonic stenosis, and occasionally pericardial effusion. Conditions associated with marked pulmonary hypertension can usually be identified by the accompanying right ventricular heave along the left sternal border; this is usually absent in tricuspid stenosis. The typical systolic murmur of pulmonic stenosis clearly separates that entity from tricuspid disease, and pericardial effusion rarely, if ever, creates prominent a waves or interferes with the y descent.

The definitive diagnosis of tricuspid stenosis ultimately requires cardiac catheterization, and even then care must be taken not to overlook the comparatively small diastolic gradient that may exist in these patients. Both in the catheterization laboratory and at the bedside it is often helpful to elevate the legs of the patient to augment venous return. This maneuver intensifies the clinical findings as well as the hemodynamic gradient.

Treatment. When stenosis is critical, surgical replacement of the tricuspid valve is the treatment of choice. Since the lesion is invariably associated with advanced disease of the mitral valve, the aortic valve, or both, the overall outcome is determined by the natural history of the associated lesions. Advances in open heart surgery in recent years permit double and even triple valve replacement with a surgical mortality only slightly greater than that in single valve replacement.

TRICUSPID REGURGITATION
As discussed earlier, incompetence of the tricuspid valve is usually secondary to right ventricular dilatation, with expansion of the tricuspid ring secondary to right ventricular failure. The commonest cause of right ventricular failure is associated left ventricular failure. The majority of patients with chronic rheu-

matic tricuspid valve disease manifest some degree of stenosis. When pure tricuspid regurgitation exists in association with other valvular lesions, it is usually secondary (functional). Isolated tricuspid insufficiency as a primary organic lesion may occur, but it is quite rare.

Natural History. Isolated tricuspid insufficiency is almost invariably the result of trauma, which can be of two types: (1) ruptured papillary muscle and (2) ruptured chordae tendineae, with or without tears in the tricuspid valve. With the first, ruptured papillary muscle, the degree of regurgitation is overwhelming and results in a rapid downhill course unless surgical repair is carried out promptly. Ruptured chordae tendineae of the tricuspid valve, on the other hand, are well tolerated and can be present for many years with no ill effect except for prominent venous pulsations in the neck.

Clinical Profile. All of the 15 cases of tricuspid regurgitation reported in the literature as of 1971 were associated with chest wall trauma, usually due to automobile accidents. Symptoms are frequently absent or mild and the onset may be delayed, particularly in regurgitation due to ruptured chordae tendineae. As mentioned, the most striking physical finding is the prominent systolic venous pulsation in the neck and an associated pulsatile liver. The systolic murmur at the lower left sternal border usually increases on inspiration (the Carvallo sign). The Valsalva maneuver is often quite helpful in distinguishing this loud systolic murmur; the murmur disappears but then returns approximately 1 second after release of the Valsalva, whereas left heart murmurs usually do not return for 3 or more seconds after a Valsalva maneuver.

X-ray and Electrocardiographic Findings. The cardiac silhouette is characterized by a prominent right heart border, which indicates right atrial enlargement. Pulmonary venous congestion is absent. The ECG usually shows incomplete right bundle branch block.

Treatment. Since isolated tricuspid insufficiency is so well tolerated, the patients should have no specific therapy until they show pronounced peripheral edema and low cardiac output. Any patient who has tolerated the lesion well for several decades may suddenly and inexplicably become symptomatic; if so, tricuspid valve replacement should be considered.

Pulmonic Stenosis and Regurgitation

Organic disease of the pulmonary valve, other than the pure congenital variety discussed elsewhere, is exceedingly rare. In the metastatic carcinoid syndrome, valvular injury is produced by a substance similar to serotonin secreted by the tumor. Since this material is inactivated in the lungs, the endocardial lesions are limited to the right side of the heart. The verrucous changes of Libman-Sacks disease found in association with systemic lupus erythematosus also have a predilection for the tricuspid and pulmonic valves.

Congenital pulmonic stenosis, when severe and uncorrected by surgery, usually results in terminal congestive heart failure between the ages of 30 and 40 years. If the degree of obstruction is mild (systolic gradient less than 70 mm Hg) the condition rarely progresses, in contrast to congenital aortic stenosis.

Clinical Profile. Estimates of the severity of pulmonic stenosis are made on the same grounds as the estimates of aortic stenosis. An ejection systolic murmur that is late in peaking is indicative of severe stenosis. The pulmonary second sound is delayed and causes wide fixed splitting; the wider the split, the more severe the stenosis. Splitting may not be appreciated because the systolic murmur from the pulmonary outflow obstruction continues after aortic valve closure, often making aortic closure inaudible. As pulmonic valve mobility decreases, the intensity of the pulmonic closure sound diminishes. Since this condition represents systolic overload to the right ventricle, it is associated with a prominent a wave in the jugular venous pulse.

X-ray and Electrocardiographic Findings. The cardiac silhouette is characterized by a prominent pulmonary conus due to poststenotic dilatation, and there is a characteristic paucity of pulmonary vascular markings when the stenosis is significant. The ECG shows typical and classic RVH.

Treatment. Surgical correction by valvotomy is the treatment of choice in childhood whenever the systolic gradient exceeds 100 mm Hg. Surgery has a low risk and a universally excellent outcome, and it should never be withheld as the treatment of choice. There is never a need to replace the pulmonary valve with a prosthesis.

Bibliography

Bland, E. F., and Jones, T. D. Rheumatic fever and rheumatic heart disease: A twenty-year report of 1000 patients followed since childhood. *Circulation* 4:836, 1951.

Eckberg, D. L., Gault, J. R., Bouchard, R. L., Karliner, J. S., and Ross, J., Jr. Mechanics of left ventricular contraction in chronic severe mitral regurgitation. *Circulation* 47:1252, 1973.

Feigenbaum, H. Clinical application of echocardiography. *Progr. Cardiovasc. Dis.* 14:531, 1972.

Frank, S., Johnson, A., and Ross, J., Jr. Natural history of valvular aortic stenosis. *Br. Heart J.* 35:41, 1973.

Jeresaty, R. M. Mitral valve prolapse – click syndrome. *Progr. Cardiovasc. Dis.* 15:623, 1973.

Morgan, J. R., and Forher, A. D. Isolated tricuspid insufficiency. *Circulation* 43:559, 1971.

Perloff, J. K., and Harvey, W. P. Auscultatory and phonocardiographic manifestations of pure mitral regurgitation. *Progr. Cardiovasc. Dis.* 5:172, 1962.

Rappaport, E. Natural history of aortic and mitral valve disease. *Am. J. Cardiol.* 35:221, 1975.

Roberts, W. C. The structure of the aortic valve in clinically isolated aortic stenosis. *Circulation* 42:91, 1970.

Ryan, T. J. Mitral Valve Disease. In H. J. Levine (ed.), *Clinical Cardiovascular Physiology*. New York: Grune & Stratton, 1976. P. 523.

Scheuer, J. Ventricular dysfunction associated with valvular heart disease. *Am. J. Cardiol.* 30:445, 1972.

Selzer, A., and Cohn, E. K. Natural history of mitral stenosis: A review. *Circulation* 45:878, 1972.

Spagnuolo, M., Kloth, H., Taranta, A., Doyle, E., and
      Pasternack, B. Natural history of rheumatic
      aortic regurgitation. *Circulation* 44:368, 1971.
Wood, P. An appreciation of mitral stenosis: Part I.
      Clinical features. *Br. Med. J.* 1:1050, 1954.
Wood, P. An appreciation of mitral stenosis: Part II.
      Investigation and results. *Br. Med. J.* 1:1113,
      1954.

31

Congestive Heart Failure

William B. Hood, Jr.

Congestive heart failure is a clinical state that may be defined pathophysiologically as one in which the load imposed on the heart exceeds the capacity of the heart to pump blood. Overloading may occur by four mechanisms: (1) pressure overload, (2) volume overload, (3) intrinsic myocardial damage resulting in inability of the myocardium to perform against normal pressure and volume loads, and (4) restriction of diastolic filling.

Pathophysiology

Since the main function of the heart is to pump blood and since it is a relatively simple matter to quantify the actions of a pump, extensive information is available about cardiac performance both in the normal state and in congestive heart failure. These data have been attained largely through cardiac catheterization, a technique ordinarily reserved for special diagnostic problems that has supplied important information over the past 30 years on the clinical manifestations of congestive heart failure. These clinical manifestations in turn often reflect the state of the myocardium and may be used to gauge the degree of congestive heart failure.

THE NORMAL CIRCULATION

To understand the genesis of congestive heart failure, it is useful to review some fundamental physiologic concepts (see Fig. 31-1). Under normal conditions the heart ejects approximately two-thirds of the blood it contains (the so-called ejection fraction). Typically the left ventricle might contain 150 ml of blood at the end of diastole and 50 ml of blood at the end of systole; therefore a stroke volume of 100 ml of blood is ejected, and the ejection fraction is 0.67. In the normal heart the end-diastolic volume is attained at a relatively low filling pressure or "preload." If the heart rate is normal, say 60 beats per minute, this 100-ml stroke volume would produce a cardiac output of 6,000 ml per minute, also normal. If the systemic vascular resistance is also normal, this

set of circumstances will lead to a normal arterial blood pressure. These concepts may be simply expressed in the following formulas: (1) ejection fraction × end-diastolic volume = stroke volume, (2) stroke volume × heart rate = cardiac output, (3) cardiac output × systemic vascular resistance = systemic arterial pressure (Fig. 31-1).

Of these parameters, only heart rate and systemic arterial blood pressure may be easily measured in the clinical setting. When either heart rate or blood pressure is markedly abnormal, it is likely that other parameters are also abnormal; however, heart rate and blood pressure measurements reflect only indirectly the underlying state of the myocardium, which is much more accurately assessed by measurement of ejection fraction or end-diastolic volume. Though the latter may not be readily measured, other available clinical information may allow an estimate to be made of them. As in other areas of clinical medicine, the history and physical examination are of great importance in assessing the functional state of the heart; they will be discussed shortly.

THE "FAILED" CIRCULATION

Intrinsic Myocardial Damage. Before delving directly into the clinical manifestations of congestive heart failure, it is important to clarify how the ejection fraction and end-diastolic volume are affected in the various forms of congestive heart failure. Consider first the situation in which intrinsic damage to the myocardium has occurred, as in acute myocardial infarction or in cardiomyopathy. A direct consequence of myocardial damage is a reduced ability of the muscle fibers to contract, resulting in a decrease in the ejection fraction. Initially this may be compensated for by ventricular dilatation, for as the heart fails to eject an adequate stroke volume, pressure builds up in the veins behind it, resulting in diastolic distention of the ventricle. Such distention, by stretching the remaining intact myocardial fibers, may improve the performance of the heart by the Starling effect (see later). However, ventricular dilatation is costly in other terms, for the dilated ventricle has a greater wall tension and consumes more oxygen than a small ventricle. This poses limitations on the utility of ventricular dilatation as a compensatory

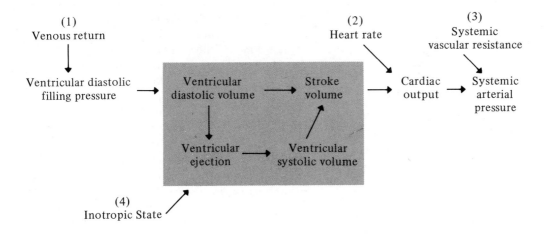

Starling's law operates in this region. With (2), (3), and (4) held constant, stroke volume increases with increases in ventricular diastolic volume

Figure 31-1. Circulatory schema. Venous return, heart rate, systemic vascular resistance, and the inotropic state of the myocardium may be regarded as the key physiologic variables that control the circulation and that determine cardiac output and systemic arterial pressure by the mechanisms shown. Starling's law of the heart (which states that the heart pumps more forcibly when progressively distended by volume loading) operates in the shaded area. This circulatory schema applies equally well to either the right or left ventricle.

mechanism, particularly when oxygen supply is limited, as it is in ischemic heart disease.

Pressure Overload. In the situation known as pressure overload, the ventricle must eject against a higher arterial pressure head, or afterload. If this afterload is sufficiently elevated, the ventricle may be unable to eject a normal fraction and blood will back up behind the overloaded ventricle, again resulting in enlargement of end-diastolic volume and partial compensation by means of the Starling mechanism. If arterial hypertension is acute and severe, left ventricular failure may occur despite an intrinsically normal myocardium. However, in chronic hypertension, intrinsic changes in cardiac muscle do occur, and the

muscle can no longer be considered completely normal.

Volume Overload. In volume overload the ventricle is subjected to high filling pressures due to an elevated venous return. This occurs in situations in which there is a reduction in peripheral vascular resistance, effectively creating a shunt between the arteries and veins by transferring some of the arterial pressure head onto the venous system. The response of the ventricle again is to dilate due to the elevated filling pressures, but in this situation there is no impairment in ejection fraction and the stroke volume is high. This is the physiologic basis for the so-called high-output states.

Restrictive Disease. A fourth situation that differs from the three above is one in which ventricular filling is compromised by increased resistance to diastolic filling. This may be due to intrinsic stiffening of the myocardium, to diseases of the pericardium that prevent the ventricle from filling adequately, or to pericardial tamponade. The ejection fraction may still be normal, but the inability of the ventricle to fill despite high filling pressures results in a low end-diastolic volume, and stroke volume must fall despite the normal ejection fraction.

LEFT-SIDED VERSUS RIGHT-SIDED
CONGESTIVE HEART FAILURE

Either ventricle may be affected when congestive heart failure is present, or both may be affected together. Congestive heart failure often begins with decompensation of the left ventricle, since this is the chamber predominantly affected by common diseases such as hypertension, coronary artery disease, and rheumatic valvular disease. Either pressure or volume overload may be present. Pressure overload is characteristic of systemic hypertension, aortic stenosis, and coarctation of the aorta. Volume overload may be caused by aortic regurgitation, mitral regurgitation, and patent ductus arteriosus, all of which result in an increased flow of blood through the left ventricle. This is true even though the forward stroke volume, that is, the volume that flows through the peripheral circulation, may be normal or even reduced. In such cases the increased volume load is a result of regurgitant valvular lesions or, in the case of patent ductus arteriosus, of a high flow state through the left ventricle, part of which is shunted back to the pulmonary artery and lungs.

Right-sided congestive heart failure may occur as an isolated event due to pressure overloading, as occurs in pulmonary hypertension due to lung disease or pulmonary emboli, or to volume overloading, as occurs in atrial septal defect, which results in a high flow state through the right ventricle. Most commonly, however, right-sided heart failure occurs as a result of left-sided heart failure; the buildup of pressure on the left side of the heart is transmitted back through the pulmonary vasculature, causing a pressure overload on the right side of the heart.

The cardiomyopathic states may affect either ventricle or both of them. Pericardial disease impedes filling of both sides of the heart, but it usually produces the clinical picture of right-sided heart failure.

COMPENSATORY MECHANISMS

Compensatory mechanisms may occur both in the myocardium and in the periphery. In the myocardium stressed by pressure overload of either the right or left ventricle, a process of hypertrophy, or increase

in mass of the ventricular musculature, develops over time. The intracavity volume of the affected ventricle may be normal or even reduced. Such a hypertrophied ventricle is capable of developing pressures in excess of those produced by the normal ventricle, and up to a point, the process of hypertrophy may be regarded as beneficial in meeting the pressure demands placed on the ventricle. However, it has been shown that the contractility of hypertrophied muscle is reduced per unit of muscle mass, so the muscle must be regarded as functionally subnormal — even though the entire ventricle, because of its increased mass, may be capable of developing the elevated pressures required. Eventually the myocardial blood flow becomes insufficient to satisfy the oxygen demands of the thick, hypertrophied ventricle. At the microscopic level, capillaries in hypertrophied ventricles are further apart than normal due to the increased mass of the interposed myocardial cells, so coronary blood flow becomes inadequate and ischemia results.

High flow states commonly result in dilatation, that is, a gradual stretching out of the ventricular myocardium so that the chamber volume becomes enlarged. Although the walls of the chamber may also hypertrophy so that the total weight of the ventricle is increased, the predominant feature is the dilatation. As in the case of simple hypertrophy, this mechanism requires time to develop. Again, the initial process of dilatation is regarded as compensatory to the large stroke volume required of the ventricle. However, dilatation, like hypertrophy, ultimately has deleterious effects on the ventricle: A markedly dilated ventricle results in an increased wall tension and oxygen consumption. Indeed, the largest and heaviest ventricles seen in any form of heart disease occur in certain of the high flow states such as severe aortic regurgitation. Typically, in the very advanced stages of ventricular dilatation due to a high flow state, the ejection fraction becomes reduced, presumably a result of the very high wall tensions that occur.

In the periphery certain other compensatory mechanisms, very important from the clinical standpoint, also occur in congestive heart failure. From the analysis presented in Figure 31-1, it is apparent that an increase in heart rate may be sufficient to compensate for a mild or modest reduction in stroke volume, allowing cardiac output to be maintained; thus, tachycardia is a common manifestation and accompaniment of congestive heart failure. Also, from the same analysis it is apparent that, in the face of a reduced cardiac output, blood pressure may be maintained by an increase in peripheral vascular resistance. In clinical heart failure, maintenance of blood pressure appears to be zealously guarded by reflex mechanisms that make an adequate pressure head available for perfusion of critical organs such as the heart and brain. In chronic congestive heart failure of severe degree, reductions in cardiac output are common despite various compensatory mechanisms including both ventricular dilatation (with the attendant Starling effect) and tachycardia. Under these circumstances a rise in peripheral resistance commonly occurs. Both the tachycardia and the increase in peripheral vascular resistance are a consequence of enhanced sympathetic activity, and patients with congestive failure are very dependent on elevated sympathetic tone for support of the circulatory system (see Ventricular Function Curves, below).

Other systemic compensatory mechanisms include salt and water retention, a consequence of reduced renal perfusion and of secondary aldosteronism. To some extent this may be considered beneficial, since expansion of intravascular volume will maintain ventricular filling pressures and enhance cardiac function by the Starling effect. Eventually, however, pulmonary congestion and peripheral edema may occur, producing serious symptoms and requiring therapy by salt restriction and diuretics.

VENTRICULAR FUNCTION CURVES

Although the concept of normal and abnormal ejection fractions is useful in understanding cardiac failure, it is also important to consider ventricular function (Starling) curves (Fig. 31-2). The normal curve shows that a normal stroke volume (approximately 100 ml) can be produced in a normal heart with a physiologic filling pressure (approximately 10 mm Hg). The shape of the ventricular function curve for the normal heart implies that a considerable reserve of function exists. This might be demonstrated by infusing fluid to increase the intravascular volume, thereby raising left ventricular end-diastolic pressure

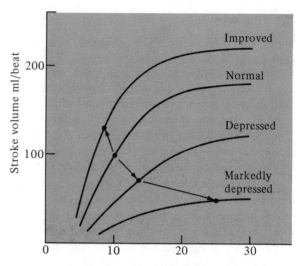

Figure 31-2. Family of ventricular function curves. The normal heart can produce a normal stroke volume (100 ml) at a normal filling pressure (10 mm Hg), and considerable functional reserve may be demonstrated if a volume load is applied. With improved ventricular function (exercise or administration of inotropic agents), an above normal stroke volume (in this example, 130 ml) may be produced with reduction of filling pressures (in this example, 9 mm Hg), and functional reserve is preserved. With depressed or markedly depressed function (intrinsic myocardial disease), stroke volume is progressively reduced in the examples shown to 70 ml and 50 ml and filling pressures progressively increase to 13 and 25 mm Hg, respectively; functional reserve is reduced or is virtually absent as the curves become flattened. For each of these curves, the actual value of stroke volume and left ventricular end-diastolic pressure obtained will, of course, depend on the existing intravascular volume load and venous return.

and volume and producing a concomitant increase in stroke volume. This is the familiar Starling effect, an expression of the ability of normal myocardium to contract more forcibly as it is progressively stretched. If measurements were made periodically during the volume infusion, points along the normal ventricular function curve would be obtained. However, the usual mechanism for increasing stroke volume in the normal heart is to shift to an "improved" ventricular function curve. Such a shift might occur, for example, during exercise. In the example shown in Figure 31-2, the shift to the left of the improved function curve has resulted in an increased stroke volume at a slightly reduced filling pressure and, of course, no Starling effect.

On the other hand, depression of ventricular function (shift to a depressed curve) may result in a decreased stroke volume and a rise in filling pressure, as is also shown in Figure 31-2. In contrast to the normal heart, the Starling effect must be invoked frequently in the depressed heart as it dilates in response to the elevated filling pressure. If depression of ventricular function is severe, congestive heart failure results. Symptoms of fatigue and weakness may occur as a result of a decrease in stroke volume; dyspnea, pulmonary vascular congestion, or edema formation follows a rise in filling pressure. The symptoms that predominate may often be altered simply by manipulating intravascular volume, a therapeutic intervention that is commonly undertaken, for example, by using diuretics. The decompensated heart is also more sensitive to volume loads than the normal heart; since the depressed curve is flatter than normal, small increases in intravascular volume result in large changes in filling pressure. This explains why patients with depressed ventricular function may be exquisitely sensitive to volume loads resulting from overingestion of salt and water, for example. Physicians usually attempt to manipulate the factors along the ventricular function curve to balance a diminished stroke volume against increased filling pressures, so that their patients are made as comfortable as possible. Unfortunately, in the advanced stages of heart disease bordering on cardiogenic shock, volume manipulation is not very helpful, as shown by the curve to the far right in Figure 31-2 (a markedly depressed ventricular function curve). The ventricular function curve is so flat that little change in stroke volume occurs despite large changes in blood volume and filling pressure.

Understanding ventricular function curves may be regarded as supplementary to the analysis presented above regarding ejection fractions. However, the ejection fraction is not related in a simple way to the Starling curves. The normal heart maintains a fixed ejection fraction in the presence of a rising filling pressure and volume, resulting in a larger stroke volume as shown by the ascending limb (upward sloping portion) of the normal ventricular function curve. The depressed heart, with ventricular function curves that lie to the right of the normal curve, has a diminished ejection fraction despite larger end-diastolic pressures and volumes, and it fails to produce a normal stroke volume. The main utility of the function curves is to emphasize the effect of volume loading on ventricular performance and to enable the physician to think physiologically when manipulating intravascular filling pressures. These function curves also do not take into account the effects of heart rate, which must be thought of as an independent reserve mechanism available to both the compensated and decompensated heart.

Chronic Congestive Heart Failure

Chronic congestive heart failure is a term applied to slowly developing cardiac decompensation over a period of time. The compensatory mechanisms of the circulatory system are such that, when a patient becomes symptomatic from chronic congestive heart failure, this indicates that most reserve mechanisms have been expended and that either the filling pressure has risen or the cardiac output has fallen to such an extent that the patient becomes symptomatic. By the time this state of affairs occurs the prospect for prolonged survival is often limited, although many exceptions exist. Much depends on which chambers of the heart are involved, the underlying cause of cardiac failure, and the possible existence of surgically remediable or other partially reversible factors.

LEFT-SIDED CARDIAC FAILURE
Left-sided cardiac failure is the most common type of clinical heart failure, and its most common causes include coronary artery disease, hypertension, and valvular heart disease. Patients with cardiomyopathy or high output cardiac failure may present with predominantly left ventricular failure, but usually their signs and symptoms are those of biventricular failure. Congenital heart disease may also present as left-sided failure, depending on the site of the lesion. The mechanism by which these forms of heart disease produce left ventricular failure varies; for example,

coronary heart disease produces attrition of muscle due to ischemia and infarction of the left ventricle, resulting in overloading of the remaining muscle. Valvular heart disease may cause either a pressure or volume overload, aortic stenosis results in a pressure overload, and aortic regurgitation or mitral insufficiency results in volume overload.

Symptoms of left-sided failure include fatigue and weakness when reductions in cardiac output and stroke volume are present, and dyspnea, orthopnea, and paroxysmal nocturnal dyspnea when elevated filling pressures are present. *Dyspnea* is a sense of difficulty in breathing, and this is usually attributable to pulmonary vascular congestion resulting from the elevated left atrial pressures. *Orthopnea* is difficulty in breathing in the supine position; this may be relieved by sitting up, which reduces the degree of pulmonary congestion by pooling blood in the lower extremities and lowering left ventricular filling pressures. *Paroxysmal nocturnal dyspnea* is a specific symptom complex in which the patient awakens short of breath at night, but often obtains relief by sitting up for a period of time. It is believed that assumption of supine posture for sleep results in resorption of extracellular fluid into the intravascular space, causing a rise in filling pressures. Sitting up reverses this process. Cough and hemoptysis occasionally may be prominent symptoms of left-sided congestive heart failure.

Certain ancillary symptoms may be specific for individual types of heart disease that lead to left ventricular failure. For example, coronary heart disease (see Chap. 28) is often characterized by precordial chest pains or by acute myocardial infarction. Aortic stenosis may be accompanied by both chest pains and syncopal attacks. Hypertension may cause headaches, dizzy spells, or evidence of hypertensive encephalopathy, as well as evidence of vascular involvement in other organs such as the kidneys.

One other form of left-sided heart failure that is not due to left ventricular failure deserves special comment. That is mitral valve stenosis, which leads to pulmonary vascular congestion and symptoms that in many respects are indistinguishable from those of true left ventricular failure. However, in this condition the left ventricle is usually normal, although pulmonary vascular congestion, dyspnea, orthopnea, and paroxysmal nocturnal dyspnea may supervene due to elevated filling pressures resulting from obstruction to blood flow at the mitral valve.

Specific physical signs of left ventricular failure that are not necessarily related to the underlying causes include left-sided gallop rhythm, pulsus alternans, and pulmonary rales. Gallop rhythms are of two types: The S_3 protodiastolic gallop, which is a low-pitched heart sound heard early in diastole, coinciding with the rapid filling phase of the ventricle, is usually indicative of severe cardiac failure; the S_4 gallop, which is heard late in diastole at a time that corresponds to atrial contraction, is much more common, but is by no means always indicative of congestive heart failure. An S_4 gallop is a frequent accompaniment of states in which the left ventricle is under strain but has not yet decompensated, as occurs, for example, in hypertension. Pulsus alternans, an uncommon finding in which alternating stronger and weaker pulse beats are detected by palpation, or are noted when inflating a blood pressure cuff, invariably indicates severe left ventricular failure. Pulmonary rales due to transudation of fluid into the lung alveoli as a result of elevated left ventricular filling pressures are extremely helpful and commonly present findings in left ventricular failure. Such rales are frequently dependent, meaning that they are heard mostly at the lung bases posteriorly. Rales due to congestive heart failure are frequently characterized as moist, and a clinician experienced in auscultation can sometimes distinguish them from pulmonary rales due to other conditions such as pneumonia or chronic lung disease. Another helpful finding is that rales due to congestive heart failure are frequently more prominent at the right than at the left lung base. Pleural effusion, which produces dullness to percussion at the lung bases, may also occur in chronic congestive heart failure. This finding is not specific for left-sided failure, however, and it may occur in right-sided failure as well.

Peripheral cyanosis, or bluish discoloration of fingertips, cheeks, tip of nose, or earlobes due to sluggish flow of blood through these tissues, may also occur. This finding should be distinguished from central cyanosis due to true unsaturation of arterial blood resulting from pulmonary disease or cyanotic congenital heart disease. Central cyanosis produces bluish discoloration of normally well-perfused tissues such as lips and mucous membranes as well as the tissues noted above. Clubbing of the fingertips is a frequent accompaniment of central cyanosis.

Other physical findings may be particularly helpful in certain types of heart disease that cause left ventricular failure. In coronary heart disease there are often no characteristic physical findings; however, on occasion, aneurysmal heaves of the left ventricle are helpful in identifying areas of focal ischemic involvement. Specific cardiac findings are often lacking in hypertension also. It is in valvular heart disease that specific physical findings are of major importance (see Chap. 30).

The electrocardiogram is sometimes useful as an ancillary tool in making a diagnosis of left ventricular failure; however, no electrocardiographic finding is specific for this disorder. The most common accompaniments of left-sided heart failure are left ventricular hypertrophy, characterized by abnormal increases in voltage of the R wave over the left precordium; and left atrial enlargement, characterized by abnormal P wave forces over the right precordium (see Chap. 32).

The chest x-ray is extremely helpful in diagnosing left ventricular failure. Specific patterns of left ventricular enlargement are often observed in the different forms of left ventricular failure. For example, in left ventricular failure due to pressure overload of the left ventricle, a rounded enlargement of the left ventricle is often present due to hypertrophy of this chamber. When volume overload is present, the ventricle is often elongated and pushed far to the left within the chest, due to dilatation of this chamber. In coronary artery disease, an aneurysm of the left ventricle is occasionally seen. Mitral valve stenosis may often be diagnosed on chest x-ray by enlargement of the left atrium, and calcification of the mitral valve can also be seen on the roentgenogram. The most helpful roentgenographic finding is the presence of pulmonary vascular congestion, which is shown on x-ray by prominent pulmonary veins, redistribution of the pulmonary venous vascular pattern toward the upper lung fields, and horizontal linear streaks located laterally at the lung bases (the Kerley B lines). Of course these roentgenographic findings do not specify the underlying cause of left ventricular failure.

RIGHT-SIDED CARDIAC FAILURE

Right-sided cardiac failure most commonly results from left-sided cardiac failure. When filling pressures on the left side of the heart increase, pulmonary arterial pressure must rise concurrently in order to maintain a perfusion gradient across the lungs. This, in effect, produces a pressure overload on the right side of the heart. Other common causes of right-sided failure are acute cor pulmonale, due to a rapid increase in pulmonary arterial pressure and right ventricular afterload, caused, for example, by pulmonary embolism or acute respiratory failure; and chronic cor pulmonale due primarily to chronic lung disease. A rarer cause is primary pulmonary hypertension. A pressure overload without pulmonary hypertension may occur in pulmonary valve stenosis. Right ventricular failure due to volume overload may occur as a part of high output states, though in general the left ventricle is affected as well. Failure of the right ventricle due to presence of a high blood flow through the right side of the heart alone, as in atrial septal defects with large left-to-right shunts, is uncommon, because the right ventricle seems remarkably capable of pumping large volume loads over long periods of time. However, if reactive pulmonary vasoconstriction occurs with rises in pulmonary arterial pressure, right ventricular failure may result. Involvement of the right ventricle in ischemic heart disease is uncommon. Presumably the thin-walled right ventricle has a more competent blood supply than the thick-walled left ventricle in myocardial ischemic states. However, primary involvement of right ventricular muscle may occur in cardiomyopathy. Isolated stenosis of the tricuspid valve may occur rarely as a feature of rheumatic heart disease; when this occurs, the physical findings are those of right ventricular failure, even though the right ventricular muscle is not directly involved.

Certain symptoms are found in isolated right ventricular failure, as is the case with left ventricular failure. When cardiac output is limited by inability of the right ventricle to pump blood, weakness and fatigue result, just as in left ventricular failure. Occasionally patients with severe right ventricular failure due to pressure overload may develop an angina type of syndrome that is commonly attributed to inadequate coronary perfusion of the hypertrophied right ventricle. Syncopal attacks may also occur. Most characteristic, however, is swelling of the soft tissues of the body, particularly in the dependent parts of the body such as the legs, sacrum, and scrotum. Though more properly classified as a sign, the patient often complains actively about this edema when questioned, or he may note it only as a gain in weight. The edema is due to a rise in venous pressure resulting in transudation of fluid into the interstitial spaces of the soft tissues. The situation is entirely analogous to that of pulmonary edema in relation to left-sided failure; however, since the interstitial fluid reservoir of the total body is quite large compared to that of the lungs, very extensive peripheral edema may occur in patients who are fully ambulatory and only moderately symptomatic. The dependent nature of the edema is occasioned by the preference of cardiac patients to maintain the upright position, and this has the effect of causing fluid to gravitate to the lower half of the body. Patients also sometimes complain of right upper quadrant discomfort that is due to a tender, distended liver.

Physical examination in isolated right ventricular failure often reveals a loud pulmonic component of the second heart sound (loud P_2) in patients with pulmonary hypertension, and the presence of S_3 and S_4 gallops emanating from the right ventricle. These gallops may be accentuated by inspiration due to the larger influx of blood into the right ventricle when intrathoracic pressure becomes more negative, an effect opposite to that usually observed with left-sided gallops. A right ventricular heave may be palpated, and if this is of the slow, lifting variety, pressure overload is suggested; when the impulse is quick and hyperkinetic, a high flow state is suggested.

Inspection of the neck veins for jugular venous distention may give an index of the filling pressure on the right side of the heart. Normally, with the patient semisupine at a $30°$ angle, the jugular veins — external, internal, or both — may be seen to pulsate just at or above the clavicles. Measured from the midchest position, a convenient reference point for measuring filling pressures of the right side of the heart, pulsation at the clavicular level corresponds to a venous pressure level of 10 cm of water or less. When the neck veins are prominent above the clavicular level, neck vein distention is said to exist. Latent right-sided failure may sometimes be detected by noting a sustained rise in the height of neck vein distention with firm pressure over the hepatic area (positive *hepatojugular reflux*). This maneuver forces hepatic blood into the venous system and transiently overloads the right ventricle, resulting in a rise in filling pressure. In extreme cases of right ventricular failure, neck vein distention may be apparent even with the patient sitting bolt upright. The level of the filling pressure of the right side of the heart may therefore be approximated by having the patient sit at different degrees of elevation and measuring the height of the neck veins above the midchest position. Furthermore, specific information may be available from neck vein pulsations about the underlying type of right ventricular failure. If a large *a* wave is present, it may be surmised that forceful atrial contraction is required to fill a compromised right ventricle; such a finding would be commonly accompanied by an S_4 gallop. If a large *v* wave is present, tricuspid regurgitation might be suspected. The experienced examiner might also be able to detect other features of the neck vein pulsations, such as a delayed *y* descent, which is suggestive of tricuspid stenosis. Paradoxical venous pulsation (positive Kussmaul sign) with reversal of the normal inspiratory fall in venous pressure may suggest the presence of constrictive pericarditis as a cause of right-sided failure (see Chap. 30).

Diffuse enlargement of the liver and tenderness of this organ are commonly observed, and ascites may also appear with severe right-sided heart failure. It is also not uncommon for *pleural effusion* to develop with isolated right-sided heart failure, even in the absence of left-sided heart failure, presumably due to inadequate drainage of lymphatic fluid from the lungs into the high-pressure venous system.

The electrocardiogram cannot be used to make a specific diagnosis of right ventricular failure. However, hypertrophy of the right ventricle may be detected as an increase in voltage of the R wave over the

right precordium. Peaking and increase of voltage of
the P waves (P pulmonale) may also be seen with right
atrial distention from increased filling pressures on
the right side of the heart. The chest x-ray may also
be useful in demonstrating specific enlargement of
chambers such as the pulmonary artery, right ventricle, and right atrium, or prominence of the
superior vena cava. Chest x-rays are particularly helpful in diagnosing congenital cardiac lesions characterized by left-to-right shunts, in which pulmonary
plethora may be observed, and in diagnosing pulmonary hypertension due to pulmonary vasconstriction,
in which pulmonary oligemia and enlargement of the
proximal pulmonary arteries may be observed.

In very advanced and long-standing cardiac failure
due to any cause, cardiac cachexia may result. Despite
the accumulation of edema, the patient loses weight
and appears gaunt and malnourished. The condition
is attributed to immobilization, to the prolonged
deleterious effects of low cardiac output on body
tissues, and possibly to severe venous congestion of
the gastrointestinal tract with resultant malabsorption.

FUNCTIONAL CLASSIFICATION OF CONGESTIVE HEART FAILURE

For the purposes of grading the degree of physical
impairment experienced by patients with congestive
heart failure, clinicians have found it useful to employ
the classification developed by the New York Heart
Association, as follows:

Class I: patients with cardiac disease but without
   resulting limitations of physical activity. Ordinary
   physical activity does not cause undue fatigue, palpitation, dyspnea, or anginal pain.
Class II: patients with cardiac disease resulting in
   slight limitation of physical activity. They are comfortable at rest. Ordinary physical activity may
   result in fatigue, palpitation, dyspnea, or anginal
   pain.
Class III: patients with cardiac disease resulting in
   marked limitation of physical activity. They are
   fairly comfortable at rest. Less than ordinary
   physical activity causes fatigue, palpitation, dyspnea,
   or anginal pain.
Class IV: patients with cardiac disease resulting in
   inability to carry on any physical activity without

discomfort. Symptoms of cardiac insufficiency or
of the anginal syndrome may be present even at rest.
If any physical activity is undertaken, discomfort
is increased.

DIFFERENTIAL DIAGNOSIS

Many of the manifestations of cardiac failure, both
symptoms and signs, are not limited to cardiac disease,
and careful attention may be required to make a
correct diagnosis. Fatigue and weakness are obviously present in many different diseases, including
endocrine disturbances, anemia, and neoplasia. Dyspnea may be due to either pulmonary or cardiac disease, which may often be confused with each other in
many other respects, as noted below. Orthopnea and
paroxysmal nocturnal dyspnea are relatively specific
for cardiac failure, although some patients with pulmonary disease may complain of orthopnea. Chest
pain due to coronary artery disease, aortic stenosis,
pulmonary hypertension, or pulmonary embolism
must be differentiated from other conditions such as
pericarditis; pleuritis; dissecting aneurysm; and esophageal, neuromuscular, or referred abdominal pain. On
physical examination, gallops are suggestive of cardiac
involvement, but when gallops are of the S_4 variety,
they do not always indicate that congestive heart
failure is present. Furthermore, an S_3 sound is
heard in many young individuals with normal
hearts. Rales may appear in pulmonary disease as
well as cardiac failure. Pleural effusion may obviously be due to noncardiac conditions such as pneumonia or tumor. Pulmonary embolism also commonly causes pleural effusion. When edema is present,
one must also consider other causes such as renal
failure with retention of salt and water; hypoalbuminemia from conditions such as hepatic disease,
malnutrition, or nephrotic syndrome; local venous
disease in the lower extremities; and intraabdominal
processes causing ascites.

It is apparent from this discussion that it is often
difficult to differentiate cardiac failure from intrinsic
pulmonary disease, particularly when right ventricular
failure is present. In fact, advanced pulmonary disease may cause the syndrome of chronic cor pulmonale, which is tantamount to right ventricular failure.
The problem is one of deciding whether pulmonary

disease is the primary cause of right ventricular failure or whether some other cause, such as concurrent left ventricular failure, exists. By careful analysis of signs and symptoms and use of ancillary laboratory tests, correct assessment of the relative importance of cardiac and pulmonary disease is usually possible.

SPECIALIZED LABORATORY TECHNIQUES

In addition to electrocardiograms and chest x-rays, which are routinely performed, certain other specialized techniques may aid in the diagnosis of congestive heart failure. In recent years it has become feasible to insert a balloon-tipped flow-directed catheter into a peripheral vein at the bedside, and direct it through the right heart chambers into the pulmonary artery. This technique may be used to monitor central venous and pulmonary arterial pressures, to measure circulation times and cardiac outputs, and to obtain so-called wedge pressures, which reflect left ventricular filling pressure and hence left ventricular failure. Central venous, pulmonary arterial, and wedge pressures are extremely useful in assessing filling pressures on the right and left side of the heart and in guiding therapeutic manipulation of intravascular volume to maximize cardiac output without overloading the circulation.

Circulation times, measured by injecting an indicator into the venous system and measuring its arrival time in the arterial circuit, may be used as an indirect assessment of the cardiac output. Most commonly the injection is dehydrocholic acid, derived from bile salts (Decholin), which can be tasted by the patient when it arrives at the tongue. The circulation time measurement is most significant when it is short; a time of less than 12 seconds is indicative of a high output state. A prolonged circulation time, however, though suggestive of a decrease in cardiac output, may be an inaccurate indicator. If accurate assessment of cardiac output is required, it is preferable to make a direct measurement using indicator dilution techniques. In patients with extreme cardiac decompensation, arterial pressure monitoring, available in intensive care units, may be used to gauge the progress of patients in cardiogenic shock. In severe left ventricular failure with marked pulmonary vascular congestion, arterial unsaturation due to shunting of blood through the lungs is commonly present, and improvement in arterial PO_2 may also be used to gauge the progress of therapy.

Certain other specialized techniques may be used to document accurately various findings in congestive heart failure. Phonocardiography may be employed to diagnose unequivocally the presence of S_3 or S_4 gallops and to identify and time various murmurs and other heart sounds. In recent years the technique of echocardiography has shown considerable promise as a noninvasive bedside method that may furnish specific data formerly obtained only at cardiac catheterization; for example, the sonarlike pictures of the heart obtained by echocardiography provide rough estimates of the ejection fraction. Cardiac fluoroscopy is frequently of use in diagnosing specific chamber enlargement not readily apparent on routine x-ray films and in determining the underlying cause of cardiac failure.

The ultimate technique for diagnosing cardiac failure is the performance of cardiac catheterization of both right and left heart chambers. Accurate measurements of ejection fractions, filling pressures, cardiac output, and other parameters of cardiac performance are readily available from this procedure, and cardiac catheterization often also permits a specific diagnosis and an assessment of the type and severity of the disease.

Treatment of Congestive Heart Failure

Treatment of congestive heart failure should be directed, first and foremost, toward reversing the underlying cause of the disturbance. Unfortunately, many forms of congestive heart failure cannot be completely reversed and must be treated symptomatically.

GENERAL MEASURES

The clinician should have uppermost in his mind a search for curable forms of disease, including the high output states caused by anemia and thyrotoxicosis; correction of abnormalities that predispose to congestive heart failure, such as extreme tachyarrhythmias or bradyarrhythmias; restoration of blood pressure toward normal in hypertensive patients; and discovery and relief of pericardial tamponade or constrictive pericarditis. Certain forms of heart disease may be cured or successfully palliated by surgery, and these include many forms of congenital heart disease, left atrial myxoma or ball-valve thrombus, and the various forms of rheumatic valvular disease.

General therapeutic measures for congestive heart failure include restriction of activity, low-salt diet, use of digitalis products to control cardiac rate and to increase the inotropic state of the heart, and employment of diuretics to relieve pulmonary and systemic venous congestion. Restriction of activity is an important form of therapy for the cardiac patient. However, in the absence of severely limiting congestive heart failure, this approach is applied less commonly today than formerly, and the emphasis has been on rehabilitation and graded activity up to the limits of comfort for the individual cardiac patient. It is clear, however, that in the presence of acute cardiac decompensation or with the more advanced degrees of chronic congestive heart failure, activity must be restricted. In addition, reduction of edema fluid is realized more easily when the patient maintains a semisupine position rather than a sitting or standing position, due to absence of hydrostatic gradients in the legs. Thus a period of bed rest and relative restriction of activity may be employed as a short-term measure to achieve diuresis. On the other hand, bed rest and immobilization are not without hazard, because these promote venous stasis and phlebothrombosis, increasing the danger of pulmonary embolism. The possibility of pulmonary embolism may be averted to some extent by having the bedridden patient periodically dangle or sit in a comfortable chair and by teaching him to exercise his legs while in bed.

Dietary restriction of salt is an effective means of counteracting the tendency toward sodium retention, which promotes edema formation in patients with congestive heart failure. However, restriction of salt to 1 or 2 gm per day may produce anorexia. With milder degrees of heart failure it is not unusual for clinicians to allow a somewhat more liberalized salt intake and to employ diuretics to control sodium balance. Such liberal use of diuretics, with the attendant loss of potassium in the urine, has made supplementation of the diet with potassium-rich foods or

with potassium salts a routine matter, provided renal failure is absent. Orange juice and bananas are foods that are both low in sodium and high in potassium, and they should be used liberally when diuretics are employed. An alternative approach is the use of salt substitutes, which are commercial preparations resembling salt in taste but which are low in sodium and high in potassium; unfortunately, many patients find these preparations unpalatable. In addition, weight reduction should be enforced in patients who are obese to reduce the amount of work done by the heart.

DIGITALIS

In chronic congestive heart failure, digitalis is the only agent with inotropic properties that has generally found acceptance. Digitalis is not a very powerful inotropic agent, but among the inotropic drugs it is the only one that has a sustained action when given by mouth and that does not accelerate the heart rate. Its chief disadvantage is that it has a narrow toxic-therapeutic ratio, and yet often it must be given to the maximum tolerated dose to exert optimal effects.

Digitalis is given to most patients with chronic left ventricular failure and hence is one of the most common cardiac drugs employed. It appears to be most useful in situations in which there is pressure or volume overload of the left ventricle, and in chronic ischemic heart disease. It appears to be less effective in treating cardiomyopathies, although it is used for this purpose. It appears to be least useful in treating pure right-sided heart failure due to, for example, cor pulmonale, although it is still often given. Digitalis is of no use in treating left-sided failure due to mitral stenosis, and it is specifically contraindicated in idiopathic hypertrophic subaortic stenosis, since it may worsen outflow tract obstruction. It should be noted that, apart from its inotropic effects, digitalis is also quite useful in treating tachyarrhythmias in which blockade of the atrioventricular node is effective in reducing the ventricular rate, such as atrial fibrillation and flutter, and it is also useful in reverting certain of the atrial tachyarrhythmias such as paroxysmal atrial tachycardia.

The clinician who employs digitalis must be intimately acquainted with both the dosage and the toxic manifestations of the drug and with the preparation he uses. In addition to provoking ventricular irritability and causing tachyarrhythmias such as junctional tachycardia and paroxymal atrial tachycardia with block, digitalis may depress atrioventricular conduction and slow the ventricular rate excessively both in atrial fibrillation and flutter. Because such rhythm disturbances could be due to intrinsic underlying heart disease, it is often difficult to decide when an excess of digitalis is present. Helpful approaches include temporarily reducing the digitalis dosage; correcting ancillary disturbances that may predispose to digitalis toxicity, such as hypokalemia, hypomagnesemia, and hypoxia; and also measuring the serum levels of digitalis. In addition to arrhythmias, some patients develop anorexia, nausea, and vomiting from digitalis excess, and, on occasion, either green or yellow vision (chromatopsia).

A number of digitalis preparations are available for use. They range from the short-acting intravenously administered agents such as ouabain or lanatoside C to the long-acting orally administered agents such as digitoxin and digitalis leaf. The short-acting preparations may be used for the treatment of acute arrhythmias or for acute pulmonary edema and the long-acting agents for long-term maintenance in stable patients. The most commonly employed compound is digoxin, which has an intermediate action time and may be given either intravenously or orally, and which has a relatively rapid onset of action, and yet is sufficiently sustained in effect to permit maintenance in adults with a single daily dose of 0.25 to 0.5 mg. For ouabain and lanatoside C, the total digitalizing doses (that amount required to achieve total digitalization) are about 0.5 and 0.8 mg, respectively, in adults. In treating arrhythmias and acute heart failure, approximately half this dose may be given intravenously as an initial amount, followed by divided doses over a period of several hours to achieve the total digitalizing dose. For digoxin, the digitalizing dose given intravenously is approximately 1.0 mg, of which one-half may be given at once, followed by the remainder in divided doses over a period of hours. For oral usage in nonemergency situations, full digitalization may be achieved by giving up to 1.5 mg in divided doses over a 24-hour period. For digitoxin and

digitalis leaf, the digitalizing doses are approximately 1 mg and 1 gm, respectively. Most commonly, initial therapy is begun with small multiples of the usual daily maintenance dose of 0.1 mg for digitoxin or 0.1 gm for digitalis leaf until the digitalizing dose has been administered.

For all these agents, considerable variability may be encountered, and lower or higher doses may occasionally be required. In patients in whom toxicity is inadvertently produced, the toxic effects of the intravenously administered agents (ouabain and lanatoside C) are usually dissipated within a matter of hours and those of digoxin within a day or two; however, because of their long biologic half-life, digitoxin and digitalis leaf may produce toxicity lasting for many days. A major consideration with employment of digoxin therapy is the status of renal function. Since digoxin is excreted primarily by the kidneys, renal failure may result in prolonged toxicity. The dosage of digoxin employed must be therefore reduced in proportion to the degree of renal failure present. Renal failure does not affect the dissipation of digitalis leaf or its active principal, digitoxin, which is primarily degraded by the liver.

Reversal of digitalis toxicity is achieved mainly by withdrawing the drug, and, in the case of ventricular and junctional tachyarrhythmias, by administration of specific antiarrhythmic drugs such as lidocaine, phenytoin sodium, or propranolol, as well as by administration of potassium salts when hypokalemia is present. For toxicity characterized by atrioventricular block, stopping digitalis is usually sufficient, although occasionally when heart rates are extremely slow, temporary pacemaking may be required.

DIURETICS

In addition to digitalis, administration of diuretics has also become a routine part of the therapy of congestive heart failure. When fluid accumulation, either in the lungs or the periphery, becomes a problem in congestive heart failure, diuretics may alleviate both symptoms and signs. However, diuretics have no intrinsic effect on ventricular function, while they do have the potential of reducing cardiac output by lowering ventricular filling pressures. For this reason, they must be employed judiciously, lest they produce a low-output syndrome, and, on occasion, even hypotension or shock. As stated above, diuretics are not a substitute for a salt-restricted diet, although they do sometimes enable less stringent salt restriction to be employed in milder degrees of congestive heart failure. All diuretics share the propensity for inducing electrolyte disturbances, especially hypokalemia and occasionally hyponatremia.

In milder degrees of congestive heart failure, milder diuretics such as the thiazides may be given orally. Doses of chlorothiazide range from 500 mg to 2 gm daily, and those of the more potent analogue, hydrochlorothiazide, from 50 to 200 mg daily. On occasion, doses given on an every-other-day basis may avoid excessive potassium depletion. Hyperuricemia and impairment of glucose tolerance may occur during therapy with thiazide diuretics, and exacerbation of gout or diabetes is not uncommon. This may require initiation or intensification of therapy for gout, or adjustment of the dose of oral hypoglycemic agents or insulin for diabetes. Patients receiving thiazide diuretics in larger amounts must receive oral replacement of potassium, either in the form of high-potassium foods such as orange juice or bananas or as potassium salts, preferably in liquid form. When control of hypokalemia proves to be a major problem, supplementation of diuretic therapy with the aldosterone antagonist spironolactone or administration of triamterene, a potassium-sparing drug, may prove successful.

More recently, highly potent diuretic agents that may be given either intravenously or orally have become available, including ethacrynic acid and furosemide. These may be given in oral doses ranging from 50 to 200 mg daily for ethacrynic acid, and 20 mg to as high as 600 mg daily for furosemide. The larger doses should be reserved for patients with refractory congestive heart failure or pulmonary edema (see later) and would be hazardous in mild or moderate congestive failure, since they can cause marked and precipitous diuresis. When given intravenously, the agents are effective within half an hour. These agents also have the propensity for producing hyperuricemia and hyperglycemia, though not as markedly as the thiazide diuretics.

The use of diuretic agents is complicated when renal failure coexists with cardiac failure. This is not an infrequent state of affairs, since certain forms of cardiac and renal disease often coexist, for example in hypertension. Advanced renal failure promotes refractoriness to diuretic therapy. At the same time, effective treatment of cardiac failure with diuretics may reduce circulating blood volume, reduce glomerular filtration rate, and worsen the degree of azotemia. In such patients, concurrent use of either peritoneal dialysis or hemodialysis has been employed, but this approach is limited to the most difficult situations.

OTHER CONSIDERATIONS

Attention to the mechanical effects of accumulation of fluids in body spaces may be required. Thus, pleural effusions may embarrass pulmonary function and accentuate dyspnea, and therefore may require repeated thoracenteses. Similarly, marked ascites may elevate the diaphragm and restrict respirations, and paracentesis may be required for relief. These palliative measures, though temporarily effective, often must be repeated indefinitely until correction of the underlying heart failure is achieved.

Care of the edematous extremities and of skin in areas of sacral and scrotal edema in bedridden patients may require special measures. Application of lanolin ointments to preserve skin softening, and use of frequent turning and soft bedclothes such as air mattresses or sheepskin, as well as application of lamb's wool between the toes, may prevent skin breakdown and decubitus ulcers. The position in bed may also be important, and a semisupine position if tolerated or elevation of the legs may promote diuresis during a period of intense diuretic therapy.

Some clinicians administer anticoagulants to bedridden patients to prevent phlebothrombosis and embolism. This is not without hazard, due to the possibility of anticoagulant-induced bleeding. Dangling, a bed-chair regimen, and leg exercises may reduce the risk of embolic disease. The value of elastic stockings or leg bandages has never been fully proved, although most clinicians order the use of such stockings; the stockings may enhance diuresis in bedridden patients by returning extracellular fluid to the central circulation.

In patients with advanced heart failure who are hospitalized, certain measurements are essential in evaluating the course of therapy. Daily weights, careful charts of intake and output, measurement of calf dimensions, and assessment of serum electrolytes and sodium balance may be of prime importance. These are especially helpful when complex electrolyte and fluid balance disturbances exist and in the presence of renal failure.

Acute Pulmonary Edema

Patients with left-sided cardiac failure from any cause may develop the syndrome of acute pulmonary edema. This may be defined as a state of acute, severe pulmonary congestion with transudation of fluid into the lung interstitium and alveoli due to elevation of filling pressures on the left side of the heart. When left-sided filling pressures exceed a mean value of approximately 20 mm Hg, pulmonary edema often results. The condition represents an advanced form of left ventricular failure, one that often has a dramatic clinical presentation and requires urgent action to avert a fatal outcome.

It is possible for patients to develop pulmonary edema when left ventricular function is only moderately impaired if a state of acute, severe pressure or volume overload arises. Thus patients with moderate left ventricular failure who ingest inordinate amounts of salt, who receive excessive volume infusions, or who develop severe systemic hypertension may develop acute pulmonary edema. The genesis of pulmonary edema under these circumstances may be visualized by examining ventricular function curves in the presence of normal, moderately, or severely depressed left ventricular function (see Fig. 31-2). In the normal ventricle it is apparent that large increases in intravascular volume may be tolerated without the development of elevated left ventricular filling pressures. With moderate impairment of left ventricular function, considerable cardiac reserve still exists, and increases in intravascular volume to some degree are tolerated without extreme elevations of left ventricular filling pressure; however, if intravascular volume is markedly increased, filling pressure may rise and pulmonary edema may nonetheless

result. With severely depressed left ventricular function, reserve cardiac function is greatly diminished, ventricular function curves are flat, and even modest volume increases may result in precipitous rises in left ventricular filling pressure. Indeed, in the most advanced left ventricular decompensation, pulmonary edema may coexist with cardiogenic shock (page 345), and it may be impossible to manipulate intravascular volume to attain a hemodynamic status in which both arterial blood pressure and ventricular filling pressure are maintained in an adequate range.

From this discussion it should be apparent that manipulation of intravascular volume constitutes a major therapeutic approach in alleviating acute pulmonary edema. Thus lowering intravascular volume directly through removal of fluid by diuresis or phlebotomy, or reducing venous return by applying venous tourniquets and by administering venodilator drugs, may make it possible to reverse clinical acute pulmonary edema quite rapidly. In patients who have coexisting systemic hypertension, acute pulmonary edema may be relieved by a rapid lowering of the systemic vascular resistance, with reduction in arterial blood pressure and afterload, and, according to the Starling mechanism, a lowering of left ventricular filling pressure.

Contemporary monitoring techniques make it possible to monitor circulatory parameters carefully in individual patients so that cardiac function may be optimized, while pulmonary edema is relieved by appropriately adjusting preload and afterload. However, it should be pointed out that pulmonary edema is a clinical diagnosis that is based on the appearance and presentation of the patient, and therefore it must be judged primarily on clinical criteria. In other words, pulmonary edema does not always occur "by the numbers," and, when encountered, must be treated in classic fashion, no matter what preload and afterload figures are recorded. Furthermore, pulmonary edema may occur quite suddenly in a patient who appears to be hemodynamically stable, that is, who has unchanging values of left ventricular filling pressures and arterial pressures. Thus, with abnormal hemodynamics the development of clinical pulmonary edema may take some time, and by the same token, resolution of pulmonary edema, that is, absorption of fluid from the lung interstitium, may lag behind correction of preload and afterload abnormalities.

CLINICAL PRESENTATION

The clinical picture of acute pulmonary edema may be characterized as follows: A patient with left-sided failure due to ischemic heart disease, systemic hypertension, aortic or mitral valve disease, or other causes such as cardiomyopathy reaches a critical stage of decompensation, either through gradual progression of disease or through some acute insult such as a new episode of myocardial ischemia, salt ingestion, or arrhythmia. He becomes acutely dyspneic and orthopneic, finds himself gasping for breath, develops a cough, and very frequently produces sputum that is either foamy and whitish or, in the most advanced cases, is tinged with blood; he becomes cyanotic, and, if the situation is allowed to progress, may eventually become weak, lethargic, and obtunded, and may die from progressive respiratory distress, hypoxia, and shock. On examination, the physician finds an agitated, tachypneic, and frequently cyanotic patient sitting bolt upright, struggling for breath. There may be audible, noisy, bubbling respirations. The blood pressure sometimes may be low if the patient is in cardiogenic shock; it may be normal, or very frequently it is elevated, presumably due to stress and concurrent sympathetic autonomic discharge. The sympathetic activity apparently aggravates pulmonary edema by increasing ventricular afterload, and it is one of the specific abnormalities that should be attacked in treating pulmonary edema. The pulse is frequently rapid due to sinus tachycardia or perhaps due to a cardiac arrhythmia, and this rapidity contributes to the pulmonary edema; the pulse also is often weak and thready due to reduced stroke volume. The cardiac sounds, if they can be auscultated, may be distant, and a gallop rhythm is frequently present. The most consistent finding is that of moist rales at the lung bases and, more frequently, throughout the lung fields even up to the apices, indicating diffuse transudation of fluid into the lung interstitium. There may be an associated element of wheezing and bronchospasm. The occurrence of this symp-

tom complex constitutes a medical emergency and demands immediate treatment by the attending physician if the patient is to survive.

DIFFERENTIAL DIAGNOSIS

The differential diagnosis of acute pulmonary edema is very important because several other common conditions may cause confusing symptomatology. Diffuse bronchopneumonia may produce rales, tachypnea, blood-tinged sputum, and respiratory distress; however, the rales are often localized; the patient may have evidence of sepsis, including a high temperature and white blood cell count; and the x-ray picture is usually characteristic, showing infiltration of localized segments of the lung rather than the symmetric pattern of perihilar pulmonary venous congestion seen in pulmonary edema. Pulmonary embolism may also produce tachypnea and dyspnea, and the patient may show hemoptysis of bright red blood, but localized rales or friction rub usually overlie the area of infarction when this follows pulmonary embolism. There is considerable debate as to whether acute pulmonary edema may accompany pulmonary embolism in certain cases; when this has occurred, it has been attributed variously to arterial hypoxemia resulting in cardiac depression; to acute distention of the right side of the heart compromising the filling of the left side of the heart; or possibly to autonomic reflexes originating from the lung. Bronchial asthma may simulate pulmonary edema, as it is accompanied by dyspnea and wheezing, and in the presence of chronic lung disease or infection, rales as well. The rales in asthma are apt to be coarser than the diffuse alveolar filling sounds heard in true alveolar acute pulmonary edema and may be accompanied by rhonchi. When an asthmatic component is found in acute pulmonary edema (so-called cardiac asthma), treatment should be directed partly toward relieving bronchospasm, as is done in true asthmatic attacks. Other conditions that may simulate pulmonary edema include aspiration of gastric contents; inhalation of toxic gases, which may create a true pulmonary edema, but by direct alveolar damage rather than left ventricular failure; and, finally, cerebral pulmonary edema, a rare condition complicating elevated intracerebral pressures. Cerebral pulmonary edema has been thought to result from autonomic reflexes and in most instances is probably caused by elevated systemic blood pressures and afterload causing acute left ventricular decompensation.

TREATMENT

Treatment of acute pulmonary edema requires a well-rehearsed and rapidly moving sequence of therapeutic maneuvers. The patient should be positioned in the reverse Trendelenburg or upright sitting or semisitting position, a position that he often attains voluntarily. Oxygen should be given by face mask or nasal prongs, but the physician should be alert to the possibility that coexisting pulmonary failure may be present and that arterial hypoxemia may represent the primary drive to respiration; the patient must be carefully watched to determine whether respirations become depressed on oxygen, resulting in hypercarbia. Morphine, 10 to 15 mg, should be promptly given intravenously to calm the patient and to sequester intravascular volume in the venous capacitance bed by the mechanism of venodilatation.

Some patients will be brought out of pulmonary edema quickly by these three measures — positioning, oxygen administration, and morphine therapy. If not, tourniquets should be applied to the limbs in rotating fashion (three limbs subjected to venous occlusion at a level of 40 mm Hg with the fourth limb unobstructed, rotating in a fixed sequence every 15 minutes). Concurrently, rapid-acting intravenous diuretics such as ethacrynic acid or furosemide may be used. This method of treating acute pulmonary edema (by using tourniquets and diuretics) has attained great popularity, but it is not without hazard, since the ensuing diuresis, sometimes massive, can readily deplete intravascular volume and result in hypotension and shock due to inadequate cardiac filling pressures. Bronchospasm should be treated by giving 250 mg of aminophylline intravenously over a 10-minute period initially and then instituting an intravenous drip to give 500 mg of the drug over a 4-hour period. Aminophylline may accelerate the cardiac rate and provoke ventricular ectopic beats, and it should be administered with this in mind.

At a convenient time after initiation of these therapeutic measures and at an early stage in refractory pulmonary edema, intravenous digitalization should be undertaken. The usual agent employed is digoxin, which is given initially as 0.5 mg intravenously and is followed by 0.25 mg as often as every 2 hours until a dose of approximately 1.0 mg is attained. More rapidly acting agents such as ouabain and lanatoside C may be employed instead of digoxin.

Meanwhile, as all these measures are being undertaken, the patient should be closely monitored for vital signs, urine output, electrocardiograms, and arterial blood gases and pH; a chest x-ray should be made to ascertain the degree of pulmonary vascular congestion and should be repeated thereafter to help gauge the results of therapy. All possible underlying causes of the acute pulmonary edema should be assiduously sought, including acute myocardial infarction, presence of unsuspected valvular lesions, pulmonary embolism, excessive salt ingestion, or hypertension. The presence of systemic hypertension represents a special case and is a frequent accompaniment of acute pulmonary edema, either as a cause (increased ventricular afterload) or as a result (stress situation, increased endogenous catecholamine secretion). If hypertension is severe and persistent, antihypertensive agents should be administered.

On occasion, acute pulmonary edema becomes refractory and does not respond to therapy; if so, efforts must move into a new phase. If not already in place, a flow-directed catheter should be inserted in the pulmonary artery to monitor left-sided filling pressures. If the patient displays persistent arterial hypoxemia, rales, tachypnea, and other evidence of cardiac decompensation, and particularly if he becomes obtunded and shows evidence of respiratory depression with carbon dioxide retention, endotracheal intubation is indicated. Instituting positive-pressure breathing not only makes it possible to control precisely the respiratory status of the patient, but also pressure gradients across the alveoli can be reversed and previously atelectatic areas can be opened up. Furthermore, by employing positive end-expiratory pressure (PEEP), further gains along this line may be achieved. Positive-pressure therapy is not without hazard, however, since it may reduce cardiac output by increasing intrathoracic pressure and reducing venous return. Nonetheless, intubation should be employed in any patient who shows evidence either of respiratory decompensation and deterioration of blood gases or of excessive fatigue during acute pulmonary edema.

In a patient with complicating disease in other organ systems, for example, hepatic failure, nephrotic syndrome, or prolonged inanition, it should be kept in mind that a diminished serum albumin may lower plasma oncotic pressure and that pulmonary edema may then occur at levels of left ventricular filling pressure below 20 mm Hg. In such cases, administration of albumin or plasma may effect at least a transient improvement, although ultimately correction of the underlying condition will be required.

It should also be kept in mind that certain forms of pulmonary edema may represent acute surgical emergencies. Prime examples are pulmonary edema due to rupture of a papillary muscle with severe mitral regurgitation, or pulmonary edema due to rupture of the interventricular septum with a left-to-right shunt following an acute myocardial infarction. Patients who present with late-stage aortic or mitral valve rheumatic heart disease with pulmonary edema may require urgent surgical replacement of the aortic or mitral valve (see Chap. 30). Finally, it should be recognized that acute pulmonary edema is but a part of the spectrum of severe left ventricular decompensation resulting from many forms of heart disease; it represents a state of volume overload relative to a decompensated left ventricle. By overzealous treatment, the patient with acute pulmonary edema may be catapulted into a state of cardiogenic shock, even though the pulmonary edema is relieved. In other instances, as discussed in the next section, pulmonary edema may be precipitated in patients with cardiogenic shock by overzealous treatment of the shock state with volume infusions. In some cases, ventricular function is so poor that shock and pulmonary edema coexist. In such cases the prognosis is grave, because left ventricular function is so marginal that neither afterload nor preload can be maintained together in a range compatible with survival. How-

ever, in some instances the physician can carefully manage the patient with marginal left ventricular function through the initial period and on to ultimate survival.

Cardiogenic Shock
When the degree of cardiac decompensation becomes so severe that arterial blood pressure can no longer be maintained, despite operation of all the available compensatory mechanisms, a state of cardiogenic shock is said to exist. This represents the most advanced form of cardiac failure, and correspondingly has a grave prognosis. Unlike pulmonary edema, which is due to the failure of the left side of the heart, cardiogenic shock may represent a preterminal event of failure of either ventricle, occurring at a time when either the right or the left ventricle is so weakened that it is no longer able to pump an adequate cardiac output to maintain blood pressure. Most commonly, however, cardiogenic shock is a consequence of left ventricular failure, and it is encountered most frequently in the syndrome of acute myocardial infarction, though occasionally it is seen in other forms of heart disease, including valvular disease and cardiomyopathy. As described earlier in this chapter, in the section on acute pulmonary edema, one of the physician's major tasks is to adjust intravascular volume to optimize ventricular filling pressures, short of producing pulmonary edema, so that maximum pumping action will be facilitated. On occasion, a patient thought to be in cardiogenic shock on clinical grounds will, in fact, respond to volume infusions, indicating that at least a part of the problem was depleted intravascular volume, whatever the underlying cardiac condition may be. On the other hand, overinfusion of fluids may transform cardiogenic shock into acute pulmonary edema, so intravenous therapy must be employed with great caution.

CLINICAL PRESENTATION
The central feature of the cardiogenic shock syndrome is a fall in arterial blood pressure accompanied by a characteristic set of shocklike clinical signs and symptoms. Decline in blood pressure per se is not an uncommon accompaniment of certain acute forms of

cardiac decompensation; hence a fall in blood pressure alone is not enough to make the diagnosis of cardiogenic shock. In general, cardiogenic shock does not occur unless systolic blood pressure falls below the level of 90 mm Hg, although previously hypertensive patients may develop the shock syndrome at higher blood pressures, presumably because they require higher pressures to perfuse their vasoconstricted vascular beds.

The symptoms and signs of cardiogenic shock are due to poor perfusion of the peripheral vasculature and to the accompanying sympathetic autonomic discharge that occurs in response to the lowered blood pressure. Symptoms include weakness, dizziness, and prostration, and signs include sweating; cold, clammy skin; and mental obtundation. On physical examination the patient often appears lethargic, his pulse is often weak and thready, and his blood pressure measured with a cuff is low and sometimes unobtainable. Signs of cardiac failure may be present, including gallop rhythm or pulmonary congestion, but these are not specific for the cardiogenic shock syndrome. Tachyarrhythmias and bradyarrhythmias are sometimes present, and if so, must be corrected, as they may contribute to the shock syndrome. Almost invariably the urine output will be low due to poor renal perfusion, and placement of an indwelling catheter and monitoring of urinary output may provide a valuable measure of the progress of therapy.

DIFFERENTIAL DIAGNOSIS

The differential diagnosis of the shock state is extremely important and must be carefully thought through by the physician in every case. Certain types of shock may be readily treated and reversed, with survival of the patient, whereas cardiogenic shock is a disorder that is usually fatal despite vigorous therapy. Therefore it is very important to determine whether potentially treatable forms of shock exist or coexist with cardiac decompensation. The most obvious and readily treatable noncardiac cause of shock is volume depletion, mentioned above. In the presence of blood loss, severe vomiting, diarrhea, or other source of volume loss, an effort to replete intravascular fluids should be undertaken. Monitoring of central venous pressure or preferably, of pulmonary arterial pres-

sures, will aid this endeavor, since intravascular volume depletion is characterized by low filling pressures. If volume replacement is required, it should be done with an appropriate fluid. For example, crystalloids should be infused if there is vomiting or diarrhea with hemoconcentration; blood should be given for blood loss; and plasma or albumin should be given for plasma loss. A diagnosis of septic shock should be considered concurrently when a septic focus exists or when there is high fever or leukocytosis, even in the presence of manifest cardiac disease. Septic shock is treated with volume infusion and appropriate antimicrobial therapy.

Other forms of shock that are not always as amenable to treatment as volume loss or septic shock and which may mimic the syndrome of acute myocardial infarction include pulmonary embolism and dissecting aneurysm of the aorta. In pulmonary embolism, pulmonary vascular obstruction is the cause of shock, while in dissecting aortic aneurysm, pain and blood loss precipitate shock. Both diseases may cause chest pain similar to that in acute myocardial infarction. Pericardial tamponade, though uncommon, may also result in the shock syndrome, and it is eminently treatable. Other treatable but less common forms of shock should be kept in mind, such as adrenal insufficiency.

TREATMENT

The treatment of cardiogenic shock remains unsatisfactory at best, and this is due to the severe degree of damage to heart muscle that is invariably present. Blood pressure must be raised at all costs. The inotropic and vasoconstrictor agents employed to achieve this may cause further damage to already injured cardiac muscle by increasing its work and oxygen requirements, but there is no recourse but to employ them, even in the presence of cardiac ischemia from acute myocardial infarction. A number of pressor agents with both alpha- and beta-adrenergic properties are available for use. In general, a severe decline in blood pressure to levels approaching the unattainable should be treated with an agent that is potent and possesses considerable alpha-adrenergic activity, such as norepinephrine. Intravenous infusions in the dosage range of 1 to 32 μg per minute are generally employed. Lesser degrees of shock in which the patient's condition is relatively stable and there is only a modest decline in blood pressure may sometimes be treated successfully with agents possessing more beta-adrenergic properties, such as dopamine. Dosages of 100 to 1,500 μg per minute given intravenously are generally employed. Agents of this sort should be started immediately when it is ascertained that the cardiogenic shock state exists, as it is thought that prolonged hypotension may accentuate the myocardial ischemia that caused it, particularly in acute myocardial infarction.

Once initial therapy has begun, it is advisable to establish a monitoring protocol. This protocol involves measuring the pulmonary arterial pressure with a balloon-flotation venous catheter, monitoring the arterial blood pressure with an indwelling arterial catheter, monitoring urinary output with an indwelling bladder catheter, and continuously monitoring the electrocardiogram. Electrolyte and blood gas measurements should be made, and if abnormalities exist, attempts should be made to correct them. This applies particularly to arterial hypoxemia and acidosis; the latter is in most instances due to lactic acidosis resulting from the low output state. Acidosis is usually not readily reversed unless cardiac pumping action is improved; however, infusions of sodium bicarbonate may at least transiently correct the acidosis. Arterial hypoxemia should be treated with oxygen administration, although when the hypoxemia is due to pulmonary congestion and shunting of blood through the lungs, such therapy may be of little avail. Tracheal intubation is indicated if the patient is not ventilating properly; however, positive-pressure ventilation must be employed with caution, since this may further lower the already depressed cardiac output. Many physicians believe that patients with cardiogenic shock should be given digitalis, although there is no convincing evidence that this measure alters the unfavorable prognosis.

Because of the extremely poor prognosis in medically treated cardiogenic shock, new approaches have been sought in recent years. Particularly promising is the use of assisted circulation in the form of intra-aortic balloon counterpulsation. This technique may be applied for short-term support of the circulation, and usually it is successful in at least partially reversing the shock state. However, it is a temporary measure and does not appear to alter significantly the ultimate prognosis unless it is supplemented by more aggressive measures, including cardiac surgery. Intra-aortic balloon counterpulsation is particularly helpful in managing patients with papillary muscle rupture or ventricular septal defects resulting from myocardial infarction, since counterpulsation can support the circulation until definitive surgical repair can be carried out. This technique also has a very modest success rate in supporting patients through surgery for coronary bypass operations, with or without infarctectomy, during the acute phase of myocardial infarction with shock. The extremely high mortality from medically treated cardiogenic shock does appear to warrant more aggressive surgical attempts at therapy.

Bibliography

Braunwald, E., Ross, J., Jr., and Sonnenblick, E. H. Mechanisms of contraction of the normal and failing heart. *N. Engl. J. Med.* 277:794, 853, 910, 962, 1012, 1967.

Duca, P., and Brest, A. N. Indications, contraindications, and nonindications for digitalis therapy. *Cardiovasc. Clin.* 6:131, 1974.

Frazier, H. S., and Yager, H. The clinical use of diuretics. *N. Engl. J. Med.* 288:246, 455, 1973.

Gunnar, R. M., and Loeb, H. S. Use of drugs in cardiogenic shock due to acute myocardial infarction. *Circulation* 45:1111, 1972.

New York Heart Association Criteria Committee. *Diseases of the Heart and Blood Vessels: Nomenclature and Criteria for Diagnosis* (6th ed.). Boston: Little, Brown, 1964.

Sarnoff, S. J. Myocardial contractility as described by ventricular function curves; observations on Starling's law of the heart. *Physiol. Rev.* 35: 107, 1955.

Scheidt, S., Wilner, G., Mueller, H., Summers, D., Lesch, M., Wolff, G., Krakauer, J., Rubenfire, M., Fleming, P., Noon, G., Oldham, N., Killip, T., and Kantrowitz, A. Intra-aortic balloon counterpulsation in cardiogenic shock: Report

of a cooperative clinical trial. *N. Engl. J. Med.*
288:979, 1973.

Smith, T. W. Digitalis glycosides. *N. Engl. J. Med.*
288:719, 942, 1973.

Swan, H. J. C., Ganz, W., Forrester, J., Marcus, H.,
Diamond, G., and Chonette, D. Catheterization
of the heart in man with use of a flow-directed
balloon-tipped catheter. *N. Engl. J. Med.* 283:
447, 1970.

Weiner, L. Rational therapeutic approach to cardiogenic shock. *Cardiovasc. Clin.* 6:223, 1974.

Wolk, M. J., Scheidt, S., and Killip, T. Heart failure
complicating acute myocardial infarction.
Circulation 45:1125, 1972.

32

Cardiac Arrhythmias and Electrocardiography

Michael D. Klein and Paul A. Levine

Technique

A conventional ECG is easily obtained. One electrode is fastened with a strap in fixed position to each of the four extremities. A movable suction electrode is placed consecutively at six prescribed sites across the anterior chest between the fourth and fifth intercostal spaces. A sequence of 12 leads is then inscribed on specially printed paper moving past a heat-sensitive stylus at 25 mm per second. The paper is marked both horizontally and vertically at 1-mm intervals, with heavier markings at 5-mm intervals. The ECG tracing is standardized so that a 1-millivolt (mV) signal gives a 1-cm deflection (Fig. 32-1).

Figure 32-1. Nomenclature for ECG waves, intervals, and time markings on ECG paper. (From G. H. Whipple et al. Acute Coronary Care. *Boston: Little, Brown, 1972. Reproduced by permission.)*

LEAD SYSTEMS

Three standard bipolar limb leads measure the cardiac voltage difference across two extremities. Three standard unipolar limb leads measure the absolute voltage from a single extremity. Each lead has a positive and negative orientation as projected onto the frontal body surface plane. Six unipolar precordial leads measure the voltage from the anterior chest wall (Fig. 32-2). As each cardiac cell depolarizes, it changes its transmembrane potential by 70 to 90 mV; at the body surface, however, the cumulative signals from all ventricular cells are attenuated to 1 to 2 mV. Atrial depolarization represented by the *P wave,* ventricular depolarization represented by the *QRS wave complex,* and ventricular repolarization represented by the *T wave* are easily discernible from the surface ECG. Atrial repolarization, represented by the *Ta wave,* is usually obscured within the larger QRS complex.

Intracardiac leads are used to amplify electrical events that are inconscpicuous or unrecordable on

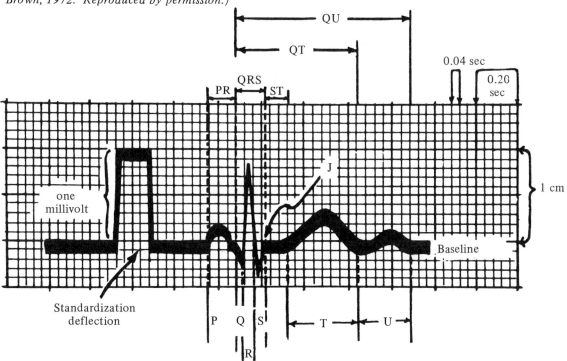

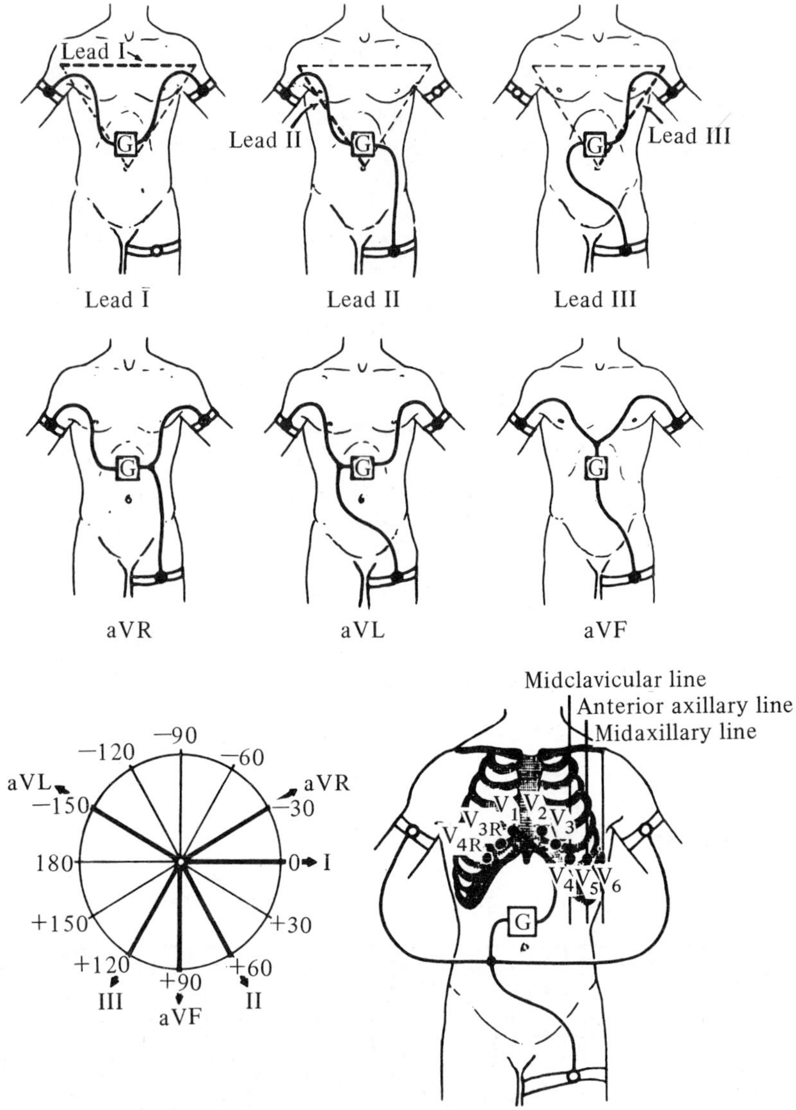

*Figure 32-2. Normal lead placement for 12-lead ECG.
G = galvanometer, which is the ECG machine. Hexaxial frontal plane reference system in lower left
corner allows one to plot direction and magnitude of
initial, terminal, mean, and maximal QRS forces.
(From G. H. Whipple et al.* Acute Coronary Care.
*Boston: Little, Brown, 1972. Reproduced by
permission.)*

the surface ECG. When applied at the bedside or, preferably, in a cardiac catheterization laboratory, these special leads may clarify obscure disorders of cardiac impulse formation and conduction (Fig. 32-3).

NOMENCLATURE
Designated waves and intervals measurable from the surface ECG are depicted in Figure 32-1. They are as follows:

1. P wave — the sum total of atrial depolarization.
2. QRS wave — the sum total of ventricular depolarization. The QRS complex is sometimes multiphasic with more than one upward (positive) or downward (negative) deflection. When a downward deflection initiates a QRS complex, it is called a Q wave if it is the dominant wave (in height), and a q wave if it is not the dominant

wave. When an upward deflection initiates a QRS complex, it is termed an R wave if it is the dominant wave, and an r wave if it is not the dominant wave. Any downward deflection that follows an R or r wave is termed an S or s wave, depending on its size. If there is more than one upward (R) deflection in the QRS complex, the second positive wave is called an R' wave. If two upward deflections are not separated by a downward deflection that crosses below the baseline, the positive wave is referred to as a notched R wave. An entirely negative QRS wave shape is usually referred to as a QS complex.
3. T wave — the sum total of ventricular repolarization.
4. U wave — late repolarization from papillary muscles, Purkinje fibers, or both.

Figure 32-3. Intraatrial electrogram (IAE) lead tracing (bottom) is compared with a standard lead II tracing from the same patient. The P wave is markedly increased in size in the IAE obtained from the right atrium. Intraatrial electrograms are helpful in verifying the presence of P waves and their relationship to the QRS complex when P waves are poorly visible on the standard ECG.

The isoelectric portion of the ECG baseline lies between the T and P waves — the TP segment. The duration of all waves is measured from the point at which the wave first leaves the baseline to the point at which it returns to the baseline. The same is true for component deflections of the QRS complex. The longest *PR interval* is calculated from a limb lead

II

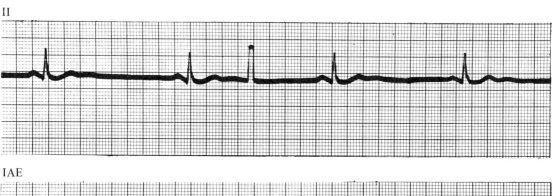

IAE

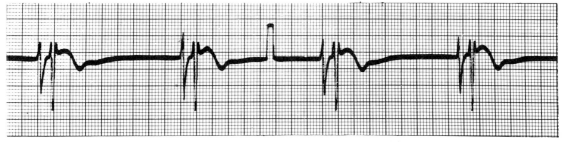

where P waves are clearly depicted, usually lead II. It is measured from the beginning of the P to the beginning of the QRS waves. The point marked *J* stands for the junction of the QRS interval with the ST segment, and it is an important reference point in exercise electrocardiography.

All of the various waves and intervals that were shown in Figure 32-1 become shorter with increasing heart rates. They are also shorter in infants and young children than in adults. Standard tables are available detailing the normal range of wave amplitudes and interval lengths for different heart rates and ages.

QRS Axis. The six limb leads can be projected onto the frontal body surface plane so as to create a hexaxial graphic system (see Fig. 32-2). Each individual axis has a positive and negative direction. By integrating the positive and negative waves of the QRS complex in any one lead, a line of force (vector) along that lead can be measured. Similar computations can be made for a second lead. By combining the measured vectors from two leads, a coordinate with magnitude and direction can be derived. This coordinate can be used to describe the mean, maximal, and early or late QRS vectors. The direction and magnitude of these vectors are useful in describing the preponderance of left or right ventricular muscle masses and in defining certain disorders of electrical conduction within the left ventricle.

Serial ECGs. The value of any ECG is enhanced by comparison with earlier tracings. Both innocuous variations from normal and variations due to disease processes are examined best with serial ECGs. Thus the evolution of a myocardial infarction may be recorded over an interval of a few days, whereas ventricular hypertrophy secondary to hypertension or valvular stenosis may be registered over many years. Consequently, the recording of an ECG should be part of a routine physical examination.

The Abnormal ECG. Electrocardiographic abnormalities are of two types: those of impulse formation and those of impulse conduction. Knowledge of the mechanisms of impulse formation and of the ana-

tomic routes of conduction is helpful in understanding cardiac arrhythmias and blocks.

Impulse Formation

Automaticity. Certain myocardial cells automatically depolarize during electrical diastole. These are the pacemaker cells, and their automaticity is caused by a time-dependent reduction in potassium efflux resulting in a net inward current and gradual depolarization of their cell membranes. Once a critical threshold potential has been attained (about −85 mV), an abrupt inward surge of sodium ions occurs, causing the cells to depolarize much more rapidly. A "sparking" action potential is generated and then propagated throughout the myocardium, inducing it to contract.

Pacemaker cells tend to be clustered in certain key regions, including the sinoatrial (SA) node, adjacent to the atrioventricular (AV) node, along the internodal atrial conducting tracts in the His bundle, and the ventricular Purkinje fiber network. Those within the SA node comprise the primary pacemaker of the heart because they have the fastest rate of discharge.

Intrinsic Control of Automaticity. The number of potential pacemakers ensures that some electrical generator activity of the heart will be preserved, even when impulse formation may be obliterated or blocked in certain areas. Two other attributes of cardiac automaticity tend to prevent competition among disparate pacemaker cells: (1) The discharge rates of atrial pacemaker cells exceed those of ventricular pacemaker cells. Similarly, within the supraventricular conducting system the SA node discharge rates are higher than those in the nonpenetrating portion of the His bundle; whereas within the ventricular conducting system, discharge rates in the penetrating portion of the bundle of His are higher than those in the Purkinje fibers. (2) There is a frequency-dependent inhibition in which the faster pacemaker sites inhibit the slower, with the degree of inhibition proportional to the differential between the two firing rates. Thus an SA pacemaker with an intrinsic rate of 75 per minute will have a greater suppressive effect on a ventricular pacemaker beating at 30 per minute than it will on a junctional pace-

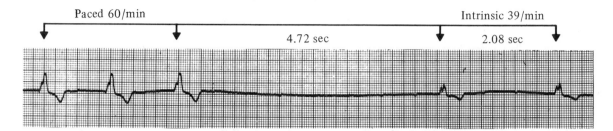

Figure 32-4. Overdrive suppression of cardiac pacemakers. Release from exogenous ventricular pacing results in a long ventricular pause in a patient with complete heart block. The pause (4.72 seconds) exceeds the expected escape interval (2.0 to 3.0 seconds) for an endogenous ventricular pacemaker whose natural frequency is 20 to 30 discharges per minute.

maker beating at 50 per minute.

Such "overdrive suppression" may be seen when the heart is suddenly released from a relative tachycardia, either spontaneous in origin or caused by an artificial pacemaker. Upon cessation of the tachycardia there is a pause of 4 or more seconds, greatly exceeding the normal escape pause of ventricular pacemakers (2 to 3 seconds) (Fig. 32-4). Overdrive suppression with failure of subsidiary pacemakers to capture the heart is also seen in the SA nodal so-called sick sinus syndrome (Fig. 32-5).

Extrinsic Control of Automaticity. The discharge rate of cardiac pacemakers can also be modified by a variety of mechanical, metabolic, and neural mechanisms. Severe acidosis, alkalosis, hypoxemia, hypokalemia, or cardiac dilatation with mechanical stretch of the heart can alter the sinus rate or promote atrial and ventricular ectopic pacemakers. The SA node is profusely innervated by both the sympathetic and parasympathetic fibers, and autonomic tone accounts in part for the wide range of SA rates observed in health and disease.

Disturbances of Automaticity. Normally pacemaker control resides in the SA node, and as the electrical impulse spreads throughout the atrial conducting system, the atrial myocardium is depolarized, giving rise to P waves. These P waves are smooth in contour and are positive (upright) in leads I, II, aVF, and the left precordium but negative in lead aVR. Then, as the electrical wave front traverses the atrial conducting system, the AV node, and the bundle of His, it creates the PR segment of the ECG. By convention, normal sinus rhythm is said to exist when the P wave rate is between 60 and 100 per minute and the PR segment is between 0.12 and 0.20 second.

Sinus Bradycardia. Sinoatrial nodal rates below 60 per minute occur in both young and old. In the young, a slow heart rate may reflect increased vagal tone and a large left ventricular stroke output, often the result of physical conditioning. In the elderly, SA nodal rates below 50 may again be associated with vagotonia and increased stroke output with a normal oxygen consumption rise during exercise. Some older individuals, however, are prone to two complicating features of sinus bradycardia: syncope and episodic tachycardia. Syncope arises when bradycardia induces cerebral hypoperfusion; episodic tachycardia occurs when bradycardia increases the dispersion of repolarization among cardiac cells, causing ectopic or reentry extrasystoles. These in turn trigger ectopic or reentry tachycardias, giving rise to the bradycardia-tachycardia syndrome.

Sinus Tachycardia. Sinoatrial rates exceeding 100 per minute arise from stress — exertional, physical, or psychological. Certain characteristic ECG features accompany sinus tachycardia and distinguish it from ectopic atrial tachycardia: (1) The atrial rate tends to vary slightly; (2) atrial depolarization occurs over an abbreviated time span and therefore the P waves, especially in lead II, tend to be large; (3) pacemaker activity shifts toward the caudal region of the SA node, and conduction across the AV node is facilitated; the PR interval therefore tends to be short

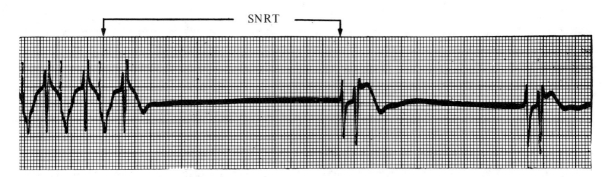

Figure 32-5. Abnormal overdrive suppression in a patient with the so-called sick or somnolent sinus syndrome. An intraatrial electrogram shows that abrupt cessation of rapid extrinsic electrical atrial pacing is followed by a prolonged sinus node recovery time (SNRT) of 2.6 seconds. The pause markedly exceeds the normally expected recovery time of 1.0 to 1.5 seconds.

(0.12 to 0.14 second); and (4) atrial repolarization also is briefer, becoming manifest as J-point depression at the beginning of the ST segment (Fig. 32-6).

Sinus Arrhythmia. Fluctuations in autonomic nervous stimulation of the SA node can cause phasic changes in heart rate, producing sinus arrhythmia. The P-wave cycle alternately shortens and lengthens by more than 0.16 second over a period of 3 to 4 seconds, but the PR interval always remains greater than 0.12 second.

The most common form of sinus arrhythmia is associated with the respiratory cycle and is often encountered in children and the elderly. Inspiration speeds and expiration slows the heart rate. Increased respiratory excursions can exaggerate the rate swings, while breath holding can abolish them. A striking form of sinus arrhythmia occurs during Cheyne-Stokes respiration, in which malfunction of the respiratory center in the brainstem causes periodic breathing over 30- to 120-second intervals. The hyperpneic phase is accompanied by bradycardia and the apneic phase by tachycardia.

Nonrespiratory sinus arrhythmia is of two types. In the first, heart rate shifts gradually over 5 to 15 seconds, but the P-wave contours remain invariable at all cycle lengths (Fig. 32-7A). Digitalis or morphine drugs may provoke this, perhaps by sensitizing the sinus node to cholinergic stimuli. In the second type, sinus arrhythmia is caused by wandering of the pacemaker within the sinus node (Fig. 32-7B). Variations in the relative proportion of sympathetic and parasympathetic tone in different regions of the sinus node presumably cause this wandering. The exact location of the pacemaker influences the egress of the atrial impulse along internodal conducting tracts. Hence, in this type of sinus arrhythmia P-wave contours vary with the site of the cell discharge that initiates the excitation.

Atrial Premature Systoles. Ectopic pacemaker cells (within atrial tissue but extrinsic to the SA node) can initiate excitation whenever they fire prematurely. Each ectopic discharge site results in a different sequence of atrial depolarization and hence in an altered P wave. If the atrial premature beat (APB) reaches the AV node when the latter is in a state of relative refractoriness, the PR interval will be greater than 0.12 second and may be more than 0.20 second. A very early APB may be blocked within the AV node and not be followed by a QRS (Fig. 32-8A, B).

The effect of APBs on cardiac rhythm depends on several variables: (1) the site of origin of the APB in relation to the SA node; (2) the speed of conduction of the APB through atrial tissue; (3) the timing of the APB during diastole (its coupling interval). Late-occurring APBs may not penetrate to the SA node before it has discharged, in which case the APB will be followed by a fully compensatory pause such that the total P-wave cycle, including the ectopic atrial focus, equals two normal P-wave cycles. An APB

L$_2$

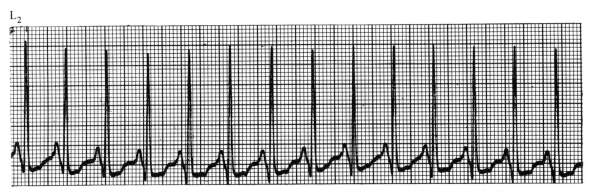

Figure 32-6. Sinus tachycardia.

II

A

II

B

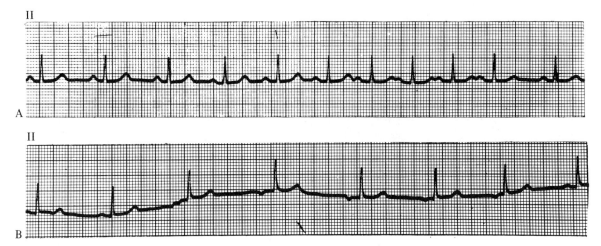

Figure 32-7. Two types of nonrespiratory sinus arrhythmia.

occurring in middiastole can enter and reset the SA node, leading to a less than fully compensatory pause following the ectopic P wave. An early diastolic APB may be blocked in the area surrounding the SA node and fail to reset it; the node then fires on time and the APB will be interpolated within a single normal P-to-P wave cycle.

Very premature atrial beats can also result in tachyarrhythmias and conduction disturbances. Atrial premature beats that have a greater than 50 percent prematurity (P-to-P'/PP < 0.50) and APBs that are closely coupled are likely to cause atrial flutter

or fibrillation (Fig. 32-8C). An atrial impulse may be conducted anomalously through the ventricular conducting system, in which case the QRS will be aberrant. Since long cardiac cycles lengthen the refractory period for the subsequent cycle, aberration of APBs is favored by a long-cycle/short-cycle sequence and the associated aberrated QRS tends to be triphasic (rSR') in lead V$_1$ (Fig. 32-8D).

Atrial Flutter. In atrial flutter, excitation recycles in a circular pathway through the atrial tissue. Atrial activity is rapid and regular, producing F waves at 250 to 350 per minute. Slower rates of atrial flutter can occur when atrial conduction is depressed by drugs such as quinidine or procainamide. The F waves have a rapid upstroke and a more gradual downstroke,

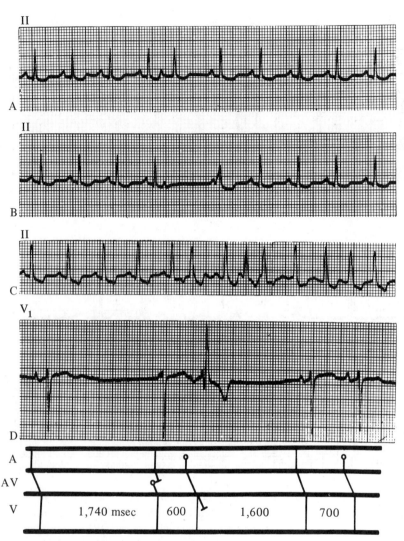

Figure 32-8. Features of atrial premature beats (APB).
A. The fifth beat is an APB conducted to the ventri-
cles. B. The fourth QRS is followed by a premature
P wave that is not associated with a QRS complex;
this APB is blocked within the atrioventricular node
or His bundle and not conveyed to the ventricles.
C. The fifth QRS is followed by a very premature P
wave. This very early APB occurs during the atrial
vulnerable period and initiates atrial fibrillation.
D. A premature P wave is associated with an altered
QRS complex because the APB is conducted aber-
rantly to the ventricles. For comparison, the fifth
beat is an APB conducted normally to the ventricles.
Designated time intervals are in milliseconds.

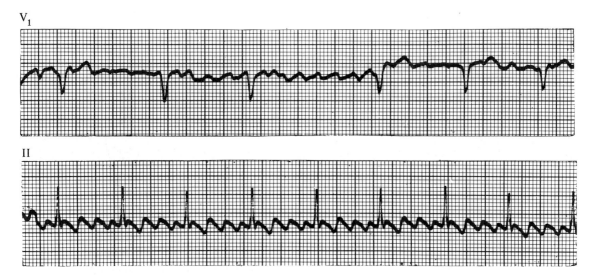

Figure 32-9. The top ECG strip shows coarse atrial fibrillation with an irregular, undulating baseline. The bottom strip shows atrial flutter with a regular, undulating (sawtooth) baseline.

giving rise to a sawtooth pattern in a continually mobile baseline. This undulating pattern is usually seen best in leads II, III, or aVF and may be accentuated by carotid sinus pressure (Fig. 32-9).

The ventricular response rate in atrial flutter is a function of both the atrial rate and the refractory period of the AV node. Usually the atrial rate is some even multiple of the ventricular rate, that is, 2:1 or 4:1 AV block exists. Wenckebach periods of conduction across the AV node can result in variations of AV block. With exertion or excitement, adrenergic facilitation across the AV node may result in a quantum rise in the ventricular response rate, emphasizing the instability of heart rate control in atrial flutter.

Atrial Fibrillation. At atrial rates in excess of 350 per minute, atrial flutter merges into atrial fibrillation, although atrial rates of up to 600 may be seen in fibrillation. In atrial fibrillation, coordinated atrial contraction is absent; multiple wavelets continually reenter and collide within various portions of atrial tissue (see Fig. 32-9). Fibrillatory waves may be either fine (< 1 mm) or coarse (> 1 mm); the fine f waves tend to be associated with atrial fibrillation

of long duration.

The ventricular response to atrial fibrillation may occasionally be regular at very fast heart rates. Generally, however, the ventricular response is irregular with no set pattern. A slow ventricular response to atrial fibrillation (< 50 per minute) suggests either intrinsic AV nodal disease or a marked digitalis effect, prolonging AV nodal refractoriness. A regularized or grouped beating pattern of ventricular complexes suggests complete entrance block into the AV node or Wenckebach (type I) exit block out of the AV node, both characteristic of digitalis intoxication.

Atrial fibrillation, like atrial flutter, usually stems from early APBs or consecutive, closely coupled APBs. Mechanisms that can engender atrial fibrillation include (1) atrial dilatation associated with congestive heart failure or mitral regurgitation; (2) atrial injury associated with ischemia or infiltrative diseases; (3) atrial hypertension associated with mitral stenosis; (4) atrial inflammation associated with pericarditis, which irritates the subjacent SA node; (5) atrial irritability associated with hyperthyroidism.

Atrial Tachycardia. Most instances of paroxysmal supraventricular tachycardia represent reentry rather than ectopic mechanisms, and they may occur in individuals without other evidence of heart disease. More commonly, however, paroxysmal atrial tachycardia with overt or covert AV block is caused by digitalis intoxication. Rarely, an ectopic atrial pace-

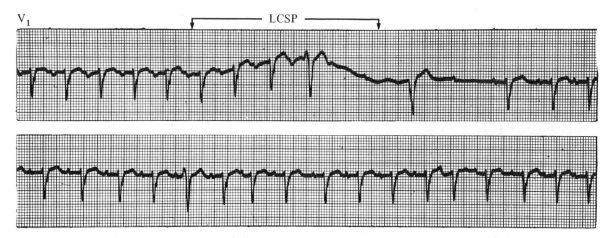

Figure 32-10. Sinus and ectopic atrial tachycardia as a manifestation of digitalis intoxication. A sinus tachycardia at 118 beats per minute with first-degree atrioventricular block (PR interval of 0.24 second) is slowed by left carotid sinus pressure (LCSP). An ectopic atrial tachycardia emerges and is identified by the change in P-wave morphology beginning with the tenth beat.

maker cell will discharge repetitively and usurp control of the heart. Though it is perceived as a sudden event, paroxysmal atrial tachycardia with block actually emerges gradually, usually from sinus tachycardia (Fig. 32-10). Its ECG features set it apart from both sinus tachycardia and atrial flutter: The P-wave rate is regular and can be as slow as 100 or as high as 240, but ordinarily it is between 120 and 220 per minute. Atrial tachycardia is accompanied by a long, rather than a short, PR interval, reflecting the direct and indirect (vagal) effects of digitalis in delaying AV nodal conduction. A 2:1 second-degree AV block can develop either spontaneously or as a result of carotid sinus pressure (see Fig. 32-11A). The P waves, consonant with their ectopic origin, are small rather than large, often appearing as triangulated diminutive forms in leads II and V_1; the baseline is isoelectric.

Multifocal Atrial Tachycardia. Patients with chronic pulmonary disease, especially during bouts of respiratory failure, can exhibit an unusual form of multifocal atrial tachycardia or chaotic atrial mechanism. Multiformed P waves from three or more ectopic foci are evident. The atrial rate varies, with multiple P-to-P

and PR intervals; the average rate exceeds 100 per minute. Multifocal atrial tachycardia probably reflects atrial ectopic activity stemming from several causes, including metabolic dyscrasias and atrial dilatation. Excessive digitalization of a heart already sensitized by cardiac and respiratory failure can transform multifocal atrial tachycardia into paroxysmal atrial tachycardia when the atrial rate speeds up and regularizes or when ventricular ectopic activity develops with AV block.

Supraventricular Tachycardia. Supraventricular tachycardia arises from ectopic beats of atrial, junctional, or ventricular origin. However, it is reentry rather than simple ectopy that sustains the tachycardia. Intracardiac electrocardiography with recordings of the bundle of His have clearly defined the sequence of atrial, bundle of His, and ventricular depolarization. The two essential ingredients for development of supraventricular tachycardia are (1) appropriately timed premature beats and (2) entrance of the premature beats into the SA or AV nodes during their relative refractory periods. Slow heart rates that foster ectopic beats and first-degree heart block with increased AV nodal refractoriness may be contributing factors. Supraventricular tachycardia usually originates in the AV node.

When premature beats enter the AV node during a critical portion of its relative refractory period, part of the wave front passes through and depolarizes the ventricles, albeit with slow conduction (prolonged AH [atrial to His] intervals). Because of nonhomogeneous refractoriness within the AV node, a portion of the antegrade impulse is blocked and reflected back to its chamber of origin. Conduction within this chamber has sufficiently recovered, however, so that the impulse is once again diverted to the AV node. Traverse of the AV node again occurs during the relative refractory period. The cycle is repeated, and supraventricular tachycardia ensues (Fig. 32-11B).

By this mechanism, supraventricular tachycardia may start and stop abruptly and last for variable periods. Neither heart rate nor the positioning of

Figure 32-11. Comparative responses of paroxysmal atrial tachycardia and supraventricular tachycardia to carotid sinus pressure (CSP). A. Paroxysmal atrial tachycardia arising from an atrial ectopic pacemaker. Carotid sinus pressure exposes a latent conduction disturbance in the atrioventricular node and second-degree atrioventricular block. B. Supraventricular tachycardia with carotid sinus pressure interrupting one limb of the reentry pathway and abolishing the arrhythmia.

P waves relative to QRS need be fixed, since cycle-to-cycle variations in antegrade or retrograde impulse passage through the AV node may exist. Heart rate itself becomes a function of AV nodal refractoriness. Therefore, maneuvers that prolong AV nodal refractoriness and slow conduction can be expected to abrogate or reduce the rate of supraventricular tachycardia. Digitalis with its cholinergic effect and beta-adrenergic blocking drugs with their antiadrenergic effect are two agents used for this purpose.

Wolff-Parkinson-White Syndrome. A distinctive variety of reentry tachycardia is seen in the Wolff-Parkinson-White (WPW) syndrome, in which anomalous conducting tracts circumvent the AV node wholly or in part. An alternative route for AV conduction exists and can bypass the normal AV nodal delay. Its ECG marker is a short or a short-normal (< 0.14 second) PR interval. When the anomalous WPW bypass tract penetrates ventricular muscle in a region remote from the AV conducting system, impulses travel slowly

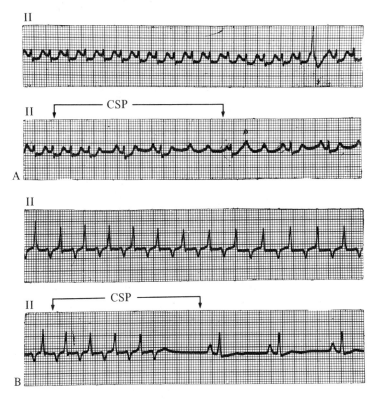

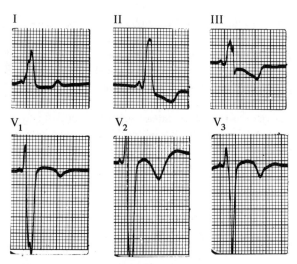
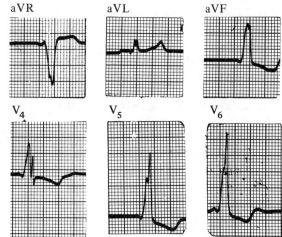

Figure 32-12. Wolff-Parkinson-White syndrome with a short PR interval and wide QRS. The wide QRS is caused by an initial slurring of the complex, called a delta wave, and is well seen in leads III and V_4.

through myocardial fibers before gaining access to the faster conducting Purkinje fiber network. The ECG reflects these events by both a short PR interval and a wide QRS that is slurred or notched at its beginning, and this is the delta wave of the WPW syndrome (Fig. 32-12).

Bypass tracts have been identified inserting into the right ventricle, the left ventricle, and the interventricular septum. In some instances several different bypass tracts may coexist. At any given moment, therefore, AV conduction may occur through the AV node, through one or more bypass tracts, or by fusion down the normal and an anomalous AV conducting system. Hence variability in delta-wave prominence and deformity of QRS complexes characterize the WPW syndrome.

The variability typical of paroxysmal tachycardias characterizes WPW. Frequency, duration, speed, and morphology of the reentry tachyarrhythmias will be determined by the precise circuit of conduction. Antegrade conduction can proceed through the AV node to the ventricles with retrograde transmission back to the atria by way of the anomalous pathway. Reversal of this loop, with antegrade conduction

down the accessory pathway and retrograde transmission through the AV node, occurs less often. When atrial fibrillation is routed through the accessory pathway, the ventricular response rate is unusually rapid. The accessory AV connection has a shorter refractory period than the AV node and transmits a larger percentage of f waves to the ventricle. Sudden onset of a tachycardia greater than 200 beats per minute, with or without aberration of the QRS, suggests the possibility of WPW syndrome. If, during digitalization, accessory pathway refractoriness shortens, the heart rate accelerates rather than slows, and the possibility of WPW should be considered.

Junctional Rhythm. The AV junction occupies a broad territory from the inferior portions of the atria, through the AV node, and including the proximal (penetrating) portion of the bundle of His. Pacemaker cells are present in various areas of this region, though not within the AV node itself. Hence ectopic rhythms originating from these areas are termed junctional rather than AV nodal in origin.

Junctional rhythms resemble conducted SA rhythms in that the QRS complexes are generally normal in width and contour. In junctional rhythm, however, the P wave approaches, lies within, or follows the QRS. Exact positioning of the P wave relative to the QRS is determined by the precise location of the junctional pacemaker and the comparative speeds of conduction, both antegrade to the ventricles and retrograde to the atria. Pacemakers situated in the penetrating portion of the bundle of His tend to exhibit P waves following the QRS, since retrograde transit to the atria is through the AV node, a site of slowed conduction. Pacemakers situated in the lower regions of the atrial tissue tend to exhibit P waves just preceding the QRS.

The natural frequency range of junctional pacemakers is 50 to 60 beats per minute. Faster rates, therefore, constitute a junctional tachycardia (Fig. 32-13). When the junctional tachycardia rate exceeds that of SA discharge, AV dissociation exists. Impulses from the two independent pacemakers collide in or near the AV node because the atria and ventricles remain under different pacemaker controls. Occasionally a premature QRS complex of identical or similar morphology interrupts an otherwise regular ventricular rhythm. This early beat reflects an SA capture beat due to momentary facilitation of antegrade AV conduction.

When AV dissociation is present and atrial and junctional pacemakers have nearly identical discharge rates, phases of SA and junctional rhythm may blend into each other. P waves may wander into and out of the QRS. *Isorhythmic dissociation* is the term used to describe this pattern. Intermittency of the sequenced AV contraction may explain isorhythmic dissociation. When the PR interval is short-normal, the atria contract in tandem with the ventricles; atrial filling of the ventricles and ventricular stroke output are maximized. Blood pressure rises, activating a baroreceptor reflex that slows the SA discharge rate, and P waves then merge into the QRS.

Ventricular Premature Systoles. Discharge of pacemaker cells within the ventricular conducting system prior to the arrival of a normally conducted sinus beat evokes a ventricular premature systole. Ventricular premature beats (VPB) also arise when a delay of unidirectional conduction occurs within the ventricular conducting system. An impulse is blocked from entering a localized ventricular area at a certain time and from a certain direction. The remaining ventricular myocardium is depolarized. The depolarization wave arrives at the region from which it had

been initially excluded, but from a different direction and later in time. Conduction through this region is now possible. The impulse then reenters the ventricle as the VPB.

Whether of ectopic or reentry origin, VPBs have the following ECG attributes: (1) premature occurrence of a QRS complex without a premature P wave preceding it; (2) a bizarre morphology of the premature QRS that is also widened to 0.12 second or more; (3) abnormal repolarization with ST-T waves usually pointing in the opposite direction from the QRS; and (4) a lengthening of the QRS cycle from the VPB itself to the next normal sinus beat (see Fig. 32-14A).

When VPBs are conducted retrograde through the AV node, they may penetrate atrial tissue and discharge the sinus node prematurely. The timing of SA discharge is thereby shifted. The QRS interval — from the last ventricular beat prior to the VPB to the first beat following the VPB — will be less than twice the normal QRS cycle length. Commonly the VPB does not reach atrial tissue, so the SA node is not discharged prematurely and SA nodal rhythm remains undisturbed. The time interval between QRS complexes flanking the VPB will be twice the normal QRS cycle length; such lengthening of the QRS cycle following the VPB is then said to be a *compensatory pause*. The presence of such a compensatory pause is not unique to VPB, however, since both atrial and junctional premature systoles can exhibit the same phenomenon.

The morphology of the QRS can provide some insight into the possible site of origin of a VPB. Ventricular premature beats arising from the branching portion of the His bundle — the left or the right common bundles — do not tend to be too bizarre. The contour of the QRS may reflect preferential conduction down the left or right common fascicle and give rise to a right or left bundle branch block pattern, respectively. By contrast, VPBs arising from distal portions of the ventricular conductioning system — the Purkinje fibers — tend to be more bizarre; their associated QRS contours may be fragmented or greatly slurred, reflecting an erratic entry into the conducting system and slow propagation through myocardial cells. Scrutiny of the QRS morphology in lead V_1 helps discriminate a VPB from an APB

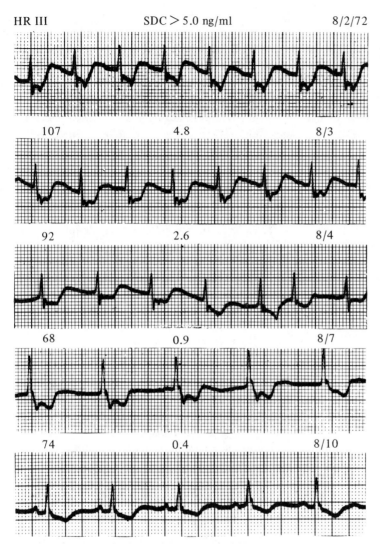

Figure 32-13. Junctional rhythm due to digitalis intoxication. Tracing 8/2 (top) demonstrates a junctional tachycardia with a narrow QRS complex not preceded by a P wave. There is a retrograde P wave in the ST segment causing a small negative deflection. As the digitalis level falls, the junctional rate slows until on 8/10 (bottom strip) sinus rhythm is restored. HR = heart rate; SDC = serum digoxin concentration.

with aberrant conduction. Ventricular premature beats are likely to be monophasic or biphasic in waveshape, exhibit a left bundle branch block configuration, and have initial deflections that are different from adjacent sinus beats. Aberrated APBs are likely to be triphasic in waveshape, exhibit a right bundle branch block configuration, and have initial deflections that may or may not resemble those of adjacent sinus beats (see Fig. 32-8D).

The key feature of a VPB is its timing, or coupling interval, relative to the T wave of the preceding beat. Ventricular premature beats occurring during middle to late electrical diastole, from the downstroke base of the T wave to the next P wave, usually present as isolated events. If middiastolic, they may be interpolated between an undisturbed sinus rhythm. If late diastolic, they may merge with a sinus beat, producing fusion QRS complexes. Ventricular premature beats arising during early diastole, within the T wave, are likely to evoke repetitive responses that can continue as ventricular tachycardia or degenerate into ventricular fibrillation (see Fig. 32-15).

The interval of 20 to 40 milliseconds bridging the apex of the T wave constitutes the vulnerable zone. Within this time span, ventricular muscle is in maximum dispersion of recovery from the preceding depolarization. Therefore, VPBs occurring during this vulnerable zone encounter an irregularly excitable electrical field. As an unstable focus, a VPB spreads outward with greater and greater conduction delay, but with a potential for single or multiple reentry. An accelerating salvo of VPBs conjoined to a progressively decreasing refractory period spreads the dysrhythmic nidus. When sufficient cellular barriers or gates are traversed, hegemony is gained over a muscle mass sufficient to launch ventricular fibrillation.

Accelerated Ventricular Rhythm. The normal discharge frequency of a ventricular pacemaker is 20 to 30 per minute. Repetitive discharge at a faster rate constitutes a relative tachycardia. At rates under 100 per minute, however, the term *accelerated ventricular rhythm* best describes the abnormality. Accelerated ventricular rhythm often emerges at rates close to 60 as the sinus node slows, especially during

sleep. Intervening fusion beats may initiate or terminate accelerated ventricular rhythm. The presence of a QRS > 0.12 second distinguishes accelerated ventricular rhythms from junctional escape rhythms (see Fig. 32-14B).

Ventricular Tachycardia. At rates between 100 and 250 beats per minute, a sustained ventricular rhythm is designated ventricular tachycardia. When both ventricular tachycardia and accelerated ventricular rhythm appear, but at different times, and the ventricular tachycardia rate is a multiple of the accelerated ventricular rhythm rate, an ectopic ventricular pacemaker with periodic exit block may be the basis for the rhythm disturbances. More commonly, ventricular tachycardia reflects a repetitive reentry within some portion of the ventricular conducting system (see Fig. 32-14C).

Ventricular Flutter. At rates exceeding 250 beats per minute, ventricular tachycardia becomes analogous to atrial flutter and can be described as ventricular flutter. These rapid types of ventricular tachycardia are particularly prone to degenerate into ventricular fibrillation (see Fig. 32-14D).

Ventricular Fibrillation. Ventricular fibrillation is analogous to atrial fibrillation in its mechanism with multiple electrical reentry sites and circulating wave fronts. Unlike atrial fibrillation, however, ventricular fibrillation represents a catastrophe during which there is no effective heartbeat (see Fig. 32-14E). Failure to revert ventricular fibrillation within 2 to 3 minutes results in irreversible brain damage unless cardiopulmonary resuscitation is administered.

Ventricular fibrillation is characterized by a distorted, irregular, rapid, and changing electrical activity of the heart. Typical QRS complexes are absent. Certain premonitory VPB patterns presage ventricular fibrillation, namely, VPBs occurring near the apex of the T wave or closely coupled consecutive VPBs (Fig. 32-15). However, ventricular fibrillation can also appear abruptly, without premonitory VPBs. It causes 75 to 80 percent of sudden cardiac deaths outside the hospital and is the major cause of cardiac arrest inside hospitals. Abolition of ventricular fibrillation requires electrical countershock to the heart.

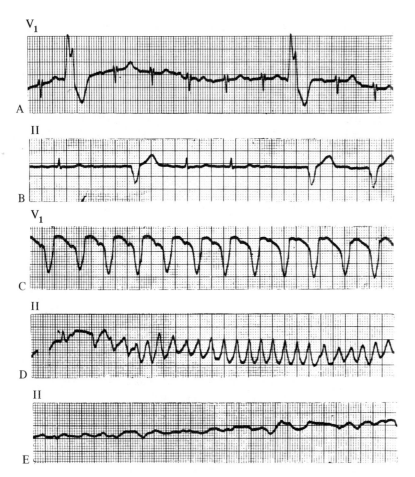

Figure 32-14. Features of ventricular beats. A. The second and eighth beats are ventricular premature beats. B. The second and fifth beats are ventricular escape beats, which are only seen when the supraventricular pacemaker slows excessively or is blocked. C. Ventricular tachycardia. Atrial activity is present as small negative P waves independent of the ventricular rhythm. D. Ventricular flutter. E. Ventricular fibrillation.

Ventricular Parasystole. Ventricular parasystole arises when a ventricular pacemaker (Purkinje fiber) is protected against being depolarized by faster discharging pacemakers. Penetration into the region of the ventricular pacemaker is prevented by a unidirectional conduction delay, known as entrance block. However, conduction outward from the parasystolic focus is possible, and invasion of the surrounding ventric-

ular muscle will occur whenever this region is not in a refractory state from a previously conducted beat. Three ECG criteria identify ventricular parasystole:

1. Ventricular ectopic beats that are independent of the dominant cardiac rhythm and show wide variations in their coupling intervals from those of the QRS complexes immediately preceding them.
2. Interectopic intervals (time between two ventricular ectopic beats) that exhibit an arithmetical relationship to each other, being either equal to or some multiple of the parasystolic pacemaker interval.
3. Periodically the region around the parasystolic focus will be jointly depolarized by the ventricular ectopic pacemaker and the conducted dominant pacemaker. A fusion QRS beat will then result.

V1

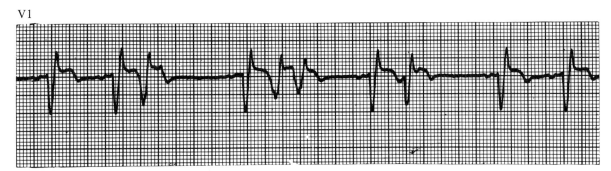

Figure 32-15. Malignant ventricular premature beats occurring on the apex of the T wave (vulnerable period) and resulting in repetitive discharge.

V1

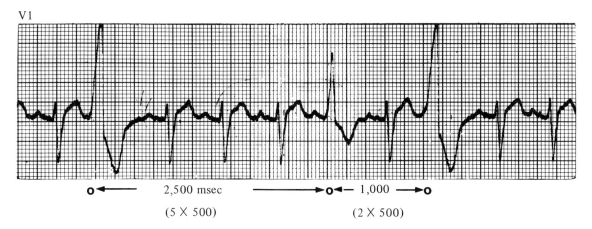

o ◄——— 2,500 msec ———►o◄— 1,000 —►o

(5 X 500)   (2 X 500)

Figure 32-16. Ventricular parasystole.

Occasionally a parasystolic ventricular ectopic beat may fail to appear as anticipated. Exit block may develop around the ectopic focus, so that although the ectopic focus discharges on time, its impulse is prevented from reaching surrounding myocardium; or, alternatively, the parasystolic focus itself may discharge intermittently. The existence of ventricular parasystole usually means that significant heart disease is present. This ventricular arrhythmia is rarely, if ever, associated with digitalis intoxication (Fig. 32-16).

Bidirectional Tachycardia. Bidirectional tachycardia is a distinctive form of ventricular tachycardia that is almost pathognomonic of digitalis intoxication. The pacemaker controlling ventricular depolarization lies within the His bundle or proximal left bundle branch. Its discharge rate and the QRS-to-QRS cycle lengths are constant. Alternate QRS complexes are opposite in direction, however, with upward and downward orientation. The bimodal QRS orientation probably reflects alternate conduction down the anterior and posterior divisions of the left bundle.

Impulse Propagation

The cardiac conducting system mediates a rapid depolarization of both atrial and ventricular muscle. It also provides an electrical filter, the AV node, that protects the ventricles against excessively fast atrial contraction rates and permits a sequenced AV con-

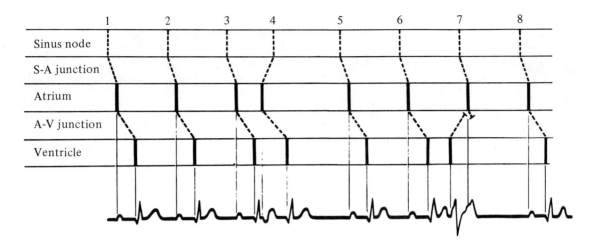

Figure 32-17. Ladder diagram demonstrating the normal sequence of atrial and ventricular activation and that associated with atrial (No. 4) and ventricular (No. 7) premature beats. (From G. H. Whipple et al. Acute Coronary Care. *Boston: Little, Brown, 1972. Reproduced by permission.)*

traction. Understanding disturbances of impulse propagation is aided by the use of ladder diagrams depicting the various phases of AV conduction (Fig. 32-17).

Atrioventricular Node. The AV node lies in the interatrial septum abutting the mitral anulus, just above the septal leaflet of the tricuspid valve. From its superior margin it extends downward and anteriorly, penetrating the central fibrous body where it gives rise to the His bundle. Conduction through the AV node is slow, 0.02 to 0.05 meter per second, and accounts for the major portion of the PR interval that demarcates atrial from ventricular depolarization. The functional refractory period of the AV node (normally 300 to 350 milliseconds) defines its properties as an output filter and prescribes a maximal ventricular rate response to atrial tachyarrhythmias. The effective refractory period of the AV node (250 to 300 milliseconds) defines its properties as an input filter. Measurement of AV nodal refractoriness provides a sensitive tool for assessing the influence of spontaneous and drug-induced changes in autonomic tone on AV nodal function. The AV node, like the SA node, is amply influenced by both cholinergic and adrenergic stimuli.

His Bundle. The bundle of His courses under the membranous interventricular septum running anteriorly and inferiorly from the lower pole of the AV node. Its proximal portion lies close to the mitral and tricuspid valve rings. Calcification and fibrosis of the central fibrous body, the mitral or the tricuspid valve rings, can disrupt AV conduction in this region. Heart block attributable to lesions in this area typically shows a narrow QRS complex.

The distal (branching) segment of the His bundle begins at a point where the posterior fascicle of the left bundle branch begins to separate from the common bundle and ends at a point where the anterior fascicle of the left bundle branch separates from the right bundle branch. This distal segment lies close to the aortic valve. Calcification or fibrosis of the aortic valve ring and injury to the summit of the muscular interventricular septum can disrupt AV conduction in this region. Heart block attributable to lesions in this area usually manifests some widening of the QRS complex.

Left Bundle Branch. The left bundle branch (LBB) emanates from the distal His bundle in a region of high pressures and turbulent blood flow. The LBB can be scarred and develop a conduction block by one of several processes: (1) invasion of a calcific process extending from the aortic valve; (2) fibrosis of the summit of the muscular interventricular septum, which occurs with aging or in coronary heart disease; (3) sclerosis of the membranous interventricular septum with aging.

Left Posterior Fascicle. The left posterior fascicle separates from the proximal LBB and turns posteriorly to reach the base of the posterior papillary muscle. It spans the inflow tract of the left ventricle, a region of low hemodynamic turbulence. The left posterior fascicle is injured when myocardial ischemia affects this area, but it tends to be protected by a dual blood supply from the right and circumflex coronary arteries.

Left Anterior Fascicle. The left anterior fascicle continues as an extension of the LBB and lies adjacent to the right bundle branch in the membranous and uppermost margin of muscular interventricular septum. Longer and thinner than the left posterior fascicle, the left anterior fascicle sweeps obliquely across the outflow tract of the left ventricle, negotiating a region of high hemodynamic turbulence. Either trauma or ischemia of the anterior left ventricular wall can cause injury to the left anterior fascicle.

Right Bundle Branch. The right bundle branch (RBB) extends from the membranous interventricular septum to the base of the anterior papillary muscle of the right ventricle, a distance of about 45 to 50 mm. Three segments of the RBB — parts I, II, and III — can be defined in relation to their surrounding anatomy and involvement in specific disease processes. Part I of the RBB runs along the left anterior fascicle in the membranous interventricular septum in proximity to the mitral and tricuspid valve rings and the summit of the muscular interventricular septum. Sclerodegenerative diseases of aging impair part I RBB conduction and may simultaneously involve conduction in the left anterior fascicle. Part II of the RBB courses within the muscular interventricular septum and is prone to ischemic injury, since its blood supply comes from the anterior descending coronary artery, a vessel frequently compromised by atherosclerosis. When ischemic injury to the interventricular septum is widespread, part II RBB conduction may be simultaneously compromised with that of the left anterior fascicle. Part III of the RBB crosses from the septum to the right ventricular free wall. Dilatation of the right ventricle can therefore stretch part III of the RBB, resulting in impaired conduction.

Purkinje Network. The ventricular conducting system is multifascicular, with a common RBB and at least two divisions of the LBB — the left anterior and left posterior fascicles. The RBB ramifies into a single extensive Purkinje fiber network. The LBB through its left anterior and left posterior fascicular divisions ramifies into two distinct Purkinje networks. Interconnections exist between the left anterior and left posterior fascicular Purkinje systems, assuring a rapid spread of excitation (3 meters per second) throughout the myocardium. The normal process of left to right interventricular septal activation may be attributable to the left posterior fascicle, which separates from the common AV bundle more proximally than either the left anterior fascicle or the RBB.

Conduction Disturbances

Impulse propagation can be disrupted at any point within the cardiac conducting system, from the SA node to the Purkinje system. When conduction is delayed or terminated at a specific point, conduction block is present. When block is abrupt and occurs over one cardiac cycle, it is termed type II block or a Mobitz pattern of conduction. When block emerges gradually over several cardiac cycles, it is termed a Mobitz type I block or Wenckebach pattern of conduction.

Sinoatrial Block. Spread of excitation from the SA node into the atria is not recorded on the ECG. However, a delay or failure of SA conduction can be deduced from certain time relationships in the P waves. Partial SA block exists when (1) the P wave rate abruptly doubles or halves, indicating 2:1 exit block from the pacemaker, or (2) the P wave rate progressively shortens, culminating in a long P-to-P interval. Sinoatrial block may be due to either myocarditis or ischemic injury in the perinodal area. It may also represent a toxic effect of digitalis.

Atrioventricular Block. Block within the AV node can be induced by a host of factors that increase its refractoriness: rapid atrial rates, premature atrial beats, and enhanced cholinergic tone induced either by ischemia or by drugs such as digitalis. Minimal degrees of AV block enhance the conduction delay that exists normally in the AV node. The PR interval then lengthens beyond 0.20 second, but a 1:1 relationship between P waves and QRS complexes still persists; first-degree heart block is then said to be present. With further increases in AV nodal refractoriness, second-degree AV block emerges; the P waves are not invariably followed by QRS complexes. A fixed ratio pertains between P wave rate and QRS wave rate, such as 2:1, 3:2, 4:1.

Second-degree AV block may become manifest as a type I Wenckebach block and may be due to digitalis intoxication. The PR interval gradually lengthens over a series of beats, while the increment in PR interval between successive beats becomes progressively smaller. As a result, the ventricular rate accelerates until a pause in the QRS cycle ensues (Fig. 32-18). The pause connotes a total block within the AV node, leading to a dropped ventricular beat. Certain other features aid in recognizing type I AV block: The pause interval is less than any two consecutive R-to-R cycles leading up to the pause, and the R-to-R cycle

after the pause is invariably longer than the R-to-R cycle before the pause.

Further increments in AV nodal refractoriness may result in third-degree AV block. Atrial and ventricular excitation are then totally separated by the barrier at the AV node. The P-wave rate is faster than and independent of QRS wave rate. P waves can be observed to migrate through the QRS complex when long rhythm strips are taken (Fig. 32-19).

In acute inferior wall myocardial infarction, AV block in its various guises may progress and regress over several days. Ischemia induces AV nodal edema and triggers cholinergic reflexes, further delaying AV conduction. When third-degree AV block evolves, the QRS complex is usually normal in contour and width, indicating that the ventricular pacemaker resides just beyond the AV node in the penetrating portion of the bundle of His.

Left Bundle Branch Block. In left bundle branch block (LBBB), the QRS interval is prolonged to 0.12 second or more. Conduction is delayed during early as well as late QRS vectors. Initial QRS forces are always changed in direction, pointing more leftward and posteriorly than normal. As a result, the usual q waves in leads I and V_6 narrow to 0.01 second or disappear entirely. Also, initial r waves in leads V_1 through V_3 become shorter and smaller. They may

Figure 32-18. Wenckebach or type I second-degree atrioventricular block.

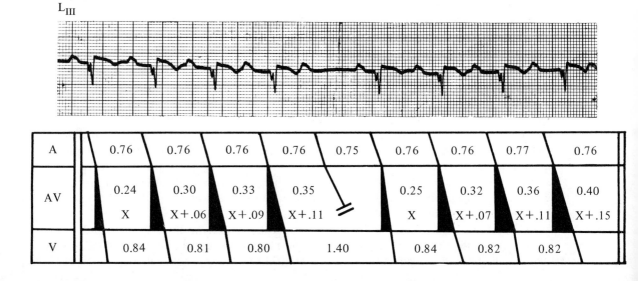

L_{III}

A	0.76	0.76	0.76	0.76	0.75	0.76	0.76	0.77	0.76
AV	0.24	0.30	0.33	0.35		0.25	0.32	0.36	0.40
	X	X+.06	X+.09	X+.11		X	X+.07	X+.11	X+.15
V	0.84	0.81	0.80	1.40		0.84	0.82	0.82	

II

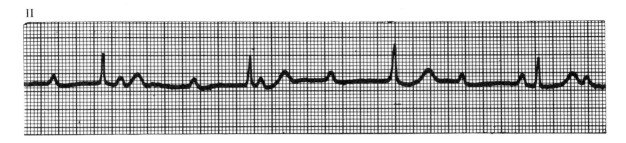

Figure 32-19. Complete heart block with an atrial rate of 85 and a ventricular rate of 38 beats per minute. The narrow QRS complex indicates the ventricular pacemaker is located in the region of the atrioventricular node and His bundle.

disappear entirely in V_1 and V_2, simulating myocardial infarction. Right precordial leads show an r, slurred S, or slurred QS pattern. Left precordial leads (V_5 and V_6) have a broad upright slurred or notched R wave (Fig. 32-20). ST-T vectors in LBBB point away from the main QRS forces; hence ST-T waves point opposite to the QRS complex in most leads.

Left bundle branch block usually connotes disease involving the LBB or its two major divisions, the left anterior fascicle and the left posterior fascicle. Discrete lesions of fibrosis or calcification can impinge upon the main LBB. Processes involving the two fascicles are more diffuse, reflecting coronary heart disease, myocarditis, or myocardiopathy.

Occasionally LBBB varies intermittently with either slow or fast heart rates as refractoriness is momentarily altered in some portion of the left conducting system. Incomplete versions of LBBB can arise from left ventricular hypertrophy. In incomplete versions the QRS is prolonged to 0.10 to 0.11 second and narrow q waves are present in leads I and V_6.

Right Bundle Branch Block. In right bundle branch block (RBBB) the QRS is also prolonged to 0.12 second or more. Contrary to LBBB, however, initial QRS vectors are not altered in direction. The q waves persist in leads I and V_6. Late QRS vectors are shifted

Figure 32-20. Left bundle branch block.

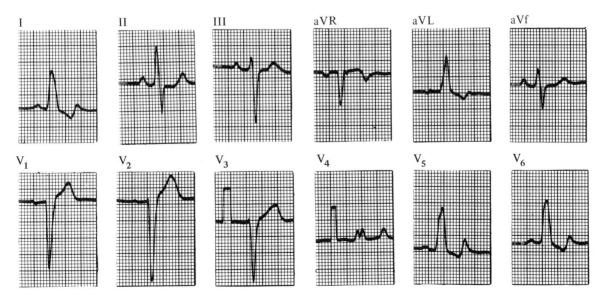

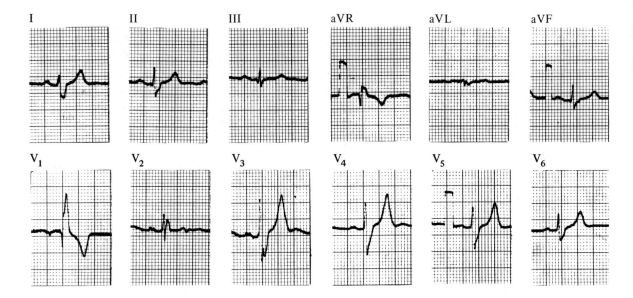

I	II	III	aVR	aVL	aVF

V_1	V_2	V_3	V_4	V_5	V_6

Figure 32-21. Right bundle branch block.

rightward and anteriorly and inscribed more slowly, however; hence a large and often slurred R' wave appears in lead V_1 with a broad S wave in leads I, V_5, and V_6 (Fig. 32-21).

Incomplete RBBB with a QRS of 0.10 to 0.11 second and a terminal R' wave in lead V_1 often accompanies right ventricular hypertrophy. Volume overloads of the right ventricle, such as occur in atrial septal defect, are associated with this pattern.

Complete RBBB usually results from ischemic or degenerative disease. When disease in the interventricular septum is either extensive or critically located, the left anterior fascicle may become involved along with the RBB, resulting in left anterior hemiblock together with RBBB.

Left Anterior Hemiblock. Selective conduction delay in the left anterior fascicle changes the sequence of left ventricular depolarization. Initial QRS vectors are directed rightward and inferiorly through the unblocked posterior fascicle. Terminal QRS vectors are shifted leftward and superiorly and are slightly delayed. Consequently in left anterior hemiblock the

QRS may be prolonged to 0.09 to 0.10 second. A qR pattern is present in leads I and aVL but with q waves 0.02 second or less in duration. S waves deepen or appear in leads II, III, aVF, V_5, and V_6. The altered sequence of depolarization diverts the mean QRS vector leftward and superiorly to −45 degrees or greater in the frontal plane, reflecting extreme left axis deviation.

Left Posterior Hemiblock. Selective conduction delay in the left posterior fascicle also changes the sequence of left ventricular depolarization. Initial QRS vectors are directed leftward and superiorly through the unblocked left anterior fascicle. Terminal QRS forces point rightward and inferiorly as conduction is delayed through the left posterior fascicle. Consequently the QRS is prolonged to 0.09 to 0.10 second. The mean frontal QRS axis is deviated to the right of +110 degrees, S waves deepen or appear in leads I and aVL, and q waves of 0.02 second or less appear in lead III.

Bifascicular Block. Bifascicular block has several forms, each of which indicates conduction delay in two of the three main ventricular conducting fascicles:

1. Right bundle branch block and left anterior hemiblock

2. Right bundle branch block and left posterior hemiblock
3. Right bundle branch block and first-degree AV block, where the prolonged PR interval reflects conduction delay in the left bundle.
4. Left bundle branch block comprised of left anterior hemiblock and left posterior hemiblock

Trifascicular Block. Trifascicular block indicates conduction delay in all three of the major conducting fascicles. Like bifascicular block, trifascicular block has several guises:

1. Right bundle branch block, left anterior hemiblock, and first-degree AV block, where the prolonged PR interval reflects additional partial left posterior hemiblock

2. Right bundle branch block, left posterior hemiblock, and first-degree AV block, where the prolonged PR interval reflects additional partial left anterior hemiblock
3. Alternating LBBB and RBBB

A major complication of trifascicular block and a possible complication of bifascicular block is the development of sudden type II (Mobitz) heart block. Because all three ventricular fascicles are blocked, residual pacemakers are lodged distally in ventricular Purkinje fibers. The natural frequency of such pacemakers is 10 to 30 discharges per minute or less, resulting in extreme bradycardia or cardiac arrest (Fig. 32-22).

Myocardial Hypertrophy
Hypertrophy of the heart muscle does not alter the electrical activity of a unit of myocardium, but hypertrophy may alter the sequence of depolarization and repolarization in various cardiac regions and can modify the relation between various cardiac chambers

Figure 32-22. Complete heart block with a ventricular rate of 20 beats per minute. The wide QRS complexes indicate that the ventricular pacemaker is located in the ventricles.

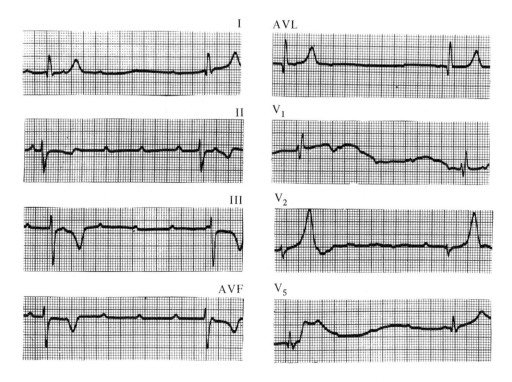

and recording electrodes. Consequently certain ECG features can be correlated with a preponderance of either left or right ventricular muscle.

Left Ventricular Hypertrophy. Left ventricular hypertrophy (LVH) can cause changes in depolarization forces (vectors) and in repolarization vectors (Fig. 32-23). Alterations in initial QRS vectors depend on the type of hemodynamic stress imposed on the left ventricle. With pressure overload (aortic stenosis, hypertension), initial QRS vectors are shifted inferiorly, foreshortening the q wave in lead I and the r wave in lead V_1. With volume overload of the left ventricle (aortic insufficiency), initial QRS vectors are increased in magnitude but are relatively unchanged in direction. Normal q waves in leads I, V_5, and V_6 become more prominent. In asymmetric septal hypertrophy (obstructive cardiomyopathy), initial QRS vectors can be increased in both magnitude and duration. Q waves resembling those in myocardial infarction may be recorded from leads reflecting regions of disproportionate hypertrophy. As LVH becomes more prominent, midterminal QRS forces shift leftward and posteriorly, pointing toward the left ventricle, which lies leftward and posterior to the right ventricle. R waves become more prominent in leads V_4 through V_6, and S waves become more prominent in leads V_1 and V_2.

Repolarization changes associated with LVH also depend on hemodynamic loading conditions. When volume overload of the left ventricle accompanies LVH, T waves in leads V_5 and V_6 become taller. In a hypertrophied left ventricle working against a pressure overload, ST-T vectors rotate away from the mean QRS vector. In leads V_5 and V_6, tall R waves of LVH plus ST-T waves that are inverted and displaced downward constitute a pattern of left ventricular strain. Strain does not imply a struggling heart; rather, the left ventricle is in an advanced state of hypertrophy.

Electrocardiographic and pathologic correlations have demonstrated that no one criterion provides a reliable marker for LVH; hence, scoring systems for LVH involve multiple items that are weighted for maximum specificity and sensitivity. The most commonly used criteria are:

I. Amplitude criteria (value of one or more items = 3 points)
    A. Largest R or S wave in a limb lead = 20 mm

Figure 32-23. Left ventricular hypertrophy with classic strain pattern.

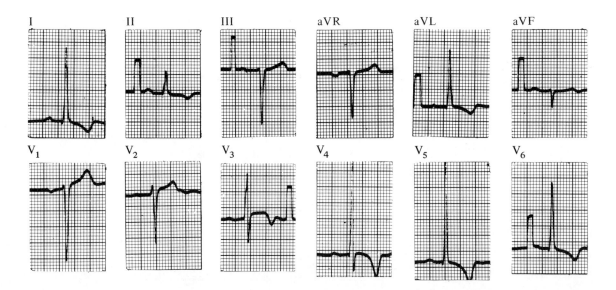

B. Largest S wave in V_1 through V_3 = 25 mm

C. Largest R wave in V_4 through V_6 = 25 mm

II. ST segment criteria (value = 1 or 3 points)

   A. Downsloping ST-T wave opposite the QRS in V_5 and V_6

      1. Left ventricular strain pattern with digitalis therapy — 1 point

      2. Left ventricular strain pattern without digitalis therapy — 3 points

III. Axis criteria (value = 2 points)

   A. Left axis deviation of −15 degrees

IV. Duration criteria (value = 1 point)

   A. QRS duration of 0.09 second

   B. Intrinsicoid deflection in V_5 through V_6 of 0.04 second

Maximum possible LVH score is 9 points; 5 or more points indicate LVH. Four points is interpreted as probable LVH.

Left Atrial Hypertrophy (LAH). Hypertrophy of the left atrium can accompany hypertrophy of the left ventricle in hypertensive, coronary, and myopathic heart disease and in mitral regurgitation. In mitral stenosis, LAH alone develops; therefore the pattern is often called P mitrale. In LAH broad and often notched P waves are present in the limb and left precordial leads. Usually lead II best shows the prolonged P waves (> 0.12 second). Left atrial components of the P wave are evident in right precordial leads. The P wave in lead V_1 becomes biphasic, upright-inverted, or entirely inverted. Duration times depth (area) of the late inverted P-wave vectors of > 0.03 mm-second reflects the posterior location of the hypertrophied left atrium.

Right Ventricular Hypertrophy (RVH). The greater muscle mass of the left ventricle usually obscures activation of the right ventricular muscle mass. In RVH, depolarization of the right ventricle becomes manifest, however (Fig. 32-24). With pressure overloading of the right ventricle (pulmonic or infundibular stenosis, pulmonary hypertension), midterminal QRS vectors are shifted toward the right ventricle rightward and anteriorly. As a result, lead I becomes more negative than positive and the S wave may exceed the R wave in amplitude. The mean frontal QRS axis is deviated rightward beyond +110 degrees. When RVH is severe, even early QRS vectors can shift in direction, reflecting right septal preponderance. Q waves deepen or appear in lead III. A qR pattern emerges in lead V_1. Discordant ST-T vectors, opposite in direction from major QRS deflections, also characterize severe RVH or right ventricular strain.

Figure 32-24. Right ventricular hypertrophy.

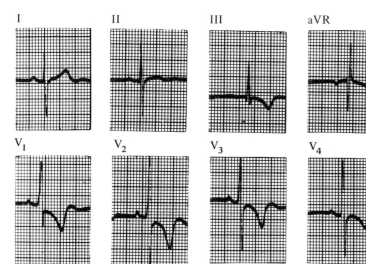

Volume overloading of the right ventricle is often accompanied by incomplete or complete RBBB. Terminal QRS vectors rotate rightward and anteriorly, deepening the S wave in leads I and V_6 and producing a terminal R$'$ deflection in leads V_1 and V_2. An R or R$'$ wave in V_1 of > 7 to 10 mm with an R/S ratio of > 1.0 and a QRS duration of < 0.12 second implies the presence of RVH. When the QRS is > 0.12, vectorcardiographic analysis may be required to diagnose RVH, even if the R$'$ wave is > 15 mm.

A third form of RVH is marked by the S_1, S_2, S_3 syndrome. Terminal QRS vectors point rightward, superiorly, and slightly anterior. Deep S waves appear in the standard leads I, II, and III; and a phasic QRS is present in the limb leads and lateral precordial leads. A small r$'$ wave appears in lead V_1. The S_1, S_2, S_3 syndrome may represent predominant hypertrophy or delayed conduction in the right ventricular outflow tract, the crista supraventricularis. It may occur in congenital heart disease (tetralogy of Fallot) or cor pulmonale; most commonly, however, it appears in young adults with no detectable heart disease.

Right Atrial Hypertrophy. Prominent P waves can be seen in right atrial hypertrophy (RAH). They are increased in amplitude (> 2.5 mm in lead II) but not increased in width (< 0.12 second). The term *P pulmonale* is used to describe this P-wave pattern because it is frequently observed with RVH in cor pulmonale associated with either chronic lung disease or congenital heart disease, such as right ventricular outflow tract obstruction and tricuspid stenosis. An unusual form of P pulmonale may be present in Ebstein's disease, in which there is downward displacement of the tricuspid valve into the right ventricle. P waves of increased duration and height are accompanied by a long PR interval in about 20 to 25 percent of cases. Left ventricular disease with abrupt development and subsidence of pulmonary edema can result in transient P pulmonale.

Myocardial Infarction (see Chap. 28)
Deprivation of blood flow to any part of the myocardium causes local changes in depolarization and repolarization and creates imbalances in the sequences by which depolarization and repolarization

sweep through ventricular muscle. A reflection of these events is readily discernible from the QRST configuration in one or more ECG leads.

T-Wave Abnormalities. The inner shell of myocardium (subendocardial layer) is in greatest jeopardy from ischemia because it is farthest removed from the compromised coronary blood vessels that lie on the outer surface of the heart. When localized myocardial ischemia is mild to moderate, the mean T-wave vector shifts away from the area of limited perfusion and the ECG leads corresponding to this region show inverted T waves. Intensification of the myocardial ischemia causes the T-wave vector to point toward the area of limited perfusion, and ECG leads corresponding to this region then manifest peaked T waves.

ST Abnormalities. ST segments may be similarly depressed or elevated in myocardial infarction, depending on the severity and extensiveness of the ischemic process. When blood flow is reduced in the inner shell of myocardium (subendocardium), ST segments become depressed, whereas when blood flow is reduced across the full thickness of myocardium (transmural), ST segments become elevated.

Q Wave Abnormalities. Q wave abnormalities appear during the later phases of myocardial infarction. They represent electrical death of cells across a variable width of regional myocardium, spreading outward from the subendocardial layer. Electrical silence in this area produces alterations in initial QRS forces. Early QRS vectors (during the first 0.04 second) tend to *point away* from the dead zone and toward the areas of still viable muscle.

Another type of QRS abnormality occurs in myocardial infarction. Late QRS forces may *point toward* the area of infarction and more or less opposite the initial QRS forces. Originally this was ascribed to impedance of the normal radial activation of the outer layers of heart muscle. Excitation of this region would therefore follow a more circuitous pathway, would be delayed, and would become manifest late in the QRS interval. It now appears more likely that such late QRS changes are related to conduction delays (blocks) within the two major subdivisions of the LBB, the left anterior and left posterior fascicles. The criteria for left anterior and posterior hemiblock were given earlier in this chapter, under Conduction Disturbances.

Topography. The regional character of myocardial infarction is best discerned from multiple ECGs taken over several days. Any selective region of myocardium can be involved with intramural, subendocardial, or transmural penetration. Typical examples of inferior and anterior transmural infarctions are shown in Figures 32-25 and 32-26.

Pericarditis

Inflammation or injury affecting the pericardium invariably involves the subjacent subepicardial myocardium. The ECG feature of this myocardial irritation is ST-segment elevation. Three attributes serve to distinguish the ST elevation of pericarditis from that of myocardial infarction (Fig. 32-27):

1. In pericarditis, the ST segment is displaced upward with a concave contour, whereas the ST segment in myocardial infarction exhibits a convex contour.
2. In pericarditis, ST segments are generally displaced upward in all leads except aVR, whereas the ST segment elevation in myocardial infarction is usually confined to leads reflecting but one region of the left ventricular muscle, that is, the anterior, posterior, inferior, or lateral region.
3. In pericarditis, T-wave inversions eventually occur, but not until the ST segments have returned to or near the baseline. Moreover, T-wave inversions are not usually so great in amplitude as those seen in myocardial infarction. In myocardial infarction, T-wave inversions appear before the ST segments have returned to the baseline.

Figure 32-25. Evolution of an acute inferior wall myocardial infarction. Day 1: hyperacute ST segment elevation and peaked T waves. Day 2: the ST segment is returning toward the baseline, the T waves are beginning to invert, and prominent Q waves are present. Day 3: symmetrically inverted T waves have occurred. The ST segments remain slightly elevated.

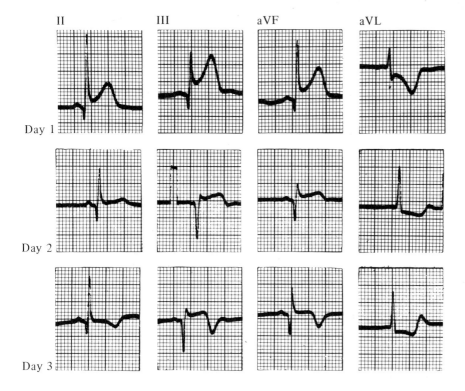

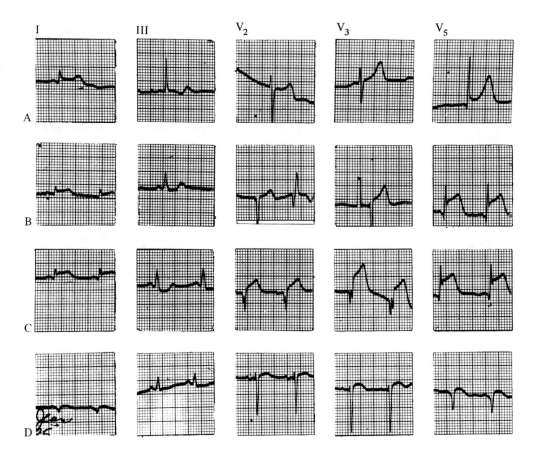

Figure 32-26. Evolution of an acute anterolateral myocardial infarction. A. ST segment elevation is present in leads I and V_5. B. ST segment elevation has increased and extends to leads V_2 and V_3. There is a premature ventricular beat in V_2. Prominent Q waves have developed in leads V_2 to V_5. C. A further increase in ST segment elevation and deepening of the abnormal Q waves is seen. D. A QS pattern is present in leads I and V_5. ST segments remain elevated in V_2 to V_5, and this finding is compatible with a ventricular aneurysm.

Exercise Electrocardiography

The use of exercise testing greatly enhances the value of the ECG as a tool for identifying and treating coronary heart disease. Abnormal tracings obtained during physical exertion may expose coronary artery disease, even when the resting ECG is normal. A markedly abnormal stress ECG may divulge a critical degree of atherosclerotic narrowing proximally in a major coronary vessel. Ventricular arrhythmias appearing or intensifying during stress testing suggest that multiple vessels are compromised in coronary patients.

Most exercise procedures are devised to impose a relatively standardized challenge to the coronary circulation. The balance between coronary blood flow and cardiac oxygen utilization (oxygen supply and demand) may be assessed by increasing the degrees of physical stress. Heart rate, which is closely related to myocardial oxygen consumption, is monitored continuously during the exercise. Comparison is made between the maximum attained heart rate and the maximum attainable heart rate, for which age is a primary determinant. Standardized tables and nomograms provide a handy reference guide for evaluating the attained versus the predicted maximal heart rate response and therefore the severity of the stress achieved.

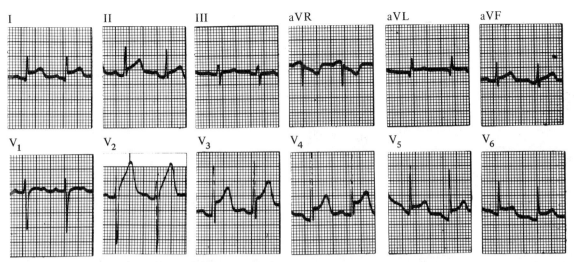

Figure 32-27. Acute pericarditis. Concave upward ST segment elevation is present in most leads of the ECG compatible with a diffuse process.

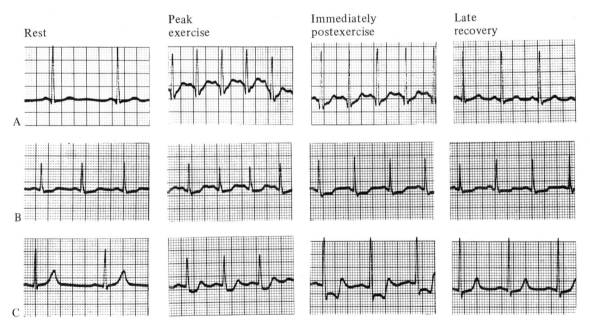

Figure 32-28. Exercise stress test. A. Normal electrocardiographic response to exercise. B. Minimally positive study for myocardial ischemia with 1-mm ST-segment depression at peak exercise and in the recovery period. C. Strikingly positive study for myocardial ischemia with 3-mm ST-segment depression in the immediate postexercise tracing.

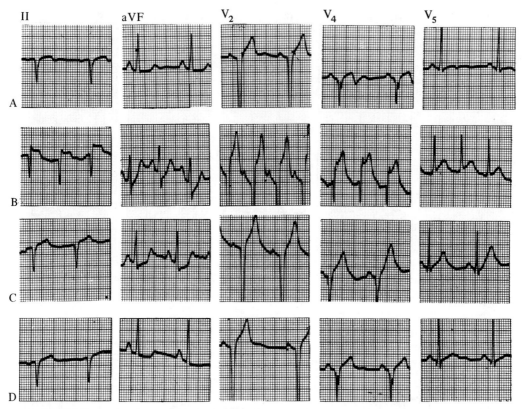

| II | aVF | V_2 | V_4 | V_5 |

Figure 32-29. Exercise test in a patient with an anterior wall aneurysm. A. Resting ECG. B. Peak exercise results in dramatic ST segment elevation in leads V_2 to V_5. C, D. Progressive return of the ST segment and T waves toward the baseline resting tracing. C was obtained 2 minutes into the recovery period and D was obtained 10 minutes into the recovery period.

Several modes of exercise testing are commonly employed. The most popular techniques involve bicycle and treadmill exercisers in which the resistance to pedaling or the work (inclination and speed) of walking is augmented at designated intervals. Sequential ECG tracings are taken at various stages during and subsequent to exertion and compared to the preexercise tracing. By choosing the appropriate ECG machine and electrode system, either a full 12-lead ECG or selected inferior and anterior leads (II, V_5) are used to detect myocardial ischemia.

The criteria by which exercise tests are judged vary among different exercise laboratories, but no single criterion has absolute specificity or sensitivity for detecting myocardial ischemia. Two items have received widespread acceptance, however, in terms of both epidemiologic follow-up of coronary events and angiographic correlation with severe obstructive coronary disease:

1. Flat or downsloping ST segment depression of 1 mm or more for at least 80 milliseconds following the J point (junction of the QRS-ST intervals)
2. A markedly depressed J point with the ST segment upsloping but remaining depressed 1.5 mm below the baseline 80 milliseconds after the J point

Patterns of normal, mildly abnormal, and markedly abnormal exercise tests are depicted in Figure 32-28. A rarer pattern of stress-related ST segment deviation, that of ST elevation, is encountered in ventricular aneurysm secondary to an old myocardial infarction (Fig. 32-29) or in localized ventricular contraction disorders associated with severe coronary stenosis (Fig. 32-30).

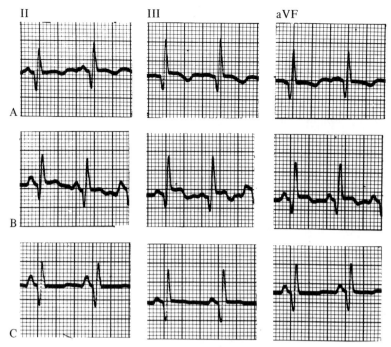

Figure 32-30. Exercise test in a patient with a prior inferior wall myocardial infarction resulted in further ST segment elevation during peak exercise (B) as compared to rest (A) and late recovery (C). This patient had inferior wall akinesis and a 95 percent occlusion of the right coronary artery demonstrated at cardiac catheterization.

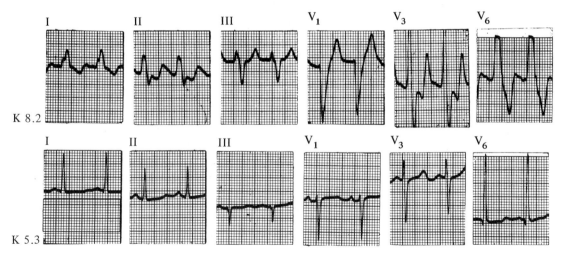

Figure 32-31. Hyperkalemia. The top tracing was obtained at a serum potassium (K) of 8.2 mEq per liter and demonstrated widened QRS, diminutive P waves, and peaked T waves. Following treatment the serum K was 5.3 mEq per liter, the QRS narrowed, P waves increased in prominence, and T waves flattened (bottom tracing).

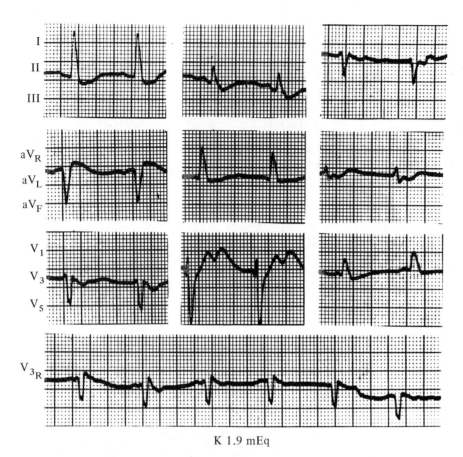

I

II

III

aV_R

aV_L

aV_F

V_1

V_3

V_5

V_{3R}

K 1.9 mEq

Figure 32-32. Hypokalemia. The ST segments are depressed and slurred with flattened T waves and prominent U waves best observed in V_3. The serum K was 1.9 mEq per liter.

Metabolic Abnormalities

Hyperkalemia. Typical ECG changes associated with hyperkalemic blood levels include the following (Fig. 32-31):

1. Tall, steep, narrow T waves (K^+ = 5.5 to 6.5 mEq per liter)
2. Diffusely widened QRS complexes (K^+ = 6.5 to 7.0 mEq per liter)
3. Prolonged PR interval (K^+ = 6.0 to 7.0 mEq per liter)
4. Flattened, prolonged P waves (K^+ = 7.0 to 8.0 mEq per liter)
5. Absent P waves (K^+ = 8.5 to 9.0 mEq per liter)

Disappearance of the P waves while QRS waves are still intact indicates that excitability of atrial muscle is abolished at a lower K^+ concentration than is excitability of ventricular muscle. Under such conditions, the cardiac pacemaker may persist in the SA node, but impulses spread directly to the AV node through internodal tracts without spilling out into atrial tissue. Alternatively the cardiac pacemaker may be displaced into the AV junction or ventricular Purkinje fibers.

Hypokalemia. The following changes occur in the ECG and are best visualized in leads II, V_2 to V_4 (Fig. 32-32):

1. Depression of ST segments by 0.5 mm or more with slow (lazy) ascent to the baseline
2. Flattening of the T waves
3. Increased amplitude of the U waves (> 0.5 mm in lead II, > 1 mm in lead V_3)

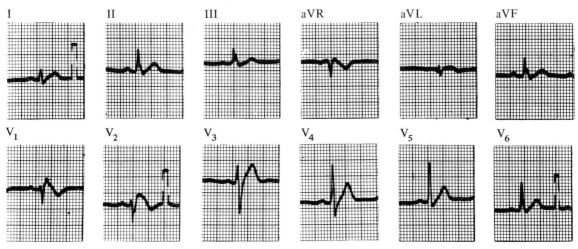

Figure 32-33. Hypercalcemia. With a serum calcium of 15 mg per 100 ml, the ST segment is markedly abbreviated with the T wave appearing to start directly from the QRS. The QRS is also widened.

These changes are usually discernible when serum K^+ is less than 3.2 mEq per liter. Since decreased extracellular potassium incites ectopic pacemakers, atrial and ventricular extrasystoles are common when serum K^+ is less than 3.0 mEq per liter. The conduction disorder of paroxysmal atrial tachycardia with block is associated with digitalis intoxication in the presence of hypokalemia.

Hypercalcemia. Hypercalcemia shortens the ST segment and consequently the QT interval. In patients with very severe hypercalcemia the QRS may widen, the PR interval may lengthen, and ventricular premature beats may occur (Fig. 32-33).

Hypocalcemia. When hypocalcemia is present, the QT interval lengthens; and with severe hypocalcemia T waves may flatten or invert, simulating myocardial ischemia or hypokalemia. The short, isoelectric ST segment then becomes a key differentiating feature of hypocalcemia.

Acidemia. Severe acidemia can seriously destabilize the heart with virulent tachyarrhythmias and bradyarrhythmias. Metabolic acidosis due, for example, to lactic acidemia with blood pH less than 7.20 evokes ventricular premature beats. The heart becomes susceptible to ventricular fibrillation that may be difficult or impossible to abolish when blood pH is less than 7.10 and advanced circulatory failure is present.

Metabolic acidemia can also result in bradyarrhythmias. Intracellular buffering of H^+ ion results in K^+ outflow from cells, so that acidemia is then accompanied by hyperkalemia. Hyperkalemia can sensitize cardiac pacemakers to cholinergic restraint, slowing the heart rate. Acidemia can also cause bradycardia by inactivating acetylcholinesterase, allowing acetylcholine to accumulate in the vicinity of pacemakers and slowing their firing rates (Fig. 32-34).

Alkalemia. Severe alkalemia also destabilizes the heart, although the concomitant presence of hypokalemia may cause additional cardiac rhythm disturbances. Alkalemia increases Purkinje automaticity and retards conduction at junctions between Purkinje and muscle fibers. Atrial and ventricular ectopic beats or tachycardias arise when blood pH is more than 7.50 to 7.55.

Electroversion

The technique of electroversion (cardioversion) is employed in abrogating tachyarrhythmias. Contemporary cardioverter machines use DC capacitor discharge of a few milliseconds' duration to depolarize the heart. Electric shocks are delivered transthoracically across the anteroposterior or anterolateral portions of the left chest. The electric discharge is triggered from the R wave of the ambient cardiac rhythm and thereby is as far removed in time as possible from

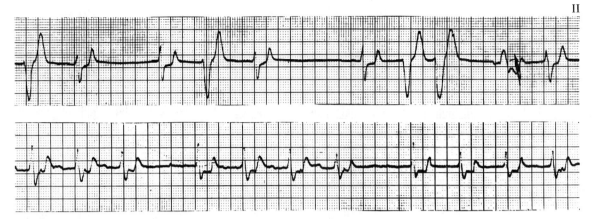

Figure 32-34. Acidosis. The top strip demonstrates sinus bradycardia and frequent premature ventricular beats. The T waves are peaked due to the hyperkalemia that accompanied the acidosis. The bottom strip was obtained following rapid correction of the acidosis with bicarbonate, resulting in an increase in the sinus rate and reduction in ventricular ectopy.

the vulnerable zone near the apex of the T wave; hence the electric shock does not incite ventricular fibrillation.

Prior to cardioversion, a full 12-lead ECG is obtained and carefully appraised for cardiac rhythm and possible drug intoxication. The patient is then anesthetized with intravenous diazepam or thiopental (Pentothal). In delivering the electric shocks, a process of energy titration is employed. Initial capacitor discharges of 1 to 50 joules (watt-seconds) are applied. If normal sinus rhythm is not restored, higher energies up to 400 joules are used in progressive increments. The magnitude of the electric shock required for successful electroversion depends on multiple factors, foremost of which are the chest thickness, type of tachyarrhythmias, and duration of tachyarrhythmia.

Electroversion is often successful in resolving atrial fibrillation when prior medical therapy with digitalis and quinidine or procainamide has failed. The risk of postreversion systemic embolism is no greater than with medical therapy alone (about 1 percent). In patients with mitral stenosis, however, cardioversion carries a higher risk of embolism (3 to 5 percent). Therefore, patients with mitral stenosis and atrial

fibrillation should have anticoagulant therapy for 2 to 3 weeks prior to and subsequent to attempted electroversion. A similar anticoagulant program should be followed for patients with atrial fibrillation of undetermined cause and prior history of embolism.

Atrial flutter is readily reversible with cardioversion shocks of 1 to 25 joules. Supraventricular tachycardias ordinarily require shocks of 50 to 400 joules for successful termination.

Ventricular tachycardia may be interrupted with very low energy shocks of 1 to 10 joules. Supraventricular tachycardias ordinarily require shocks of 50 to 400 joules for successful termination. The very low energy shocks of 1 to 10 joules needed to interrupt ventricular tachycardia represent a range equivalent to mechanical blows to the chest, which are also known to dispel ventricular tachycardia. Safe, low-energy cardioversion of ventricular tachycardia requires that the physician's eye and the cardioverter machine can clearly distinguish QRS from T waves. At ventricular tachycardia rates of 180 or less, this should be feasible. At higher rates, QRS-T complexes take on patterns similar to sine waves, and this may make it impossible to identify the apex of the T wave. In this situation even low-energy capacitor discharges may trigger the vulnerable period and precipitate ventricular fibrillation. In cardioverting fast ventricular tachycardia, therefore, shocks of 100 joules or more should be employed because such higher energy discharges will not induce ventricular fibrillation.

Sinus rhythm may be restored immediately following the electric shock. Sometimes, however, a warm-

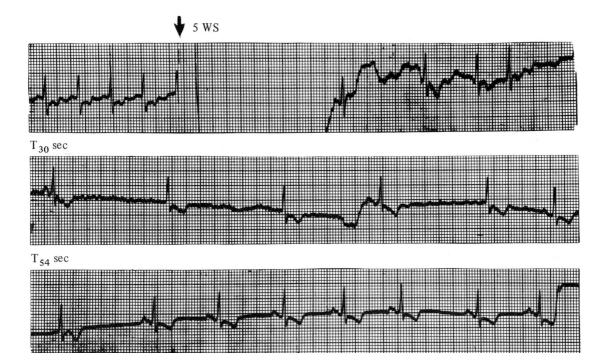

↓ 5 WS

T₃₀ sec

T₅₄ sec

Figure 32-35. Cardioversion. Atrial tachycardia was
converted to sinus rhythm with a 5-joule (watt-second)
discharge. Following the electrical discharge there
was a period of marked bradycardia before sinus
rhythm was established.

up period of minutes or hours ensues before sinus
rhythm is reestablished; in the warm-up interim,
atrial ectopic or junctional bradycardia prevails (Fig.
32-35).

The emergence of ventricular ectopic beats during
cardioversion strongly suggests the possibility of
digitalis intoxication. Digitalis and electricity have
additive effects on the heart in terms of cardiac irritability. The use of energy titration as a safeguard
against shock-induced ventricular fibrillation when
covert digitalis intoxication is present has not been
fully appreciated. Lower energy discharges provoke
ventricular premature beats and short volleys of ventricular tachycardia that are reversible with intravenous lidocaine, 50 to 100 mg. Attempts to use
higher energy shocks in a vain effort to restore SA
rhythm can only result in catastrophe and irreversible
ventricular fibrillation.

Spontaneously occurring ventricular fibrillation
demands prompt countershock therapy. For defibrillation, the machine is turned up to its highest discharge capacity of 400 joules, and repeated shocks
may be required when circulatory collapse has lasted
for a few minutes. Interim measures such as cardiopulmonary resuscitation; intravenous sodium bicarbonate, 44 mEq every 5 minutes; intravenous catecholamine or calcium infusion; and endotracheal
intubation may permit improvement of heart failure,
acidemia, and hypoxemia so as to permit successful
defibrillation.

Elective cardioversion is not likely to be successful
in certain situations. A careful appraisal of the cause
or causes of supraventricular tachyarrhythmias should
suggest the reasons: severe congestive heart failure
with pulmonary edema, pericardial inflammations,
and immediate postoperative states of heightened
adrenergic discharge. All of these may perpetuate
atrial tachyarrhythmia. Cardioversion can then, at
best, achieve only momentary restoration of sinus
rhythm. Under these conditions, antiarrhythmic
therapy with digitalis and other agents may help

stabilize the heart. Reversion to normal sinus rhythm may then ultimately occur or be possible with cardioversion.

Bibliography

Bellet, S. *Clinical Disorders of the Heartbeat* (3rd ed.). Philadelphia: Lea & Febiger, 1973.

Constant, J. *Learning Electrocardiography.* Boston: Little, Brown, 1973.

Grant, R. P. *Clinical Electrocardiography: The Spatial Vector Approach.* New York: McGraw-Hill, 1957.

Katz, L. N., and Pick, A. *Clinical Electrocardiography: The Arrhythmias.* Philadelphia: Lea & Febiger, 1956.

Lipman, B. S., Massie, E., and Kleiger, R. E. *Clinical Scalar Electrocardiography* (6th ed.). Chicago: Year Book, 1972.

Marriott, H. J. L. *Practical Electrocardiography* (5th ed.). Baltimore: Williams & Wilkins, 1973.

Narula, O. S. *His Bundle Electrocardiography and Clinical Electrophysiology.* Philadelphia: Davis, 1975.

Rosenbaum, M. B., Elizari, M. V., and Lazzari, J. *The Hemiblocks.* Oldsmar, Fla.: Tampa Tracings, 1970.

Samet, P. *Cardiac Pacing.* New York: Grune & Stratton, 1973.

Scherf, D., and Schott, A. *Extrasystoles and Allied Arrhythmias* (2nd ed.). Chicago: Year Book, 1973.

33

Diseases of the Pericardium, Myocardium, and Endocardium

David C. Hueter

From a tissue viewpoint the heart is basically muscle lined by endothelium and surrounded by a serous tissue sac. As such, these tissue components are susceptible to involvement in multisystem disorders of virtually every variety, and the number of underlying causes is nearly as great as the number of systemic diseases. Tables 33-1 and 33-2 outline the major disorders that affect the heart and also indicate how each may involve the pericardium, the myocardium, and the endocardium, separately or in any combination. Obviously a presentation of each of these disorders is beyond the scope of this text, but acute rheumatic fever, which is described in this chapter, is an example of a specific systemic disease that may involve any or all of the tissue components of the heart. Involvement of the various tissue components of the heart, regardless of underlying etiology, is manifest in a relatively few general categories of cardiac dysfunction, and the focus of this chapter will be on the basic clinical and pathophysiologic syndromes produced by these disorders.

Pericardial Diseases

PERICARDIAL INFLAMMATION (PERICARDITIS)
Inflammation of the pericardium from any cause is signaled by a fairly characteristic pain syndrome. The pain is typically substernal or parasternal, occasionally subxiphoid or epigastric, and it may radiate into the neck, shoulder, or back, usually on the left side. Radiation down the arm and forearm is rare and should raise the question of an associated myocardial process. The pain is generally sharp and pleuritic, with intensification on deep inspiration or coughing. It is often worsened in the recumbent or lateral decubitus positions and improved in the upright position. Its intensity may vary from mild to severe, and it may wax and wane with time. Systemic symptoms frequently include fever, chills, sweats, and malaise.

On physical examination the hallmark of pericarditis is the pericardial friction rub, typically a superficial, coarse, scratchy, or grating sound heard along the left sternal border. The rub is frequently quite localized, is generally loudest in the third or fourth left intercostal spaces, and requires careful auscultation of the precordium to be heard best. Specific patient maneuvers may be necessary to hear the sound, such as held expiration, held full inspiration, leaning forward in the sitting position, or even assuming a hands-and-knees position. The typical pericardial friction rub has three distinct components corresponding to the timing of atrial systole, ventricular systole, and early ventricular filling. It is not uncommon to hear only one of these components, and a rub may be quite evanescent; it may appear, disappear, and reappear over a period of hours.

The ECG (see Chap. 32) in acute pericarditis characteristically demonstrates ST-segment elevations with preservation of normal upward concavity that evolve over a period of days; these are usually followed by T-wave inversions. As opposed to the epicardial injury current seen in myocardial infarction, reciprocal ST depressions are not seen (except in aVR, the intracavitary lead) and Q waves do not appear. Atrial ectopic rhythms (especially atrial fibrillation) are frequent. Laboratory findings reflect the acute inflammatory process (elevated sedimentation rate and leukocytosis) as well as manifestations of any associated disease. There are no specific chest x-ray or echocardiographic findings of pericardial inflammation, although these tests may be useful to detect an accompanying pericardial effusion (see below).

PERICARDIAL EFFUSION
Pericardial effusion means simply excessive fluid within the pericardial space. A small amount of fluid is normal within the pericardial sac to provide lubrication. This amount may increase in any disease in which a transudate, exudate, lymphatic fluid (chylopericardium), blood (hemopericardium), and even air (pneumopericardium) accumulates. Since the parietal pericardium is relatively inelastic, such an accumulation may result in an increase in intrapericardial pressure and thereby interfere with normal diastolic filling of the heart. This produces a specific

Table 33-1. Noninfective Cardiac Disorders: Classification and Sites of Involvement

Disorder	Site		Disorder	Site		Disorder	Site
Physical agents			**Inflammatory**			**Inborn errors of metabolism**	
Trauma	PME		Postinfective			Mucopolysaccharidoses	M
Heat stroke	M		Posttrauma	PME		Pompe's disease	M
Radiation	PM		Postpericardiotomy	P		Refsum's disease	M
Chemical toxins			Postinfarction	PM		Niemann-Pick disease	M
Heavy metals			**Connective tissue diseases**			Glycogen storage disease	M
Cobalt	M		SLE (Libman-Sacks)	PME		Hemochromatosis	M
Arsenic	M		Scleroderma	PM		**Neoplasm**	
Antimony	M		Polyarteritis nodosa	M		Primary	
Ethanol	M		Rheumatoid arthritis	PM		Myxoma	ME
Drugs			Acute rheumatic fever	PME		Sarcoma	M
Emetine	M		Dermatomyositis	M		Secondary	
Daunamycin	M		**Neuromuscular diseases**			Metastatic, e.g.,	
Anesthetic agents			Muscular dystrophy	M		Ca breast	PME
Halothane	M		Myotonic dystrophy	M		Ca lung	
Chloroform	M		Friedreich's ataxia	M		Leukemia	
Cyclopropane	M					Lymphoma	
Uremia	P					Local invasion	PME
Endocrine							
Thyrotoxicosis	PM						
Myxedema	PM						
Acromegaly	M						
Pheochromocytoma	M						
Carcinoid	E						
Degenerative							
Amyloidosis	M						
Calcification	PME						
Granulomatous							
Giant cell myocarditis	M						
Sarcoid	M						
Nutritional							
Beriberi (thiamine deficiency)	M						
Sensitivity							
Serum sickness	M						
Postvaccinal	M						
Dressler syndrome	P						
Pregnancy							
Peripartum cardiomyopathy	ME						

Note: P = pericardial involvement; M = myocardial involvement; E = endocardial involvement; SLE = systemic lupus erythematosus; Ca = cancer.

Table 33-2. Infective Cardiac Disorders: Classification and Sites of Involvement

Viral diseases		Mycotic diseases		Bacterial diseases		Spirochetal diseases	
Coxsackie	PME	Actinomycosis	PME	Brucellosis	PME	Leptospirosis	PME
Cytomegalovirus	M	Aspergillosis	PM	Diphtheria	M	Syphilis (tertiary)	ME
ECHO	PM	Blastomycosis	PM	Gonococcal	ME		
Herpes simplex	PM	Coccidioidomycosis	PM	Melioidosis	M	Helminthic diseases	
Herpes zoster	M	Cryptococcosis	M	Meningococcal	PM	Ascariasis	M
Infectious hepatitis	M	Histoplasmosis	PME	Pneumococcal	PME	Cysticercosis	M
Infectious mononucleosis	PM	Moniliasis	ME	Salmonella infection		Echinococcosis	PM
Influenza	M	Sporotrichosis	M	Typhoid fever	M	Filariasis	PME
Lymphocytic choriomeningitis	PM			Staphylococcal	PME	Heterophyiasis	ME
Mumps	PM	Protozoal diseases		Streptococcal	PME	Paragonimiasis	M
Poliomyelitis	M	Amebiasis	PM	Rheumatic fever	PME	Schistosomiasis	M
Primary atypical pneumonia	PM	Balantidiasis	M	Scarlet fever	M	Strongyloidiasis	M
Psitticosis	PM	Chagas disease	ME	Tuberculosis	PM	Trichinosis	M
Rabies	M	Leishmaniasis	M	Tularemia	PM	Visceral larva migrans	M
Rubella	PM	Malaria	M	Tetanus	M		
Rubeola	PM	Sarcosporidiosis	M				
Varicella	PM	Toxoplasmosis	PM	Rickettsial diseases			
Variola	M	Trypanosomiasis	M	Rocky Mountain	M		
Viral encephalitis	PM	(sleeping sickness)		spotted fever			
				Typhus	M		
				Q fever	PME		

*Note: P = paricardial involvement; M = myocardial involvement; E = endocardial involvement.

hemodynamic dysfunction known as cardiac tamponade. It is important to note that tamponade is a function of the intrapericardial pressure rather than the absolute volume of pericardial effusion. Thus a very large volume of effusion may accumulate gradually over a long period of time, allowing the parietal pericardium to stretch and accommodate the fluid without the development of cardiac tamponade. Conversely, a relatively small amount of fluid, if acquired rapidly, can raise intrapericardial pressure sufficiently to produce life-threatening tamponade. Therefore, clinical assessment of pericardial effusion and cardiac tamponade should be separated.

There are usually no subjective symptoms directly ascribable to pericardial effusion per se. Dyspnea may occur with a large effusion; the pathogenesis of the dyspnea is uncertain, but mechanical compression of the airways and diminished vital capacity have been suggested to play a role. Physical findings reflect the large, fluid-filled pericardium; by percussion, there is an increase in the cardiac dullness both in its area and in its flatness of tone. Palpation of the precordium reveals diminished or absent impulses, and auscultation usually reveals distant heart sounds. With very large pericardial effusions, an area of dullness, bronchial breathing, and/or egobronchophony is found over the left posterior chest below the angle of the left scapula (the Ewart sign) due to compression of the base of the left lung.

The characteristic ECG finding with significant pericardial effusion is low QRS voltage. In addition there may be nonspecific ST- and T-wave abnormalities. Alternations in the QRS amplitude in various leads (electrical alternans) may be seen in some patients with voluminous pericardial effusion; it has been postulated that this is due to periodic motion or rotation of the heart within the fluid-filled pericardial sac. The x-ray appearance of pericardial effusion is that of cardiomegaly with a characteristic pear-shaped or water-bottle cardiac silhouette and obliteration of the normal cardiac outlines, especially along the left heart border. As opposed to cardiomegaly from heart failure and chamber enlargement, the lung fields are normal with no evidence of pulmonary vascular congestion. Serial chest x-rays showing rapid changes in cardiac size and silhouette

may be of great value in the diagnosis. Chest fluoroscopy shows diminution or absence of the normal visible cardiac pulsations. Effusion can be definitely diagnosed by demonstrating an increased distance between the right border of the cardiac silhouette and the right atrial cavity boundary either by carbon dioxide angiography or by the position of a catheter within the right atrium. Echocardiography has become a most valuable and reliable tool in assessing pericardial effusion.

CARDIAC TAMPONADE
Cardiac tamponade results when an increase in intrapericardial pressure interferes with the normal diastolic filling of the heart. This results in a rise in central venous pressure and a fall in cardiac output that can progress to shock and cardiovascular collapse. The physical findings reveal evidence of low output and shock with pallor; cool, clammy skin; rapid, feeble pulse; and low arterial blood pressure. The hallmark of pericardial tamponade is a paradoxical pulse, in which the peak systolic arterial pressure during inspiration is considerably lower than during expiration. An inspiratory fall of up to 10 mm Hg in systolic blood pressure may be seen in normal individuals during quiet respiration. Cardiac tamponade produces much greater degrees of inspiratory decline. It is also important to remember that conditions associated with increased ventilatory effort (e.g., asthma) will also produce a paradoxical pulse. Elevation of central venous pressure is manifested by engorgement of the neck veins. Careful examination will reveal a characteristic abnormally prominent X descent of the jugular venous pulse. Chronic passive congestion may occur, producing an enlarged, smooth, tender, and sometimes pulsatile liver and peripheral edema. There are no specific associated ECG, chest x-ray, or echocardiographic findings except for those of pericardial effusion already mentioned.

CHRONIC PERICARDIAL CONSTRICTION
Pericardial constriction is a chronic disorder caused by dense, fibrous thickening of the pericardium, usually the result of a prior inflammatory process. The pericardium is leatherlike with involvement of both the parietal and the visceral surfaces and frequently extending down into the superficial layers

of the myocardium. The heart becomes encased in an inelastic, constrictive shell that interferes with normal diastolic filling of both ventricles and thereby embarrasses normal cardiac function. The resultant hemodynamic abnormalities produce a characteristic clinical syndrome sometimes known as Pick's disease. The general clinical presentation is frequently insidious, with a very gradual development of systemic venous hypertension producing symptoms resembling those in chronic right heart failure. Symptomatically there is fluid retention with ascites frequently out of proportion to peripheral edema. Easy fatigability and exertional dyspnea frequently occur but are generally mild. Anorexia and epigastric discomfort, probably due to visceral engorgement, may be striking.

The most notable physical findings in chronic pericardial constriction include venous distention, fluid retention in the form of ascites and edema, and hepatomegaly. The ascites and hepatomegaly may so dominate the clinical presentation that they are often considered to be due to cirrhosis of the liver. The Kussmaul sign (an inspiratory increase rather than the normal inspiratory fall in jugular venous distention) is commonly seen. The jugular venous pulse contour shows a characteristic early diastolic collapse (the Friedreich sign), namely an abnormally sharp, deep y descent. Arterial blood pressure is usually slightly diminished with a narrow pulse pressure and, frequently, a paradoxical pulse. Long-standing, severe hepatic congestion is sometimes associated with jaundice.

Examination of the heart reveals a small to slightly enlarged area of cardiac dullness. The precordium is quiet with a reduced or absent apical impulse. The heart sounds are normal and slightly diminished. The most distinctive feature is a palpable and sometimes an audible sharp pericardial "knock" occurring in early diastole, when rapid filling of the ventricle encounters the nondistensible pericardium. This sound is similar to the third heart sound, but it occurs slightly earlier.

The ECG in pericardial constriction frequently shows low QRS voltage, diffuse T-wave flattening or inversion, and atrial fibrillation. The cardiac silhouette on x-ray may be slightly enlarged, but it is usually normal in size. Pericardial calcification is frequently seen, and though highly suggestive, is not diagnostic of chronic constrictive pericarditis. Cardiac fluoroscopy demonstrates diminished to absent cardiac pulsations. Echocardiography can be quite useful by demonstrating multiple dense echoes from the pericardium. Cardiac catheterization is required to definitively establish the diagnosis of pericardial constriction and to distinguish it from restrictive cardiomyopathy, which may produce a similar clinical picture. In pericardial constriction there is a distinctive equalization of diastolic pressures on both sides of the heart.

MANAGEMENT

In general, treatment of pericardial inflammation is directed against the underlying etiology (e.g., antibiotics are given for bacterial pericarditis). Various antiinflammatory drugs have been used in the treatment of noninfective pericardial inflammation. Salicylates, corticosteroids, or indomethacin may provide relief in many cases. Pericardiocentesis, the removal of pericardial fluid percutaneously through a needle, is performed on an emergency basis when severe and life-threatening cardiac tamponade is present, and in such a situation the removal of even a few hundred milliliters of fluid may produce rapid and dramatic clinical improvement. Pericardiocentesis may also be useful for diagnostic analysis of the fluid and for instillation of chemotherapeutic agents against infectious or malignant processes. Recurrent pericardial effusion with tamponade requires surgical intervention to create a pericardial "window" for continued drainage into the pleural space. Pericardiectomy for constrictive pericarditis is a more major surgical undertaking, but it frequently results in significant relief. The degree of myocardial involvement in the chronic fibrotic process is an important determinant of the amount of postoperative cardiac impairment.

Myocardial Diseases

As in the case of the pericardium, a great number of diseases (see Tables 33-1 and 33-2) may involve the myocardium, either primarily or in association with other organ systems, but each expresses itself pathophysiologically in only a limited number of ways.

These can be roughly categorized as systolic contraction failure, diastolic relaxation failure, obstruction to flow, and arrhythmia.

Systolic Contraction Failure. Diminished systolic contraction or pump failure of the heart is the most frequent final common pathway of diseases affecting the heart. It is due to progressive loss or replacement of effectively contracting myofibrils, resulting in progressive chamber dilatation and overall cardiomegaly, producing the syndrome of low cardiac output and congestive heart failure. The clinical manifestations of congestive heart failure are covered in Chap. 31.

Diastolic Relaxation Failure. This is caused by either abnormally hypertrophied muscle or myocardial infiltrative processes that produce a poorly compliant or stiff ventricle. In this case, the myocardial as opposed to pericardial constrictive pathology prevents normal diastolic filling and impairs cardiac function.

Obstruction to Flow. A few diseases of the myocardium result in obstruction to blood flow within the cardiac chambers. Thus septal hypertrophy may result in left ventricular outflow obstruction, whereas atrial tumors may obstruct ventricular inflow.

Arrhythmia. The myocardium is an electrical as well as a mechanical tissue; thus diseases affecting the myocardium may disturb the normal syncytial depolarization and repolarization and produce virtually any type of arrhythmia or conduction disturbance. Chapter 32 discusses the various cardiac arrhythmias.

MYOCARDITIS

Myocarditis is an inflammatory disease that occurs as a reaction to a wide variety of disease processes (see Tables 33-1 and 33-2). Frequently the pericardium, the endocardium, or both may also be involved (e.g., viral myopericarditis). Usually the heart is affected incidentally as one of many organs involved in a widespread disease. Thus myocarditis may occur in virtually every known bacterial, viral, mycotic, or parasitic disease. It also occurs in many of the collagen, vascular, or autoimmune diseases, the most notable of which is acute rheumatic fever. Occasionally there

is an isolated inflammation of the heart of unknown etiology, which then carries the eponym of Fiedler's myocarditis.

Acute myocarditis is often clinically silent. When symptoms do occur, they include precordial discomfort that is atypical of angina pectoris and is often only a mild, continuous sensation of pressure or soreness. A pleuritic component generally indicates associated involvement of the pericardium or pleura. If systolic contraction failure occurs during the acute process, right- and left-sided congestive heart failure may appear. Physical findings may include cardiomegaly; tachycardia, often out of proportion to the associated febrile illness; arrhythmias; and evidence of congestive heart failure. Ventricular and atrial gallops may be heard, and the first heart sound is frequently diminished. With progression of left ventricular failure and dilatation, a murmur of mitral regurgitation may appear due to papillary muscle dysfunction. The ECG may show diffuse, nonspecific ST- and T-wave abnormalities, prolongation of the PR interval, severe degrees of heart block, and prolongation of the QT interval. Virtually any form of arrhythmia may be seen.

Acute myocarditis is generally self-limited. Sequelae are common only after acute rheumatic fever, in the form of chronic valvulitis (Chap. 30). In some instances, acute myocarditis may result in significant residual systolic contraction failure known as congestive cardiomyopathy; and some cases of apparently idiopathic congestive cardiomyopathy may be the result of prior undetected myocarditis.

CARDIOMYOPATHIES

The term *cardiomyopathy* literally means heart muscle disease, and the term has been variably applied to describe diseases in which pathology of the myocardium (and sometimes of the mural endocardium) constitutes the primary cardiac defect. In its broadest sense, cardiomyopathy includes ventricular dysfunction of any etiology, including coronary disease (coronary cardiomyopathy); valvular disease (e.g., myopathic left ventricle of end-stage aortic regurgitation); and inflammatory processes (the myocarditides). In its narrowest use, the term is confined to disorders with no known etiology or associated disease. The most common usage of the term *cardiomyopathy* in this country includes diseases involving the myocardium (and sometimes the endocardium) in the absence of associated significant coronary atherosclerosis, valvular disease, or hypertension. Within the group of diseases thus defined, some are clearly secondary to specific etiologic agents, some are strongly correlated with certain noncardiac diseases, some occur in certain recognized clinical settings with no established causal relationship, and some are truly idiopathic with no recognizable etiology or associated disease. Table 33-3 outlines a clinically useful nomenclature that divides the cardiomyopathies into four basic pathophysiologic groups.

Congestive Cardiomyopathy

Congestive cardiomyopathy is a clinical syndrome resulting from myocardial cell damage or dysfunction that produces systolic contraction failure. As the ejection force of the ventricle is reduced, the chambers dilate, producing cardiomegaly. There is usually some degree of associated ventricular hypertrophy, but the dilatation is out of proportion to the hypertrophy. The hypertrophy appears to be a compensatory mechanism, and patients with a relatively greater degree of hypertrophy appear to have a better survival.

The clinical picture is primarily that of congestive heart failure (see Chap. 31), which is usually gradual and insidious in onset; the disease is usually well advanced before coming to clinical attention. Almost any form of cardiac arrhythmia may occur, and both atrial and ventricular ectopic rhythms are frequently seen. Heart block, though less common, is also seen. Sudden death, presumably due to ventricular fibrillation or asystole, is common.

Most patients with congestive cardiomyopathy have areas of endocardial thickening and fibrosis, usually patchy in distribution. Mural thrombi are found at autopsy in roughly half of the patients, most commonly in the left ventricle, and these thrombi usually occur at sites of endocardial scarring. Both pulmonary and systemic emboli frequently arise from these thrombi. Mild systolic hypertension is frequently seen, even in the face of severe congestive heart failure. This association has led to the speculation that chronic silent hypertension may be the underlying cause of congestive cardiomyopathy in many cases.

The chest x-ray shows generalized cardiomegaly, though in early or compensated cases this may be relatively subtle. X-ray evidence of pulmonary congestion appears as the disease progresses. The ECG is usually abnormal, often showing evidence of left ventricular hypertrophy, bundle branch block, and fascicular block. Pseudoinfarct patterns with pathologic Q waves are sometimes seen, and coronary angiography in such cases may help to exclude significant coronary disease. Echocardiography has proved diagnostically valuable by indicating abnormal chamber sizes, abnormal wall motion and thickness, and reduced ejection fraction. Left ventriculography demonstrates left ventricular dilatation with diffuse hypokinesis and poor ejection fraction.

Therapy of congestive cardiomyopathy is supportive: Digitalis and diuretics are used for the congestive failure, antiarrhythmic drugs are given to suppress ventricular and atrial arrhythmias, and anticoagulants may be used to reduce the risk of mural thrombi and embolism. There appears to be some improvement in both hemodynamic and clinical parameters after long-term vasodilator therapy with, for example, long-acting nitrates. Prolonged bed rest has been shown to result in substantial reductions in heart size and clinical symptoms. However, lasting benefits have not been conclusively demonstrated, and many patients are unwilling to accept long-term bed rest. Abstinence from alcohol is required, especially in patients with a history of chronic alcohol abuse.

Hypertrophic Cardiomyopathy

Hypertrophic cardiomyopathy is a distinct pathologic entity characterized by ventricular hypertrophy that appears to be primary, not secondary, to an increase in ventricular work load. Disproportional or asymmetric septal hypertrophy (ASH) is the characteristic anatomic feature of this disease, but much of the left ventricular free wall and even the right ventricular free wall may also be involved. Both ventricular cavities are small, and the internal anatomic relationships of the papillary muscles, mitral valve, and left ventricular outflow tract are distorted. When the anatomy is sufficiently disturbed, obstruction to the

Table 33-3. Classification of Cardiomyopathies: Pathology, Physiology, and Clinical Findings

Type of cardiomyopathy	Pathology	Physiology	Clinical
Congestive	Dilated chambers, especially LV; myocardial fibrotic replacement; secondary hypertrophy; patchy endocardial fibrosis; mural thrombi	Systolic contraction failure	CHF, mostly left sided; dysrhythmia; emboli
Hypertrophic	Whorls of disorganized muscle bundles, myofibrils, and myofilaments; primary hypertrophy of all chambers with disproportionate septal involvement; small to normal chamber size; distortion of internal ventricular geometry; secondary fibrosis of endocardium of outflow tract and mitral valve	Diastolic relaxation failure; end-stage systolic contraction failure; mitral regurgitation	Dysrhythmia, dyspnea; frank CHF is a late sign; angina. Emboli rare (occur with atrial fibrillation).
With obstruction (IHSS)	Distorted geometry results in LV outflow obstruction between hypertrophied septum and abnormally moving mitral valve	Mitral regurgitation, dynamic LV outflow gradient	emboli rare (occur with atrial fibrillation)
Restrictive	Chamber size normal to moderately enlarged, generally due to an infiltrative process of the myocardium (e.g., amyloid)	Diastolic relaxation failure dynamically similar to pericardial constriction; variable degree of associated systolic contraction failure	CHF, may be mostly right sided; dysrhythmia
Obliterative (endomyocardial disease)	Severe focal fibrosis of the endocardium and underlying myocardium, may affect one or both ventricles; sparing of ventricular outflow tracts; fibrosis may involve chordae tendineae and bind down mitral or tricuspid valves; mural thrombi; end-stage obliteration of ventricular cavity	Combined systolic contraction and diastolic relaxation failure, mitral and/or tricuspid regurgitation	CHF, right and/or left sided; emboli

*Note: IHSS = idiopathic hypertrophic subaortic stenosis; LV = left ventricle; CHF = congestive heart failure.

left ventricular outflow occurs between the hypertrophied septum and the distorted anterior leaflet of the mitral valve. This obstructive form of the disease was the first to be generally recognized and emphasized as idiopathic hypertrophic subaortic stenosis. As nonobstructive variants became known, the disease was categorized into obstructive and nonobstructive forms.

Pathologically, abnormal whorls of fragmented, thick muscle fibers with large perinuclear halos and nuclei are scattered throughout the myocardium in hypertrophic cardiomyopathy. This abnormal tissue appears to be associated with ventricular compliance dysfunction, regardless of whether obstruction is present or not. Variable amounts of fibrosis are frequently seen in this abnormal tissue. The disease appears to have a familial transmittance, although sporadic forms frequently occur. Familial inheritance has been further suggested in recent years by echocardiographic demonstrations of asymmetric septal hypertrophy in the asymptomatic relatives of patients with hypertrophic cardiomyopathy. The course of the disease appears to be largely a function of progression of diastolic filling failure with elevation of left ventricular end-diastolic pressure. In a given patient, the degree of obstruction can wax and wane over time, and the obstruction may even disappear with progression of the disease. In advanced stages there also appears to be some impairment in systolic contraction function of the ventricle. Mural thrombi may form and lead to pulmonary or systemic embolism. As the disease progresses, congestive heart failure predominates the clinical picture. Atrial fibrillation is not uncommon, and its development with loss of the normal augmentation in ventricular filling from atrial contraction can precipitate a rapid deterioration that should be approached as a medical emergency. As in congestive cardiomyopathy, sudden death is not uncommon and is generally presumed to have an arrhythmic basis.

Hypertrophic obstructive cardiomyopathy, or idiopathic hypertrophic subaortic stenosis (IHSS), as it is frequently referred to in this country, presents a characteristic clinical syndrome. Though generally diagnosed during adult life, the underlying pathology has most likely been present since childhood. The

appearance of symptoms and the diagnosis in childhood occurs in severe cases and carries a poor prognosis. In addition to the reduced compliance of the ventricle seen in the nonobstructive form of hypertrophic cardiomyopathy, the abnormal muscle bundles in IHSS distort the internal anatomy of the ventricle to such an extent that ventricular outflow obstruction occurs. The presenting features of IHSS include atypical angina pectoris, dyspnea, and exertional syncope. In the absence of symptoms, however, identification of the typical cardiac murmur may constitute the initial sign.

The dynamic nature of the systolic obstruction in IHSS produces certain characteristic physical findings. The distortion of the papillary muscles results in abnormal motion of the mitral valve apparatus such that in many cases the anterior leaflet both participates in the left ventricular outflow obstruction and causes some degree of mitral regurgitation. As opposed to the slow upstroke found in valvular aortic stenosis, the arterial pulse shows a rapid upstroke that plateaus or even falls in early systole. The heart may be slightly enlarged, but frequently it is within normal limits. A presystolic impulse corresponding to atrial contraction is frequently palpable over the apex. The systolic outflow murmur characteristically starts shortly after the first heart sound and ends before the aortic sound. It is generally heard best between the apex and lower left sternal border, and frequently it is transmitted to the axilla and base but is transmitted poorly to the carotids. The murmur of IHSS increases with the Valsalva maneuver and decreases in the squatting position. Normally the pulse generated by the beat following a compensatory pause of a premature ventricular contraction is augmented, but in IHSS this pulse is often diminished. A ventricular gallop is occasionally heard at the apex and generally reflects associated mitral regurgitation. The second sound may be paradoxically split.

The ECG typically shows evidence of left ventricular hypertrophy with disproportionate hypertrophy of the ventricular septum frequently producing abnormally prominent septal Q waves, creating a pseudoinfarct pattern. These Q waves are characteristically found in the anterolateral leads, but they may also be seen in the inferior leads. As with other forms of cardiomyopathy, virtually any form of arrhythmia may be seen, the most serious of which is an ectopic ventricular tachyarrhythmia. The chest x-ray may show mild to moderate cardiomegaly, but more often than not it is normal. The echocardiogram may reveal a pathognomonic picture, namely, an asymmetrically hypertrophied and poorly contractile septum, an abnormal systolic anterior motion of the anterior leaflet of the mitral valve, and a premature systolic closure of the aortic valve leaflets. Cardiac catheterization reveals a gradient below the aortic valve that is exacerbated by positive inotropy such as occurs with isoproterenol or after the pause following a premature ventricular contraction. Left ventricular angiography demonstrates thickening of the ventricular wall, especially of the septum, and a characteristic distortion of the internal ventricular anatomy that is frequently associated with mild to moderate mitral regurgitation.

Treatment with either medical or surgical procedures may achieve limited success. The mainstay of medical therapy is beta-adrenergic blockade with propranolol, which has been demonstrated to increase ventricular volume, reduce left ventricular end-diastolic pressure, and reduce the outflow gradient. Digitalis and other positive inotropic agents generally have a deleterious effect in IHSS, and for this reason it is important to make a proper differentiation of IHSS from the other causes of congestive heart failure in which these agents are of benefit. Similarly, vasodilators, notably nitroglycerine, may exacerbate the obstruction; and before nitroglycerine is given to any patient with angina, the possibility of IHSS should be considered. Surgical procedures have been aimed at relieving the outflow tract obstruction and the mitral regurgitation. Operations have varied from extensive muscle resections combined with mitral valve replacement to simple ventriculomyotomy. Recent experience suggests that ventriculomyotomy effectively abolishes the abnormal systolic anterior motion of the mitral valve, relieving both the outflow obstruction and the mitral regurgitation. Though the clinical and hemodynamic results of surgery are generally good, a significant surgical mortality in these patients dictates

that only those who remain symptomatic on adequate medical therapy be operated on.

Restrictive Cardiomyopathy

A number of cardiomyopathies produce a rigid, noncompliant ventricular wall associated with diastolic filling failure. These diseases include some of known cause (e.g., amyloid heart disease), some with known disease associations (e.g., Friedreich's ataxia), and some that are truly idiopathic. The infiltrative cardiomyopathies, including those due to the presence of iron, calcium, lipids, mucopolysaccharides, granulomas, amyloid, or neoplasms, constitute an important subgroup of these diseases.

The restriction created by the noncompliant left ventricle produces a clinical picture that may be quite similar to that seen in constrictive pericarditis. Systolic contractile function is usually relatively well preserved, and the left ventricle is generally not enlarged. Symptoms are variable, depending on the underlying etiology. Atypical angina is not infrequently seen. Many patients have a normal exercise tolerance; they increase their cardiac output by tachycardia, thus compensating for their inability to increase stroke volume. The ECG may show only nonspecific repolarization changes; chest x-ray and echocardiographic findings are frequently normal. Cardiac catheterization may reveal hemodynamics quite similar to those in constrictive pericarditis. The left ventricle is generally more affected than the right, resulting in higher diastolic pressures in the left than in the right ventricle; this contrasts to constrictive pericarditis, in which right- and left-sided diastolic pressures are more or less equal. Nevertheless, in patients in whom the diagnosis remains sufficiently uncertain and the possibility of surgically remediable constrictive pericarditis cannot be entirely excluded, exploratory thoracotomy for possible pericardiectomy is undertaken. Endomyocardial fibrosis and Loeffler's endocarditis are rare entities in this general group of restrictive cardiomyopathies. They are notable for the predominant fibrosis and thrombosis found in the endocardium, and they can progress to involve the mitral and tricuspid valves, producing regurgitation. In the end stages virtual obliteration of the ventricular cavity may occur and the term *obliterative cardiomyopathy* is often applied to these entities.

Endocardial Diseases

NONINFECTIVE (MARANTIC) ENDOCARDITIS

Marantic endocarditis is a noninfective thrombotic lesion that is often seen as an incidental finding at the time of autopsy, but it is also capable of producing clinically significant embolic phenomena. Originally described as Libman-Sacks disease associated with systemic lupus erythematosus, it may be seen in the setting of a number of chronic disease states, cachexia, and various malignancies, notably in malignant carcinoid, in which it involves primarily the right side of the heart. There is no specific therapy for noninfective endocarditis.

INFECTIVE (BACTERIAL) ENDOCARDITIS*

Though infective endocarditis may be caused by various fungal and rickettsial organisms, most cases of infective endocarditis are due to bacteria. In the preantibiotic era, when bacterial endocarditis was uniformly fatal, the rate of progression of disease was the basis for making a distinction between the more fulminant course of acute bacterial endocarditis and the more indolent form, subacute bacterial endocarditis. As a general rule, organisms capable of primary invasion such as the pyogenic cocci, *Staphylococcus aureus,* pneumococci, and gonococci produce the more fulminating course of acute bacterial endocarditis that is associated with rapid destruction of valves, local abscesses in the area of the anulus, the metastatic abscesses seeded by septic emboli. Organisms of low pathogenicity such as viridans streptococci and enterococci produce a more insidious disease with less valvular destruction and ulceration, but they may cause large vegetations resulting in widespread systemic embolisms. The introduction of effective antimicrobials makes differentiation between acute and subacute forms less clear, since these agents are often curative or modify the course of the disease, even in ultimately fatal cases.

*This section was written by David C. Hueter and William R. McCabe.

Although low-grade bacteremia is a common day-to-day occurrence, certain clinical settings may produce significantly higher degrees of bacteremia, thereby increasing the chances of infection. These include surgery of any form, but most importantly gynecologic or genitourinary, and dental procedures (including even the cleaning of the teeth).

Host mechanisms play a most important role in the pathogenesis of endocarditis and certain clinical groups of patients are at increased risk. The development of endocarditis requires the combination of a significant bacteremia with an endocardium susceptible to invasion by the particular organism. The virulent organisms of acute bacterial endocarditis frequently involve the normal heart, whereas subacute bacterial endocarditis invariably involves only an abnormal heart. Though the precise mechanism is still poorly understood, experimental studies and clinical observations suggest that nonlaminar or turbulent blood flow along a given endocardial surface predisposes the endocardium at that point to bacterial infection. Significant congenital or acquired structural cardiac disease is the most frequent setting producing such turbulent blood flow, although the hemodynamic lesion itself may be quite insignificant (e.g., a small ventricular septal defect or a prolapsing mitral leaflet) and may come to clinical attention only after the development of bacterial endocarditis. In addition to local factors, any condition or chronic disease that suppresses general host defenses to infection may predispose to the development of endocarditis.

Combinations of the various predisposing factors frequently coexist, as in the case of patients on long-term hemodialysis for chronic renal failure. Both right- and left-sided acute bacterial endocarditis are being seen with increasing frequency in narcotic addicts, presumably because of the bacteremias produced by nonsterile intravenous injections. Patients who have had cardiac surgery with implantation of prosthetic heart valves are also at increased risk to develop bacterial endocarditis, either in a period of weeks following surgery, representing infection acquired in the perioperative period, or in the late postoperative period. Treatment of early endocarditis following cardiac surgery sometimes fails to eradicate the infection, and removal of the infected prosthesis is required. Endocarditis can also occur late after valve implantation and is similar to typical endocarditis with respect to predisposing factors and causative agents and, generally, in its satisfactory response to appropriate antibiotic therapy.

Infectious endocarditis becomes clinically manifest through three basic pathophysiologic mechanisms: generalized infection, valvular destruction, and peripheral embolism. Systemic infection accounts for the fever; weight loss; malaise; anorexia; leukocytosis; and mild normochromic, normocytic anemia. Valvular destruction is signaled by the appearance of new murmurs, generally regurgitant in character. As valve dysfunction progresses, signs of congestive heart failure appear and can progress in a fulminating course over a short period of time. Embolism of fragments of vegetation produce embolic manifestations. Secondary inflammatory reaction frequently occurs at the site of the embolic infarct. Septic involvement at the embolic site also occurs with the more virulent organisms of acute bacterial endocarditis, but it is uncommon in subacute bacterial endocarditis. Fungal endocarditis generally produces larger emboli, and an occlusion of a large artery should always raise the question of a fungal etiology. Septic pulmonary infarcts commonly accompany the right-sided endocarditis seen in drug addicts. Systemic septic embolism from left-sided lesions may produce a great number of signs and symptoms, depending on the organ involved. Thus embolic strokes, myocardial infarction, renal infarction, glomerulonephritis, and splenic infarction may be seen. Embolism to the skin, retina, and mucous membranes produces certain classic physical findings, namely conjunctival hemorrhages; retinal hemorrhages (Roth spots); subungual or splinter hemorrhages; and tender, erythematous papules in the pulp of the fingers (Osler's nodes). Emboli may continue for weeks after cure and should not be construed as an indication of treatment failure.

Effective therapy of endocarditis depends on early diagnosis, identification of the causal organism, and institution of appropriate antibiotic therapy. Since early manifestations of endocarditis may be quite subtle, persistent fever, especially in patients at increased risk of endocarditis, should raise the question of endocarditis and instigate a prompt collection of blood cultures. The bacteremia of endocarditis is continuous, and the etiologic agent is usually obtained in the first three to four blood cultures. Preceding antibiotic therapy can mask a bacteremia; therefore, antibiotics ideally should be discontinued for several days prior to collection of cultures. Culture-negative endocarditis has been reported to occur in from 5 to 20 percent of patients with subacute endocarditis, and in such cases the diagnosis must rest on clinical and laboratory findings. In acute bacterial endocarditis the diagnostic problem is often reversed, with bacteremia but no obvious valvular involvement until relatively late in the illness. For this reason, staphylococcal bacteremia requires prolonged treatment to ensure adequate therapy of unrecognized endocarditis.

To insure optimal therapy of endocarditis, the bacteriocidal levels of the antibiotic in the patient's serum against the specific organism (serum bacteriocidal test) should be determined and confirmed to be adequate. As a general rule, bacteriocidal rather than bacteriostatic antibiotics are chosen. In viridans (alpha-hemolytic) streptococcal endocarditis, daily parenteral doses of from 4 to 6 million units of penicillin for 4 weeks, or alternatively, 2.4 million units of penicillin and 2.0 gm of streptomycin for 2 weeks, are usually adequate. Staphylococcal endocarditis usually requires daily parenteral doses of 10 to 12 gm of nafcillin or oxacillin or 18 gm of methicillin for 6 weeks. Enterococcal endocarditis is usually treated for 6 weeks with daily parenteral doses of 20 million units of penicillin plus one of the aminoglycosides, which act synergistically with penicillin. In the face of penicillin allergy, treatment is more difficult but other agents, depending on the causative organism, may be effective.

Although blood cultures rapidly become negative with antibiotic therapy, low-grade fever, anemia, and an elevated sedimentation rate may persist for a considerable time, making the clinical assessment of the effectiveness of therapy difficult. Usually, however, general clinical improvement is apparent. Increasing valvular incompetence can lead to progressive congestive heart failure, which may require prosthetic valve replacement. Although it is generally preferable to delay such surgery until a maximum duration of antibiotic treatment has been achieved, emergency prosthetic valvular replacement is sometimes required when congestive failure cannot be controlled by medical therapy.

From a public health viewpoint, prophylactic antibiotic therapy is perhaps the most important therapeutic measure against endocarditis. Patients with underlying predispositions to endocarditis, especially those with organic heart disease, should receive antibiotic prophylaxis prior to surgical procedures associated with significant bacteremia, especially dental, oropharyngeal, genitourinary, gynecologic, or gastrointestinal surgery or manipulation. The rapidity with which antibiotic-resistant bacteria may appear in the oral or gastrointestinal flora after antibiotic administration makes it necessary that the prophylactic antibiotic not be given prior to the day of the procedure. For dental work, a parenteral dose of 600,000 units of procaine penicillin should be given the same morning of the procedure, another 600,000 units of aqueous penicillin immediately before the procedure, and a third 600,000 units of procaine penicillin the day after the procedure. Since patients receiving long-term penicillin prophylaxis for rheumatic fever usually harbor penicillin-resistant streptococci, a different antibiotic, usually erythromycin, must be used. Prophylaxis to prevent bacteremia associated with urologic, gynecologic, or gastrointestinal procedures is directed against the enterococcus; thus larger doses of penicillin combined with an aminoglycoside are required.

ACUTE RHEUMATIC FEVER

Although acute rheumatic fever is a systemic disease with a name that emphasizes involvement of the joints, its clinical importance is related to its involvement of the heart, including the pericardium, myocardium, and endocardium. Accordingly acute rheumatic fever is more properly considered here rather than in the section on rheumatic disease.

Rheumatic fever is an inflammatory disease that occurs as a sequel some 1 to 3 weeks following an infection with group A beta-hemolytic streptococci, usually acute pharyngitis. It may occur at any age, but it is extremely rare in infancy and is usually a disease of children and young adults, in whom

streptococcal infections are most frequent. The incidence of disease following streptococcal infections is greatly increased in patients who have had previous attacks of rheumatic fever, and recurrences occur well into the adult years. A variety of pathophysiologic causes have been proposed, including autoimmunity through cross-reactivity of streptococcal and human tissue antigens as well as toxic factors produced by the streptococcus. Nevertheless, the underlying mechanism by which the tissue damage of rheumatic fever occurs as a sequel to group A streptococcal infection remains obscure.

Certain characteristic clinical features occur in acute rheumatic fever; however, the infection and rheumatic manifestations often remain subclinical. The course of the attack may persist over weeks or months. Systemic manifestations include fatigue, malaise, and fever. Acute migratory polyarthritis occurs, most frequently involving the large joints of the extremities and sometimes with transient joint effusions. Erythema marginatum is a characteristic but infrequent finding consisting of an evanescent painless, nonpruritic erythema of the trunk and proximal extremities that is more evident with local heat such as after a hot bath. Subcutaneous nodules of rheumatic fever are transient, small, painless swellings over the bony prominences; these are often overlooked. Sydenham's chorea is generally a late manifestation occurring months after the streptococcal infection, and though once a common feature of rheumatic fever, appears to be increasingly infrequent. Abdominal pain is not uncommon and is thought to be the result of hepatic engorgement or of inflammatory serositis involving the peritoneum; sometimes the pain leads to unnecessary exploratory laparotomy.

As previously mentioned, acute rheumatic carditis may involve the pericardium, myocardium, and endocardium. Pericardial involvement is marked by inflammation with the associated typical clinical findings described previously in this chapter. There is an associated serofibrinous effusion of variable degrees. The myocarditis of acute rheumatic fever, characterized histologically by the presence of Aschoff bodies, can result in significant systolic pump failure that is manifested by cardiomegaly and frank congestive heart failure. Endocardial involvement primarily involves the valvular endocardium with swelling, erosions, and vegetations of the valve leaflets and relative sparing of the mural endocardium. The mitral, aortic, and tricuspid valves are involved in that order of frequency, while the pulmonary valve is only rarely involved. Cardiomegaly and congestive heart failure are often seen. The ECG shows prolongation of the PR interval, and this delay in atrioventricular conduction probably accounts for the muffled first heart sound frequently found. An apical holosystolic murmur of mitral regurgitation is common and is sometimes accompanied by a short middiastolic sound, the Carey-Coombs murmur. Aortic valve involvement is indicated by the typical blowing early diastolic decrescendo murmur of aortic regurgitation. As the valvular endocardial lesions heal, they will evolve in time to produce the characteristic findings of chronic rheumatic valvular disease described in Chapter 30. Laboratory findings in acute rheumatic fever consist of elevated erythrocyte sedimentation rate, an increased antistreptolysin O titer, and the appearance of C-reactive protein as well as of many other so-called acute-phase reactants.

There is no specific cure for rheumatic fever, but good supportive therapy can reduce the mortality and morbidity. Effective antibiotic treatment to eliminate group A streptococci (e.g., 1.2 million units of benzathine penicillin G intramuscularly) is advisable, even if throat cultures are negative for streptococci, and continuous antibiotic prophylactic coverage should be initiated. Salicylates are of considerable value in controlling fever, anorexia, and joint pain and swelling. Corticosteroids are more potent antiinflammatory agents than salicylates and are preferred by many physicians, especially if the clinical response to salicylates is suboptimal. However, careful studies have failed to show that steroids, even when administered early and in large doses, have a beneficial effect in preventing acute or chronic damage to the heart, and the use of corticosteroids for acute rheumatic fever with carditis varies with the convictions of the individual physician. Historically, prolonged bed rest was considered a cornerstone of therapy; however, it has not been shown to have any proved value in reducing morbidity or mortality. Recurrences are prevented by providing continuous antibiotic prophylaxis

against group A streptococci, for which the most efficient regimen is monthly intramuscular injections of 1.2 million units of benzathine penicillin G. Initial attacks of rheumatic fever can be prevented by prompt and adequate treatment of respiratory infections due to group A streptococci. The spread of streptococcal infections can be prevented or markedly modified by appropriate diagnostic throat cultures and adequate antibiotic treatment, ideally in the form of a single intramuscular injection of benzathine penicillin G of 600,000 units in children or 1.2 million units in adults.

Bibliography

Black, S., O'Rourke, R., and Karliner, J. Role of surgery in the treatment of primary infective endocarditis. *Am. J. Med.* 56:357, 1974.

Caluss, R. H. Pericardial disease. *Cardiovasc. Clin.* 3:45, 1971.

Fowler, N. O. Diagnosis of the myocardial diseases. *Cardiovasc. Clin.* 4:77, 1972.

Fowler, N. O., and Manitsas, G. T. Infectious pericarditis. *Progr. Cardiovasc. Dis.* 16:323, 1973.

Goodwin, J. F. Hypertrophic diseases of the myocardium. *Progr. Cardiovasc. Dis.* 16:199, 1973.

Linde, L. M., and Rao, P. S. A modern view of infective endocarditis. *Cardiovasc. Clin.* 5:15, 1973.

Oakley, C. M. Clinical definitions and classifications of cardiomyopathies. *Postgrad. Med. J.* 48:703, 1972.

Perloff, J. K. The cardiomyopathies — current perspectives. *Circulation* 44:942, 1971.

Roberts, W. C., and Ferrans, V. J. Pathologic aspects of the idiopathic cardiomyopathies. *Adv. Cardiol.* 13:349, 1974.

Rodnan, G. P. (ed.). Rheumatic Fever. In *Primer on the Rheumatic Diseases. J.A.M.A.* 224 (Suppl.): 5, 1973.

Shabetai, R., Fowler, N. O., and Guntheroth, W. G. The hemodynamics of cardiac tamponade and constrictive pericarditis. *Am. J. Cardiol.* 26: 480, 1970.

Shah, P. M. Idiopathic hypertrophic subaortic stenosis — changing concepts — 1975. *Chest* 68: 814, 1975.

Weinstein, L., and Schlesinger, J. S. Pathoanatomic, pathophysiologic, and clinical correlations in endocarditis. *N. Engl. J. Med.* 291:832, 1122, 1974.

Wenger, N. K. Infectious myocarditis. *Cardiovasc. Clin.* 4:167, 1972.

VI The Gastrointestinal Tract

34

The Esophagus

Lauran D. Harris

The esophagus is a unique part of the digestive tract. The most obvious example of its uniqueness is purely anatomic – it is located in the chest, whereas the rest of the digestive system is isolated in the abdomen. The functions of the esophagus are also unique. It does not alter the contents entrusted to it either chemically or physically, but rather performs two deceptively simple functions: transporting its contents to the stomach and preventing the return of gastric contents.

Anatomy

The more important anatomic features of the esophagus having clinical relevance are illustrated in Figure 34-1. The esophagus is a muscular tube, about 25 cm long in the adult, which is fixed only at its proximal and distal ends. In its course through the superior and posterior mediastinum, it lies in proximity first to the thyroid gland, the trachea, and the carotid arteries and then to the aorta, the left main stem bronchus, and the left atrium. Distally, the esophagus passes through the esophageal hiatus of the diaphragm and terminates by joining the cardiac portion of the stomach. It is innervated by the vagus nerves and by sympathetic nerves forming the esophageal plexus. As described elsewhere in this book, the anastomosis between portal and systemic venous systems located in the distal esophagus can be of considerable clinical importance when pressure in the portal venous system becomes abnormally increased. The fact that the esophagus is composed of both skeletal and smooth muscle makes it vulnerable to generalized diseases primarily affecting either kind of muscle.

Physiology

The act of swallowing triggers a beautifully coordinated sequence of events affecting both skeletal and smooth muscles, and requiring carefully integrated contraction and relaxation of these muscles. The result of this cooperation – primary peristalsis – is to transport material from pharynx to stomach. Figure 34-2 is a diagrammatic representation of the events involved in swallowing. The distally progressive peristaltic wave of increased pressure (a band of contraction some 3 to 4 cm long) sweeps down the esophagus at a rate of 3 to 5 cm per second until it reaches the already relaxed lower esophageal sphincter (LES) and ends by restoring LES tone. This progressive obliteration of the esophageal lumen effectively "milks" the esophageal contents into the stomach. The restoration of LES tone acts to prevent retrograde flow. If initiated by swallowing, the sequence is called *primary peristalsis.* However, stimulation of the esophageal mucosa, either by material remaining after inefficient primary peristalsis or by refluxed gastric contents, can initiate an apparently identical process called *secondary peristalsis.* A misnomer, *tertiary peristalsis,* has been applied to local, nonpropulsive, ineffective esophageal contractions. The term *esophageal peristalsis* is appropriate only to the entire integrated process, which includes properly timed relaxation of both upper and lower esophageal sphincters as well as the distally progressive wave of contraction.

The LES is a specialized area responsible for the very important function of preventing gastroesophageal reflux. This small segment (3 to 5 cm) of distal esophagus has been the subject of much more interest than all the rest of the esophagus. Naturally, controversy has been generated in proportion to this interest. The following statements about LES function seem now to be backed by solid data:

1. The barrier to gastroesophageal reflux resides in the LES alone and does not depend on mechanical factors such as various acute angulations or resultant flap valves, or on compression by surrounding organs.
2. The LES can prevent gastroesophageal reflux as efficiently when it is located in the chest as when it is located in the abdomen.
3. The major, and perhaps the sole, responsibility for maintaining LES tone resides in the enteric hormone gastrin. Thus gastrin release, triggered by a meal, not only stimulates gastric hydrochloric acid release but also increases LES strength.

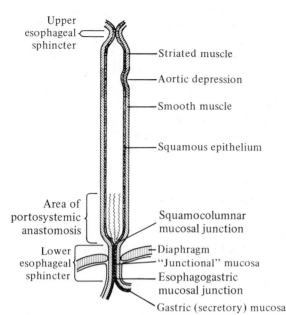

Figure 34-1. *Clinically important anatomy of the esophagus.*

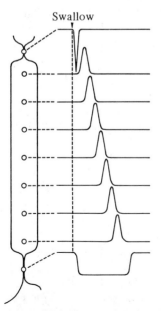

Figure 34-2. Sequential changes in pressure (primary peristalsis) that occur upon swallowing.

4. As an additional mechanism for preventing gastro-esophageal reflux, LES strength increases as gastric pressure increases. The greater the resting or base-line LES strength is, the greater is the LES response to a given increase in gastric pressure. This mechanism is probably neurogenic (reflex) rather than hormonal in origin, but its precise details have not yet been worked out.

Symptoms of Esophageal Origin

DYSPHAGIA

Dysphagia literally means only difficulty in swallowing. As the term is presently used, however, it is much more restricted and precise in meaning. Dysphagia can best be defined as a subjective awareness that a *particular bolus,* solid or liquid, is not pursuing its orderly progression from mouth to stomach and becomes "stuck." The sensation may either be painless or be accompanied by pain *(odynophagia),* but pain is an entirely separate component and need not be present in dysphagia. Used in this proper, restrictive sense, dysphagia is perhaps the most significant and specific symptom arising from the esophagus. In part, the symptom derives its importance from the fact that it is *never* emotional or psychogenic in origin; thus one should never make a diagnosis of "psychogenic" dysphagia. The symptom of dysphagia derives additional significance from the fact that a careful history alone can lead the physician to a correct diagnosis of its cause in about 85 percent of cases. With the use of a few relatively simple additional procedures, the correct diagnoses should approximate 95 to 100 percent. It should be emphasized that these statements apply only if the term is used with discrimination. A patient with a "lump in the throat" sensation (globus hystericus) can actually swallow a bolus perfectly well and thus does not have dysphagia. Similarly, the symptom of substernal fullness or heaviness after eating cannot properly be called dysphagia. The patient must be aware that a particular bolus does not move smoothly from mouth to stomach before he is said to have dysphagia. Any patient with true dysphagia may, of course, also have substernal fullness postprandially (or may experience globus hystericus, for that matter), but these symptoms themselves cannot be called dysphagia.

The type of bolus that causes dysphagia can be of

considerable help in determining the type of lesion responsible for it. Two types of abnormalities can cause dysphagia: defective propulsion or esophageal motor disorders, and lesions obstructing the lumen of the esophagus. Patients with an esophageal motor disorder usually experience dysphagia with solids, but they also have dysphagia with liquids alone. On the other hand, an obstructive lesion does not cause dysphagia for liquids but only for solids. If the obstruction becomes complete or nearly complete, or if a solid bolus is already lodged at the obstruction, the patient may then experience total dysphagia. Therefore, the diagnostic clue afforded by the symptom of dysphagia for liquids is particularly valuable early in the course of a patient's dysphagia. A patient's subjective sensation of the anatomic site of obstruction is usually quite accurate, particularly when the site of obstruction is described as being in the low substernal area near the xiphoid.

ESOPHAGEAL PAIN

Three types of pain arise from the esophagus: (1) pain accompanying disorders primarily affecting the mucosa, (2) pain accompanying disorders of esophageal muscle, and (3) heartburn. Each of these types of pain is sufficiently characteristic as to be of considerable diagnostic value.

Mucosal Pain

Mucosal pain always accompanies swallowing; thus it is properly called *odynophagia*. It usually lasts from seconds to a minute or two, and is described as sharp, sticking, knifelike, or stabbing. An occasional patient may also describe a burning component. The severity is described as varying from only moderate annoyance to extremely severe pain. The variation in severity seems to be among different individuals, with each patient's pain always tending to be approximately equal in severity. The pain is usually located substernally, but it is often described as seeming to go straight through to the back, and occasionally a patient describes the pain as being located primarily, or solely, in the back. The correspondence of the location of the pain (near the xiphoid or near the manubrium) to the location of the lesion responsible for it is fairly good. The most characteristic feature of mucosal pain is its temporal relationship to swallowing; that is, the patient describes pain as

occurring a constant, predictable time (usually a few seconds) after swallowing a bolus.

By far the most common process responsible for mucosal pain is esophagitis resulting from gastroesophageal reflux, but a rare esophagitis of infectious origin or one resulting from ingestion of corrosive liquids may also be responsible. On occasion, pain of this type — particularly when it is felt only in the back — may be a very early symptom of a carcinoma of the esophagus.

The mechanism by which mucosal pain arises is unknown. From the preceding description, one would expect the mechanism to be local stimulation of mucosal pain fibers. Pain fibers potentially responsible for this kind of pain, however, are not found in the esophagus. In fact, the absence of pain fibers is usually considered to be the explanation for the well-established clinical observation that multiple biopsies of esophageal mucosa can be obtained quite painlessly.

Muscular Pain

In contrast to mucosal pain, muscular pain is usually described by the patient as cramping, constricting, crushing, or squeezing; "like a heavy weight"; "like someone sitting on my chest." There is often a vaguely ominous quality to the pain, conveying the impression that it is serious or life-threatening. The duration varies from minutes to as long as an hour or two, although the pain tends to wax and wane in severity when it is of long duration. Muscular pain is also usually located primarily substernally, but it tends to be rather diffuse and to cover a larger area than does mucosal pain. In addition, muscular pain often radiates laterally and occasionally up into the neck or the arms (or both). It is frequently triggered by eating, but it may occur at various times during the day and may even wake the patient from sleep.

It is obvious that many features of muscular esophageal pain also apply to angina pectoris; this similarity and the resultant difficulty in separating the two conditions have been emphasized in many articles. Actually, the resemblance is only superficial, and the physician should experience relatively little difficulty separating them. Not only does angina pectoris have important features of its own such as a temporal relationship to bodily exercise, but pain of esophageal origin is frequently accompanied by other symptoms that are clearly esophageal in origin, such as dysphagia.

Evidence that the mechanism of muscular esophageal pain is spasm of esophageal muscle is compelling, if not absolutely conclusive. This type of pain is usually a feature of disorders of esophageal motor function such as achalasia or diffuse esophageal spasm.

Heartburn

Heartburn combines many of the features of both mucosal and muscular pain. Most patients describe it as a burning sensation, often with a superimposed cramping or squeezing quality. The sensation is primarily located deep substernally, near the xiphoid, but it usually spreads proximally in a wavelike fashion. Occasionally, heartburn extends proximally into the neck, and in these instances the patient often notes the arrival of sour, "burning," or bitter liquid in the mouth, usually in relatively small amounts. On occasion, the liquid may even contain partially digested particles of food. Some patients describe a sudden increase in salivation just before they experience heartburn, and the increased salivation usually continues during the heartburn. Rarely, this increased salivation is so sudden and of such large volume that the patient describes fluid "gushing" into his mouth. When it is this extreme, the increased salivation is often called waterbrash.

The most characteristic feature of heartburn, however, is its relationship to meals and to conditions favoring gastroesophageal reflux. It is often precipitated by bending or stooping over, especially soon after a meal. Heartburn seems to occur at two distinct times after eating: (1) within half an hour, and (2) from 1½ to 2½ hours after eating. Onset of symptoms in the interval (one-half to 2 hours after a meal) seems to be relatively uncommon. Patients with severe or very frequent heartburn tend to have it soon after a meal, and they often have both early and late heartburn. On the other hand, patients with only occasional or infrequent heartburn usually have only the late-onset type of heartburn. Patients — particularly those with early pain — tend to implicate a wide variety of foods. Highly seasoned, spicy foods are often mentioned, but perhaps the most frequently blamed are those rich in carbohydrates and fat — desserts and pastries. Sweet foods containing chocolate (fudge, cake with abundant chocolate frosting) are particularly likely to precipitate heartburn in sus-

ceptible persons. There is experimental evidence that these foods decrease LES strength (or decrease the ability of the LES to prevent gastroesophageal reflux) in both normal persons and in those prone to heartburn. The mechanism of this effect is unknown.

Prompt (if often temporary) relief of heartburn follows ingestion of appropriate amounts of acid-neutralizing substances (commercial antacids, baking soda, or milk) and is so characteristic that failure of these substances to provide relief should make one doubt that the pain is actually heartburn. When heartburn is complicated by esophagitis, however, acid-neutralizing substances may relieve the symptom of heartburn while leaving a residual substernal soreness or a "raw" sensation.

A cause-and-effect relationship between the presence of irritating material in the esophagus (usually from gastroesophageal reflux) and the symptom of heartburn is generally assumed but is only partially supported by experimental evidence. Since irritating material in the esophagus is not always accompanied or followed by heartburn, it is clear that some other factor must also be operative. It seems fair to say that the precise mechanism whereby gastroesophageal reflux produces heartburn is not completely understood.

ESOPHAGEAL BLEEDING

The symptoms just described are highly specific for the esophagus. Bleeding, however, is entirely non-specific and will be mentioned as appropriate in each section dealing with specific diseases of the esophagus. The relative frequency with which various symptoms are found in the common esophageal diseases is summarized in Figure 34-3.

Diagnostic Procedures

A careful, detailed history is by far the most useful diagnostic procedure, allowing the physician both to suspect the presence of esophageal disease and to make a correct, specific diagnosis. Of course, it is important to seek confirmation by other means. The procedures considered to be the most useful are x-ray, endoscopy, cytology, and manometry (Fig. 34-4).

X-RAY

X-ray, when properly performed — whether in the conventional manner using a combination of fluoros-

	Chest Pain	Odynophagia	Dysphagia Solids	Liquids	Heartburn	Bleeding	Regurgitation of undigested food
Achalasia	X	X	X X	X X X			X X X
Diffuse esophageal spasm	X X X	X X X	X	X X X			X
Scleroderma		X	X X	X	X X X	X	
Lower esophageal ring			X X X				X
Benign stricture		X	X X X		X	X	X X
Incompetent LES					X X X		
Esophagitis	X	X X X			X X X	X	
Carcinoma	X	X	X X X			X X X	X X
Zenker's diverticulum			X	X		X	X X X
Esophageal varices						X X X	

Figure 34-3. Relative frequency of symptoms in common esophageal disorders.

copy and spot films, or by the more recently introduced cineradiography techniques — is potentially the single most useful procedure in the diagnosis of esophageal disease. As with many procedures, however, its actual usefulness largely depends on the skill and experience of the person performing the examination. The type of contrast medium used may vary depending on what is seen or anticipated, but certainly the most commonly employed medium is a suspension of barium sulfate in water. As adjuncts to the barium sulfate suspension, various more or less solid boluses are often employed. These boluses may be either radiopaque (e.g., barium sulfate compressed into a wafer, a gelatin capsule containing barium sulfate powder, gelatin containing a radiopaque iodine solution) or radiolucent (e.g., a marshmallow swallowed whole and unchewed, a bolus made of lightly compressed fresh bread). Radiolucent boluses are usually "washed down" by a small amount of barium sulfate suspension.

The potential usefulness of x-ray studies in the diagnosis of lesions of the esophageal mucosa or lesions that are likely to compromise the esophageal lumen (ranging from benign or malignant strictures to esophageal varices) is obvious. Moveover, since cineradiography techniques allow movements to be carefully studied and restudied, they are also often valuable in the diagnosis of motor disorders of the esophagus. Radiology would also seem to be an ideal way to document the presence or absence of gastroesophageal reflux. Despite the many maneuvers designed to facilitate reflux that have been described, this use of radiology has proved to be disappointing. The number of false-positive and false-negative results is so high that little reliance can be placed on either the presence or the absence of radiologically demonstrated gastroesophageal reflux.

ENDOSCOPY
In selected cases (e.g., for diagnosis of esophagitis, evaluation of obstructing lesions, attempts to find the site of upper gastrointestinal bleeding), direct visualization of the esophageal lumen may be of considerable value. The opportunity to obtain a mucosal biopsy under direct vision is also an obvious advantage of this technique. At present, practically all diagnostic endoscopies are performed with flexible fiberoptic

	X-ray	Esophagoscopy	Biopsy	Cytology	Manometry
Achalasia	+ + +	+ +		+	+ + + +
Diffuse esophageal spasm	+ + +				+ + + +
Scleroderma	+ + +				+ + + +
Lower esophageal ring	+ + + +	+ + + +	+ +		
Benign stricture	+ + +	+ + +	+	+	+
Incompetent LES	+ + +	+ + +			+ + + +
Esophagitis	+ +	+ + + +	+ + + +		+ +
Carcinoma	+ + +	+ + + +	+ + + +	+ + + +	+
Zenker's Diverticulum	+ + + +				+ + +
Varices	+ + + +	+ + + +			

+ + + + − May be diagnostic
+ + + − May strongly suggest diagnosis
+ + − May be useful by helping to confirm diagnosis
+ − May be useful by helping to rule out another lesion

Figure 34-4. Relative usefulness of various procedures in the diagnosis of common esophageal disorders.

instruments; rigid endoscopes are now usually reserved for special procedures such as removal of impacted foreign bodies. The procedure can be performed with such relative ease and safety using the flexible fiberoptic instrument that indications for its use are rapidly being expanded. Relative contraindications to endoscopy (even using fiberoptic instruments) include (1) severe bony abnormalities of the cervical spine, (2) large aortic aneurysms, (3) pharyngeal diverticula or strictures, and (4) lack of patient cooperation.

Since endoscopy requires only topical anesthesia and mild sedative premedication, it is not strictly necessary that the patient be hospitalized. The incidence of complications is very low, the most frequent being reaction to the topical anesthesia or the sedation. The most common serious complication of the procedure itself (less than 0.01 percent) is perforation, usually at the cricopharynx. Thus fiberoptic esophagoscopy is a relatively safe procedure, usually involves only minimal discomfort for the patient, and is capable of providing information not otherwise available. As with many methods of investigation, there is good correlation between the skill and experience of the endoscopist and the value and safety of the procedure.

CYTOLOGY

The usefulness of cytology in diagnosing esophageal disease is confined to the diagnosis of neoplasms of the esophagus. Cytology is so highly accurate for this purpose, however, that it has become one of the most reliable and valuable procedures available for investigating the esophagus. In expert hands, a positive diagnosis can be made in over 90 percent of esophageal neoplasms, with a false-positive rate of less than 1 percent. Material for study is acquired either by lavage or by direct brushing of a suspected lesion. Again, the skill, experience, and dedication of the individual performing the procedure are of paramount importance in cytologic diagnosis. Carefully performed, cytology is a highly accurate and valuable method for the diagnosis of esophageal malignancy; performed with carelessness or indifference, the procedure is potentially more harmful than valuable.

ESOPHAGEAL MANOMETRY

Originally a research tool used by physiologists to define normal functions of the esophagus and its sphincters, this technique of measuring pressures from within the esophagus has been shown to be capable of providing clinical information not otherwise available. In particular, manometry can provide precise quantitative data rather than the descriptive information provided by most other methods used to investigate esophageal function. In the most commonly used clinical procedure, pressure is transmitted by thin water-filled plastic tubes to a transducer located outside the patient. Usually, pressures are recorded simultaneously from three different sites that are 5 cm apart. In addition to the three pressure measurements, the usual recording also incorporates separate records of both the patient's respiration and swallowing. The entire tube assembly, consisting of three separate pressure-transmitting tubes fused together, is about 0.5 cm in external diameter. Recently, miniature transducers have been developed that are small enough to be swallowed by the patient, thus eliminating the need for the pressure to be transmitted by a column of fluid. Elimination of the fluid also avoids potential hydrostatic error and possible "damping" of rapid oscillations in pressure. However, the miniature transducers have not yet been shown to be as stable, reliable, and accurate as are the external transducers now in general use. Presumably, future generations of miniature transducers will eliminate the shortcomings of the ones currently available.

In the usual procedure, the pressure-transmitting tube assembly is first advanced until all three pressure-transmitting orifices are in the stomach. The tube assembly is then withdrawn by increments of 0.5 to 1.0 cm, and the effects of both a "dry" swallow (swallowing the small amount of saliva present in the mouth) and a "wet" swallow (swallowing 2.0 to 5.0 ml of water) are recorded. The tube assembly is thus withdrawn step by step until three separate records have been obtained successively from the LES, the body of the esophagus, and the upper esophageal sphincter (UES). It is usually possible to obtain only two measurements from the pharynx.

When the procedure is properly performed, the record obtained provides both quantitative data about strength of the sphincters and graphic evidence of esophageal activity (e.g., peristaltic and nonperistaltic activity, segmental abnormalities). In addition, the degree of coordination between the pharynx and the UES can be studied. Esophageal manometry is most valuable for study of the various motor abnormalities of the esophagus and its sphincters. It cannot provide positive evidence of an obstructive disorder such as a benign or malignant stricture, but it can be helpful in such a case by ruling out a motor disorder having a similar clinical picture.

Diseases of the Esophagus

ACHALASIA

Symptoms

Dysphagia — usually insidious, even intermittent in onset — is the primary symptom of achalasia. Often the dysphagia appears so gradually that the patient cannot really be certain when it began. In fact, after successful treatment some patients cannot remember *ever* having swallowed with so little difficulty. The most important feature of the dysphagia, however, is that it occurs with liquids as well as solids. Many patients seem to have particular difficulty with very cold liquids. The dysphagia cannot be said to be progressive (it does not occur with foods having a progressively finer consistency), but it usually does become more troublesome (or less tolerable) to the patient. There is usually only minimal to moderate weight loss, but often weight is maintained only when the patient spends several hours a day eating slowly. Naturally, social dining must be virtually eliminated. Pain — substernal, varying in intensity, usually cramping or squeezing in character — is common, but this symptom is usually so overshadowed by the dysphagia that patients seldom mention it spontaneously. Pain may occur at any time during the day or night, but it seems to occur most often while the patient is eating.

Other relatively rare symptoms include lung abscess or repeated bouts of pneumonia (presumably secondary to aspiration of retained esophageal material), excess salivation, and painless enlargement of the parotid glands.

Pathophysiology

There is now unanimous agreement that the myenteric plexus is virtually absent in an esophagus afflicted with achalasia. Changes interpreted as being vagal degeneration have also been described, but it is uncertain whether these changes are primary or secondary. The etiology of the absence of the myenteric plexus — or even whether the myenteric plexus has degenerated or has simply never been present — is unknown. There is also evidence that the esophagus is not the only organ involved in achalasia. For example, it has long been known that the achalasic esophagus responds with a tetanic contraction to very small doses of methacholine chloride (Mecholyl). This response is so strong that it has been interpreted as an example of Cannon's law of denervation. However, anyone performing this test cannot fail to note that marked extraesophageal effects, such as profuse salivation, tachycardia, or peripheral vasodilatation, also follow these small doses of methacholine chloride. In fact, the response of the parotid gland to methacholine chloride in achalasia is typical of a denervated gland. It is of interest that a virtually identical esophageal lesion, both functionally and pathologically, is found in association with infection by some strains of trypanosomiasis (Chagas' disease). In Chagas' disease, however, abnormalities of the myenteric plexus are also found in the small bowel and colon, and degenerative lesions are found in the heart. None of these features has been found in achalasia.

The functional esophageal abnormalities in achalasia are striking: The LES is tightly closed and does not relax normally with swallowing; motor activity in the body of the esophagus may be totally absent, but even if some activity is present, it is never peristaltic.

Diagnosis

In most cases of achalasia, the x-ray findings are striking and are not readily confused with any other conditions. Indeed, the diagnosis can often be suspected even from an ordinary posteroanterior chest film (widened mediastinal shadow with an air-fluid level in the esophagus produced by retained contents). Absence of the gastric air bubble is often mentioned as a sign that should make one suspect achalasia, but this sign is unreliable and of little diagnostic value. Barium swallow makes visible the classic, smoothly tapered narrowing or "beak" interposed between the esophagus and the stomach, which is about 5 cm long. This narrowing (representing the LES) is often almost horizontal and points to the patient's left side. The esophagus is often greatly widened (10 to 12 cm) and contains large quantities of a mixture of secretions and previously eaten food. Motor activity may be entirely absent, but if present it is random, seemingly purposeless, and nonperistaltic. Occasionally, the esophageal lumen may be essentially normal in diameter; however, the characteristic beak and the uncoordinated motor activity will practically always be present.

The differential diagnosis between achalasia and a stricture (either benign or malignant) may at times be difficult or impossible to determine. In particular, a carcinoma originating in the gastric fundus and growing submucosally into the distal esophagus may mimic the x-ray picture of achalasia almost exactly.

Esophagoscopy is not of primary diagnostic value in achalasia, but it may be quite valuable in helping to rule out benign stricture or carcinoma (by appearance and because in achalasia the endoscope can easily pass through the narrowed area into the stomach). It is not unusual in achalasia to find that the distal esophagus has the appearance of esophagitis, presumably secondary to the almost constantly retained esophageal contents.

Biopsy and cytology are not of primary diagnostic value in achalasia. They may, however, be valuable in helping to rule out a carcinoma.

Esophageal manometry is the only procedure capable of providing a primary diagnosis of achalasia. The manometric pattern is easily recognized: Resting LES pressure is elevated (35 mm Hg to more than 100 mm Hg, as opposed to the normal pressure of 12 to 30 mm Hg); even more important, the drop in LES pressure with swallowing is incomplete. Normally, resting LES pressure drops by 90 percent or more with swallowing; in achalasia, the drop in pressure is usually only about 50 percent, and often less. Findings in the body of the esophagus are equally clear-cut: Resting esophageal pressure is often, but not invariably, increased; motor activity is variable — there may be either practically no activity or almost continuous uncoordinated activity. The important fact is that coordinated, peristaltic activity is never present. Both the UES and the pharyngeal pressure patterns are normal.

Treatment

As yet there is no satisfactory purely medical therapy for achalasia. Although the function of the body of the esophagus cannot be restored (one cannot restore the absent myenteric plexus), treatment nevertheless is highly satisfactory. All efforts are directed at weakening the LES, either by a direct surgical approach or by rapidly distending the LES mechanically and thus tearing some of its muscle fibers. In the former approach (the Heller procedure) an incision is made through the circular muscle fibers down to the mucosa over the entire length of the LES. The latter approach, a much simpler procedure, consists in the rapid distention of the LES by a firm balloon or other mechanical device to a diameter of about 3.0 to 3.5 cm. Since proper placement of the device is crucial, the procedure is usually done under continuous fluoroscopic guidance. The choice of procedure is largely dictated by the physician's surgical orientation. Both procedures yield satisfactory results in the vast majority of cases, although if one compares the results of a single attempt, the direct surgical approach is perhaps followed by a greater percentage of successes. The simpler distention, however, may be easily repeated, and the ultimate results are comparable. In the rare instance in which rapid distention fails, the direct surgical approach is still available. On the other hand, if surgery is unsuccessful, it is not then advisable to attempt distention but rather to repeat the surgery.

Complications are rare with either method of treatment. A rare patient (probably less than 3 to 5 percent) has a tear into the mediastinum when the distention method is used. Although a few of these tears may require surgical repair, most can be treated satis-factorily by nonsurgical methods. A most serious functional derangement of the esophagus — an incompetent LES allowing free gastroesophageal reflux — may follow the direct surgical approach. This is a dreaded event. In contrast to the normal esophagus in which refluxed gastric contents are rapidly returned to the stomach by secondary peristalsis, in achalasia secondary peristalsis is absent and the refluxed material simply stays in the esophagus until returned by gravity. Thus achalasic patients usually develop severe, intractable esophagitis. This complication is reported to vary from about 5 percent to as high as 25 to 30 percent, but the more experienced surgeons seem to have fewer instances of it. Since rapid distention yields excellent results and is seldom if ever followed by the complication of gastroesophageal reflux, it would seem to be the preferable method of treatment.

DIFFUSE ESOPHAGEAL SPASM

Symptoms

The primary symptom of diffuse esophageal spasm, a relatively rare disorder, is chest pain. The pain is substernal, usually severe, and typical of the muscular esophageal pain described earlier. Pain usually occurs with eating but may also occur at other times, often at night. Cold liquids are usually described as most likely to precipitate the pain. Although pain seems to be the symptom most important to these patients, they also have dysphagia which, not unexpectedly, occurs with both solids and liquids.

Obviously, there is considerable overlap in the symptoms of achalasia and diffuse esophageal spasm, and one cannot always separate these patients on purely clinical grounds. In general, however, patients with achalasia are more troubled by dysphagia, whereas patients with diffuse esophageal spasm are more troubled by pain. Although occasionally a teenage patient is seen, most patients with diffuse spasm are in their forties and fifties.

Pathophysiology

Diffuse esophageal spasm is thought by some authorities to be either an early state of or a precursor to achalasia. Cases have been described in which an individual patient has been followed through what appeared to be typical diffuse esophageal spasm to what appears to be typical achalasia. Such cases, however, are extremely rare. The following facts make it likely that achalasia and diffuse esophageal spasm are actually separate disorders:

1. Achalasia is a relatively common disorder, whereas diffuse esophageal spasm is relatively rare.
2. Patients with achalasia do not give a history suggesting previous diffuse esophageal spasm, although that might be expected if diffuse esophageal spasm regularly led to achalasia. The symptoms of diffuse esophageal spasm are certainly not trivial, easily overlooked, or quickly forgotten.
3. Patients with diffuse esophageal spasm have been followed for years with no change in their clinical, radiologic, or manometric studies.

Surprisingly few pathologic studies have been done in patients with diffuse esophageal spasm, and these studies have yielded conflicting results. Some studies describe an abnormal myenteric plexus, some an entirely normal pathologic picture; in short, the cause is unknown.

Diagnosis
X-rays show considerable random activity, often producing striking patterns colorfully described as "corkscrew" or "rosary bead esophagus," "ladder spasm," and "spastic pseudodiverticulosis." Equally striking is the fact that one cannot correlate the radiologic with the clinical picture; most patients with these colorful radiologic diagnoses are entirely asymptomatic. In short, whereas a patient with clinical diffuse esophageal spasm has an abnormal x-ray picture, the majority of patients with what appears to be the same abnormal x-ray picture do not have clinical diffuse esophageal spasm.

Esophagoscopy is not often done in diffuse esophageal spasm, but when it is performed, the findings are normal. Biopsy and cytology are rarely done, but the findings are also normal.

Esophageal manometry occasionally shows resting LES pressure to be slightly elevated (30 to 50 mm Hg as opposed to the normal pressure of 12 to 30 mm Hg), but LES pressure is usually normal, with a nor-

mal drop in pressure on swallowing. Resting or baseline pressure in the body of the esophagus is normal. The esophageal response to a swallow, however, is grossly abnormal: The postswallowing increases in pressure are both elevated and prolonged (both usually several times greater than normal), repetitive, and nonperistaltic. Occasional, apparently identical, pressure increases occur spontaneously (not preceded by a swallow). In the course of the study, however, a few perfectly normal peristaltic complexes will be seen. The upper esophageal sphincter and pharynx are normal.

Treatment
Treatment of diffuse esophageal spasm is difficult and often disappointing. The therapeutic agents usually employed are local mucosal anesthetics and sympathomimetics. If the patient's symptoms occur primarily with eating (or at other predictable times), pretreatment with long-acting nitrites is often helpful. Recently, a surgical approach consisting of a long esophageal myotomy has been advocated. The myotomy (cutting circular muscle down to mucosa) usually extends from just above the LES to about the aortic arch. Obviously, such a drastic operation should be reserved for the few patients having symptoms sufficiently severe and intractable as to leave no alternative. When the procedure is performed by an experienced surgeon, results are usually excellent. (Incidentally, since only a small percentage of patients with this relatively rare disorder require surgery, there are very few experienced surgeons.)

SCLERODERMA
Symptoms
In this chapter only the esophageal manifestations of scleroderma or systemic sclerosis will be discussed (see Chap. 46).

Heartburn, gradually increasing in frequency and severity, is the most common initial gastrointestinal complaint with scleroderma. When questioned carefully, however, most patients also admit to occasional dysphagia for liquids and solids, the dysphagia often preceding even the heartburn. Later, symptoms of esophagitis and stricture usually appear. With the development of a stricture, the symptom of heartburn often becomes less troublesome. An occasional patient, however, may have well-advanced, clearly diagnostic findings of esophageal scleroderma with minimal or no symptoms.

Pathophysiology
The functionally important lesions of scleroderma are located in the esophageal smooth muscle (the distal two-thirds to three-quarters of the esophagus). Early in the disease, there are small, patchy areas of muscle necrosis and fibrosis; later, these scattered areas become larger and confluent, with resultant extensive necrosis and fibrosis of much of the smooth muscle portion of the esophagus. The striated muscle portion of the esophagus is entirely spared. The early lesions of scattered necrosis and fibrosis of smooth muscle may produce virtually no symptoms. When the muscle necrosis becomes sufficient, however, dysphagia for liquids and solids may develop simply from inadequate motor activity. When the LES also becomes affected, gastroesophageal reflux and the symptoms of heartburn appear and are soon followed by esophagitis and stricture.

Diagnosis
X-ray fails to show the early, scattered lesions by a barium swallow, even when they are known to be present. Later, when there is free gastroesophageal reflux and motor failure of the distal two-thirds to three-quarters of the esophagus, the abnormalities become obvious. The radiologist can rarely suggest scleroderma until the full-blown picture is present.

Esophagoscopy is normal early in the disease; later the complications of esophagitis and stricture will, of course, be seen, but a specific diagnosis of scleroderma cannot be made. Biopsy and cytology do not provide a specific diagnosis of scleroderma. As with esophagoscopy, early results are normal, whereas evidence of esophagitis may be found later in the course of the disease.

Esophageal manometry is diagnostic, often while the patient is still asymptomatic and even before a specific diagnosis of scleroderma can be made from the peripheral findings. Early in the disease, the esophagus is completely normal except for a segment in the body of the esophagus some 1 to 2 cm long in

which no activity is recorded — in essence a "dead" area. Later in the course of the disease, the LES becomes incompetent, allowing free gastroesophageal reflux. Still later, the dead area extends to the entire distal two-thirds to three-quarters of the esophagus, and the LES becomes virtually nonexistent. The proximal esophagus, upper esophageal sphincter, and pharynx, which are all composed of striated muscle, remain normal.

Treatment
Treatment is lacking for the disease itself, and treatment of the esophageal manifestations is limited to attempts at minimizing complications. By far the most serious functional derangement in esophageal scleroderma is the incompetent LES. Whereas gastroesophageal reflux alone may be serious even to a patient without scleroderma, the combination of reflux and a dead distal esophagus may be devastating. Under these conditions, refluxed gastric contents are not returned to the stomach so that esophagitis, ulceration, and stricture formation are almost guaranteed. Attempts to prevent these complications (and to treat them if they are already present) involve the use of frequent antacids and mechanical measures such as making certain that the head of the patient's bed is elevated. Surgical attempts to strengthen or bolster the LES are seldom made because of the danger that the weak or virtually absent esophageal motor activity may be unable to overcome any added barrier from esophagus to stomach. There is no treatment for the necrosis and fibrosis found in the body of the esophagus.

LOWER ESOPHAGEAL RING
Symptoms
A lower esophageal ring produces only one symptom — intermittent dysphagia for solids. Typically, the dysphagia is for elastic solids such as bread or meat. In fact, these solids are so commonly responsible that the condition has been labeled "steak-house syndrome." Unless a solid bolus is already lodged, causing temporary complete obstruction, there is never dysphagia for liquids. In a typical attack, the patient notes first that a given bolus has become stuck. Often, the patient is able to wash down the stuck bolus by a

combination of frequent swallowing attempts and drinking liquids. If these measures are unsuccessful, he is usually able to dislodge the bolus by induced gagging or vomiting. Once the bolus is dislodged, the patient is usually able to return to the table and continue his meal without difficulty. The presence or absence of dysphagia for any given bolus seems to be related only to its size. Although emotional tension has been cited as a precipitating cause of the dysphagia, this seems unlikely unless the presumed emotional tension can somehow influence the size of the bolus the patient attempts to swallow.

Pathophysiology

A lower esophageal ring is a weblike esophageal constriction in the distal esophagus, usually at the junction of squamous and columnar epithelia. The underlying tissue is a varying mixture of fibrous, areolar, and muscular tissues. The ring probably represents hypertrophy or exaggeration of a normal structure, but its actual cause is unknown. Functionally, the lower esophageal ring marks the junction of the distal esophagus and the proximal extent of the LES. The fact that the lower esophageal ring is located at the squamocolumnar mucosal junction (and is located radiologically some 2 to 3 cm above the diaphragm) is often cited as evidence that all patients with a lower esophageal ring must therefore have a hiatus hernia. However, the distal esophagus (primarily the LES) is normally lined by nongastric columnar epithelium called *junctional epithelium*. This fact together with the studies that have shown the area just distal to a lower esophageal ring to function as LES, not stomach, makes untenable the often-repeated statement that all patients with a lower esophageal ring have a hiatus hernia.

Diagnosis

X-rays of a lower esophageal ring show it as a sharply defined narrowing located some 2 to 3 cm above the shadow of the diaphragm. This narrowing or constriction is about 0.5 cm long, with the residual lumen varying from 3 or 4 mm to 20 mm or more. Most symptomatic lower esophageal rings leave a residual esophageal lumen less than 12 to 15 mm in diameter. The area immediately distal to the ring often looks like a hiatus hernia (but see the preceding section on pathophysiology). Since a lower esophageal ring can be found in at least 20 percent (probably 60 to 80 percent if carefully looked for) of "normal" asymptomatic individuals, it is important to prove that a lower esophageal ring found on x-ray is actually responsible for a given patient's dysphagia. This is done by giving the patient a large, solid bolus (bread, a whole marshmallow) and demonstrating that it obstructs at the ring and that this obstruction reproduces the patient's spontaneous symptoms.

Esophagoscopy using the older, semirigid endoscopes rarely visualizes the lower esophageal ring; however, it is routinely seen with the newer fiberoptic instruments. Its appearance is about as one would expect — a smooth, mucosa-covered, weblike narrowing with a concentric opening.

Biopsy and cytology are rarely done. Biopsy shows that the lower esophageal ring is usually located at the squamocolumnar mucosal junction. Esophageal manometry, not unexpectedly, shows normal findings.

Treatment

By the time a patient is recognized as having a symptomatic lower esophageal ring, he has usually become convinced that his symptoms are emotional in origin. Probably the most important aspects of treatment, therefore, are assurance and demonstration that an organic lesion is responsible for the symptoms, together with reassurance that the lesion is not a cancer and will not shorten the patient's life. Once the patient understands the mechanism of his symptoms, he is usually able to control them simply by more careful chewing. In an occasional patient, the residual lumen is so small that these simple measures are insufficient; in such patients, the ring may either be stretched (or torn) by rapid distention of a balloon (as with achalasia), or surgically incised or removed. Overall, the results of treatment are gratifying.

BENIGN STRICTURE

Symptoms

A benign stricture causes only one symptom — dysphagia for solids. Any associated symptoms are the result of the process responsible for the esophagitis that preceded the stricture.

Pathophysiology

A benign stricture represents fibrosis secondary to esophagitis. The esophagitis may be infectious in origin, or it may follow ingestion of corrosive liquids, but both of these causes are exceedingly rare. In the overwhelming majority of cases, the esophagitis responsible for benign stricture follows gastroesophageal reflux. However, gastroesophageal reflux is much more frequent than esophagitis which, in turn, is much more frequent than fibrosis or benign stricture. While quantitative differences in the degree of reflux are clearly important, it is unlikely that this is the only factor involved in causing esophagitis. Variations in the degree of esophageal mucosal resistance and in the corrosiveness of the refluxed material are probably at least as important as is variation in the amount or frequency, or both, of gastroesophageal reflux. Thus, some patients give a history of frequent heartburn or daily regurgitation (or both) for many years and do not have even minimal esophagitis, whereas other patients with severe esophagitis and stricture give a clinical history suggesting that gastroesophageal reflux has been present for only a few weeks. In the majority of cases, however, patients with a benign stricture have a history of long-standing gastroesophageal reflux.

Diagnosis

X-ray (barium swallow) typically shows a smoothly tapered, concentric narrowing of the distal end of the esophagus. Occasionally, however, the narrowing is sufficiently eccentric or has enough edema and, perhaps, ulceration, that it is difficult or even impossible to differentiate it from a carcinoma. The degree of narrowing varies considerably; on occasion, the esophageal lumen may be almost completely obliterated.

Esophagoscopy makes a stricture and any associated esophagitis easily visible, but the degree of confidence with which the endoscopist can differentiate a benign from a malignant lesion varies. Essentially, absence of signs suggesting malignancy are considered points in favor of a benign stricture.

Biopsy and cytology, as with endoscopy, cannot make a positive diagnosis of a benign stricture; they can only show lack of evidence of a malignant one.

In the proper hands, repeatedly negative cytology can be considered excellent evidence against the presence of a malignant lesion.

Esophageal manometry provides no specific findings pointing to a benign stricture. A weak LES is usually found, but this means only that the patient is likely to have gastroesophageal reflux.

Treatment

From the preceding discussion, two things should be obvious: (1) No single diagnostic procedure can positively differentiate a benign from a malignant stricture, and (2) proper treatment requires that this be done. Fortunately, the combination of a good clinical history and a properly performed x-ray examination (plus, in selected patients, esophagoscopy and cytology, and, rarely, esophageal manometry) almost always allows the diagnosis of a benign stricture to be made with considerable confidence.

Once the diagnosis of a benign stricture has been made, treatment theoretically should be directed at two levels: (1) the stricture itself, and (2) the underlying gastroesophageal reflux and esophagitis. Even if one could reliably stop all further gastroesophageal reflux, it would seem unreasonable to expect a fibrotic stricture to dilate by itself. The fact that strictures occasionally seem to do just that suggests that some apparent strictures are really edematous, not fibrotic. Generally, a benign stricture will require dilation with a series of mercury-filled bougies, starting with one small enough to just pass through the stricture and slowly increasing the size to bougies more than an inch in diameter. The bougies are not forced; only the weight of the mercury column serves to dilate the stricture. It is usually necessary to repeat the dilation at intervals. Medical treatment of the gastroesophageal reflux consists in the frequent use of antacids and measures such as elevating the head of the patient's bed, which is designed to make gravity decrease the likelihood of gastroesophageal reflux.

Few would disagree with the treatments outlined above. However, an appreciable number, if not a majority, of these patients will be found on careful x-ray examination to have a hiatus hernia; hence, it is widely believed that a hiatus hernia predisposes to or creates a weak LES. If this were the case, it would seem logical to repair all hiatus hernias surgically — or at least those demonstrably responsible for enough LES weakness to cause esophagitis and a stricture. On the other hand, careful studies designed to show if and how a hiatus hernia may produce LES weakness have failed to find any relationship between LES weakness and hiatus hernia. Since a high percentage of all persons have a hiatus hernia (probably more than half the population over age 50), one would expect a high percentage of those with gastroesophageal reflux and stricture to have a hiatus hernia also. Therefore, one may ask, why repair surgically something that is a (statistically) normal structure? Obviously, there is some merit in both points of view, and the following approach seems a reasonable compromise. As long as nonsurgical treatment of a patient yields clinically satisfactory results, it should be continued. The majority of patients with a benign stricture will do relatively well on a combination of intermittent dilation and medical management of the gastroesophageal reflux. In an occasional patient, however, either the stricture cannot be satisfactorily dilated or medical management fails to provide adequate control of gastroesophageal reflux. In others, the stricture is already so narrow that it cannot be adequately dilated (or it cannot be adequately dilated for some other reason). In these cases, surgical dilation of the stricture under direct vision (usually from below) seems reasonable. While the operation is in progress, of course, the hiatus hernia can be repaired at the same time, and one of the various wraparound procedures may also be performed.

INCOMPETENT LOWER ESOPHAGEAL SPHINCTER

Symptoms
Heartburn is the only primary symptom of an incompetent LES. This symptom has been fully described. Esophagitis and stricture (also discussed earlier in this chapter) are common complications.

Pathophysiology
It is a common misconception that the LES displaced into the chest by a hiatus hernia is necessarily weaker than one in its normal location below the diaphragm

and in the abdomen (but see the section on treatment of benign stricture). Recent evidence strongly suggests that the most important factor in maintenance of LES strength is the hormone gastrin, and that an incompetent LES is the result of a defect in this mechanism. The precise nature of the defect (whether faulty LES response to endogenous gastrin, quantitative or qualitative defects in the release of endogenous gastrin, or the presence of a gastrin inhibitor) is not yet known.

Diagnosis
X-ray may reveal gastroesophageal reflux in patients complaining of reflux, but it also frequently reveals reflux in patients having no symptoms at all. Moreover, x-ray evidence of gastroesophageal reflux cannot be found in many patients known to have severe clinical gastroesophageal reflux. In short, there are so many false-positive and false-negative results that x-ray evidence of gastroesophageal reflux must be considered an unreliable sign of clinical gastroesophageal reflux.

Esophagoscopy may show a patulous gastroesophageal junction, allowing free reflux, but this cannot be considered a reliable indicator of a weak LES. The complication of esophagitis is better evidence but is not a sufficiently sensitive index.

Biopsy and cytology may show evidence of esophagitis even though the mucosa appears normal to the endoscopist; thus biopsy may be a much more sensitive indicator of this complication of an incompetent LES than simple endoscopy alone. Clinically significant gastroesophageal reflux may occur, however, without the complication of esophagitis.

Esophageal manometry is the only method available for quantitating LES strength. Practically all patients with symptoms of severe gastroesophageal reflux have LES pressures below 8 to 10 mm Hg and often below 5 to 6 mm Hg (the lower limits of normal are 10 to 12 mm Hg). The remainder of the esophagus is functionally normal. On rare occasions, a patient having no symptoms suggesting an incompetent LES will be found to have LES pressures below 8 to 10 mm Hg, and despite the lack of symptoms, the patient can be shown by other means to have frequent gastroesophageal reflux.

Treatment

At the present time, frequent antacids are the mainstay of treatment for an incompetent LES. Incidentally, recent evidence suggests that antacids do not exert their beneficial effect simply by neutralizing the refluxed material, but rather by releasing endogenous gastrin, thereby actually increasing the strength of the LES. Is there any other way that knowing about the gastrin mechanism for maintaining LES strength can help to improve the treatment of an incompetent LES? Certainly, this knowledge can provide a rationale for *not* using some previously advised but unsuccessful methods of treatment. For example, since both a surgical vagotomy and anticholinergic agents (in essence, a medical vagotomy) actually decrease endogenous gastric secretion, they should not be used. Similarly, operations designed to decrease acid production by the stomach (removing the gastric antrum) actually serve to remove the source of most endogenous gastrin, so they would also seem to be an irrational form of therapy for an incompetent LES. Why not, then, administer gastrin itself? Several factors make the presently available forms of gastrin unsatisfactory: (1) They must be given by injection; (2) they have a functional life measured in minutes; and (3) their gastric acid—stimulating properties would result both in inhibition of endogenous gastrin release by the gastric antrum and, possibly, in production of a peptic ulcer. Preliminary studies with the cholinergic agent bethanechol chloride (Urecholine) show that it is effective in increasing LES strength in patients with an incompetent LES; it is possible that longer-acting cholinergic agents will be even more effective.

CARCINOMA

Symptoms

The primary symptom of an esophageal neoplasm is dysphagia. The dysphagia is typically progressive, starting with solids but later including semisolids and finally liquids. The sequence from the initial dysphagia only for solids to virtual total dysphagia and an inability to swallow even saliva may take only a few weeks. Obviously, weight loss may be considerable. Pain is usually not a prominent symptom; most patients describe only a dull, deep, substernal ache of mild to moderate degree, which is sometimes aggravated by swallowing. An occasional patient describes a sharp, "sticking" pain felt only in the midback, between the shoulder blades. This pain occurs only with swallowing and at a uniform interval after each bolus is swallowed; it has been described as feeling as if each swallow irritates a "raw" area. Although this symptom is rare, its importance lies in the fact that it may appear very early, preceding even the dysphagia.

Pathophysiology

The lesions adenocarcinoma and squamous cell carcinoma, which are primarily obstructive, occur with approximately equal frequency. Most adenocarcinomas actually arise from the stomach and affect the esophagus by local invasion.

Diagnosis

X-ray usually provides the first confirmatory evidence of a suspicion gained from the clinical history. The lesion is usually seen as an irregular mass, often completely encircling the esophagus, leaving an eccentric lumen. Adenocarcinomas arising from the gastric fundus may be difficult — or impossible — to differentiate from benign strictures unless a primary site in the fundus is sought and found.

Esophagoscopy usually reveals the irregular, often ulcerated, mass. Occasionally, however, the endoscopist sees only esophagitis proximal to a stricture that he is unable to pass, and thus he may be unable to determine whether the stricture is benign or malignant.

Biopsy and cytology obviously may be diagnostic of carcinoma. A biopsy showing only esophagitis, however, cannot be considered to be reliable negative evidence. On the other hand, repeated, properly performed cytologic examinations are highly reliable and are of almost equal value whether positive or negative.

Esophageal manometry may occasionally be of value in helping to differentiate between achalasia and carcinoma. This procedure, however, has no direct value in the diagnosis of esophageal carcinoma.

Miscellaneous Disorders of the Esophagus

The abnormalities described in the preceding sections

make up the vast majority of clinically significant disorders affecting the esophagus. Other abnormalities are either so rare or so poorly understood that they are described only briefly here. Most have a clinical history and diagnostic signs that are only minor variations of the abnormalities already described. These miscellaneous disorders are grouped under three headings.

MOTOR DISORDERS

Only three motor disorders of the esophagus (achalasia, diffuse esophageal spasm, and scleroderma) are adequately characterized; patients are seen, however, who do not fulfill the criteria for any of these disorders and yet who clearly seem to have an esophageal motor disorder. Symptoms are highly variable but usually include occasional dysphagia for both solids and liquids (predominantly solids) and vague substernal chest pain. Diagnostic procedures (the most important of which is esophageal manometry) either have completely normal results or exhibit only minor changes. These patients are designated as having a *nonspecific motor disorder of the esophagus;* treatment is symptomatic, and the prognosis seems excellent.

A variety of diseases affect only esophageal skeletal muscle (the opposite of scleroderma); these disorders include both dermatomyositis and a variety of myopathies (varying from the myopathy seen rarely in thyrotoxicosis to the myopathy seen with malignant disease and that seen in myasthenia gravis). Although the esophagus is usually involved as only part of the generalized muscle disorder, esophageal involvement may occasionally dominate the picture.

OBSTRUCTIVE DISORDERS

Both *leiomyomas* and *leiomyosarcomas* can arise from the esophagus. Patients usually complain of dysphagia for solids, but the clinical history is often not specific enough to allow the correct diagnosis to be even suspected. Rarely, an aberrant right subclavian artery may arise directly from the aortic arch and pass posterior to the esophagus, compressing it against the trachea anteriorly. Although this abnormality is obviously congenital, symptoms (dysphagia lusoria) of dysphagia for solids may not be noted until the

patient reaches age 30 or even later. This abnormality cannot be suspected from the history alone, but it may be suggested by a barium swallow and confirmed by aortography.

A web arising anteriorly at the level of the cricopharyngeal muscle has occasionally been described in association with chronic iron-deficiency anemia (the Plummer-Vinson syndrome). This lesion is so poorly understood that many authorities even question its existence.

OTHER DISORDERS

A *diverticulum* arising anteriorly from the pharynx just proximal to the upper esophageal sphincter (Zenker's diverticulum) has been ascribed to pharyngocricopharyngeal incoordination. The symptoms, which are usually not characteristic enough to allow a diagnosis from the history alone, include effortless regurgitation of undigested food, occasional dysphagia, and a vague sensation of "heaviness" and "gurgling" in the neck or high substernal area. The diverticulum can be confirmed by careful radiologic examination and by finding incoordination between the pharynx and the upper esophageal sphincter on careful esophageal manometry. Treatment includes surgical excision of the diverticulum and surgical section of the upper esophageal sphincter. Diverticula may also arise from the esophagus proper, particularly just proximal to the lower esophageal sphincter.

A variety of *traumatic esophageal tears or lacerations* may occur; the best known is the Mallory-Weiss syndrome, a linear mucosal tear at the esophagogastric junction that occurs following prolonged vomiting, particularly in alcoholics. Hematemesis is the cardinal feature of the syndrome, and the diagnosis is confirmed by endoscopic demonstration. In most patients bleeding stops spontaneously, and surgical intervention is unnecessary.

Bibliography

Castell, D. O., and Harris, L. D. Hormonal control of gastroesophageal sphincter strength. *N. Engl. J. Med.* 282:886, 1970.

Cohen, S., and Harris, L. D. Does hiatus hernia affect competence of the gastroesophageal sphincter? *N. Engl. J. Med.* 284:1053, 1971.

Cohen, S., and Harris, L. D. The lower esophageal sphincter. *Gastroenterology* 63:1066, 1972.

Cohen, S., and Lipshutz, W. Hormonal regulation of human lower esophageal sphincter competence: The interaction of gastrin and secretin. *J. Clin. Invest.* 50:449, 1971.

DiMarino, A. J., and Cohen, S. Characteristics of lower esophageal sphincter function in symptomatic diffuse esophageal spasm. *Gastroenterology* 66:1, 1974.

Ellis, F. H., Jr., and Olsen, A. M. (eds.). *Major Problems in Clinical Surgery.* Vol. 9, *Achalasia of the Esophagus.* Philadelphia: Saunders, 1969.

Harris, L. D. Dysphagia. *Adv. Intern. Med.* 15:203, 1969.

Ingelfinger, F. J. Esophageal motility. *Physiol. Rev.* 38:533, 1958.

Payne, W. S., and Olsen, A. M. (eds.). *The Esophagus.* Philadelphia: Lea & Febiger, 1974.

35

Gastroduodenal Disorders

Thomas A. O'Gorman

Gastroduodenal Symptoms

Gastric mucosal lesions are generally silent and give rise to symptoms only if they breach the mucosa, or if they are so located anatomically that they can cause obstruction, for example, at the cardia or at the pylorus. When there is a tear, erosion, or ulceration of mucosa the patient may have gastrointestinal bleeding.

The most common presenting syndrome is the so-called peptic ulcer equivalent, in which pain is the most constant and important feature. The pain is frequently of such low intensity that the patient will deny it, but on direct questioning he will admit to discomfort. This sensation of pain is localized to the epigastrium, and its most characteristic feature is that it is relieved by anything that raises the gastric pH above 3.0; thus vomiting, nasogastric suction, administration of antacids, or ingestion of food will all relieve the symptom.

Anorexia, nausea, and vomiting may be caused by a local gastric lesion. It is important to quantitate the volume of the vomitus, and particularly to inquire if the patient has recognized any food eaten 4 or more hours previously. Voluminous vomiting and the presence of undigested food suggest a problem with gastric emptying. A gastric lesion must always be considered in any patient presenting with significant weight loss. Lesions at the cardia often produce dysphagia.

Although the symptoms just discussed require an investigation of the upper gastrointestinal tract, they have no specificity in etiologic diagnosis. As mentioned, dysphagia and delayed vomiting of ingested material may be of aid in localizing the lesion. Computer analyses of the symptoms of patients with gastric ulcer, gastric cancer, gastritis, and duodenal ulcer have not differentiated these disorders.

PHYSICAL SIGNS

Physical findings are few in patients with gastroduodenal disorders. An epigastric mass may suggest a very late gastric carcinoma. Point tenderness on deep palpation is sometimes found in patients with peptic ulcer. The most valuable finding is the presence of a succussion splash more than 4 hours after the last ingestion of food or liquid; it usually means that there is a disorder of gastric emptying. If in addition peristaltic waves are visible crossing the epigastrium, then outlet obstruction rather than defective motility is likely.

SPECIAL STUDIES

Radiology: The Upper Gastrointestinal Barium Study
Radiologic examination using barium as the contrast material remains the mainstay of gastroduodenal investigation. An upper gastrointestinal barium study (UGI) shows the relationship of the stomach and duodenum to the surrounding organs; it demonstrates the distensibility of the stomach; and it is particularly useful in detecting gastric ulcers and mass lesions that are not confined to the mucosa. Unfortunately, a UGI is less accurate in detecting lesions that are confined to the gastric mucosa. Recently, however, the study of this area has been improved by means of a modified technique using both gas and barium — the so-called double-contrast examination.

Endoscopy
In recent years the introduction of flexible, fiberoptic endoscopes combined with "target" cytology and biopsy (that is, cytology and biopsy of a lesion under direct vision through an endoscope) has greatly improved gastroduodenal diagnosis. In all gastric lesions (e.g., an ulcer, a mass, or thick mucosal folds), the radiologist's impression should be confirmed by these methods.

Cytology
Wash cytology is performed in a fasting patient. The stomach is first emptied via a nasogastric tube and is then lavaged with 300 ml of saline solution, whereupon the aspirated wash is rapidly processed by a cytology laboratory. In good hands a single gastric wash yields positive cytology in 85 percent of patients with proved gastric cancer. Wash cytology is also valuable in any patient in whom endoscopy is not

possible, or in whom target cytology is negative despite an endoscopic appearance of malignancy.

Acid Studies

The process of measuring gastric acid secretion has undergone many changes during the years. At present acid output is measured both in the basal state and after stimulation of the parietal cells by a maximal, parenteral dose of an acid-secretagogue. The secretagogue of choice is now pentagastrin. A number of acid determinations are made:

1. Basal acid output (BAO); this refers to the acid produced during 1 hour by the fasting, unstimulated stomach.
2. Maximal acid output (MAO); this refers to the highest hourly output of acid after stimulation with a maximal dose of secretagogue. It is obtained by adding together the milliequivalents of acid in each of the four highest consecutive 15-minute samples.
3. Peak acid output (PAO); this is the summation of the two highest consecutive 15-minute samples after maximal stimulation, and it gives the peak acid output in 30 minutes. It is usually doubled and expressed as the PAO per hour.
4. Achlorhydria; a patient is said to be achlorhydric if his fasting gastric pH is above 6.0 and does not fall below 6.0 or more than one pH unit after maximal stimulation.

The MAO is directly proportional to the number of parietal cells in the stomach, and it approximates the acid output after a protein meal. Acid output is generally low in patients with gastric cancer, low or normal in those with gastric ulcer, normal or high in patients with duodenal ulcer, and high in those with the Zollinger-Ellison syndrome. Since there is considerable overlap in these conditions, certain other facts are useful:

1. Twenty percent of symptomatic gastric cancer patients are achlorhydric at the time of diagnosis.
2. If the MAO is greater than 20 mEq per hour, the patient is extremely unlikely to have a gastric cancer.

3. If the MAO is less than 12 mEq per hour, the patient does not have an active duodenal ulcer.

In every patient with a gastric lesion one should quickly establish whether or not the stomach makes acid. A gastric ulcer in a patient who is achlorhydric must be considered malignant. Acid studies should be performed in all patients prior to surgery for peptic ulcer disease, in order to identify any who may have an unsuspected Zollinger-Ellison syndrome (see later in this chapter), and to establish baseline data in a patient who might return postoperatively with an ulcer. In addition, acid studies should be obtained in every patient with a postoperative recurrent ulcer and in all those suspected of being acid hypersecretors. The latter group includes (1) patients with a complication of duodenal ulcer; (2) patients with postbulbar or jejunal ulcers; (3) patients with bulbar ulcers who have thick gastric folds, a "wet stomach," and an abnormal small-bowel pattern on UGI; and (4) patients with secretory diarrhea, with or without peptic ulcer disease.

Serum Gastrin Levels

Radioimmunoassay now permits the accurate determination of serum levels of the immunologically homogeneous forms of the hormone gastrin, which is normally produced in the antrum and stimulates the parietal cells to produce acid. The stimuli for gastrin secretion include peptide ingestion, vagal stimulation, and local cholinergic reflex responses to antral distention. The release of gastrin is inhibited by acid within the antrum. High serum gastrin levels have been noted in the Zollinger-Ellison syndrome; in the retained antrum syndrome (in which antral mucosa remains at the proximal end of the duodenal stump, and since it is excluded from an acid milieu, there is no inhibition of gastrin release); in achlorhydric or hypochlorhydric persons (again, no acid); in pyloric outlet obstruction (antral distention); and in the short bowel syndrome. It should be clear that a serum gastrin level cannot be evaluated without making acid studies. At present, a fasting serum gastrin level should be obtained in (1) all patients about to undergo peptic ulcer surgery; (2) all patients with a postoperative recurrent ulcer; (3) all patients suspected of having the Zollinger-Ellison syndrome on clinical grounds; and (4) all patients with a BAO greater than 10 mEq per hour, or with a BAO/MAO ratio of 0.4 or greater. (For additional details see Table 35-1, which shows acid and gastrin levels in various disorders, and the discussions on the Zollinger-Ellison syndrome and postoperative recurrent ulcer later in this chapter.)

Mucosal Biopsy

Blind suction mucosal biopsy is useful in the examination of the stomach only in those disorders in which the mucosa is diffusely abnormal, such as diffuse gastric atrophy (see later in this chapter, under Atrophic Gastritis and Gastric Atrophy).

Nasogastric Suction and Tests of Gastric Emptying

In any patient in whom a disorder of gastric emptying is suspected, residual fasting gastric volume should be measured by nasogastric suction. This volume is normally less than 150 ml.

SEQUENCE OF STUDIES

In an elective workup of a suspected gastroduodenal lesion, an upper gastrointestinal barium study should be the first investigation. Subsequent investigations, if any, are then determined by the findings on the UGI. The role of endoscopy in a symptomatic patient with a negative UGI remains controversial. Any patient over age 40 with a recent onset of symptoms and a negative UGI should have an endoscopic search made for gastric cancer or an ulcer. On the other hand, a patient with many negative UGIs who has been complaining about vague pains for years generally does not warrant endoscopy unless there has been a recent change in his symptomatology.

Chronic Peptic Ulcer Disease

In the gastrointestinal tract, the term *ulcer* is reserved for lesions in which there is loss of superficial epithelium and in which the depth of the lesion involves or extends below the muscularis mucosae. Similar lesions that remain superficial to the muscularis mucosae are called *erosions*. A *peptic ulcer* is defined as a benign ulcer that arises in a part of the gastrointestinal tract bathed by acid-peptic juice. Peptic ulcers can therefore be found in the esophagus (with reflux of gastric juice), the stomach, the duodenum, or the jejunum (in hypersecretors who may have the Zollinger-Ellison syndrome; at gastrojejunal anastomoses; and in a Meckel's diverticulum, ectopic gastric mucosa in a congenital ileal diverticulum). The duodenum and the stomach are by far the most common sites of ulcers, as will be discussed in detail later.

EPIDEMIOLOGY

The annual prevalence rate for all peptic ulcer disease in a London general practice was 16 per 1,000. A prevalence rate of 17.2 per 1,000 was obtained in a health interview survey in the United States. In Massachusetts, 10 percent of physicians over age 45 have, or have had, a duodenal ulcer. Duodenal ulcers are more frequent than gastric ulcers in men. In women the frequency of duodenal ulcers is about equal to that of gastric ulcers. Mortality rates, incidence of complications, prevalence rates in health surveys, and disability rates for peptic ulcer disease are all declining in the United States, indicating a true regression of the disease. The reasons for this decline are not known.

Although duodenal ulcer may occur at any age, its incidence peaks in the third and fourth decades, while the peak incidence of gastric ulcer is one decade later; thus the latter disease is predominant in the middle-aged and the elderly.

DUODENAL ULCER

The etiology of duodenal ulcer is unknown, but certain facts about the disease have been established:

1. As a group, patients with duodenal ulcer have a higher than normal BAO and MAO.
2. The total parietal cell count is greater than normal.
3. The pH of the duodenal bulb is lower than normal.
4. There is increased responsiveness to pentagastrin in patients with duodenal ulcer, so that a smaller dose than in normal persons is required to produce a 50 percent maximal secretion.
5. Fasting serum gastrin levels are normal, but the total gastrin output in response to a protein meal is increased.
6. In addition, patients with duodenal ulcer have a diminished sensitivity in the negative feedback, pH inhibition of antral gastrin release.

Table 35-1. Acid and Gastrin Studies in Various Disorders

Type of study	Normal levels	Gastric adenocarcinoma	Gastric ulcer	Duodenal ulcer	ZE syndrome	Retained antrum	Hyper-secretor	Gastric atrophy
BAO (mEq/hr)	0–5	0–5	Varies	0–18	> 10	Varies	> 10	0
MAO (mEq/hr)	15–35	< 20	Varies	> 12	Varies	Varies	> 45	0
BAO/MAO	< 0.6	< 0.6	< 0.6	< 0.6	> 0.4	> 0.4	> 0.4	Not applicable
Gastrin (fasting)	Depends on lab	Normal or ↑↑a	Normal or ↑↑a	Normal	> Lab mean × 3	> Lab mean × 3	Normal	> Lab mean × 3
Gastrin (IV secretin)	↓	↓	↓	↓	↑↑	↓	↓	↓
Gastrin (IV Ca++)	↑	....	↑	↑	↑↑↑ Increase > 500 pg/ml	....	↑	....
Gastrin (on acid infusion into antrum)	No change or ↓	No change or ↓↓↓a	No change or ↓↓↓a	No change or ↓	No change	Infusion in retained antrum ↓↓↓↓	No change	↓↓↓

aAt MAO < 12 mEq/hour there is an inverse ratio between acid output and gastrin level in serum.

7. Smoking is positively associated with duodenal ulcer disease, and smokers have lower serum secretin levels after perfusion of the duodenum with acid. In addition, the pancreatic output of bicarbonate is reduced in smokers as compared to nonsmokers.

Clinical Features

The patient with a duodenal ulcer usually presents with epigastric pain or discomfort, which commences approximately 2 hours after the last meal and not infrequently awakens him in the early hours of the morning. The discomfort, often described as a burning or gnawing sensation, is relieved by food and antacids. The patient typically has a good appetite and does not vomit or lose weight. In fact, if a patient with known duodenal ulcer disease develops anorexia, nausea, or vomiting or begins to lose weight, one should suspect a complication such as penetration, obstruction, or an associated gastric ulcer, and a UGI should be obtained promptly. The pain is cyclical in nature; that is, it may be present for 2 to 3 weeks and then remit spontaneously, only to recur several months later. The course is chronic and recurrent; once a patient develops a duodenal ulcer he has a 95 percent likelihood of recurrence. In some patients duodenal ulcer disease is painless and may present first as a complication (see under Complications of Chronic Peptic Ulcer).

Management

Although duodenal ulcer is a clinical diagnosis, a UGI provides objective evidence and should be performed soon after the patient presents with symptoms. There is no need to follow the ulcer to radiologic healing, and radiologic studies need to be repeated over the years only if the symptoms change or a complication develops. A fasting serum calcium level should be obtained to exclude overt hyperparathyroidism, which may be associated with duodenal ulcer disease. Acid studies should be performed in any patient with a complication or in whom Zollinger-Ellison syndrome is suspected on clinical grounds, and also in all patients scheduled for elective surgery.

Patients with duodenal ulcer can be treated easily as outpatients. All therapy aims at lowering gastric,

and hence duodenal, acidity. It is well established that reducing acidity does relieve symptoms, but there are few controlled studies to show that any form of medical management actually affects ulcer healing. Neutralization of acid is the mainstay of treatment; antacids may be administered hourly during waking hours when the patient is symptomatic. The most popular antacids are combinations of magnesium and aluminum hydroxides. Once the symptoms have been controlled, antacids are administered 1 hour after meals for several weeks; administration at that time supplements the buffering capacity of the meal. The dietary regimens recommended for duodenal ulcer have varied widely; some are designed to neutralize acid, others to limit stimulation of acid output. There are now a number of well-controlled studies showing that dietary manipulations have no effect on the ultimate outcome of duodenal ulcer disease. In fact, frequent small feedings of milk and milk products have been shown to allow the intragastric pH to remain below 3.0 for much longer periods than when three regular meals a day are eaten.

Atropine is as effective as vagotomy in reducing gastric acid output. Unfortunately, the dose of atropine that is effective also produces side effects that are at the very least quite uncomfortable and in most cases unacceptable. Thus anticholinergics are not often utilized, but in a patient who is being awakened each night by ulcer pain, administration of an anticholinergic at bedtime usually allows an uninterrupted night's sleep.

Smoking should be discouraged in patients with duodenal ulcer since it reduces pancreatic bicarbonate output and may retard healing. Alcohol damages the gastric mucosal barrier and in animals, but not in humans, stimulates acid output; because of the former factor, patients with peptic ulcer are usually advised to avoid alcohol. Coffee, both caffeinated and decaffeinated, stimulates acid production. The mechanism is unclear, but it may be mediated via gastrin release induced by the peptides in coffee. For this reason, patients should be advised not to drink either regular or decaffeinated coffee. Ulcerogenic drugs, such as aspirin, should be avoided.

Elective surgery for duodenal ulcer is both safe and effective. For example, vagotomy and antrectomy have both a mortality rate and a recurrence rate of less than 1 percent and give about 90 percent patient satisfaction. Elective surgery is usually recommended for patients with significant complications, such as obstruction, penetration, recurrence of symptoms after simple closure of a perforation, or two major hemorrhages. In addition, surgery may be necessary in a patient who for social, personal, or occupational reasons will not adhere to a medical regimen. Modern ulcer surgery is directed primarily at the physiologic stimulants of the parietal cell, that is, the vagus and gastrin; thus some form of vagotomy or gastric resection which includes the antrum, the site of gastrin production, or both, is currently acceptable.

The type of operation performed will depend on many factors, including the patient's general condition, the anatomic findings at operation, and the personal experience of the surgeon. A vagotomy reduces MAO by 60 to 70 percent, and an antrectomy reduces it by 50 to 60 percent. The mortality rate from vagotomy with or without a drainage procedure is lower than that from a partial gastric resection, although the rate of recurrent ulcer is much higher after vagotomy without resection.

GASTRIC ULCER

The cause of gastric ulcer is not known. There are two popular theories; the first theory postulates that there is interference with gastric emptying (caused by duodenal ulcer disease for example), which results in stasis and distention of the antrum followed by release of gastrin and increase in acid secretion. This acid is slowly emptied, and in the end a gastric ulcer may develop. The second theory contends that reflux of bile through the pylorus damages the mucosal barrier, allowing hydrogen ion [H^+] to diffuse back into the mucosa, resulting in an ulcer. In support of the second theory, it has been demonstrated that patients with gastric ulcer have a higher bile salt concentration in their gastric juice than do control patients; in addition, patients with gastric ulcer reflux barium and other markers more readily from the duodenum. Their pyloric sphincter pressure does not increase with duodenal acidification as it does in normal patients, and this abnormality persists even after healing of the ulcer. Bile salts and lysolecithin

have been shown to damage the gastric mucosal barrier.

These two theories are not necessarily exclusive, since scarring in a patient with a duodenal ulcer can lead to anatomic distortion and persistent patency of the pylorus.

Clinical Features

Epigastric pain or a discomfort similar to that in duodenal ulcer is the main symptom of gastric ulcer. The pain commences sooner after a meal than with duodenal ulcer, and its pattern of occurrence is less consistent than in duodenal ulcer. The pain is relieved by food, antacids, and vomiting. Anorexia, nausea, vomiting, and weight loss are common in patients with gastric ulcer, unlike those with uncomplicated duodenal ulcer. Sometimes the patient has no pain and presents first with a complication.

Management

Unlike duodenal ulcers, gastric ulcers may be malignant; this fact leads to major differences in their management. A UGI will permit detection of more than 90 percent of gastric ulcers, and endoscopy should pick up the remainder. Once identified, the ulcer must be definitely diagnosed as either benign or malignant. On a statistical basis, more than 90 percent of gastric ulcers in the United States are benign. In most cases the radiologist is able to give a definite opinion; such opinions are more than 95 percent accurate. In a minority of cases the radiologist is uncertain, and his accuracy in these cases is about 70 percent. Endoscopy with target biopsy and cytology has an accuracy of more than 98 percent in the differentiation of benign from malignant ulcers; a physician should have this level of assurance about the benignity of an ulcer before embarking on medical therapy. In addition, the physician should establish that gastric acid is present, since an achlorhydric ulcer must be considered malignant. In cases in which target biopsy and cytology are indeterminate despite a radiologic or endoscopic suspicion of malignancy, gastric lavage cytology may be valuable. A controlled course of medical therapy is appropriate in a patient who produces acid, whose biopsy and cytology are benign, and who has the radiologic and endoscopic features of a benign ulcer.

In controlled studies the only treatments that have been demonstrated to accelerate the healing of gastric ulcers are bed rest in the hospital, cessation of smoking, and the use of a drug called carbenoxolone, which is not presently available in the United States (a major side effect of this drug is retention of salt and water). Antacids relieve symptoms, but there is only one controlled study showing that they promote healing. The comments made about diet, coffee, alcohol, and ulcerogenic drugs in the discussion of duodenal ulcers are also applicable to gastric ulcers. Anticholinergics are contraindicated in gastric ulcer, in contrast to duodenal ulcer, as they impair gastric emptying and may delay healing.

A patient with a gastric ulcer should be hospitalized, placed on hourly antacids while awake, and asked to stop (1) smoking, (2) imbibing alcohol and coffee, and (3) ingesting ulcerogenic drugs such as aspirin. After the patient has been in the hospital for 3 weeks, the UGI should be repeated to assess healing. Although there have been reports of malignant gastric ulcers that temporarily healed with medical management, failure of a gastric ulcer to show adequate healing (usually defined as a 50 percent decrease in size after 3 weeks) increases the probability that it is malignant, and such a patient should undergo surgery. If healing is adequate at 3 weeks, the patient is discharged on the same medical regimen, and the x-ray studies are repeated at 6 to 12 weeks to ensure that healing is complete. Seventy-five percent of benign gastric ulcers will heal with medical management. Unfortunately, at least 40 percent will have a recurrence, usually in the same area. In these cases, investigation and management as already outlined must be reinstituted. It is for this reason that many physicians recommend surgery after a single recurrence and that most gastroenterologists agree after a second recurrence.

Surgery is recommended for gastric ulcers that fail to heal with medical management, for recurrent ulcers, and for ulcers complicated by bleeding (usually two major hemorrhages), penetration, or obstruction. The usual operation consists of a distal resection with inclusion of the ulcer site, either through a proximal

tonguelike extension or through a wedge resection. The resection may be accompanied by a vagotomy; the vagotomy is more important if there is associated duodenal ulcer disease. Recurrence of gastric ulcer after this type of resectional surgery is very unusual.

RECURRENT ULCER AFTER PEPTIC ULCER SURGERY
A recurrent ulcer may occur in the duodenum, rarely in the stomach, and on the jejunal side of a gastrojejunal anastomosis, where it is referred to as a *marginal* or *anastomotic ulcer*. The symptoms of a marginal ulcer are often vague and nonspecific. The major complaint is pain, but its location may be unusual and it may not be relieved by food or antacids. Not infrequently the patient presents first with a complication such as bleeding, obstruction, or perforation. Gastrojejunocolic fistula is a rare but well-known complication which, in addition to pain, may cause weight loss, diarrhea, and often steatorrhea. The steatorrhea occurs when the small bowel is contaminated by colonic contents, resulting in bacterial overgrowth. Diagnosis of a fistula is best made by a barium enema examination.

In any patient in whom a recurrent ulcer is suspected, the first investigation should be a UGI. Because an anastomosis is difficult to evaluate radiologically, many marginal ulcers are missed. Even when an abnormality is demonstrated one must decide whether it is a result of the operation or caused by an ulcer. In this decision postoperative x-ray films are invaluable, and therefore all patients who undergo peptic ulcer surgery should have a UGI between 6 weeks and 3 months after the operation. After the UGI all patients with any likelihood of a recurrent ulcer should also be evaluated with endoscopy.

When the diagnosis of a recurrent ulcer is established, the following conditions must be excluded before any further surgery is performed:

1. The Zollinger-Ellison syndrome, which can be excluded with acid and serum gastrin studies (see next page).
2. Retained antrum; acid and serum gastrin studies are also helpful in the case of retained antrum, because they are both elevated when there is no feedback to inhibit gastrin release from the unre-

sected, excluded antrum, which is not exposed to acid. To confirm that no antrum was left behind, the sections of the distal margin of the original gastrectomy specimen should be reexamined for the presence of a cuff of duodenal mucosa.

3. Incomplete vagotomy; if the original surgery included a vagotomy, one must demonstrate by acid studies that the vagotomy was complete. Insulin-induced hypoglycemia (less than 40 mg glucose per 100 ml) causes strong vagal stimulation and, if there are residual vagal fibers, will produce acid secretion. Hypoglycemia is not without risk, and it should be induced only with a physician in attendance, an intravenous line in place, and 50 ml of 50% glucose solution at hand in a syringe for administration in case symptoms of hypoglycemia should develop. This test should never be performed in a patient with cerebral or coronary vascular disease, or in a patient with deficient growth hormone production. If baseline, preoperative acid studies are available, they can be compared with postoperative studies. The finding that the MAO has not been reduced by at least 50 percent after surgery suggests that the vagotomy was incomplete.

Management

Recurrent ulcers should be managed surgically, since they respond poorly to medical therapy and are prone to complications. If the original operation consisted only of a gastric resection, then a vagotomy should be added. If the first operation included a vagotomy that is shown to be complete, then a distal gastric resection should be performed. If the original vagotomy is functionally incomplete, a transthoracic vagotomy is appropriate.

THE ZOLLINGER-ELLISON SYNDROME

The Zollinger-Ellison (ZE) syndrome is caused by the autonomous production of gastrin, either from a malignant or benign tumor of gastrin-producing cells (gastrinoma), or from diffuse islet cell hyperplasia of the pancreas. Nonbeta islet cell tumors are found in the pancreas, but extrapancreatic tumors (most often in the duodenum) may also be responsible for the syndrome. In 60 percent of cases the tumor is malignant; however, the malignancies are biologically low grade, and with hepatic metastases patients may survive even 8 to 10 years. As a result of the chronic overproduction of gastrin, the parietal cells increase their acid output. In addition, the trophic effect of gastrin leads to an increased parietal cell mass, which further augments acid production. All the clinical features of the syndrome are caused by excess acid production. Because ZE may be part of a multiple endocrine adenoma syndrome (type 1), hyperparathyroid, pituitary, adrenal, and other islet cell tumors should be excluded.

Clinical Features

In ZE the symptoms of peptic ulcer or one of its complications are the usual presenting features. Ulcers in unusual sites, such as the postbulbar duodenum or jejunum, should suggest the diagnosis; however, the majority of patients have bulbar duodenal ulcers. Postbulbar and jejunal ulcers may also be seen in hypersecretors of acid who do not have ZE. The radiologist often suggests the diagnosis of ZE when he finds peptic ulcers in association with large gastric folds, a "wet stomach," and thickened duodenal and jejunal folds. As stated in the preceding section, all patients with recurrent postoperative ulcers and especially those with complications, such as bleeding or perforation in the early postoperative period, should be studied for gastrinoma.

Diarrhea is present in approximately 50 percent of patients with ZE and may be associated with steatorrhea. The diarrhea can be relieved by nasogastric suction. The steatorrhea is caused by a lowering of the duodenal and jejunal pH below the level at which lipase is active, thus resulting in relative pancreatic insufficiency. Between 5 and 10 percent of patients with a gastrinoma have diarrhea without peptic ulcer disease.

Diagnosis

All the clinical features of ZE result from the hypersecretion of acid; therefore, patients with high acid output and the clinical features just outlined should be considered as hypersecretors, with the diagnosis of gastrinoma to be excluded. As this implies, patients have been described having these same clinical features, but with normal serum gastrin levels and no tumor.

Acid Studies. The indications for acid studies have already been discussed. In patients with a gastrinoma the parietal cells are under constant high gastrin stimulation, even in the resting state, and the patients therefore have a high BAO. Administration of a maximal dose of a secretagogue will produce little additional increase in acid output. Thus patients with a gastrinoma have a high ratio of BAO to MAO. The criteria currently accepted for identifying hypersecretors (and, therefore, patients in whom a gastrinoma should be excluded by further investigation) are a BAO greater than 10 mEq per hour or a BAO/MAO ratio greater than 0.4. It should be emphasized that these criteria have been somewhat arbitrarily defined and that better, statistically derived criteria should be sought.

Serum Gastrin Studies. If a patient is a hypersecretor in the absence of either the short bowel syndrome, a retained antrum, or pyloric outlet obstruction, and if he has a fasting serum gastrin level greater than 10 times the laboratory's fasting mean level, then the diagnosis of ZE is established. For hypersecretors with intermediate values (that is, a fasting gastrin level between 3 and 10 times the normal mean), some form of provocative test is necessary; for example, intravenous secretin administered to normal patients causes a fall in the serum gastrin level, whereas in patients with gastrinoma there is a paradoxical rise. In another test, intravenous calcium salts infused over a 3-hour period lead to a marked increase in the serum gastrin level in patients with gastrinoma, whereas normal patients have only a moderate rise.

Management of the Patient
with an Established Gastrinoma
Islet tumors are vascular and may be identified by angiography in about 50 percent of cases. Angiography may also be useful in revealing hepatic metastases or the rare solitary, localized tumor. Since fewer than 20 percent of tumors are localized and potentially resectable, therapy is directed against the target organ in an effort to reduce the hypersecretion

of acid responsible for the clinical features; at present this approach means a total gastrectomy. Gastrectomy should always be performed even in patients with obvious hepatic metastases, since death is more likely to result from the complications of ulcer disease than from metastatic disease in these patients, unless they have a total gastrectomy. If a localized gastrinoma is suspected at operation, a total gastrectomy should be performed, unless it can be demonstrated intraoperatively that acid studies have returned to normal after resection of the tumor. Moreover, even when acid studies return to normal, many of the patients subsequently prove to have tumor remaining and require a total gastrectomy.

COMPLICATIONS OF CHRONIC PEPTIC ULCER
The complications of chronic peptic ulcer disease, listed in order of decreasing frequency, are as follows:

1. Bleeding; this is discussed later in this chapter in the section on upper gastrointestinal bleeding. It occurred in 14 percent of patients with peptic ulcer followed over a 15-year period by a general practitioner.
2. Perforation; this is a surgical emergency. It occurred in 6 percent of the same group of patients.
3. Penetration; this occurs when the ulcer extends beyond the stomach or duodenal wall into an adjacent structure such as the pancreas, liver, or bile duct. The pattern of pain often changes, with a new location or radiation, and antacid may fail to relieve the pain. Barium studies show the ulcer extending beyond the confines of the stomach or the duodenum.
4. Pyloric obstruction; this is also discussed later in the chapter. It is the least common complication.

Acute Peptic Ulcer Disease
Under the heading of acute peptic ulcer disease, a number of disorders will be discussed which, despite different names, have many features in common. These disorders include erosive gastritis, hemorrhagic gastritis, acute gastritis, alcoholic gastritis, acute gastroduodenal ulceration, and stress ulceration. In contrast to chronic peptic ulcer disease, the incidence of these acute diseases and the mortality resulting from them have markedly increased in recent years.

CLINICAL FEATURES

Hematemesis is the only valuable clinical clue to the presence of the acute peptic ulcer diseases, and those patients with hematemesis represent only a small fraction of the total number. Free perforation may be the presenting feature when these disorders are accompanied by acute ulcerations, as distinct from erosions.

The macroscopic (and hence the endoscopic) features that are shared by all these acute diseases include erythema, swelling, and friability of the mucosa, often accompanied by mucosal or submucosal petechiae. If these features are accompanied by erosions, the entity is called *erosive gastritis;* if they are accompanied by ulceration, it is called *stress gastritis* or *stress ulceration;* and finally, if there is neither erosion nor ulcer but only blood weeping through the mucosa, it is known as *hemorrhagic gastritis.* Mucosal biopsies show marked edema with or without hemorrhage into the tissue, and there is frequently a polymorphonuclear infiltrate in the lamina propria. The surface cells may be lost (an erosion), or if still present, they are often appreciably flattened when compared with their usual columnar shape. Collections of polymorphonuclear cells may also be found in the gastric pits, forming pit or crypt abscesses.

THE MUCOSAL BARRIER

In the normal stomach a barrier prevents the back-diffusion of hydrogen ion into the mucosa — the so-called mucosal barrier. In the disorders just described, this barrier is lost and H^+ back-diffuses (this has been demonstrated experimentally in man by using lithium as an isotopic marker). There is also a transmucosal potential difference in the stomach of approximately 50 millivolts, the mucosal surface being more negative than the serosal. This difference is thought to result from chloride secretion into the lumen, and it is intimately associated with the mucosal barrier so that when the latter is lost, the potential difference also falls. Agents that disrupt the barrier and reduce the potential difference include aspirin, alcohol, short-chain fatty acids, bile salts, lysolecithin, and urea. The barrier is also damaged in stressed patients; it has been suggested, but not yet proved,

that ischemia is the factor mediating this effect. In animal studies, disruption of the barrier alone is not sufficient to produce gastritis; acid must also be present. Based on this observation, the major prophylactic and therapeutic endeavors in man have been directed toward raising the gastric pH, which is usually accomplished by removing acid via nasogastric suction or by employing monitored neutralization, in which sufficient alkali is added to the stomach to raise the pH to 7.0. There are no controlled studies to show which method is more effective. Both methods are being applied prophylactically to stressed patients considered to be at high risk of developing gastritis; controlled studies are not yet available.

TREATMENT

If gastric bleeding persists despite neutralization or removal of acid, the next mode of therapy is usually perfusion with the vasoconstrictor drug vasopressin (Pitressin) via a catheter, which is placed angiographically in the left gastric artery. Although a controlled series demonstrating the efficacy of such therapy is not available, the general clinical impression is that it arrests the bleeding, at least temporarily.

Surgery is undertaken only if the bleeding continues after all other modes of therapy have failed. The reluctance to operate results from the belief that the only definitive operation is a total gastrectomy, which carries a high surgical mortality in emergency situations. The procedure of vagotomy and drainage has been used but is associated with a high frequency of rebleeding.

Good statistics relative to the prognosis for gastric bleeding in these disorders are not available. It is clear that gastritis in a stress situation is associated with a high mortality rate, reported to be between 20 and 60 percent. The actual number of patients who die because of bleeding is uncertain. Gastritis associated with alcohol intake probably has a much lower mortality. It appears that survival may be related to the underlying general condition of the patient.

OTHER VARIANTS OF ACUTE PEPTIC ULCER DISEASE

Curling's Ulcer

Curling originally described an acute duodenal ulcer

in patients with extensive burns. It is now recognized that patients with burns are subject to the whole spectrum of acute mucosal lesions, of which duodenal ulcer is only one.

Cushing's Ulcer

The ulcers described by Cushing are acute, full-thickness ulcers that occur in neurosurgical patients who have had recent intracranial surgery or a brain injury. The presenting feature may be bleeding but, according to Cushing, free perforations are common. Cushing also noted a peculiar softness of the stomach wall, to which he applied the term *gastromalacia*. Patients with Cushing's ulcer differ from those with the acute lesions previously discussed in that they have high acid output and their mucosal barrier is often intact. They are managed in the same way as a patient who has a bleeding or perforated chronic ulcer. Methods of prophylaxis include antacid administration or acid removal via nasogastric suction. Anticholinergic agents may be of value in this situation by reducing the acid output.

Gastric Cancer

When confined to the mucosa, adenocarcinoma of the stomach is associated with a five-year survival rate of greater than 90 percent; yet in the United States, the overall five-year survival rate of patients with gastric cancer is only 10 to 15 percent. The reason for this low survival rate is that mucosal lesions are "silent," and patients do not present themselves until there is advanced extramucosal involvement. The techniques available to make the diagnosis in the pre-symptomatic stages include endoscopy, double-contrast radiologic examination, and gastric wash cytology. The patients most at risk are the middle-aged and the elderly; the disease is uncommon in patients under age 40 — in fact, 90 percent of patients are 45 or more years old.

In the United States the death rate for gastric carcinoma in men is presently 8 per 100,000, down from the 1950 rate of 18 per 100,000. This rate is continuing to fall. There are five times as many cases of cancer of the colon and rectum as cases of cancer of the stomach in the United States population. The dimensions of the problem and the overall cost make a mass screening program for gastric cancer impractical in the United States; the physician must therefore identify those patients having an increased risk of cancer of the stomach, for whom he should institute individual long-term screening programs. These patients include those with pernicious anemia or gastric adenomatous polyps, and those who have survived 15 or more years after partial gastrectomy. All these entities have the associated features of atrophic gastritis, gastric atrophy (with achlorhydria), and intestinal metaplasia. Although the risk in such patients is five to ten times that of the general population, only about 1 percent per year will develop carcinoma. A program of annual wash cytology, together with double-contrast radiology alternating yearly with endoscopy, is an appropriate screening method.

ETIOLOGY

The etiology of gastric cancer is unknown. Epidemiologic studies suggest that environmental (probably dietary) factors are much more important than genetic ones. Among these are studies showing that Japanese immigrants in the United States have a death rate from gastric cancer close to the high rate found in Japan (69 per 100,000), whereas their children have a death rate closer to that found in the United States.

PATHOLOGY

Macroscopically, gastric cancer presents in three forms: (1) the *malignant ulcer,* (2) the *polypoid* or *mass lesion,* and (3) the *infiltrating lesion,* wherein the tumor spreads submucosally and encases the stomach (linitis plastica). More than 90 percent of primary gastric cancers are adenocarcinomas. The other primary lesions are *lymphoma,* which presents as either an ulcer, a mass, or an infiltrating lesion; *leiomyosarcoma,* which presents as a submucosal or ulcerating mass, and *carcinoid,* which presents as a polypoid mass. Metastases to the stomach most commonly come from primary foci in the breast or lung, and less frequently from malignant melanomas and hypernephromas.

CLINICAL FEATURES

When symptoms of gastric cancer develop they are frequently vague; weight loss is characteristic and is usually associated with anorexia. Early satiety, when the patient has eaten only part of his usual meal, suggests extensive involvement of the stomach. Pain, indistinguishable from that in peptic ulcer, may also be present. A lesion at the cardia may cause dysphagia, while a lesion at the pylorus may present with features of pyloric obstruction, and a gastric succussion splash may be found on physical examination. A mass found on palpation of the abdomen suggests a late lesion.

DIAGNOSIS

The UGI study will usually show an ulcer, a mass, or a rigid stomach. The differentiation of a benign from a malignant ulcer has already been discussed in the section on gastric ulcer. The same procedure should be followed in the evaluation of any other gastric lesion (that is, endoscopy with target biopsy and target cytology should be done after the UGI). The combination of target biopsy and cytology is highly accurate (approaching 100 percent) in diagnosing malignant ulcers and polypoid or fungating adenocarcinomas; however, the accuracy falls to 50 percent in the case of infiltrating lesions. In systemic lymphoma with gastric involvement the accuracy is 70 percent; good statistics are not available for primary lymphoma. Acid studies should be performed, since 20 percent of patients with adenocarcinoma are achlorhydric at the time of their presentation. Gastric wash cytology may be useful when endoscopy is not possible and when, despite a negative target biopsy and cytology, the clinical suspicion of malignancy remains high. In patients over age 40 with suggestive symptoms but a negative UGI, an endoscopy should be performed.

MANAGEMENT

The definitive therapy in all primary gastric malignancies is surgical resection. In the case of lymphoma, the resection should be followed by postoperative radiation. Radiation and chemotherapy have not been very effective for late or recurrent adenocarcinoma. In the near future, trials of adjunctive radiotherapy and chemotherapy are planned for the early postoperative period in patients with adenocarcinoma; it is hoped that such adjunctive therapy will eliminate any malignant cells that remain either locally or systemically after surgical resection. In addition to patients in whom there is a definite tissue diagnosis

of cancer, surgery should also be undertaken in patients whose radiologic and endoscopic features are suggestive of cancer, despite negative biopsies and cytology.

PROGNOSIS

At present, 60 percent of patients who have a laparotomy for gastric adenocarcinoma have a resectable lesion. Surgical mortality is approximately 7 percent, and the overall five-year survival rate is less than 15 percent. For primary gastric lymphoma the five-year survival rate ranges between 20 and 50 percent. In the case of adenocarcinomas, primary resection may fail because of recurrence locally at the anastomosis, or because of metastases to the peritoneum, to the abdominal, thoracic, and cervical lymph glands, and to the liver.

Benign Gastric Tumors

The two main types of benign gastric tumors are the *mucosal adenoma* and the *submucosal leiomyoma.* These tumors must be distinguished from inflammatory polyps, ectopic pancreatic tissue, and polypoid carcinomas. The only certain way of making the distinction is to submit the whole lesion to the pathologist. Thus, whenever possible these lesions should be totally removed; the procedure of choice is a gastrotomy with enucleation of the tumor for submucosal lesions, and removal via an endoscope or gastrotomy for mucosal lesions.

Atrophic Gastritis and Gastric Atrophy

Atrophic gastritis is a disorder in which mononuclear cells heavily infiltrate the lamina propria of the gastric mucosa, and the gastric glands, although present, are reduced in number. By contrast, in *gastric atrophy* there is minimal or no mononuclear infiltration, and there are no gastric glands remaining. Patients with gastric atrophy therefore secrete neither acid nor intrinsic factor. Both disorders are clinically silent but are important because they predispose the patient to pernicious anemia, gastric adenoma, and gastric adenocarcinoma. It has been estimated that for each case of pernicious anemia there are 10 to 20 cases of gastric atrophy. The frequency of adenocarcinoma in atrophic gastritis and gastric atrophy is variously reported at between four and ten times that in the general population. These carcinomas develop in the stomach at points where the gastric mucosa has been replaced by an intestinal type of mucosa. An individual screening program for identifying cancer in these patients has been outlined in the section on gastric cancer.

Upper Gastrointestinal Bleeding

In the emergency condition of upper gastrointestinal bleeding, the patient presents with hematemesis or melena. He may be in shock and may have a bloody nasogastric aspirate. The bowel movements are either bloody or black and tarry in character. Restoration and stabilization of the intravascular volume must precede all attempts to make an etiologic diagnosis. An intravenous line should be placed; blood should be cross-matched; and saline and blood should be administered. A nasogastric tube should be passed, and the stomach should be lavaged with iced saline solution until the return is clear.

A history of previous peptic ulcer disease, gastric surgery, alcohol or aspirin intake, liver disease, previous gastrointestinal bleeding, recent abdominal pain or heartburn, and a clear vomitus preceding the bloody vomitus should be sought. Tenderness in the epigastrium, a pulsatile or nonpulsatile mass, and evidence of liver disease should be searched for on physical examination. However, the diagnosis arrived at from this information is at best only an educated guess. To make an accurate diagnosis one of the following four procedures, or a combination thereof, is necessary: endoscopy, UGI, angiography, or surgery. The particular choice and sequence of diagnostic procedures must be individualized in each case. The aim should be to identify patients with peptic ulcer disease first, since they benefit from early rather than late surgery; endoscopy followed by UGI will identify most of these cases. The common causes of upper gastrointestinal bleeding include gastritis, duodenal ulcer, gastric ulcer, esophageal varices, gastric cancer, mucosal tears at the gastroesophageal junction (Mallory-Weiss syndrome), and esophagitis.

Therapy obviously must be individualized. The treatment for gastritis has already been outlined in the section on acute peptic ulcer disease. A peptic ulcer that continues to bleed or that bleeds a second time should be managed surgically. Variceal bleeding is very difficult to control. Among the present therapeutic modalities is the lowering of portal pressure by infusing vasopressin into a systemic vein or into the superior mesenteric artery. Local tamponade may be achieved by inflating a balloon in the lower esophagus; however, this procedure is fraught with many dangers. Emergency surgery may be necessary but has a very high mortality rate.

Pyloric Obstruction

The clinical syndrome of pyloric obstruction develops when there is a disorder of gastric emptying secondary to a mechanical obstruction at the pylorus or in the proximal duodenum. The most important clinical feature is voluminous vomiting, occurring approximately once or twice a day, in which undigested food eaten at least 4 hours previously is identified. Ninety-five percent of cases are a result of peptic ulcer disease, most often duodenal ulcer. The next most frequent etiology is antral carcinoma. Other causes are rare but include pancreatitis with or without pseudocyst, pancreatic carcinoma, duodenal carcinoma, gallbladder carcinoma, Crohn's disease of the duodenum, traumatic duodenal stricture, a gallstone lodged in the duodenal bulb, and a prolapsing gastric polyp. On physical examination a succussion splash and visible gastric peristalsis should be looked for. Disordered gastric emptying should be confirmed by measuring residual volume (see earlier in this chapter, under Special Studies).

Nasogastric suction should be instituted and continued for several days prior to barium studies, in order to empty the stomach and reduce the mucosal edema. Intravenous fluid replacement is very important to correct the dehydration and the hypokalemic metabolic alkalosis that are usually present. Intravenous feeding to restore positive nitrogen balance and to replenish the protein losses is usually necessary, especially if the obstruction has been prolonged.

Barium studies will outline the obstructing lesion. Additional information can be obtained from endoscopy, biopsy, cytology, and acid studies. Early elective surgery is usually required after the nutritional status has improved and the inflammatory response associated with the ulcer has subsided.

Future Outlook

The management of acid-peptic disease may well be revolutionized in the coming years by the introduction of potent inhibitors of acid secretion. These inhibitors include analogues of histamine that block acid secretion by combining with histamine receptors on the parietal cells. These receptors, which are not blocked by ordinary antihistamines, are known as histamine-2 (H-2) receptors; thus the histamine analogues that reduce acid secretion are called H-2 blockers.* A second group of drugs is comprised of the prostaglandin analogues, which are not destroyed by gastric juice and are potent acid inhibitors. Like the H-2 blockers, they are undergoing extensive investigation at present.

Bibliography

Colcher, H. Current concepts — Gastrointestinal endoscopy. *N. Engl. J. Med.* 293:1129, 1975.

Current concepts in cancer: Gastric cancer diagnosis. *J.A.M.A.* 228:883, 1974.

Grossman, M. I., Guth, P. H., Isenberg, J. I., et al. A new look at peptic ulcer. *Ann. Intern. Med.* 84:57, 1976.

Isenberg, J. I., Walsh, J. H., and Grossman, M. I. Zollinger-Ellison syndrome. *Gastroenterology* 65:140, 1973.

Littman, A., and Pine, B. H. Antacids and anticholinergic drugs. *Ann. Intern. Med.* 82:544, 1975.

Malt, R. A. Control of massive upper gastrointestinal hemorrhage. *N. Engl. J. Med.* 286:1043, 1972.

Morrisey, J. F. Gastrointestinal endoscopy — A review. *Gastroenterology* 62:1241, 1972.

Morrisey, J. F., and Barreras, R. F. Antacid therapy. *N. Engl. J. Med.* 290:550, 1974.

Schiller, K. F. R., Truelove, S. C., and Gwyn Williams, D. Hematemesis and melaena, with special reference to factors influencing the outcome. *Br. Med. J.* 2:7, 1970.

Stabile, B. E., and Passaro, E. Recurrent peptic ulcer. *Gastroenterology* 70:124, 1976.

Veterans Administration Cooperative Study on Gastric Ulcer. *Gastroenterology* 61:567, 1971.

Walsh, J. H., and Grossman, M. I. Gastrin. *N. Engl. J. Med.* 292:1324, 1377, 1975.

Winawer, S. J., Posner, G., Lightdale, C. J., et al. Endoscopic diagnosis of advanced gastric cancer. Factors influencing yield. *Gastroenterology* 69:1183, 1975.

*Cimetidine, the first H-2 blocker available for general use, has just been released by the F.D.A.

36

Diseases of the Small Intestine

Sander J. Robins and John A. Hermos

General Anatomic and Functional Considerations

The most remarkable feature of the small intestine is its enormous surface area, which is conferred not so much by its length as by its circumferential convolutions and the villous projections that extend into its lumen. The anatomic regions of the small intestine, designated as *duodenum, jejunum,* and *ileum,* have no clear boundaries with regard to absorptive cell characteristics, and the functional similarities are greater than the differences in these regions. Indeed, strict regional specialization exists only with respect to vitamin B_{12} and conjugated bile salts, which are both absorbed in the distal ileum. Although absorption of all other nutrients appears to be greater in the proximal than the distal sites, absorption takes place along the entire length of the intestine. In addition, the small intestine has an enormous reserve capacity and can fully compensate for losses of up to one-half its length.

The intestine must be regarded as more than a conduit for nutrients. Although most of the enzymatic digestion of carbohydrates, proteins, and lipids takes place in the intestinal lumen prior to their intestinal uptake, optimum absorption of both protein and carbohydrate is closely linked to an ultimate phase of hydrolysis that occurs within the intestinal brush border. Dietary fat that is digested in the lumen is not further hydrolyzed in the intestinal cells. However, within these cells, absorbed fat is resynthesized to complex lipids and combined with transport proteins for delivery into the lymph.

Symptoms and Signs of Small Bowel Disease

The consequences of malabsorption are reflected chiefly by nutritional deficiencies and by an increase in stool mass. Malabsorption will usually result in weight loss associated with either no decrease or an actual increase in dietary intake. A variety of specific nutritional deficiencies may result, singly or in combination, and on occasion may be more prominent than the weight loss. For example, malabsorption of iron, of vitamin B_{12}, or of folate may produce a significant anemia; malabsorption of vitamin D and calcium may lead to clinically apparent osteomalacia; and malabsorption of vitamin K may produce an increase in prothrombin time with a hemorrhagic diathesis.

Malabsorption of food, especially of fat, results in increased stool bulk without necessarily an increase in stool frequency. Therefore, although malabsorption of osmotically active nutrients may be accompanied by increased water secretion into the small bowel, diarrhea will not ordinarily ensue, provided water absorption in the colon remains normal. The stools of a patient with malabsorption are characteristically light in color, soft, and large in volume (and thus difficult to flush). When fat is excessive, the stools may indeed float, but normal stools may also float when containing an excess of trapped air. When malabsorption of fat is pronounced, the stool may be coated with obvious oil.

Frank diarrhea may occur as a result of small bowel disease in two general circumstances. First, as in cholera, the disease process may produce small bowel hypersecretion, with fluid volumes that simply overwhelm the absorptive capacity of the colon. Second, as in the case of ileal resection, the products of malabsorption (both long-chain fatty acids and bile salts) may directly impair the colonic absorption of water and electrolytes.

Pain is not a usual symptom of small bowel diseases that produce malabsorption. However, transient periumbilical discomfort occurs in many diarrheal illnesses, and severe abdominal pain, typically colicky, occurs in intestinal obstruction or infarction.

Certain generalized diseases of the small intestine that are often, though not invariably, accompanied by malabsorption are also associated with a significant transudation of plasma proteins into the intestinal lumen. A protein-losing enteropathy (specific examples are enumerated later in the chapter) is encountered in extensive inflammatory, ulcerative, or neoplastic disorders of both the surface epithelium and the deeper bowel wall, and it is especially pronounced when the mesenteric lymphatics are obstructed. Loss of plasma protein is not confined to the albumin fraction; thus, although dependent edema resulting from albumin loss may be the most clinically apparent feature, plasma concentrations of the immunoglobulins, lipoproteins, fibrinogen, and all other proteins are also reduced. A number of tests have been designed to demonstrate a protein-losing enteropathy. These tests involve the injection of a radiolabeled protein (such as ^{51}Cr albumin) into the systemic circulation and subsequent measurement of the radioactivity excreted in the stool.

Diagnostic Procedures

A great variety of laboratory tests have been proposed for evaluating patients with presumed malabsorption. Some of these tests have remained strictly research tools; many have not been generally adopted because they measure discrete functions that can be just as reliably assessed by the few readily available clinical procedures described below.

EXAMINATION OF STOOL

The single most meaningful test of malabsorption is the gross and microscopic examination of stool for excess fat and undigested meat fibers. Although the microscopic estimation of steatorrhea clearly is not quantitative, it can be strongly correlated with more tedious chemical estimations of fecal fat. As conventionally performed, a microscopic stool examination can reveal only the magnitude of malabsorption; it cannot indicate the degree of dietary triglyceride hydrolysis. However, pancreatic disease should be strongly suspected when the stool contains an excess of undigested meat fibers and visible oil droplets.

D-XYLOSE ABSORPTION-EXCRETION TEST

The pentose sugar, D-xylose, is absorbed in the proximal small intestine; within 5 hours after a 25-gm oral dose, more than 4 gm is normally excreted in the urine. Urinary excretion of the pentose is impaired not only in the presence of proximal mucosal disease but also as a result of renal insufficiency, delayed gastric emptying, or retention of the pentose within ascites.

SCHILLING TEST

Vitamin B_{12}, combined with intrinsic factor, is absorbed only in the distal ileum after its binding to the intestinal brush border. In the absence of renal insufficiency, a diminished urinary excretion within 24 to 48 hours after the test dose occurs as a result of either ileal mucosal dysfunction or competitive binding by increased concentrations of intraluminal bacteria. Although the phenomenon is as yet unexplained, many patients with pancreatic insufficiency have abnormal absorption of vitamin B_{12} and intrinsic factor, but this abnormality may be corrected by pancreatic enzymes.

RADIOLOGIC PROCEDURES

The most useful of the x-ray studies continue to be plain films of the abdomen to disclose pancreatic calcifications, and barium studies of the small intestine. In the presence of malabsorption secondary to intestinal disease, two general radiologic patterns emerge: Either the intestine may be dilated, with thin plications, while the column of barium is segmented and diluted with intraluminal fluid; or, alternatively, the intestinal folds may be thickened and appear nodular. The first pattern usually indicates a diffuse mucosal destructive disease such as celiac sprue, whereas the second pattern usually represents an infiltrative disease involving primarily the lamina propria and submucosa.

PERORAL JEJUNAL BIOPSY

The peroral jejunal biopsy, which is usually performed after the diagnosis of malabsorption has been confirmed and the intestine implicated, has proved to be a safe and reasonably specific diagnostic measure for identifying mucosal diseases. In general, a biopsy is most productive when involvement is diffuse and primarily proximal in location. Three general patterns of abnormalities may be observed. First, in diseases such as celiac sprue there are combined changes in the villous and crypt architecture, the surface epithelial cells, and the cells within the lamina propria. Although many diverse processes may produce what superficially appears to be an identical intestinal response, better differentiation can be made by examining epithelial cell characteristics and, in particular, the extent of mitotic activity (for example, to distinguish sprue from radiation enteritis or from the intestinal lesion produced by vitamin B_{12} or folate deficiency). Second, infiltrative or immunologic disturbances (such as lymphoma, eosinophilic gastroenteritis, Whipple's disease, or agammaglobulinemia) may involve only the cells of the lamina propria. Finally, parasitic infections of the intestine associated with malabsorption may be diagnosed by identifying the parasites in histologic sections or in intestinal secretions.

A general scheme for employing these several tests to identify diseases producing malabsorption is provided in Table 36-1. The first task is to demonstrate by stool examination the presence of excessive fat, and once this is accomplished, to determine if the process is intraluminal (that is, the result of pancreatic or biliary disease) or intrinsic (the result of intestinal malfunction).

Diseases of the Small Intestine that Produce Malabsorption

In some diseases, both a definite histologic lesion and a precise physiologic mechanism for malabsorption are readily apparent; in others, multiple or unknown mechanisms may exist. The diseases that produce malabsorption may be categorized as follows: (1) disorders of the surface absorptive cells, (2) proliferative disorders of the crypt epithelium, (3) infiltrative diseases (largely involving the lamina propria and submucosa), (4) immunoglobulin deficiency syndromes, (5) small intestinal resections, (6) stasis syndromes, and (7) parasitic infections.

Malabsorption resulting directly from abnormalities of intraluminal digestion, as in pancreatic enzyme deficiency, will not be discussed in this chapter. However, other abnormalities of intraluminal digestion that occur as an immediate consequence of intestinal disease will be considered. These disorders arise mainly from anatomic changes in the intestine (categories 5 and 6) that either disturb the mixing of intraluminal contents (following gastric resection and gastrojejunostomy) or allow intraluminal bacterial overgrowth (such as blind loops and fistulas).

DISORDERS OF THE SURFACE ABSORPTIVE CELLS

Celiac Sprue

Celiac sprue, which is also referred to as gluten-sensitive enteropathy, celiac disease, or nontropical sprue, is an important mucosal disease characterized by (1) malabsorption, (2) a characteristic microscopic lesion of the intestinal mucosa, and (3) clinical and histologic improvement upon removing from the diet the gluten-containing cereal grains (wheat, rye, barley, and oats). Celiac sprue may occur in infants and young children, remit in adolescence, and then reappear in adult life. However, cases frequently occur in adults who have had no apparent childhood disease. Although the disease appears to be confined to the intestine, a curious and unexplained fact is that patients with dermatitis herpetiformis invariably have the intestinal lesion of celiac sprue. Patients with sprue may present with either severe malabsorption that involves all nutrients, a selective malabsorption, or a latent disease that becomes clinically manifest only after a gluten challenge. Typically, the patient with sprue will have moderate steatorrhea, an abnormal D-xylose test, abnormal small bowel x-rays, and an increased net secretion of intestinal fluid, electrolytes, and protein. Peroral biopsy of the proximal intestine will show a characteristic lesion: The mucosal surface is flat, villi are absent, and crypts are hypertrophied with increased mitotic figures; the surface epithelial cells are cuboidal or flattened, are vacuolated, and have a decreased brush border; and the lamina propria contains increased plasma cells, lymphocytes, and polymorphonuclear leukocytes. Gluten, gliadin (an alcohol-extracted protein of gluten), and a glutamine-rich polypeptide digest of gliadin all produce the typical mucosal injury in patients with sprue. However, these cereal fractions in high concentrations do not adversely affect normal persons, and it seems likely that host immunologic and genetic factors play a central etiologic role in this disease. Treatment consists of a gluten-free diet, with the substitution of rice, soybean, and corn products for the toxic cereals. With this therapy, which ordinarily must be continued throughout the patient's life, the clinical symptoms remit and the histologic lesion improves. In intractable cases, corticosteroids have proved beneficial.

Tropical Sprue

Tropical sprue is a syndrome of unknown etiology, characterized by general malabsorption, that occurs in residents of or visitors to certain tropical regions. The Indian subcontinent and the Caribbean have

Table 36-1. Diagnostic Findings in Diseases Producing Steatorrhea

Etiology	Xylose	Schilling test (B$_{12}$ & intrinsic factor administered)	Correction of Schilling test	Other laboratory results
Pancreatic insufficiency	Normal	Abnormal in 40%	Pancreatic	Abnormal x-ray may show pancreatic calcifications. Meat fibers in stool
Bile salt insufficiency				
Bile duct obstruction	Normal	Normal	.....	Increased serum bilirubin
Bacterial overgrowth	Borderline	Abnormal	Antibiotics	Increased intraluminal bacteria. X-ray evidence of stasis, blind loops, or fistula
Ileal resection	Normal	Abnormal	None	(History of surgery)
Intrinsic intestinal disease				
Surface cell (diffuse)	Abnormal	Abnormal	Specific therapy	Abnormal barium pattern (dilatation, thin folds). Abnormal peroral biopsy
Infiltrative	Borderline	Normal	.....	Abnormal barium pattern (nodularity, thick folds). Abnormal peroral or surgical biopsy

historically been major endemic areas, but cases have occurred in North Africa, the Middle East, and most Asian countries. Epidemics of acute tropical sprue have been documented, and sporadic cases may occur in individuals several years after leaving endemic areas. Diagnosis requires, in particular, exclusion of parasitic infections, severe protein-calorie malnutrition, and celiac sprue. The biopsy is not specific and may show a spectrum of changes ranging from a severe villous lesion to simply a moderate infiltrate in the lamina propria. Although the etiology of this disease is unknown, the probable pathogenic mechanism involves an infectious or "toxic" injury to the mucosa. Recently, studies have indicated that increased numbers of aerobic coliform organisms in the intestine may be of pathogenic significance. Most cases of tropical sprue respond to oral tetracycline and folic acid.

It is noteworthy that, in tropical and subtropical populations, small intestinal morphology ordinarily differs from that of North Americans and Europeans. Moreover, many persons in these regions have mild malabsorption but no overt diarrhea or clinical illness. Whether this widespread and largely subclinical state represents a mild form of tropical sprue or whether these two conditions are unrelated is not known.

Acute Nonbacterial Gastroenteritis
Acute nonbacterial gastroenteritis, which is of viral etiology, is characterized by various combinations of nausea, vomiting, diarrhea, headache, abdominal cramps, and fever of 24 to 48 hours' duration. In addition to watery diarrhea, malabsorption of fat, D-xylose, and lactose have been demonstrated. With acute infections in man (experimentally induced), a distinct mucosal lesion occurs in the proximal intestine consisting of shortened villi, hyperplastic crypts, inflammatory cells in the lamina propria, and extensive vacuolation of the epithelial cell cytoplasm. These changes revert to normal with clinical resolution of the illness. It is of interest that the gastric mucosa appears unaffected histologically, despite the frequency of nausea and vomiting. Clinically, viral gastroenteritis is self-limited and requires only symptomatic treatment.

Disaccharidase Deficiencies
The microvillous membrane (brush border) of the intestinal absorptive cells may be deficient in the disaccharidases necessary for the hydrolysis of lactose, sucrose, and maltose. These enzyme deficiencies may be primary (either congenital or acquired) or they may be secondary to other mucosal diseases of the small bowel. The lactase deficiency syndromes are the most important clinically. Congenital lactase deficiency becomes manifest in infants shortly after the initiation of milk feedings, with symptoms of diarrhea, bloating, and — if milk feedings are prolonged — growth impairment. In adults, primary acquired lactose intolerance occurs commonly in blacks and Orientals (about 80 percent), less commonly in Mediterraneans and other Asians, and infrequently in Northern Europeans (about 10 percent). Secondary lactase deficiency is combined with other microvillous enzyme deficiencies and occurs in most mucosal diseases associated with absorptive cell damage. Diarrhea occurs as a result of bacterial fermentation of unabsorbed sugars to organic acids which, by an osmotic effect, produces increased secretion of colonic water.

The diagnosis of lactase deficiency can be made in several ways: (1) by a history of milk and milk-product intolerance in a high-risk person; (2) by a lactose tolerance test, in which an oral lactose load fails to produce a rise in blood glucose and may precipitate diarrhea with stool pH of 5.0 to 6.0; (3) by a small bowel biopsy that is normal histologically but shows diminished or absent lactase activity; or (4) by increased breath hydrogen, which results from fermentation of unabsorbed lactose by colonic bacteria. In most cases, the history is adequate for diagnosis, and the treatment involves removing milk and milk products from the diet and supplementing calcium as needed. Other isolated disaccharidase deficiencies (such as sucrase-isomaltase deficiency) are uncommon and present problems only in pediatric nutrition.

Abetalipoproteinemia
Abetalipoproteinemia is a rare familial disease characterized by inability of the absorptive cells to synthesize the protein moiety of chylomicrons. Thus, while digested lipid is taken up by the cells and resynthesized to triglyceride, newly synthesized triglycerides (as chylomicrons) are not secreted. Although the resulting steatorrhea is mild and the absorption of

water-soluble nutrients remains unimpaired, the peroral intestinal biopsy reveals a distinctive abnormality.
When obtained after prolonged fasting, the biopsy
reveals absorptive cells laden with fat droplets,
whereas no fat is apparent within the lymphatics of
the lamina propria and submucosa. Systemic manifestations may be present and include spiculated red
blood cells (acanthocytes), hypolipidemia, cerebellar
ataxia, and retinitis pigmentosa. Treatment of steatorrhea is symptomatic and usually involves both
reduction of dietary fat and substitution of medium-
chain triglycerides which, after absorption, can be
transported out of the epithelial cells as water-soluble
fatty acids without reesterification to triglyceride.

PROLIFERATIVE DISORDERS OF THE CRYPT EPITHELIUM

The intestinal epithelium is normally renewed rapidly
by proliferative activity confined to the intestinal
crypts. After cell division in the crypts, absorptive
cells progressively differentiate as they migrate onto
the base of the villi and toward the villous tips, where
old cells are shed into the intestinal lumen. In diseases such as celiac sprue and nonbacterial gastroenteritis, absorptive cell injury is accompanied by crypt
hyperplasia and increased mitotic activity, apparently
to compensate for increased cell losses. In contrast to
these hyperplastic states, true villous atrophy may be
produced by certain nutritional deficiencies or by
drugs that inhibit mitosis and cell proliferation.

In untreated pernicious anemia and severe nutritional folate deficiency, DNA synthesis is impaired in
the intestine, as it is in the bone marrow. The histologic consequences in the intestine are a reduction in
mitoses, production of megalocytic crypt epithelial
cells, and shortening of villi. Many investigators believe that in chronic tropical sprue the mucosal lesion
is intensified by the development of folate or vitamin
B_{12} deficiency, and that treatment with these agents
effects a partial remission by improving intestinal
morphology. True villous atrophy may also be encountered in severe protein-calorie malnutrition or
kwashiorkor, and also after therapy with methotrexate and 5-fluorouracil, which are antimetabolites that
impair DNA synthesis and crypt cell division.

Irradiation for pelvic or abdominal malignancies
can produce another intestinal disorder with diminished cell proliferation in both an acute and a chronic
stage. The histologic changes of early radiation enteritis consist of decreased mitosis, short crypts and villi,
and an inflammatory infiltrate in the lamina propria.
Chronic radiation injury is characterized by vascular
changes, with fibrosis and thickening of the submucosa. Malabsorption may occur in either stage of this
disorder and may be accentuated by diarrhea secondary to coexistent radiation-induced disease of the
colon. Malabsorption in this setting is difficult to
treat, but when complicated by bacterial overgrowth
(see the section on stasis syndromes), it may respond
to antibiotics.

INFILTRATIVE DISEASES OF THE LAMINA PROPRIA AND SUBMUCOSA

Whipple's Disease

Whipple's disease is a rare, systemic, potentially fatal
disease that responds dramatically to antibiotic
therapy. Its classic manifestations are fever, arthritis,
lymphadenopathy, and steatorrhea. The small intestine is invariably involved, and thus the diagnosis is
usually established by intestinal biopsy. The lamina
propria of the intestine is infiltrated with large, foamy
macrophages that stain positively with the periodic
acid–Schiff (PAS) technique. On electron microscopy, bacilli are present in the lamina propria and
within the macrophages. Additional histologic findings are clubbing of the villi due to the infiltrate and
dilatation of the lymphatic vessels. Extraintestinal
PAS-positive macrophages have been identified in the
heart, lungs, liver, spleen, endocrine glands, central
nervous system, bone, kidneys, synovium, and lymph
nodes. Clinically, malabsorption of fat is moderate
to severe, and proteins leak into the gut lumen; but
absorption of xylose and vitamin B_{12} is not markedly
impaired. The responsible bacterial organism (or
organisms) has not yet been identified. Recent evidence indicates a possible defect in host cell–mediated
immunity. Treatment with antibiotics, penicillin or
tetracycline results in definite improvement within
several months. Relapses may occur but again respond
to antibiotics.

Intestinal Lymphoma

Lymphoma of the small intestine may be primary
(with an unusually high incidence in Arabs and Mid-

dle Eastern Jews) or it may be secondary to systemic disease. Primary intestinal lymphoma may present as localized disease, in a multifocal and segmental distribution, or as a diffuse process. Although all intestinal lymphomas can cause pain, obstruction, perforation, or bleeding, primary diffuse lymphoma is the most common malignancy that causes malabsorption. Such lesions usually cause a significant protein-losing enteropathy. Barium studies often show an infiltrative pattern, and a surgical biopsy will demonstrate the lymphoma if a peroral biopsy fails to do so. Therapy for localized disease has consisted primarily of surgical resection. In the treatment of diffuse intestinal lymphoma both radiotherapy and chemotherapy have been employed, but with uniformly poor results.

Intestinal Lymphangiectasia

Dilatation of the intestinal lymphatics may be congenital, and if so, it is associated with widespread lymphatic disease elsewhere. Lymphangiectasia may be acquired and localized to the intestine as a result of primary retroperitoneal diseases causing mesenteric lymphatic obstruction. In both conditions a protein-losing enteropathy is prominent, but malabsorption is only minimal. Intestinal biopsy will ordinarily reveal dilated lymphatics within the lamina propria and submucosa, and blunted and distorted villi. In acquired disease, treatment should, of course, be directed against the underlying cause.

Eosinophilic Gastroenteritis

Acute manifestations of allergic phenomena are relatively uncommon in the intestine, except in celiac sprue. Eosinophilic gastroenteritis with primary intestinal mucosal involvement represents a treatable allergic syndrome in which there are acute, severe symptoms, as well as malabsorption. The key diagnostic features are (1) nausea, vomiting, abdominal cramps, and diarrhea following food ingestion; (2) peripheral eosinophilia; and (3) intestinal biopsy findings of collections of eosinophils in the lamina propria, as well as patchy abnormalities of the villi and epithelial cells. In addition to abdominal symptoms, moderate malabsorption of both fat and D-xylose occurs, together with significant losses of plasma proteins into the gut lumen. Barium x-rays of the small bowel show an infiltrative pattern. The offending foods are usually not identified, and the illness requires short- or long-term treatment with corticosteroids.

Other Infiltrative Diseases

Other disorders that cause diffuse or localized infiltration of the lamina propria or the submucosa, or both, include amyloidosis, mast cell disease, tuberculosis, carcinomatosis, and regional enteritis (Crohn's disease). The pathologic features of regional enteritis in the small intestine are essentially the same as in the colon; these features are described in Chapter 37. The other disorders listed are largely systemic and are also discussed elsewhere.

IMMUNOGLOBULIN DEFICIENCY SYNDROMES

The immunoglobulin deficiencies produce a variety of complex, poorly understood lesions of the intestine, some of which are associated with diarrhea or malabsorption. About half of the patients with congenital *agammaglobulinemia* or severe *hypogammaglobulinemia* have gastrointestinal symptoms, chiefly diarrhea. A consistent feature on mucosal biopsy is an absence of plasma cells in the lamina propria. The villous architecture may vary from normal, to intermediate, to flat. Some patients have *Giardia lamblia* infections that respond to treatment. In *dysgammaglobulinemia,* IgA deficiency is constant, IgM may be depressed, and diarrhea and malabsorption are frequent. Barium contrast x-rays show a nodular pattern, and biopsies reveal abundant, hyperplastic lymphoid follicles with scanty plasma cells (nodular lymphoid hyperplasia). The villous architecture is usually normal, and *Giardia* are almost always present. Treatment of giardiasis in these patients generally improves the symptoms (see the section on parasitic infections).

MALABSORPTION RESULTING FROM
SURGICAL RESECTION

The *short bowel syndrome* is usually a consequence of massive intestinal resection undertaken as a life-saving procedure for bowel infarction, strangulation, radiation damage, trauma, or neoplasm; however, it may be induced by intestinal bypass surgery, as for morbid obesity. When more than 50 percent of the intestine is resected, malabsorption of fat and water-soluble nutrients becomes clinically apparent; with losses of 75 percent or more, malabsorption is profound and life-threatening. When only the jejunum is resected, adaptation occurs as a result of compensatory ileal hyperplasia and a corresponding increase in ileal absorptive capacity. Nutritional losses are generalized following large resections, and replacement therapy must often include long-term parenteral supplementation of all nutrients and vitamins.

In contrast, *ileal resection* is accompanied by malabsorption that more specifically affects fat and fat-soluble vitamins and that is not reversed by adaptive changes in the residual bowel. The principal consequence of an ileal resection is bile salt malabsorption, which results in an insufficient bile salt pool and inadequate micellar solubilization of the lipid products of pancreatic hydrolysis. Not only does steatorrhea result, but both the unabsorbed bile salts and the dietary fatty acids induce a net secretion of colonic water and electrolytes, leading to diarrhea ("cholereic enteropathy"). Cholestyramine, an anion-exchange resin that binds bile salts, reduces the colonic water secretion, while substitution of medium-chain triglycerides for dietary (long-chain) fatty acids has been found to ameliorate the steatorrhea. An additional consequence of the diminished bile salt pool is ineffective solubilization of biliary cholesterol together with an increased frequency of gallstones. Moreover, after ileal resection the absorption of vitamin B_{12} complexed to intrinsic factor is abnormal, and patients require lifelong therapy with parenteral vitamin B_{12}. A recently observed consequence of ileal resection is enhanced oxalate absorption and an increased formation of urinary oxalate stones. Treatment should be preventive — simply a reduced intake of high oxalate foods.

A common example of steatorrhea that is caused at least in part by surgical resection is that occurring after gastrectomy and gastrojejunostomy (a Billroth II anastomosis). After such surgery, food enters the bowel distal to pancreatic and biliary secretions, with which the food is poorly mixed. Moreover, since food bypasses the duodenum, pancreatic and biliary secretions may be inadequately stimulated. Malabsorption, however, is usually mild in this situation and requires no treatment. If therapy is necessary one may try either pancreatic enzyme replacement or additional surgery to restore normal intestinal continuity (conversion to a gastroduodenostomy). A possible complication of gastrojejunostomy is bacterial overgrowth occurring in an excessively long, although not necessarily obstructed, afferent limb of the anastomosed small bowel segment. Antibiotic therapy may suffice in this situation, but usually the afferent limb will need to be shortened by further surgery.

STASIS SYNDROMES CAUSING
BACTERIAL OVERGROWTH
A disruption in intestinal continuity and flow results from (1) surgically (and often inadvertently) created blind or self-filling loops, (2) interluminal fistulas, (3) multiple diverticula, or (4) chronic intestinal obstruction. Primary impairment of intestinal motility often has the same consequences as frank obstruction; the former condition may occur as a complication of scleroderma involving the bowel wall, or as a result of a severe visceral autonomic neuropathy caused by diabetes mellitus. In intestinal stasis syndromes, bacterial overgrowth occurs in the proximal small intestine; it is predominantly anaerobic and qualitatively similar to colonic flora. The principal consequences of bacterial overgrowth are (1) bile salt deconjugation, which renders bile salt unavailable for micelle formation and intraluminal lipid solubilization; and (2) vitamin B_{12} malabsorption resulting from bacterial binding of the vitamin. In most cases of bacterial overgrowth, antibiotic therapy eliminates both the steatorrhea and the malabsorption of vitamin B_{12}. However, surgery will often be necessary to correct the underlying anatomic abnormality. Surgery must always be undertaken for a gastrojejunocolic fistula (the result of a perforated anastomotic ulcer), in which colonic bacterial contamination of the proximal small bowel is both continual and massive and, consequently, resistant to antibiotics.

PARASITIC INFECTIONS OF THE INTESTINE
Although many parasitic infections occur in patients who are already malnourished, certain intestinal parasites are clearly capable of producing a malabsorption syndrome.

Giardia lamblia is a flagellated protozoan parasite that proliferates in the proximal intestine; it may be associated with an acute or chronic diarrheal illness, generally accompanied by steatorrhea. *Giardia* have worldwide distribution; they are more frequently found in the stools of children than of adults; and in most affected persons, they cause no apparent symptoms. Epidemics of giardiasis have been reported in travelers, yet cases also occur in apparent nonendemic areas with no obvious epidemiologic explanation. As noted previously, giardiasis is frequently associated with hypogammaglobulinemia, particularly nodular lymphoid hyperplasia. Although the organism can be invasive and may be associated with a nonspecific mucosal lesion, the mechanism by which steatorrhea is caused is not known. Diagnosis of giardiasis requires identification of the organism either in the stool, in the duodenal drainage, or in mucus smears and histologic sections from mucosal biopsies. Treatment with either quinacrine hydrochloride or metronidazole is usually effective.

Coccidiosis, a parasitic infection that occurs rarely in humans, is caused by the sporozoa *Isospora belli, I. hominis,* and *I. natalensis.* Coccidiosis is a common intestinal infection in many wild and domestic animals, and infections in man probably result from contact with animal hosts. In man, coccidiosis is usually a self-limited diarrheal illness, but cases have been seen with chronic malabsorption and have even resulted in death. Coccidia are invasive organisms, and the various sexual and asexual forms of the organism can be identified on surface epithelial cells or in intestinal secretions. The mucosal lesion may be severe, resembling that of celiac sprue with a flat mucosal surface and crypt hypertrophy, or the mucosa may show only mild changes. There has been one report of successful treatment of chronic coccidiosis with pyrimethamine and sulfadiazine.

Capillariasis, infection with the intestinal roundworm *Capillaria philippinensis,* is recognized as a prominent medical problem in the Philippines. The offending parasite is a small roundworm that proliferates within the lumen of the intestine and burrows into the intestinal mucosa. Clinical features include bloating, abdominal cramps, vomiting, diarrhea, weight loss, and malaise. Fat and D-xylose are malabsorbed, fluids are secreted into the gut, and there is a significant protein-losing enteropathy. Examination of

duodenal secretions is the most effective diagnostic procedure, and thiabendazole provides effective treatment.

Strongyloidiasis, infection with the roundworm *Strongyloides stercoralis,* still occurs in warm, rural areas of the United States and has a wide distribution in tropical and subtropical areas. Severe intestinal infections may cause nonspecific abdominal symptoms, diarrhea, and steatorrhea. On occasion, systemic migration of the organism causes fever as well as acute hepatic and pulmonary symptoms. Diagnosis is made by the identification of rhabditoid larvae in the stools or duodenal secretions. Thiabendazole is the most effective available treatment.

Infections with *Ascaris,* hookworm, and the tapeworms are usually asymptomatic. However, in areas in which the dietary intake of iron is marginal, chronic blood loss resulting from heavy hookworm infection may cause anemia. In addition, *Ascaris,* hookworm, and tapeworm infections may all be associated with diarrhea and weight loss, but the mechanisms producing clinical disease are probably multiple and largely unknown.

Tumors of the Small Intestine

BENIGN TUMORS

Involvement of the small intestine with either benign or malignant tumors is uncommon. Of the tumors that do occur, the majority are benign, are of little clinical import, and are usually discovered only at autopsy. These growths include adenomatous polyps, leiomyomas, fibromas, hemangiomas, and lipomas. On rare occasions benign polyps may bleed, or they may intussuscept, causing acute intestinal obstruction. Certain hereditary polypoid syndromes involve the small intestine. The *Peutz-Jeghers syndrome* is characterized by multiple hamartomas of the intestine, stomach, and colon, and by brownish mucocutaneous pigmentation, primarily of the lips and buccal mucosa. Multiple *juvenile polyps* of the stomach, intestine, and colon occur as an isolated inherited disease, or they may appear in the *Canada-Cronkhite syndrome* associated with alopecia, nail dystrophy, and hyperpigmentation. The risk of intestinal malignancy is not increased in these hereditary syndromes.

MALIGNANT TUMORS

Adenocarcinoma of the small intestine is rare, occurs primarily in persons over 50 years, and is usually located in the duodenum or proximal jejunum. These tumors may occasionally arise from large adenomatous polyps or from villous adenomas. Patients with adenocarcinoma can present with pain, bleeding, obstruction, or constitutional symptoms. About half the patients will have either local or distant metastases at the time of diagnosis. The surgical cure rate is approximately 20 percent. *Lymphoma* has been discussed in a previous section of this chapter. It is noteworthy that, in contrast to adenocarcinoma, intestinal lymphoma occurs primarily in younger patients and is generally located in the distal intestine. *Leiomyosarcoma* occurs predominantly in older men and can be found anywhere in the intestine. Abdominal pain and bleeding are the most common presenting symptoms and may be accompanied by a palpable abdominal mass. Surgery is the only effective treatment, with cure rates for resectable lesions being close to 50 percent.

CARCINOID TUMORS

Gastrointestinal carcinoid tumors may arise anywhere, from the proximal stomach to the rectum, but they occur most frequently in the appendix and terminal ileum. By histologic criteria alone, carcinoid tumors are difficult to classify as either benign or malignant; appendiceal carcinoids are virtually all benign, whereas half of the intestinal and colonic carcinoids may be malignant with metastatic lesions. Carcinoid tumors originate from enterochromaffin cells and produce several pharmacologically active polypeptide substances, among them 5-hydroxytryptamine (serotonin), 5-hydroxytryptophan, bradykinin, catecholamines, and histamine. When carcinoid tumors metastasize to the liver, the *carcinoid syndrome* becomes manifest as episodes of flushing and cyanosis, abdominal cramps, diarrhea, bronchoconstriction, and continuous cardiac murmurs. Presumably, the vasoactive polypeptides secreted by these tumors produce the systemic effects. The diagnosis is suspected with the detection of increased urinary 5-hydroxyindolacetic acid and is established by liver biopsy. Treatment includes resection of the primary tumor if it is large,

together with chemotherapy, radiotherapy, the use of various serotonin antagonists, and antihistamines for symptomatic relief. Despite the presence of metastases, patients with malignant carcinoid tumors may have a prolonged survival.

Ischemic Diseases of the Small Intestine

Vascular disorders involving the splanchnic circulation can be broadly categorized as occlusive or nonocclusive. Occlusive diseases are responsible both for the acute symptoms of frank infarction of the bowel, and for the chronic, recurrent symptoms of transient ischemic episodes. Whether the symptoms are acute or chronic, occlusive vascular disease usually occurs in elderly patients with manifestations of ischemic disease elsewhere, and most often as a result of atherosclerosis, which produces narrowing of one or more of the three major abdominal arteries just after their origin in the aorta. Less frequently, acute occlusive disease is secondary to an embolic episode occurring in patients with atrial fibrillation or other known heart disease. Embolic occlusion almost always occurs in the distribution of the superior mesenteric artery, which appears particularly predisposed to occlusion because of its relatively narrow caliber and its oblique takeoff from the aorta.

The predominant symptom of *acute occlusive disease* is sudden, severe abdominal pain, which initially is apt to be periumbilical and colicky, and only later becomes more generalized and constant, when associated with peritonitis. Although tachycardia, hypotension, and leukocytosis are generally profound when pain first begins, the abdominal examination is usually not abnormal, and gastrointestinal bleeding is not apparent until bowel necrosis and peritonitis supervene. A plain abdominal x-ray often shows evidence of ileus with air-fluid levels, but it may also reveal an asymmetrically thickened bowel wall, the result of intramural edema and hemorrhage. Abdominal angiography is the most useful diagnostic procedure and should be undertaken to determine the site of occlusion, unless the procedure would delay necessary surgery unduly. If the patient's condition permits, surgery must be undertaken to resect any gangrenous bowel and to attempt revascularization. Furthermore, a second laparotomy must often be performed within 30 hours of the first, to determine whether or not the unresected bowel remains viable. Survival of the patient often depends not so much on the extent of bowel loss but on the magnitude of associated, complicating illness, especially in the elderly.

Chronic occlusive disease may occur in two distinct patterns. The syndrome of *abdominal angina,* which is by far the more common, is often a harbinger of acute disease, whereas the syndrome of *celiac axis compression* is actually rare but appears readily amenable to surgery. Pain is a prominent feature in both conditions. When secondary to abdominal angina, pain typically occurs 15 to 30 minutes after a meal, leading the patient to avoid food and thus to lose much weight. Bruits may or may not be audible, but angiography typically shows stenosis greater than 50 percent in at least two of the three major abdominal arteries and demonstrates collateral flow. Revascularization surgery, consisting of bypass grafts, endarterectomies, and vessel reimplantations, has been used with variable success. Compression of the celiac axis results from entrapment of this single vessel by contiguous structures (usually the median ligament of the diaphragm), and patients have benefited symptomatically by surgery to free this vessel.

Nonocclusive vascular disease ordinarily occurs in the elderly but is not accompanied by demonstrable arterial stenosis. The precipitating event appears to be diminished cardiac output, usually secondary to shock, congestive heart failure, or drugs that produce splanchnic vasoconstriction (such as digitalis). The process may involve only the mucosa, resulting in a hemorrhagic necrosis, but it may terminate in transmural infarction. Treatment is most often expectant and supportive, with replacement of fluid losses. However, when there is a high suspicion of bowel gangrene, surgical intervention should be employed.

Bibliography

Ament, M. D., and Rubin, C. E. Relation of giardiasis to abnormal intestinal structure and function in gastrointestinal immunodeficiency syndromes. *Gastroenterology* 62:216, 1972.

Donaldson, R. M., Jr. Small bowel bacterial overgrowth. *Adv. Intern. Med.* 16:191, 1970.

Gardner, J. D., Brown, M. S., and Laster, L. Medical progress: The columnar epithelial cell of the small intestine. Digestion and transport. *N. Engl. J. Med.* 283:1196, 1264, 1317, 1970.

Lindenbaum, J. Tropical enteropathy. *Gastroenterology* 64:637, 1973.

Maizel, H., Ruffin, J. M., and Dobbins, W. O. Whipple's disease: A review of 19 patients from one hospital and a review of the literature since 1950. *Medicine* 49:175, 1970.

Marshak, R. H., and Lindner, A. E. Malabsorption syndrome. *Semin. Roentgenol.* 1:138, 1966.

Rubin, C. E., Brandborg, L. L., Phelps, P. C., and Taylor, H. C., Jr. Studies of celiac disease. 1. The apparent identical and specific nature of the duodenal and proximal jejunal lesion in celiac disease and idiopathic sprue. *Gastroenterology* 38:28, 1960.

Trier, J. S. Current concepts: Diagnostic value of peroral biopsy of the proximal small intestine. *N. Engl. J. Med.* 285:1470, 1971.

Waldman, T. A. Protein-losing enteropathy. *Gastroenterology* 59:422, 1966.

Williams, L. F. Vascular insufficiency of the intestines. *Gastroenterology* 61:757, 1971.

Wilson, F. A., and Dietschy, J. M. Differential diagnostic approach to clinical problems of malabsorption. *Gastroenterology* 61:911, 1971.

37

Diseases
of the Colon

Charles J. Schwartz and Philip Kramer

The major functions of the large intestine are (1) to receive the intestinal fluid from the ileum, (2) to absorb water and electrolytes from this fluid, (3) to store the residua temporarily, and (4) to evacuate the fecal waste. Approximately 600 ml of fluid is delivered each day through the ileocecal valve into the large bowel. This ileal fluid contains about 75 mEq sodium, 5 mEq potassium, 36 mEq chloride, and 44 mEq bicarbonate. Since fecal excretions average daily about 100 ml water and contain about 4 mEq sodium, 9 mEq potassium, 2 mEq chloride, and 3 mEq bicarbonate, simple calculation reveals that the colon absorbs 500 ml water, 71 mEq sodium, 34 mEq chloride, and 41 mEq bicarbonate and secretes 4 mEq potassium. These daily processes require only about 20 percent of the normal ability of the colon to absorb water and electrolytes; thus the reserve capacity of the colon is significant.

The large bowel may be subdivided into three principal areas: the right colon (cecum, ascending colon, hepatic flexure, and proximal half of the transverse colon); the left colon (distal transverse colon, splenic flexure, descending and sigmoid colon); and the rectal and anal canals. The rectum, comprising the distal 15 cm of the large bowel, terminates at the anus, which maintains fecal continence by contraction of its internal and external sphincters.

Symptoms of Large Bowel Disease

Important symptoms of colonic and rectal disease include diarrhea, constipation, abdominal pain, and colonic or rectal bleeding. Each of these symptoms may also be produced by noncolonic disorders; however, a careful history can frequently distinguish between colonic and noncolonic diseases. It is important to understand the patient's own definition of a symptom, since the norm for one individual may be abnormal for another; that is, some patients complain of diarrhea with one bowel movement a day whereas others complain of constipation with the same frequency of bowel evacuation.

Diarrhea means abnormal frequency or liquidity of bowel movements. A colonic origin for diarrhea is suggested by frequent, small fecal discharges, especially if accompanied by rectal urgency, tenesmus, or lower abdominal pain that is relieved by defecation. Nocturnal diarrhea awakening the patient is rarely seen in individuals with only functional bowel disease and usually implies organic disease.

Constipation may be defined as the difficult evacuation of feces. The frequency is not important; some normal persons have only a soft bowel movement once a week. Constipated patients may complain bitterly of passing one to two stools a day consisting of small, dry, hard balls known as scybala. Constipation associated with tenesmus usually implies rectal disease. A variant of constipation is the sense of incomplete evacuation often noted in patients with a rectal lesion. Any recent change in either bowel habits or frequency must be investigated.

Abdominal pain — localized to the suprapubic area or to the right or left lower quadrant, and especially when it is relieved by passage of flatus or stool — suggests disease in the large bowel; however, pain may be felt anywhere along the course of the large bowel. *Tenesmus,* which is painful (and often ineffective) straining at stool, is specific for rectal or anal canal disease. Frequent causes of tenesmus include proctitis, thrombosed hemorrhoids, and anal fissures.

Colonic or rectal bleeding can be either overt or occult. *Hematochezia,* the passage of bright red blood per rectum, usually originates from lesions of the large bowel but rarely may appear from upper gastrointestinal hemorrhage (e.g., a bleeding duodenal ulcer combined with rapid intestinal transit). Occult blood in stools can result from a lesion anywhere in the intestinal tract. A formed stool streaked with blood suggests a lesion in the left colon, whereas blood on the toilet paper implies a rectal or anal lesion.

Diagnostic Studies

STOOL EXAMINATION

Microscopic examination of the stool is important for the diagnosis of both parasitic disease and inflammatory disease (see Chap. 39). For example, amebiasis may be diagnosed by demonstration of trophozoites or cysts. Fifty percent of patients with giardiasis pass cysts in the stool. The presence of fecal leukocytes can be used to differentiate the inflammatory causes of diarrhea — including ulcerative colitis and granulomatous colitis as well as infectious colitis with *Shigella, Salmonella,* and amebae — from viral or toxicogenic diarrhea, in which fecal leukocytes are absent. A Gram's stain of the stool can aid in the diagnosis of staphylococcal or clostridial enterocolitis or of gonococcal proctitis in the appropriate clinical setting. Other important stool studies include occult blood tests and bacteriologic cultures.

ENDOSCOPY

Endoscopic studies include anoscopy, proctosigmoidoscopy, and colonoscopy. These procedures should always be preceded by a digital examination of the rectum to detect lesions that may preclude these examinations. Proctosigmoidoscopy is used to evaluate the integrity of the anal canal and rectosigmoid mucosa as well as to exclude mass lesions that are beyond digital examination and should always be performed prior to barium enema x-ray examination. Microscopic evaluation of tissue obtained by rectal biopsy may confirm the presence of disease even in an area that appears normal on inspection. Colonoscopy is used to evaluate suspicious lesions disclosed by barium enema in the right or left colon that are proximal to the reach of the sigmoidoscope. Occult neoplasms or polyps not seen with the barium enema may also be visualized. In addition, biopsies or polypectomies can be performed through the colonoscope, thereby avoiding unnecessary surgery.

RADIOLOGIC STUDIES

A plain film of the abdomen can reveal abnormal collections of air within the lumen or outside of the bowel; it is a key aid in the diagnosis of toxic megacolon. Abnormal calcifications may be seen in the pancreas, gallbladder, lymph nodes, or adrenal glands. Barium enema occasionally detects obstructing carcinoma, polyps, abnormal mucosa, strictures, and fistulas or demonstrates displacement due to a mass. Air contrast studies with barium enema improve the diagnosis of small carcinomas or polyps. Abdominal angiography is helpful in demonstrating hemorrhage from diverticula and cecal angiodysplasia.

OTHER STUDIES

Ultrasound study may confirm the presence of an intraabdominal mass and distinguish solid from cystic lesions. Elevated serum levels of carcinoembryonic antigen (CEA) are found in a number of malignant diseases (e.g., carcinoma of the stomach, pancreas, and colon) as well as in benign inflammatory disorders. CEA is not helpful as a primary screen for malignancy but may assist in monitoring cancer therapy.

Clinical Syndromes

MECHANICAL OBSTRUCTION OF THE INTESTINE

Mechanical obstruction of the small or large bowel can occur with or without interference with its blood supply. The obstruction may be either intraluminal, mural, or extramural. Intraluminal causes include polyps, bezoars, gallstones, foreign bodies, congenital diaphragms, meconium, or fecal impaction; mural etiologies include diverticulitis, hematomas, and strictures due to malignancy, irradiation, or inflammatory bowel disease; extramural etiologies include adhesions, nonstrangulated hernias, or rarer entities such as an annular pancreas. Mechanical obstruction associated with secondary intestinal circulatory interference may result from intussusception, volvulus, strangulated hernias, and closed loop obstruction due to adhesions. About 70 percent of cases of mechanical obstruction are caused by hernias or adhesions. The frequency of any cause varies with age; for example, in the neonate, mechanical obstruction is most commonly caused by meconium ileus, intestinal atresia, malrotation, or a congenital band. In childhood, hernias are the most common cause of obstruction. In geriatric patients, colorectal carcinoma and diverticulitis are more frequent causes.

Clinical Features

During the history taking, one should elicit predisposing factors such as previous abdominal surgery or episodes of pelvic inflammatory disease, regional enteritis, or diverticulitis, all of which may lead to the development of adhesive bands. In the initial stage of proximal uncomplicated, mechanical intestinal obstruction, vomiting is an early complaint and abdominal distention is rare. On the other hand, vomiting is less constant as an early symptom of distal bowel obstruction whereas abdominal distention is common. Other symptoms of mechanical obstruction include obstipation or the failure to pass either gas or feces, and feculent vomitus resulting from stagnation of intestinal contents and bacterial overgrowth. Patients with partially obstructing lesions of the rectum can present with paradoxical diarrhea (discussed later in this chapter). The presence of a fever or leukocytosis in a patient with a mechanical obstruction suggests strangulation, perforation, or an abscess.

Diagnosis

The undisturbed abdomen should be observed closely. Visible peristalsis can sometimes be seen in the distended abdomen while the patient is complaining of crampy abdominal pain. At the same time one may hear borborygmi and peristaltic rushes. Laboratory tests frequently show evidence of dehydration as fluid accumulates in the bowel, indicated by a rise in hematocrit and blood urea nitrogen. Plain films of the abdomen, taken in the supine and upright positions, are helpful in revealing air-fluid levels in the small bowel in a stepladder pattern. Little or no air is seen distal to an obstructing lesion of the colon. Volvulus is suspected from the flat plate alone. With a cecal volvulus, a markedly distended viscus is seen in the left upper quadrant, and little or no gas in the remainder of the colon; in a sigmoid volvulus, an inverted U arising from the pelvis is noted, with air in the remainder of the colon. A barium enema should always be done first to rule out an obstructing lesion of the colon. If a colonic lesion is suspected, upper intestinal barium studies are contraindicated because of the possibility that inspissation of barium might cause obstruction.

Treatment

Treatment of intestinal obstruction depends on the cause. Surgery is indicated for persistent obstruction. If vascular compromise is suspected, the patient should be operated on immediately regardless of his preoperative condition. Patients with simple mechanical obstruction of less than 24 hours' duration usually have a good fluid and electrolyte balance and can undergo early surgery. Other patients with obstruc-

tion of greater than 24 hours' duration may benefit from a delay sufficient for preoperative colloid and electrolyte replacement.

Functional Colonic Disorders

Disorders of the colon and rectum can produce symptoms without any detectable organic lesion; these conditions apparently arise as a result of alteration in physiology or function, and are therefore called functional colonic disorders. The dysfunction may be in muscular contraction (e.g., tone, peristalsis, excretory activity), absorption, secretion, or any combination of these. However, the role of these specific colonic dysfunctions is poorly defined. Consequently, the development and perpetuation of such functional disorders are classified on the basis of their clinical manifestations rather than on their etiology, pathology, or pathophysiology.

IRRITABLE COLON SYNDROME

The term *irritable colon* is used to describe a symptom complex characterized by abdominal pain that is presumably of colonic origin, with constipation or diarrhea or alternating constipation and diarrhea, and sometimes with the passage of mucus. *Mucus colitis* and *spastic colitis* are commonly used synonyms for this disorder. None of the terms is entirely correct because inflammation is absent (hence the condition is certainly not colitis), and although motility studies suggest hyperirritability of the colon, normal persons have similar alterations in motility. In spite of the latter objection, the term *irritable colon syndrome* is preferred for this common disorder, which is seen in about 30 to 50 percent of private or clinic patients with gastrointestinal disorders.

Observations of patients with clinical manifestations of this entity suggest certain possible etiologic factors: (1) psychological or emotional causes in about 80 percent of patients, (2) preceding attacks of infectious diarrhea in 25 percent of patients, and (3) laxative abuse in 30 percent of patients. Most often the symptoms appear to be in response to stress and to frustrating life situations. However, some patients date their disorder to an attack of amebiasis, shigellosis, salmonellosis, or a similar disease. Others attribute their disease to bad bowel habits, that is, failure to have regular bowel movements by inhibiting the urge to defecate because of (1) emotional problems, (2) allowing insufficient time for a movement, or (3) being too busy at the time the urge is present. Repeated inhibition of the urge causes loss of rectal sensibility and hence constipation; a variety of laxatives or enemas may then be taken to produce an evacuation. The unanswered question is whether or not patients who develop the irritable colon syndrome have a true predisposition to this disorder. Once the syndrome has been initiated, secondary factors may play a precipitating or perpetuating role in an attack. Thus, diet (e.g., onions, cabbage, beans, condiments, or highly seasoned foods), roughage, laxatives, and other physical or chemical irritants, as well as intercurrent infections, are often implicated by patients.

Clinical Features

Women are afflicted more commonly than men (2:1) by the irritable colon syndrome. About three-quarters of affected patients are between the ages of 20 and 50 at the time of diagnosis, but they may have had their symptoms for years. Onset above the age of 60 is rare. Patients generally can be grouped into several categories depending on their dominant complaints: (1) patients having abdominal pain with abnormal bowel habits, (2) those having painless diarrhea, and (3) those with pain but no change in bowel function. The pain of irritable colon may be constant, griping, or colicky, and it is most often felt in the left lower quadrant or hypogastrium; however, it may be located anywhere along the course of the colon. If the pain is in the left upper quadrant and radiates to the shoulder and left arm, the pattern has been described as the *splenic flexure syndrome.*

Bowel habits of patients vary considerably. Constipation is usual; sometimes there is diarrhea, but at other times constipation alternates with diarrhea. The constipation is characterized by the passage of scybala and is often associated with the feeling of distention and flatulence. In approximately half the patients, temporary relief of pain occurs with the expulsion of feces or gas. Diarrheal stools, whether or not they are associated with pain, are usually semiliquid or mushy and small in quantity. Only rarely is a patient awakened from sleep by pain or stools. The patient's first bowel movement on arising in the morning or after breakfast is often solid, but the stool becomes progressively less formed on subsequent movements during the day. Excessive passage of mucus, increased abdominal gurgling and rumbling, anxiety, headache, insomnia, and weakness are common. In spite of such multiple, extensive complaints, the patients appear healthy. Tenderness over some part of the colon, particularly in the left lower quadrant or over the cecum, is elicited in about 60 percent of cases. The sigmoid is often palpable.

Diagnosis

No single objective test is diagnostic. Sigmoidoscopy is usually normal but occasionally shows hyperemia or excessive mucus secretion, although the same abnormalities may be observed in asymptomatic persons. The stools do not contain blood or show evidence of malabsorption. It should be emphasized that only about half the patients are relieved of pain by bowel movements, and a significant number have no change in their bowel habits. Consequently, other colonic disorders, infectious diarrheas, other diarrheal and malabsorptive syndromes, other causes of abdominal pain, such as pancreatic or biliary tract disease, and even cardiac disease have been considered in the differential diagnosis. Patient evaluation should include (1) routine blood examinations, (2) stool examinations for blood, leukocytes, fat, pathogenic bacteria, and parasites, (3) sigmoidoscopy, and (4) radiographic examination of the gastrointestinal tract.

Treatment

Most patients with irritable colon syndrome are afraid that they have a serious or life-threatening disease. Hence, a thorough diagnostic investigation as outlined in the preceding section should be conducted first; then reassurance, derived from the fact that no organic disease is found, is the second step in treatment. Success is directly proportional to the patient's confidence in the physician, which is gained by a sympathetic attitude and careful study on the part of the physician. In the patient with constipation, elimination of irritant laxatives must be attempted and satisfactory bowel habits must be reestablished; pain is often eliminated by these methods. A bowel training program should be initiated: The patient is instructed to have a bowel movement at times when he or she is not rushed, particularly in the morning after breakfast. Instead of laxatives, a high fiber diet is recommended, consisting of fresh fruits and vegetables, both twice a day; prune juice, 7 ounces per day at breakfast; and coarse or unprocessed bran, 2 heaping teaspoons three times a day. Additional measures that may help to alleviate pain are applications of heat to the abdomen and oral anticholinergic agents. If diarrhea is the predominant symptom, fresh fruits and vegetables should then be interdicted, and antidiarrheal agents such as diphenoxylate hydrochloride with atropine (Lomotil), 2.5–5.0 mg four times per day, may be given. Hydrophilic colloids are of value for diarrhea, or for alternating diarrhea and constipation, since they make hard stools soft and diarrheal stools firm. Sedatives and antidepressants may also be employed in patients with underlying anxiety or depressive states.

MEGACOLON

Megacolon, or enlargement of the colon, is not a single entity but a manifestation of many diseases, some functional, others organic. It does not lend itself to simple classification and is included here under functional disorders because intrinsic organic intestinal disease is often not demonstrable. Megacolon can be divided into two categories: *congenital* (Hirschsprung's disease or aganglionic megacolon) and *acquired*. Both types are characterized by marked colonic enlargement and by the filling of the colon with large quantities of puttylike feces (in fecal impaction the colon is not enlarged). Although constipation (or infrequency of bowel movements) is the major symptom, it may be obscured by "overflow diarrhea," that is, a leakage of liquid or mushy feces around the fecal mass with soiling of underclothes. Other symptoms and findings may include abdominal distention, palpable fecal masses, cramping abdominal pain, borborygmi, and occasionally nausea and vomiting.

In congenital megacolon there is an absence of Auerbach's (myenteric) and Meissner's (submucosal) plexuses; the aganglionosis usually involves the rectum only, but it may extend proximally for a variable distance and, at times, may even include the entire colon and rarely the small intestine. Skip lesions have been observed, with normal colon intervening. As a consequence of the neurologic defect, the colonic contents are not propelled distally. Subsequently the colon dilates and the feces become static proximal to the aganglionic segment. Peristalsis in the dilated colon is normal or often exaggerated. The disease is more common in males, and a familial tendency has been reported.

Aganglionosis is usually detectable at birth and presents clinically as meconium ileus. Some infants may remain completely obstructed and require early surgery; others may be relieved by rectal manipulation, with an outpouring of fecal material. Rarely, the diagnosis is delayed until childhood, and then it may be confused with acquired or psychogenic megacolon of children. In the latter, the child has a history of having had normal bowel movements at some time during infancy, whereas in the congenital disease constipation is present from birth. Rectal examination in the congenital disease reveals a normal rectal size, but in acquired megacolon the rectum is markedly dilated and full of feces. Barium enema provides confirmation: In acquired megacolon the colonic dilatation extends to include the rectum as far as the anus, whereas in congenital megacolon the rectum is normal in shape and size, the colonic dilatation being proximal. A full-thickness biopsy of the rectum demonstrating absent plexuses is diagnostic of aganglionosis. Motility studies show abnormal motor activity in the aganglionic segment.

Acquired megacolon in the adult may be either psychogenic in origin or secondary to organic disease. The multiple causes include (1) inflammatory bowel disease with obstruction (e.g., Crohn's disease with stricture); (2) pelvic irradiation resulting in proctitis; (3) neurologic disease (e.g., diabetic neuropathy, Chagas' disease); (4) metabolic disorders (e.g., acute intermittent porphyria, lead poisoning); (5) smooth muscle atrophy (e.g., scleroderma, myotonia dystrophica, congenital myotonia); (6) abuse of cathartics; (7) drugs (e.g., antimotility drugs such as anticholinergics or opiates; in Parkinson's disease, megacolon is often produced by trihexyphenidyl [Artane]; and (8) endocrine disease (e.g., myxedema).

Treatment

Once the diagnosis of congenital megacolon is made with certainty, treatment is surgical, with resection of the aganglionic segment and anastomosis of proximal normal bowel to the anal area. Psychogenic acquired megacolon in children should be treated initially with cleansing enemas in order to shrink the dilated bowel; thereafter, attempts are made to establish spontaneous bowel movements by administering increasing amounts of mineral oil. If a specific treatable cause exists (e.g., inflammatory bowel disease, myxedema) then appropriate therapy is directed at the underlying disorder. Otherwise treatment is largely symptomatic and is aimed at establishing spontaneous bowel evacuation (see Treatment, under Fecal Impaction).

FECAL IMPACTION

Fecal impaction is characterized by an absence of bowel movements and the finding on rectal examination of a large fecal mass that is puttylike or hard. The impaction is usually of recent origin, but it may have been present for months in certain predisposed persons. Although the fecal masses are often confined to the rectum and sigmoid, they may extend as far back as the cecum. Certain features are common to most patients regardless of the cause: (1) The rectum is full of feces and (2) the patient has little desire to move his bowels, that is, there is loss of rectal sensitivity. Incontinence (often misinterpreted as diarrhea by both patient and physician) is frequent, with leakage of liquid feces around the impaction with the result that the patient may keep soiling his underclothes, or if bedridden, his bed sheets.

Fecal impaction results from multiple causes, the common denominator being constipation, and it occurs in a variety of situations and patients. The elderly and the debilitated, especially those who are institutionalized, are most susceptible, particularly if they are being treated with tranquilizing drugs, narcotics, or other agents that cause constipation. Fecal impaction may also be observed in the following: (1) patients confined to bed for any reason, but especially for heart disease or orthopedic problems; (2) emotionally disturbed persons, particularly children, who for some reason are upset by having bowel movements; (3) patients for whom defecation is painful because of anal fissures, perirectal abscesses, anal cryptitis, fistula in ano, or ruptured intervertebral disk disease; (4) patients who recently have been given barium, either as an enema or for a gastrointestinal series; and (5) gastrointestinal bleeders who have received constipating preparations (e.g., aluminum hydroxide or calcium carbonate), in whom the intraluminal combination of blood and antacid forms a sticky, nonexpulsive mass.

Diagnosis

The diagnosis of impaction should be suspected in any patient in the above categories, especially if he is in a hospital and has asymptomatic constipation and fecal incontinence. Complaints of a sensation of fullness or incomplete evacuation of the rectum and cramping abdominal discomfort, as well as symptoms produced by the underlying disease, may be described at times. The abdominal discomfort is much less severe than that of patients with irritable colon syndrome, in whom it is often incapacitating and of long duration. On physical examination rectal disease, if present, can be noted, together with fecal masses along the course of the colon and mushy or inspissated feces in the rectum. The extent of fecal accumulation may be seen on a plain film of the abdomen.

Treatment

Therapeutic measures depend in part on the conditions causing the impaction; that is, a patient with a recent myocardial infarction has to be handled differently from one who is elderly or demented. Anorectal disease, especially if painful, needs to be corrected or alleviated to permit other procedures. Large volume saline enemas to stimulate peristalsis and thereby bowel evacuation, or oil retention enemas to soften the stool followed by saline enemas, should be tried first. If these methods are unsuccessful, digital disimpaction is necessary. Fecal impaction beyond the reach of the finger may require the use of a sigmoidoscope and irrigation of the fecal mass via a large-bore rectal tube passed up the sigmoidoscope. In the elderly patient who is confined to bed with loss of rectal sensitivity, stimulating laxatives (e.g., anthraquinone derivatives) may be needed. If the impaction is hard, a combination of mineral oil, 30 ml, and milk of magnesia, 15 ml, may have to be given by mouth several times a day to soften the fecal mass.

Diverticular Disease: Diverticulosis and Diverticulitis

DIVERTICULOSIS

Colonic diverticula of clinical importance are, with rare exceptions, false diverticula; that is, they are saccular outpouchings lacking a muscular coat and consisting of a mucosal layer covered by serosa. Herniations of the mucosa occur through defects in the circular muscle layer, where the intestinal arteries penetrate and form diverticula between the teniae coli, especially on the lateral surfaces of the colon. Although the diverticula are multiple and may be located anywhere along the colon, 95 percent are sigmoidal.

Certain experimental and epidemiologic evidence suggests that diverticulosis is caused by a deficiency in dietary fiber intake (roughage or bulk). Thus, the disorder is rare in rural black Africans, who consume a high fiber diet (it is also rare in Koreans, Japanese, and Russians, who also consume a high fiber diet). However, when black Africans migrate to urban centers and eat a low fiber diet, their incidence of diverticular disease approaches that of the white urban population. A high fiber diet results in large, soft bowel movements. It is postulated by some investigators that diverticulosis is caused by hypersegmentation and excessive intraluminal pressures in the sigmoid colon, resulting from the small fecal flow induced by fiber deficiency. The small fecal flow causes the sigmoid colon to contract more vigorously to move the feces distally, which results in high pressures and mucosal herniations. Other investigators have shown that emotional stress can cause hypersegmentation and increased pressures in the sigmoid colon.

The reported frequency of diverticulosis varies with age and the method used for its detection. It is rare below the age of 30; radiologic studies show the incidence to be 20 to 50 percent in patients above age 60.

Diverticulosis has been classified into three types: (1) *single diverticulum,* (2) *simple massed diverticulosis,* in which there are no muscle changes, and (3) *spastic diverticulosis* or *painful diverticular disease,*

in which both the circular and longitudinal muscle layers are greatly thickened and contracted, and the mucosa is thrown into folds. In the third type, the colon has a sawtooth appearance on barium enema. Spastic diverticulosis is said by some physicians to cause symptoms (e.g., left lower quadrant pain and constipation) but in the opinion of these authors, diverticulosis is asymptomatic, and any associated symptoms are caused by concomitant irritable colon syndrome (discussed earlier in the chapter). When pain is caused by diverticular disease, the patient may be said to have diverticulitis rather than diverticulosis.

Complications of Diverticulosis

Hemorrhage. Diverticulosis is the most common cause of acute, extensive lower gastrointestinal hemorrhage; patients with diverticulitis, by contrast, may ooze but rarely bleed massively. In diverticulosis, hemorrhage results from ulceration of the mucosa, and the bleeding may be profuse because of the large concentration of intramural vessels in the area of a diverticulum. In the preangiographic era, whenever emergency operations were performed one had to accept a surgical mortality rate of 20 to 50 percent since the patients were elderly with other complicating disease, and the site of bleeding was not localized. Consequently, the wrong area (e.g., the sigmoid colon) was often resected and the patient would bleed again. Modern angiography has demonstrated that 75 percent of patients bleed from a diverticulum in the right colon, not in the sigmoid colon. The diagnosis is made by the history of passage of red blood by rectum, the absence of blood in the gastric aspirate, negative sigmoidoscopy (except for red blood coming from above), demonstration of the site of active bleeding by angiography, and failure to find other disease on barium enema. In most patients bleeding stops spontaneously. If bleeding persists, blood replacement may be necessary to maintain blood volume. Vasopressin infusion through the angiography catheter leading to the bleeding site often halts blood loss. Surgery is indicated when the bleeding cannot be controlled by these means.

DIVERTICULITIS

The exact incidence of diverticulitis is uncertain.

About 12 percent of patients with diverticulosis show the inflammatory pathologic changes of diverticulitis. On the other hand, 25 to 37 percent of patients with diverticulosis who are followed for 10 to 15 years develop clinical evidence of inflammatory disease. Diverticulitis is not caused by intraluminal obstruction as is appendicitis (see later in the chapter) but rather is thought to be caused by a microperforation or macroperforation of an involved diverticulum. This concept is extremely important because it means that patients with diverticulitis have varying degrees of peritonitis. The perforation may result in inflammation of the serosa, pericolic fat, intestinal wall, and peritoneum. Diverticulitis may be either acute or chronic. Recurrent episodes may lead to fibrosis, muscular hypertrophy with thickening of the intestinal wall, and narrowing of the bowel lumen.

Clinical Features

The two major complaints of patients are typically pain in the left lower quadrant and a change in bowel habits consisting of either frequent loose movements, constipation, or diarrhea followed by severe constipation. Evidence of peritoneal irritation may be indicated by an increase in left-sided pain on walking or riding over a bumpy road in a car. Tenderness in the left lower quadrant (that is, the sigmoid colon) and peritoneal rebound are often noted, with variable abdominal muscle guarding and spasm. A mass is palpable in 25 to 50 percent of the patients. During severe attacks, the abdomen is distended and may be tympanitic, depending on the degree of mechanical or paralytic ileus (or both). Fever, tachycardia, and leukocytosis will vary with the severity and extent of inflammation.

Sigmoidoscopy is of value primarily to rule out other diseases, but occasionally a red, edematous mucosa may be observed proximal to the rectosigmoid. Helpful or diagnostic procedures include a plain film of the abdomen and a barium enema. The flat film may demonstrate a soft tissue mass, air under the diaphragm in the case of free perforation, or intestinal distention in the presence of obstruction and ileus. A cautiously performed barium enema without excessive pressure (some physicians believe that this procedure is contraindicated in acute attacks) is of

great help in the diagnosis of diverticulitis. The diagnostic findings are (1) rupture of a diverticulum as demonstrated by the presence of extraluminal barium (extravasation), (2) a filling defect due to external pressure by a mass, (3) fistula formation, (4) circumferential narrowing of the sigmoid colon, (5) complete obstruction of the sigmoid colon, and (6) a dissecting intraluminal fistula.

Diagnosis

The diagnosis of diverticulitis should be considered in any patient, especially an elderly one, who has left lower quadrant pain, a change in bowel habits, and signs of an inflammatory process predominantly localized in the left lower quadrant. The irritable colon syndrome and carcinoma of the sigmoid colon are the principal diseases that may be confused with diverticulitis. Clinical evidence of inflammatory disease and the radiographic findings previously discussed will rule out a functional bowel disorder. Carcinoma is usually characterized by a longer history of symptoms, blood in the stools, and barium enema findings different from those of diverticulitis (see later in this chapter, under Carcinoma). If obstruction is complete, it may not be possible to differentiate carcinoma until follow-up x-ray studies have been performed or until the resected specimen is examined microscopically. Ulcerative colitis, Crohn's colitis, and ischemic colitis also have to be considered in the differential diagnosis.

Complications of Diverticulitis

The complications discussed below should be suspected in patients who have clinical evidence of diverticulitis and who then develop the symptoms and signs described under each complication.

Obstruction. Partial obstruction is seen in most patients with diverticulitis; however, the obstruction can also be complete. Narrowing of the sigmoidal lumen results from changes in the gut wall or from external compression of the lumen by a perisigmoidal mass. Cramping pain, severe constipation, abdominal distention, and tympany on percussion are the principal clinical findings. Occasionally a coexisting carcinoma will be the cause of the obstruction.

Perforation. As mentioned previously, some degree of perforation is considered to be the fundamental pathologic process in diverticulitis. Macroperforation may lead to pericolic abscesses, local or diffuse peritonitis, or fistula formation. Perforation or abscess formation is suggested by the presence of exquisite abdominal tenderness and peritoneal rebound in addition to other signs and symptoms of inflammation in an acutely ill patient.

Fistula. The most common fistulous communication is between the colon and the urinary bladder (colovesical fistula), found in 6 to 28 percent of patients operated on for diverticulitis. Other communications are to the small bowel (coloenteric), colon (colocolic), skin (colocutaneous), perineum (coloperineal), vagina (colovaginal), and uterus (colouterine). Urinary frequency, urgency, and dysuria may precede colovesical fistula by months and should alert the physician to this potential complication. Pneumaturia, fecaluria, chills, and fever, in addition to the preceding symptoms, signal the presence of a fistula. The diagnosis is confirmed by urinary findings (mixed bacteriology), cystoscopy, and barium enema.

Dissecting Diverticulitis. Multiple microabscesses within the bowel wall that communicate with each other can form a long tract under the mucosa parallel to the long axis of the intestine. This process is known as dissecting diverticulitis; it may be confused with Crohn's colitis on barium enema.

Treatment

Diverticulosis per se requires no therapy except when the patient has associated constipation (see the section on treatment of irritable colon syndrome earlier in the chapter). The treatment of diverticulitis depends on the acuteness and severity of the attack and the presence of complications. Acute, uncomplicated diverticulitis is best treated medically. The basic forms of therapy in mild attacks are bed rest, a soft or liquid diet, hot packs applied to the abdomen for comfort, and mineral oil taken orally to soften the stools behind the partial obstruction. Since perforation is presumably present in all diverticulitis, antibiotic therapy is indicated, for example, ampicillin,

500 mg four times a day. With more severe attacks (as indicated by high fever, pain, tenderness, distention, and obstruction), nasogastric suction should be instituted, and intravenous ampicillin, 1 gm every 4 hours, should be administered.

Approximately 50 percent of patients with acute diverticulitis will have one attack and will not require any additional therapy. Urgent surgical intervention is indicated in patients with (1) generalized peritonitis, (2) increasing or persistent intestinal obstruction, (3) enlarging mass, or (4) evidence of abscess. Since surgery in acute diverticulitis carries a mortality rate of 15 to 23 percent, and the mortality rate in elective surgery, on the other hand, is only 1.5 percent, operation should be deferred whenever possible unless urgently required. Elective surgery is indicated in patients with (1) recurrent attacks (especially in patients under the age of 50), (2) a persistent, tender mass, (3) narrowing or marked deformity of the colon seen on x-ray, (4) dysuria and evidence of colovesical fistula or any fistula, (5) persistent blood in stools, and (6) clinical or x-ray suspicion of carcinoma. The type of operation depends on the pathologic process, that is, whether primary resection should be attempted or whether a multiple staging procedure is necessary.

Diseases of the Vermiform Appendix

MUCOCELE AND CARCINOID

The appendix is rarely involved by tumors, either benign or malignant. A benign mucocele may be caused by chronic luminal obstruction in the absence of bacteria. A malignant mucocele is a manifestation of a mucous cystadenocarcinoma. Pseudomyxoma peritonei, or accumulation of mucin in the peritoneal cavity, occurs as a complication of malignant and even of benign mucocele either because of spontaneous appendiceal rupture or following spillage of appendiceal contents at the time of emergency surgery. It is thought that the mucin acts as an irritant or that there is implantation of tumor within the peritoneum with subsequent mucin production.

Carcinoid is the most frequent neoplasm of the appendix and is found in 0.15 percent of appendixes removed surgically. However, in most instances it is an incidental microscopic finding and is without clinical significance. Rarely, carcinoid may produce symptoms simulating appendicitis and may result in an appendectomy. In patients with carcinoid tumor the appendix is the most common site of origin, the incidence in some series being as high as 60 percent. Although appendiceal carcinoids invade the wall of the appendix and metastasize, disagreement exists in the literature as to whether they cause the so-called carcinoid syndrome.

APPENDICITIS

Acute inflammation of the appendix is believed to start as an obstruction of its lumen by inspissated contents, followed by spasm, edema, impaired blood supply, bacterial proliferation, and mural inflammation. If the process continues unchecked, the wall of the appendix becomes necrotic, and either a localized appendiceal abscess or a diffuse peritonitis results. Acute appendicitis affects all age groups and has such a high incidence (1 to 3 per 1,000 per year in the United States, though apparently declining) that it should be suspected whenever a previously healthy person suddenly has abdominal complaints, irrespective of their nature.

Clinical Features

The classic early symptom of appendicitis is a vague periumbilical or epigastric distress associated with anorexia, nausea, and sometimes vomiting. Within hours the distress shifts to the right lower quadrant of the abdomen, becoming severe and more sharply localized. The bowels are usually inactive. The oral temperature ranges between 100 and 102°F (37.8 to 38.9°C). Physical examination reveals maximum tenderness in the right lower quadrant associated with muscular guarding or spasm, the intensity of which depends on the stage and acuteness of the appendicitis. Tenderness in the right iliac fossa may also be elicited on rectal examination in about one-half of patients. Rebound tenderness referred to the area of the affected appendix is a classic manifestation. The outstanding finding on laboratory examination is leukocytosis, usually ranging between 10,000 and 16,000 cells.

Diagnosis

In half the patients the classic features of acute appen-

dicitis may not obtain, in that the pain may be atypical, the physical findings minimal, and fever and leukocytosis absent. In the elderly and the very young, in particular, the early symptoms of acute appendicitis may be deceptively mild and nonspecific. Another cause for atypical symptoms is a retrocecal appendix that points upward behind the cecum; in such cases the patient may complain of distress in the right upper abdominal quadrant and present few physical findings. In some cases, because either the inflamed appendix or an appendiceal abscess is contiguous to the bowel, motility is stimulated and the patient has diarrhea rather than constipation.

Acute appendicitis, therefore, must be considered whenever a patient has an acute illness with abdominal symptoms and the systemic signs of an inflammatory process. The differential diagnosis includes acute enteritis of viral or bacterial etiology, ovarian and tubule disease in women, mesenteric adenitis (which may mark the onset of some acute infectious diseases), diverticulitis affecting Meckel's diverticulum or the ascending colon, Crohn's disease, some cases of biliary tract disease, and disease affecting the right genitourinary tract. The last condition can usually be differentiated from acute appendicitis by the urinary findings, but occasionally appendiceal inflammation near the right ureter will lead to the appearance of moderate numbers of white cells in the urine. Major abdominal catastrophes such as mesenteric vascular occlusion or perforated viscus are less apt to be confused with uncomplicated acute appendicitis, since appendicitis is characterized by relatively moderate reactive phenomena: moderate pain, moderate tenderness, moderate fever, and moderate leukocytosis.

Treatment

The treatment of acute appendicitis is immediate surgical removal. In cases of diagnostic doubt, appendectomy is also indicated if the patient's operability is not impaired by other disease. By and large, it is not hazardous to carry out an appendectomy during the course of another disease producing symptoms that cannot be differentiated from those of acute appendicitis.

Medical management pending surgical treatment consists in withholding food and fluid by mouth and administering fluids and electrolytes parenterally if the patient has had pronounced vomiting or diarrhea or both. If the abdomen is distended, gastric suction is advisable. Antibiotics are usually not necessary at this stage. The prime duty of the physician is *not* to administer a laxative, because it may aggravate the inflammatory process and possibly cause perforation. This obligation should not be hard to meet, since there are no acute abdominal situations that warrant the administration of laxatives.

Complications

Necrosis of the appendiceal wall may lead to diffuse peritonitis; to abscesses that localize in the right peritoneal gutter, under the right hemidiaphragm, or about the liver; or to pylephlebitis and liver abscesses. Perforation with local abscess formation is characterized by intensification of the symptoms, physical findings, and laboratory abnormalities. In particular, increased spasm or masses may be detected in the right lower quadrant, and the white blood cell count may mount to or above 20,000. X-ray examination may reveal a pressure defect in the small or large bowel in the right lower quadrant. If the complications of acute appendicitis are suspected or evident, antibiotic therapy is indicated (see Chap. 43).

Chronic Appendicitis

Chronic appendicitis, in the sense of a process that causes chronic right lower quadrant pain (and perhaps tenderness) day after day, without any other findings, probably does not exist; such symptoms have other causes. On the other hand, a recurrent appendicitis, consisting of intermittent bouts of pain with spontaneous subsidence of each recurrent inflammatory reaction, is occasionally seen and should be considered in the differential diagnosis when right lower quadrant pain is episodic.

Benign Polyps of the Colon and Rectum

Polyps are pedunculated or sessile tumors that project into the lumen of the bowel. Most occur within reach of the sigmoidoscope. Polyps usually are asymptomatic, although some can give rise to overt or occult rectal bleeding, crampy abdominal pain, or a change in bowel habits. It is difficult to distinguish a benign colonic polyp from the rarer polypoid adenocarcinoma. Some polyps have a high incidence of malignant transformation.

There are four main types of colonic polyps, varying in clinical importance: (1) neoplastic polyps, including adenomatous polyps and villous adenomas; (2) hamartomas; (3) inflammatory polyps; and (4) hyperplastic or metaplastic polyps. The last three groups are nonneoplastic and have no malignant potential.

NEOPLASTIC POLYPS

Adenomatous polyps are by far the most common neoplastic lesion of the colon and rectum. The incidence rises steeply after age 50 and reaches a peak in the seventh decade; there is a slight predominance in men. In 35 to 40 percent of cases the polyps are multiple. Three-quarters of polyps are within reach of the sigmoidoscope. Polyps proximal to the rectosigmoid area are best diagnosed with an air contrast barium enema or colonoscopy.

Adenomatous polyps are characterized microscopically by branching tubular glands lined with mature, mucus-secreting goblet cells. They are usually pedunculated and have a smooth surface. Whether or not these polyps are premalignant remains controversial. Most lesions under 1 cm remain benign, while those larger than 2 cm may be cancerous and should be removed. Polyps that can be reached through the sigmoidoscope should be excised. Proximal large lesions should be removed by colonoscopic polypectomy or by direct surgical intervention.

Multiple familial polyposis and Gardner's syndrome (multiple familial polyposis with osteomas and sebaceous cysts) are diseases transmitted by an autosomal dominant gene. In both disorders, the incidence of malignancy approaches 100 percent by age 40. Adenomatous polyps are distributed fairly evenly throughout the large bowel and may number in the hundreds or thousands. When carcinoma develops it is frequently multifocal. The diagnosis is usually made in asymptomatic persons by investigating the families of known patients. Children at risk must be followed with routine sigmoidoscopy at 6-month intervals, and by barium enemas once a year. If adenomatous polyps develop, confirming the disease, total colectomy in the late teens or early twenties is recommended.

Villous adenomas account for 1 to 3 percent of surgically removed neoplasms of the colon. Sixty percent of villous adenomas arise in the rectum, 30 percent are located in the sigmoid or rectosigmoid area, and the remainder are distributed proximally. Villous adenomas are most commonly found in the sixth decade and are usually asymptomatic. Presenting symptoms, when they occur, include a change in bowel habits, with either constipation or diarrhea; lower abdominal cramps; and the passage of large amounts of mucus, occasionally mixed with blood. Rarely, villous adenomas may cause a protein-losing enteropathy or may produce secretions containing large amounts of potassium, sodium, and chloride. Hypokalemia or severe dehydration may be a prominent feature. The lesion is premalignant, with a reported incidence of carcinomatous transformation ranging between 40 and 60 percent.

The typical villous adenoma is usually large and sessile with a shaggy surface made up of fingerlike projections. Microscopically, projections of loose vascular stroma covered by a single layer of epithelial cells are seen. Glands and mucus-producing cells are absent. All villous adenomas should be excised.

NONNEOPLASTIC POLYPS

Nonneoplastic polyps have no malignant potential; they include hamartomas (see Chap. 36), inflammatory polyps, and hyperplastic polyps. A variety of inflammatory polyps with differing histology have been described, but the edematous, polypoid, mucosal type (the *pseudopolyp*) is the best known and is seen most frequently in ulcerative colitis. Hyperplastic (metaplastic) polyps are also common; they are made up of elongated tubules showing cystic dilatation. Although hyperplastic polyps are occasionally mistaken for adenomatous polyps, they do not produce symptoms and do not increase in size on follow-up.

Carcinoma of the Colon and Rectum

Colorectal carcinoma is the second most common malignant disease in the United States, following only skin cancers. Ninety-five percent of malignant colonic tumors are adenocarcinomas. Colorectal carcinoma is usually a disease of older persons, with a peak incidence in the sixth decade. Carcinoma of the rectum tends to occur more frequently in men than in women (2:1), whereas in colonic carcinoma the ratio is equal. Seventy percent of colorectal tumors occur within reach of the sigmoidoscope, and half can be palpated on rectal examination. Predisposing factors include ulcerative colitis, multiple familial polyposis, villous adenoma, some adenomatous polyps and, to a lesser extent, granulomatous colitis. Colorectal carcinoma spreads by lymphatic or bloodstream dissemination, by direct extension, by gravitational seeding, or by implantation during surgery.

CLINICAL FEATURES

The signs and symptoms of colonic carcinoma may be nonspecific; weight loss, abdominal pain, and a change in bowel habits are frequent. In many instances the presenting features are related to the location and extent of the tumor. For example, *right-colon carcinomas* tend to present insidiously and are discovered late in the course of the disease. An abdominal mass is noted in 60 percent of such patients, and occult blood in the stools together with anemia is present in about 75 percent. *Rectal carcinoma* is rarely associated with a mass that is palpable per rectum. Ten to forty percent of adenocarcinomas of the colon, particularly those of the left colon, present with intestinal obstruction. The classic radiologic finding on barium enema is an "apple-core" lesion.

DIAGNOSIS

Sigmoidoscopy with biopsy and barium enema or air contrast barium enema usually establish the diagnosis. The diagnosis of colorectal carcinoma should be considered in any elderly patient who presents with a change in bowel habits, overt or occult rectal bleeding, weight loss, or an abdominal or rectal mass. Patients with predisposing factors should be closely followed for the development of colonic carcinoma by an annual barium enema and semiannual sigmoidoscopy. The differential diagnosis includes disorders associated with strictures and mass lesions noted on barium enema. Colonic strictures can result from inflammatory bowel disease, ischemic colitis, diverticulitis, lymphogranuloma venereum, endometriosis, pancreatitis, or an ameboma. Lesions simulating polypoid adenocarcinoma include adenomatous polyps, villous adenomas, or rarely, giant pseudopolyps. If the lesion is beyond the reach of the sigmoidoscope, colonoscopy with biopsy can confirm the diagnosis.

TREATMENT
In the absence of distal metastases, the treatment for colorectal carcinoma is surgical resection. The resectability of colonic tumors is said to be 95 percent, with an overall operative mortality rate of 4 percent. In an acutely ill patient with colonic obstruction the critical treatment of choice may be a diverting colostomy. The 5-year survival rate is 75 percent in patients having carcinoma limited to the bowel wall and with no documented metastasis. With disseminated disease, less than 5 percent live for 5 years. Including all stages, the absolute 5-year survival rate is 37 percent. Following surgical resection, 18 percent of patients are discovered to have recurrent tumor in the suture line. With documented metastasis, chemotherapy with 5-fluorouracil may provide palliation.

Sarcoma
Lymphomas rarely arise in the colon or rectum. Secondary involvement of the large bowel occurs in about 6 percent of patients with lymphosarcoma. Treatment is by surgical excision when possible, associated with x-ray therapy.

Bibliography
Berman, P. M., and Kirsner, J. B. Current knowledge of diverticular disease of the colon. *Am. J. Dig. Dis.* 17:741, 1972.

Chaudhary, N. A., and Truelove, S. C. The irritable colon syndrome: A study of the clinical features, predisposing causes and prognosis in 130 cases. *Q. J. Med.* 31:307, 1962.

Copeland, E. M., Miller, L. D., and Jones, R. S. Prognostic factors in carcinoma of the colon and rectum. *Am. J. Surg.* 116:875, 1968.

Fagin, R. R., and Kirsner, J. P. Ischemic diseases of the colon. *Adv. Intern. Med.* 17:343, 1971.

Fleischner, F. G. Diverticular disease of the colon: New observations and revised concepts. *Gastroenterology* 60:316, 1971.

Fordtran, J. S. Speculations on the pathogenesis of diarrhea. *Fed. Proc.* 26:1405, 1967.

Morson, B. C., Dawson, I. M. P., and Jones, F. A. *Gastrointestinal Pathology.* Oxford: Blackwell, 1972.

Painter, N. S. Diverticular disease of the colon: A disease of western civilization. *DM,* June 1970.

Williams, L. F., and Wittenberg, J. Ischemic colitis. *Ann. Surg.* 182:439, 1975.

38

Inflammatory Bowel Disease

Charles J. Schwartz and Philip Kramer

Ulcerative Colitis

Ulcerative colitis or *proctocolitis* is an inflammatory disease affecting primarily the mucosa and submucosa of the rectum and colon. The etiology is unknown. Host factors — for example, an altered immune state or a characteristic personality type — and exogenous agents such as bacteria, bacterial products, viruses, and chemicals have been implicated in the disease. The evidence is largely circumstantial, however, and the role of any one factor in the pathogenesis of ulcerative colitis remains uncertain.

In the United States the annual incidence of ulcerative colitis is about 3 to 6 cases per 100,000 and the prevalence rate is approximately 40 to 70 per 100,000 persons. Most new cases are recognized in persons between the ages of 15 and 25, although there is a small secondary peak in incidence between ages 55 and 60. The disease is more common in whites, in women, in urban centers, in highly educated persons, and in the higher socioeconomic level groups. Approximately 40 percent of patients are Jewish, but strangely, ulcerative colitis is unusual in Israel.

The rectum and colon are involved in continuity with the disease, starting in the rectum and progressing proximally in the colon. The pathologic changes are usually limited to the mucosa and submucosa. Microscopic features of acute and chronic inflammation — ulcerations, hemorrhage, and crypt abscesses — are characteristic but nonspecific. Although crypt abscesses are often considered a hallmark of ulcerative colitis, they may also be found in Crohn's (granulomatous) colitis, ischemic colitis, and infectious colonic diseases. Granulomas are rarely seen in ulcerative colitis. Goblet cell depletion with a corresponding decrease in mucus is considered specific for ulcerative colitis. *Ulcerative proctitis* is a mild form of ulcerative colitis in which the previously described pathologic changes are limited to the rectum.

CLINICAL FEATURES

Rectal bleeding and diarrhea with the daily passage of 10 to 30 small fecal discharges of blood and mucus,

associated with tenesmus, constitute the common presentation of ulcerative colitis. Fever is frequent, and abdominal pain may be present but is less common than in Crohn's colitis. Surprisingly, constipation with one bowel movement of stool every other day may be seen in about 10 percent of patients with proctosigmoiditis although these same individuals may complain of frequent, even hourly, rectal discharges of blood and mucus.

Occasionally the onset of illness is insidious, and the extracolonic manifestations (discussed later) may be more prominent than the colonic symptoms. The patient will complain of fatigue and anorexia, and weight loss may occur. Ten to fifteen percent of patients have a fulminant course, with toxic megacolon, perforation, or massive hemorrhage, and require a colectomy during their first attack. Most patients (60 to 70 percent) have intermittent symptoms with long periods of complete remission; a few have continuous distress. Five to ten percent of patients will have no symptoms for as long as 15 years after a single episode.

Abdominal tenderness may be elicited over the colon. Sigmoidoscopy reveals diffuse involvement of the rectal mucosa with friability, multiple small ulcerations, fine granularity, purulent exudate, inflammatory pseudopolyps, blunted rectal valves, and loss of the normal vascular pattern. The rectum almost always is involved. Anemia and hypoalbuminemia indicate a poor prognosis. Flat plate of the abdomen may reveal varying amounts of air with either toxic dilatation or "thumbprints" representing submucosal edema outlined by air. Radiologic findings on barium enema include decreased rectal distensibility, contraction and shortening of the colon, and symmetrical serration of the wall of the colon, indicating ulceration. Pseudopolyps are noted in 15 to 30 percent of patients and are usually seen in the rectum and descending colon. "Backwash" ileitis, a dilatation of the terminal ileum with loss of normal mucosal markings, is found in 20 to 30 percent of patients; this finding is distinguished from the scarred and contracted terminal ileum seen in regional enteritis. The fistulas often seen in Crohn's colitis are not present.

COMPLICATIONS

The complications of ulcerative colitis may be either

local, involving diseased bowel, or systemic, with protean manifestations. Colonic complications include anorectal lesions, massive hemorrhage, perforation, toxic megacolon, pseudopolyposis, benign strictures, and carcinoma. Anal and perianal disorders, including hemorrhoids and fissures occur frequently in ulcerative colitis (25 percent of patients), but in contrast to Crohn's colitis, where similar problems are more frequent, perianal abscesses and fistulas are unusual. Massive hemorrhage and free perforation rarely occur.

Toxic megacolon occurs in only 3 percent of patients with ulcerative colitis, but it has a case fatality of about 13 percent that increases threefold when associated with free perforation. The pathologic features of toxic megacolon include deep ulceration and inflammation involving the muscularis and serosa; this involvement is an exception to the usual mucosal and submucosal limitation of disease in ulcerative colitis. Patients with toxic megacolon are generally very ill, with fever, tachycardia, abdominal distention, rebound tenderness, and diminished bowel sounds. *Flat plate of the abdomen* in toxic megacolon is diagnostic and reveals (1) a dilated transverse colon exceeding 5.5 cm in diameter, (2) a scalloped contour of the bowel lumen, and (3) numerous broad-based polypoid projections in the lumen. Barium enema is contraindicated in this condition since it may precipitate perforation.

In ulcerative colitis the incidence of colorectal carcinoma is markedly increased over that of the general population. In patients presenting with ulcerative colitis before age 14, the incidence of cancer is about 3 percent after 10 years of active disease and increases about 2 percent each year thereafter. Benign strictures may simulate carcinoma, and present a difficult differential.

Systemic complications of ulcerative colitis are common and occasionally precede the primary diagnosis by several years. Hepatobiliary complications are discussed in Chapter 41. Associated musculoskeletal disorders include peripheral arthritis (5 to 10 percent of patients), sacroiliitis (8 percent), and digital clubbing (5 percent). Skin lesions include erythema nodosum (5 to 10 percent), aphthous ulcers of the mouth and, rarely, pyoderma gangrenosum. Ocular involvement may take the form of conjunctivitis, iritis, or uveitis. Nephrolithiasis and renal amyloidosis occasionally occur. Other important general complications are an increased frequency of thromboembolic disease and growth retardation in children.

DIAGNOSIS
The differential diagnosis includes Crohn's colitis, ischemic colitis, and pseudomembranous colitis; the infectious colitis produced by *Salmonella, Shigella,* or amebae; and the proctitis that occurs rarely with either lymphogranuloma venereum or gonococcus. In Crohn's colitis fever, weight loss or perianal disease often antecedes bowel symptoms; rectal sparing is noted in 50 percent of patients; skip lesions and fistulas are common, whereas gross rectal bleeding is not prominent. Ischemic colitis is usually a disease of the elderly, presenting with a sudden onset of bloody diarrhea; unlike ulcerative colitis, it does not usually involve the rectum. In amebic disease, the mucosa between ulcers is frequently normal on sigmoidoscopy, and amebae may be seen in the stool. *Shigella, Salmonella,* gonococcus, and lymphogranuloma venereum may be excluded by appropriate cultures and serologic tests (see Chap. 39).

TREATMENT
Mild cases of ulcerative colitis are treated with bed rest and the judicious use of antispasmodics. Salicylazosulfapyridine (Azulfidine), in a maintenance dose of 3 to 6 gm per day, has been shown to both induce remissions and decrease the frequency of exacerbations in this disease. Side effects of salicylazosulfapyridine are common (5 to 45 percent of patients) and include headache, nausea, vomiting, rash, abdominal pain, and hemolysis in glucose 6-phosphate dehydrogenase—deficient patients. Ulcerative proctitis may remit spontaneously without any treatment or, if persistent, may respond to salicylazosulfapyridine or to rectal steroids. More severely ill patients will require hospitalization, oral or parenteral corticosteroid treatment, and meticulous management of nutrition, fluid, and electrolyte balance. Patients with toxic megacolon should receive nasogastric suction, parenteral feeding, broad-spectrum antibiotics as in peritonitis, and parenteral corticosteroids. Methylprednisolone,

60 mg per day given intravenously, and in some cases corticotropin, 60 units per day given intravenously in divided doses, are commonly employed. With clinical improvement, parenteral steroid treatment may be switched to an equivalent oral dose and then tapered slowly over several months. Surgical intervention with total colectomy may be required in patients with toxic megacolon if there is evidence of progression or lack of response within a few days. Other indications for surgery in patients with ulcerative colitis include perforation, massive hemorrhage, intractability with maximum medical therapy, suspicion of carcinoma, retardation of growth in children, and severe systemic complications not responsible to medical therapy.

Crohn's Disease

Crohn's disease (regional enteritis) is a chronic disease of unknown etiology characterized by transmural inflammation of the bowel. Although the terminal ileum is the most commonly involved area, any part of the gastrointestinal tract may be affected from the mouth to the anus with "skip" areas of normal intervening mucosa. Among patients with small bowel involvement, approximately half will exhibit colonic disease. In other patients, Crohn's (granulomatous) colitis occurs without associated small bowel disease. Crohn's disease is most common in persons between the ages of 10 and 30; the sex ratio is equal. As in ulcerative colitis, there is a significantly higher incidence (3 to 6 times) in Jews. Crohn's disease is uncommon in American blacks, American Indians, and Orientals.

In Crohn's disease, the involved bowel wall and mesentery are edematous and thickened, with narrowing of the intestinal lumen. Mesenteric fat is found extending over the antimesenteric side of the bowel, and mesenteric lymph nodes are prominent. The mucosa typically has a "cobblestone" appearance produced by deep transverse and longitudinal fissures. Occasionally these fissures extend to form blind sinus tracts or fistulas to other organs. Noncaseating granulomas, usually in the submucosa, are found in 50 percent of resected specimens. Other histologic features include transmural edema, fibrosis and lymphoid hyperplasia, and lymphangiectasia.

CROHN'S DISEASE OF THE ILEUM

Clinical Features

In Crohn's disease of the ileum (regional enteritis), spontaneous remissions and exacerbations are characteristic, and a history of intermittent episodes of right lower quadrant or periumbilical cramping pain with diarrhea is common. There is frequently a preceding history of perianal disease (anal fissures, fistula-in-ano, or perianal abscesses), weight loss, unexplained fever or anemia, arthralgias, erythema nodosum, or renal stones. Stools tend to be large and frequent with three to five bowel movements per day; occult bleeding is common, but hematochezia is unusual, and massive hemorrhage is rare. Children may come to medical attention because of growth retardation. An occasional patient will present with malabsorption or manifestations of an enterocutaneous fistula. Partial or complete intestinal obstruction is a late feature. Occasionally a mass may be noted in the right lower quadrant.

Sigmoidoscopy is abnormal in 50 percent of patients with mild granularity and friability of the mucosa and longitudinal and transverse fissures. Anal and perianal disease including perianal abscesses and fistulas as well as hemorrhoids and anal fissures is found in more than 80 percent of these patients. The most common radiologic finding on the small bowel series is the "string sign," or marked narrowing of the lumen of the terminal ileum. Early radiologic changes include thickening and distortion of the mucosal pattern; other features are a cobblestone mucosa, blind sinus tracts, enteric fistulas, skip areas with normal intervening bowel, and displacement of loops of intestine suggesting a mass effect.

Diagnosis

A history of abdominal pain, diarrhea, and perianal disease in a young patient who, in addition, may also complain of fever and weight loss, suggests Crohn's disease. Rarely a patient may present with a right lower quadrant mass and fever, suggesting an appendiceal abscess, only to have the correct diagnosis confirmed at laparotomy. Radiologic features of Crohn's ileitis may be seen in other diseases, such as lymphoma, mesenteric vascular disease, intestinal tuberculosis, carcinoid tumors, actinomycosis, and chronic fungal diseases.

CROHN'S DISEASE OF THE COLON

Clinical Features
The presentation in Crohn's disease of the colon (Crohn's colitis, transmural colitis, or granulomatous colitis) may be similar to that in Crohn's disease of the ileum. Nonbloody diarrhea with frequent loose stools and colicky suprapubic pain are cardinal symptoms. Grossly bloody stools are seen less commonly than in ulcerative colitis. In about 15 percent of cases, a history of perianal disease, fever, weight loss, or other systemic complications of Crohn's disease may precede the overt bowel disease by several years. The rectum is spared in 50 percent of patients with Crohn's colitis. When affected, the rectum shows asymmetric involvement of the mucosa, skip segments, or a cobblestone mucosa. Occasionally the proctoscopic findings may simulate those of active ulcerative colitis. Rectal biopsy may help to differentiate the two conditions; noncaseating granulomas or the presence of goblet cells with a normal mucus content in the presence of active inflammation suggest Crohn's colitis. The flat film of the abdomen is usually normal, although thumbprinting may be seen; very rarely, the dilated, ahaustral transverse colon of toxic megacolon may complicate Crohn's colitis.

A barium enema will demonstrate the segmental nature of the disease, showing skip areas, cobblestone mucosa, and deep linear ulcerations. Blind sinus tracts and colonic fistulas may be seen. Localized strictures may be confused with carcinoma of the colon. The differential diagnosis is the same as that in ulcerative colitis.

COMPLICATIONS OF CROHN'S DISEASE
Small bowel obstruction occurs in 25 to 30 percent of patients. Fistulas are present in at least half of the patients and may lead to a variety of symptoms. An enteric fistula may produce malabsorption from the short bowel syndrome, as a result of bypass of most of the small bowel, or from bacterial overgrowth in a blind loop or in multiple intestinal strictures. Occasionally a blind sinus tract ends in an intraabdominal abscess. Rarely, an enterovesical fistula develops. Perianal disease occurs in 80 percent of patients.

Free perforation, toxic megacolon, massive bleeding, and adenocarcinoma are rare complications. Systemic complications of Crohn's disease are similar to those mentioned in the section on ulcerative colitis. In addition, renal stones composed of calcium oxalate are noted in patients with either a resected or diseased terminal ileum; an increased intestinal absorption of oxalate appears to be responsible.

TREATMENT OF CROHN'S DISEASE
The treatment of Crohn's disease depends on the patient's condition, presentation, and complications. Mild cases can be treated with bed rest, a low residue diet, and the judicious use of antispasmodics. Although the efficacy of salicylazosulfapyridine in Crohn's disease has not been established, a trial therapy with the administration of 3 to 6 gm per day is warranted. Symptoms of obstruction should be treated with continuous nasogastric suction and intravenous fluids. An occasional patient with significant weight loss will require hyperalimentation. Corticosteroid therapy may be required if the patient does not respond to conservative therapy; however, corticosteroids are contraindicated in patients suspected of having an intraabdominal abscess. In the acutely ill patient without these complications, parenteral corticosteroids should be given in the form of methylprednisolone, 60 mg per day in divided doses. With clinical improvement, parenteral steroids may be switched to the equivalent oral dose and slowly reduced over a period of months. Surgery is indicated in the acutely ill patient with persistent obstruction, enterovesicular fistula, perforation, massive hemorrhage, or a suspected abscess. Other indications for surgical treatment include intractability despite maximum medical therapy, retardation of growth, and severe anal and perianal complications that are unresponsive to local measures or medical therapy. Unfortunately, the recurrence rate following surgery ranges between 50 and 90 percent.

Ischemic Colitis
Ischemic colitis may result either from nonocclusive vascular disease in which the vessels of the entire colon and rectum can be demonstrated to be patent or from occlusive arterial or venous lesions. Arterial

causes of occlusive vascular disease include embolization or thrombosis of the inferior mesenteric artery (both of which are rare in comparison to superior mesenteric artery occlusions), volvulus and intussusception, aortic dissection, and surgical ligation. Rarely, amyloidosis, vasculitis, and colonic carcinoma are associated with arterial occlusion. Factors predisposing to mesenteric vein thrombosis include abdominal sepsis, hypercoagulable states (polycythemia vera, essential thrombocytosis, and sickle cell anemia), mechanical compression (volvulus, intussusception, or tumor), and portal hypertension. Most patients with ischemic colitis have nonocclusive disease with such predisposing conditions as hypotension, congestive heart failure, and digitalis intoxication. Patients usually range between the ages of 50 and 90, but younger patients are being reported with increasing frequency. Both men and women are affected.

The most commonly involved area (in about three-quarters of patients) is the splenic flexure, the watershed area between the superior and inferior mesenteric arteries. The incidence of involvement of other areas of the colon is as follows: the transverse colon (with or without involvement of either flexure), 15 percent; the right colon, 10 percent; and the rectum and rectosigmoid, 5 percent.

Based on the severity of disease, ischemic colitis may be subdivided into two distinct clinical groups. The group comprises patients with mild disease in whom clinical manifestations of ischemia resolve within 2 weeks, and also those with bowel wall stricture. The severe disease group includes patients with either localized or generalized peritonitis, as well as those whose ischemic process has not resolved within 2 weeks. Thus, an episode of ischemic colitis may resolve completely, leaving no residue; it may result in stricture formation; or it may progress to transmural infarction and peritonitis. Approximately 70 percent of patients fall into the mild disease group, in which the prognosis is good.

CLINICAL FEATURES

The sudden onset of mild, crampy, or constant lower abdominal pain and bloody diarrhea in an elderly patient is characteristic of ischemic colitis. In more fulminant cases, the patient presents in shock with bloody diarrhea, fever, and tachycardia. Severe diffuse abdominal pain accompanied by rebound, tenderness, and rigidity, which is indicative of peritonitis, can be striking. Rectal involvement is uncommon, and sigmoidoscopy is usually normal. If the rectum or rectosigmoid is involved, cyanotic cystlike masses, representing submucosal hemorrhages, are seen protruding into the lumen. In several days these cysts are replaced by ulcerations. The surrounding mucosa appears friable and often cyanotic. These same submucosal hemorrhages in the colon appear as "thumbprints" outlined by air in a plain film of the abdomen or noted in a barium enema. In addition, air may be seen in the wall of the bowel, indicating transmural necrosis or impending perforation. Toxic megacolon, a rare complication, is occasionally noted. Several months after an episode of ischemic colitis, it is important to obtain a barium enema to rule out the development of strictures. Since most cases of ischemic colitis are associated with nonocclusive causes, mesenteric angiography is usually negative and is not indicated.

DIAGNOSIS

The differential diagnosis includes both ulcerative colitis and granulomatous colitis, various forms of bacterial or amebic colitis, carcinoma of the colon or, more rarely, diverticulitis and pseudomembranous enterocolitis. Both ulcerative colitis and granulomatous colitis involve a younger age group. Rectal involvement is more common in ulcerative colitis than in ischemic colitis. A preceding history of abdominal pain, diarrhea, or perianal disease is characteristic of granulomatous colitis, in which hematochezia is unusual. The presence of amebae is excluded by stool examination and serologic tests; appropriate cultures should be obtained for *Shigella* and *Salmonella*. Carcinoma is usually excluded by sigmoidoscopy and barium enema. A mass is frequently palpable in diverticulitis, and frank rectal bleeding is unusual. Pseudomembranous enterocolitis is excluded by the absence of a history of previous antibiotic therapy and by appropriate Gram's stains and cultures of the stool.

TREATMENT

Many cases of ischemic colitis probably resolve spontaneously and are never seen or recognized by a physician. Mild cases of ischemic colitis are best treated with nasogastric suction, intravenous feeding, and broad-spectrum antibiotics. Surgery is indicated for patients with signs of localized or diffuse peritonitis or those with fulminant disease. Bloody diarrhea with active disease persisting beyond 2 weeks indicates a poor prognosis. The treatment of an ischemic stricture is controversial; many surgeons favor resection of ischemic stricture because of the likely development of colonic obstruction, and because it may be extremely difficult to differentiate stricture from carcinoma.

Bibliography

Dukes, C. E. The surgical pathology of ulcerative colitis. *Am. R. Coll. Surg. Engl.* 14:389, 1954.

Kirsner, J. B., and Shorter, R. G. *Inflammatory Bowel Disease.* Philadelphia: Lea & Febiger, 1975.

Morson, B. C., Dawson, I. M. P., and Jones, F. A. *Gastrointestinal Pathology.* Oxford: Blackwell, 1972.

39

Gastroenteritis and Infectious Diarrheas

William R. McCabe and Neil R. Blacklow

Gastrointestinal infectious agents may be pathogenic in two ways: (1) direct invasion of the intestinal mucosa by bacteria or viruses and (2) production of toxins that act upon the intestinal tract. Infectious diseases of the gastrointestinal tract are usually manifested as one of two relatively distinct clinical syndromes: gastroenteritis or diarrheal disease. Although there is some overlap of both the clinical features and the etiologic agents, the syndromes often can be distinguished sufficiently to indicate the nature of the etiologic agent.

Gastroenteritis

The onset of the syndrome of gastroenteritis is relatively abrupt, with salivation, nausea, vomiting, and abdominal cramps. Diarrhea of variable severity may or may not occur. The severity of both vomiting and diarrhea may vary from mild to extremely profuse; if they are severe, blood and mucus may appear in the vomitus or stool. Fever is usually not observed in gastroenteritis resulting from ingestion of bacterial toxins in food, except in staphylococcal food poisoning, and therefore fever usually suggests bacterial or viral invasion. Rarely, hypotension may occur. The course of the illness is usually self-limited and the outcome is rarely fatal, only in the very young and the elderly. Symptoms usually begin within 24 hours after ingestion of the offending food and subside after another 24 hours.

BACTERIAL GASTROENTERITIS

"Food poisoning" is the most frequent cause of gastroenteritis. This type of illness is solely an intoxication; the ingestion and invasion of viable bacteria are not required. The illness results from the contamination of food with enterotoxin-producing bacteria (coagulase-positive *Staphylococcus aureus, Clostridium perfringens, Clostridium botulinum,* or enterococci) during processing and the subsequent production of

the enterotoxin. Usually the food product has been heated inadequately to kill the bacteria and spores or to inactivate the toxins and has been subsequently maintained at a temperature sufficient to allow further toxin generation. Although individual cases of food poisoning may be recognized, the diagnosis is made most often when an outbreak results from communal dining such as picnics or banquets.

Staphylococcal food poisoning is caused almost exclusively by members of bacteriophage groups III and IV, with bacteriophage types 6/47 and 42-D predominating. The incubation period is from 2 to 6 hours, and the gastrointestinal symptoms are considerably more severe than those observed with other types of food poisoning.

Botulism is appropriately classified as a form of food poisoning, although the major clinical findings are neurologic. The onset of signs and symptoms may vary from a few to 26 hours after ingestion, with the severity of manifestations usually paralleling the brevity of the incubation period. Gastrointestinal symptoms may be slight or absent. Neurologic manifestations usually consist of diplopia, dysarthria, dysphagia, nystagmus, dilated pupils, and symmetrically depressed deep-tendon reflexes, without sensory or pyramidal involvement. Six antigenically distinct types, A through F, of botulinal toxin have been identified. There is a tendency for individual serotypes to be associated with specific foods.

Food poisoning caused by *C. perfringens* or enterococci has incubation periods ranging from 8 to 24 hours and is much milder than staphylococcal food poisoning.

VIRAL GASTROENTERITIS

The majority of cases of acute, self-limited, infectious enteritis in older children and adults are of unknown etiology; hence, these extremely common illnesses have masqueraded under such descriptive labels as "winter vomiting" and "intestinal flu." Since the disease has been transmitted experimentally in man by the oral administration of bacteria and toxin-free fecal filtrates derived from several different disease outbreaks, the etiologic agents are currently thought to be unidentified viruses. One such filtrate contains the Norwalk agent, a small virus that appears to belong to the parvovirus group. Viral gastroenteritis is characterized by diarrhea or vomiting, or both, and can be accompanied by nausea, abdominal cramps, headache, low-grade fever, myalgias, and malaise. The illness lasts 24 to 48 hours, with spontaneous recovery; complications of dehydration and even death may occur in elderly debilitated patients and in newborns. The disease is accompanied by a transient histopathologic lesion of the upper small intestine, but the large bowel is uninvolved; hence, fecal leukocytes are not seen in diarrheal stools.

In approximately one-half of infantile (under age 2) enteritis patients requiring hospitalization because of dehydration, the illness has recently been shown to be produced by a ubiquitous reoviruslike agent. This illness of infants occurs primarily during the winter months, and the etiologic agent is felt to be the cause of many common mild diarrheas in young children. The agent infects small intestinal epithelial cells, and the diarrheal stools from infants with the illness lack fecal leukocytes. Most older children and adults possess serum antibodies against the reoviruslike agent, indicating prior infection. The disease potential of this agent in reinfection of older children and adults remains to be assessed. Gastroenteritis may also result from infections with *Salmonella, Shigella, Vibrio parahaemolyticus,* and certain strains of *Escherichia coli.* Diarrhea is usually the most prominent sign in such infections.

Infectious Diarrhea and Dysentery

Several species of bacteria may produce diarrheal disease, which tends to be of two types. First, bacteria that produce enterotoxins, such as *Vibrio cholerae,* the noncholera vibrios, and toxicogenic *E. coli,* cause an illness characterized primarily by watery diarrhea. The severity of this diarrhea may vary from a few stools per day to an explosive, almost continuous passage of liquid stools, which in cholera may exceed 20 liters per day. The second type of diarrhea is the "dysentery syndrome," which tends to be associated with chills, fever, severe cramping abdominal pain, and the passage of only small quantities of blood and mucus-tinged, liquid stools. Bacteria that produce mucosal invasion tend to cause the dysentery syn-

drome, although some may cause either a diarrheal or a dysentery syndrome.

SALMONELLOSIS

Salmonellosis is the most frequent of the identified causes of bacterial diarrheal disease among adults in the United States, and its frequency has increased progressively over the past few decades with the expansion of food processing. Almost all animal species, especially cattle, hogs, and poultry, may harbor *Salmonella,* and even one infected animal or egg can lead to contamination of large quantities of processed food. Most strains of *Salmonella* can be isolated from animals as well as from humans, but certain strains (e.g., *S. typhosa, S. paratyphi A,* and *S. schottmülleri [paratyphi B]*) are limited almost exclusively to man. *Salmonella* differs from the other bacterial causes of gastrointestinal infection in that it may cause a variety of clinical infections. The four major types of *Salmonella* infection are discussed in the following sections.

Diarrhea and Gastroenteritis

After an incubation period of 8 to 48 hours following ingestion of contaminated food, symptoms appear. Usually there is an initial chill, fever, and sometimes nausea and vomiting. Colicky abdominal pain and diarrhea of variable severity are usually prominent. The small intestine and colon are sites of bacterial multiplication and invasion, which results in enlargement and ulceration of the lymphoid follicles. The stool often contains flecks of blood and mucus. Leukocytosis is infrequent, but blood cultures may be positive. Spontaneous remission usually occurs within 5 days, but rarely fever and diarrhea may persist as long as 2 weeks.

Carriers of Salmonella Infection

Carriers of infection — patients with continued excretion of *Salmonella* for 2 weeks following diarrhea — are frequent, but they decline to 10 to 15 percent of cases by the end of 4 weeks. Such "convalescent carriers" constitute less of a public health problem than the so-called chronic carriers, who usually carry *S. typhosa* or *S. paratyphi A* or *B.* Chronic carriage of *Salmonella* occurs after recovery in approximately 3 percent of cases of typhoid or enteric fever.

Bacteremia and Focal Infections

As mentioned previously, bacteremia is not infrequent in uncomplicated *Salmonella* diarrhea and usually subsides spontaneously. In a small number of patients, bacteremia may persist and produce prolonged, intermittent fever, with chills, anorexia, and weight loss. Salmonellae also have a predilection for localizing in sites of prior tissue injury and may produce local lesions such as bronchopneumonia, empyema, pericarditis, renal abscess, osteomyelitis, mycotic aneurysms, and other abscesses.

Typhoid or Enteric Fever

Several species of *Salmonella* (in addition to *S. typhosa* and *S. paratyphi A* and *B*) may produce the syndrome of prolonged, enteric fever, although the illness caused by these other strains tends to be less severe and of shorter duration than true typhoid. The incubation period is from 8 to 14 days. The initial symptom is a stepwise increase in temperature accompanied by anorexia, lethargy, malaise, and generalized aches. A nonproductive cough is also frequent. After the first week, the fever becomes continuous; if untreated, it may persist for 6 to 8 weeks. Diarrhea almost never occurs, but abdominal tenderness and distention are frequent. Splenomegaly is found in approximately two-thirds of patients, and crops (20 to 30) of small (2 to 5 mm), red, maculopapular lesions or "rose spots" are frequently found over the abdomen. Delirium often supervenes, and gastrointestinal perforation or hemorrhage may occur. The pulse rate tends to be low in proportion to the fever, and a relative leukopenia is common. The absence of localizing findings often results in typhoid or enteric fever being called a fever of undetermined origin (FUO) in nonendemic areas.

SHIGELLOSIS (BACILLARY DYSENTERY)

Each of the four serologic groups of *Shigella (S. dysenteriae, S. flexneri, S. boydii,* and *S. sonnei)* produces diarrheal disease in man. In contrast to *Salmonella, Shigella* bacilli are limited to man and primates, almost never cause bacteremia, are unasso-

ciated with infections other than diarrhea, and are rarely associated with chronic carriage. *Shigella* bacilli also tend to be more infective than *Salmonella*, with as few as 200 bacilli constituting an infective dose[25] for man in contrast to the approximately 100,000 *Salmonella* bacilli required for equal infectivity. Following an incubation period of 36 to 72 hours, the initial symptoms — usually fever and cramping abdominal pain — are followed by diarrhea, which often contains blood and mucus. In general, shigellosis tends to have a more explosive onset and a more severe course than *Salmonella* diarrhea, and infections caused by *S. dysenteriae* are more severe than those produced by the other species of *Shigella.*

CHOLERA AND NONCHOLERA VIBRIOS

Although cholera has long been both endemic and epidemic in the Far East, an outbreak in 1973 extended to Asia Minor, Italy, and Portugal, demonstrating the potential of this disease for spread into all areas of the world. Cholera is characterized by massive diarrhea, which may be as great as 24 liters per day in severe cases. Initially, the stool is brown but rapidly becomes clear with small flecks of mucus ("rice water" stools). Severe dehydration followed by hypovolemic shock with acute renal failure ensues, unless there is adequate hydration. Fatality rates as high as 50 to 75 percent have occurred in the absence of adequate fluid therapy. Cholera is a self-limited disease, however, provided dehydration and shock do not prove fatal. A similar but less severe disease is produced by other vibrios which, collectively, are termed *noncholera vibrios.*

In contrast to salmonellosis and shigellosis, cholera vibrios do not invade the intestinal mucosa or produce any inflammatory reaction. The diarrhea results solely from the production of an enterotoxin that causes a massive outpouring of isotonic fluid from the small intestinal mucosa. The toxin binds preferentially to gangliosides in the cell membrane and initiates an increase in adenyl cyclase activity. This increased adenyl cyclase activity catalyzes the conversion of adenosine triphosphate (ATP) to adenosine monophosphate (AMP) and is followed by a marked increase in cyclic AMP levels, which results in the active secretion of chloride and bicarbonate ions along with large volumes of water into the intestinal lumen, exceeding the reabsorptive capacity of the intestinal mucosa. Glucose given orally in a 2 to 5% solution enhances the reabsorptive capacity of the intestine — a finding of considerable therapeutic value.

ESCHERICHIA COLI
Strains of *E. coli* have been associated with several types of diarrheal disease; some strains have been shown to produce mucosal invasion similar to that seen in shigellosis, while an even larger number have been shown to produce an enterotoxin similar to but less potent than that of *V. cholerae.*

Certain strains of *E. coli* (e.g., 0111:B4, 055:B5, 026:B6, 086:B4) were first associated with outbreaks of fatal gastroenteritis and diarrhea in infants in the 1940s. Those outbreaks tended to occur in newborn nurseries and rarely involved adults. The pathogenesis of this type of *E. coli* infantile diarrhea has not been elucidated. More recently, both invasive *E. coli* and enterotoxin-producing strains have been implicated in diarrheal disease in adults.

AMEBIC DYSENTERY
Although amebic dysentery is more frequent in the tropics, it does occur in the temperate zones. Acute amebic dysentery has an abrupt onset, with headache, nausea, chills, fever, and abdominal cramps. There may be as many as 15 to 20 liquid stools per day containing flecks of bloody mucus. Pathologically, lesions are limited to the large intestine and consist of shallow mucosal ulcers with a necrotic base which may extend into the submucosa and rarely may perforate. A more frequent type of amebiasis is characterized by intermittent episodes of constipation and diarrhea.

PSEUDOMEMBRANOUS ENTEROCOLITIS
Pseudomembranous enterocolitis is an acute, inflammatory, necrotic lesion diffusely affecting the mucosa of the large bowel, where the destroyed epithelium is covered by a yellowish-gray membrane. At one time this condition was a frequent complication of abdominal surgery in patients who had received prolonged broad-spectrum antibiotic therapy, and antibiotic-resistant staphylococci were found to be the causative agents. The onset of the disease is sudden, with watery diarrhea, and it is often of sufficient severity to produce dehydration and collapse resulting from hypovolemia. During the past decade, the incidence of staphylococcal enterocolitis has decreased markedly. A similar but less severe type of pseudomembranous enterocolitis of uncertain etiology has been observed after treatment with lincomycin or clindamycin.

TUBERCULOUS ENTERITIS
Tuberculous enteritis has become an extremely rare disease in the United States with the disappearance of bovine tuberculosis; it is currently seen only in patients with cavitary tuberculosis who swallow large numbers of tubercle bacilli. The disease presents as an ulcerative or infiltrative granulomatous mass in the ileocecal region that may cause abdominal cramping, diarrhea, or even intestinal obstruction.

Differential Diagnosis of Gastroenteritis and Infectious Diarrheas
Distinguishing gastroenteritis from food poisoning is often done readily when there are multiple cases in which a single food source can be identified, but diagnosis is much more difficult with a single case. In general, clinical symptoms are so similar with different agents that they are of little assistance in making an etiologic diagnosis. Moreover, certain noninfectious inflammatory bowel diseases may produce signs and symptoms indistinguishable from those caused by infections of the gastrointestinal tract.

Microscopic examination of the stool is of great assistance in making a tentative etiologic diagnosis. The finding of large numbers of polymorphonuclear leukocytes and erythrocytes in stained preparations of fresh diarrheal stool specimens suggests infection with either *Shigella, Salmonella,* or invasive *E. coli.* Similar findings may also occur in acute ulcerative colitis and Crohn's (granulomatous) colitis. In amebic colitis, erythrocytes are found but the predominant inflammatory cells are mononuclear leukocytes. In addition, the finding of motile amebic trophozoites of *Entamoeba histolytica* establishes the diagnosis of amebic colitis. Leukocytes are absent in stool specimens from patients with diarrhea caused by enterotoxin-producing pathogens, such as toxin-producing *E. coli* and *V. cholerae.* Since the usual enteric pathogens cannot be distinguished from the gram-negative bacilli normally present in the bowel, examination of Gram's stains of the stool are of little diagnostic value in most cases of diarrheal disease. In staphylococcal enterocolitis, on the other hand, Gram's stains are of value, since the large numbers of staphylococci seen are not normally present in the stool.

Stool culture is the only method for establishing the etiology of diarrheal disease with certainty. Routine stool culture techniques allow ready identification of *Salmonella* and *Shigella,* but modification of standard techniques used in the United States may be required for isolation of *V. cholerae* and noncholera vibrios. The tendency toward spontaneous recovery in salmonellosis and, to a lesser degree, in shigellosis frequently results in the patient's recovering before the results of stool cultures become available. Greater difficulty is encountered in diagnosing diarrheal disease caused by *E. coli,* since *E. coli* are normally found in the stool. The *E. coli* strains that produce diarrhea in infants can be identified, since they are of specific serologic types, but this does not hold true for the invasive types or for enterotoxin-producing *E. coli.* Moreover, there are no simple techniques suitable for routine laboratory use that test either invasiveness or toxin production. Two to three blood cultures should also be obtained in patients with fever and severe diarrhea.

Early diagnosis of typhoid and enteric fevers is dependent on isolation of *Salmonella* from blood cultures, since the organism does not begin to appear in the stool until the second or third week of this type of *Salmonella* infection. Rising antibody titers to O and H antigens begin in the third week of illness and may be of diagnostic value. Antibody titers may also be of assistance in the chronic type of amebic colitis. Sigmoidoscopic and x-ray examination of the large bowel are of little diagnostic assistance. The changes seen in severe, protracted shigellosis or salmonellosis may mimic those seen in acute ulcerative colitis or Crohn's colitis.

Treatment of Diarrheal Diseases

The most important aspect of the treatment of all diarrheal disease is the correction of fluid and electrolyte abnormalities. The paramount importance of adequate fluid and electrolyte replacement is most convincingly demonstrated in cholera (discussed previously), where such treatment reduces the fatality rate from 50 or 75 percent to 5 percent or less. Intravenous administration of fluids is usually preferable, but the discovery that oral administration of 2 to 5% glucose solution promotes electrolyte and water reabsorption in the intestine has provided an important breakthrough in the treatment of diarrheal disease in areas with limited medical facilities.

The self-limited nature of many diarrheal diseases often makes antimicrobial therapy unnecessary. Even in *Salmonella* and *Shigella* infections, fever and diarrhea often abate before the results of stool cultures are available. However, antibiotic therapy materially shortens the course of shigellosis. Parenteral ampicillin, 15 mg/kg/body weight every 6 hours, is the most effective agent if the infecting organism is susceptible, but other parenterally administered or orally absorbable antibiotics are also effective. Nonabsorbable antimicrobials are ineffective in shigellosis. In contrast, antibiotics are contraindicated in uncomplicated *Salmonella* diarrhea, both because they do not shorten its course and because they increase the duration of fecal excretion of *Salmonella.*

Chloramphenicol is the most effective agent for the treatment of typhoid and enteric fevers, but ampicillin is only slightly less effective. Chloramphenicol is usually given parenterally in a dose of 50 mg/kg/day for 5 days, discontinued for 7 days, and then readministered for 5 additional days. Ampicillin is given intravenously in a dose of 100 mg/kg/day for 14 days. Response is not always prompt, and fever may persist for as long as 7 to 8 days after initiation of antibiotics. Recently, a combination of sulfamethoxazole and trimethoprim has been shown to be effective in the treatment of typhoid caused by chloramphenicol-resistant bacilli. Chloramphenicol is ineffective in the treatment of chronic *Salmonella* carriers, but long-term administration (4 to 6 weeks) of high-dose oral ampicillin may be curative.

The treatment of both shigellosis and typhoid has been complicated by the appearance of ampicillin-resistant *Shigella* and chloramphenicol-resistant *S. typhosa.* This type of antibiotic resistance has been shown to be mediated by extrachromosomal genetic material termed *episomes,* which may be transferred between bacteria of different species, resulting in the rapid spread of antibiotic resistance among gram-negative bacilli. Outbreaks of bacillary dysentery caused by ampicillin-resistant *S. dysenteriae* and of typhoid caused by chloramphenicol-resistant *S. typhosa* in which episomal-mediated antibiotic resistance was demonstrated have occurred in Central America and Mexico in recent years.

Bibliography

Blacklow, N. R., Dolin, R., Fedson, D. S., et al. Acute infectious nonbacterial gastroenteritis: Etiology and pathogenesis. *Ann. Intern. Med.* 76:993, 1008, 1972.

Carpenter, C. C. J. Cholera and other enterotoxin-related diarrheal diseases. *J. Infect. Dis.* 126: 551, 1972.

Drachman, R. H. Acute infectious gastroenteritis. *Pediatr. Clin. North Am.* 21:3, 1974.

Grady, G. F., and Keusch, G. T. Pathogenesis of bacterial diarrheas. *N. Engl. J. Med.* 285:831, 891, 1971.

40

Diseases of
the Biliary Tract
and Gallbladder

Donald M. Small

Diseases of the biliary tract and gallbladder may be divided simply into two areas: diseases involving gallstones and their sequelae, and disorders that are unrelated to gallstones. To the practicing physician, by far the most important are the diseases related to gallstones, which extend from the "silent" stone to ascending cholangitis. Among the disorders that are unrelated to gallstone disease are primary tumors, sclerosing cholangitis, and uncommon infections leading to cholecystitis or cholangitis.

The Enterohepatic Circulation and the Gallbladder
Molecules that are secreted into the bile by the liver, absorbed by the intestine, and then resecreted by the liver are said to have an *enterohepatic circulation (EHC)*. Quantitatively the most important class of compounds undergoing EHC are bile salts, which are synthesized in the liver from cholesterol and are then conjugated with glycine or taurine to produce detergent-like molecules resistant to the acid pH of the duodenum. Conjugated bile salts are secreted by an active transport mechanism into the bile canaliculi and progress down the biliary tract to enter the duodenum and gallbladder. Studies in baboons show that during fasting about half the secreted bile salts enter the gallbladder, while the rest pass into the duodenum to be recycled; as fasting continues, the bile salts recycle repetitively, and nearly all eventually pass into the gallbladder. Since the volume of bile entering the gallbladder during a 12-hour fast may be 300 to 600 ml in man, the gallbladder must reabsorb considerable fluid and electrolytes to maintain its volume of about 25 to 50 ml. Thus during gallbladder filling, sodium bicarbonate, chloride, and water are reabsorbed to leave a bile about 10 times as concentrated as the original hepatic bile with respect to bile salts and bilirubin.

During eating, specific amino acids and fatty acids stimulate the duodenal mucosa to release cholecysto-

kinin-pancreozymin (CCK-PZ), causing the gallbladder to contract, Oddi's sphincter to open, and concentrated gallbladder bile to enter the duodenum. Bile salts aid in the digestion of dietary fats by augmenting the action of pancreatic lipase and by removing the products of lipolysis (fatty acids and monoglycerides) from the reaction site. Bile salts solubilize fatty acids and monoglycerides in mixed micelles and bring them in contact with the mucosa of the small intestine, where they are absorbed. Conjugated bile salts, however, are not readily absorbed in the upper intestine, and so they progress to the ileum to be reabsorbed efficiently by an active transport process. The bile salts then enter the portal vein, are bound by albumin, and are transported to the liver, where they are rapidly extracted. Normally, of the total bile salts secreted into the intestine, at least 95 percent is reabsorbed and less than 5 percent is excreted in the feces. Furthermore, about 95 percent of the bile salts passing through the liver is extracted in a single passage. Thus, as a result of efficient ileal absorption and hepatic extraction, bile salts are largely contained in the EHC (liver, biliary tract, gallbladder, intestine, and portal vein), and only very small amounts are present in the rest of the body (estimated at about 2 percent of the total). This fact accounts for the very low concentration of bile salts in the systemic circulation. In the presence of liver disease, hepatic extraction and secretion may be impaired, leading to increased concentrations of serum bile salt. Thus, measurement of bile salt concentration may be considered to be a liver function test, but further study is required to determine its clinical utility.

A normal 70-kg person has a total pool of bile salts of 2 to 4 gm and a 24-hour liver-to-duodenum bile salt secretion of 15 to 35 gm. For example, assume that a typical person has a bile salt pool size of 3 gm and that he secretes 24 gm of bile salt per 24 hours. These figures imply that his 3-gm pool must circulate, on the average, about 8 times in 24 hours, or about 2 to 3 times per meal. Of the 24 gm secreted, he will reabsorb about 23.5 gm and lose 0.5 gm into the feces. During a 24-hour period the liver synthesizes an amount equal to the loss, thereby maintaining a normal pool size. Of the 24 gm of bile salts secreted, 23.5 gm (98 percent) is recycled, and only 0.5 gm (2 percent) is newly synthesized.

If a person suddenly loses his bile salt pool (for example, by ingesting the drug cholestyramine resin, which binds bile salts in the gut and prevents their reabsorption), the rate of bile salt return to the liver will markedly decrease. The liver senses the low return rate of bile salts and responds by increasing bile salt synthesis. A normal person can augment synthesis tenfold to about 5 gm per 24 hours; this high synthetic rate will persist until the liver senses a high return rate and slows synthesis. Thus bile salt synthesis is effectively controlled by the rate of bile salt return to the liver.

The secretion of bile salts varies throughout the day; it is highest in the morning following gallbladder contraction as the ejected pool recycles to the liver. Secretion remains relatively high throughout the day, since gallbladder filling is minimal until the stomach is empty and gallbladder contraction ceases. At this point, part of the secreted bile is directed to the gallbladder, and the hepatic return diminishes. Therefore secretion decreases at night and reaches a low level early in the morning. It is obvious that dietary habits may greatly affect the temporal aspects of the secretion rate of bile salts and their EHC.

Many other substances are secreted in the bile and some, including certain drugs and hormones, have an important EHC. Other substances that are secreted into bile and that play a role in diseases of the biliary tract include cholesterol, phospholipid, and bilirubin. Normally a 70-kg person secretes about 750 mg of cholesterol, 8 gm of phospholipid, and 250 to 300 mg of bilirubin daily.

Diagnostic Assessment of Biliary Tract and Gallbladder Disease

CLINICAL FEATURES

The history and physical examination of the patient together with standard laboratory tests aid in establishing the correct diagnosis and help in assessing the severity of the disorder. For example, the appearance of *biliary colic* (a persistent, severe pain in the right upper quadrant, often radiating to the tip of the scapula, sometimes increasing in severity for a period of minutes or hours and then gradually declining),

accompanied by an enlarged and tender gallbladder, is a good indication of a stone impacted in the cystic duct. If the stone dislodges or is passed into the duodenum, the pain abates and the patient recovers. Persistent pain accompanied by chills, fever, and leukocytosis suggests that *cholecystitis* has developed in an obstructed gallbladder. The appearance of jaundice and bilirubin in the urine, with similar bouts of pain, suggests *choledocholithiasis,* that is, a stone lodged in the common bile duct. Continuing chills, fever, leukocytosis, increasing jaundice, and impaired liver function tests indicate the presence of *ascending cholangitis,* a bacterial infection and inflammation of the biliary tract extending into the liver; this complication has a more serious prognosis than does cholecystitis. Intermittent partial biliary tract obstruction is often accompanied by right upper quadrant pain with little or no jaundice, but the presence of a high serum alkaline phosphatase level should lead the physician to suspect a stone partly blocking the common duct. Chronic intermittent biliary obstruction may lead eventually to *secondary biliary cirrhosis.* Complete biliary obstruction accompanied by steady pain located deep in the epigastrium or in the back suggests a tumor of the head of the pancreas or of the biliary passages. Finally, intermittent small bowel obstruction in an elderly patient whose abdominal x-ray shows air in the biliary tract should lead to the diagnosis of a *fistula* between the gallbladder or common duct and the small bowel and the presence of *gallstone ileus.*

SPECIAL DIAGNOSTIC PROCEDURES

To identify patients at high risk for gallstones that are not clinically apparent, to demonstrate "silent" or asymptomatic stones, or to pinpoint the specific position of an obstructing lesion, more sophisticated diagnostic procedures are necessary.

Flat Plate of the Abdomen

The flat plate may reveal calcified gallstones, calcified wall of the gallbladder, or "milk of calcium bile," in which the gallbladder fluid appears to be more radiopaque than the surrounding tissues. Air in the biliary tree may be the result of a fistula between the biliary tract and the intestines, or it may be produced by gas-forming bacteria such as *Clostridium* or *Escherichia coli* that are infecting the gallbladder or biliary passages. Occasionally, during barium studies of the upper or lower intestinal tract, a distended gallbladder may be identified as a mass pressing on the duodenum or the colon, or a distended common duct may be seen impressing the duodenum. Finally, in a case of intestinal obstruction, one may be able to identify a calcified gallstone as the cause.

Oral Cholecystogram (Gallbladder Series)
In an oral cholecystogram, an oral dose of 2 to 4 gm of an iodinated compound (iopanoic acid) is given in tablet form the night before the study. This compound is absorbed by the intestine, extracted by the liver, secreted into the bile, and concentrated in the gallbladder. The high electron density of the iodine scatters the x-ray beam and allows the gallbladder lumen to be visualized as an underexposed (radiopaque) area on the film. Radiolucent stones are seen as filling defects within the opacified gallbladder lumen; they may be differentiated from polyps and other tumors because stones usually change position when the patient is turned.

Nonvisualization of the gallbladder in cholecystography may be caused by a number of conditions that are not related to gallbladder pathology, such as failure to swallow the pills, inability to absorb the ingested pills (for example, in a patient with gastric retention), poor liver function due to intrinsic liver disease and, rarely, selectively impaired biliary secretion of iopanoic acid (the Dubin-Johnson syndrome). Blockage of the cystic duct by a stone, acute pyogenic cholecystitis or cholangitis, acute and chronic cholecystitis with reabsorption of the contrast material from the gallbladder, and inability of the gallbladder to concentrate the contrast medium may all result in nonvisualization and indicate disease of the gallbladder or biliary tract. As a general rule, a patient with normal liver function tests who absorbs the contrast material, but whose gallbladder does not fill on two successive tests in a 48-hour period, has a 95 percent chance of having gallbladder disease and at least a 90 percent chance of having gallstone disease. It is helpful to do an upright film of the gallbladder, since stones occasionally layer evenly in a

single-density band and may be obscured in the ordinary supine views of the gallbladder. Finally, it may be helpful to give a fatty meal or CCK-PZ and then observe contraction of the gallbladder. Occasionally symptoms are produced during the contraction that may aid in the diagnosis of intermittent obstruction of the cystic duct, or of biliary dyskinesia if stones are absent (see later in the chapter).

Cholangiography

Intravenous Cholangiography. In patients with serum bilirubin levels of 3 mg per 100 ml or less in whom partial obstruction of the biliary tract is suspected, an iodine-labeled contrast material may be given either as an intravenous bolus injection or as an infusion during a 30- to 60-minute period. This material is taken up by the liver and secreted into the ducts, allowing the biliary tree, but usually not the gallbladder, to be opacified. Stones, tumors, and strictures may be identified as filling defects or narrowings. Since occasional idiosyncratic reactions to iodinated compounds have been observed, these tests should be performed with care.

Percutaneous Transhepatic Cholangiography. In patients whose serum bilirubin level is higher than 4 mg per 100 ml, visualization of the biliary tract by oral cholecystography or intravenous cholangiography usually fails. In such instances it is possible to pass a thin needle through the skin to the liver substance, locate a bile duct by exploration with fluoroscopy, and then inject contrast material directly into a hepatic bile duct. The entire biliary tract may be visualized, and the site (and in some cases the cause) of a complete or partial obstruction may be identified. The success rate in demonstrating the site of the obstruction is close to 90 percent. This procedure is usually followed by definitive surgery. Transjugular passage of a catheter that traverses the superior vena cava and a hepatic vein before puncturing through the liver into a bile duct has been employed in patients with impaired hemostasis; however, experience with this technique is limited.

Transduodenal Cholangiography. In transduodenal cholangiography, a side-viewing endoscope is first passed into the duodenum; the ampulla of Vater may then be identified and a catheter inserted into the common bile duct. Retrograde injection of contrast material then permits visualization of the biliary tree. Although this test is both difficult to perform and time-consuming, experienced endoscopists perform successful cannulations in 70 to 80 percent of the cases attempted. Transduodenal cholangiography is the procedure of choice when transhepatic percutaneous cholangiography cannot be performed.

Intraoperative Cholangiography. Intraoperative cholangiography may be performed just prior to removal of the gallbladder by injecting the contrast material directly into the common duct, or after cholecystectomy and T tube insertion, by injecting it into the T tube. This procedure identifies tumors, strictures, or retained stones in the common and hepatic bile ducts.

Duodenal Intubation and Bile Collection
In the duodenal intubation procedure, a tube is placed in the duodenum and a secretagogue such as CCK-PZ is given to produce gallbladder contraction. Bile is collected before giving the secretagogue, during the ejection of gallbladder bile, and after completion of gallbladder contractions. The finding of cholesterol crystals and bilirubin granules in the aspirate correlates well with the presence of gallstones. Gallbladder bile may be collected for chemical determinations of cholesterol saturation (see the following section).

Epidemiology of Gallstone Disease
For many years it was taught that one should suspect cholelithiasis in females who are "fair, fat, forty, and fertile"; or in other words, in light-skinned, obese, middle-aged, and multiparous women. Recently, the true prevalence of cholelithiasis (as determined by cholecystography) has been established in a random population of Pima Indians living in Arizona. Gallstones are extraordinarily prevalent among these dark-skinned people: 70 percent of the females have gallstones by the age of 30, and males have the same prevalence in later decades. In nearly all the females, the stones appear between the ages of 20 and 30; in males, they develop gradually from ages 30 to 60.

Comparison of the true prevalence of gallstone disease in the Pima Indians to the clinical prevalence shows that symptoms do not appear until several years after the development of the stones, and that about half the women and two-thirds of the men with gallstones *never* have any clinical symptoms. The true prevalence of gallstone disease in the general population is unknown; however, on the basis of data reported in the Framingham study, an estimated 15 million women and 5 million men in the United States have gallstones. In about half of the approximately 800,000 new cases of cholelithiasis each year, surgery is ultimately performed. About 6,000 deaths per year are attributed to gallstone disease, and the total cost of morbidity approaches $1 billion annually.

In the United States and other high-prevalence countries, gallstones are mostly of the cholesterol type. Japan and India, on the other hand, have a lower prevalence, and gallstones in these countries are mainly the pigment variety. Certain populations, such as the Masai tribe of East Africa, do not have gallstones at all.

Pathogenesis of Gallstone Disease
Human gallstones fall into two chemically different categories: those composed of *bile pigments* or their derivatives, and those composed primarily of *cholesterol*. In the former case, the pathogenesis involves bile pigment metabolism and in the latter, cholesterol and bile salt metabolism. Although each category will be considered separately, the fact that cholesterol stones often contain a small pigment center and that *mixed pigment-cholesterol stones* occur suggest that, in a given patient, both disorders may be present at some time.

PIGMENT STONES
Pigment stones probably form only when excess unconjugated bile pigments or their derivatives are present in bile and precipitate to form insoluble, polymerlike complexes with calcium and copper (see Fig. 40-1). These stones are dark brown or black, do not contain cholesterol, and as far as is known, cannot be dissolved in vivo or in solutions of artificial bile. Since pigment stones contain calcium, they are usually seen on x-ray films of the abdomen. The source of excessive free pigment may involve increased hepatic secre-

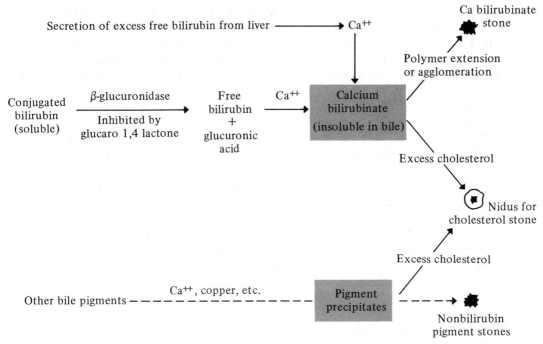

Figure 40-1. Mechanisms of pigment stone formation. True calcium bilirubinate stones result from excess secretion of free bilirubin or deconjugation of conjugated bilirubin in bile. Other pigment stones of unknown chemical structure (not bilirubin) may also result from secretion of these pigments from the liver or their production from known pigments such as bilirubin in the bile. Substances such as calcium and copper may be important in the precipitation process of both true calcium bilirubin stones and nonbilirubin pigment stones. Pigment stones may also form a nidus for precipitation of cholesterol from cholesterol-supersaturated bile. (Adapted from D. M. Small. Gallstones: Current concepts. N. Engl. J. Med. 279:588, 1968.)

tion of bilirubin in disorders associated with rapid hemoglobin breakdown, or chemical alteration of conjugated bilirubin followed by the precipitation of calcium bilirubinate or related compounds in the biliary tract or gallbladder by the action of bacterial deconjugating enzymes.

Since little is known of the chemical and physical makeup of pigment stones, and nothing of the solubility of the precipitating molecules, one cannot discuss the early stages of this disorder, nor can one

predict from bile composition whether or not a patient will develop such stones. One can, on epidemiologic grounds, suggest that patients with increased pigment production resulting from severe chronic hemolytic anemia (e.g., sickle cell anemia, thalassemia, spherocytosis) and infants with severe erythroblastosis fetalis will tend to get stones. Pigment stones are more common than cholesterol gallstones in alcoholic cirrhosis. Pure pigment stones comprise about 10 percent of all gallstones in Western countries. The true prevalence of pigment stone disease may be much higher than is indicated by the prevalence of pure pigment stones, since predominantly cholesterol stones often have a small pigment stone at their center. Strictly speaking, such patients first have pigment stone disease, which acts as a nucleus for the precipitation of cholesterol during a subsequent bout of cholesterol stone disease.

CHOLESTEROL GALLSTONES

Cholesterol stones (that is, stones of pure cholesterol or those having cholesterol as the major chemical component) account for most of the gallstone disease in the Americas, Europe, and South Africa. Gallstones usually present clinically as a medical or surgical emergency, or they may be an incidental radiologic finding in an asymptomatic person. However, the silent or asymptomatic gallstone is virtually the end stage in the pathogenesis of cholelithiasis; the disease begins much earlier in life and proceeds through a number of stages that culminate in stone formation.

Bile Composition and Cholesterol Solubility
Normal bile is a liquid, whereas bile from patients with cholesterol cholelithiasis also contains cholesterol in crystalline form that has precipitated from solution. The solubility of cholesterol in bile is limited and depends on the three major lipid components of bile: conjugated bile salts, phospholipids, and cholesterol. These components make up about 90 percent of the dry weight of gallbladder bile.

Bile salts are water-soluble, detergent-like molecules which, in aqueous solution, form small aggregates called micelles. At least 90 percent of the phospholipid in bile is phosphatidylcholine (lecithin), which is insoluble in aqueous systems but can be dissolved by bile salts in micelles. Cholesterol is also insoluble in water, but it becomes soluble when incorporated into the lecithin–bile salt mixed micelle, whose capacity to dissolve cholesterol is related to their relative contents of lecithin and bile salts.

Triangular coordinates were used by Admirand and Small to define the maximum solubility of cholesterol in lecithin–bile salt mixtures in a system containing 90% water and 10% bile salts together with phospholipids and cholesterol (Fig. 40-2). The line *ABC* represents the effective maximum solubility of cholesterol in varying mixtures of bile salt and lecithin. A mixture in the zone below line *ABC* forms a single homogeneous liquid from which cholesterol does not readily precipitate. A mixture that has a composition falling above line *ABC* contains readily precipitable excess cholesterol. In physical terms, bile with excess cholesterol may present either as a single, liquid phase that is supersaturated with cholesterol or as a two-phase system of liquid bile and solid crystalline cholesterol. The crystals may be either very small or large enough to be called stones. As a general rule, patients with cholesterol gallstones have a bile that contains excess cholesterol, whereas subjects without stones have a bile composition lying below line *ABC*.

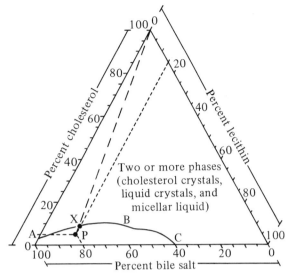

Figure 40-2. Three major components of bile plotted on triangular coordinates. The percent of total moles of bile salt, lecithin, and cholesterol constituted by each of the separate components is shown on the scales along the sides of the triangle. Since the sum of the three components equals 100 mol, the composition of any bile can be represented as a single point within the triangle. For instance, point P represents a bile consisting of 80% bile salt, 5% cholesterol, and 15% lecithin. Line ABC represents the maximal effective solubility of cholesterol in varying mixtures of bile salt and lecithin as determined by Admirand and Small. P falls below line ABC and within the zone of a single phase of micellar liquid, and is less than saturated with cholesterol. To calculate the percentage saturation of a bile having composition P, draw a line through to cholesterol apex. The intersection of this line with line ABC (point X) gives relative cholesterol concentration at 100 percent effective saturation, in this case, 8% cholesterol. Percent saturation of point P is percent saturation = 5/8 (100) = 62.5 percent saturated.

Stages of Cholesterol Gallstone Disease
The first diagnosable abnormality of cholesterol gallstone disease becomes apparent when the patient begins to secrete bile containing an excessive proportion of cholesterol relative to bile salts and phospholipids; that is, a bile composition falling above line *ABC* in Figure 40-2. Whereas all normal persons may secrete such a bile occasionally during fasting, the potential gallstone patient secretes a bile in which the

Table 40-1. Stages of Cholesterol Gallstone Formation

	Stones Absent			Stones Present	
	I	II	III	IV	V
Stage	Genetic-metabolic	Chemical	Physical	Growth	Clinical
Abnormality		Bile becomes super-saturated with cholesterol	Nucleation, flocculation, and precipitation of cholesterol crystals	Growth to macro-scopic stones	Blockage of cystic duct, cholecystitis, and/or jaundice
Diagnosis		Duodenal drainage shows that gallbladder bile has excess cholesterol (estimated from triangular plot as in Fig. 40-2) but no crystals by microscope	Duodenal drainage shows cholesterol crystals by microscope. No stones by cholecystography	Cholecystography reveals stones or nonfunctioning gallbladder. Usually cholesterol crystals and/or abnormal bile are found by duodenal drainage. Patient is asymptomatic	Signs and symptoms are present; positive cholecystography

Source: From D. M. Small, Advantages of a Varied and Individualized Approach. In Ingelfinger, Ebert, Finland, and Relman (eds.), *Controversy in Internal Medicine II.* Philadelphia: Saunders, 1974. Reproduced by permission.

mean 24-hour bile composition contains excess cholesterol. The gallbladder bile from these patients thus
becomes supersaturated with cholesterol. If the level
of supersaturation is very marked, precipitation of
cholesterol may occur rapidly and spontaneously and
result in a large number of small stones. If only a
moderate degree of supersaturation is present, nucleation may be necessary to initiate precipitation. Many
small cholesterol crystals may flocculate to produce
aggregates, or a single crystal may grow to form an
individual stone. The rate of growth depends on the
degree of supersaturation: The greater the supersaturation, the more rapid is the growth.

The pathogenesis of cholesterol gallstones can be
subdivided into five stages (Table 40-1). Stage I involves the genetic, biochemical, or metabolic defect
that leads to the production of gallbladder bile supersaturated with cholesterol. Stage II, the chemical
stage, involves the production of an abnormal, supersaturated bile. Stage III, the physical stage, involves
a change in the physical state of bile from a single,
liquid phase that is supersaturated with cholesterol to
a system containing both a liquid bile phase and
cholesterol crystals. The key processes in this stage
are nucleation, flocculation, and precipitation of
cholesterol from the supersaturated bile. Stage IV
involves the growth of the small crystals into macroscopic stones; and the final stage (stage V) involves
the appearance of clinical symptoms.

The diagnosis of cholesterol gallstone disease may
currently be made as early as stage II, using duodenal
intubation and collection of bile discharged from the
gallbladder after administration of CCK-PZ. If the
bile is supersaturated (by the criteria shown in Fig.
40-2) but contains no crystals, the patient can be
considered to be in stage II. Stage III may be diagnosed by finding cholesterol crystals in a patient who
has a normal cholecystogram; stage IV by finding, in
addition, stones on cholecystography; and stage V by
the presence of signs and symptoms.

Pathophysiologic Types of
Cholesterol Gallstone Disease
Cholesterol gallstone disease is not a single entity;
there are at least six different categories of pathophysiologic abnormalities that may lead to abnormal

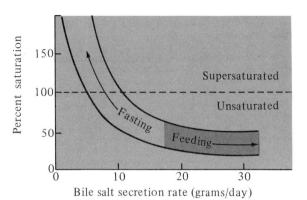

Figure 40-3. The relationship between bile salt secre-
tion rate and cholesterol saturation in bile. The esti-
mated normal relationship between bile salt secretion
rate in grams per 24 hours per 70-kg human is plotted
against the effective percent saturation of cholesterol
in bile as calculated from line ABC according to
method described in Figure 40-2. The zone between
the two curved lines approximates the normal relation-
ship. Bile composition fluctuates within this zone
depending on the hour to hour secretion rate. During
fasting the secretion rate decreases and bile becomes
more saturated and even supersaturated if secretion
rate is below 5 gm per 24 hours (200 mg per hour).
When the subject is eating, the bile salt secretion rate
is high due to cycling of the bile salt pool in the EHC
and bile is quite unsaturated. Since very little bile is
secreted during fasting, the mean bile salt secretion
rate over an average 24-hour period is also high
(stippled zone) and the bile composition is unsatu-
rated. Either low mean 24-hour bile-salt secretion
rates, or an abnormal relationship between bile salt
secretion and percent cholesterol saturation, gives
rise to supersaturated (lithogenic) bile. [From D. M.
Small. The Formation and Treatment of Gallstones.
In L. Schiff (ed.), Diseases of the Liver *(4th ed.).*
Philadelphia: Lippincott, 1975. Reproduced by
permission.]

bile and ultimately to cholesterol gallstones (see the
following section). All these abnormalities result in
an excess quantity of cholesterol relative to bile salt
and phospholipid so that gallbladder bile becomes
supersaturated. An understanding of these different
mechanisms requires knowledge of the normal relationship between the bile salt secretion rate and bile
composition. The relationship between the saturation
percentage of cholesterol in bile and the bile salt
secretion rate is illustrated schematically in Figure
40-3. At high bile salt secretion rates, a bile is less

saturated with cholesterol, but as the secretion rate decreases, the percentage of cholesterol saturation increases. Since the bile salt secretion rate decreases during fasting, some normal persons have a bile that is supersaturated with cholesterol for short periods of time; however, stones are not produced in this instance because the small amount of supersaturated bile mixes with large amounts of normal bile in the gallbladder to give a mean composition that is unsaturated.

The application of techniques for measuring bile acid pool size, synthetic rate, secretion rate, and hepatic return rate, as well as cholesterol secretion rates, permits a tentative classification of gallstone disease resulting from disorders of bile salt and cholesterol metabolism into six types (Table 40-2).

Type 1: Excessive Bile Salt Loss. Excessive bile salt loss, such as occurs in ileectomy, certain kinds of ileal disease, and perhaps in ileal bypass, results in a decrease in the bile salt pool and a very low hepatic return rate. Bile salt synthesis increases to its maximum of about 5 gm per 24 hours, but it cannot make up for the loss; thus the pool remains decreased, the bile salt secretion rate is low, and the bile becomes supersaturated. This mechanism probably accounts for the increased prevalence of gallstones in patients with ileectomy and ileal disease.

Type 2: Oversensitive Bile Salt Feedback. When hepatic return rate falls below a certain level, bile salt synthesis increases to augment the secretion rate and thus return it to normal. If the decreased hepatic return is the result of an increased loss, bile salt pool size and secretion rate can be maintained provided the loss does not exceed the ability of the liver synthesis to compensate. Minor bile salt loss, such as occurs with cholestyramine feeding, a small ileal resection, or a partial ileal bypass, is compensated by increased synthesis, while bile composition remains unsaturated. However, certain patients develop a low pool size and a low return rate without the compensation of increased synthesis; they appear to have an oversensitive feedback mechanism in which even relatively low rates of hepatic return act to depress bile salt synthesis. Assuming that type 2 patients start with a normal

secretion rate and pool size, as oversensitive feedback develops the patient makes less bile salt than he loses, and a period of negative bile salt balance ensues. In time, a new steady state is reached characterized by a decreased pool size, decreased bile salt secretion rate, and a decreased hepatic return. As a result of the decreased secretion rate, bile composition becomes supersaturated. This appears to be the main cause of gallstones in Caucasians of normal weight.

Type 3: Excessive Cholesterol Secretion. Some patients whose bile salt pools and estimated bile salt secretion rates are within the normal range nevertheless have supersaturated bile, because they have a cholesterol secretion rate that is higher than normal. Obesity, which increases the synthesis of cholesterol in man, has been shown to augment cholesterol secretion into bile and lead to supersaturation. Clofibrate, estrogens, and other similarly acting drugs that appear to mobilize cholesterol pools and increase biliary cholesterol secretion probably induce cholesterol stones in some chronic users. Rapid weight loss enhances cholesterol secretion and induces supersaturation. Increased cholesterol intake may also be implicated in increased cholesterol secretion.

Type 4: Mixed Defect. Most American Indians of the Southwest and some Caucasians who are cholesterol stone formers have a double defect that is a combination of type 2 and type 3 defects. These patients have a decreased bile salt secretion rate and a high cholesterol secretion rate. It has been postulated that there may be a defect in the conversion of cholesterol to bile salt in these patients resulting in excessive cholesterol secretion and inadequate synthesis of bile salt.

Type 5: Rapid Bile Salt Circulation with Decreased Pool Size. It has been suggested that the bile salt secretion rate might be normal in some patients with gallstones and that stones could result from a primary disorder in the EHC. This disorder might develop as follows: First, an excessive stimulus for gallbladder contraction or intestinal motility arises and causes a rapid circulation of the pool. Bile salt secretion would increase and result in excessive return of bile salts to the liver. Hepatic synthesis would then decrease and give rise to a period of negative bile salt balance until a new steady state developed, characterized by a decreased but rapidly circulating pool and a normal secretion rate. Under these circumstances the mean 24-hour bile composition would not be supersaturated. However, during fasting the small bile salt pool would mix with a relatively large amount of potentially supersaturated bile coming from the liver; thus, the gallbladder bile composition following fasting might be supersaturated, even though the mean 24-hour bile was not. This hypothesis is intriguing but needs further evaluation.

Type 6: Primary Disorders of the Gallbladder, Ducts, or Sphincters. Extrahepatic mechanisms by which the gallbladder, the sphincter of Oddi, and the bile ducts might be implicated in the formation of gallstones include primary cholecystitis and the biliary dyskinesia syndromes. First, inflammation associated with primary cholecystitis might cause the gallbladder to absorb bile salts abnormally or might even cause a chemical degradation of bile salts and biliary lipids, thus converting a normal hepatic bile into a supersaturated bile within the gallbladder. These mechanisms have not been investigated in man, but bile salt reabsorption in the gallbladder appears to be the cause of stones in mice that are fed cholesterol and cholic acid. Certainly, cholecystitis that is secondary to existing stones, by causing bile salt absorption or by chemically altering biliary lipids, may make gallbladder bile composition even more supersaturated, which could result in the formation of cholesterol stones around existing pigment stones (see Fig. 40-1) or accelerate the growth rate of existing stones. Second, more subtle defects may result from abnormal biliary dynamics. If, for instance, the cystic duct failed to open when the gallbladder contracted, cholecystitis might be produced. Furthermore, if the Oddi's sphincter failed to open when the gallbladder contracted, a condition of intermittent biliary obstruction would result, which could lead to the production of supersaturated bile.

Treatment of Uncomplicated Gallstone Disease
There are two established modes of dealing with un-

complicated gallstones. One is cholecystectomy; the other is a "wait and see" attitude. Patients who have had intermittent episodes of biliary colic should have a cholecystectomy. Patients with asymptomatic gallstones should be followed carefully and be considered for surgery if they develop symptoms.

Pharmacologic therapy is still in the clinically experimental stage and will offer new therapeutic approaches in the future. The oral ingestion of two naturally occurring bile salts, chenodeoxycholic acid and ursodeoxycholic acid, alters biliary lipid metabolism and secretion in such a way that the bile becomes unsaturated. Chenodeoxycholic acid, in doses of 0.75 to 4.0 gm per day, and ursodeoxycholic acid in lower doses have been shown to dissolve radiolucent (presumably cholesterol) gallstones in patients with *functioning* gallbladders. The efficacy and safety of these drugs are now being tested. These and other drugs that alter bile composition, such as phenobarbital, might also be used in the early stages of stone development (stages II and III) to prevent the formation of stones in high-risk patients.

Complications of Gallstone Disease

CHOLECYSTITIS
Most patients with acute cholecystitis have gallstones. Symptoms may result either from local irritation caused by the gallstones within the gallbladder, or more likely from obstruction of the cystic duct by the gallstones, causing edema and consequent inflammation. An acute attack of cholecystitis is characterized by prolonged biliary colic, chills, fever, leukocytosis, and tenderness in the right upper quadrant. The attack either may abate spontaneously, or may persist, leading to perforation of the gallbladder into the peritoneum or into a contiguous organ. Early in the attack the gallbladder contents are often sterile, but if obstruction continues beyond a week, the gallbladder and its contents often become infected with enteric bacteria. Acute cholecystitis rarely occurs in the absence of gallstones. Chronic cholecystitis, either as a microscopic diagnosis or as fibrosis of the gallbladder, accompanies most cases of chronic cholelithiasis and probably has little clinical importance.

The diagnosis of acute cholecystitis is made primarily from the clinical symptoms. The flat plate of

Table 40-2. Classification of Cholesterol Stone Disease

Type of disorder	Hepatic return rate	Bile acid synthetic rate	Bile acid pool size	No. of circulations of pool/24 hr
Normal values (estimated for 70-kg man)	14–34 gm/24 hr	350–550 gm/24 hr	2–4 gm	5–15 gm
Disorders of the EHC and liver affecting bile acid and cholesterol metabolism				
Type 1: Excessive bile salt loss	Decreased (very low)	Increased to maximum level	Decreased	. . . .
Type 2: Oversensitive bile acid feedback	Decreased	Normal to low	Decreased	Normal
Type 3: Excessive cholesterol secretion	Normal	Normal	Normal	Normal
Type 4: Mixed (types 2, 3)	Decreased	Normal to low	Decreased or normal	As in type 2
Disorders primarily extrahepatic in origin				
Type 5: Rapid bile salt circulation	Normal	Normal	Decreased	High
Type 6: Disorders of gallbladder, ducts, or sphincters	. . . .	. . . .	. . . .	. . . .

Source: From D. M. Small, The Formation and Treatment of Gallstones. In L. Schiff (ed.), *Diseases of the Liver* (4th ed.). Philadelphia: Lippincott, 1975. Reproduced by permission.

Bile salt secretion rate	Cholesterol secretion rate	Primary defect	Examples
15–35 gm/24 hr	0.5–1 gm/24 hr	....	....
Decreased	Normal to low	Loss of mechanisms to absorb bile salts results in decreased pool and bile salt secretion rate. Synthesis cannot fully compensate loss	Occurs in ileectomy, ileal bypass, ileal disease; congenital loss of ileal active transport system of bile salts
Decreased due to small pool circulating normally	....	A relative depression in bile acid synthesis. Decreased hepatic return excessively inhibits bile acid synthesis	Occurs in many of the cholesterol stone cases in Caucasians, especially those who are not obese
Normal	High	Excessive cholesterol is secreted into bile despite normal bile salt secretion rate	Occurs in obese patients
Decreased	High	Mixture of types 2 and 3	American Indians, perhaps some Caucasians
Normal	Normal	Small pool of normal bile collecting in gallbladder cannot compensate for abnormal bile entering gallbladder during fasting	May occur in some patients with decreased bile acid pool but further proof is needed
....	....	Absorption of bile salts and/or phospholipids or secretion of cholesterol by gallbladder; chemical alteration of normal hepatic bile in the gallbladder to produce supersaturated gallbladder bile	Cholecystitis, aseptic or bacterial, may secondarily complicate other types of gallstone disease, including pigment stone disease

the abdomen occasionally shows either air in the gallbladder or radiopaque stones. Despite normal liver function tests, the gallbladder fails to visualize on oral cholecystography. The presence of either jaundice or abnormal liver function tests indicates partial obstruction of the common duct resulting from severe inflammatory disease, abscess formation, or stones in the common duct. Treatment consists in supportive therapy for dehydration, nasogastric suction, and antibiotic therapy if the course extends beyond 1 week. In patients with a severe attack and suspected perforation, surgery should be performed immediately; less severely ill patients should have a cholecystectomy after the acute attack has subsided.

CHOLEDOCHOLITHIASIS

Gallstones often pass through the cystic duct into the common duct, where they must pass through the ampulla of Vater and into the duodenum to be eliminated. Stones retained in the common duct constitute choledocholithiasis. Patients with choledocholithiasis may be asymptomatic with normal laboratory findings; they may have an occasional bout of colic-like pain with intermittent signs and symptoms of biliary tract obstruction; or they may develop complications — specifically, ascending cholangitis and secondary biliary cirrhosis. Choledocholithiasis with partial, intermittent biliary tract obstruction is characterized by intermittent bouts of abdominal pain, intermittent jaundice, and often a strikingly elevated serum alkaline phosphatase level. Occasionally, an impacted stone causes mild, chronic, partial obstruction; in such cases the patient may be asymptomatic, with a normal or only slightly increased bilirubin. The diagnosis is made by one of the cholangiographic techniques mentioned earlier. The treatment is surgical removal of the stone and exploration of the common duct for other retained stones.

CHOLANGITIS

A serious complication of choledocholithiasis is cholangitis, or inflammation of the biliary tree above a partially obstructed common duct. The major cause is the presence of gallstones, but rarely tumors, polyps, or parasitic inflammation (common in the Orient) may be responsible. The symptoms of biliary colic,

jaundice, fever, and chills indicate inflammation of the biliary tree. If the obstruction is removed (for example, by the passage of the stone), the symptoms may abate. However, if obstruction is not relieved, bacterial infection ascends the biliary tree, and the patient becomes more severely ill and may develop septicemia with enteric organisms. The condition may progress rapidly to severe toxic delirium with high fever. Diagnosis often must be established at some risk, by percutaneous cholangiography. Occasionally, pus rather than bile may be aspirated from the liver during this test. Suppurative cholangitis requires emergency surgical drainage of the biliary tree. Cholangitis may lead to abscesses within the liver, a condition with a very high mortality rate. Except for parasitic infestations, nearly all cholangitis is related to an obstructing lesion in the ductal system. Surgical removal of the obstruction is the ultimate therapy; however, treatment with antibiotics that are effective against enteric organisms may permit stabilization of the patient prior to surgery.

SECONDARY BILIARY CIRRHOSIS

A late complication of chronic choledocholithiasis, with or without cholangitis, is secondary biliary cirrhosis. This condition may follow several attacks of acute cholangitis, but it may also develop silently in a patient with chronic, asymptomatic, partial biliary tract obstruction due to a stone. Diagnosis is made by liver biopsy to establish the presence and severity of the biliary cirrhosis, and by appropriate cholangiographic tests to locate the obstructing stone. Occasionally biliary cirrhosis may lead to hepatic failure or to portal hypertension and bleeding. Once secondary biliary cirrhosis has developed, removal of the obstructing lesion may fail to stop the progression of the cirrhosis.

POSTCHOLECYSTECTOMY COMPLICATIONS

A serious complication of gallbladder surgery is injury to the common duct. Occasionally the common duct is unknowingly completely severed, and the bile drains into the peritoneum to form a local chemical peritonitis, requiring a second surgical intervention. In the absence of complete transection, trauma to the common duct may lead, after a period of weeks, months, or years, to stricture formation and result in partial or complete biliary tract obstruction. The symptoms that develop are related to biliary tract obstruction, with or without infection, and include abdominal pain, jaundice, increased serum alkaline phosphatase level, and fulminant cholangitis. A rare surgical complication, ligation of the common duct, results in an identical clinical syndrome, which begins, however, within a day or two postoperatively and is characterized by progressively increasing jaundice. An important consideration in the differential diagnosis is the presence of stones that have been retained since the operation, or of stones that have formed in the biliary tree as a result of persistent cholangitis. Therefore, the diagnostic tests include an appropriate type of cholangiography. The problem of removing the retained or reformed stones is difficult; it may be helpful in this regard to place a large T tube in the duct at operation. The duct can then be cannulated and the stones removed or irrigated with stone-dissolving solutions. Some success in stone fragmentation and dissolution has been reported with the use of infusions of sodium cholate into the common duct. If a stricture is found, surgical reconstruction is necessary. Occasionally it is necessary to attach the gallbladder to the duodenum if the common duct is so badly damaged that it cannot be repaired. Such patients are often difficult to manage and develop relapsing cholangitis, often complicated by septicemia and subsequent biliary cirrhosis.

FISTULAS AND GALLSTONE ILEUS
During acute cholecystitis, the gallbladder may rupture not only into the peritoneum or locally to form an abscess, but also into one of the hollow organs, such as the stomach, duodenum, or colon. The most common place of perforation is the duodenum. If the patient does not undergo surgical repair, he may be left with a chronic choleduodenal fistula. Occasionally, a gallbladder containing large stones may erode, with few or no symptoms, into the duodenum or colon and result in a chronic fistula. These chronic fistulas rarely produce symptoms; occasionally, however, a large gallstone that passes from the gallbladder to the duodenum will cause intermittent intestinal obstruction as it moves down the small bowel and will lodge at the ileocecal sphincter to produce complete small bowel obstruction (gallstone ileus). This diagnosis is strongly suspected in a patient without previous abdominal surgery who develops small bowel obstruction and has air in the biliary tree. In some instances a radiopaque stone may be seen at the site of the obstruction. Gallstone ileus represents a surgical emergency.

GALLSTONE PANCREATITIS
A major cause of acute pancreatitis in nonalcoholic persons is a gallstone lodged in the common channel that drains both the pancreas and the biliary system. The diagnosis may be made by cholangiography, and the treatment is surgical (see Chap. 42).

Other Disorders Affecting the Gallbladder and Biliary Tract

TUMORS
Benign or malignant tumors may affect the biliary tree. Polyps of the gallbladder are usually benign and are rarely associated with cholecystitis. Malignant tumors of the gallbladder are often accompanied by stones, but there is no proof that one leads to the other. Certainly a tumor may alter bile composition and precipitate stones in the gallbladder, and conversely, stones may possibly irritate the gallbladder in such a way that a tumor forms. Symptoms from cancer of the gallbladder are often minimal until either the cystic duct or the common duct becomes involved, producing signs of obstruction. Tumors of the head of the pancreas, the common duct, or the large hepatic ducts often produce progressive, unrelenting jaundice; enlargement of the gallbladder (in the absence of chronic cholecystitis); steady, deep, epigastric pain; and anorexia and weight loss. These tumors are rarely complicated by cholangitis. Metastases to the liver are common. Whereas persistent or progressive obstructive jaundice is common in carcinoma of the ampulla of Vater, this lesion may also produce intermittent or fluctuating jaundice associated with occult bleeding into the intestinal lumen. Necrosis and sloughing of the tumor mass, temporarily relieving the obstruction of the bile duct, appears to be responsible for these phenomena. Surgical intervention to relieve obstruction may reduce the clinical symptoms, but prolonged survival is uncommon.

CHOLESTEROSIS OF THE GALLBLADDER

Cholesterosis of the gallbladder is a pathologic entity in which the wall of the organ is infiltrated with small flecks of lipid, presumably cholesterol esters. This condition is often found in association with chronic cholecystitis and cholelithiasis, but it is rarely seen in patients without gallstones. Its clinical significance is uncertain.

BILIARY DYSKINESIA

Some patients who complain of colic-like biliary pain have a normal cholecystogram and at operation are found to have a normal gallbladder without gallstones. Although it is conceivable that such a patient had a stone and passed it, it is also possible that alterations in the pressure dynamics of the biliary tract might be responsible for the pain. It has been suggested that a dose of CCK-PZ given during oral cholecystography may show that the gallbladder contracts but does not discharge its contents. The development of pain at the same time would suggest the presence of spasm of the cystic duct. The clinical significance of biliary dyskinesia is not known, but it is possible that alterations in biliary dynamics may be related to the formation of certain types of gallstones (see the section on gallstone disease).

SCLEROSING CHOLANGITIS

Sclerosing cholangitis is a rare disease of unknown etiology resulting in chronic inflammation and stenosis of the common bile duct, the hepatic bile ducts, or the intrahepatic radicles, in the absence of gallstone disease or prior biliary tract surgery. It may be associated with ulcerative colitis, retroperitoneal fibrosis, thyroiditis, or other autoimmune disorders. The initial symptom is a slowly progressive jaundice, often without pain or fever. Cholangiography, either percutaneous, retrograde, or operative, is necessary to establish the diagnosis. The possibility of sclerosing bile duct carcinoma must always be considered, and because histologic diagnosis is extremely difficult, malignancy can be excluded only by the passage of time. Although surgical decompression of the biliary tract and immunosuppressive treatment with corticosteroids and azathioprine have been attempted, the prognosis is generally poor, with death resulting from secondary biliary cirrhosis.

Bibliography

Admirand, W. H., and Small, D. M. The physicochemical basis of cholesterol gallstone formation in man. *J. Clin. Invest.* 47:1043, 1968.

Danzinger, R. G., Hofmann, A. F., Schoenfield, L., and Thistle, J. L. Dissolution of cholesterol gallstones by chenodeoxycholic acid. *N. Engl. J. Med.* 286:1, 1972.

Glenn, F., and McSherry, C. K. Calculous Biliary Tract Disease. In M. M. Ravich (ed.), *Current Problems in Surgery.* Chicago: Year Book, 1975. P. 4.

Grundy, S. M., and Bennion, L. J. Effects of obesity and caloric intake on biliary lipid metabolism in man. *J. Clin. Invest.* 56:996, 1975.

Grundy, S. M., Metzger, A. L., and Adler, R. Pathogenesis of lithogenic bile in American Indian women with cholesterol gallstones. *J. Clin. Invest.* 51:3026, 1972.

Maki, T. Pathogenesis of calcium bilirubinate gallstones: Role of *E. coli,* β-glycuronidase and coagulation by inorganic ions, polyelectrolytes and agitation. *Ann. Surg.* 164:90, 1966.

Redinger, R. N., and Small, D. M. Bile composition, bile salt metabolism and gallstones. *Arch. Intern. Med.* 130:618, 1972.

Sampliner, R. E., Bennett, P. H., Commess, L. J., et al. Gallbladder disease in Pima Indians: Demonstrations of high prevalence and early onset by cholecystography. *N. Engl. J. Med.* 283:1358, 1970.

Shaffer, E. A., and Small, D. M. Biliary lipid secretion in cholesterol gallstone disease: The effect of cholecystectomy and obesity. *J. Clin. Invest.* 59:828, 1977.

Small, D. M. The formation of gallstones. *Adv. Intern. Med.* 16:243, 1970.

Small, D. M. Advantages of a Varied and Individualized Approach. In F. J. Ingelfinger et al. (eds.), *Controversy in Internal Medicine II.* Philadelphia: Saunders, 1974. P. 545.

Small, D. M. The Formation and Treatment of Gallstones. In L. Schiff (ed.), *Diseases of the Liver*
(4th ed.). Philadelphia: Lippincott, 1975.
P. 146.

Small, D. M., Dowling, R. H., and Redinger,
R. N. The enterohepatic circulation of bile
salts. *Arch. Intern. Med.* 130:552, 1972.

41

Diseases of the Liver

Raymond S. Koff

The liver, the largest internal organ of the body, receives approximately one-quarter of the cardiac output and plays a fundamental role in the metabolism of protein, carbohydrate, and fat. It is solely responsible for the production of albumin and for the synthesis of a number of coagulation factors. It serves as a site of drug detoxification and of inactivation of both steroid and nonsteroid hormones. In early fetal life the liver is a hematopoietic organ, and it may resume this function in some abnormal conditions. Bilirubin metabolism is subserved by the liver, which is also responsible for the secretion of bile. In addition to its secretory and excretory functions, the liver stores vitamins and minerals, and the Kupffer cells (hepatic mononuclear macrophages) represent an important element in the body's defense mechanisms. Furthermore, the liver is endowed with a remarkable reserve; its regeneration and complete functional restoration have followed the removal of up to 90 percent of the organ.

Although studies of the function and structure of the normal liver have led to important advances in our understanding of hepatic metabolism, much basic information concerning the etiology, epidemiology, pathogenesis, and natural history of hepatic diseases is still limited, frustrating efforts at prevention and treatment. In recent years acute and chronic disorders of the liver have been recognized as sources of increasing morbidity and mortality throughout the world. As basic knowledge of these disorders accrues, the concepts presented here will need continued revision.

Disorders of Bilirubin Metabolism

Bilirubin, a lipid-soluble yellow pigment, is formed chiefly (80 percent) from the heme of senescent red blood cells, with a daily production of 250 to 300 mg; the so-called early-labeled fraction of bilirubin is derived from the hemoglobin of immature red cells and from other hemoproteins, for example, the cyto-

chromes. The conversion of heme to biliverdin by the microsomal enzyme, heme oxygenase, occurs in the spleen, kidney, and liver. Biliverdin is subsequently reduced to bilirubin by the soluble enzyme biliverdin reductase.

In plasma, bilirubin is bound to albumin in a molar ratio of 2:1; however, the first of the two bilirubin molecules is more tightly bound than the second. Production of bilirubin in excess of binding capacity, or displacement of bilirubin from albumin by changes in pH or by organic anions (e.g., sulfonamide drugs), permits the pigment to diffuse from the plasma into the tissues. In jaundiced newborns such transfer of bilirubin into the central nervous system may produce kernicterus (bilirubin encephalopathy).

Bilirubin in plasma is delivered to the surface of the hepatocytes, where the pigment is rapidly taken up, presumably by means of a specific carrier mechanism. Within the hepatocytes most of the bilirubin is bound to two soluble cytoplasmic protein acceptors, ligandin, and Z. These proteins also bind other organic anions, which can compete with bilirubin for binding sites. Intracellular lipid-soluble bilirubin is then converted to water-soluble conjugates, which are readily excreted in bile. Bilirubin conjugation is catalyzed primarily by the microsomal enzyme, bilirubin glucuronyl transferase. The activity of this enzyme may be stimulated by phenobarbital treatment. Most of the conjugated bilirubin formed is bilirubin diglucuronide, but both a monoglucuronide and several nonglucuronide sugar conjugates have also been described. The conjugated pigment is secreted into bile against a concentration gradient, probably by a carrier-mediated, energy-utilizing process, which is still poorly understood. Conjugated bilirubin traverses the biliary system and small intestine and is reduced in the colon by bacterial enzymes to a group of compounds called urobilinogen. Although most of the urobilinogen is excreted in the feces, a small fraction is reabsorbed and is subsequently reexcreted by the liver into bile (enterohepatic circulation). Trace amounts appear in urine.

Alternate pathways of bilirubin excretion have been identified, in which bilirubin is degraded directly to water-soluble derivatives without conjugation. The mechanisms of this process, its physiologic importance, and its promotion by blue or white light (phototherapy) are now under investigation.

The serum of normal adults contains 1 mg or less of bilirubin per 100 ml. Two pigment fractions are present: a water-soluble, conjugated fraction consisting predominantly of bilirubin diglucuronide and giving a direct Ehrlich's diazo reaction, and a lipid-soluble, unconjugated fraction giving an indirect diazo reaction. In healthy adults the direct fraction is usually less than 0.25 mg per 100 ml. Measurement of both fractions may be helpful in identifying certain disorders of bilirubin metabolism that cause jaundice or hyperbilirubinemia in the absence of intrinsic liver diseases.

UNCONJUGATED HYPERBILIRUBINEMIA
An increase in serum unconjugated bilirubin may be a result of increased pigment production. Either increased hemolysis from any source (for example, extravasated blood in tissues) or ineffective erythropoiesis (as in thalassemia and pernicious anemia) may overload the liver with unconjugated pigment, causing hyperbilirubinemia without bilirubinuria. Hemolysis, except when massive, results in bilirubin levels of 2 to 4 mg per 100 ml.

Unconjugated hyperbilirubinemia may also result from an impaired or an absent hepatic conjugation of bilirubin. Two variants of this condition have been described. In the first, the classic Crigler-Najjar syndrome, bilirubin is absent from bile. Both bilirubin glucuronyl transferase and bilirubin glucuronide formation are completely absent, and phenobarbital has no effect. Genetic studies suggest an autosomal recessive mode of inheritance. Severe jaundice is life-long, but it is usually associated with kernicterus and leads to early death. In the other variant, an autosomal dominant transmission has been suggested; hyperbilirubinemia is less marked, brain damage is not clinically apparent, some conjugated bilirubin is present in bile, and phenobarbital treatment does lower the serum bilirubin level.

Gilbert's syndrome is a common disorder characterized by unconjugated hyperbilirubinemia in the absence of any recognized liver disease. A reduced bilirubin clearance and an impaired conjugating ability appear to be present, resulting in hyperbilirubinemia;

the mechanism of this process is unknown. Except for an increase in lipofuscin in liver biopsy specimens in some patients, the liver appears to be structurally normal. Liver function tests are usually within normal limits, although clearance of sodium sulfobromophthalein (Bromsulphalein) may be reduced in a few patients. Patients with Gilbert's syndrome are not clinically ill, although they may have nonspecific gastrointestinal symptoms and mild fatigue. The hyperbilirubinemia may be most marked after either stress or prolonged fasting (longer than 48 hours). No treatment other than explanation and reassurance is required. Phenobarbital may be used to reduce the serum bilirubin level for cosmetic purposes.

CONJUGATED HYPERBILIRUBINEMIA
Increased serum levels of predominantly conjugated bilirubin are observed in the Dubin-Johnson syndrome. In this familial disorder, there is a defect in the transport of a number of organic anions (including bilirubin, sodium sulfobromophthalein, and cholecystographic contrast media) from the hepatic cells into the bile. Liver biopsy specimens are usually, but not always, dark as a result of the accumulation of a melanin pigment. A variant of the Dubin-Johnson syndrome without hepatic pigmentation is called Rotor's syndrome. Defects in porphyrin metabolism and excretion have been described in these two syndromes. Patients with either disorder may be asymptomatic, but about half of them have mild abdominal pain and hepatomegaly.

Cholestatic Syndromes
The term *cholestasis* is used to describe the clinical picture resulting from a decrease in the flow of hepatic bile into the duodenum, including both diminished bile flow resulting from parenchymal liver disease, and that caused by either intrahepatic or extrahepatic obstruction of the bile ducts. Diminution of bile flow is accompanied by increased blood levels of bile acids, bilirubin, cholesterol, and alkaline phosphatase (the increase in alkaline phosphatase is due to increased hepatic synthesis of the enzyme). A unique lipoprotein, termed *lipoprotein-X,* which consists of a 1:1 molar mixture of free cholesterol

and phospholipid, appears to be responsible for hyper-lipemia in the clinical syndrome of cholestasis. Pruritus, which can be correlated with the levels of bile salts in the skin, and low-grade steatorrhea resulting from inadequate intestinal micelle formation, may also be prominent features of cholestasis. Malabsorption of the fat-soluble vitamins (A, D, E, and K) may result, and hypoprothrombinemia, responsive to parenteral vitamin K administration, is characteristic. By contrast, in severe parenchymal liver disease the prolongation of the prothrombin time is not responsive to vitamin K, except to the extent that cholestasis may be present.

Functional impairment of bile excretion (intra-hepatic cholestasis) may occur in a variety of medical conditions, including acute viral, drug-induced, or alcoholic hepatitis; primary biliary cirrhosis; gram-negative septicemia; Hodgkin's disease; recurrent jaundice of pregnancy; benign familial recurrent cho-lestasis; and following surgery. This functional im-pairment must be distinguished from anatomic or mechanical bile duct obstruction caused by stones, tumors, strictures, or compression of the biliary tree. Since patients with intrinsic liver disease carry an increased risk during both anesthesia and surgery, a precise diagnosis is desirable to avoid unnecessary operations. Laboratory, radiographic, and other specialized diagnostic procedures should be obtained within a few days of admission and prior to laparot-omy. If signs of ascending cholangitis are present, surgery is indicated, and operative cholangiography will quickly determine the presence and site of biliary obstruction. Frequently the history and physical examination suggest a nonsurgical cause of choles-tasis, and additional diagnostic procedures may be employed during a 2- to 4-week period of observation. These procedures include barium meals and hypo-tonic duodenography for defining the area surround-ing the ampulla of Vater. Transhepatic "skinny-needle" cholangiography may demonstrate anatomic abnormalities of the biliary tree, but if this procedure is not available, transduodenal retrograde cholangi-ography may reveal the site of obstruction, which should be immediately attacked by laparotomy. If intrahepatic cholestasis is likely and cholestasis per-sists during the observation period, needle biopsy of the liver may confirm a primary liver disease. How-ever, without the hallmarks of extrahepatic obstruc-tion (bile "lakes" and polymorphonuclear leukocytes intimately associated with the portal tract bile ducts), morphologic differentiation of extrahepatic from intrahepatic cholestasis may be extremely difficult.

Viral Hepatitis

DEFINITION

Hepatitis, if defined simply as injury to hepatic cells and infiltration of inflammatory cells into the liver, is not an uncommon manifestation of a variety of sys-temic infectious processes. In such instances, histo-pathologic changes are minimal and liver involvement is usually clinically silent, and thus there is little con-fusion with viral hepatitis. *Viral hepatitis* is the term used to describe at least three common, clinically similar systemic diseases caused by three, and possibly four distinct agents, hepatitis A, B, and non-A, non-B viruses, which affect the liver predominantly. Heterogenous immunity does not develop between these types. Hepatitis A has also been called infec-tious hepatitis, and hepatitis B was formerly called serum hepatitis. Non-A, non-B hepatitis viruses (at least two are postulated) are an important cause of transfusion-associated hepatitis; their identity and properties are not yet established.

ETIOLOGY

The agent of hepatitis A has been identified during the early acute phase of the disease in the stools of affected patients. It is 27 nm in diameter, appears to be an enterovirus (RNA), and reacts with an antibody found in both convalescent hepatitis A sera and im-mune serum globulin. The marmoset, a South Amer-ican monkey, and the chimpanzee appear to be sus-ceptible to hepatitis A. The hepatitis B virus is about 42 nm in diameter and contains antigenic materials both on its surface (the hepatitis B surface antigen [HB_sAg]) and in its core (the hepatitis B core antigen [HB_cAg]). Both DNA and DNA polymerase activity are associated with HB_cAg. A third antigen, the "e" antigen, is a nonparticulate material closely associated with the hepatitis B virus. This antigen appears to be a marker of infectivity, and its persistence in serum may indicate the progression of acute to chronic hepatitis. HB_sAg appears in the circulation of patients affected with acute hepatitis B, and persistent HB_sAg is found in 0.1 to 1.0 percent of apparently healthy persons in the United States. It is more prevalent in subtropical and tropical climates and in immunosuppressed patients. HB_sAg is an indicator of hepatitis B but is not infectious by itself. Chimpanzees have been infected with hepatitis B. Neither the virus of hepatitis A nor that of hepatitis B has been propagated in tissue culture.

EPIDEMIOLOGIC FEATURES
Both hepatitis A and B are transmissible by oral and parenteral routes. The incubation period of hepatitis A is usually about 30 days (15 to 50 days), whereas that of hepatitis B is longer — up to 180 days. The incubation period of parenterally transmitted non-A, non-B viral hepatitis resembles that of hepatitis B. Viremia occurs during both the incubation period and the acute phase of both hepatitis A and B, but it is short-lived in hepatitis A and is rare after the first few days of illness. Five to ten percent of patients with hepatitis B continue to have circulating HB_sAg 3 months after the onset of illness. Although many patients seem to recover completely, some have chronic hepatitis. Fecal shedding of hepatitis A occurs during the latter half of the incubation period through the first few days of the illness. Fecal excretion of HB_sAg is uncommon. Neither urinary nor nasopharyngeal excretion of virus A or B has been clearly demonstrated, but HB_sAg has been identified in saliva and a variety of other body fluids and secretions.

Person-to-person transmission by the fecal-oral route is the predominant means of spread of hepatitis A. Transmission of hepatitis B by the oral route can occur, and it is more likely to occur under poor sanitary conditions (although the importance of this is uncertain). Venereal transmission appears to be a means of spread in hepatitis B and possibly may occur in hepatitis A. Respiratory spread and arthropod vectors have been suggested for both hepatitis A and B, but again, their significance is uncertain. In all forms of viral hepatitis, anicteric infections are more common than icteric disease. Intimate exposure to persons with anicteric cases of hepatitis A or B or to certain asymptomatic carriers of HB_sAg may be a significant mode of spread.

Common-source outbreaks of hepatitis A have been traced to the ingestion of contaminated water and foods, including milk, and raw or inadequately cooked clams or oysters; hepatitis B has not been associated with this mode of transmission. Hepatitis A, B, and non-A, non-B can be spread parenterally by the injection of minute amounts of contaminated blood, serum, or blood products made from large donor pools but not inactivated either by heating or by ethanol fractionation. Non-A, non-B hepatitis are the most important hazards of blood transfusion, and the risk depends on the number of units transfused and the donor sources (paid donors are more hazardous than volunteers). Contamination of needles, syringes, and other intravenous infusion equipment, as well as of tattooing needles, has led to outbreaks of hepatitis. Sporadic cases and outbreaks of hepatitis are common among parenteral drug users.

PATHOLOGY
Hepatitis A, B, and non-A, non-B viral hepatitis produce identical histologic changes in the liver. The characteristic lesions include diffuse areas of hepatocyte necrosis or degeneration (manifested as cell dropout), ballooning of cells, free acidophilic bodies, or a combination of these, accompanied by thickened liver cell plates, binucleated liver cells, and occasional mitotic figures. A mononuclear cell infiltrate is present in areas of necrosis and in the portal zones. Kupffer cells are usually prominent and may contain lipofuscin pigment. Cholestasis is variable, but fatty infiltration is not usually seen. Anicteric hepatitis usually results in similar but more subtle changes. Electron microscopic studies reveal diffuse organelle injury and may show viruslike particles in hepatocytes in patients with hepatitis.

CLINICAL FEATURES
The illness typically begins with constitutional symptoms such as anorexia and malaise, accompanied by nausea, vomiting, diarrhea, and in about one-third to one-quarter of patients, diffuse arthralgia. A weight loss of 2 to 4 kg is not unusual during this phase. Right upper quadrant discomfort and a distaste for

cigarettes are commonly reported during this prodromal period, which may last from 2 to 14 days.
Patients with hepatitis A often experience fever with
an influenzalike illness of abrupt onset, but this is less
frequent in hepatitis B. A syndrome resembling serum
sickness and consisting of urticaria, angioneurotic
edema, skin eruptions, polyarthritis, and, rarely,
hematuria may be the initial manifestation of hepatitis B; this syndrome appears to result from the
deposition of immune complexes of HB_sAg and antibody with complement. Patients with anicteric hepatitis may have only transient fever, gastrointestinal and
respiratory symptoms, malaise, and anorexia, with an
abbreviated course. In such patients the diagnosis
may be difficult unless appropriate laboratory tests
are obtained.

When jaundice does appear, it is often preceded
for a few days by darkening of the urine (bilirubinuria)
and lightening of the stool color. Transient pruritus is
common during this preicteric phase. Physical examination reveals hepatic enlargement and mild liver
tenderness on palpation. Punch tenderness may be
elicited over the lower right rib cage. Transient
splenomegaly and lymphadenopathy are found in
approximately 20 percent of patients. With the
development of jaundice, many of the prodromal
symptoms and the fever, if present, subside. The
jaundice is usually maximal by the second week after
onset; it then decreases, disappearing by 6 to 8 weeks
or earlier in most cases, while stool color darkens
again. Full clinical recovery may be expected in more
than 80 percent of patients by the end of the six-
teenth week, and in 90 to 95 percent by the end of
6 months. In about 1 to 5 percent of patients a recurrence of symptoms, transaminase elevation, and jaundice may occur following an apparently complete
recovery. This relapse usually occurs within 6 months
of the original illness, is short-lived and milder in
severity, and does not affect the prognosis. In a few
patients, vague functional complaints (asthenia,
malaise) may be noted following viral hepatitis,
although liver function tests and liver biopsy reveal
no abnormalities.

Anicteric disease is rarely, if ever, fatal. Case fatality rates of hepatitis are highest in transfusion-associated hepatitis with jaundice (approaching 10 percent),
and lowest[1] in orally transmitted hepatitis A (0.1 percent). Debility, malignancy, and increased age diminish the survival rate of affected patients.

Infrequently, mild steatorrhea may occur during
the icteric phase of hepatitis, resulting from a deficiency of bile salts. Glomerulonephritis, pancreatitis,
myocarditis, pericarditis, acute myelitis, aseptic
meningitis, and peripheral neuropathy have all been
reported to occur rarely in viral hepatitis.

LABORATORY FEATURES

Serologic detection of HB_sAg and antibody to the
core antigen (anti-HB_c) during the acute phase, and of
antibody to HB_sAg (anti-HB_s) in convalescent sera,
permits specific identification of hepatitis B infection.
Hepatitis A infection may be identified by demonstration of seroconversion using immune adherence,
complement fixation, or radioimmunoassay techniques. Non-A, non-B viral hepatitis are diagnosed
by exclusion.

Leukopenic or low-normal leukocytic counts with
relative lymphocytosis are common during the prodromal and early acute phases. Atypical lymphocytosis
may occur, and mild hemolytic anemia is rarely observed. Occasional patients with sickle cell anemia or
others with a glucose 6-phosphate dehydrogenase
deficiency may develop severe hemolysis (with marked
hyperbilirubinemia) when they have viral hepatitis.
Rarely, a fatal aplastic anemia may occur during
convalescence.

Serial liver function tests reveal a progressive rise of
serum transaminase levels beginning during the prodromal period. The elevations of serum glutamic-
pyruvic transaminase (SGPT) are often higher than
those of serum glutamic-oxalacetic transaminase
(SGOT); peak values of 400 to 4,000 units or higher
may be observed. Elevation of serum transaminase
levels may be the only abnormality present in anicteric hepatitis, although the serum conjugated bilirubin level is also often increased. Total serum bilirubin may reach peak levels of between 5 and 20 mg
per 100 ml in icteric cases. Serum alkaline phosphatase and serum globulin levels are usually normal or
mildly elevated. Serum albumin may decrease slightly,
and the prothrombin time may be slightly to moderately increased.

TREATMENT

No specific treatment is available for viral hepatitis. Although the disease is usually mild, hospitalization may be required for clinically severe cases. Such patients generally desire rest and occasionally require parenteral feeding if they vomit persistently. When possible, a palatable, balanced diet is desirable. High-protein diets offer no specific benefit and may be hazardous in a patient with severe hepatitis and impending coma. Drugs should be used only with caution, and elective surgery should be avoided during the acute phase. Both at home and in the hospital, separate toilet facilities are desirable for patients with hepatitis A during the first days of the acute phase of illness. Relapses of hepatitis are treated similarly.

VARIANTS OF VIRAL HEPATITIS

Cholestatic Hepatitis

Infrequently, patients with viral hepatitis present a clinical picture of intrahepatic cholestasis closely resembling extrahepatic bile duct obstruction. Liver studies typically reveal severe hyperbilirubinemia — total serum bilirubin may reach levels as high as 30 mg per 100 ml or more, and serum alkaline phosphatase activity may rise to two to six times normal. Serum transaminase levels are elevated. On liver biopsy, bile stasis, hepatocyte necrosis, and a portal inflammation rich in polymorphonuclear leukocytes are found. Severe pruritus and deep jaundice may persist for weeks, but in time these symptoms subside. Surgery may be extremely hazardous in these patients.

Bridging Necrosis

Bridging necrosis, also called subacute hepatic necrosis, an infrequent variant of viral hepatitis, may occur more often in hepatitis B than in type A. The disease usually begins insidiously, but the presenting features may be indistinguishable from those of classic acute viral hepatitis. The subsequent course, however, is often strikingly different. Jaundice persists or increases during the first few weeks, and total serum bilirubin levels fluctuate at values usually greater than 20 mg per 100 ml. The patient continues to feel ill during this period, with persistent nausea, vomiting, and malaise as prominent features. Serum transaminase levels remain elevated, and significant hypo-albuminemia and hyperglobulinemia are often noted. The prothrombin time may be prolonged. Physical findings include persistent hepatosplenomegaly, multiple spider angiomas, and signs of fluid retention. Liver biopsy, if not contraindicated by coagulation abnormalities, discloses confluent, intralobular hepatic necrosis "bridging" adjacent portal tracts, or situated between the portal tracts and the central veins. A predominantly mononuclear infiltrate may be present in areas of necrosis and in the portal tracts.

The course of the disease is variable. About half the patients recover completely after many weeks or months, but as many as 30 percent may go on to have postnecrotic cirrhosis. Some of these patients pass through a phase of illness resembling chronic active hepatitis. Death may result from liver failure, hemorrhage resulting from esophageal varices, or infection. Although corticosteroids have been given for bridging necrosis, their effectiveness has not been proved and they may be hazardous.

Massive Hepatic Necrosis

Massive hepatic necrosis (fulminant hepatitis, acute yellow atrophy) in acute viral hepatitis is manifested by a rapid downhill course characterized by the development of hepatic coma, a diminution of liver size, and in 65 to 95 percent of patients, death within a few weeks. It should be emphasized that sudden shrinking of the liver is an ominous finding and is never to be interpreted as a sign of recovery. Serum bilirubin levels are variably elevated; serum transaminase may be only moderately increased (occasionally it is near normal immediately before death), but the prothrombin time is profoundly abnormal, and bleeding is common. Hypoglycemia may be present in 5 percent of patients and may contribute to the encephalopathy. Sepsis, renal and respiratory failure, hypotension, and cerebral edema are common in terminal cases. Liver tissue, obtained either at postmortem or by biopsy in survivors, reveals massive interlobular necrosis affecting most liver lobules. In survivors, nearly normal liver tissue may subsequently be found.

Treatment is directed at maintenance of vital functions, correction of hypoglycemia, and control of fluid and electrolyte balance until liver regeneration occurs. Minimally absorbed antibiotics or lactulose is administered to reduce intestinal putrefaction and lower stool pH, and dietary protein is restricted. Corticosteroids in large doses, L-dopa administration, and other methods have been tried, but their efficacy has not been established. Exchange transfusions are not effective.

PREVENTIVE MEASURES

Immune Serum Globulin

Immune serum globulin (in a dose of 0.02 ml/kg/ body weight), when given intramuscularly to household members or other intimate contacts of patients with hepatitis A, will modify the disease to a subclinical form. Globulin has no effect when administered *after* the actual onset of illness or more than a few weeks after exposure. Immune serum globulin is also indicated for persons exposed to identified common-source vehicles of hepatitis A. A larger dose (0.10 ml per kilogram) will produce a modifying effect for a period of up to 6 months and is indicated in travelers who require prolonged protection in endemic areas.

Although available data are conflicting, standard immune serum globulin probably does not modify parenterally transmitted hepatitis A or B; however, hyperimmune globulin containing large amounts of antibody to HB_sAg appears to reduce the incidence of both parenterally and nonparenterally transmitted hepatitis B. Trials of a purified HB_sAg containing vaccine are under consideration for prophylaxis in hepatitis B.

Other Control Measures

The incidence of parenterally transmitted hepatitis may be decreased by the use of disposable parenteral injection equipment, but scrupulous attention must be directed even to the disposal of these "throwaways," to prevent accidental inoculations. The avoidance of unnecessary blood transfusions and the use of noninfective blood products or of lower-risk frozen red cells instead of whole blood will lessen the incidence of such cases. The risk of posttransfusion hepatitis may also be significantly reduced by the elimination of commercial blood donors.

Liver Disease Associated with Other Infectious Agents

Infrequently during the course of infection with a number of viral or nonviral agents, for example, cytomegalovirus, herpes simplex, enteroviruses, toxoplasmosis, Q fever, psittacosis, or secondary syphilis, clinical evidence of liver injury resembling viral hepatitis is present. Accurate diagnosis is dependent on appropriate isolation and serologic studies. Usually the hepatic manifestations of infection are overshadowed by signs and symptoms of other organ involvement. Differentiation of hepatitis associated with infectious mononucleosis (Epstein-Barr virus) is a frequent problem. Although only about 10 percent of patients with mononucleosis have clinical jaundice, they usually have laboratory evidence of hepatic dysfunction. The signs and symptoms of liver disease in infectious mononucleosis are usually short-lived, and hepatic fatalities are very rare. Clinical differentiation of the hepatitis associated with mononucleosis from viral hepatitis may be difficult in some instances, but pharyngitis, prominent cervical lymphadenopathy, fever, and (in more than half the cases) splenomegaly all point to mononucleosis. Measurement of acute and convalescent serum levels of EB virus antibody, together with the differential heterophil agglutination test, may help to confirm the diagnosis of mononucleosis.

Jaundice is noted in approximately 40 percent of leptospirosis cases in the United States. It is most frequent in *Leptospira icterohaemorrhagiae* infections, but it may be seen with other serotypes. Diffuse myalgia, fever, headache, conjunctivitis, and severe malaise are common. Leukocytosis is often striking, and renal damage is characteristic, in contrast to the leukopenia and the usually normal renal function of patients with viral hepatitis. Serial measurement of leptospiral agglutinins will usually confirm the nature of the disease process.

Chronic Hepatitis

CHRONIC ACTIVE HEPATITIS

Chronic active hepatitis is a disorder characterized by hepatic necrosis, inflammation, and fibrosis, progressing in some patients to postnecrotic cirrhosis. Synonyms for the disease include *autoimmune hepatitis, lupoid hepatitis,* and *plasma cell hepatitis.* Immune mechanisms are thought to be involved in the initiation or progression of this disorder, since abnormal immunologic reactions and other conditions suspected of having an immune basis are not uncommon in affected patients. Inciting factors include viral infections, particularly hepatitis B; drugs (e.g., oxyphenisatin, methyldopa, isoniazid); and possibly other unknown agents. Genetic susceptibility has been postulated.

Pathology

Affected liver lobules show a dense infiltration of mononuclear and plasma cells in the portal zone, extending into the surrounding parenchyma. Individual lobules may be spared. *Piecemeal necrosis* refers to the characteristic necrosis of liver cells occurring at the periphery of the liver lobule adjacent to the portal zone. Septa of connective tissue extend from the portal zone into the parenchyma. Postnecrotic cirrhosis may be found at postmortem examination. In some patients the histologic features of bridging necrosis or primary biliary cirrhosis may also be observed.

Clinical Features

Men and women of all ages are susceptible. The disease develops insidiously in about two-thirds of patients, whereas an abrupt onset resembling viral hepatitis occurs in the remainder; the features of chronic active hepatitis develop within 6 months. In other patients the disease may be discovered incidentally, or it may come to light because of extrahepatic features or complications of cirrhosis. Fatigue is usually the most salient symptom. Abdominal pain, polyarthralgia or polyarthritis, pleurisy, acne, amenorrhea, diarrhea, and fever may be presenting features drawing attention away from the liver. However, persistent or intermittent jaundice develops in 80 percent of patients with the classic syndrome, and hepatomegaly is found in a similar proportion. Splenomegaly is present in about 50 percent of patients, and ascites and spider angiomas may be present or may develop with progression of the disease. Wedged hepatic venous pressure is usually elevated and reflects

portal hypertension. Skin lesions commonly observed include acne vulgaris, erythema nodosum, urticaria, striae, ulcerations, and maculopapular eruptions. About 30 percent of patients have chronic diarrhea, and 10 percent have a disease similar to ulcerative colitis (in true ulcerative colitis, the incidence of chronic active hepatitis is under 5 percent). Hematuria, the nephrotic syndrome, and renal tubular acidosis may be noted.

The course of the disease, although variable, is usually progressive in the classic case, with inactive phases occurring in approximately 20 percent of patients. The histologic lesion may become quiescent before the establishment of cirrhosis. Mortality is high in patients with bridging necrosis during the early years of illness, with death usually resulting from hepatic failure. In later years, death may be a result of the complications of cirrhosis. The entity known as cryptogenic cirrhosis is believed in some cases to be a sequel of unrecognized chronic active hepatitis. The natural history of asymptomatic patients with chronic active hepatitis is uncertain.

Laboratory Studies

Anemia, leukopenia, and thrombocytopenia may reflect either hypersplenism or an immune-mediated process. Serum bilirubin levels may be moderately elevated but are usually less than 20 mg per 100 ml. SGOT levels range from 100 to 1,000 units in most cases, although both nearly normal and exceedingly high values have been occasionally observed. Gamma globulin levels above 2.0 gm per 100 ml are not unusual, and depressed albumin levels are found in patients with active or advanced disease. The prothrombin time may be prolonged. As many as one-quarter of patients have positive tests for HB_sAg, in low titer. The L.E. cell phenomenon, antinuclear antibodies, and smooth muscle antibodies are commonly found and may be most frequent in those patients who are negative for HB_sAg. Antimitochondrial antibodies are present in 10 to 20 percent of patients, usually in low titer.

Diagnosis

The early course of the disease may resemble acute

viral hepatitis; however, disease activity continuing for longer than 6 months indicates chronic active hepatitis, which must be distinguished from slowly resolving or persistent hepatitis (see the following section). Liver biopsy is required for definitive diagnosis.

Treatment

Rest may be beneficial during active phases of the disease, and 20 percent of patients may remit spontaneously with only supportive care. Therapy with corticosteroids (e.g., prednisolone, 15 to 20 mg daily) is effective in prolonging life expectancy during the early years of illness in severely ill patients with bridging necrosis. Symptomatic relief resulting from steroids occurs within weeks, whereas biochemical improvement may occur over a period of months. Histologic regression may be delayed for as long as 2 years. Azathioprine treatment combined with corticosteroids is effective, although azathioprine alone is not beneficial. It is not yet known whether such treatment is beneficial in patients with mild or asymptomatic disease.

PERSISTENT HEPATITIS

The term *persistent hepatitis* is synonymous with a slow resolution of and a delayed convalescence from viral hepatitis. Although the disorder is recognized in 5 to 10 percent of patients with viral hepatitis, only 70 to 80 percent of patients with persistent hepatitis give a history of a preceding acute episode suggestive of viral hepatitis. It seems probable that the remainder have had anicteric or asymptomatic viral hepatitis.

Pathology

The characteristic histopathologic change in persistent hepatitis is a portal mononuclear cell infiltration with preservation of lobular architecture. Portal fibrosis, if present, is slight, and progression to cirrhosis does not occur. Hepatocyte degenerative changes are minimal, and nodular regeneration and confluent necrosis are not seen.

Clinical Features and Course

Many patients are asymptomatic and do not seek medical attention. Elevation of serum transaminase levels may be the only recognizable abnormality. Persistent circulating HB_sAg is found in high titer in 10 to 40 percent of cases, and in some patients other liver function tests may be mildly abnormal. Moderate hepatomegaly may be noted. Recurrent acute episodes of viral hepatitis-like illness occur but are infrequent. In about two-thirds of patients the disease lasts for up to 8 months; in the remainder the disease may persist for years. Evidence of extrahepatic involvement is rare; wedged hepatic vein pressure is normal; and the prognosis is invariably good.

Treatment

No specific treatment is indicated. Reassurance of the patient is necessary to make it clear that a serious disorder is not present and full recovery is to be expected.

Abscess of the Liver

PYOGENIC ABSCESS

The primary sources of infection leading to *pyogenic abscess* of the liver are intraperitoneal sepsis, biliary obstruction, and generalized septicemia. The predominant pathogens include nonspore-forming, anaerobic gram-negative rods; anaerobic or microaerophilic streptococci; and typical enteric, aerobic gram-negative rods. Aerobic streptococci and staphylococci may be etiologically identified, particularly in cases beginning with septicemia.

Clinical Features

Symptoms may be present for 2 or 3 months before the diagnosis of pyogenic abscess is established. The typical clinical picture is that of sepsis, with fever, chills, and profuse sweating. Malaise, anorexia, and weight loss exceeding 4 kg are present in about 50 percent of patients; diarrhea is a feature in more than one-third. Dull, constant, right upper quadrant abdominal pain with or without pleuritic pain is common. Hepatomegaly and liver tenderness are characteristic, and a right pleural effusion may be observed. Jaundice is unusual (about 10 percent) in a solitary abscess, but it is more frequent in multiple abscesses. The latter are most commonly associated with biliary tract obstruction and have a high mortality rate.

Laboratory Studies
Polymorphonuclear leukocytosis is often striking, with a shift to the left; anemia is common, particularly in disease of prolonged duration. The serum alkaline phosphatase level is usually elevated, although serum transaminase levels are either normal or only minimally elevated. Moderate to high serum transaminase levels suggest acute suppurative cholangitis with miliary abscesses.

Diagnosis
The diagnosis of pyogenic abscess should be suspected in any patient with either sepsis following recent abdominal or rectal surgery, known bowel or biliary tract disease, endocarditis, or fever of unknown origin. Hepatic scintiscans may reveal a space-occupying lesion, which may be confirmed by angiography. Plain films of the chest and abdomen may reveal elevation of the diaphragm, right pleural effusion, and in some instances, an air-fluid level in an abscess cavity. Repeated aerobic and anaerobic blood cultures are mandatory, and the fluid aspirated by needle biopsy must be cultured promptly for anaerobes to avoid a false report of a "sterile" abscess. Hemagglutinin or complement fixation tests for amebiasis are necessary in all patients with liver abscesses.

Treatment
The mainstays of therapy consist of antibiotics and surgical drainage. The choice of antibiotics may be based on the susceptibility pattern of the organisms isolated from the blood or abscess cavity, and on the predicted susceptibility of organisms seen on Gram's stain. In the latter instance, antibiotics effective against anaerobes should be included, since mixed infections are common. Foul-smelling pus or gas in the abscess cavity is suggestive of anaerobic infection. Antibiotics should be continued for at least 4 months in patients with multiple abscesses and for at least 1 month in those with a solitary lesion. Surgical drainage is indicated for a single abscess but may be technically impossible for multiple abscesses. Mortality rates of 55 to 80 percent have been reported in recent series.

AMEBIC ABSCESS OF THE LIVER
While there are significant regional and socioeconomic

variations, the overall prevalence rate of *Entamoeba histolytica* infections in the United States is somewhat under 5 percent. Most of the affected persons are asymptomatic intestinal carriers. Amebic abscess of the liver is observed in about 2 to 5 percent of patients with intestinal amebiasis. A large proportion of these infections are acquired in foreign endemic areas, for example, Mexico. Amebic abscess is a disease predominantly of middle-aged men, although women, infants, and the elderly may also be affected.

Clinical Features
The symptoms of an amebic abscess of the liver resemble those just described for a pyogenic hepatic abscess, namely, an acute inflammatory process of a few weeks' duration, or less commonly, a chronic disease of several weeks' duration. Fever is characteristic, chills are present in about one-third of patients, and right upper quadrant abdominal pain, presumably resulting from distention of the liver capsule, is noted in about two-thirds. Pleuritic pain is present in about 10 percent of patients. Amebic abscess in the left lobe is less common than in the right, and may produce an epigastric mass or elevation of the left hemidiaphragm. A left lobe abscess is more likely than a right to rupture into either the abdominal cavity or the pericardial space. Amebic abscess in the right lobe is more likely to involve the pleura and lung. Laboratory features are similar to those found in pyogenic abscess.

Jaundice is present in 10 to 30 percent of patients and is a poor prognostic sign, but chemical studies are usually only mildly abnormal. Although single abscesses are typical of amebiasis of the liver, multiple abscesses have been reported in 10 to 20 percent of patients and are often associated with signs of peritonitis. Mortality rates vary between 10 and 20 percent.

Diagnosis
Amebic abscess should be suspected in any traveler returning from hyperendemic areas, but the absence of such a history does not exclude the diagnosis. The diagnostic finding of *Entamoeba histolytica* in the stool, associated with colonic ulceration, is uncommon; the most useful tests are the indirect hemag-

glutination, complement fixation, and gel diffusion procedures, the first being the most sensitive. The value of skin tests employing amebic antigens remains to be determined.

Needle aspiration may reveal "anchovy sauce" fluid with motile trophozoites that are either in the fluid or, more commonly (about 50 percent of cases), in the wall of the abscess cavity. The therapeutic value of multiple needle aspirations of amebic abscesses remains to be established. Treatment consists of metronidazole, 750 mg three times daily for 10 days, or chloroquine, 500 mg daily for 10 weeks.

Schistosomiasis and Echinococcosis

Schistosoma ova are transported from the bowel to the portal veins of the liver, where they induce an endophlebitis. A granulomatous eosinophilic response ensues, followed by periportal fibrosis; the latter results in presinusoidal portal hypertension and secondary splenomegaly. The liver may be enlarged, but liver chemistries, with the exception of sodium sulfobromophthalein (BSP) clearance, are frequently normal. Cirrhosis, if present, is caused by other conditions. Serologic tests (complement fixation) may reveal exposure to schistosomal antigen. The demonstration of *Schistosoma* eggs in fresh liver biopsy material crushed between glass slides is a quick diagnostic procedure and is more reliable than histologic studies of the same material. Treatment consists of antimonial compounds. Portacaval anastomosis may be required for repeated variceal hemorrhage.

A calcified and slowly progressive cystic lesion within the liver is the hallmark of echinococcal liver disease. Only a small number of cases are detected in the United States, but infection is frequently found in regions producing sheep and cattle. Although commonly asymptomatic in man, a cyst may present with the clinical picture of pyogenic liver abscess resulting from secondary bacterial invasion. Diagnosis is based on the roentgenographic appearance of the calcified lesion, and on skin and serologic testing. Percutaneous aspiration of the cyst is contraindicated because of the risk of a fatal anaphylactic reaction occurring after leakage of cyst contents. Surgical resection is curative.

Drug-induced Hepatitis

Injury to the liver may result from the percutaneous absorption, the inhalation, the ingestion, or the parenteral administration of a number of chemicals, including systemic poisons, which may be classified as direct hepatotoxins. The major group of drugs causing hepatitis are not direct hepatotoxins but rather certain pharmacologic agents classified as "sensitizing" agents, because their adverse hepatic effects appear to be related to poorly defined host susceptibility factors unique to man.

LIVER INJURY CAUSED BY HEPATOTOXINS

Direct hepatotoxin-induced liver injury is not unique to man because it can regularly be produced by the administration of the same toxins to other species. Hepatotoxin-induced injury is both predictable and dose-dependent; that is, all persons who are exposed to a sufficient quantity of a hepatotoxic agent will be affected and will have manifestations of toxicity shortly (within hours) after exposure. Agents responsible for hepatotoxin-induced liver injury include carbon tetrachloride, yellow phosphorus, and the cyclic peptides of the poisonous mushrooms (e.g., *Amanita phalloides*). Carbon tetrachloride, although it has been particularly well studied in experimental animals, is now an infrequent cause of liver disease in man (actually carbon tetrachloride itself is not an active hepatotoxin, but it is converted within the liver to toxic metabolites).

A characteristic morphologic pattern of hepatic injury is induced by each of the direct hepatotoxins. Thus, carbon tetrachloride produces centrilobular necrosis, yellow phosphorus typically causes periportal hepatic necrosis, and other agents may produce massive necrosis. Damage to other organs is to be expected, and in some instances liver injury may be inapparent until jaundice is evident. The clinical picture may be entirely similar to that of severe hepatic necrosis, as seen in viral hepatitis, but it is often complicated by evidence of dysfunction of other organs (for example, acute tubular necrosis of the kidney).

LIVER INJURY CAUSED BY SENSITIZING AGENTS

The liver injury induced by sensitizing agents, on the other hand, is unpredictable in that most persons can tolerate the responsible drugs without difficulty. Occasional patients give a history of other allergic reactions or drug sensitivities. This form of drug-induced hepatitis is not dose-dependent and may occur at various intervals during or after administration of the offending agent, although most cases are seen within the first few months. Infrequently and inexplicably, hepatic function and morphology may return to normal despite the continued administration of the responsible agent.

Extrahepatic allergic clinical manifestations, which are common in sensitivity hepatitis, include urticaria, rash, arthralgia, fever, leukocytosis, and eosinophilia. Both the liver injury and the accompanying allergic features are believed to be immunologically mediated, although this has not been proved. For some drugs, hepatitis appears to be more closely related to unique metabolic reactions controlling the disposition of the agent than to immunologic mechanisms. Two major patterns of liver pathology may be induced by sensitizing agents: One resembles viral hepatitis, with hepatocellular necrosis and inflammation, and the other resembles bile duct obstruction with cholestasis, with or without inflammatory changes in the portal zones. An example of the first condition is the viral hepatitis-like disease associated with isoniazid (INH) therapy; an example of the second is the intrahepatic cholestasis produced by chlorpromazine.

Approximately 10 percent of patients receiving INH will develop mild increases in serum transaminase levels, which return to normal within a few weeks whether or not therapy is continued. In contrast, about 1 percent of patients receiving INH develop an illness resembling viral hepatitis, with characteristic symptoms, signs, and biochemical abnormalities. Allergic manifestations are rare. In this illness, liver biopsy reveals hepatocellular damage, with infiltration of mononuclear, polymorphonuclear, and eosinophilic leukocytes in the areas of necrosis; these findings are frequently indistinguishable from those in viral hepatitis or bridging necrosis. Rechallenge with INH may precipitate acute elevations of serum transaminase levels. In some patients the disease is severe, and in 10 percent it has been reported to be fatal. Other drugs associated with a viral hepatitis-like illness include halothane, phenytoin, and methyldopa, to name but a few.

Chlorpromazine produces intrahepatic cholestasis with jaundice in about 1 percent of those taking the drug, usually during the first weeks of treatment. The illness begins with fever, rash, joint pains, nausea and vomiting, and abdominal pain. Pruritus may be striking and usually precedes the development of jaundice. Peripheral eosinophilia is common. Bile stasis is observed on liver biopsy, and chemical studies are compatible with cholestasis. Interruption of chlorpromazine usually relieves pruritus and jaundice within a few weeks to months; however, jaundice may persist for months or years, and in a few patients a syndrome resembling primary biliary cirrhosis has been described. Similar cholestatic drug reactions have been observed following administration of erythromycin estolate, methimazole, para-aminosalicylic acid, chlorpropamide, and other drugs.

In a few patients, sensitivity hepatitis may result in the production of granulomas within the liver (see the following section on granulomatous disorders). Drugs inducing this lesion include sulfonamides, phenylbutazone, and allopurinol.

LIVER DAMAGE CAUSED BY OTHER DRUGS
Other adverse hepatic drug reactions occur which cannot be classified as either toxic or sensitizing. Agents inducing these reactions include anabolic steroids, 17-alpha-alkyl-substituted testosterone derivatives, and oral contraceptives. The hepatic dysfunction produced by these agents is dose-related. For example, a combination of estrogen and progesterone regularly produces hepatic dysfunction in a large proportion of recipients, but it only infrequently causes jaundice. The dysfunction is most often observed in women who have recurrent, idiopathic jaundice or severe pruritus during successive pregnancies. Signs of extrahepatic hypersensitivity are absent. Liver biopsy reveals cholestasis without hepatocellular damage or inflammation. The disease subsides on withdrawal of the agent or on cessation of pregnancy. Rarely, hepatic vein occlusion or hemoperitoneum from focal nodular hyperplasia of the liver or hepatic

adenoma may occur in women treated with oral contraceptive agents.

DRUG-INDUCED CHRONIC LIVER DISEASE

As noted previously, a syndrome resembling primary biliary cirrhosis has occurred rarely after cholestatic reactions to chlorpromazine, tolbutamide, and methyltestosterone. A disease that is clinically and morphologically indistinguishable from chronic active hepatitis has been described after prolonged use of laxatives containing oxyphenisatin, and after treatment with methyldopa or isoniazid. Withdrawal of these drugs has resulted in clinical and histologic improvement. Prolonged administration of the antimetabolite methotrexate has been associated with the development of hepatic fibrosis and cirrhosis, but in these cases disturbances of liver function tests correlate poorly with the degree of damage found on liver biopsy. A rare, malignant tumor, angiosarcoma of the liver, has been identified following exposure to arsenic, thorium dioxide, or vinyl chloride.

The recognition that chronic as well as acute liver disease can follow the use of a wide variety of chemical agents emphasizes the importance of documenting drug exposure in every patient with jaundice or abnormalities of liver function.

Infiltrative, Granulomatous, and Metabolic Disorders

The liver may be affected by a number of systemic diseases and metabolic disorders. Although evidence of liver involvement may be subtle, signs and symptoms reflecting hepatic dysfunction may be among the first manifestations of a systemic illness. The liver may also be infiltrated by either materials or cells not normally present there, in diseases such as amyloidosis, extramedullary hematopoiesis, Hodgkin's disease, and leukemia. In galactosemia, abetalipoproteinemia, and diabetes, triglycerides accumulate in the liver, whereas in Tangier disease and cholesterol ester storage disease, cholesterol esters are increased. Hepatic phospholipids are present in excessive amounts in Gaucher's disease, Niemann-Pick disease, Wolman's disease, and Fabry's disease. Glycogen accumulation is observed in diabetes and hepatic glycogen storage disorders, and mucopolysaccharides are increased in the liver in Hurler's syndrome and

other related syndromes. Hepatic amyloid deposition is characteristic of both primary and secondary amyloidosis. Hepatomegaly is characteristic of the infiltrative diseases, and splenomegaly is occasionally observed. Liver function test abnormalities, although common, are usually nonspecific; the earliest abnormality may be a retention of sodium sulfobromophthalein (BSP) and an increase in serum alkaline phosphatase. Biopsy of the liver is the best means of diagnosis.

Granulomatous diseases may similarly affect the liver, producing hepatomegaly, and in some instances, signs of portal hypertension and postnecrotic cirrhosis. Examples of systemic diseases producing hepatic granulomas include sarcoidosis, berylliosis, and drug reactions. Among the infectious diseases, granulomas have been described in Q fever, infectious mononucleosis, syphilis, brucellosis, schistosomiasis, histoplasmosis, and tuberculosis. However, the bulk of hepatic granulomas are caused either by sarcoidosis or by tuberculosis, or they simply go undiagnosed. Liver biopsy alone rarely furnishes a specific diagnosis. Although cultures and special stains of liver tissue are occasionally helpful, other tissues must often be studied, and intensive clinical and laboratory investigations must be made for an absolute diagnosis.

THE PORPHYRIAS

The porphyrias are a group of genetic or acquired disorders affecting the regulation of the heme biosynthetic pathways. They are characterized by excessive production of porphyrin, porphyrinogens, or porphyrin precursors. These metabolic defects arise in either the bone marrow (erythropoietic porphyria), the liver (the hepatic porphyrias), or both (erythrohepatic protoporphyria). The pathophysiologic mechanisms responsible for the clinical manifestations of the porphyrias are incompletely understood. Photosensitivity, a feature of all the porphyrias except acute intermittent porphyria, is evoked by the accumulation of porphyrins, which absorb light, emit fluorescence, and induce photo-oxidative effects. Hemolysis in erythropoietic porphyria may be the result of a similar mechanism, that is, porphyrin-induced fluorescence in maturing red cells in the marrow. Excess excretion of porphyrins and their precursors may occur without symptomatic porphyria in cirrhosis, Hodgkin's disease, solid tumors, and other conditions.

Erythropoietic Porphyria

Erythropoietic porphyria is a rare, autosomal recessive disorder characterized by the onset in infancy and early childhood of photosensitivity, hirsutism, dermatitis, severe scarring of the skin from mutilation, red staining of the teeth, bones, and urine, and hemolytic anemia with splenomegaly. The accumulation and increased urinary excretion of uroporphyrinogen and coproporphyrinogen I have been attributed to impaired conversion of porphobilinogen to uroporphyrinogen III in the bone marrow.

Acute Intermittent Porphyria

Acute intermittent porphyria is an autosomal dominant disorder resulting from an incomplete block in the conversion of porphobilinogen to uroporphyrinogen in the liver. Uroporphyrinogen I synthetase activity is reduced by about 50 percent. Derepression of delta-aminolevulinic acid (ALA) synthetase leads to the increased production of ALA and porphobilinogen followed by their increased excretion in the urine. Drugs known to induce hepatic ALA synthetase, such as barbiturates, sulfonamides, or estrogens, may precipitate attacks and should be avoided. Attacks are marked by severe, acute abdominal pain, frequently accompanied by vomiting and constipation. Striking neurologic and psychiatric abnormalities (e.g., peripheral neuropathy, flaccid paralysis, psychosis) may be associated with the acute episodes, and transient hypertension is common. Inappropriate secretion of antidiuretic hormone has been described. Between attacks, patients appear normal, although excessive amounts of porphobilinogen and ALA may be present in the urine. Treatment of the acute attacks is symptomatic. Chlorpromazine is used to suppress pain, and the administration of glucose, given orally or parenterally to inhibit the induction of ALA synthetase, may be effective in suppressing acute episodes. Propranolol has also been used. Prompt clinical and chemical remission may result in addition from the intravenous administration of

hematin, which also represses induction of ALA synthetase.

Variegate Porphyria and Hereditary Coproporphyria

Variegate porphyria (mixed hepatic porphyria) is an autosomal dominant disease marked by moderate photosensitivity, abnormal mechanical fragility of the skin leading to blister formation, erosions, and scarring, and in many patients, symptoms of acute intermittent porphyria, which can be precipitated by the drugs mentioned in the previous section. Cirrhosis and hepatic dysfunction may be observed. Excessive coproporphyrin and protoporphyrin are consistently excreted in the feces; urinary ALA and porphobilinogen may be markedly increased during the acute attacks only. The defect responsible for this disorder is uncertain but impaired heme synthetase activity has been suggested. Treatment is the same as that for acute intermittent porphyria, together with avoidance of sunlight.

Hereditary coproporphyria appears to be closely related to variegate porphyria in its clinical features, but in the former, fecal protoporphyrin excretion is low.

Porphyria Cutanea Tarda and Toxic Porphyria

Uroporphyrin excretion is markedly increased in patients with porphyria cutanea tarda, in association with photodermatitis, skin blisters, dermal fragility, and hirsutism. Decreased activity of uroporphyrinogen decarboxylase and uroporphyrinogen III cosynthetase has been demonstrated. Most patients have underlying alcoholic liver disease, and iron overload may be a prominent finding. Phlebotomy may result in clearing of cutaneous lesions and a decrease in uroporphyrin excretion. Abdominal pain and neurologic involvement are absent. A toxic porphyria that resembles porphyria cutanea tarda has been induced by the ingestion of hexachlorobenzene, estrogens, chloroquine, and polychlorinated phenols.

Erythrohepatic (Erythropoietic) Protoporphyria

In erythrohepatic protoporphyria, an autosomal dominant disorder of childhood, photosensitivity is punctuated by the development of urticaria or eczema without blisters or dermal fragility. Protoporphyrin levels are elevated in the plasma, red blood cells, and feces. Urinary porphyrins are normal. Cholelithiasis, cirrhosis, and progressive hepatic failure are common. Avoidance of sunlight and β-carotene treatment to reduce photosensitivity are the only available prophylactic measures.

Liver Disease Accompanying Inflammatory Bowel Disease

Hepatic involvement has been found frequently in both Crohn's disease and ulcerative colitis. Although the hepatic histologic alterations in these two conditions are qualitatively similar, the liver disease associated with ulcerative colitis is of greater clinical importance. In both diseases the most characteristic morphologic changes are enlargement and edema of the portal tracts associated with a mononuclear cell infiltration. In some patients a picture resembling chronic active hepatitis ensues, and cirrhosis may result. Fatty infiltration of the liver is commonly found in debilitated or malnourished patients with inflammatory bowel disease, but this condition may diminish with clinical improvement. Cholelithiasis is especially common in patients with Crohn's disease, possibly as a result of impaired absorption of bile salts in the diseased terminal ileum.

Liver disease may be silent in some patients, whereas in others recurrent bouts of fever, chills, and jaundice, with intrahepatic cholestasis, have been noted. Advanced liver disease reflected by portal hypertension, portasystemic encephalopathy, or liver failure is uncommon. Rarely, bile duct carcinoma, sclerosing cholangitis, and amyloidosis have been reported in ulcerative colitis.

The etiology of hepatic involvement in inflammatory bowel disease is uncertain, and liver function tests do not correlate well with the extent of the liver disease. Specific therapy has not been determined. Attempts to alter the course of the liver disease by administration of corticosteroids and antibiotics have not proved effective. The efficacy of colectomy in interrupting the progression of liver disease in ulcerative colitis is disputed; it is certain that in the majority of cases, the liver disease itself is not of sufficient severity to warrant surgery.

The Liver in Congestive Heart Failure, Shock, and Hypoxemia

During either congestive failure, shock, or hypoxemia, regardless of the underlying cause, hepatic blood flow and oxygen supply are diminished. As a consequence, hepatic parenchymal degeneration or necrosis occurs in the most distal part of the liver lobule, that is, the centrilobular area. Derangements in BSP and bilirubin excretion may be early manifestations of these circulatory disturbances.

Clinical features include mild hyperbilirubinemia, BSP retention, and moderate to marked increases in serum transaminase levels. Serum alkaline phosphatase levels are either normal or slightly increased. Clinically detectable jaundice is uncommon in congestive failure per se; when present, it raises the suspicion of associated pulmonary infarction.

Cardiac cirrhosis is an uncommon manifestation of prolonged, severe, valvular heart disease, cor pulmonale, or constrictive pericarditis. The natural course of these conditions is usually so short that most patients do not live long enough to develop cirrhosis.

Hepatic Vein Occlusion (Budd-Chiari Syndrome)

ETIOLOGY

Hepatic vein occlusion is an uncommon lesion that may result from a number of diseases. Established causes include (1) hematologic disorders: polycythemia vera, paroxysmal nocturnal hemoglobinuria, sickle cell anemia, and leukemia; (2) intraabdominal malignancies: hypernephroma, primary liver cell cancer, and metastatic diseases of the liver; (3) congenital or acquired lesions of the inferior vena cava or hepatic veins: webs, strictures, leiomyomas, or leiomyosarcomas; (4) intraabdominal sepsis; (5) poisoning by the pyrrolizidine alkaloids present in the "bush-teas" of Jamaica; and (6) a miscellaneous group of causative factors, including pregnancy, oral contraceptive medication, trauma, and rarely congestive heart failure. Unfortunately, in a significant proportion of patients, no etiologic factor can be identified. In almost half of recognized cases the site of obstruction is in the inferior vena cava, at or near the entrance of the hepatic veins.

SIGNS AND SYMPTOMS

The principal presenting features of hepatic vein

occlusion are gross ascites, liver enlargement and tenderness, and abdominal pain. Occasional patients have hematemesis, or they may present in shock with signs of an acute abdominal catastrophe. Leg edema, distended superficial abdominal veins, and mild jaundice are not uncommon.

LABORATORY FEATURES
The serum bilirubin level is mildly increased, usually less than 4 mg per 100 ml; BSP retention is almost invariably increased, and the serum alkaline phosphatase level is moderately increased. Serum transaminase levels may be increased during the acute phase. The serum albumin level is decreased, and prothrombin time is near normal or mildly prolonged. Ascitic fluid protein is high (more than 2.5 gm per 100 ml) in two-thirds of patients.

DIAGNOSIS
Liver biopsy reveals centrilobular congestion with dilated sinusoids filled with masses of red blood cells, and moderate centrilobular necrosis. Late in the course of the illness, central fibrosis may be observed. Diagnosis usually requires hepatic venous and inferior vena caval catheterization to establish the site of obstruction. Hepatic scanning may reveal enlargement of the caudate lobe. Superior mesenteric arteriography may be useful to demonstrate esophageal varices, since the portal vein may drain the hepatic venous outflow. This procedure will also provide information about the patency of the portal vein if surgical decompression of the portal hypertension is being contemplated, as for recurrent hemorrhage from varices.

Although prolonged survival has been reported, presumably as a result of venous recanalization, the prognosis is poor for patients with total occlusion of the hepatic veins. Death usually results from hepatic coma, variceal hemorrhage, intercurrent sepsis, or portal or mesenteric thrombosis with intestinal infarction. Even if the patient survives these conditions, the problem of the primary disease remains.

Cirrhosis
The term *cirrhosis* describes chronic, diffuse, hepatic pathology, presumably resulting from recurrent or low-grade hepatocyte necrosis followed by fibrosis.

Although the term is often applied loosely, it refers to a specific histologic diagnosis, the sine qua non of which is nodular regeneration of surviving liver parenchyma with disorganization of lobular architecture (the latter feature indicates that the normal spatial relationships of portal tracts and central veins are lost). Diffuse connective tissue proliferation and inflammation are usually associated findings. In general, the presence of cirrhosis implies irreversible damage, since restoration of normal hepatic architecture occurs rarely, if ever.

Cirrhosis is a major health problem in the United States and is one of the 10 leading causes of death (more than 30,000 deaths annually are attributed to cirrhosis). Cirrhosis has been found in 2 to 10 percent of routine postmortem examinations, and of these cases, 25 to 50 percent were clinically latent.

PATHOLOGY
Most classifications of cirrhosis are based on the presumed etiology, which may be incorrect. Morphologic classifications are also subject to errors, including those due to sampling of the biopsy specimens. Nevertheless, a morphologic classification is useful in understanding the common variants of cirrhosis. Two major patterns are recognized: *portal* or *micronodular cirrhosis,* and *postnecrotic* or *macronodular cirrhosis.*

In portal or micronodular cirrhosis, the liver lesion is uniformly distributed. Fine, narrow bands of connective tissue (scarring) are present, enclosing small nodules (micronodules) of regenerating hepatic parenchyma. Normal lobular architecture is totally lacking, and intralobular bands of connective tissue divide the lobule into multiple pseudolobules without central veins. Postnecrotic or macronodular cirrhosis is characterized by coarse scarring of the liver, which is irregularly distributed through the liver. Regenerative nodules are irregular in shape, varying in size from microscopic to grossly visible nodules. In some areas, lobular architecture may be nearly intact but the central veins may be markedly displaced or absent.

Etiologic correlations have been attempted but are far from perfect. Alcoholic liver disease is characteristically associated with portal (Laennec's) cirrhosis, whereas in Wilson's disease, hemochromatosis, biliary cirrhosis, and chronic active hepatitis the cirrhosis is typically of the postnecrotic pattern. However, there is some justification for considering postnecrotic cirrhosis to be a final common pathway of almost all cirrhotic processes. Serial liver biopsies have, in fact, revealed the conversion of portal to postnecrotic cirrhosis in some alcoholic patients. A mixture of both portal and postnecrotic cirrhosis is very common in patients with alcoholic liver disease. Although the distinctions between the two are arbitrary, portal and postnecrotic cirrhosis will be discussed separately, the former in the context of alcoholic liver disease.

ALCOHOLIC LIVER DISEASE

Alcoholic Hepatitis and Fatty Liver

Although nutritional and other factors may contribute importantly, an excessive intake of alcohol clearly can produce hepatic injury in man as well as in other species. Excessive alcohol intake regularly causes accumulation of fat in the liver on both short- and long-term ingestion, but it does not seem to lead directly to cirrhosis since only about 10 to 15 percent of alcoholic patients develop cirrhosis. Both hepatitis and cirrhosis resulting from alcohol ingestion have been reported to occur in nonhuman primates, but this has not yet been confirmed. Most patients with alcoholic hepatitis, with or without cirrhosis, have consumed large amounts of alcohol for a long time (more than 70 gm daily for at least 10 years).

Definition and Pathology

As just indicated, alcoholic liver disease can be divided into three components: alcoholic fatty liver, alcoholic hepatitis, and alcoholic cirrhosis. Although at any one time a single component may predominate, a mixed picture is usually observed in man. Present evidence suggests that a fatty liver, even when histologically striking, is less likely to lead to the development of cirrhosis than is the acute liver lesion termed *alcoholic hepatitis*. This disease is characterized histologically by hepatic cell degeneration and necrosis, often with ballooned hepatocytes, accompanied by an inflammatory infiltrate consisting of polymorphonuclear leukocytes and lymphocytes. Irregular, dendritic, or globular intracytoplasmic hyaline material (called Mallory's bodies or alcoholic hyaline) is often present within the hepatocytes, which may be sur-

rounded by both polymorphonuclear leukocytes and frankly necrotic liver cells. However, intracellular hyaline is not specific for alcoholic hepatitis; morphologically similar material has been seen in Indian childhood cirrhosis, in Wilson's disease, in primary biliary cirrhosis, in the liver lesion that may follow jejunoileal bypass surgery, and in some hepatomas. Fibroblasts may be found at the sites of injury — in the portal, or less prominently, in the centrilobular zones, where collagen may accumulate between two portal zones, or between a portal and a centrilobular zone, bisecting the hepatic lobule.

Clinical Features

Patients with alcoholic liver disease often give no history of a recognized illness compatible with hepatitis and, in fact, may not even admit to drinking. However, the clinical spectrum of alcoholic hepatitis is wide, varying from asymptomatic cases to severe illnesses that may be fatal. Presenting complaints in symptomatic patients include anorexia, nausea and vomiting, weakness, abdominal distress, and weight loss, with fever in about 50 percent of patients. Hepatomegaly is the most common physical finding, but spider angiomas, jaundice, and ascites are frequently observed, and the spleen is enlarged in about a third of patients.

Laboratory Studies

Hematologic abnormalities are common in alcoholic liver disease (see also the section on laboratory studies under Portal Cirrhosis): anemia is present in 60 to 70 percent of patients, leukocytosis in about 40 percent, and platelet counts under 100,000 in 10 to 15 percent; marked leukocytosis (leukemoid reaction) has also been occasionally observed. Total serum bilirubin and the direct fraction are elevated, but the ranges are extremely variable. The serum alkaline phosphatase level is usually mildly to moderately raised, although levels compatible with bile duct obstruction are not infrequent. The SGOT is usually higher than the SGPT, with levels varying between near normal and 250 to 300 units in most patients. The serum albumin level may be decreased and the prothrombin time prolonged.

Course

Although the course of occasional patients worsens inexplicably during the first few weeks of hospitalization, jaundice, signs of portal hypertension, fluid retention, and other evidence of liver dysfunction often subside some weeks after alcohol ingestion is halted. A few patients die in hepatic failure, with coma, deepening jaundice, and gastrointestinal bleeding. A number of patients experience a cholestatic syndrome, which ultimately disappears during the course of treatment; this syndrome must be distinguished from extrahepatic bile duct obstruction caused by alcoholic pancreatitis or choledocholithiasis. The severity of the clinical illness is probably correlated at least in part with the degree of cirrhosis.

Treatment

No specific treatment is available for alcoholic liver disease. Alcohol is forbidden, and a nutritious diet is given. Corticosteroids have been used in severe cases, but their efficacy is uncertain. Treatment of complications such as portal hypertension, ascites, and hepatic encephalopathy is described later in the chapter. Rare patients with severe pruritus during the cholestatic phase of alcoholic hepatitis may require oral cholestyramine resin therapy.

The administration of drugs is hazardous in acutely intoxicated alcoholic patients or in those with severe liver disease in whom hepatic drug-metabolizing activity may be deranged. The danger lies in the fact that drugs can have either a heightened or (occasionally) a decreased action, depending on the patient's hepatic drug-metabolizing activity; this activity, which is usually decreased, may be increased in a sober chronic alcoholic with minimal hepatic dysfunction.

PORTAL CIRRHOSIS

Clinical Features

Portal cirrhosis (alcoholic cirrhosis, Laennec's cirrhosis) is uncommon in the first decades of life, since the disease is usually not discovered until after 10 or more years of continued alcohol ingestion. Affected men outnumber women by about 2:1, presumably reflecting different rates of alcoholism. Presenting complaints include nausea and vomiting, weakness,

fatigue, anorexia, and mild weight loss. Jaundice is present in a variable proportion of patients, particularly those with acute alcoholic hepatitis, but it is also seen in advanced cases with deteriorating liver function resulting from diminished liver cell mass. Ankle edema and increasing abdominal girth due to ascites are common in patients with portal hypertension. Decreased libido is a frequent complaint.

Physical examination reveals an enlarged liver with a rounded, firm edge. Spider angiomas, gynecomastia, and testicular atrophy are common. Other signs include an emaciated appearance, muscle wasting of the extremities, splenomegaly, and prominent venous collaterals in the superficial abdominal wall. Palmar erythema, parotid gland enlargement, and clubbing of the fingers are less commonly observed. Dupuytren's contracture is not uncommon in alcoholics, irrespective of whether or not they have cirrhosis. Low-grade fever is frequent.

Late in the course of the disease, signs of portal hypertension and hepatic encephalopathy may become prominent. Patients with advanced cirrhosis usually die in hepatic coma, which is frequently precipitated by bleeding esophageal varices and the associated functional renal failure, or by intercurrent sepsis. Spontaneous peritonitis, gram-negative septicemia, and primary hepatic cell cancer are not infrequent terminally. Although the incidence of pigment gallstones is increased in alcoholic cirrhosis, presumably as a result of the chronic hemolysis of hypersplenism, the incidence of cholecystitis and extrahepatic bile duct obstruction is low.

Laboratory Studies

Leukopenia is common in patients with hypersplenism or in those with recent alcohol ingestion, since alcohol may suppress white blood cell precursors in the bone marrow. Leukocytosis, if present, reflects either acute alcoholic hepatitis or an associated infection. However, the presence of normal or decreased white cell counts by no means excludes the possibility of septicemia in patients with portal cirrhosis. Direct effects of alcohol on the hematopoietic system may be evident: the myeloid precursors may be vacuolated, and the adult polymorphonuclear leukocytes may have impaired mobilization and phagocytic activity. Iron deficiency anemia may be secondary to gastrointestinal bleeding from gastritis, esophagogastric varices, or peptic ulcer disease. Megaloblastic anemia commonly results from folic acid deficiency. Ring sideroblasts are seen in the marrow in some instances, presumably because of impaired conversion of pyridoxine to pyridoxal phosphate, especially in the presence of folate deficiency. Thrombocytopenia is not unusual even in the absence of hypersplenism; evidence for a direct effect of alcohol on marrow megakaryocytes and on the circulating platelets has been reported. Platelet counts usually rise during the second week following cessation of alcohol ingestion.

Liver function tests are useful in establishing the severity of the disease, but they may be normal despite definite histologic alterations. Hyperbilirubinemia, mild to moderate elevations of serum alkaline phosphatase, and mild increases in serum transaminase levels are frequently observed. Prolongation of the prothrombin time and depression of the serum albumin level are common in severe cases. Serum globulins and the gamma globulin fraction may be mildly elevated. Hyponatremia and low blood urea nitrogen levels are characteristic, reflecting starvation and also vascular dilution. Glucose tolerance is often impaired without overt diabetes; this may be related to hypokalemia or to a deficiency of total body potassium. Cirrhosis may be complicated by renal tubular acidosis or renal failure (see The Hepatorenal Syndrome, page 514).

Respiratory alkalosis secondary to CNS-mediated hyperventilation is a common feature. Arterial hypoxemia (PO_2 lower than 80 mm Hg) is not infrequent in cirrhotic patients; recurrent pulmonary infections and cardiomyopathy may contribute to the hypoxemia. Lung volumes may be reduced when the diaphragm is elevated by ascites; this reduction in volume may occur with or without pleural effusion, which is noted in about 10 percent of cirrhotics with ascites. Arterial hypoxemia occurring in the absence of ascites or cardiopulmonary disease has been attributed to intrapulmonary or portopulmonary shunting or, more frequently, to ventilation-perfusion imbalance in the lower portions of the lungs. A hyperkinetic circulation, presumably resulting from arteriovenous shunting, from anemia, and possibly from circulating vasoactive peptides, is not uncommon in cirrhosis, but it has also been described in acute, severe liver disease and in thiamine deficiency in alcoholics.

Diagnosis and Prognosis

The diagnosis of portal cirrhosis can usually be made on clinical grounds. A satisfactory liver biopsy may be difficult to obtain because in severely cirrhotic livers, fragmentation of the tissue is common during biopsy and the diagnostic fibrous tissue may be left behind. In the absence of histologically unequivocal cirrhosis, the diagnosis may be suspected from the biopsy if evidence of regenerating nodules is found. The prognosis in cirrhosis depends on the stage of the disease and on whether or not alcohol consumption continues. Five-year survival rates of 40 to 60 percent are observed, the higher rates being in patients who abstain. Only 10 to 30 percent of patients survive five years after the onset of ascites, and only 5 to 20 percent of patients are alive five years after the onset of esophageal variceal hemorrhage.

Treatment

Hospitalization may be required for diagnosis, for management of complications, or for treatment in severely ill patients. Alcohol is contraindicated. No specific therapy is available, but supportive care is given while the natural healing and regenerative processes are occurring.

A balanced diet is prescribed except for patients with hepatic precoma, in whom protein restriction is necessary. Vitamin supplements should be given to patients with clinically apparent vitamin deficiency syndromes, and thiamine should be given to all hospitalized alcoholic patients. Bed rest and salt restriction (250 to 500 mg sodium daily) are indicated for patients with fluid retention; this regimen is often sufficient to produce diuresis. Patients with tense ascites that produces respiratory embarrassment or threatens to rupture an umbilical hernia may require a therapeutic paracentesis. However, excessive fluid removal may be hazardous, causing hypovolemia and renal insufficiency.

The anemia may require extensive study to establish a precise etiologic diagnosis and to permit specific therapy (e.g., iron and folic acid). Infectious complications may or may not be signaled by spiking fever or shaking chills (quite apart from the low-grade or moderate fever of alcoholic hepatitis), warranting a careful evaluation for occult sepsis. The detailed treatment of ascites, hepatic coma, portal hypertension, and the hepatorenal syndrome will be described later in the chapter.

POSTNECROTIC CIRRHOSIS

Clinical Features
Patients with postnecrotic cirrhosis are usually younger than those with alcoholic cirrhosis, and in contrast to the preponderance of males in the latter disease, postnecrotic cirrhosis affects women at least as often as men. Latent postnecrotic cirrhosis may be diagnosed at surgery performed for unrelated diseases, or at postmortem examination. Although many of the clinical features of the disease are identical with those described in alcoholic cirrhosis, there are some noteworthy differences. The patient with postnecrotic cirrhosis typically presents with complications of portal hypertension, especially hematemesis due to ruptured esophagogastric varices, whereas the patient with alcoholic cirrhosis typically presents with features of hepatocellular insufficiency. Splenomegaly may be the only sign of postnecrotic cirrhosis; persistent jaundice is commonly an early sign, whereas ascites is a relatively late one. Pruritus is present in about 15 percent of postnecrotic patients, and episodic abdominal pain occurs in a large proportion. In contrast to alcoholic cirrhotics, at least one-third of patients with postnecrotic cirrhosis are well nourished and have no muscle wasting.

Laboratory Features
Anemia, if present in postnecrotic cirrhosis, reflects either hypersplenism or iron deficiency due to bleeding from varices. Leukopenia with or without thrombocytopenia, if present, is indicative of splenic sequestration. The liver function tests resemble those seen in alcoholic cirrhosis, except that hyperglobulinemia is often more striking and hyperbilirubinemia may be more persistent.

Diagnosis, Prognosis, and Treatment
Postnecrotic cirrhosis should be suspected in nonalcoholic patients who present with features of portal hypertension. Needle biopsy of the liver may provide a definitive diagnosis, but the nonuniformity of the pathologic process often results in confusing sampling errors. Although the disease is latent in some patients, those with persistent jaundice or recurrent variceal hemorrhage have a poor prognosis; they may die in hepatic coma, after an exsanguinating hemorrhage, or from primary liver cell cancer. Treatment of postnecrotic cirrhosis is similar to that for alcoholic cirrhosis.

PRIMARY BILIARY CIRRHOSIS

Definition and Etiology
Primary biliary cirrhosis is a progressive disorder affecting the intrahepatic bile ducts, leading to the syndrome of prolonged intrahepatic cholestasis and eventual cirrhosis. The etiology is unknown. The actual disease may be confirmed in some family members, whereas in other members only nonspecific tissue antibodies are identified. In a small number of patients, a disease resembling and perhaps identical to primary biliary cirrhosis has appeared following the administration of chlorpromazine, tolbutamide, methyltestosterone, or oral contraceptive agents.

Pathology
Early in the course of the disease, the interlobular (portal) bile ducts are surrounded by dense accumulations of mononuclear and plasma cells often resembling follicles. At this stage there is no cirrhosis. Granulomatous changes and epithelioid cells may be seen in the portal tracts or within the follicles. At this early stage, the hallmark of the disease is distortion, degeneration, necrosis, or hyperplasia of the interlobular bile duct epithelium. Later, a paucity of interlobular bile ducts is characteristic, with proliferation of atypical ductules, expansion of portal tracts, and deposition of portal fibrosis. The end-stage histologic picture is one of postnecrotic cirrhosis with prominent cholestasis. In a few patients, a dense portal inflammatory infiltration, with "piecemeal" necrosis, suggests chronic active hepatitis.

Clinical Features

Primary biliary cirrhosis affects predominantly women between the ages of 35 and 65, although 10 to 15 percent of patients are men. The disease usually has an insidious onset, and the first — or the major — early symptom is slowly progressive pruritus, related to increased concentrations of bile salt in the skin. Months to years later, jaundice may appear, and the diagnosis of chronic intrahepatic cholestasis may be made. As a result of a deficiency of bile salts in the intestinal lumen, steatorrhea is common, often associated with osteomalacia. Hepatomegaly is found in most patients, splenomegaly in about half, and increased skin pigmentation, with or without xanthoma, in approximately one-third. Clubbing of the digits is not uncommon. Despite the distressing pruritus, most patients feel reasonably well and do not seek early medical aid. The terminal phase of the disease is marked by the usual complications of advanced, postnecrotic cirrhosis and portal hypertension. A small number of patients have cutaneous calcinosis, Raynaud's phenomenon, sclerodactyly, and telangiectasia (CRST syndrome), or various components of this syndrome.

Laboratory Studies

Hyperbilirubinemia is noted in over 90 percent of patients, and chemical studies typically reveal moderate to very high elevations of serum alkaline phosphatase, cholesterol, and serum globulin. The antimitochondrial antibody test is positive in 85 to 95 percent of patients with proved primary biliary cirrhosis (it is usually negative in extrahepatic bile duct obstruction). The increased hepatic copper content found in primary biliary cirrhosis may result from impaired biliary excretion of this metal, but it is also found in other forms of chronic obstructive liver disease.

Diagnosis

The major diagnostic problem is the differentiation of primary biliary cirrhosis from secondary cirrhosis due to prolonged extrahepatic obstruction resulting, for example, from sclerosing cholangitis, carcinoma or stricture of the bile ducts, or gallstones. Although a diagnostic laparotomy with operative cholangiog-

raphy is the method commonly employed, a percutaneous transhepatic or a retrograde cholangiogram, together with a liver biopsy, may provide the diagnosis. As indicated previously, definitive diagnosis may be difficult because elements of chronic active hepatitis may be found in primary biliary cirrhosis.

Treatment

Therapeutic corticosteroids and immunosuppressive agents (e.g., azathioprine) have been used in the treatment of primary biliary cirrhosis, but these agents appear to be ineffective. Since corticosteroids may accelerate the development of osteomalacia and may lead to bone fractures in these patients, they are extremely hazardous and should be avoided. Pruritus may be relieved by oral cholestyramine resin, an anion-exchange resin that exchanges chloride ions for bile salts in the intestinal lumen; unfortunately, however, this agent may increase steatorrhea. If cholestyramine resin therapy is ineffective, pruritus may be controlled in some patients by the use of phenobarbital. The long-term effectiveness of the latter agent remains to be established. Parenteral fat-soluble vitamins may be given to prevent deficiency of vitamins A, D, and K. Penicillamine, a copper-chelating agent, may be beneficial, but further studies are needed.

Hemochromatosis

DEFINITION AND ETIOLOGY

Hemochromatosis may be defined as an abnormal, widespread accumulation of iron in tissues, associated with certain structural changes that presumably result from iron overload. Hemosiderosis is also an abnormal tissue accumulation of iron, but it is usually quantitatively less extensive and is often not associated with pathologic reactions which, if present at all, may have preceded the accumulation of iron. The total body iron level in hemochromatosis may be 5 to 10 times the normal levels (3 to 5 gm). These definitions remain controversial, however, and some authors have also used the designations *primary* and *secondary hemochromatosis*. The first term refers to a genetic disorder of metabolism, in which an unexplained increase in iron absorption from the intestine has been demonstrated. An increased tissue avidity for iron has been postulated to be responsible for the iron overload in this disorder, in which a dominant mode of inheritance has been occasionally documented. The second form of hemochromatosis, called secondary hemochromatosis or hemosiderosis, occurs in diseases such as thalassemia minor, sideroblastic anemia, and atransferrinemia. In these diseases, no increased tissue avidity for iron is postulated; the iron overload results from either hemolysis, multiple transfusions, or both, and may or may not cause tissue damage.

PATHOLOGY

Hemochromatosis is characterized by portal fibrosis, progressing to portal cirrhosis and, in the late stages, to postnecrotic cirrhosis with large quantities of histologically demonstrable iron in the hepatocytes. Iron may also be present in Kupffer cells and in the bile duct epithelium, and lipofuscin, a noniron yellow pigment, may also be prominent. In the early stages of the disease, almost all the excess iron is localized to the liver. In more advanced cases, excessive iron may also be present in the pancreas, which is fibrotic with reduced islets, and in the spleen, gastric mucosa, pituitary, myocardium, and skin. The dark tan pigmentation of the skin is caused primarily by melanin deposition. Primary hepatoma as a terminal complication is observed three times more often in hemochromatosis than in Laennec's cirrhosis. It must be emphasized that 5 to 10 percent of patients with alcoholic cirrhosis have excessive hepatic iron deposition which, although less severe, may be histologically indistinguishable from that in hemochromatosis.

CLINICAL FEATURES

An asymptomatic period of many years is characteristic, during which iron gradually accumulates but physical findings are absent. During this period, tissue iron and iron absorption are increased but plasma iron concentration may be within the normal range. Hemochromatosis is about 10 to 15 times more common in men than in women. Symptoms usually begin between the ages of 40 and 60, although a number of cases in young adults have been described. Initial symptoms include weakness, weight loss, and decreased libido. Diabetes mellitus is present in about three-quarters of patients, and gray, dark tan, or bronze hyperpigmentation of the skin in about 90 percent. Congestive heart failure or arrhythmias may be present in one-third of patients. Symptoms of cirrhosis are common, and splenomegaly is found in about half the patients. Portal hypertension and ascites may occur, and testicular atrophy is common. Acute polyarthritis caused by chondrocalcinosis is not unusual. Death usually results from complications, which may include diabetes, cirrhosis, primary liver cell cancer, congestive heart failure, or arrhythmia.

LABORATORY FEATURES

The most helpful laboratory tests are the measurements of plasma iron and iron-binding capacity. The plasma iron concentration is typically elevated (in the range of 175 to 300 μg per 100 ml), and total iron-binding capacity may be decreased to levels below 300 μg per 100 ml. The unsaturated iron-binding capacity is usually less than 50 μg per 100 ml. Serum ferritin levels are elevated.

DIAGNOSIS AND TREATMENT

The syndrome of biopsy-proved cirrhosis together with excessive iron deposition, diabetes mellitus, skin pigmentation, polyarthritis, and congestive heart failure favors the diagnosis of hemochromatosis. Early in the course of the disease, deposition of hemosiderin in the bone marrow is usually considerably less extensive than that in the liver. Occasionally the diagnosis cannot be established by measurements of plasma iron and transferrin, so either iron-kinetic studies or the response to phlebotomy must be employed. Measurements of plasma iron and transferrin concentrations in family members may reveal some affected persons.

Available iron-chelating agents are of little therapeutic value. Treatment consists of repeated phlebotomy until a mild iron deficiency anemia results. With this regimen, insulin requirements may decrease, cardiac symptoms may disappear, pigmentation may lighten, and signs of liver disease may regress. Phlebotomy significantly increases life expectancy when it results in iron depletion in hemochromatotic patients, but it does not improve the morbidity or mortality rate in patients with excessive iron deposition secondary to alcoholic cirrhosis.

Wilson's Disease

DEFINITION AND ETIOLOGY

Wilson's disease is an inherited autosomal recessive disorder of copper metabolism that leads to the accumulation of excessive amounts of copper. In time, this accumulation results in or is associated with pathologic alterations in the liver, central nervous system, kidney, cornea, and bones. A deficiency of serum ceruloplasmin, an increase in urinary excretion of copper, and an elevated hepatic copper concentration may precede the appearance of structural alterations and clinical manifestations. It has been suggested that the major defect in Wilson's disease is the impairment of biliary excretion of copper, but the mechanism is unexplained.

PATHOLOGY

The earliest histopathologic change in the liver consists of fatty metamorphosis, followed by hepatocyte necrosis, round cell infiltration, and fibrosis (resembling the findings in chronic active hepatitis). Ultimately either micronodular or macronodular cirrhosis develops. Large numbers of atypical, vacuolated, glycogen-rich nuclei are common but not specific, and cytoplasmic hyaline (Mallory's) bodies have also been observed. Degenerative changes are found in the brain, particularly in the basal ganglia. Copper is deposited in Descemet's membrane of the cornea, causing the characteristic Kayser-Fleischer ring. Renal tubular dysfunction has been demonstrated in many cases. Abnormal renal phosphate clearance may be responsible for the osseous abnormalities, which include osteomalacia, osteochondritis dissecans, and cystic bone changes.

CLINICAL FEATURES

About 60 percent of patients with Wilson's disease present with neuropsychiatric symptoms, although in the pediatric age group, symptomatic liver disease often precedes neurologic involvement. Liver disease may be insidious but is almost always present and progressive. Presenting features may be jaundice, unexplained hepatosplenomegaly, complications of portal hypertension or, rarely, hepatic failure. Ascites and hepatic coma are usually late phenomena. Sudden episodes of jaundice may reflect acute hemolysis resulting from an abrupt release of copper from the tissues into the circulation. Neurologic symptoms include dysphagia, dystonia, dysarthria, chorea, tremors, pronounced behavioral abnormalities (suggesting schizophrenia), seizures, and hemiplegia. Kayser-Fleischer rings are characteristic, but their absence in younger patients does not exclude the diagnosis.

LABORATORY FEATURES

Liver function tests are usually abnormal and are similar to those found in cirrhosis or chronic hepatitis from other causes. Anemia, leukopenia, and thrombocytopenia are manifestations of hypersplenism. The creatinine clearance may be decreased, and albuminuria is commonly present. Aminoaciduria, uricosuria, glycosuria, phosphaturia, and renal acidifying defects have been observed in association with low serum levels of uric acid and phosphate, reflecting defective renal tubular function. A serum ceruloplasmin below 20 mg per 100 ml is found in 95 percent of patients. Hepatic copper concentration exceeds $250\,\mu g$ per gm dry weight of liver, and urinary copper excretion exceeds $100\,\mu g$ per day.

DIAGNOSIS

The demonstration of Kayser-Fleischer rings is diagnostic of Wilson's disease, provided primary biliary cirrhosis and chronic active hepatitis can be excluded, since corneal rings have also been reported, rarely, in those disorders. Slit-lamp examination is necessary when Kayser-Fleischer rings are not grossly visible. The findings of low serum ceruloplasmin and increased urinary copper are highly suggestive of Wilson's disease; high hepatic copper concentration determined quantitatively on tissue obtained by biopsy confirms the diagnosis.

Patients with primary biliary cirrhosis and other liver diseases may also have elevated hepatic copper concentrations; their ceruloplasmin levels are normal, however. The liver biopsy is usually characteristic in Wilson's disease. When the diagnosis is suspected but ceruloplasmin levels are normal (5 percent of cases) and a liver biopsy cannot be obtained, measurements of intravenously administered radioactive copper kinetics may reveal impaired incorporation of copper into ceruloplasmin, thus confirming the diagnosis.

TREATMENT

The goal of therapy in Wilson's disease is the depletion of copper stores. This goal is accomplished by the avoidance of copper-rich foods, the ingestion of potassium sulfide to reduce the intestinal absorption of copper, and most importantly, the long-term administration (indefinitely) of D-penicillamine, a chelating agent that enhances urinary copper excretion. Such treatment is also indicated for asymptomatic siblings of patients with Wilson's disease in whom ceruloplasmin is decreased and hepatic copper concentration increased.

With treatment, improvement in hepatic, neurologic, and renal functions can be expected in most patients. Toxic reactions that are associated with D-penicillamine, presumably immunologically mediated, include skin rashes, leukopenia, and thrombocytopenia; most importantly, the nephrotic syndrome; and rarely, a lupuslike syndrome and Goodpasture's syndrome. Triethylene tetramine dihydrochloride, another chelating agent, may be useful in patients who develop serious toxic reactions to D-penicillamine.

Rare Forms of Cirrhosis

ALPHA$_1$-ANTITRYPSIN DEFICIENCY

Alpha$_1$-antitrypsin is a glycoprotein (an alpha$_1$-globulin) that inhibits a number of proteolytic enzymes. A deficiency of this glycoprotein, which is synthesized in the liver, is associated with the development of pulmonary emphysema. Rapidly progressive cirrhosis and primary hepatic cell cancer have also been observed in some patients with the homozygous deficiency. Examination of liver tissue from patients with this disease and from others with emphysema has revealed distinctive intracytoplasmic, PAS-positive diastase-resistant globules that react with antibodies to alpha$_1$-antitrypsin. It has been suggested that these globules reflect an impaired export of the enzyme from the liver. The mechanism of the induction of cirrhosis in affected patients is as yet unknown.

OTHER DISORDERS ASSOCIATED WITH CIRRHOSIS

Diverse disorders have been associated with the development of cirrhosis, including (in addition to alpha$_1$-antitrypsin deficiency) galactosemia, glycogen storage diseases, sarcoidosis, ulcerative colitis, regional enter-itis, cystic fibrosis, and abetalipoproteinemia. Although a variable proportion of patients with these diseases have cirrhosis, they comprise only a minute fraction of the total cirrhotic population.

Complications of Advanced Liver Disease

PORTAL HYPERTENSION

A portal venous pressure above 20 mm Hg (normal pressure is 7 to 14 mm Hg) indicates *portal hypertension,* which is caused by an increase in either intrahepatic resistance or extrahepatic resistance, or both, to portal venous blood flow. Portal venous pressure may also be increased in a number of hematologic disorders associated with massive splenomegaly; increased portal blood flow has been postulated to be responsible in these disorders, but the exact pathogenesis remains to be determined. Irrespective of the nature of the underlying disease and the anatomic site of the obstruction, extensive collateral venous channels develop to return the portal blood to the systemic circulation. Collateral flow between the coronary and azygos veins may cause gastroesophageal varices; collateral flow through the hemorrhoidal veins may cause hemorrhoids; and increased flow through the umbilical vein remnant, the retroperitoneal veins, and the veins of the capsule of the liver and diaphragm may cause these veins to become grossly distended. Congestive splenomegaly, ascites, and portasystemic encephalopathy are the other major consequences of portal hypertension.

Although portal hypertension may temporarily be associated with any acute liver disorder (for example, alcoholic hepatitis), the most common cause of persistent portal hypertension in the United States is cirrhosis. By contrast, infiltrative or vascular diseases of the liver are only occasionally responsible for persistent portal hypertension. Compression of the hepatic venules by regenerative, fibrotic tissue with obstruction of blood flow from the sinusoids (so-called postsinusoidal hypertension) is thought to be the major cause of portal hypertension in cirrhosis, although excessive hepatic artery—portal vein and portal vein—hepatic vein anastomoses also contribute to portal hypertension. Deposition of intrasinusoidal collagen, as well as swelling due to necrosis and inflammation, may produce portal hypertension in alcoholic hepatitis even when there is no cirrhosis. Both thrombosis of the major hepatic veins (the Budd-Chiari syndrome) and thrombosis of the small hepatic veins within the liver (resulting either from pyrrolizidine alkaloid poisoning or from irradiation of the liver) typically cause portal hypertension of the postsinusoidal type. *Presinusoidal portal hypertension* refers to impedance of blood flow within the portal vein itself, which is usually a result of thrombosis but may also be caused by schistosomiasis, congenital hepatic fibrosis, vitamin A intoxication, chronic arsenic poisoning, and other conditions. Liver function is usually not impaired in this type of portal hypertension, even when it is severe.

Clinical Features

Patients with portal hypertension may be asymptomatic for prolonged periods and may not come to medical attention until they have extensive hemorrhage from esophageal or gastric varices. Fatal hemorrhage is not uncommon in cirrhotic patients with severe varices, but patients with presinusoidal portal hypertension tolerate hemorrhage better than those with postsinusoidal hypertension, since the former have little or no intrinsic liver disease. Variceal bleeding into the small or large bowel or into the retroperitoneal space is less frequent than bleeding into the esophagus or stomach. Gastrointestinal hemorrhage may precipitate portasystemic encephalopathy, or encephalopathy may appear spontaneously, particularly in patients with extensive collaterals between the portal and systemic venous systems. Signs of portal hypertension include distended collateral vessels on the abdomen or around the umbilicus (caput medusae), with blood flow directed centrifugally from the umbilicus. Splenomegaly, with or without hypersplenism, occurs frequently.

Diagnosis

Portal hypertension should be considered in patients with unexplained splenomegaly, upper gastrointestinal hemorrhage, or known cirrhosis. Esophagogastric varices may be demonstrated by barium swallow x-ray examination or by endoscopic visualization. Selective arteriography may confirm varices, portal hypertension, and the patency of the portal, splenic,

and left renal veins — all crucially important findings if surgery is being considered.

Treatment

A prophylactic, surgical portacaval anastomosis for the decompression of varices in patients who have not yet bled is unwarranted, since it has no effect on the mortality due to the underlying cirrhosis; however, the anastomosis may prevent death from bleeding varices (provided it remains patent). The operation, or one of several available variants (for example, distal splenorenal anastomosis), is therefore reserved for patients who have already bled from varices, and it is better when performed electively after a period of stabilization of the patient's clinical condition. When performed as emergency treatment for actively bleeding varices, the operation is associated with a mortality rate of 20 to 50 percent.

The management of acute, bleeding esophagogastric varices is difficult. Ice water lavage may be attempted, but it commonly fails; if so, esophageal-gastric tamponade with the triple-lumen, double-balloon Sengstaken-Blakemore tube may be undertaken. Because mortality and morbidity rates associated with the use of such tamponade are often high, pharmacologic control of bleeding is now favored for the temporary control of hemorrhage. The intravenous administration of aqueous vasopressin may reduce portal venous pressure (and flow) by its vasoconstrictive action on the splanchnic arterioles. Unfortunately, vasopressin may also constrict the coronary arteries, and tachyphylaxis to vasopressin may develop after repeated systemic injection. Another, though more difficult method is the selective catheterization of the superior mesenteric artery and the continuous infusion of intraarterial vasopressin, which may arrest bleeding more often and with fewer adverse reactions than its intravenous administration. Elective surgical decompression may then be considered.

Prognosis of Shunt Surgery

As indicated earlier, emergency shunt surgery for persistently bleeding varices may be inordinately dangerous in an unstable cirrhotic patient. Elective shunt surgery has a lower operative mortality rate (less than 10 percent) and reduces to nearly zero the recurrence of bleeding varices. However, long-term survival is only slightly better in shunted than in nonshunted patients. Either portacaval or standard splenorenal anastomosis will decompress portal hypertension and may also correct hypersplenism; the splenorenal shunt is more likely to thrombose but is less likely to cause postshunt encephalopathy, which occurs in about 20 to 33 percent of shunted patients and may be incapacitating. A selective, distal splenorenal shunt with portal-azygous disconnection, which decompresses varices without altering portal pressure, is currently under evaluation. A late and infrequent complication of shunt surgery is hepatic iron deposition. Rarer complications include mild unconjugated hyperbilirubinemia and a transverse myelitis syndrome of uncertain etiology.

PORTASYSTEMIC ENCEPHALOPATHY (HEPATIC COMA)

Definition and Etiology

Portasystemic encephalopathy (PSE) is a neuropsychiatric syndrome resulting from impaired cerebral metabolism, which may complicate any severe, acute, or chronic liver disease, or may follow portasystemic shunting. Its precise cause is unknown, although failure of the liver either to remove noxious factors from the blood, or to add normal substances to the blood, may be involved. Although available evidence favors the former concept, it has not disproved the latter. Nitrogenous substances such as ammonia that are derived from the intestine are probably involved in PSE, but other materials (e.g., amines, short-chain fatty acids, and methionine derivatives) may also play a role. It has been proposed that amines formed in the gut may accumulate in the general circulation as a result of their bypassing the liver, where they would normally be degraded. These compounds may then be taken up by neurons of the peripheral and central nervous systems, where they act as false neurotransmitters. Excessive production of these materials may also occur in brain tissue. Elevated plasma levels of aromatic amino acids associated with depressed branched-chain amino acids have also been implicated in the pathogenesis of PSE. Regardless of its causative factors, PSE is associated with abnormal oxygen utilization in the brain. In acute PSE the brain may appear histologically normal, but in chronic, nonreversible PSE, glial hyperplasia and loss of nerve cells in the cortex, the cerebellum, and the lenticular nuclei are frequently observed.

Clinical Features

PSE may begin either abruptly or insidiously, with disturbances of mental function leading to progressive obtundation and coma. The early stages of the syndrome (hepatic precoma) are characterized by intermittent or fluctuating personality changes, confusion, and slowing of both speech and mental reactions. Constructional apraxia is usually demonstrable, and asterixis, the flapping tremor (which is best elicited with the wrists hyperextended and forearms fixed), is usually present, although it is not specific. Electroencephalograms show a slowing of wave frequency, with characteristic high voltages, and symmetrical waves in the delta range. A sweetish, musty odor of the breath, known as fetor hepaticus, may be observed. The fluctuating neurologic picture includes rigidity, pyramidal tract signs, and occasionally seizures. Patients with chronic PSE, who typically are stable cirrhotics with large spontaneous or surgically-induced shunts, may present with organic psychosis, choreoathetosis, intellectual deterioration, and in some instances, signs of myelopathy. Sensorineural hearing losses may be observed, whether or not neurotoxic antibiotics have been used in therapy. Elevated arterial blood levels of ammonia may be found, particularly in patients with chronic liver disease, but in severe, acute liver disease these levels are less well correlated with PSE.

Precipitating Factors

A number of factors may precipitate or potentiate PSE; among the most important is the administration of opiates, sedatives, or tranquilizers. An increase of nitrogenous substances in the intestinal lumen, caused by gastrointestinal bleeding, a high-protein diet, or constipation, may also precipitate PSE. Ammonia is released by the action of bacterial enzymes on these substances in the lower ileum and colon. Renal failure will increase the quantity of urea in the intestine; bacterial ureases will then break down this urea and further contribute to hyperammonemia. Increased ammonia production by the kidney itself can be provoked by the use of diuretics, or by renal tubular acidosis, hypokalemia, or metabolic alkalosis. Alkalosis per se appears to potentiate the effects of hyperammonemia by shifting the dissociation of ammonium ion to freely diffusible ammonia gas. Other precipitating factors of PSE include infection, hypotension, hypoxemia, surgery, and therapeutic paracentesis.

Treatment
The management of PSE is directed at therapy of the underlying liver disease, elimination of any precipitating factors, and control of encephalopathy before deep coma supervenes. Treatment must be initiated at the first sign of mental deterioration, which can be detected only by repeated bedside testing of the mental status, the handwriting, and the constructional ability. Patients at risk should be so tested at least once daily and the results recorded in the hospital chart. A search for correctable precipitating events should continue while treatment is started.

Dietary protein is reduced to zero. Caloric intake and fluid and electrolyte balance are maintained by the intravenous infusion of glucose, appropriate fluids, and electrolytes. Protein and blood in the intestine are removed by the use of laxatives, such as magnesium citrate, and by cleansing enemas. Concomitantly, oral administration of *either* neomycin in a divided dose of 4 to 8 gm daily or lactulose 30 to 45 ml three to four times a day is initiated. Neomycin will decrease the intestinal bacterial production of ammonia. Unfortunately, occasional patients who are treated with neomycin for prolonged periods develop steatorrhea or staphylococcal enteritis, and since up to 1 percent of the drug is absorbed, nerve deafness and, rarely, renal toxicity may also occur. Lactulose, a synthetic disaccharide, which produces acidic stools and may favor the fecal excretion of ammonia as nonabsorbable ammonium ions, is not associated with important side effects other than diarrhea and abdominal cramping. The exact mechanism of lactulose's action is not clear, however.

Once improvement is noted, protein is gradually added to the diet until nearly normal levels are reached; neomycin or lactulose therapy may be dis-

continued if possible. Patients with chronic PSE may require low daily dosages (1 to 2 gm) of neomycin or maintenance lactulose treatment to permit nearly normal protein intake.

ASCITES

Definition and Pathogenesis
In most cirrhotic patients, excessive peritoneal fluid results primarily from the combined effects of portal hypertension and hypoalbuminemia, although secondary hyperaldosteronism, impaired "third" factor activity, and other poorly understood mechanisms may contribute importantly. Hypoalbuminemia results in decreased plasma oncotic pressure and readily leads to ascites when portal hypertension is present; when the hypoalbuminemia is extreme, even slight portal hypertension may cause ascites. The site of the portal venous obstruction also plays a role in ascites formation. For example, portal vein thrombosis with portal hypertension rarely causes ascites, whereas hepatic vein occlusion regularly does so. In the latter condition, as well as in the postsinusoidal obstruction of cirrhosis, hepatic lymph production is increased, and the leakage of this lymph into the peritoneal space may contribute to the ascites. Thus in hepatic vein occlusion, ascitic fluid protein concentrations are high, indicating a significant contribution from the hepatic lymphatics. In most cirrhotics, however, the ascitic fluid protein levels are low, suggesting that fluid loss from the mesenteric capillaries is more important than the leakage of hepatic lymph. Direct albumin transport from the liver to ascitic fluid has been described; although this factor may contribute to ascites, the mechanism is poorly understood.

Other factors probably contribute to the perpetuation of ascites. The role of depletion of "effective" plasma volume is controversial; this depletion has been thought to be responsible for the characteristic avid renal retention of sodium, through the mechanism of decreased renal glomerular filtration and plasma flow. When measured, however, renal filtration and plasma flow have not been significantly impaired, except terminally.

Regardless of its origin, secondary hyperaldosteronism, presumably initiated by the renin-angiotensin system, leads to increased distal tubular sodium reabsorption. Present data indicate that the secretion of aldosterone is markedly increased in cirrhotics, but its metabolism may also be impaired. Another theoretically important mechanism may be a decrease in "third" or "natriuretic" activity, which normally blocks tubular reabsorption of sodium in response to expansion of extracellular volume. A reduced free water clearance has also been observed in cirrhotics with ascites; it is presumed to be caused, at least in part, by excessive antidiuretic hormone activity.

Diagnosis

Ascites can usually be detected clinically when about 500 ml of fluid is present in the peritoneal cavity. Diagnostic paracentesis with removal of 50 to 100 ml of fluid is indicated to determine the nature of the fluid. Typical cirrhotic fluid is a transudate with a specific gravity of less than 1.018, a protein content of 2.5 gm per 100 ml or less, and a cell count of fewer than 300 mononuclear cells per cubic millimeter. The presence of an exudate suggests either a cause other than cirrhosis or a superimposed complication. However, in about 20 percent of cirrhotic patients no other etiology can be determined.

Prognosis

The development of ascites is an ominous sign in cirrhosis, since the 5-year survival rate then decreases to only 10 to 30 percent. Similarly, ascites associated with chronic active hepatitis indicates a poor prognosis. In alcoholic hepatitis, ascites may herald a rapid demise, but abstinence and prolonged treatment may be followed by the disappearance of ascites. Ascites is uncommon in fulminant hepatitis, and its development in severe hepatitis is highly suggestive of bridging necrosis.

Treatment

It must be emphasized that ascites is a manifestation of underlying liver disease, which itself must be the primary concern in treatment. In many instances an improvement of liver function alone will result in a spontaneous diuresis and a disappearance of ascites and edema. In rare cases in which respiratory embarrassment is severe or rupture of an umbilical hernia is imminent, therapeutic paracentesis with removal of

1 to 2 liters of fluid may produce symptomatic improvement.

The success of treatment depends on the cooperation of the patient and on the stage of the disease. Attempts at vigorous therapy in the severely ill cirrhotic patient with jaundice or hepatic precoma, or both, frequently lead to further deterioration of hepatic function, frank hepatic coma, or the hepatorenal syndrome. The most important therapeutic measures are designed to diminish sodium retention. Rigid restriction of dietary sodium to 250 to 500 mg per day is necessary. Fluid restriction to 1,500 ml per day may also be required in some patients to prevent severe dilutional hyponatremia resulting from impaired free water clearance. Careful daily measurements of weight, fluid intake, urinary output, and urine sodium concentration are necessary to monitor the effectiveness of therapy. Drug therapy may be initiated in the stable cirrhotic patient with ascites when a spontaneous diuresis has not occurred within 2 weeks of hospital observation. Spironolactones, which antagonize aldosterone, and diuretics such as the thiazides, which impair tubular reabsorption of sodium, may be used. However, these and the more potent diuretics (for example, furosemide) may promote hypokalemia, plasma volume depletion, and encephalopathy. Ascitic patients with no peripheral edema are even more prone than those with edema to develop encephalopathy and plasma volume contraction after diuresis, because the diuresis may exceed the mobilization of ascitic fluid into the vascular space. In such patients diuresis should not exceed 0.2 to 0.3 kg per day, whereas in ascitic patients with edema one may aim for about 1 kg daily.

Other measures, for example, the infusion of salt-free albumin or of the osmotic diuretics, such as mannitol, are only temporarily effective and rarely produce a sustained diuresis. Moreover, these agents may produce pulmonary edema in patients with normal or high central venous pressures. Finally, they may result in excessive portal venous pressure and thus precipitate variceal rupture. Side-to-side portacaval shunt surgery has been advocated for the rare patient with nonresponsive ascites, but this procedure is associated with such a high operative mortality rate that it cannot be enthusiastically recommended.

Surgically constructed peritoneovenous shunting procedures have also been attempted; their value is uncertain.

DEFECTIVE BLOOD COAGULATION IN LIVER DISEASE
Bleeding is a common complication of cirrhosis, and bleeding from esophageal varices, peptic ulcer, or gastritis is a principal mode of exitus. Impaired hemostasis may contribute to bleeding in the cirrhotic patient. Depression of the clotting factors synthesized in the liver may play a role, but rarely is this so profound as to be considered of primary importance. In the presence of advanced liver disease, the clearance of activated blood-coagulation products is impaired, leading to disseminated intravascular coagulation (DIC), which is often but not always clinically unimportant. Fibrinolytic activity is increased to compensate for the accelerated coagulation. Thus, laboratory evidence of DIC may be associated with low levels of clotting factors, thrombocytopenia, and secondary fibrinolysis. Defective platelet aggregation may contribute another coagulation defect in some cirrhotics. Treatment of DIC with heparin and antifibrinolytic drugs, together with replacement of clotting factors and platelet concentrates, has been advocated, but in general the results of such therapy have not been impressive.

THE HEPATORENAL SYNDROME

Definition and Pathogenesis
The development of oliguria, impaired water clearance, and progressive azotemia is of grave prognostic significance in a patient with severe liver disease, and this syndrome is rarely reversible. Present evidence suggests that the basic defect is an alteration in hemodynamics, with a decrease in both renal plasma flow and glomerular filtration rate (that is, increased renal vascular resistance in the face of decreased systemic resistance). Although tubular injury may be evident terminally in some patients, the excretion of urine that is low in sodium, that is lacking tubular cells, and that has adequate urine-to-plasma ratios for osmolarity and creatinine suggests that renal tubular function is adequately preserved, distinguishing this syndrome from acute tubular necrosis. Xenon washout studies and renal arteriography have revealed a marked reduc-

tion in renal cortical perfusion, with a relative increase in medullary blood flow. The functional nature of the defect is evident both in the failure to find significant histopathologic or ultrastructural alterations in affected kidneys, and in the fact that these kidneys function normally when they are transplanted into patients with severe kidney disease. The mechanism by which the altered renal hemodynamics develop is uncertain.

Diagnosis and Treatment
The diagnosis of the hepatorenal syndrome is dependent on excluding other causes of renal failure, such as underlying intrinsic kidney disease, prerenal azotemia, acute tubular necrosis, or diminished effective blood volume. Exclusion of the last condition often requires a trial with volume expanders, which unfortunately may be hazardous for the patient with portal hypertension, since hemorrhage from esophageal varices may be precipitated. Although beneficial effects have been claimed with L-dopa, adrenergic amines, corticosteroids, salt-free albumin infusions, portacaval anastomosis, and hepatic transplantation, the efficacy of any of these treatments remains unproved by controlled trials. In general, management of the hepatorenal syndrome is usually similar to that for oliguria in any patient.

Congenital Liver Disease

POLYCYSTIC LIVER DISEASE
Polycystic liver disease is an uncommon embryologic defect that is transmitted genetically as a mendelian dominant trait, with a reported incidence of 1 in 1,000. Approximately 50 percent of patients with polycystic liver disease also have multiple renal cysts; however, only one-fifth to one-third of patients with polycystic kidney disease also have liver cysts. The cysts, which may represent the residue of defective intrahepatic bile ducts, vary in size from minute to 15 cm in diameter and may contain clear or brown-stained fluid. Otherwise the bile ducts are normal, and cholestasis is not seen.

Clinical Features
Most persons affected with polycystic liver disease are asymptomatic, although rarely patients may present

with abdominal discomfort resulting from stretching of the liver capsule by an enlarging cyst. Infrequently, a cyst may rupture or become infected. Chemical studies are usually normal, and portal hypertension is uncommon. The diagnosis may be suspected from hepatomegaly and from multiple defects found on hepatic scintiscan or on arteriography. The diagnosis can be confirmed by visualization of the liver through the peritoneoscope or by biopsy of a portion of a cyst. Death may result from associated polycystic kidney disease or from hemorrhage of an associated intracerebral aneurysm, and it rarely results from involvement of the liver. No treatment is usually necessary. Puncture of a large cyst may be required to relieve abdominal discomfort, and very rarely, portacaval anastomosis may be needed to control hemorrhage from esophageal varices.

CONGENITAL HEPATIC FIBROSIS

Congenital hepatic fibrosis is primarily a disease of children, transmitted as a recessive trait. The lesions are multiple bile duct hamartomas or adenomas, accompanied by dense portal tract fibrosis. Presenting features include hepatosplenomegaly and upper gastrointestinal hemorrhage from esophageal varices. Since portal hypertension in this disorder is presinusoidal, jaundice is unusual; the liver function tests may be within normal limits; and the clinical course is usually mild. Diagnosis requires biopsy of the liver. The kidney may be normal, but polycystic disease or medullary sponge kidney may also be found in a few patients. Portacaval anastomosis may be necessary to control variceal hemorrhage.

Neoplasms

PRIMARY CANCER OF THE LIVER

There are two major pathologic forms of primary cancer of the liver: *hepatocellular carcinoma* (hepatoma), in which the neoplastic cells resemble hepatic parenchymal cells, and *cholangiocarcinoma* (cholangioma), in which the neoplasm resembles bile duct epithelium. Rarely, a mixed type is observed. Malignant involvement of the littoral cells (angiosarcomas) has also been described. Hepatoma is four to five times more common than cholangioma. Clinically, there are no

features to distinguish the two conditions, although it has been suggested that survival may be somewhat longer in cholangioma. Except in the Far East and Africa and among very young children, most cases of primary liver cancer occur in cirrhotics. Hepatoma is considerably more frequent in patients with either postnecrotic cirrhosis or hemochromatosis than in those with alcoholic cirrhosis. The etiology of primary cancer of the liver is not known, although mycotoxins, parasitic infestations, and viral infections (hepatitis B) have all been postulated to play a role. Thorium dioxide, arsenic, and exposure to vinyl chloride have been associated with the development of angiosarcoma.

Clinical Features

Generalized abdominal pain (or pain in the right upper quadrant or epigastrium) and weight loss are the presenting complaints in about two-thirds of patients. A few patients have signs of distant metastases. About 25 percent of hepatomas are manifest as a sudden and unexplained deterioration in the clinical condition of a patient with known cirrhosis or hemochromatosis. A smaller number of patients present with fever of unknown origin or an acute abdominal catastrophe (for example, a hemoperitoneum caused by erosion of a vessel on the surface of the liver).

Rare systemic manifestations of hepatoma include erythrocytosis, hypoglycemia, hypercalcemia, hyperlipidemia, dysfibrinogenemia, and precocious puberty in childhood. Spread of tumor to the hepatic veins may result in the Budd-Chiari syndrome. In approximately 10 percent of patients, the hepatoma is asymptomatic and is discovered only at laparotomy or at postmortem examination.

Hepatomegaly is present in most patients. The liver may be tender and massively enlarged, with an irregular surface or a palpable mass. Ascites is present in about 50 percent of patients. The ascitic fluid either may be blood-stained with an increased protein concentration, or it may be typical of a transudate. Jaundice is present in less than half the patients. Signs of chronic liver disease usually reflect the presence of underlying cirrhosis.

Laboratory Studies

Mild anemia is common except in rare patients who present with polycythemia. Leukocytosis is present in about a third of the patients, and the serum alkaline phosphatase level is elevated in a large proportion. The serum alkaline phosphatase level is often very high, and this factor, together with a normal or minimally elevated serum bilirubin level, suggests a space-occupying or infiltrative lesion. Alpha-fetoprotein is present in the serum of about 75 percent of patients, but it is not specific for hepatoma. Hepatitis B surface antigen is detected in a variable proportion of patients.

Diagnosis

Antemortem clinical recognition of primary cancer of the liver is often dependent mainly on clinical suspicion. Chest films may reveal abnormal elevation or bulging of the right hemidiaphragm. A major difficulty is in distinguishing between primary and secondary neoplastic involvement of the liver. Hepatic scintiscanning with technetium sulfur colloid is useful in confirming the presence of focal defects. Gallium scanning may be useful in patients with hepatoma and underlying cirrhosis by demonstrating the accumulation of the radionuclide within tumor masses. Hepatic arteriography may reveal the presence of vascular cuffing or a tumor blush in primary lesions, whereas metastatic lesions, with few exceptions, are avascular. Needle biopsy will confirm the diagnosis in approximately 75 percent of patients. Peritoneoscopy may provide a diagnosis when the lesion is on the surface of the liver.

Treatment

In occasional patients in whom the tumor is limited to one lobe and the function of the remainder of the liver is not impaired, subtotal hepatectomy may be successful. However, most tumors are inoperable, and chemotherapy has been generally disappointing. Although transplantation of the liver has been performed, the occurrence of metastases in the transplanted liver has discouraged this approach.

METASTATIC LIVER DISEASE

Approximately 40 percent of patients dying of malignancy have hepatic metastases at postmortem examination. The primary sites may be in organs that are adjacent to the liver and that drain into the portal vein, or they may be elsewhere. The most common sites of origin are in the gastrointestinal tract, breast, and lung, but tumors at any site (except the brain) may metastasize to the liver.

Clinical Features

Patients may present with nonspecific complaints, abdominal pain, or less commonly, with symptoms of liver disease. Hepatomegaly is common; the liver is typically very firm to stone-hard on palpation and is often nodular. Jaundice is a late manifestation.

Diagnosis

Liver function tests may be abnormal but are rarely diagnostic. Striking increases in serum alkaline phosphatase levels and BSP retention may be the only abnormalities seen early in the course of metastatic liver disease. There is a positive correlation between the extent of metastatic involvement, the degree of hepatomegaly, and the frequency and degree of liver function abnormalities. Liver scans may suggest a space-occupying mass, but liver biopsy, directed at the probable site of the lesion as indicated by palpation, scan, or direct vision through a peritoneoscope, is necessary for confirmation. A single blind needle biopsy will establish metastatic disease in over 50 percent of patients in whom it is strongly suspected, and a repeat biopsy will improve this percentage.

Treatment

Although systemic chemotherapy, regional perfusion chemotherapy through the hepatic artery, and hepatic resection of metastases have prolonged life in some instances, the outlook for most patients with metastatic carcinoma in the liver is exceedingly poor.

HYPERNEPHROMA AND LIVER DYSFUNCTION

Infrequently, in patients with renal cell carcinoma but without hepatic metastases, hepatomegaly and abnormal liver function tests have been observed. BSP retention, elevation of serum alkaline phosphatase, hypoprothrombinemia, increased serum globulins, and decreased serum albumin are the major abnormalities noted. Mild hyperbilirubinemia and splenomegaly are inconstant features. The liver is histologically normal in most cases or shows only nonspecific changes. Since hepatomegaly and hepatic dysfunction may disappear following nephrectomy, the elaboration of a hepatotoxic humoral factor by the hypernephroma has been postulated, but the nature and mechanism of action of this factor have not been established.

BENIGN HEPATIC TUMORS

Previously regarded as extremely rare, two pathologically distinct forms of benign hepatic tumors have been reported with increased frequency in recent years. These lesions, termed *hepatic adenoma* and *focal nodular hyperplasia,* have been associated with oral contraceptive use. The hepatic adenomas are encapsulated, lack bile ducts, ductules, nodularity, and central scarring. The lesions of focal nodular hyperplasia have no capsules, but do have bile ducts, ductules, nodularity, and a central scar. Patients with either lesion may present with nonspecific abdominal pain, an abdominal mass or hepatomegaly, or intraperitoneal bleeding with shock. The latter complication may be fatal and requires surgical resection of the ruptured mass. Hepatic arteriography may be diagnostic in patients seen before the onset of hemorrhage. Liver biopsy is contraindicated. In some patients discontinuation of oral contraceptive use has been accompanied by a regression of the lesions.

Bibliography

BILIRUBIN METABOLISM

Bissell, D. M. Formation and elimination of bilirubin. *Gastroenterology* 69:519, 1975.

Schmid, R. Bilirubin metabolism in man. *N. Engl. J. Med.* 287:703, 1972.

HEPATITIS (VIRAL, DRUG-INDUCED, AND CHRONIC)

Black, M., Mitchell, J. R., Zimmerman, H. J., Ishak, K. G., and Epler, G. R. Isoniazid-associated hepatitis in 114 patients. *Gastroenterology* 69:289, 1975.

Ishak, K. G., and Irey, W. S. Hepatic injury associated with the phenothiazines; clinicopathologic and follow-up studies of 36 patients. *Arch. Pathol.* 93:283, 1972.

Karvountzis, G. G., Redeker, A. G., and Peters, R. L. Long-term follow-up studies of patients surviving fulminant viral hepatitis. *Gastroenterology* 67:870, 1974.

Proceedings of a symposium on viral hepatitis. *Am. J. Med. Sci.* 270:1, 1975.

Ritt, D. J., Whelan, G., Werner, D. J., Eigenbrodt, E. H., Schenker, S., and Combes, B. Acute hepatic necrosis with stupor or coma: An analysis of thirty-one patients. *Medicine* 48:151, 1969.

Robinson, W. S., and Lutwick, L. I. The virus of hepatitis, type B. *N. Engl. J. Med.* 295:1168, 1238, 1976.

Summerskill, W. H. J. Chronic active liver disease re-examined: Prognosis hopeful. *Gastroenterology* 66:450, 1974.

Ware, A. J., Eigenbrodt, E. H., and Combes, B. Prognostic significance of subacute hepatic necrosis in acute hepatitis. *Gastroenterology* 68:519, 1975.

ALCOHOLIC LIVER DISEASE AND CIRRHOSIS

Conn, H. O. A rational approach to the hepatorenal syndrome. *Gastroenterology* 65:321, 1973.

Conn, H. O., Ramsby, G. R., Storer, E. H., Mutchnick, M. G., Joshi, P. H., Phillips, M. M., Cohen, G. A., Fields, G. N., and Petroski, D. Intraarterial vasopressin in the treatment of upper gastrointestinal hemorrhage: A prospective, controlled clinical trial. *Gastroenterology* 68:211, 1975.

Grace, N. D., and Powell, L. W. Iron storage disorders of the liver. *Gastroenterology* 67:1257, 1974.

Lieber, C. S. Liver adaptation and injury in alcoholism. *N. Engl. J. Med.* 288:356, 1973.

Powell, W. J., and Klatskin, G. Duration of survival in patients with Laennec's cirrhosis. *Am. J. Med.* 44:406, 1968.

Resnick, R. H., Iber, F. L., Ishihara, A. M., Chalmers, T. C., Zimmerman, H. C., and the Boston Inter-Hospital Liver Group. A controlled study of the therapeutic portacaval shunt. *Gastroenterology* 67:843, 1974.

Schenker, S., Breen, K. J., and Hoyumpa, A. M.

Hepatic encephalopathy: Current status. *Gastroenterology* 66:121, 1974.

Sherlock, S., and Scheuer, P. J. The presentation and diagnosis of 100 patients with primary biliary cirrhosis. *N. Engl. J. Med.* 289:674, 1973.

Strickland, G. T., and Leu, M. L. Wilson's disease: Clinical and laboratory manifestations in 40 patients. *Medicine* 54:113, 1975.

HEPATIC NEOPLASIA

Kew, M. C., Dos Santos, H. A., and Sherlock, S. Diagnosis of primary cancer of the liver. *Br. Med. J.* 4:408, 1971.

Margolis, S., and Homcy, C. Systemic manifestations of hepatoma. *Medicine* 51:381, 1972.

MISCELLANEOUS

Barbour, G. L., and Juniper, K., Jr. A clinical comparison of amebic and pyogenic abscess of the liver in sixty-six patients. *Am. J. Med.* 53:323, 1972.

Cohen, H. G., and Reynolds, T. B. Comparison of metronidazole and chloroquine for the treatment of amebic hepatic abscess. A controlled trial. *Gastroenterology* 69:35, 1975.

Simon, H. B., and Wolff, S. M. Granulomatous hepatitis and prolonged fever of unknown origin: A study of 13 patients. *Medicine* 52:1, 1973.

Tavill, A. S., Wood, E. J., Kreel, L., Jones, E. A., Gregory, M., and Sherlock, S. Budd-Chiari syndrome: Correlation between hepatic scintigraphy and the clinical, radiological and pathological findings in nineteen cases of hepatic venous outflow obstruction. *Gastroenterology* 68:509, 1975.

42

Diseases of the Pancreas

Elihu M. Schimmel

Physiologic Considerations

The pancreas, which develops from the embryonic intestinal tube, functions in the alimentary tract in the digestion and assimilation of food. Hormonal interrelationships link the pancreatic digestive secretions to the flow of nutrients through the stomach and duodenum. In addition, the endocrine secretions of the pancreas (insulin, glucagon) play major homeostatic roles in the metabolism of the absorbed products of digestion. The normal sequence of digestion and absorption depends on the anatomic and physiologic integrity of the upper gastrointestinal tract, and when this system is disrupted, disorders of digestion and absorption ensue. The following discussion is a simplified formulation of this system.

FUNCTIONING OF THE
UPPER GASTROINTESTINAL TRACT
Under the stimulus of a meal, the pancreatic acini produce polypeptides — digestive enzymes — for excretion via the major pancreatic ducts (the ducts of Wirsung and Santorini) into the descending duodenum. One of these ducts and the main bile duct share a common opening (the ampulla of Vater) into the gut. Not only is the anatomic drainage coincident, but also bile flow and pancreatic flow are stimulated by the same hormones, secretin and CCK-PZ (the current designation of a single polypeptide, formerly identified as two different hormones, cholecystokinin and pancreozymin). Furthermore, a simultaneous flow of bile and pancreatic lipase is necessary for normal fat digestion. It is noteworthy that this common pathway may play a role in the pathogenesis of pancreatitis secondary to gallstone disease, and also of cholestatic jaundice that occurs incidental to a pancreatic mass.

CCK-PZ stimulates the flow of pancreatic secretions that are rich in proteolytic enzymes (e.g., trypsin), lipolytic enzymes (e.g., lipase), and the carbohydrate hydrolytic enzyme, amylase. After the first wave of pancreatic enzymes enters the intact gut,

there is probably a secondary response to the resultant increase in peptides and fatty acids, stimulating a continued elaboration of duodenal CCK-PZ and augmentation of pancreatic synthesis of digestive enzymes. The clinical importance of these circular pathways is twofold. First, in acute inflammatory disorders, a primary therapeutic goal is to interrupt these pathways in order to rest the organ and prevent the release of additional proteolytic enzymes (these disorders are discussed in the section on pancreatitis). Second, in pancreatic insufficiency, a lack of enzyme and hormone production may lead to various deficiency states resulting from malabsorption.

After ingestion, nutrients stimulate the gastric antrum and duodenal mucosa, where specialized cells release gut hormones with the following primary functions related to the pancreas:

1. Gastrin stimulates the secretion of hydrochloric acid and pepsin, which in turn initiate the process of peptic digestion of proteins to amino acids and peptides.
2. Secretin is released (by duodenal mucosa) in response to luminal stimuli (particularly acid), which are secondary to gastrin-mediated effects on the stomach. In turn, secretin stimulates the pancreatic secretion of a large volume of fluid rich in bicarbonate.
3. CCK-PZ is released in response to the presence of food in the duodenum, especially in response to peptide-rich chyme, which is induced by gastrin-mediated, acid-peptic digestion of protein in the stomach. Fatty acids are also potent stimuli of release of CCK-PZ.

The Islets of Langerhans

Interspersed within the pancreas are several hundred thousand islets of Langerhans with different cell types that produce hormones related to the cellular processes of energy metabolism. Primary insulin deficiency, a defect in juvenile diabetes mellitus, is discussed in Chapter 59. Often the islets are damaged or destroyed by an inflammatory or a malignant process of the surrounding tissue, and insulin therapy may be required as part of the management of several pancreatic disorders. Malignant tumors of the islets

519

of Langerhans may produce either insulin (beta cells), glucagon (alpha cells), or gastrin (cell type uncertain). These tumors are discussed in the chapters on endocrine disorders (insulinomas and glucagonomas) and gastroduodenal disorders (gastrinomas, or the Zollinger-Ellison syndrome) (Chaps. 35, 55 to 61).

General Diagnostic Considerations
Clinical studies of diseases of the pancreas can be considered under several different categories.

TESTS
Unfortunately there are only a few specific tests for a particular pancreatic disease. One example is the sweat test in cystic fibrosis.

NONSPECIFIC SYMPTOMS
Nonspecific manifestations of intraabdominal inflammation or neoplasia (e.g., pain, fever, or weight loss) usually bring the patient to the physician. These symptoms rarely indicate the pancreas specifically as the cause.

EFFECTS ON THE ENDOCRINE ISLETS
Coincidental effects on the endocrine islets, though nonspecific, help to identify the pancreas as the site of disease; an example is hyperglycemia.

EXOCRINE INSUFFICIENCIES
Pancreatic exocrine insufficiencies (e.g., steatorrhea) are useful in terms of diagnosis, but they become apparent only after nearly total loss of function.

STUDIES OF ENZYME ACTIVITY
Biochemical studies of pancreatic enzyme activity (e.g., serum or urine assays of amylase or lipase) are the most reliable methods for clinical diagnosis. Unfortunately, enzyme changes may be minimal or transient, and they may be found in other diseases included in the differential diagnosis such as intestinal infarction or perforated peptic ulcer. Recent studies have reawakened interest in modifications of the amylase test to increase its sensitivity and specificity, namely, the amylase clearance test and the simultaneous amylase-creatinine clearance ratio in serum and urine. The clinical usefulness of the latter test has not as yet been established in a prospective study.

ANATOMIC STUDIES
Anatomic studies of the diseased pancreas have been difficult to obtain and hitherto limited to surgical and fatal cases. In the last decade, however, a number of techniques have been developed to outline the size and position of the organ, its duct system, and its patterns of blood flow. Since the biliary tree is intimately associated with the pancreas, secondary information may be gained from anatomic studies of the bile ducts. Finally, pancreatic form and function may be studied by radioisotope scanning, using the phenominal amino acid uptake and protein synthesis of this exocrine gland. Several of these methods are still in evolutionary stages, and their benefits relative to cost are as yet unknown.

Radiology
Conventional radiology of the abdomen either may show pancreatic calcification or may reveal a mass impinging on and displacing adjacent barium-filled viscera.

Double-Contrast Studies
Double-contrast studies of the duodenum may be performed (see Chap. 35) after motor tone has been inhibited by anticholinergics or glucagon (hence the term *hypotonic duodenography*). This technique has few serious side effects, but in diagnosing pancreatic disease, it is useful only for lesions of the head of the pancreas.

Abdominal Angiography
Abdominal angiography may be used in selective studies of the celiac axis and the superior mesenteric artery. Such studies may also visualize the portal system (in the venous phase). Inflammatory and neoplastic processes are often signaled by arterial distortions or venous occlusions; pseudocysts and tumors may also displace vessels. Tumors often show characteristic vascular patterns (avascular in adenocarcinoma; occasionally intensely vascular in islet cell tumors) and may lack the physiologic response of vasoconstriction after epinephrine infusion. Primary pancreatic neoplasms as well as liver metastases usually share similar patterns on angiography.

Cholecystography and Cholangiography

Oral cholecystography and intravenous cholangiography are low-risk, high-yield approaches to the biliary tree, but their successfulness is limited by even minimal elevation of serum bilirubin levels or moderate biliary obstruction. Invasive cholangiography can be carried out by percutaneous, transhepatic needle puncture, with fluoroscopic exploration for a branch of the biliary tree. The procedure can be made quite safe by the use of needles of very small diameter, and the diagnostic information is valuable in over 95 percent of cases, which represents a great improvement in safety and yield over older versions of the technique. An alternate approach to the biliary system by angiographic technique is one using a transjugular puncture and a catheter that traverses the superior vena cava, right atrium, and hepatic vein and then punctures through the liver into a biliary duct. Either method may reveal biliary obstruction and distinguish between choledocholithiasis or a pancreatic mass as the cause. Jaundice does not preclude successful study by either of these puncture methods.

Endoscopy

Fiberoptic endoscopic techniques (see Chap. 35) permit transduodenal visualization of the ampulla of Vater and retrograde cannulation of the papilla. Radiographic contrast material can be injected to visualize the biliary and pancreatic ducts with an average success rate of 70 to 80 percent by experienced operators. This technique is the only available preoperative method for studying the morbid anatomy of the pancreatic ducts to assess the possibility of inflammatory strictures, stones, occlusive tumors, or complicating pseudocysts. Additional diagnostic findings available by endoscopic retrograde cannulation include the collection of pancreatic exfoliative cytology, the accurate assessment of pancreatic secretion as a functional test, and the measurement of secretory pressures.

Radionuclide Scanning

Radionuclide scans of the pancreas have been largely disappointing in sensitivity and accuracy. Selenomethionine is given as a gamma-emitting radioactive amino acid, which is incorporated into pancreatic protein and thus outlines the gland. However, the liver parenchyma may mask much of the pancreas because of its overlapping function and position. Double-isotope studies using I^{131}-labeled rose bengal may allow computerized "subtraction" of the liver uptake and give an acceptable image of the pancreas. Moderate-sized tumors may be recognized by this technique.

Computerized Axial Tomography

Computerized axial tomography has been used primarily in neuroradiology. However, several small series have been reported using the technique for abdominal organs, and a number of pancreatic tumors have been dramatically portrayed.

Sonar Echography

Sonar echography has had its greatest usefulness in the identification of pancreatic pseudocysts and allows an assessment of their response to nonsurgical management. Tumors and inflammatory masses may also be delineated by this method, but with less precision.

Summary

In summary, the pancreas is now accessible to anatomic visualization, and with future refinements of available techniques, it may become a more satisfactory organ to study. However, complications are still too common and the necessary expertise is difficult to achieve.

Pancreatitis

The pathologic diagnosis of pancreatitis includes a wide spectrum of diseases in which diffuse inflammation is associated with a complaint, usually pain, that brings the patient to the physician. Based on its outcome, pancreatitis is often classified as acute or chronic (recurring, relapsing, or persistent). The pathologic findings in milder cases are limited to interstitial edema and minimal necrosis; more severe episodes may progress to hemorrhagic necrosis with extension of the necroinflammatory process to adjacent structures. Liquefaction of a necrotic mass may fail to resolve and may result in a pancreatic pseudo-cyst. In chronic, or recurrent, pancreatitis there is progressive destruction of both exocrine and endocrine tissue, calcification of acini, and stone formation within the duct system.

Certain *predisposing factors* may be significant in the etiology of pancreatitis, although the pathogenesis is poorly understood. In populations where *alcoholism* is prevalent, a heavy, continuous intake or an alcoholic binge often precedes an episode of acute pancreatitis. There is usually a delay in the onset of clinical symptoms, with the result that Monday morning is a common time for patients to present after a weekend of heavy drinking. Nutrition tends to be better than in alcoholics with cirrhosis, but this clinical impression is hard to substantiate. Most characteristic of an alcohol-related disease is the slow, gradual destruction and fibrosis of the pancreas, often considerably before the onset of pain.

In private patients, particularly the elderly and women, *gallstone disease* is the most common cause of a painful attack. The attack is usually acute, and the clinical features of pancreatitis may mask the underlying gallstones. Cholecystectomy with removal of the common duct stone or stones is curative, and there is no expectation of recurrence or of pancreatic fibrosis. Mortality ranges from 5 to 50 percent.

Direct injury to the gland or its ducts is easily recognized, provided the physician considers pancreatitis as a possible cause of an unexpected, painful complication of conditions such as penetrating peptic ulcer, surgical injury in the neighborhood of the pancreas, or other abdominal traumas.

Metabolic and systemic disorders associated with pancreatitis include hyperparathyroidism, hyperlipidemia, hereditary pancreatitis with aminoaciduria, pregnancy, side effects of drugs (including thiazides and corticosteroids), mumps, and ascariasis.

ACUTE PANCREATITIS

The pathogenesis of an acute attack of pancreatitis remains unknown, but there are several factors of probable importance:

1. Gallstones in the distal common bile duct may make the patient vulnerable to obstruction of the pancreatic duct or may allow bile to reflux into the pancreas.
2. Alcohol, which is known to be toxic to many tissues, may precipitate bouts of alcoholic pancreatitis. It has been postulated that alcohol may lead to direct damage of the acini with secondary obstructive phenomena in the small and large ducts. Similar damage may account for pancreatitis induced by drugs or viruses.
3. An inflamed pancreas may be further damaged by its own enzymes, which can digest any tissue, including the pancreas itself.

The classic features of acute pancreatitis are easily recognized, once the diagnosis is considered. Positive proof of the diagnosis is more difficult, and response to therapy plays an important role in management. With an occasional exception, pain is usually the complaint bringing the patient to the physician. The pain is typically severe and steady; it is most severe in the upper abdomen, often to the left, and commonly penetrates to the midback. Occasionally, the patient prefers a bent-over position, either flexed forward or with his knees drawn upward. Surprisingly, the abdomen usually is not boardlike; tenderness and guarding may be the only physical findings. If the patient demands narcotics, and particularly if he has done so in the past, he may pose difficult management problems. The remaining secondary features of acute pancreatitis are discussed in the following section.

Pathophysiology of Clinical Manifestations

A great variety of symptoms, signs, and laboratory features are present in acute pancreatitis. The clinical features of acute pancreatitis, arranged here according to organ function, are as follows:

1. A large, inflammatory mass is present in the abdomen, usually accompanied by nonspecific pain, fever, and leukocytosis; the patient feels sick and may appear toxic when the signs are severe.
2. There is contiguous involvement of adjacent organs by the pancreatic inflammatory mass, accompanied by disturbed function in the organs, as follows:
   a. Common bile duct obstruction, partial or com-

plete, may occur; it is accompanied by jaundice (in about 20 percent of patients), cholestatic enzyme changes (e.g., elevated alkaline phosphatase level), and a nonvisualizing cholecystogram (in about 10 percent of patients).

b. Distention of the stomach and anorexia may occur.

c. The duodenum and jejunum may also be distended, and radiologic signs of a dilated, isolated "sentinal" loop may be present. The distended, atonic viscera may be responsible for much of the accompanying nausea and vomiting.

d. The transverse colon may be involved by the necroinflammatory mass, either directly or by extension through the mesocolon over the pancreas. Either a dilated colon or diarrhea from irritative effects may be prominent.

e. Pleural fluid collections and pulmonary atelectasis, especially on the left side, may result from pancreatic inflammation operating across the diaphragm. Pleuritic pain, however, may occur without effusion.

f. Abnormalities of the urinary sediment may be related to direct extension of the pancreatic mass to the left kidney.

g. Adjacent veins, especially the splenic or portal, may be occluded by thrombosis. Extension of the mass to the retroperitoneal nerve plexus may contribute to the pain.

h. Peritoneal surfaces may be contaminated by enzyme-rich exudates, leading to an ascites that is high in protein, cells, and amylase activity. This noninfectious peritonitis may also contribute to the pain and abdominal tenderness. The peritoneal effusion is usually small. When the disease has a large hemorrhagic component (which is rare), there may be blue or purple discoloration of the flanks (Grey-Turner sign) or of the umbilical area (Cullen's sign).

3. In addition to the nonspecific signs just listed, the pancreatic inflammation may also result in the release of a variety of specific pancreatic digestive enzymes. Lipolytic enzymes can lead to extensive fat necrosis locally or at distant sites, with calcium deposition (as fatty acid soaps) in the peritoneal

cavity, the omentum, or the pancreas itself. The release of proteolytic enzymes presumably contributes to the persistence of the autodigestive destruction of the pancreas and may be a prelude to pseudocyst formation. These complications are particularly prominent in alcoholic pancreatitis.

4. Distant organs are occasionally involved in necrosis of fat or other tissue, suggesting the possibility of widespread dissemination of destructive enzymes. Infarcts and fat necrosis may be seen in the skin, long bones, and periarticular tissues, or even in the brain, myocardium, or lungs. The hematuria or proteinuria seen in 20 percent of cases may reflect similar damage of the glomeruli.

5. The hormonal effects of inflammatory damage of the islets commonly present as hyperglycemia, which has been attributed to both low insulin levels and high glucagon levels.

6. Other metabolic effects of pancreatitis include hypocalcemia; when the serum calcium level is lower than 7 mg per 100 ml, there is a high mortality rate (50 percent). The likely causes of hypocalcemia include (a) calcium deposition as insoluble soaps in areas of fat necrosis; (b) calcium deposition in bone as a result of thyrocalcitonin release in response to elevated levels of glucagon; or (c) a parathormone-resistant state contributed to by coincidental hypomagnesemia, especially in alcoholic patients. Hyperlipidemia is occasionally a transient finding, with increased triglycerides producing a cloudy serum. The mechanisms are unclear, and no consistent pattern of hyperlipoproteinemia has been elicited. Associated alcoholic hepatitis may contribute to the finding. Rarely, hyperlipidemia associated with chylomicronemia (types I and V) may produce recurrent pancreatitis. In such patients, reduction of serum triglycerides may help to reduce the frequency of attacks.

7. Profound early circulatory collapse may be a life-threatening complication of acute pancreatitis; the principal manifestations are hypovolemia and hemoconcentration. A variety of contributory factors have been implicated, including myocardial depressant factors, bradykinin, serotonin, and other humoral agents that damage capillary endo-

thelial integrity and lead to a shift of fluid from the plasma to an extravascular "third space." A high hematocrit and a concentrated urine are indicative of this process and serve as guides to therapy.

8. The surgical complications of pancreatitis include abscess and pseudocyst, each of which may present as a mass with pain, fever, and leukocytosis. The differentiation between these entities and a large necroinflammatory process is difficult at the bedside and needs to be resolved radiologically or surgically.

9. The ultimate consequence of severe, recurrent pancreatitis is destruction of functioning tissue. At first fibrotic, the gland may progress to calcification (in 30 percent of cases) with intraductal stones and with dystrophic deposition of calcium in necrotic tissue. Hormonal deficiencies may result in diabetes (30 percent of cases) and a broad maldigestion syndrome (60 percent of cases), in which steatorrhea is the most prominent feature.

Special Diagnostic Methods

A clear clinical diagnosis can be confirmed when pancreatic enzyme levels are elevated in the serum or in other biologic fluids (such as urine, ascites, or pleural effusion). Amylase and lipase are the most accessible to measurement. With recurrent disease and progressive destruction of the gland, elevations of serum enzyme levels become less common.

Amylase clearance, expressed as a percentage of the simultaneous creatinine clearance, may provide a more sensitive and specific test for acute pancreatitis.

Therapy of Acute Pancreatitis

Since an early death and much of the morbidity resulting from acute pancreatitis are related to hypovolemia, the first therapeutic obligation is to restore effective plasma volume with parenteral saline solution or plasma. Clinical guides to replacement therapy are pulse rate, blood pressure, and urine output. The second therapeutic requirement is relief of pain; narcotics such as meperidine hydrochloride are often necessary. Since drug addiction is an occasional complication of prolonged analgesic treatment, narcotics should be withdrawn as soon as feasible. The third

measure is the institution of antral decompression by means of low-pressure, nasogastric aspiration; ordinarily pancreatitis should be so treated for several days after symptomatic relief has been achieved. The main purpose of nasogastric suction is to interrupt all stimuli to pancreatic exocrine secretions. Withholding food obviously prevents peptides and fatty acids from entering the duodenum. Continuous aspiration is instituted after the nasogastric tube has been fluoroscopically positioned in the most distal portion of the antrum. The aspiration inhibits pancreatic stimulation by two effects: (1) Antral distention is precluded and a major stimulus to gastrin release is thus avoided; and (2) gastric acid is eliminated and, consequently, the stimulation of duodenal secretin and CCK-PZ is prevented.

A second purpose of nasogastric suction is to decompress the distended stomach and, indirectly, the small bowel, thereby providing symptomatic relief. In many cases of recurrent pancreatitis, patients who have previously experienced relief from nasogastric suction ask for the tube. However, controlled studies have not proved the superiority of gastric decompression over a simple restriction of oral intake. Theoretically, anticholinergics might complement suction by inhibiting vagal stimulation of pancreatic flow. Unfortunately the side effects of anticholinergic therapy are more apparent than their possible benefits, and these drugs are not consistently used. In any event, anticholinergics should not be used without gastric suction, since alone they could aggravate the distention of the antrum and small bowel and thus allow continued hormonal drive of the pancreas. Antibiotics have been occasionally recommended to prevent secondary infection, but this therapy has no sound rational basis and has not gained wide acceptance.

Surgery

The patient with acute pancreatitis often presents with an "acute abdomen," which may not be clinically distinguishable from an intraabdominal process requiring surgery (such as perforated peptic ulcer, appendicitis, bowel infarction, or acute cholecystitis). The response to gastric suction may be helpful diagnostically if the course can be followed for a few days. When there is diagnostic uncertainty, surgical exploration is warranted, with one caveat: If pancreatitis is discovered with no other complications, the abdomen should be closed without handling or mobilizing other organs and without surgical biopsy of the inflamed pancreas. Peritoneal lavage has often been recommended if the exploration reveals a necroinflammatory mass or pancreatic ascites. An abscess or pseudocyst should be drained, and cholecystostomy may be the only procedure possible in gallstone pancreatitis.

Associated Problems

Particularly in an alcoholic, pancreatitis is often associated with other major problems, such as alcoholic hepatitis, hemorrhagic gastritis, and various neurologic manifestations of alcoholism. Obviously, each associated disease entails its own management, but it generally worsens the prognosis.

CHRONIC PANCREATITIS

Chronic pancreatitis refers to pancreatic disease that persists or recurs. With the passage of years, the pancreas undergoes progressive destruction, fibrosis. calcification, and loss of endocrine and exocrine functions. Patients with such a chronic, progressive pancreatitis experience a wide spectrum of clinical features. At one extreme, up to 20 percent of patients with calcifications and functional impairment have no history of painful episodes. Many patients, however, have repeated painful episodes, each lasting days to weeks and only occasionally coming to medical attention. Some attacks are managed at home by the patient's limiting his food intake for a few days (or, to his detriment, by his increasing alcohol consumption to relieve pain). An unfortunate minority of patients have continuous pain for periods of weeks or months and, rarely, unremitting pain leading to narcotic addiction, frustrating encounters with the physician, and often a variety of surgical procedures providing little or only short-lived relief. These surgical procedures, even when well-conceived and given physiologic support, are without controlled evaluation. At the present time, some procedures have been wholly abandoned, namely, vagotomy, pyloroplasty, distal gastrectomy, gastrojejunostomy, sphinc-

terotomy, sphincteroplasty, cholecystectomy (in the absence of gallstones), partial pancreatectomy, pancreaticojejunostomy, and even bilateral sympathectomy (for relief of pain). Surgical procedures currently employed include resection of pseudocysts, cyst drainage into the nearby duodenum or jejunum, and the "fringe" pancreatic resection (95 percent of the organ), which preserves minimal tissue surrounding the common bile duct.

Relentless, painful pancreatitis is often associated with changes in other organs to which the pain is wrongly attributed. Thus, patients with chronic pancreatitis may be diagnosed as having pleurisy, idiopathic pleural effusion, gastritis, gastroenteritis, hepatitis, or similar conditions. Such patients may have had ulcer surgery for intractable pain (attributed to duodenal deformity), neurosurgery for back pain (attributed to herniated nucleus pulposus), cholecystectomy (because of nonvisualization on cholecystogram) or, commonly, at least one exploratory laparotomy for acute "surgical" abdomen.

As discussed previously, surgery is most useful in the treatment of gallstone pancreatitis and should prevent recurrences and pancreatic fibrosis. Surgery is also indicated to drain or resect a pseudocyst or abscess. Unfortunately, the patient still remains at risk of developing these complications in another portion of the pancreas.

Other Diagnostic Approaches

The documentation of calcification, late onset diabetes, and steatorrhea support the diagnosis of chronic pancreatitis. The once-popular pancreatic secretory test (measuring the response to intravenous secretin) is rarely needed for clinical diagnosis, but it may prove useful when collections can be made by peroral pancreatic cannulation, a method that avoids loss or contamination of the secretions. The best methods are the newer anatomic studies outlined earlier in this chapter.

Treatment

Replacement therapy for pancreatic insufficiency is relatively simple, but it is often complicated by the patient's poor eating habits and noncompliance with the prescribed regimen. Diabetes is usually mild and responds to small doses of insulin. Enzymes extracted from animal pancreas are available commercially, but they vary greatly in potency and palatability. Steatorrhea is treated by the administration of these enzymes with each meal. The patient should also take antacids to protect the exogenous enzymes from inactivation by gastric acidity. Occasionally, fat digestion is enhanced by additional doses of sodium bicarbonate tablets to help provide an alkaline medium for intraluminal lipolytic activity. The primary goal of enzyme replacement therapy is the promotion of weight gain and general nutrition. Occasionally, diarrhea is alleviated, presumably through a reduction of hydroxy-fatty acids in the colon. A decrease in fecal fat is only an indirect measure of therapeutic success and need not be followed carefully.

Early in the course of chronic pancreatitis, withdrawal from alcohol may benefit the patient. Late in the disease, when there are secondary changes in the duct system, abstinence from alcohol does not consistently arrest progressive pancreatic destruction. However, after 10 to 15 years painful episodes seem to abate in many patients, presumably due to the extensive loss of pancreatic function.

Carcinoma of the Pancreas

The incidence of carcinoma of the pancreas has continued to increase over the past decade, and in many tumor registries it has exceeded new cases of carcinoma of the stomach. Attention has focused on dietary and environmental risk factors such as alcohol, cigarette smoking, and food additives. The clinical features of the disease are similar to those of chronic pancreatitis and have a similar pathophysiologic basis. The major aspects are pain, weight loss, and a rapid course leading to death within a year of recognition. Impingement on adjacent organs may facilitate delineation of the tumor mass, and the newer anatomic diagnostic methods are the most useful in identifying the lesion.

A special feature of carcinoma of the head of the pancreas is the dilated, nontender gallbladder seen in a jaundiced patient, known as Courvoisier's gallbladder. This condition contrasts with jaundice caused by choledocholithiasis, in which the gallbladder is usually thickened and shrunken rather than dilated;

it also differs from an empyema of the gallbladder, which is tender and painful. The patient with a septic gallbladder is also acutely ill.

Another feature of pancreatic carcinoma is the development of mild diabetes. This metabolic abnormality is usually *not* explained by extensive loss of the islets of endocrine cells. Metastases to the liver, the peritoneum, the bones, and the thoracic organs are common.

SPECIAL DIAGNOSTIC FEATURES

The tumor mass and its invasion of adjacent structures may be outlined radiologically; pancreatic cells for cytologic study may be collected by duodenal intubation or by direct cannulation of the pancreatic duct. Unfortunately the yield by this technique is quite low, and adequate specimens may be difficult to collect. The assay of blood for carcinoembryonic antigen (CEA) is now commercially available and is positive in a high proportion of cases; however, it is also positive in chronic benign pancreatitis as well as in other malignancies.

DIFFERENTIAL DIAGNOSIS

Metastatic lesions occasionally appear before the discovery of primary carcinoma in the tail or body of the pancreas, but these lesions are not amenable to therapy and usually do not warrant even palliative surgery. When it presents as obstructive jaundice, carcinoma in the head of the pancreas must be differentiated from choledocholithiasis and tumors of the ampulla of Vater, since both of these conditions are readily accessible to surgery. Furthermore, some patients with ampullary and bile duct malignancies have a reasonable five-year survival rate after resection.

Ampullar tumors generally obstruct both the pancreatic and the common bile ducts; they also tend to bleed. The tumor may thus be suspected when the patient passes the characteristic silvery, slate-gray stools, which are the result of pancreatic and biliary insufficiency. The stools are acholic (pale) and contain excess fat (greasy), and a small amount of changed blood contributes a gray cast.

TREATMENT

Even in surgical circles, debate continues as to the efficacy of radical surgical excision of malignancies of the pancreas. Lesions of the tail, which are more easily encompassed, are usually discovered only after metastases have developed. Resection of tumors of the head is performed either with total pancreatectomy or with Whipple's operation, in which the antrum, duodenum, and common bile duct are resected with the pancreatic head; gastrojejunostomy and biliary-enteric fistula are part of the extensive reconstruction and contribute to palliation by relieving jaundice and itching. In spite of improvements in surgical techniques, a simple diversion of bile into the small intestine may give palliation with a lower surgical mortality rate. Five-year cures are rare, regardless of the treatment chosen.

Diseases of the Pancreas in Childhood

Developmental anomalies of the pancreas include *annular pancreas* and *heterotopic rests.* Annular pancreas may be clinically silent, or it may present as an obstruction of the descending duodenum. This complication may be treated by incision or resection in most cases. However, if the glandular tissue has grown into the full thickness of the duodenal wall, a bypass procedure (such as gastroenterostomy) may be required.

Heterotopic pancreatic tissue is usually clinically silent and may be discovered only incidentally during gastrointestinal radiologic study, endoscopy, or at autopsy. The most frequent site is the duodenum, followed by the stomach and the jejunum; a Meckel's diverticulum may also harbor an island of pancreatic exocrine gland. The most common complication is acid-peptic ulceration presenting as occult gastrointestinal hemorrhage.

Cystic fibrosis of the pancreas is a familial disorder with an autosomal recessive inheritance. About 80 percent of patients with cystic fibrosis have pancreatic exocrine insufficiency. Infants may present with meconium ileus, in which abnormal intestinal secretions are inspissated and cause obstruction. In older children maldigestion and undernutrition are the chief problems. The sweat glands are also involved in all patients with cystic pancreatic disease; thus the basis for the most reliable test for the disorder is the finding in the sweat of a high concentration of salt under the provocation of pilocarpine iontophoresis.

Virtually all patients have pulmonary obstructive disease and respiratory infections, which formerly precluded survival to adult life. However, newer antibiotic therapy and increased clinical sophistication now permit many patients to survive into the third decade of life. These patients usually require pancreatic enzyme replacement therapy but only rarely need insulin therapy. Pathologic secretions and anatomic anomalies may also be found in the liver, gallbladder, salivary glands, and secondary sexual apparatus in both males and females.

Viral pancreatitis can be seen in children, most commonly with mumps but occasionally in other poorly defined systemic viral diseases. Manifestations and therapy are similar to those of acute pancreatitis in the adult.

Bibliography

Banks, P. A. Acute pancreatitis. *Gastroenterology* 61:382, 1971.

Bouchier, I. A. D. The Pancreas. In *Clinical Investigation of Gastrointestinal Function.* Oxford: Blackwell, 1969. P. 149.

Brooks, F. P. Testing pancreatic function. *N. Engl. J. Med.* 286:300, 1972.

Brusilow, S. W. Cystic fibrosis in adults. *Annu. Rev. Med.* 21:99, 1970.

Child, C. G., Frey, C. F., and Fry, W. J. A reappraisal of removal of 95 percent of the distal portion of the pancreas. *Surg. Gynecol. Obstet.* 129: 49, 1969.

Crile, G., Jr. The advantages of bypass operations over radical pancreatoduodenectomy in the treatment of pancreatic carcinoma. *Surg. Gynecol. Obstet.* 130:1049, 1970.

Ferrucci, J. R., Jr., and Eaton, S. B. Radiology of the pancreas. *N. Engl. J. Med.* 288:506, 1973.

Levitt, M. D., Rapoport, M., and Cooperband, S. R. The renal clearance of amylase in renal insufficiency, acute pancreatitis, and macroamylasemia. *Ann. Intern. Med.* 71:919, 1969.

Ogoshi, K., Niwa, M., Hara, Y., and Nebel, O. T. Endoscopic pancreatocholangiography in the evaluation of pancreatic and biliary disease. *Gastroenterology* 64:210, 1973.

Silverberg, M., and Davidson, M. Pediatric gastro-
    enterology: A review. *Gastroenterology* 58:
    229, 1970.
Strum, W. B., and Spiro, H. M. Chronic pancreatitis.
    Ann. Intern. Med. 74:264, 1971.
Warshaw, A. L., and Fuller, A. F., Jr. Specificity of
    increased renal clearance of amylase in diag-
    nosis of acute pancreatitis. *N. Engl. J. Med.*
    292:325, 1975.
Watson, D. W. Pancreatic carcinoma. *Am. J. Dig.
    Dis.* 15:767, 1970.

43

Diseases of the Peritoneum and Mesentery

Raymond S. Koff

The linings of the abdominal cavity and the intra-abdominal viscera are contiguous, semipermeable membranes through which water and electrolytes diffuse rapidly. As a result, only a very small amount of free fluid is present in the normal peritoneal space. *Ascites,* the accumulation of excessive fluid in the peritoneal space, may result from increased peritoneal capillary permeability due to inflammation or neoplasia of the peritoneum. However, most patients with ascites do not have peritoneal disease, but other conditions associated with marked increases in hepatic sinusoidal hydrostatic pressure, for example, cirrhosis, inferior vena cava or hepatic vein obstruction, constrictive pericarditis, or severe congestive heart failure. Marked hypoalbuminemia, such as that occurring in the nephrotic syndrome or in severe malnutrition, results in diminished plasma oncotic pressure and may also produce ascites. Ascites may also be associated with myxedema or with diseases of the ovary.

The parietal peritoneum, which covers the walls of the abdominal cavity, is supplied by spinal nerves, while the subdiaphragmatic peritoneal surface is supplied by intercostal nerves and the phrenic nerve. Irritation of the parietal peritoneum results in pain localized to specific dermatomes, whereas subdiaphragmatic irritation causes pain referred to the top of the shoulder or to the chest or abdominal wall. The visceral peritoneum, which lines the intraperitoneal organs and the suspending mesentery, has no pain receptors. Pain caused by irritation of the visceral peritoneum is poorly localized and ill defined because it is mediated by the visceral autonomic nervous system.

Peritonitis

ACUTE PERITONITIS

Acute inflammation of the peritoneal surface may result from the introduction of chemical or bacterial agents into the peritoneal space. For example, chemical peritonitis due to pancreatic enzymes is observed in acute pancreatitis, or when a pseudocyst leaks or a pancreatic duct ruptures. Similarly, bile peritonitis may follow the rupture of the gallbladder or of a bile duct. Exposure to blood (for example, from a ruptured spleen) or to urine (from a perforation of the bladder) may also produce chemical peritonitis. Peritonitis resulting from bacterial infection is more common; most episodes are caused by enteric organisms that enter the peritoneal space through defects in the gut wall. Such defects may result from ulceration, neoplasm, infarction, obstruction, perforation by foreign objects, or an inflammatory disease such as severe ulcerative colitis. In addition to bacterial peritonitis following bowel surgery, nonbacterial granulomatous inflammation of the peritoneum may occur if a foreign body (e.g., a surgical sponge or surgical glove powder) is left there. Recurrent, sterile *paroxysmal peritonitis* associated with pleurisy and arthritis is a familial disease of uncertain cause. In Middle Eastern and Eastern Mediterranean populations it may lead to amyloidosis. Drug-induced peritonitis caused by the beta-adrenergic receptor blocking agent, practolol, resulted in the withdrawal of this drug from clinical practice in England.

Leakage of bacteria from the intestinal tract into the peritoneum is by far the most common cause of peritonitis. In these instances, multiple bacterial species are involved. The bacteria that are of pathogenic importance in the development of peritonitis include anaerobic gram-negative bacilli, *Bacteroides* species, *Clostridium,* anaerobic and aerobic cocci, and aerobic coliform bacilli *(Escherichia coli, Klebsiella-Enterobacter* species, and species of *Proteus).* Numerically, anaerobic bacilli predominate in the feces and in peritonitis, but aerobic gram-negative bacilli are also pathogenetically important. Spontaneous infection of the peritoneum without recognizable bowel leakage is considerably less frequent, but it does occur in cirrhotic patients with ascites, in patients with the nephrotic syndrome, and in patients during and after peritoneal dialysis.

Clinical Features

The patient with acute peritonitis appears ill, is usually febrile, and complains of persistent, severe abdominal pain that is intensified by movement. Nausea and vomiting are common. Spasm of the abdominal muscles and acute abdominal tenderness are usually striking. The tenderness may be localized to a specific area, where an abdominal mass may be evident. With extension of the inflammatory process, boardlike rigidity may be observed, together with signs of paralytic ileus. Rectal and vaginal examinations may reveal localizing signs in patients with pelvic peritonitis. Exudation of large quantities of fluid into the peritoneal space may lead to depletion of intravascular volume with hypotension and oliguria. Leukocytosis (a count higher than 15,000) is characteristic.

Diagnosis and Management

Radiologic examination may reveal free air in the peritoneal cavity following perforation of a hollow viscus or it may confirm the expected paralytic ileus; the absence of free air does not exclude perforation of a viscus, however. Aspiration of peritoneal fluid for cell count, Gram's stain, and culture is important for both diagnosis and determination of antibiotic therapy. The finding of multiple types of bacteria on Gram's stain and culture indicates leakage of bacteria from the intestinal tract, whereas the presence of only one type of organism suggests one of the types of spontaneous peritonitis. The presence of blood-stained or bile-stained fluid, and the simultaneous measurement of amylase, bilirubin, and creatinine levels in both the fluid and the peripheral blood, may aid in determining the etiology. Concomitantly with these diagnostic maneuvers, the parenteral administration of fluids, electrolytes, and colloids is usually necessary to restore intravascular volume and maintain electrolyte balance. Antibiotic therapy, which is directed at anaerobic bacteria and aerobic gram-negative bacilli, usually consists of clindamycin and an aminoglycoside. Analgesics are used to control pain. Surgical intervention is often required, but a decision to operate will depend on the underlying disease process, the operative risk, and whether or not the peritonitis has localized. Attacks of paroxysmal peritonitis may be suppressed by the administration of colchicine.

TUBERCULOUS PERITONITIS

Tuberculous infection of the peritoneum may present as an acute peritonitis but more often occurs as a chronic illness with ascites and vague abdominal distress. Examination of ascitic fluid may reveal a protein level greater than 2.5 gm per 100 ml and a white blood cell count greater than 300 cells per cubic millimeter, with a predominance of lymphocytes. Cultures of the ascitic fluid for tubercle bacilli may be rewarding, but most often the diagnosis is made either by percutaneous peritoneal needle biopsy or by peritoneoscopy.

SPONTANEOUS BACTERIAL PERITONITIS IN CIRRHOTIC PATIENTS

Bacterial peritonitis in cirrhotic patients with ascites is not rare, occurring in up to 10 percent of cases. Although the typical syndrome includes fever, chills, abdominal pain, ileus, and often impending hepatic coma and hypotension, the process may be silent and its diagnosis difficult. Paracentesis may reveal an exudate, but in the majority of patients the ascitic fluid protein level ranges between 0.5 and 2.0 gm per 100 ml. Culture reveals bacteria in the ascitic fluid, and about 50 percent of patients have positive blood cultures. Responsible organisms include *E. coli* and members of the *Klebsiella-Enterobacter* family in about two-thirds of cases, and gram-positive organisms, especially pneumococci, in as many as one-third. Although antibiotic therapy is often successful, the prognosis is grave (less than 5 percent of such patients survive) because of the severity of the underlying liver disease.

SPONTANEOUS BACTERIAL PERITONITIS IN NEPHROSIS

Bacterial peritonitis in nephrosis, a rare complication of the nephrotic syndrome, occurs almost solely in patients with ascites. Pneumococci and group A streptococci are the usual etiologic agents. Appropriate antibiotic therapy is curative.

BACTERIAL PERITONITIS FOLLOWING PERITONEAL DIALYSIS

Bacterial infection of the peritoneum may occur during the course of peritoneal dialysis. Coliform bacilli and staphylococci are the most frequent causative agents. Clinical symptoms tend to be less severe than in other types of bacterial peritonitis, although bacteremia is a not infrequent complication. There is a prompt response to appropriate antibiotic therapy, and a fatal outcome is rare if the infection is recognized.

Neoplasms of the Peritoneum

The peritoneal surfaces are commonly involved in metastatic disease. Adenocarcinoma of the ovary, stomach, pancreas, and colon is found most frequently, but primary liver cell carcinoma as well as sarcomas and lymphomas may be responsible. The peritoneal fluid may be an exudate (with the protein level greater than 2.5 gm per 100 ml) and may be either grossly bloody or chylous. The latter finding, when confirmed by a high triglyceride content, usually indicates lymphomatous disruption of the abdominal lymphatics. Cytologic study of aspirated fluid, peritoneal biopsy, or peritoneoscopy will indicate the presence of tumor in most patients with peritoneal metastases.

Rupture of a primary mucinous cystadenoma or cystadenocarcinoma of the ovary or appendix (malignant mucocele) results in abdominal distention due to accumulation of mucinous material in the peritoneal space. Surgical treatment and intraperitoneal chemotherapy have been used to control this unusual form of peritoneal disease.

Primary mesothelioma of the peritoneum may be associated with pleural mesothelioma; it presents with an insidious onset of abdominal pain, weight loss, and ascites. Diagnosis is dependent on cytologic study and peritoneal biopsy. The prognosis, regardless of therapy, is extremely poor.

Other Diseases of the Mesentery

Primary inflammatory diseases of the mesentery are poorly understood. Among these, *mesenteric panniculitis* is characterized by recurrent abdominal pain and signs of intestinal obstruction, and *retractile mesenteritis* by chronic intestinal obstruction and continuous pain, fever, and ascites. Primary mesenteric cysts and tumors are rare and are discovered only after rupture, hemorrhage, or infection, unless they produce prior symptoms related to their position or compression of adjacent organs. Treatment is by surgical excision.

Bibliography

Bender, M. D., and Ockner, R. K. Diseases of the Peritoneum, Mesentery, and Diaphragm. In M. H. Sleisenger and J. S. Fordtran (eds.), *Gastrointestinal Disease.* Philadelphia: Saunders, 1973. P. 1578.

Correia, J. P., and Conn, H. O. Spontaneous bacterial peritonitis in cirrhosis: Endemic or epidemic. *Med. Clin. North Am.* 59:963, 1975.

Singh, M., Bhargava, A., and Jain, K. Tuberculous peritonitis. *N. Engl. J. Med.* 281:1091, 1969.

Sohar, E., Jafni, J., Pras, M., and Heller, H. Familial Mediterranean fever: A survey of 470 cases and review of the literature. *Am. J. Med.* 43:227, 1967.

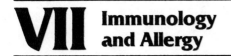

VII Immunology and Allergy

44

Immunology and Immunodeficiency Diseases

Sidney R. Cooperband

Immunology originated from the observation that patients who had recovered from an infectious illness could not generally be reinfected with that same disease. In the hundred-odd years since that beginning, it has become apparent that the immune response is a complex, multicellular, and genetically controlled series of biologic phenomena involving interrelationships between different cells, unusual reactions, and continuing differentiations, including the unique phenomenon of recognition of self and nonself. It is now well understood that there are two essentially independent but interrelated aspects of immunity: humoral immunity (or antibody) and cell-mediated immunity (or delayed hypersensitivity). Both aspects ultimately function through a nonspecific (nonimmunologic) host resistance apparatus that includes most reticuloendothelial tissues, which can phagocytize and destroy organic materials and produce an inflammatory response. These nonspecific inflammatory and phagocytic responses are essential parts of all immune reactions. It is now appreciated that immunity protects not only against infection but also against the development of cancer, and it prevents an individual from accepting grafts of tissue from other persons. Immunologic reactions may be harmful as well as beneficial to the host: They may be etiologically involved in the production of diseases (the so-called autoimmune diseases), and there may be detrimental immunities to foreign substances (anaphylaxis or allergy).

The immune response is first concerned with the recognition of a foreign substance. In order to be recognized as foreign, a substance must be a protein or polysaccharide of relatively large molecular weight. Lipids and polynucleotides generally are not antigenic, although they may become antigens in certain autoimmune diseases. The smallest protein unit that is recognized as foreign is a 7-8 amino acid fragment, about 1,000 daltons in molecular weight. However,

molecules of much lower molecular weight may become antigenic if they are covalently linked to a macromolecular carrier molecule. Thus dinitrofluorobenzene, with a molecular weight of 203 daltons, is a potent immunogen, but only if it is bound to a protein carrier. Such antigens are called haptens.

Ontogeny of T and B Cell Development

Lymphocytes and other cells of the lymphoid tissues are the host cells responsible for the immune response. Embryologically, the precursors of these cells arise during the third through sixth weeks of fetal life, first in the yolk sac, then in the liver, and finally in the bone marrow. During the eighth through tenth weeks, some of the stem cells take the form of small lymphocytes, but these cells are not yet immunologically competent. These incompetent lymphocytes migrate from the bone marrow into the developing thymus. In birds, a second key lymphoid organ, called the bursa of Fabricius, forms at the same time at the other end of the intestinal tract just posterior to the cloaca. Current evidence is that lymphoid cells become immunocompetent, while the thymus or the bursa of Fabricius becomes able to recognize antigens and develops a humoral or a cell-mediated immune response. Cells that have matured in the thymus, called T lymphocytes, give rise to cell-mediated immunity; cells that have matured in the bursa of Fabricius, called B lymphocytes, give rise to antibody-producing cells and humoral immunity. A bursa of Fabricius has never been clearly defined morphologically in mammals, including man; some analogous structure, probably the bone marrow, must generate B lymphocytes. The mechanism by which T and B cells differentiate is not fully understood, but some observations suggest that locally produced peptide hormones may be involved.

A small percentage of T and B cells migrate from the thymus or bursa into the lymph nodes or spleen. By the middle of the twentieth week, the immune apparatus is almost fully differentiated. B lymphocytes, however, do not normally become plasma cells or secrete large quantities of antibody until triggered by an antigen; thus there are few plasma cells in newborn infants. A schema of differentiation is shown in Figure 44-1. Within peripheral lymphoid tissue,

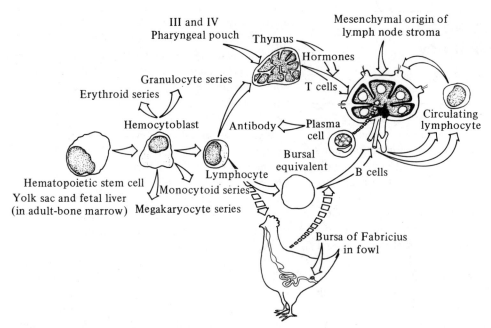

Figure 44-1. Differentiation pathway for the production of T and B lymphocytes.

T and B lymphocytes reside in defined regions. The cortex of the lymph node, which receives afferent lymph, contains the B cells, whereas T lymphocytes are mostly located in the paracortical area inside the cortex. Plasma cells, when present, are usually found in the medulla, from which lymph leaves the node. When the host is exposed to antigen, B and T cells in lymphoid tissues divide and rapidly produce large numbers of clonal daughter cells. The B cells form germinal nodules in the cortex of the lymph node. As these new B cells are transformed into plasma cells, they begin to secrete immunoglobulins and migrate into the medulla. The mature plasma cells live only 4 to 6 days in the medulla; during this period they produce and secrete antibody at maximal rates. Cellular immunity is activated when a population of competent T cells is exposed to an antigen. The reactive T cell population proliferates and develops new functional capabilities. The most important new capability is the ability to destroy nucleated cells, which is the prime function of a subpopulation called killer cells. Other functional roles are those of helper cells, which "help" T and B cells respond to antigen; suppressor cells, which can "suppress" both killer cell function and antibody production; and memory cells, which are long-lived cells that respond rapidly to rechallenge with the same antigen.

The mechanism by which lymphocytes recognize antigens and are activated is currently an active area of research. Both T and B lymphocytes have surface receptors capable of binding to foreign antigens. Each cell produced during differentiation in the thymus or bursa can recognize only one antigenic determinant and becomes the source of all similar daughter cells formed during an immune response. On B cells, the surface receptors appear to be IgG or IgM molecules (or both). The receptors on T cells are a matter of dispute, but they appear to be immunoglobulinlike. The body appears to have a "fail-safe" mechanism in the activation of lymphoid cells; a single signal, such as the binding of antigen, is usually not enough to cause activation. For B cells, the required second signal may be a humoral factor produced and secreted by T cells. In this case, T cells assume a helper function in humoral immunity; the antigens involved are said to be thymus-dependent, since antigen recognition by thymocytes must precede antibody formation. Other antigens are thymus-independent; in this case, the second signal may be a cleavage product of the third component of complement, C3b. Such antigens produce C3b by activating the alternative pathway of complement (properdin). Most B lymphocytes appear to have specialized receptors for C3b. An additional control mechanism involved in B cell activation, a humoral factor produced by suppressor T lymphocytes, has the ability to inhibit B cell activation.

Humoral Immunity

Immunoglobulins are a group of glycoproteins that circulate in body fluids and share certain similarities of structure. There are five different classes of immunoglobulins, designated Immunoglobulins (Ig) G, M, A, D, and E (see Table 44-1). Immunoglobulin M, present primarily in the bloodstream, is the first antibody formed after challenge with an antigen. The second immunoglobulin produced is G, the predominant immunoglobulin, which is present in serum and extracellular fluid in approximately equal concentrations. Current evidence is that immunoglobulin A is produced primarily in submucosa, mainly to protect the mucous membranes from infection. Immunoglobulin E, which is responsible for allergic manifestations and for anaphylaxis, is present in trace quantities in serum but predominantly is bound to tissue mast cells. The function of immunoglobulin D, also present in trace quantities in serum, is not known.

All immunoglobulins share certain structural features. They are made of two amino acid chains that are labeled "heavy" and "light," because the first is roughly twice the size of the second. The two chains are held together by disulfide bridges to form one antigen-binding macromolecule. All immunoglobulins can bind at least two antigen molecules by forming a second heavy/light chain complex that is bound to the first pair by disulfide bridges. Thus, the basic unit has two heavy chains in a symmetrical molecule, which has the shape of a letter H (see Fig. 44-2). Differences among the various classes of Ig are the result of variations in the amino acid sequence of heavy chains. The light chains of all classes of Ig are identical: In each class there may be either of two antigenically different light chains, called λ and κ, which vary in amino acid sequence at the carboxy-terminal end of the protein. Immunoglobulin M is

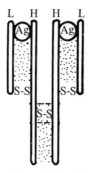

Figure 44-2. Basic structure of immunoglobulins; IgG protein composed of two identical "heavy" chains (H) of amino acids and two identical "light" chains (L) of amino acids.

composed of five repetitions of IgGlike molecules linked by a peptide chain called the J fragment. In immunoglobulin A, two IgGlike units are joined by a J fragment and another peptide, the T fragment, which helps transport the molecule across the mucosal cell.

The time sequence of antibody appearance in the blood is important in understanding the pathogenesis of infections and immunologic diseases. Antibody first appears in the blood 2 to 3 days after exposure to antigen. During the lag period, B cell proliferation is maximal. The first antibody, an IgM, is produced for 5 to 6 days. IgG antibody appears only after the first week, but secretion continues for longer periods. Both types of antibody disappear if a second "booster" exposure to antigen (or the continued presence of a bacterial infection) does not stimulate a secondary response. The secondary response produces many more activated B and plasma cells, which produce IgG antibody for longer periods of time.

Complement and Nonspecific Host Resistance

By themselves, antibodies are not capable of protecting a host. Either of two additional mechanisms is required: (1) complement, which can lyse bacterial cell walls, or (2) enhancement of phagocytosis. The complement system, a complex of at least nine protein components with a number of regulatory cofactors, is shown in Figure 44-3. The combination of antibody with antigen alters the antibody molecule sterically so that it can bind the first component of

Table 44-1. Some Properties of Classes and Subclasses of Human Immunoglobulins

Property	IgG				IgA		IgM	IgD	IgE
	IgG-1	IgG-2	IgG-3	IgG-4	IgA-1	IgA-2			
Sedimentation coefficient (S)	7	7	7	7	7−13	7−13	18−32	7	8
Molecular weight ($\times 10^{-3}$)	150	150	150	150	150−600	150−600	900	?	190
Heavy chains	$\gamma1$	$\gamma2$	$\gamma3$	$\gamma4$	$\alpha1$	$\alpha2$	μ	δ	ϵ
Carbohydrate (% approx.)	3	3	3	3	7	7	12	13	11
Average concentration in normal serum (mg/ml)	8	4	1	0.4	3.5	0.4	1	0.03	0.0001
Half life in serum (days in vivo)	23	23	8	23	6	(6?)	5	3	2.5
Effector Functions									
Active in complement fixation	++	+	++	0	0	0	++	?	0
Sensitizes human mast cells for anaphylaxis (homocytotropic)	0	0	0	0	0	0	0	0	+
Binds to macrophages	++	+	++	±	....	....	0	....	....

complement. The first component of the complement sequence (actually a mixture of peptide molecules labeled the C1 qrs complex) thereafter activates a cascade of reactions, which results finally in the production of hydrolytic enzymes. In addition, a variety of pharmacologically active products are released, causing local inflammation. These substances include anaphylatoxin, leukocyte chemotactic factors, and substances that nonspecifically enhance phagocytosis. As the sequence proceeds through complement components 7, 8, and 9, these activated components become proteolytic and lipolytic, capable of "punching holes" in cell walls and membranes and thus destroying bacteria. Macrophages then ingest the dead organisms. Complement proteins are produced by a variety of cells in the body, including intestinal mucosal cells and macrophages.

In the past few years, an alternative route has been discovered that activates C3 and the subsequent complement sequence. This pathway (originally called properdin) may be activated without antigen by plasmin or other proteolytic enzymes via interaction of a plasma protein (component D) with poly-saccharides or aggregated immunoglobulin. This alternate pathway facilitates nonspecific host resistance by activating the several factors that enhance inflammation and phagocytosis.

Antibodies also enhance phagocytosis and the destruction of bacterial dead cells and large molecules. Most organs contain fixed and wandering macrophages, which are the principal phagocytes of the body. Antibodies enhance phagocytosis in two ways. First, they coat foreign particles and, with the help of complement, render them recognizable to macrophages as foreign. This process is called opsonization. Second, antibodies may also function as cytophilic antibodies, binding onto the surface of the macrophage and holding foreign substances (antigens) that contact the phagocyte. Once the antibody-antigen complex is formed at the surface of the macrophage, the complex is engulfed.

Cell-mediated Immunity (Delayed Hypersensitivity)
Delayed hypersensitivity was first observed by Robert Koch, who discovered that guinea pigs injected with tubercle bacilli developed an inflammatory response

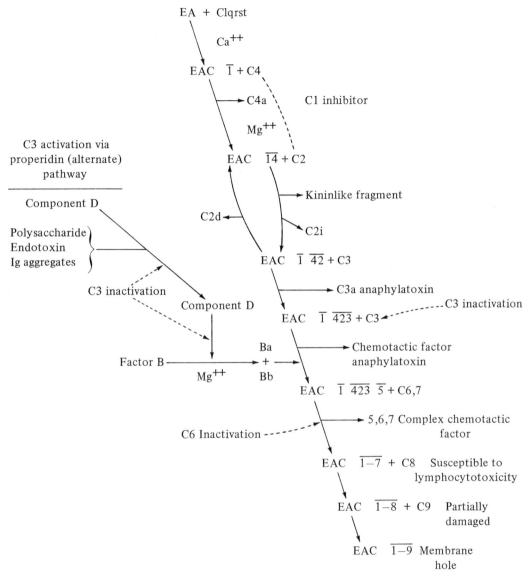

Figure 44-3. Sequence of events in the activation of the complement system. E = *erythrocyte,* A = *antibody,* C = *complement.*

at the site of injection which required 24 to 48 hours to reach maximum intensity. A knowledge of the histopathologic sequence of events in delayed hypersensitivity is essential to understanding the biologic events. Upon *primary* challenge, an antigen (generally administered intradermally or subcutaneously) slowly finds its way to the draining lymph node and stimulates a very rapid increase in size. The increase occurs as a result of two events: trapping of cells migrating in from the afferent lymph stream, and proliferation of T cells. Four or five days following antigen exposure, the node cells begin to appear in the blood; at this time, skin hypersensitivity can be demonstrated. Within 2 to 3 hours after a *second* antigenic challenge, morphonuclear leukocytes infiltrate the injected area. Within 5 to 6 hours, mononuclear cells begin to accumulate in perivascular zones. Within 6 to 24 hours, one finds a massive accumulation of mononuclear cells, the development of erythema, vasodilatation, vascular endothelial retraction, and local edema, which together cause a swollen, red lesion at the site of injection — the classic induration and erythema of delayed hypersensitivity. At the node draining the site of injection, proliferation similar to that which occurred after the first challenge occurs again.

The production of delayed hypersensitivity is mediated by T lymphocytes. When a sensitized T lymphocyte recognizes an antigen as foreign, increased cytoplasmic protein synthesis and cell mitosis occur. The cell undergoes morphologic transformation (differentiation) to a "blast-transformed" lymphocyte, which ultimately replicates its DNA and then divides. The daughter cells morphologically revert to small lymphocytes. These cells respond to the continuous presence of antigen by repeating the cycle as often as every 6 to 8 hours, thus producing a clonal enlargement of the antigen-responding cells. The ability to produce a delayed hypersensitivity response also depends on production by these cells of a large variety of humoral mediators, called lymphokines. One type of lymphokine acts to "amplify" the initial immune response, that is, to augment its intensity several thousandfold; the other type, the so-called effector substances, alters the tissues and cells involved in the delayed hypersensitivity reaction. Among the amplifying factors are (1) a skin reactive factor, which initiates an inflammatory response in skin vessels; (2) a chemotactic factor, which attracts mononuclear cells; (3) a macrophage inhibitory factor (MIF), which inhibits migration of mononuclear cells; (4) a blastogenic factor, which converts nonreactive lymphocytes to a stage of blast transformation; (5) a macrophage spread inhibitory factor; and (6) a transfer factor, which confers antigen recognition on nonimmune T cells. Among the effector substances are (1) interferon, which has a direct antiviral effect and also is cytostatic; (2) a proliferation inhibiting factor (or colony inhibitory factor), which inhibits the synthesis of DNA in tumor cells and graft rejected cells; (3) a lymphotoxin, which is cytotoxic to nucleated cells; and (4) a macrophage arming factor (perhaps the same substance as MIF), which converts benign macrophages to a "killer" state with the capacity to destroy adjacent normal cells and intracellular parasites. In addition to these known humoral effector substances, there is a very important direct cellular component of delayed hypersensitivity. This component involves "contact" cytotoxicity, a process mediated by T cells and activated macrophages that come in contact with eukaryotic cells residing at the site of an antigenic reaction. Sensitized macrophages or lymphocytes bind to and ultimately destroy target cells by mechanisms as yet unknown.

The relatively prolonged, sequential events associated with blast transformation, the production of lymphokines, recruitment of cells into the reaction, and the cell contact necessary for cell death cause the delay in response that is typical of cell-mediated immunity. This type of immunity is a unique reaction in that normal host cells are destroyed as part of an immune response. As in the humoral immune response, it is the nonspecific macrophage that is the destructive agent. Ultimately, macrophages destroy or remove foreign antigen.

In recent years, the complex events and cell cooperation necessary to develop a cell-mediated immune reaction have become understood. Within the T cell population, at least four subpopulations of lymphocytes are generated following an antigen exposure: helper cells, killer cells, suppressor cells, and memory cells. Each type of cell is capable of recognizing the antigen. In order that T cells may develop the capacity to produce the event which is recognized as delayed hypersensitivity or graft tumor rejection, it appears that the participation of at least helper cells and killer cells in a cell-to-cell interaction is required. Two signals are necessary for activation of killer T cells: antigen binding, and contact of a killer cell with a helper T cell of appropriate histocompatibility and surface configuration. The histocompatibility antigens are under genetic control; within this complex genetic regulatory system, there exists a series of immune-response genes that permit cooperation to occur when two cells recognize a specific antigen.

The complexities of antigen recognition are increasingly relevant to our understanding of autoimmune diseases and immune mechanisms in cancer. Preliminary data suggest that some abnormality in a two-cell cooperation may cause autoimmune disease, and that the capacity to recognize tumor antigens as foreign and to reject the tumor cells also involves a series of responses to histocompatibilitylike antigens.

Clinical Measurement of Immune Functions

Humoral immunity is estimated by counting B cells or by measuring immunoglobulins, which are the products of B cells. B lymphocytes in blood are identified either by their unique capacity to bind the C3b component of complement or by the relatively high density of IgG or IgM on their surfaces. C3b receptors are usually measured by the number of rosette formations that occur when lymphocytes are incubated with erythrocytes that have been coated with antibody and minimal quantities of complement; the coating is sufficient to cover the surface with C3b fragments but not sufficient to carry out complete lysis of the red cell population. These coated erythrocytes, called EAC cells (erythrocyte-antibody-complement) are mixed with washed peripheral blood cells, sedimented in the centrifuge, and gently resuspended. B lymphocytes gather clusters of erythrocytes around their surfaces to form rosettes. Immunoglobulin-binding B lymphocytes are usually detected by fluorescence after incubation with antisera against human IgG and IgM and with antirabbit gamma globulin to which fluorescein has been linked.

Antibody or immunoglobulin in the serum may be determined by a number of techniques. The most frequently used is simple electrophoresis, in which the serum is placed on an inert support and subjected to an electrophoretic voltage difference. The gamma globulins are neutral or slightly positively charged at pH 8.6 and thus tend either to migrate very slowly or to remain at the origin, forming the "gamma globulin peak." The quantity of gamma globulin is determined spectrophotometrically after the proteins have been stained. The individual immunoglobulins may be quantitated by electrophoresis in agarose that contains antibody (electroimmunodiffusion). A precipitin arc is formed, the area of which is proportional to the concentration of the individual immunoglobulin. There are also a number of immunodiffusion techniques for estimating the quantity of individual immunoglobulins, all of which depend on precipitation with antibody that is specific for the individual protein. Antibody response is most simply and directly measured by determining the antibody titer to a specific antigen (for example, blood group antibodies by agglutination of erythrocytes). One may test ability to develop a primary antibody response by challenging a patient with a bacterial toxoid to which he has never been exposed and measuring antibody titer 2 to 3 weeks later.

Cell-mediated immunity in man is estimated by eliciting delayed hypersensitivity reactions. Most often, skin sensitivity is tested to an antigen to which a person is likely to have already been exposed in nature. For example, more than 90 percent of the normal population will have a delayed hypersensitivity reaction to *Candida (Monilia), Trichophyton, Streptococcus,* and mumps antigens administered intradermally. Another test of cell-mediated immunity is to produce a primary immunization with a potent antigen. For example, a hapten such as dinitrochlorobenzene will elicit a delayed hypersensitivity reaction some 7 to 10 days after application to the skin in more than 95 percent of the population. It is also possible to estimate human T cells by a number of in vitro procedures. T cells in blood may be counted directly, taking advantage of the observation that these cells spontaneously form rosettes when they are centrifuged with washed sheep erythrocytes. Lymphokine production can be assayed by measuring macrophage inhibitory factor, that is, the ability of antigen to inhibit the migration of macrophages from a capillary tube in the presence of immune T cells. Another test makes use of the fact that T lymphocytes undergo blast transformation and mitosis upon culture with a variety of plant lectins, such as phytohemagglutinin. The intensity of cell proliferation is roughly proportional to the number of competent T cells in the blood sample.

Complement is usually estimated from the hemolytic capacity of whole serum. In this test, erythrocytes are sensitized with antibody from serum that has been heated to inactivate endogenous complement. Thereafter, varying dilutions of the serum containing an unknown quantity of complement are added, and a hemolysis curve is determined. The individual proteins of the complement sequence are measured by electroimmunoassay, in which the serum is electrophoresed on agarose containing antibodies specific to the individual proteins; the proteins may also be measured by microprecipitation tests or by complement fixation assays.

Certain aspects of macrophage function can be estimated clinically on preparations of human blood macrophages or monocytes. Phagocytic activity can be tested directly by noting ingestion of inert particles or indirectly by measuring metabolic changes induced by phagocytosis, such as reduction of the dye nitroblue tetrazolium (NBT). A test for the ability of leukocytes to kill bacteria is important in the diagnosis of macrophage deficiencies. Surviving intracellular bacteria are usually estimated by separating and lysing the phagocytes, and then enumerating the viable organisms by colony count.

Immunodeficiency Diseases

Large numbers of diseases, mostly genetic in origin, are now recognized which involve either a deficiency in one or another part of the human immune response, or a nonspecific resistance, such as complement and phagocytosis. These diseases, which are enumerated in the following list, may generally be classified by the specific cells or molecules responsible for the deficiency; thus they are grouped into the primary and secondary immune cell deficiencies, the macrophage deficiencies, and the complement deficiencies.

Primary Immune Cell Defects	*Cell Type Involved*
X-linked agammaglobulinemia	B lymphocyte
Common variable (acquired) hypogammaglobulinemia	B lymphocyte
X-linked immunodeficiency with increased IgM	B lymphocyte
Selective immunoglobulin deficiencies	B lymphocyte
Selective deficiencies of IgG subclasses	B lymphocyte
Selective IgA deficiency	B lymphocyte
Transient hypogammaglobulinemia of infancy	B lymphocyte
Transcobalamin II deficiency and agammaglobulinemia	B lymphocyte
Severe combined immunodeficiency disease	B and T lymphocytes and marrow stem cells
With generalized hematopoietic hypoplasia	B and T lymphocytes and marrow stem cells
With dysostosis	B and T lymphocytes and marrow stem cells
With adenine deaminase deficiency	B and T lymphocytes
Congenital thymic aplasia (DiGeorge's syndrome)	T lymphocyte
Immunodeficiency with ataxia-telangiectasia	B and T lymphocytes
Immunodeficiencies with thrombocytopenia and eczema (Wiskott-Aldrich syndrome)	B and T lymphocytes
Immunodeficiency with thymoma	B lymphocyte; ? T lymphocyte
Immunodeficiency with normal gamma globulin or hypergammaglobulinemia	B and T lymphocytes

Episodic lymphopenia with lymphocytotoxins	T lymphocytes

Secondary Immune Cell Defects	*Cell Type Involved*
Malignancy	T lymphocyte
Granuloma (e.g., leprosy, sarcoid)	T lymphocyte
Viral infection (e.g., varicella, measles)	T lymphocyte
Aging	T lymphocyte
Nutritional deprivation	T lymphocyte
Surgery	T lymphocyte
Lymphoreticular malignancy	T lymphocyte
Increased catabolism of Ig (e.g., myotonic dystrophy)	B lymphocyte
Increased loss of Ig (e.g., burns, enteropathy)	B lymphocyte
Increased synthesis of pathologic Ig (e.g., multiple myeloma, macroglobulinemia)	B lymphocyte

Deficiencies and Nonspecific Host Resistance (Phagocytosis)	*Cell Type Involved*
Primary Defects	
Chronic granulomatous disease of children	Macrophages and other phagocytic cells
Chédiak-Higashi syndrome	Macrophages
Myeloperoxidase deficiency	Macrophages
Defective chemotaxis ("lazy leukocyte syndrome")	Macrophages
Chronic mucocutaneous candidiasis	Macrophages; ? T cells
Job's syndrome	Macrophages

Deficiencies Secondary to Other Diseases

Drug-related influences (e.g., narcotics, steroids, alcohol)
Liver disease
Rheumatoid arthritis
Sepsis
Burns
Congenital or acquired neutropenia
Tuftsin peptide deficiency

Complement Deficiencies

C_1 inhibitor deficiency (hereditary angioneurotic edema)
C1r deficiency
C2 deficiency
C3 deficiency
C3b inactivator deficiency
C4 deficiency
C5 deficiency
C6 deficiency
C7 deficiency

In general, these deficiencies manifest an inability of the host to resist infectious organisms. Animals with B cell defects are particularly prone to infections with pyogenic organisms. Patients with T cell deficiencies are more susceptible to infections with gram-negative bacteria, viruses, or fungi. Both macrophage dysfunctions and complement deficiencies are usually associated with pyogenic infections. Interestingly, many patients with complement deficiencies also suffer from autoimmune phenomena.

Since most immunodeficiency diseases are prominent only in children, they will not be considered in detail here. References to the uncommon disorders in the preceding list are provided in the bibliography at the end of this chapter. However, a few syndromes that occur in adults are described here as examples of this class of disorders.

COMMON VARIABLE HYPOGAMMAGLOBULINEMIA
Common variable (acquired) hypogammaglobulinemia is the most common form of immunodeficiency. It occurs in either sex, at any age, without any known causative factor, and it may be either genetic or acquired (although a predisposition may be inherited). It is probably a mixture of a number of diseases. The predominant infections are sinusitis and pneumonia, often leading to bronchiectasis. A spruelike malabsorption syndrome and pernicious anemia are often present; the malabsorption syndrome is frequently associated with *Giardia lamblia* infection of the duodenum. Autoimmune phenomena are common, especially hemolytic anemia, thrombocytopenia, and neutropenia. Blood gamma globulin levels, usually less than 500 mg per 100 ml, are not as low as those seen in hereditary X-linked agammaglobulinemia. There may be either normal or reduced numbers of B cells, which do not respond to mitogenic stimulation and do not synthesize immunoglobulin. Treatment with parenteral γ-globulin may be beneficial, but in some cases autoimmunity against the administered γ-globulin develops. Steroids may also be effective. Appropriate antibiotic therapy is essential in the treatment of all these disorders.

DEFECTS IN T CELL OR B CELL FUNCTION ASSOCIATED WITH OTHER DISEASES
Decrease in T cell or B cell function may occur in a variety of clinical disorders; the mechanisms of the decrease are not well understood. Chronic anergy occurs in certain granulomatous diseases, such as sarcoidosis and leprosy. Viral infections (such as rubella and rubeola) and parasitic diseases may produce acute or chronic defects in T cell function. The number of competent T cells and their functional capacity decrease with age; thus, anergy is common in the elderly. Nutritional deprivation is a potent immunosuppressant, interfering with many steps in the immune response, especially T cell function. Surgery is also immunosuppressive, partly because anesthetics can inhibit T cell activation. Cancer may be associated with loss of delayed hypersensitivity (anergy) and defective T cell function, particularly when a tumor disseminates or increases in size. A number of lymphoreticular malignancies may be associated with T or B cell abnormalities. Chronic lymphocytic leukemia may suppress B cell function, while T cell deficiencies may occur in Hodgkin's disease and in chronic lymphocytic leukemia. In some of the paraproteinemias (multiple myeloma, macroglobulinemia), the increased production of the abnormal M spike characteristic of these disorders may be associated with a decreased production of normal immunoglobulin; patients with these disorders may be unable to produce adequate quantities of antibody upon challenge with a new antigen. The deficiency of circulating antibody in myotonic dystrophy results from increased catabolism of immunoglobulin. Increased losses of IgG account for reduction in levels of these proteins in protein-losing gastroenteropathy, burns, and the nephrotic syndrome.

IMPAIRED PHAGOCYTOSIS
Phagocytosis may be impaired in a number of disorders, including sickle cell disease, rheumatoid arthritis, burns, liver disease, and severe bacterial infections. Various drugs may also inhibit phagocytic function, including narcotics, barbiturates, steroids, chloramphenicol, sulfonamides, iron, phenylbutazone, and alcohol.

C_1 INHIBITOR DEFICIENCY (HEREDITARY ANGIONEUROTIC EDEMA)
Alpha-2-neuraminoglycoprotein (C_1 inhibitor) in the serum acts on the first component of complement to

prevent its subsequent participation in the complement cascade. This protein is capable of inhibiting a number of other plasma enzymes such as kininogenase, plasmin, activated Hageman factor, and thromboplastin. Activation of these other enzymes may deplete the available quantities of C_1 inhibitor if there is a quantitative deficiency of this protein. C_1 inhibitor deficiency results in a clinical picture of episodic, acute, nonpainful edema of the subcutaneous tissues and of the mucosa of the respiratory and alimentary tracts. One or many areas may be involved in an attack; the affected areas may be painful, especially if the intestine is involved. Attacks can be life-threatening if the larynx is involved. The attacks are caused by kininlike fragments that are released during C2 activation by the C14 complex. Once the C1 inhibitor in a local site is exhausted, the reaction becomes autocatalytic and continues until all C2 is consumed. The disease is autosomal dominant and usually begins in early childhood; it is exacerbated at adolescence and finally tends to subside during the sixth decade of life. Prophylaxis with epsilon-aminocaproic acid (EACA) and its analogues has been partially successful in preventing activation of plasma proteases, thereby preventing the consumption of the small quantities of the inhibitor that are present in these patients. Recently a new drug, danazol, has been found to stimulate the production of C1 inhibitor in these patients, and now appears to be the drug of choice in this disorder.

Bibliography

Back, F. H., and Good, R. A. *Clinical Immunobiology.* Vol. 1 (1972) and Vol. 2 (1974). New York: Academic.

Benacerraf, B. (ed.). *Immunogenetics and Immune Deficiency.* Baltimore: University Park Press, 1975.

Bloom, B. M., and Glade, P. R. (eds.). *In Vitro Methods in Cell Mediated Immunity.* New York: Academic, 1971.

Gordon, B. L. (ed.). *Essentials of Immunology* (2nd ed.). Philadelphia: Davis, 1975.

Lawrence, H. S. Transfer factor and cellular immune deficiency disease. *N. Engl. J. Med.* 283:411, 1970.

Park, B. H., and Good, R. A. (eds.). *Principles of Modern Immunobiology.* Philadelphia: Lea & Febiger, 1974.

45

Allergy

Merrill D. Benson

Allergy is a term coined by von Pirquet in 1906 to describe a state of altered immunologic reactivity to foreign material. Over the past 50 years, the term *allergy* has been used mainly to describe immunologic reactions to foreign substances that are mediated by humoral antibodies. The term *hypersensitivity reaction* has been used to encompass all types of immunologically mediated reactions to foreign substances.

Classification of Hypersensitivity Reactions

The present classification of hypersensitivity reactions was proposed by Gell and Coombs, who grouped them into four categories (Table 45-1). *Type I* hypersensitivity includes reactions that have been termed *immediate* in the past; these reactions are mediated by reaginic antibody. *Type II* hypersensitivity reactions are those in which the antigen is fixed to cells, where it combines first with circulating antibody and subsequently with complement. *Type III* reactions involve the formation of free or circulating antigen-antibody complexes, and subsequent complement fixation and activation, causing tissue injury. *Type IV* reactions, which were previously termed *delayed* or *cellular* hypersensitivities, include the allergic disorders caused by the reaction of antigen with sensitized lympho-

Table 45-1. Classification of Hypersensitivity Reactions

Type	Name	Immunologic mediator	Clinical example
I	Anaphylactic	IgE	Allergic rhinitis
II	Cytotoxic	IgM or IgG	Transfusion reactions Hemolytic disease of newborn
III	Toxic-complex	IgM or IgG	Serum sickness
IV	Cellular (delayed)	T lymphocytes	Contact dermatitis

Adapted from P. G. H. Gell and R. R. A. Coombs (eds.), *Clinical Aspects of Immunology* (2nd ed.). Philadelphia: Davis, 1969.

cytes. A more detailed discussion of each of these categories is given below to show how (1) types of immunoglobulins, (2) characteristics of classes of immunoglobulins, (3) cellular mechanisms, and (4) chemical mediators relate to the various clinical syndromes.

TYPE I OR ANAPHYLACTIC REACTIONS

Type I hypersensitivity reactions include those denoted by the previously used terms, *anaphylactic hypersensitivity, immediate-type hypersensitivity,* and *reaginic hypersensitivity.* The clinical syndromes in type I include extrinsic asthma, allergic rhinitis, immediate reactions to insect venoms, some food and drug allergies, and perhaps some cases of urticaria. The factor unifying these various clinical syndromes is that they all involve IgE antibody. The original terms, *reagin* and *skin-sensitizing antibody,* were used prior to the demonstration that a very small amount of a unique immunoglobulin is present in normal serum with the ability to fix to basophils and mast cells. This IgE antibody has a molecular weight of approximately 200,000, a larger amount of carbohydrate than does IgG, and a sedimentation coefficient of 8S. While its original identification was made by finding an IgE-producing myeloma, this immunoglobulin has now been demonstrated in the serum of all normal persons. The fact that its serum concentration is only 5 to 800 ng per milliliter explains why its discovery was delayed. While the IgE molecule can fix to basophils and mast cells because of its unique heavy chain, it cannot cause complement fixation. IgE does not cross the placental barrier and has been shown to be destroyed by heating to 56°C.

Studies have shown that IgE attaches to cells through the Fc portion of the heavy chain of the immunoglobulin molecule, leaving the Fab end (the antibody combining region) exposed to react with antigen. It is necessary, however, for the antigen molecule to combine with more than one IgE molecule on the cell surface so as to create "bridging" between adjacent IgE molecules, in order to trigger the mast cells or the basophils to release mediators that in turn cause all the clinical manifestations of type I reactions. Within minutes of the combination of antigen with cell-bound IgE antibody, the cell releases histamine, slow-reacting substance of anaphylaxis (SRS-A), and possibly certain kinins causing vasodilatation, increased capillary permeability, and contraction of smooth muscle. These mediators then lead to the bronchospasm, hypotension, angioedema, and urticaria seen in these immediate-type reactions. Table 45-2 lists the known mediators involved in type I reactions and some of their biologic properties.

IgE is known to be synthesized in large part in the upper respiratory tract and therefore is felt perhaps to be related to the prevention of sinopulmonary infections. Certain clinical observations, such as an increased number of pulmonary infections in patients with immunodeficient diseases (for example, ataxia-telangiectasia), tend to support this impression. However, it is not settled that IgE is an important antibody in the prevention of infections. High levels of IgE in parasitic diseases have also been noted, but the significance of this observation is not clear. IgE levels may be elevated in allergic diseases such as seasonal allergic rhinitis, discussed later in this chapter.

Chemical Mediators of Type I Reactions

Histamine is the most prominent mediator of the allergic response. It is stored in granules within the basophils and mast cells; it can be shown to be released by IgE-mediated antigen-antibody reactions; and when administered to humans, it can be shown to give virtually all the features of anaphylaxis. Furthermore, mast cells can be shown to be depleted of histamine after they are challenged by allergen. Histamine causes both contraction of smooth muscle and the increased vascular permeability found in the typical wheal and flare reaction. Both of these effects can be prevented by the use of antihistamines.

Slow-reacting substance of anaphylaxis (SRS-A) is also released from sensitized mast cells challenged with allergin. Like histamine, SRS-A causes contraction of smooth muscle and increased vascular permeability, but it does so more slowly than histamine and is not antagonized by antihistamines. In fact, the actions of histamine and SRS-A on smooth muscle are additive. Whereas histamine is preformed and stored within mast cells, the formation of SRS-A requires a metabolic step after allergen challenge and does not occur if cell metabolism has been stopped.

Eosinophil chemotactic factor of anaphylaxis (ECF-A) is also released from sensitized mast cells that are challenged with allergen. It is a small peptide with molecular weight of about 500, and it causes the migration of eosinophils into the area of its release. The importance of eosinophils in the allergic response is not clear; however, recent studies have shown that eosinophils contain histaminase, an enzyme that degrades histamine, as well as an arylsulfatase that presumably degrades SRS-A.

The cellular mechanisms involved in release of mediators from sensitized mast cells are not completely understood, but it is thought that they involve the cyclic AMP system. Triggering of the cell by the combination of antigen and cell-surface-bound IgE is felt to cause a decrease in membrane-associated adenyl cyclase, with a resultant change in the level of cyclic AMP. Therefore, all the ancillary systems that have an effect on the cyclic AMP level can effect the release of histamine. Figure 45-1, which is a schematic presentation of the release of chemical mediators, shows the different factors that may modulate the release of histamine, SRS-A, and ECF-A. Elevation of cyclic AMP levels by beta-adrenergic stimulation, as with drugs such as isoproterenol or epinephrine, causes a relative blocking of mediator release. On the other hand, a decrease in the cyclic AMP

Table 45-2. Chemical Mediators of Type I (Immediate) Reactions

Mediators	Physiochemical characteristics	State in tissues	Functional activities
Histamine	β-imidazolylethylamine	Preformed	Constricts bronchial smooth muscle, increases vascular permeability
Slow-reacting substance of anaphylaxis (SRS-A)	Acidic sulfate ester, m.w. < 500	Precursor	Constricts bronchial smooth muscle, increases vascular permeability
Eosinophil chemotactic factor of anaphylaxis (ECF-A)	Tetrapeptides Val-Gly-Ser-Glu Ala-Gly-Ser-Glu	Preformed	Attracts and deactivates eosinophils

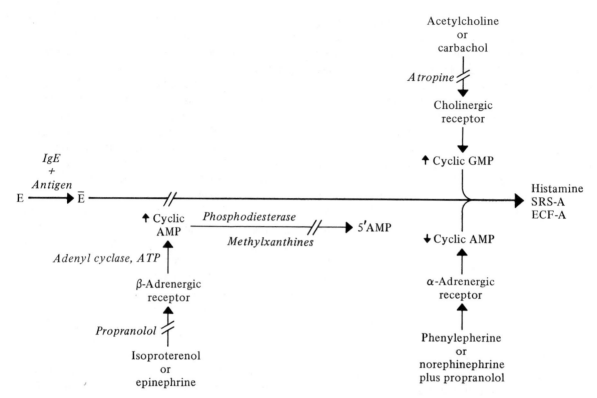

Figure 45-1. Schematic presentation of the pharmacologic controls of the immunologic release of chemical mediators of type I reactions. (Courtesy of Dr. K. F. Austen.)

level, as by alpha-adrenergic stimulation with phenylephrine hydrochloride or norepinephrine, can increase the release of histamine, SRS-A, and ECF-A. Cholinergic stimulation can cause elevation of cyclic GMP, which has been shown to have the reverse effect of cyclic AMP. Atropine can block the cholinergic effect, whereas propranolol can block the beta-adrenergic effect. The levels of cyclic AMP can also be modulated by inhibiting phosphodiesterase, an enzyme that degrades cyclic AMP to 5'AMP. The schema in Figure 45-1 helps in understanding the mediators of allergic responses and will be referred to later, in the section on the rationale of drug therapy for allergic asthma.

TYPE II REACTIONS

Type II hypersensitivity reactions are called cytotoxic or cytolytic. Major mediators of this type of

reaction are (1) humoral antibody and (2) antigen fixed to tissue cells. The antigen may be part of the structure of the cell (for example, a surface protein) or it may be an antigen or hapten that has become fixed to the tissue cells. After the primary reaction of antigen with antibody, complement is usually necessary for the production of cell damage, although this is not always the case. The importance of the complement system in tissue injury is discussed elsewhere in this text. While the primary effect of this system appears to be cell lysis, there are other associated aspects of complement activation that should be mentioned. It appears that the $C3_a$ and the $C5_a$ fragments that are split off during complement activation can cause histamine release and increased vascular permeability; this release of anaphylatoxin by the complement system can result in clinical features similar to those in type I reactions. The chemotactic properties of the $C3_a$ and $C5_a$ fragments may also be important in the tissue injury seen in both type II and type III reactions.

Type II reactions may be considered in two clinical

groups, depending on whether the antigen involved is autologous or exogenous. Examples of the first group include transfusion reactions, in which there is antibody against surface determinants on blood cells; hemolytic disease of the newborn and autoimmune hemolytic anemias also fall into this group. Diseases in which antibodies are produced against exogenous bacterial antigens, but then in turn cross react with normal autologous tissue antigens, are also regarded as type II. Examples of this group may be rheumatic fever and acute poststreptococcal glomerulonephritis. In the latter disease, it is felt that antibody to streptococcal antigen combines with glomerular basement membrane containing autologous cross-reacting antigenic determinants. Tissue injury then occurs via complement fixation.

The second group of type II reactions includes reactions in which antigens from outside the body are attached to tissue cells. An example of this type of reaction may be Coombs-positive hemolytic anemia, which is seen in association with the use of alpha-methyldopa, although there is some evidence in this disease that there is also antibody against intrinsic structures of the red blood cell membrane.

TYPE III REACTIONS

Type III hypersensitivity reactions include such toxic complex reactions as serum sickness, the experimental Arthus reaction, and the immunologic reactions seen in systemic lupus erythematosus and systemic vasculitis, (felt in both to be due to antibody complexes). Current thinking about immune complex disease holds that soluble antigen-antibody complexes are important in the resultant tissue injury. IgG, the principal antibody involved in type III reactions, is bivalent; in the presence of either an excess of antibody or equivalent amounts of antigen and antibody, IgG will cause precipitation of the antigen-antibody complexes and subsequent clearance of these large aggregates. In the presence of only slight antigen excess, however, the antigen-antibody complexes remain in the circulation, where they may subsequently be deposited in the walls of blood vessels and in glomerular basement membranes. Complement fixation may then lead to polymorphonuclear leukocyte infiltration with subsequent release of proteolytic enzymes. There is some evidence that activation of the kallikrein system may also play a part in the tissue injury found in this type of immune hypersensitivity reaction.

The mechanisms just described are thought to explain the Arthus reaction, an experimental model of type III reactions. The Arthus reaction is a local phenomenon of tissue injury produced when an animal is given an intradermal injection of an appropriate antigen to which the animal has been previously sensitized. In this model, circulating antibody appears in the serum, and after injection of the antigen, antibody can be demonstrated within the lesion. Histologically, infiltration by inflammatory cells, occlusion of blood vessels, and tissue necrosis can be seen at the injection site. Similar reasoning can be used to explain systemic type III reactions, such as experimental serum sickness. In this model, an animal is sensitized with heterologous serum proteins and subsequently is given an intravenous challenge of serum protein. Resultant inflammatory lesions are seen in many tissues, and antigen, antibody, and complement can all be demonstrated within these lesions. Glomerulonephritis, synovitis, and generalized vasculitis may all be part of this syndrome. The occurrence of these lesions has been shown to correlate with the appearance of soluble antigen-antibody complexes in the serum when there is an excess of antigen. Clinical examples of type III reactions include systemic lupus erythematosus, polyarteritis nodosa, serum sickness, and reactions to the administration of tetanus antitoxin. Drug reactions, in which the drug functions as a hapten bound to serum proteins, also represent a form of this type of reaction.

TYPE IV REACTIONS

Type IV hypersensitivity reactions in the Gell and Coombs classification involve cellular hypersensitivity (delayed hypersensitivity). This type of reaction cannot be transferred by serum, as the other three types can, and it is dependent on effector lymphocytes. The term *delayed* was given to this type of reaction because after injection of an antigen to which an individual is sensitized, a period of at least 48 to 72 hours is required before any signs of inflammation (erythema and induration) are observed. This reaction involves the migration of sensitized lymphocytes into the area of antigen challenge and the local release of factors that attract a host of lymphocytes and macrophages, which themselves are not sensitized. Giant cell formation and necrosis of the central portion of the lesion cause a typical granuloma.

Clinical examples of type IV reactions include tuberculin hypersensitivity, contact dermatitis, allograft rejection, and immunity to many viral antigens. The properties of an antigen that cause it to stimulate cellular immunity are not clear. This type of hypersensitivity reaction is thymus-dependent; it is specifically absent in the athymic immunodeficiency syndromes. In these syndromes major problems are encountered with fungal and viral agents, and tissue graft rejection is absent. In the case of contact dermatitis, the hapten must be bound to proteins present within the skin before it can cause sensitization; challenge with hapten then may produce all the characteristic inflammatory reactions of delayed hypersensitivity.

Evidence has accumulated on how the inflammatory tissue response is initiated and sustained in type IV reactions. In vitro, sensitized lymphocytes exposed to specific antigen undergo a blast-transformation reaction, in which cell division, DNA synthesis, and protein synthesis are observed. These sensitized lymphocytes have been shown to give rise to several factors that have effects on nonsensitized lymphocytes and macrophages. *Transfer factor,* originally described by Lawrence, is a low-molecular-weight substance that can be obtained from sensitized lymphocytes and can cause activation of lymphocytes in another individual not previously sensitized to the antigen. *Macrophage inhibiting factor (MIF)* is another mediator that is produced by sensitized small lymphocytes in minute quantities and is capable of inhibiting the motility of macrophages. Presumably the effect of MIF in type IV (delayed hypersensitivity) reactions is to cause an accumulation of macrophage cells within the area of antigen challenge. MIF may also be important in the accumulation of mononuclear cells seen in contact dermatitis, and at the site of graft rejection. The majority of the mononuclear cells found in a delayed hypersensitivity reaction are not antigen-specific sensitized cells, but it appears that

they play a large role in the tissue injury. The tissue injury presumably results from cell-to-cell membrane phenomena, and perhaps also from humoral factors called lymphotoxins.

Diagnostic Tests in Allergic Diseases

Each of the four types of hypersensitivity reaction lends itself to certain diagnostic tests that may be helpful in evaluating allergic diseases. Some of these tests are relatively crude, while others, though highly sophisticated, have only recently been applied to clinical medicine.

TYPE I HYPERSENSITIVITY TESTS

Type I hypersensitivity tests should be capable of measuring specific IgE antibody. The classic test for immediate hypersensitivity uses the skin as the target organ where IgE antibody is affixed to mast cells. Two techniques can be used either separately or in combination. The *scratch test* is done by scarifying or abrading the skin with a needle or small rotating blade. A dilute solution of the antigen (allergen) to be tested is then applied to the abraded area, and after 20 minutes the area is observed for a wheal and flare reaction. This test is usually used to detect sensitivity to tree, grass, and weed pollens; animal danders; house dusts; molds; and some foodstuffs, such as milk and egg proteins. The test requires the cooperation of the patient and, therefore, is not generally applicable to children under age 5. *Intradermal skin testing* is more sensitive but perhaps slightly more dangerous, in that systemic reactions can be provoked by the intradermal injection of even dilute solutions of allergen. In intradermal tests, wheal and flare reactions are again observed and measured. In many clinics, the standard procedure is to do the scratch tests first, and if the patient shows a highly positive reaction to any one allergen, it is not included in subsequent intradermal tests. Allergens that give negative scratch tests, however, may be used in appropriate dilutions for intradermal testing. Similar in vivo testing can be performed in a hay fever patient by applying allergen solutions to the nasal mucosa, or in asthmatic patients by having the patient inhale aerosolized allergens. The latter method of allergy testing is considered hazardous by many physicians, although when carefully performed, it may have more clinical significance than skin testing.

After IgE immunoglobulin was discovered, many investigators sought a correlation between the level of this immunoglobulin and the degree of type I hypersensitivity. However, in general they did not find a good correlation. IgE serum concentrations vary considerably; they usually range between 5 and 800 ng, with increasing median concentrations during the first decade or so of life. In some parasitic diseases, the IgE level can be very high.

The *radioallergosorbent test* (RAST) is now available to measure specific antibodies to a number of clinically significant allergens. In this test the antigen (allergen) to which antibody is to be measured is coupled to a solid-phase substance (a paper disk or gel). The patient's serum is then applied to the solid-phase substance, which has the allergen bound to it. Nonspecific proteins, including nonspecific IgE, are washed away, and then the disk or gel is exposed to ^{125}I-labeled anti-IgE antibody. After the solid-phase absorbent has been thoroughly washed, the amount of radiolabeled antibody bound to IgE is quantitated by determining the counts per minute emitted by the labeled antibody fixed to the solid-phase reactant. Using known standards, it is then possible to determine the concentration of the allergen-specific IgE in the serum of the patient. In this way specific IgE antibodies against animal danders, egg white, ragweed pollen, trees, grasses, several yeasts or molds, house dust, and other commonly encountered allergens can be tested. Although it is not as easy to perform as skin testing, the RAST test may become increasingly important in the evaluation of type I hypersensitivity diseases.

TYPE II HYPERSENSITIVITY TESTS

The most commonly used immunologic test for type II hypersensitivity reactions is the *Coombs test.* Diagnostically, this test is used to evaluate hemolytic anemias by testing for antibody on the surface of red blood cells. Before routine blood transfusions, such tests may be used to measure antibodies to red cell antigens. This type of immunologic test for type II or cytotoxic reaction may be very important in the field of organ transplantation, where circulating anti-

bodies in the recipient against major blood group antigens, and possibly also against serologically detected (HL-A) antigens, may be responsible for an acute rejection of the graft.

TYPE III HYPERSENSITIVITY TESTS

Tests to evaluate type III hypersensitivity reactions are used mainly to detect circulating antibody. A common one is the *fluorescent antinuclear antibody test,* in which cell substrate is used to demonstrate antinuclear antibodies in the serum of patients with connective tissue disease. In both hypersensitivity pneumonitis and allergic alveolitis, circulating precipitating antibody can be shown by the Oüchterlony technique of double diffusion in agar gel. In this test the allergen to be tested (e.g., the *Micromonospora* or *Thermoactinomyces* antigens in farmer's lung or in mushroom picker's disease, or the bird serum proteins in bird fancier's disease) are placed in an empty well in agar gel and allowed to diffuse toward another well containing serum from the patient to be tested. The development of precipitin lines between the wells indicates that the patient is sensitized to the allergen being tested. Similar precipitins can be seen in bronchopulmonary aspergillosis. In this disease, an intradermal skin test may also be done to evaluate immediate, late, and delayed hypersensitivity reactions in the skin.

TYPE IV HYPERSENSITIVITY TESTS

The classic test for type IV hypersensitivity is the *intradermal test.* The prime example of this type of test is the tuberculin or purified protein derivative (PPD) test, in which cellular products of *Mycobacterium tuberculosis* are injected into the skin. Observations at 48 and 72 hours in a tuberculin-positive patient may reveal an area of erythema and induration typical of a delayed hypersensitivity reaction. Similar tests are used for systemic fungal infections (histoplasmosis and coccidioidomycosis). Patients can also be tested in this manner for sensitivity both to skin fungi such as *Trichophyton* and *Candida,* and to certain viral infectious agents (e.g., mumps).

In-vivo testing for hypersensitivity to contact allergens is often done by *patch testing.* In this technique the suspected offending substance is applied to the skin and held in place by a cloth patch. Usually 2 or more days are required for the skin to give the reaction of contact dermatitis. Allergens tested in this fashion include nickel, rubber, and any chemical substance suspected of causing a contact allergy.

Clinical Allergic Diseases

Allergic diseases are common; indeed, a majority of people suffer at some time from one or several allergic conditions, such as allergic rhinitis, urticaria, drug reactions, or sensitivity to bee stings or foods. Most such patients have no clinically significant allergic symptoms most of the time. On the other hand, some individuals are chronically afflicted with allergic diseases; they may have asthma and eczema in infancy and subsequently suffer from allergic rhinitis, chronic urticaria, or drug allergies. The term *atopy* has been applied to the condition of these unfortunate individuals, implying that they have a heightened immunologic reactivity or a tendency to develop allergic diseases.

Atopy is felt to be genetically determined because of the familial occurrence of diseases such as eczema, allergic rhinitis, and extrinsic asthma. The mode of inheritance of the atopic state is not known, but recent evidence shows that certain HL-A (histocompatibility antigen) tissue types are found more frequently in families with seasonal allergic rhinitis than in unaffected families, suggesting that genetic factors are important in the control of immunoglobulin synthesis. It is known from animal studies that the ability to synthesize antibody to any given antigen is controlled by immunoregulatory genes (Ir), and this system is assumed to be functional in human beings. The idea that an atopic person may synthesize IgE at higher levels than normal persons is not supported by controlled studies in the two groups. There is evidence that the basophils and mast cells of atopic persons are able to bind a greater number of IgE molecules to their cell surfaces than normal cells can. Measurements of circulating basophils in allergic persons have shown them to have between 15,000 and 60,000 IgE molecules per cell, as compared with 5,000 to 30,000 molecules per basophil in nonallergic persons. It is not known whether this difference is a result of cell surface phenomena or whether it is even

important in the pathogenesis of allergic disease. Other possible explanations of a genetic basis of atopy include the idea that atopic persons preferentially make IgE (reaginic) antibody on sensitization to certain antigens, whereas normal persons make a different class of immunoglobulin molecule.

Another possible explanation for the atopic state is the beta-adrenergic blockade hypothesis. This idea focuses on the chemical mediator mechanisms of the allergic state rather than on the production of antibody. It is known that beta-adrenergic stimulation has an effect on the release of the chemical mediators of type I reactions, and there is evidence that in extrinsic asthma there is decreased cell responsiveness to beta-adrenergic stimulation. Exogenous beta-adrenergic-stimulating agents used in the treatment of allergic asthma are believed to help restore the normal balance of contraction and relaxation of bronchial smooth muscle.

In the following sections, some of the important allergic diseases will be discussed, along with their clinical presentation, pathophysiology, diagnosis, and treatment.

ALLERGIC RHINITIS

Allergic rhinitis is caused by an allergic response of the nasal mucosa to pollens or to other allergens in the air. It is termed *seasonal allergic rhinitis* when it refers to an allergic response to plants with a characteristic seasonal pollination. The syndrome, however, may not be seasonal but may persist throughout the year if the patient is sensitized equally to a number of pollens that succeed each other in the spring, summer, and fall. This latter situation is to be expected because atopic persons are prone to develop sensitivities to a multiplicity of allergens. The onset of allergic rhinitis is greatest in childhood and young adult life, and often there is a family history of allergic rhinitis. The familial nature of atopic diseases requires an evaluation of the family history for rhinitis, asthma, and infantile eczema.

In the usual case, 2 or more years of exposure to a seasonal allergen are necessary before symptoms appear. It is not unusual for a patient to become free of rhinitis for 2 to 4 years after moving to a new location but then to develop sensitivity to the new local pollens. Once allergic rhinitis has become established the clinical syndrome will usually persist, although it may vary from year to year, depending on numerous factors. The allergens responsible for allergic rhinitis include various pollens from trees, grasses, or weeds; spores from molds; animal danders; house dust; and a variety of other small, particulate antigens in the patient's environment. Most trees, grasses, and weeds produce pollens that are airborne and can cause sensitization after inhalation. Flowering plants such as roses, dandelions, and fruit trees that depend on insects for pollination do not usually cause allergic rhinitis. Times of pollination of most plants vary geographically, but they are usually predictable for each species in any one place. In the northern and eastern parts of the United States, tree pollens are prevalent in April and May; grass pollens appear in May and persist through June; June and July may be times of pollination for English plantain; and ragweed usually starts pollinating in the third week of August and persists until autumn frost. Pollination of such plants is usually greatest in the morning and, therefore, symptoms of allergic rhinitis are often most severe in the morning. Pollen counts are one way of measuring the amount of pollination at any given time; they can be affected by factors such as wind and humidity. In other parts of the United States, seasonal factors may be less important. In the Southwest, for example, grass pollination may occur all summer and therefore may cause persistent symptoms.

Allergic rhinitis is not just a disease of the warm summer months. Rhinitis persists in many patients throughout the winter, and appropriate tests may reveal allergies to house dust and molds. Molds can also be a problem in the summer months in warm, damp weather. The properties of airborne allergens will not be discussed further here; however, certain points should be made about environmental allergens other than pollens and molds. Epidermal allergens from dogs, cats, and horses are present in the dander of the animal and not in the hair. Therefore, the impression often held by the owner of a pet that a short-haired animal is safer than a long-haired one for an allergic person is not true. Feathers are also epidermal appendages and must be considered whenever a patient is suffering from allergic rhinitis or asthma.

House dust is a collection of many potential allergens, but most attention recently has been focused on the mites in house dust. *Dermatophagoides farinae* (dust mites) may well be the source of sensitizing antigens in many allergic persons. The molds *Hormodendrum* and *Alternaria* frequently cause sensitization and grow during the entire year. Significant sensitivity to these molds may cause a vexing perennial rhinitis.

Clinical Syndrome

Allergic rhinitis is characterized by sneezing, watery rhinorrhea, and swelling of the nasal mucous membranes. A concomitant conjunctivitis, with erythema and itching, is relatively common. Often nasal blockage occurs, requiring breathing by mouth and circumventing the normal functions of the nose to filter, warm, and humidify the inspired air. Postnasal discharge, especially during sleep, can cause hoarseness and pain in the pharyngeal and laryngeal areas. Persistent nasal blockage can lead to sinusitis with bacterial infection, as well as to recurrent otitis media. The qualities of phonation are frequently affected by the nasal blockage. Physical examination will show an erythematous, swollen nasal mucosa with copious, clear (or sometimes thick) discharge. Nasal polyps tend to occur after prolonged allergic rhinitis and appear as "grapelike" structures in the posterior parts of the nasal passages. Polyps cannot usually be seen on initial examination, unless the mucosa is treated with a dilute aerosolized vasoconstrictor, such as ephedrine, to shrink the boggy nasal mucosa.

Diagnosis

The diagnosis of allergic rhinitis starts with a thorough history, including questions about the seasonal nature of symptoms, family history of atopic disease, and exposure to allergens (e.g., pets, dust). Initially, allergic rhinitis can be confused with coryza or vasomotor rhinitis. Tests for type I hypersensitivity are the mainstay of diagnosis in allergic rhinitis; they include skin testing and serologic tests for specific IgE antibody (RAST tests), as discussed previously. A very good correlation between positivity on these tests and seasonal symptomatology is often found and may be helpful in both the diagnosis and the subsequent treatment of this disease. Atopic patients often show positive results on both skin tests and RAST tests to more than one allergen, although only one or two of these may prove to be clinically significant.

Some patients appear to have all the clinical findings of allergic rhinitis more or less continuously, but on testing they are not found to have reactivity to any of the common allergens. This finding is most common in children and is then often associated with chronic middle ear infection or sinusitis. The patient may have persistent nasal discharge, mouth breathing, and snoring. Drying of the nasal mucosa may lead to epistaxis. Some of these children are probably allergic to substances not routinely evaluated, whereas others have no demonstrable allergy. In adults, chronic rhinitis may be associated with cigarette smoking and other kinds of air pollution. In the differential diagnosis of allergic rhinitis it is important to consider iatrogenic conditions such as the nasal stuffiness caused by the use of reserpine. Some women have this symptom while taking birth control pills.

Treatment

Avoidance Therapy. The treatment of allergic rhinitis falls into three categories: avoidance therapy, drug therapy, and immunotherapy. Strict avoidance by a patient of a specific allergen can completely abrogate the reactions seen in the same patient when exposed to this allergen. This is true, of course, in all types of antigen-antibody mediated reactions, but on the basis of frequency alone, it is of most importance in type I reactions, such as allergic rhinitis and extrinsic asthma. Therefore, an attempt should be made with hypersensitive patients to minimize contact with the offending allergen. Patients who are allergic to feathers should have pillows stuffed with synthetic material. Meticulous housekeeping, including the avoidance of dust collecting on rugs or venetian blinds, can significantly lower dust allergens in the patient's house. Similarly, control of humidity can lessen a patient's exposure to mold spores. Patients who are sensitive to airborne allergens found outside the house have a more perplexing problem. If sensitive to molds, they should avoid raking leaves and other activities that may expose them to smuts. Total avoidance of plant pollens is nearly impossible. Inside the house, air conditioners and filters may help to reduce the pollen

count. During any particular pollinating season the patient may get relief of symptoms by leaving the area. For example, patients with ragweed hay fever who live in the northeastern United States may be able to take their August or September vacations in Europe, where there is no ragweed.

Drug Therapy. A number of chemical compounds that counteract histamine are available. Most of these antihistamines are substituted ethylamines, which presumably inhibit the actions of histamine (beta-imidazolylethylamine) by combining with histamine receptors in the body. They block the increased capillary permeability caused by histamine, the major symptom-producing mechanism in allergic rhinitis. The most commonly used antihistamines include diphenhydramidine hydrochloride (Benadryl), chlorpheniramine maleate (Chlor-Trimeton) and tripelennamine (Pyribenzamine). All these compounds are effective when given orally. They may be more effective therapeutically when given prior to exposure to an allergen; in other words, antihistamines block histamine effects, not histamine release, and therefore have no effect on histamine effects that have already occurred. Side effects of the antihistamines include somnolence and drying of mucous membranes. Initially, the sedative effect of antihistamines may be marked and therefore patients should avoid hazardous activities such as driving an automobile or piloting an airplane when starting these drugs. The sedative effect often becomes less pronounced after antihistamine therapy has been continued for some time. Also, for unknown reasons, a patient may respond much better to one particular antihistamine than to another.

Since the major pathophysiologic mechanisms in allergic rhinitis are vasodilatation and increased permeability, sympathomimetic agents that cause vasoconstriction can be effective in modifying the symptoms. Judicious use of nose drops or nasal sprays containing sympathomimetic agents such as phenylephrine hydrochloride can relieve symptoms, but they often cause a problem when used for more than 2 or 3 weeks because of the "rebound" phenomenon; that is, after such prolonged use of a nasal spray, the mucous membranes may become *more* congested after each use of the drug. Discontinuance of the nasal spray for 2 to 4 weeks usually allows the nasal mucosa to recover its normal state of responsiveness. Phenylephrine, ephedrine, and isoephedrine may also be given in conjunction with oral antihistamines, enhancing the clinical benefits. Unfortunately, many patients find that sympathomimetic agents cause undue nervousness and drying of mucous membranes.

When all other drug therapy fails, local use of a corticosteroid can be effective in relieving the symptoms of allergic rhinitis. The steroids have potent effects on the edema and the capillary permeability effector mechanisms of type I reactions. The use of dexamethasone sodium phosphate in a Freon nasal spray can give good relief of symptoms in allergic rhinitis if used no more than twice a day, and it is not likely to give any systemic side effects. The use of the dexamethasone spray has also been reported to reduce the size of the nasal polyps often seen in allergic rhinitis. Finally, local injection of a steroid into nasal polyps may avert the necessity for surgery.

Immunotherapy. Immunotherapy (hyposensitization) has been tried since 1911 when it was first introduced by Noon, who observed that repeated immunization caused a reduction in rhinitis symptoms during the grass pollen season. This form of therapy became prominent in the treatment of allergy, although arguments continued concerning its efficacy. Within the last 10 years, controlled studies have shown that this form of therapy is effective in both allergic rhinitis and allergic asthma.

The basis for the effectiveness of immunotherapy in ragweed hay fever is thought to be induction of antiragweed (IgG) antibody (blocking antibody). Unlike IgE, the IgG does not fix to cell membranes, but it is capable of combining with the allergen in the fluid phase before it can couple with IgE. The basophils and mast cells are then not triggered and therefore the clinical mediators are not released. It has also been shown that both IgA and IgG antibodies are increased in the nasal secretions in patients on immunotherapy. IgE serum levels may decline slightly during immunotherapy but of more significance is the marked lessening of the usual sharp increase in antiragweed IgE antibody seen in untreated patients during the ragweed season. At the same time, IgG antibodies to ragweed antigen can be shown to increase. It is felt that the tying up of the ragweed allergen by IgG or IgA antibody may prevent subsequent stimulation of IgE synthesis. When immunotherapy is discontinued, patients can be shown to have decreasing amounts of IgG antibodies, and then in the next ragweed season to have sharply rising levels of IgE, with a resumption of clinical symptoms.

The major secret of success in the use of immunotherapy appears to be in the selection of patients. The results described above are those observed in patients who are definitely positive on skin testing and who have increased levels of specific IgE antibody on RAST tests. If every patient with rhinitis symptoms is treated with immunotherapy, whether or not he is positive on allergy testing, the overall results will be disappointing. Therefore, in both allergic rhinitis and allergic asthma, it is important to correlate symptoms and allergy tests before starting immunotherapy.

Indications for the use of immunotherapy in allergic rhinitis are relative. If a patient has rhinitis symptoms for a few weeks during only one season of the year, it may be best to use symptomatic therapy. If, however, the patient is allergic to a number of different pollens and has symptoms lasting for months, or if he has an occupation that prohibits the use of antihistamines because of their sedative effects, it may be best to use immunotherapy. Cost can be an important consideration, since weekly visits to the physician's office may be much more expensive than medications. Immunotherapy should usually be restricted to patients who are sensitive to environmental allergens that cannot be avoided. It is dangerous, and rarely necessary, to treat a patient sensitive to animal danders with immunotherapy when his livelihood is not dependent on continued contact with animals.

The usual method of immunotherapy is to give injections of very small and slowly increasing amounts of the offending allergen on a weekly basis. The practical details of immunotherapy will not be discussed here, but certain factors should be noted. First, it usually takes 6 months before the weekly dosage reaches the maximum that can be tolerated by the patient. Second, commercially available allergin extracts are not standardized and therefore a patient cannot switch back and forth from one commercial preparation to another. Because of the time involved in bringing the sensitive patient up to the maximum effective dose, one must expect to start therapy approximately 6 months prior to the expected pollen season. It is now felt that continuous injection therapy throughout the year is more effective than starting and stopping immunotherapy each year. After a patient is on the full dose of allergen, it is often possible to spread out the injections to every 2 weeks and then every 3 weeks, and often to once a month. The patient should be informed that it will take a minimum of 3 years to evaluate fully whether or not this form of therapy is effective. Repeated skin tests and RAST tests for specific IgE antibody can be helpful in evaluating the effectiveness of therapy. If no clinical improvement is noted after two seasons of immunotherapy, the treatment should probably be discontinued. The question of how long the therapy should be continued in a patient who has a favorable response is not easily answered. Occasionally a patient will be able to discontinue immunotherapy and not have any exacerbation of symptoms; the usual situation is that the next season brings mild to moderate rhinitis symptoms, and the following year, a return of the full syndrome. Immunotherapy is generally considered to be safe during pregnancy, when all other types of drug therapy should be employed with great caution.

VASOMOTOR RHINITIS

Vasomotor rhinitis is a syndrome that is easily mistaken for allergic rhinitis. It is not immunologically mediated but appears to result from autonomic nervous system responses to changes in temperature, emotional stimuli, or humidity. The clinical features include chronic nasal congestion, sneezing, and watery rhinorrhea. These symptoms typically occur whenever the patient is subjected to a draft, such as from an open window or air conditioner, or they may appear early in the morning when the patient first puts his feet onto a cold floor. Although more patients suffer from vasomotor rhinitis during the cold than the warm months, the appearance of symptoms seems to depend more on fluctuations of tem-

perature than on background patterns. Treatment of vasomotor rhinitis with antihistamines and oral nasal decongestants may be satisfactory in some patients. Avoidance of precipitating factors may also be helpful; for example, a patient who has symptoms of vasomotor rhinitis in the morning may be instructed to sleep with the windows closed, to wear slippers, or to have rugs on the floor of his bedroom and bathroom. The chronic topical use of nasal sprays or steroids should be discouraged because of their side effects. Vasomotor rhinitis that starts in the second trimester of pregnancy usually disappears soon after parturition.

ASTHMA

The term *asthma* describes a syndrome of episodic bronchospasm in association with other pathophysiologic processes. The general subject of bronchial asthma is treated elsewhere in this text (Chaps. 9, 10), but it is important to discuss here certain aspects of the diseases grouped under this heading from the vantage point of immunology and allergy. Bronchial asthma is often classified simplistically as *extrinsic* when type I hypersensitivity reactions can be shown to be important in its pathogenesis, and *intrinsic* when they cannot.

Extrinsic asthma can be precipitated by the inhalation of allergens and sometimes by the parenteral administration of these allergens. The disease commonly occurs in atopic persons and can be shown to be mediated by IgE. There is often a strong family history of atopic diseases, including childhood eczema or allergic rhinitis. The adult who has extrinsic asthma often gives a history of childhood asthma or of eczema in the first 2 or 3 years of life. There is a strong correlation of the asthmatic attacks with childhood episodes of bronchopneumonia. The patient may have asthma that began early and persisted throughout life; or his condition may improve for several years, only to have an exacerbation of the disease later. This waxing and waning of asthmatic symptoms has led to a common misconception that the child with asthma will "outgrow it." However, we know that the lymphocyte has an extremely long memory, and it is unlikely that its sensitization to an allergen will be "forgotten" in a normal human life span. There are, however, many factors that do affect the clinical expression of type I hypersensitivity reactions. Among these factors are (1) the amount and frequency of exposure to antigens, (2) variations in the release of chemical mediators (histamine and SRS-A), (3) autonomic nervous system control of smooth muscle, and (4) infections.

Patient Evaluation

Clinical evaluation of the asthmatic patient should always include a thorough check of possible allergic aspects of his disease, which means performing tests for type I hypersensitivity, as outlined in the section on allergic rhinitis. The demonstration of an allergic basis for a patient's asthma should strongly influence the therapeutic strategy for that patient.

Treatment

Avoidance Therapy. The treatment in allergic asthma falls into the same three categories as that in allergic rhinitis, namely, avoidance therapy, drug therapy, and immunotherapy. When one specific allergen can be shown to be the causative factor in asthma, removal of this allergen from the patient's environment will give relief of symptoms. This is rarely the case, however, both because most allergic patients are found to be sensitive to multiple allergens, and because the allergens that cause asthmatic attacks are usually inhaled and are fairly ubiquitous. Even so, exposure to certain allergens can be controlled to a certain extent, provided the asthmatic patient can be shown to have a single sensitivity. The amount of dust in the patient's house should be kept at a minimum. This is especially true in the bedroom, since the patient spends more time there than anywhere else and because asthmatic symptoms often are most severe during the night-time. Draperies, rugs, and upholstered furniture should not be used in the bedroom. Mattresses and pillows should be enclosed in plastic covers. Humidity in basements and heating systems should be controlled to reduce mold spores. The patient with allergic asthma should avoid animal danders and thus should not have cats, dogs, or birds in his house. If the atopic patient does not already have a sensitivity to animal danders, there is a good chance that he will develop it in the future.

Drug Therapy. The rationale for drug therapy in allergic asthma is based on a knowledge of the factors influencing the release and function of the chemical mediators of type I reactions. Reference to Figure 45-1 shows that the level of cyclic AMP is the major determinant of the release of histamine, SRS-A, and ECF-A. A relative increase in cyclic AMP decreases the release of the mediators, whereas a decrease in cyclic AMP will enhance their release. The level of cyclic AMP can be increased by two mechanisms: (1) by increasing adenyl cyclase, the enzyme necessary for the production of cyclic AMP from ATP; this can be accomplished by the stimulation of beta-adrenergic receptors by giving sympathomimetic agents such as isoproterenol or epinephrine (this effect is blocked by propranolol, which is therefore contraindicated in asthma); or (2) by inhibiting the enzyme phosphodiesterase, which is necessary for the degradation of cyclic AMP; this can be accomplished by giving the methylxanthines, which include the theophylline compounds. The various therapeutic agents that modulate the cyclic AMP level, namely, epinephrine, isoproterenol, and the theophylline compounds, have been used empirically in the treatment of asthma for years as bronchodilators.

Reference to the schema in Figure 45-1 also explains why agents causing alpha-adrenergic stimulation and those causing cholinergic stimulation may be deleterious in asthma. It is generally believed that since the beta-adrenergic stimulators and the phosphodiesterase inhibitors act by different mechanisms and therefore theoretically complement each other, various combinations of these two types of agents might be more effective than either one alone in the treatment of asthmatic bronchospasm. Therefore, numerous preparations are available containing one or several of these drugs, including some of the newer sympathomimetic agents (metaproterenol and terbutaline sulfate) that produce both more specific beta-adrenergic stimulation and fewer side effects.

Corticosteroids are effective in the treatment of asthma and are often necessary during prolonged attacks. They have an effect on vascular permeability and mucosal edema, as well as on the inflammatory response. One of the more obvious benefits of corticosteroids is to restore the patient's responsiveness to bronchodilator drugs; this may be accomplished by activation of the adenyl cyclase system. Therefore, when a patient no longer responds to the conventional bronchodilator therapy, corticosteroids may be tried in the hope of restoring the patient's responsiveness. Prolonged use of corticosteroids in asthmatics, as in all patients with chronic conditions, should be discouraged because they can cause hyperadrenocorticism, and in children, growth retardation. Most patients with severe, acute asthma can be rapidly weaned from corticosteroids without an exacerbation of the disease, after the acute attack has subsided.

Disodium cromoglycate (chromolyn sodium) is a new compound that has proved to be effective in treating some cases of asthma by inhibiting the release of histamine and SRS-A. The drug is inactivated when taken orally and therefore at present must be taken by inhalation of the powder. Preliminary studies have shown it to be most effective in pediatric patients and in young adults suffering mainly from extrinsic asthma.

Immunotherapy. The earlier discussion of immunotherapy for allergic rhinitis applies equally to extrinsic asthma. Studies have now shown that there is definitely a place for immunotherapy in the treatment of allergic asthmatic patients. Immunotherapy must be instituted in these patients with extreme caution, however, since systemic reactions and iatrogenically induced bronchoconstriction can occur. Treatment of a patient with frequent, acute asthmatic attacks requires patience and persistence, since injection therapy often has to be delayed because of recurrent attacks. Patients who respond to immunotherapy probably should remain on it for prolonged periods of time.

Aspirin-Sensitive Asthma

Aspirin-sensitive asthma is a syndrome that should be included in this discussion of asthma, even though it probably has nothing to do with immunologic mechanisms. This syndrome is often seen in patients who do not have an atopic history. After the ingestion of aspirin, the patients develop very persistent bronchospasm within one-half to one hour. Not uncommonly, these patients also have chronic rhinitis with nasal polyposis and a peripheral blood eosinophilia. There is no evidence of true allergy to aspirin. In a patient with the aspirin-sensitive syndrome, other drugs, including indomethacin, mefenamic acid, and other nonsteroid antiinflammatory agents, can induce a similar bronchospasm. The syndrome may also be seen after ingestion of the coal tar dye tartrazine, which is found in many foodstuffs and medications. The mechanism of the reaction is not clearly understood, but it is thought to be related to inhibition of prostaglandin synthesis. Prostaglandin E_2 can be shown to cause bronchial dilatation, whereas prostaglandin F_{2a} can cause bronchial constriction. Since antiinflammatory drugs such as aspirin and indomethacin probably function by interfering with prostaglandin synthesis, this seems a logical explanation of their bronchoconstrictor effect. Patients with the aspirin-sensitive syndrome should avoid all such compounds, because the bronchospasm they induce usually proves to be extremely resistant to conventional therapy.

URTICARIA

Urticaria is a common disorder, occurring as a single, self-limited episode in up to 20 percent of persons, and occurring in a much smaller proportion in its chronic form. Urticarial lesions appear as papular wheals of varying sizes and shapes, each surrounded by an erythematous base. These lesions may be found anywhere on the body and are frequently exacerbated by scratching. The term *chronic urticaria* is used when the lesions last for more than 2 weeks. The mechanisms involved in the production of urticarial lesions are not known, but there is evidence that histamine or histaminelike substances are the major mediators of the reaction. Lesions identical to those in urticaria can be reproduced by the intracutaneous injection of histamine, and drugs that cause release of endogenous histamine, such as morphine, frequently produce urticarial reactions. Another indication that histamine is the mediator of urticaria is the fact that urticaria is often a prominent feature of type I hypersensitivity reactions. Allergic syndromes that are mediated by type I reactions, with urticaria as one of the presenting features, include stinging insect reactions, allergic rhinitis, allergic asthma, and allergic reactions to crustacea or to animal danders.

Clinical Picture

As mentioned previously, urticarial lesions may occur anywhere on the body; they appear as papular wheals surrounded by an erythematous base with a tendency to coalesce, sometimes producing single lesions up to 10 cm or more in diameter. The lesion is generally pruritic, and it becomes larger and more pruritic when scratched. Dermatographia is frequently found in patients with urticaria, seen as a wheal and flare reaction after the skin is stroked. The urticarial lesions seen under tight clothing or after scratching are probably manifestations of this phenomenon. Urticarial lesions may resolve within hours, or they may persist for days. Some patients may have urticaria for years, with the lesions waxing and waning, whereas other patients with chronic urticaria may have urticarial lesions for several months, followed by freedom for several years before another episode occurs.

Etiologic Diagnosis

The cause of urticaria cannot be found in the majority of patients despite extensive evaluation. In patients with persistent urticaria, a search for an etiologic agent may be fruitless; however, several possible factors should be considered. Food sensitivities are common causes and sometimes can be disclosed by an adequate history and the use of an elimination diet. Foods that frequently cause urticaria include seafoods (e.g., lobster, shrimp), strawberries, tomatoes, nuts, eggs, milk, and grains. Making a diagnosis from a dietary history alone may be difficult, however, since certain foodstuffs (e.g., tomato paste) may be used as ingredients in many foods without the patient's being aware of it. Urticarial lesions may also be caused by many drugs, including common compounds such as aspirin and laxatives, that may be overlooked in the routine medical history. As mentioned previously, drugs such as morphine can cause liberation of histamine and hence urticaria without invoking any immunologic mechanism; this is probably also true of certain foods, such as strawberries, which can cause histamine release. The acute allergic reaction to penicillin often includes urticaria, and the possibility

that this antibiotic may contaminate foods such as milk may explain urticaria in some persons. Other etiologic factors to be considered in the diagnosis of urticaria include inhalation of animal danders, use of cosmetics, and stinging by insects.

Cold urticaria is a term used to describe a syndrome found in certain persons on exposure to cold. In the few cases evaluated, both IgE and IgM humoral factors have been shown to mediate the syndrome. Urticaria is also seen occasionally in the prodromal phase of serum hepatitis.

Treatment

The subcutaneous injection of epinephrine is usually quite effective in acute urticaria and is certainly indicated when the urticaria is part of an anaphylactic syndrome. Ephedrine given orally, with or without antihistamines, may also give relief. Antihistamines (e.g., diphenhydramine and chlorpheniramine maleate) are the most commonly used agents, and some patients who do not respond well to the usual antihistamines may respond to hydroxyzine. Even though these drugs may not suppress the urticaria completely, they usually relieve the pruritus. Some patients with a large psychogenic contribution to their symptom complex may benefit more from the use of sedatives or tranquilizers.

SERUM SICKNESS
The use of heterologous antiserums for the treatment of infectious diseases such as diphtheria, tetanus, and pneumococcal pneumonia may be followed by a syndrome of fever, polyarthralgia, generalized lymphadenopathy, and skin rash, occurring usually from 8 to 12 days after the administration of the serum. This syndrome, called serum sickness, represents a typical type III hypersensitivity reaction. Immunologically speaking, there are three phases of the syndrome. The first is sensitization, which occurs after the heterologous serum proteins are administered. A latent period of 8 to 12 days follows, during which IgM antibodies to the foreign proteins are being synthesized. When sufficient antibodies are produced to form circulating antigen-antibody complexes, the clinical syndrome appears. This is a time of slight antigen excess, when immune complexes remain

within the circulation instead of being precipitated and cleared by the reticuloendothelial system. At this point there is usually a mild depression in serum complement levels, indicating that the reaction is complement-mediated. The third phase occurs when there is an excess of antibody; the antigen-antibody complexes become precipitated and are cleared by the reticuloendothelial system, with a resolution of the clinical syndrome. After this phase, any subsequent injection of the same foreign proteins can produce one of two clinical manifestations. The first is an immediate anaphylactic reaction, which would indicate that reaginic or IgE antibodies are present. The second clinical picture may be the same as the original serum sickness, but starting this time about 4 days after the injection of the foreign proteins. This more rapid response coincides with the anamnestic state of the immune system with respect to synthesized IgG antibody, which can produce the same antigen-antibody complex disease as in the original serum sickness.

Clinical Picture

As stated previously, serum sickness syndrome usually has an onset 8 to 12 days after the administration of serum and begins with a pruritic, urticarial, or morbilliform skin rash. Fever to 103°F (39°C), malaise, nausea, and abdominal pain are not uncommon. Generalized lymphadenopathy occurs, and the majority of patients develop migratory polyarthritis. Peripheral neuritis and other evidence of systemic vasculitis may appear and may be confused with other diseases such as polyarteritis nodosa. The syndrome is usually self-limited, and spontaneous recovery begins within 1 week after the onset.

The incidence of serum sickness declined sharply with the advent of antibiotics and the decrease in injections of specific antisera. Antibacterial vaccines such as tetanus and diphtheria toxoid have also markedly decreased the need for specific antisera. Antitetanus antiserum is still occasionally used in a patient who has never received primary immunization. Antisera are also available for clostridial infections and, similarly, antisnake venom antisera are sometimes used; if obtained from heterologous sources, both of these antisera can cause serum sickness. In the case of tetanus, there is now available an antitetanus antiserum of human origin that obviates the development of sensitivity and, therefore, avoids the serum sickness syndrome.

Before a patient is given heterologous antiserum, he should be questioned about prior reactions to serum and should be tested by an intracutaneous injection of the antiserum, usually diluted 1:10 or 1:20. If there is an immediate hypersensitivity reaction with a wheal and flare, the patient is considered to have homocytotropic antibody (IgE), and his chance of having an immediate anaphylactic-type reaction is significant. If it is nevertheless absolutely necessary to give antiserum, as in the case of snake bite, a desensitization procedure can be instituted. One method of desensitization is to give 0.1 ml of 1:100 dilution of the antiserum subcutaneously and, if no reaction occurs, the amount can be doubled every 15 minutes until a subcutaneous dose of 1.0 ml of this dilution is given. If no reaction has occurred, the injections can be repeated intravenously, first with the diluted antiserum and then with the undiluted antiserum, doubling the volume every 15 minutes until a full dose of 1.0 ml of undiluted antiserum is given. Epinephrine for parenteral administration should be available at all times during this procedure.

The treatment of serum sickness includes the use of antihistamines for the control of pruritus and the use of antipyretics. In severe cases, a short course of corticosteroids may give good symptomatic relief.

BEE STING ALLERGY

Anaphylactic reactions to the stings of members of the Hymenoptera species (honey bees, yellow jackets, hornets, and wasps) cause more deaths in the United States than do all the other venomous animals and insects combined. These reactions are IgE-mediated, and specific antibody to the sensitizing venom can be demonstrated in the patient's serum by the RAST test. For many years it was thought that there were cross-reacting antigens in the venoms of the members of the Hymenoptera species; however, this supposition was based on evidence obtained from testing patients with whole body extracts of bees. More recent work has suggested that each venom has specific antigens. Treatment of the acute anaphylactic reaction includes the immediate administration of parenteral epinephrine followed by an oral antihistamine. Blood pressure should be maintained if hypotension tends to persist.

Hyposensitization to whole body extracts of bees is the accepted method of preventing systemic reactions in the bee-sensitized person; however, the efficacy of this method is being seriously questioned. The use of allergenic extracts of each specific bee venom may prove to be more efficacious. Sensitized patients should take every precaution against stings. They should never go barefoot outdoors, they should not wear clothes with floral patterns, and they should not use scented cosmetics. Carrying a syringe and a solution of epinephrine may be difficult, but most patients can carry epinephrine for inhalation or isoproterenol sublingual tablets, both of which are effective. The patient should always go immediately to the closest emergency room or physician when he is stung by a bee; he should *not* wait for symptoms to appear.

A less life-threatening complication of bee sting allergy is a syndrome resembling serum sickness. In this case, the patient often develops arthralgias, fever, and urticarial skin rash several days after being stung. This is a self-limited syndrome that may be treated with antiinflammatory drugs. Allergy testing of these patients often discloses IgE antibody, although the serum sicknesslike syndrome is felt to be IgG-mediated. The presence of IgE antibodies signifies that the patient could suffer an anaphylactic reaction on any subsequent contact with the venom.

FOOD ALLERGY

Many people have gastrointestinal or systemic syndromes associated with intolerance to certain foods. Few of these syndromes, however, have been definitely shown to involve immunologically mediated reactions. A few of the immunologically mediated reactions to ingested materials have been discussed earlier, in the section on urticaria. Greater significance should be placed on food allergies that frequently precipitate anaphylactic reactions and that, therefore, are potentially fatal. The most dramatic reactions are those associated with the ingestion of crustacea (e.g., lobster, shrimp) or nuts. It appears that crustacea

contain cross-reacting antigen or antigens that can precipitate anaphylactic type I reactions in a sensitized person. A similar picture may be seen after the ingestion of nuts. The anaphylactic reaction usually occurs within minutes after ingestion of the allergenic food, resulting in hypotension and laryngeal edema. There may or may not be generalized urticaria. Treatment consists in administration of parenteral epinephrine. Obviously, persons who are sensitive to these substances should go to great lengths to avoid them.

Although sensitized persons may show only urticaria on their second exposure to an allergenic food, they may also have a generalized anaphylactic reaction. Attempts to use immunotherapy in this disorder are to be discouraged because of the great danger involved. It is difficult, but important, for any child with a sensitivity to peanuts to avoid all related substances such as peanut oil and peanut butter.

ATOPIC ECZEMA

Atopic eczema is an inflammatory reaction in the skin; it is discussed here because of its frequent association with asthma and allergic rhinitis. It is characterized by an erythematous, pruritic eruption, which is often generalized in infancy but which occurs in the flexure distribution (the antecubital and popliteal areas) in late childhood or adulthood. On biopsy, there is spongiosis of the epidermis and infiltration of the dermis with chronic inflammatory cells. Despite the occurrence of atopic eczema in patients with atopic diatheses, no immunologically mediated mechanism has been described. The treatment is symptomatic and often includes the use of steroid creams applied to the skin. Fortunately, there is often a spontaneous regression after age 20. The association of childhood atopic eczema and subsequent asthma can give a valuable clue in the diagnosis of bronchospastic disease in the young adult.

PHOTOSENSITIVITY

Two types of reactions can result from abnormal photosensitivity. The first type is the phototoxic reaction, which is nonimmunologic and can be precipitated either by endogenous substances such as porphyrins, or by exogenous substances such as tetracyclines and psoralens. It is postulated that in this type of reaction the photosensitizing molecule absorbs light and then causes cell damage by dissipating its absorbed energy through biologic mechanisms such as free radical formation.

The second type of photosensitivity reaction has been observed with compounds such as phenothiazines, sulfonamides, sulfonylureas, thiazide diuretics, griseofulvin, and sensitizing soap additives. The pathogenic mechanisms are believed to involve first the patient's exposure to the photocontact allergen, and next, exposure to appropriate wavelengths of light. The haptenic compound is altered by the light exposure and then combines with a carrier protein to form the complete antigen. This disease is typically expressed as a straightforward contact dermatitis (see the following section), but it can occur in a sensitized patient on exposure to light alone. The photoallergy usually persists after the eruption resolves and, although avoidance of the photoallergen may prevent further dermatitis in some persons, exposure to light alone may cause an exacerbation in others.

ALLERGIC CONTACT DERMATITIS

Allergic contact dermatitis represents a type IV hypersensitivity reaction. Cell-mediated hypersensitivity is caused by the combination of an appropriate hapten with dermal proteins during the sensitizing exposure to the allergen. The *Rhus* antigen of poison ivy is typical of the chemical haptens that cause contact dermatitis, but many commonly used chemicals can cause sensitization (e.g., paraphenylenediamine, nickel, pyrethrum, phenyl-beta-naphthylamine). After sensitization, exposure to the offending chemical causes an inflammatory, pruritic dermatitis, usually progressing to vesiculation. Although contact with poison ivy is usually easily determined, allergic dermatitis caused by nickel, commonly found in watch casings, or by chemicals found in the rubber used in footwear, often escapes detection. The diagnosis of a specific sensitivity can be aided by patch testing, using the suspected allergen. The treatment of contact dermatitis includes local therapy with drying agents such as calamine or with steroid creams. Avoidance of the offending allergen is the most important therapeutic measure. In severe cases of contact dermatitis or when there is involvement of the conjunctivas, a short course of an orally adminis-

tered corticosteroid in large doses can be very effective. Whenever oral steroid therapy is used, the dosage should be discontinued abruptly after 3 to 5 days, because tapering the dosage will often cause the dermatitis to flare.

DRUG ALLERGIES

Adverse reactions to therapeutic agents are common and often play a significant role in the final effectiveness of a treatment. However, very few of these adverse reactions have been shown to have an immunologic basis. Certain reactions have been shown to be genetically controlled, such as the hemolytic anemia that occurs in patients with deficiency of glucose 6-phosphate dehydrogenase. The acetylation of isoniazid (INH) is also a genetically controlled process and may be the basis of unwanted high serum levels of this drug when the dosage is not carefully adjusted. Idiosyncratic reactions, such as an aplastic anemia after administration of phenylbutazone and a hypotensive reaction after intravenous use of radiocontrast materials containing iodide, also have not been shown to be immunologic in origin.

Drug Reactions Involving Immunologic Mechanisms
Examples of drug reactions that do involve immunologic mechanisms include the Coombs-positive hemolytic anemia associated with the administration of α-methyldopa (Aldomet), and the thrombocytopenia seen with the use of quinidine or quinine. Humoral antibody can be demonstrated in these syndromes. A drug-induced systemic lupus erythematosus (SLE) syndrome may follow the use of hydralazine hydrochloride, procainamide, or rarely, isoniazid. It is felt that the major manifestations of this syndrome are expressed through the induction of antinuclear antibodies; however, circulating antibodies to some of these therapeutic agents have also been described. One possible mechanism of drug-induced SLE is that the drugs may alter nucleoprotein in such a way as to render it autoantigenic. The syndrome usually resolves soon after the offending agent is stopped, but it may persist for months.

Many other drugs may cause adverse reactions that involve immunologic mechanisms. It is most important in making a proper diagnosis of a drug allergy to explore all the therapeutic agents that the patient may be taking, and what their possible adverse effects may be. The most common symptoms caused by allergy to therapeutic agents include pruritus, urticaria, exfoliative dermatitis, fever, and some variation of the serum sickness syndrome.

Penicillin Allergy

Because of its clinical importance, allergy to penicillin compounds will be discussed here in some detail. Penicillin and its congeners can cause many clinical manifestations, including anaphylaxis, serum sickness, skin rash, fever, hemolytic anemia, vasculitis, and nephropathy. Approximately 500 deaths per year in the United States are associated with acute reactions to penicillin.

There are three possible mechanisms by which penicillin may become a complete antigen: (1) The penicillin can combine with a carrier protein, (2) a breakdown product of penicillin such as penicilloyl acid can combine with a carrier, or (3) a contaminant in the penicillin preparation can combine with a carrier. All three of these mechanisms have been shown to occur. Actually, hemagglutination tests can show that most humans treated with penicillin will develop antibodies to penicilloyl derivatives; thus the demonstration of such antibodies is not helpful clinically in patients with possible hazardous penicillin reactions. What is needed is an assay for IgE antibodies that is specific for penicillin. At the present time three types of compounds can be used to do immediate hypersensitivity skin tests: (1) penicilloyl polylysine (PPL), (2) penicilloic acid, and (3) penicillin itself. PPL is available commercially for skin testing, whereas penicillin and penicilloic acid can be mixed fresh for each skin test. By using all these compounds, the physician can identify between 98 and 99 percent of patients with allergy to penicillin without risking anaphylaxis. Since PPL is not immunogenic, it can be used without sensitizing the patient. About 90 percent of patients who are sensitive to penicillin respond to PPL on skin testing, whereas about 5 percent of the general population will react to PPL.

If a patient is found to be sensitive to penicillin, the drug should be completely avoided, if possible, and another therapeutic agent should be chosen instead. Up to one-third of patients with penicillin allergy, however, have been shown to have cross reactivity with the cephalosporins. If it is absolutely imperative to use penicillin, one can usually treat the patient with a desensitization procedure; the patient is started on small intradermal doses of penicillin (e.g., 1 to 10 units), which are increased every half hour as long as no reaction occurs. An alternative method is to give 500 to 1,000 units of penicillin orally for the first dose and then to increase the dosage over a number of hours. This mode of desensitization may avert an anaphylactic type I reaction, but the appearance of a late manifestation of penicillin allergy, such as serum sickness or fever, may necessitate that the drug be discontinued.

While caution should always be used in administering penicillin, many patients who give a history of penicillin hypersensitivity do not really have a penicillin allergy. A good history may help to resolve the question, but unfortunately it is not always reliable. There is little justification for testing a patient for possible penicillin allergy unless there is a need to use the drug at that time, because the tests that are presently available involve a degree of risk. The further development of the RAST test may provide an in vitro method of identifying persons with IgE antipenicillin antibodies, but this test probably will not be available for the general physician's use for some time.

Bibliography

Ishizaka, K., and Ishizaka, T. Mechanisms of reaginic hypersensitivity: A review. *Clin. Allergy* 1:9, 1971.

Norman, P. S. Symposium on allergy in adults. *Med. Clin. North Am.* 58:111, 1974.

Norman, P. S. Immunotherapy (desensitization) in allergic disease. *Annu. Rev. Med.* 26:337, 1975.

Norman, P. S., Lichtenstein, L. M., and Ishizaka, K. Diagnostic tests in ragweed hay fever. *J. Allergy Clin. Immunol.* 52:210, 1972.

Parker, C. W. Practical aspects of diagnosis and treatment of patients who are hypersensitive to drugs. In M. Samter and C. W. Parker (eds.), *Hypersensitivity to Drugs.* Vol. 1. New York: Pergamon, 1972. P. 367.

Wide, L. Clinical significance of measurement of reaginic (IgE) antibody by RAST. *Clin. Allergy* 3(Suppl.):583, 1973.

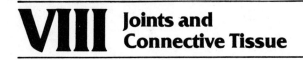

VIII

Joints and Connective Tissue

46

Arthritis and Connective Tissue Disorders

Alan S. Cohen, Edgar S. Cathcart,
and Kenneth D. Brandt

For centuries connective tissue was regarded as having a static and purely structural function. It is only within the past 40 years that the concept of the connective tissue as an organ has taken hold and that diseases involving portions of the connective tissue in a diffuse fashion have been clearly described. Since then a variety of descriptive terms, including collagen diseases, hypersensitivity diseases, autoimmune diseases, connective tissue diseases, and mesenchymal diseases, have been used to describe a group of syndromes with similar clinical, pathologic, and serologic manifestations. The major disorders included in this classification have been rheumatic fever, rheumatoid arthritis, systemic (disseminated) lupus erythematosus (SLE or DLE), dermatomyositis (polymyositis), scleroderma (progressive systemic sclerosis), and polyarteritis nodosa. In the past 20 years several other diseases (various types of vasculitis, thrombotic thrombocytopenic purpura, Sjögren's syndrome, possibly idiopathic pulmonary fibrosis, and others) have been related to these primary disorders of connective tissue. There are a number of reasons for grouping these diseases together:

1. They are multisystemic, usually involve joints, and often involve other areas such as the skin, blood vessels, kidney, lung, gastrointestinal tract, or heart.
2. They have similar and very often overlapping histopathologic lesions.
3. They share many abnormal serologic reactions, and there is an overlap in the incidence of unusual serum proteins such as rheumatoid factors and antinuclear antibodies in the various syndromes.
4. They overlap in families — that is, one may see one or more of these syndromes in a single family kinship.
5. They share a therapeutic response to certain anti-

inflammatory agents, such as salicylates, adrenocortical steroids, and antimalarial drugs.
6. They are all disorders in which the basic etiology is unknown.

Characteristics of Connective Tissue

Clearly an understanding of the nature of connective tissue itself is essential to the understanding of diseases that may manifest themselves in this particular organ. The connective tissue of the body develops from the middle layer of cells of the embryo, the mesoderm. In particular, it develops from a subdivision of the mesoderm called the mesenchyme, which is typically a loose, soft tissue infiltrating the various structures of the body, consisting of cells and intercellular substances. Since mesenchymal cells have great potentiality to differentiate into any one of several lines, mature connective tissue may contain not only differentiated cells but also undifferentiated cells that are capable, under certain pathologic conditions, of developing in any one of a number of ways.

CELLS

In the adult the cellular elements of connective tissue are *fibroblasts* (and osteoblasts and chondroblasts), which elaborate the extracellular substances collagen and mucopolysaccharides; *histiocytes,* or macrophages, which are capable of phagocytosis; *plasma cells,* which are the chief antibody producers; *mast cells,* which form heparin and contain large amounts of histamine and serotonin that are known to affect vascular permeability; and *lymphocytes,* which also produce antibodies and play an important role in cell-mediated immunity.

EXTRACELLULAR MATERIAL

Structural Proteins

The predominant structural protein is *collagen,* a fibrous protein characterized by an axial periodicity that repeats at intervals of 640–700Å, a characteristic low and wide-angle x-ray diffraction pattern, a high hydroxyproline and glycine content, a low aromatic amino acid content, and a low sulfur amino acid content. Collagen is unique in that it is the major body protein that contains hydroxyproline (elastin contains small amounts). The principal constituent of collagen is tropocollagen, a three-stranded coiled rod that participates in fiber formation and contributes to the electron microscopy periodicity by its quarter stagger overlap. Tropocollagen is made up of three 1,000 amino acid polypeptide chains, two of which are similar (α1) and one different (α2). The proportions of the α1 and α2 chains and minor variations in their composition permit the differentiation of the collagens found in different parts of the body and possibly in different diseases (see Table 46-1).

The second structural protein is *elastin,* which is a refractile fibril with an x-ray diffraction pattern differing from that of collagen. It is characterized by a high content of nonpolar amino acids, particularly valine, and recently desmosine and isodesmosine have been described as unique components. The third structural protein is *reticulin,* which many believe to represent merely young or immature collagen, since it has a similar appearance on electron microscopy. Others classify reticulin as a separate fiber on the basis of its light microscopic tinctorial properties (that is, positive staining with the periodic acid–Schiff reagent and positive silver staining).

Nonstructural Matrix or Ground Substance

Nonstructural matrix or ground substance is primarily mucopolysaccharide. Mucopolysaccharides are high-molecular-weight carbohydrate-containing compounds that are made up of equimolecular parts of hexosamine and hexuronic acids. Most of the mucopolysaccharides are sulfated, but one very common one, hyaluronic acid, is not. Electrolytes, proteins, carbohydrates, and other substances are also present in the extracellular matrix.

Blood Vessels

Another major component of the connective tissue is its vascular bed — blood vessels of various types whose reactivity is significant in many of the connective tissue diseases.

The Synovial Space

The synovial space and its lining, both of mesenchymal origin, are specialized types of connective tissue. The synovial membrane is an imperfect lining and allows a direct connection between synovial fluid and the connective tissue to be maintained throughout life.

Table 46-1. Classification of Collagen into Types

Type	Location	Composition
Type I collagen	Bone, skin, and tendon	$[\alpha 1\ (I)]_2\ \alpha 2$
Type II collagen	Cartilage	$[\alpha 1\ (II)]_3$
Type III collagen	Fetal skin, aorta, and uterus	$[\alpha 1\ (III)]_3$
Type IV collagen	Basement membrane	$[\alpha 1\ (IV)]_3$

Etiology of Connective Tissue Diseases

All diseases of connective tissue manifest themselves in the system of cells, structural proteins, nonstructural matrix, blood vessels, and joints just described. It is because of the ubiquitous nature of these elements that the various clinical disorders are indeed often systemic and overlapping. The etiology of the various connective tissue diseases is unknown. Numerous concepts, however, have been considered.

DISORDERS OF METABOLISM

It was believed for a short time (especially when the rapid suppression of these disorders by the adrenocortical steroids became evident) that a hormonal deficiency might be present in one or more of the connective tissue diseases. Studies to date have not demonstrated this to be the case. Abnormalities in the metabolism of tryptophan, and recently in that of histidine, have been suggested in rheumatoid arthritis, but their significance is not known.

INFECTION

For years many of the rheumatic disorders were regarded as infectious diseases, and indeed rheumatoid arthritis was first known as chronic infectious arthritis. There is no evidence at present that infection has a direct role in any of the inflammatory connective tissue diseases. There is suspicion, however, that the ultimate trigger that causes the production of rheumatoid factors, antinuclear antibodies, and other antibodies found in the blood of these patients may indeed be an infectious agent such as a virus or *Mycoplasma.* While there is no proof of this theory, it is interesting to compare the history and clinical picture of a disease such as syphilis with those of rheumatoid arthritis or SLE. Syphilis, a disorder affecting skin, heart, nervous system, and many other organs and characterized by a positive serologic reaction (Wassermann antibody), is known to be secondary to infection with a spirochete. Much of the same (except for the identification of a specific agent) can be said about rheumatoid arthritis.

ALLERGY

Immune mechanisms may be involved in the pathogenesis of the connective tissue diseases, although there is some controversy as to whether primary hypersensitivity (production of humoral antibody) or delayed hypersensitivity (tuberculin-type allergy) has the more important role (see Chap. 45).

Primary hypersensitivity has been shown to be the principal mechanism involved in experimental serum sickness. Antigen-antibody complexes tend to localize on the basement membranes of blood vessels and renal glomeruli. Complement is then activated, and the peak severity of the vascular lesions corresponds in time to the elimination of circulating antigen. The varied patterns of involvement mimic features of polyarteritis nodosa, rheumatoid arthritis, and SLE, although in these conditions there is no confirmation of a causative antigen and the clinical course is more protracted. Acute rheumatic fever also shares many features in common with experimental serum sickness, in that foreign antigens (streptococci) invade the host, vasculitis and fibrinoid lesions develop in connective tissue, specific circulating antibodies are produced following a latent period, and finally, the lesions heal when immune complexes are eliminated from the system.

Cell-mediated or delayed hypersensitivity represents a second type of immunologic reaction in which, in contrast to serum sickness, humoral antibody may not be present and the lesions become manifest within 24 to 48 hours after injection of the antigenic material. Plasma cells and bone-marrow-derived lymphocytes (B cells), which are mainly responsible for immunoglobulin synthesis, do not appear to be primarily involved in the production of delayed hypersensitivity. On the contrary, cell-transfer studies have demonstrated that viable thymus-derived lymphocytes (T cells) are mediators in this reaction. Several investigators have now confirmed that the ability to produce tuberculin-type reactions against foreign antigen is retained by agammaglobulinemic subjects. Support for the theory that delayed hypersensitivity

plays an important pathogenetic role in certain diseases is found in the observations that rheumatoid arthritis, dermatomyositis, scleroderma, and diffuse vascular inflammatory disease all occur with increased frequency in patients with agammaglobulinemia, and further, that specific alterations in delayed hypersensitivity and in T cell function occur in certain of the connective tissue disorders.

AUTOIMMUNITY

The concept that autoimmunity may be related to the etiology of the connective tissue diseases deserves consideration. The presence of antibodies to autologous immunoglobulin G (rheumatoid factors) in rheumatoid arthritis, and the presence of antibodies to cell membrane nuclear and cytoplasmic components in SLE, may indicate some derangement of the "self-recognition" mechanism in these diseases. Studies in animals have demonstrated that autoimmune disease can be produced by sensitization with an appropriate antigen under certain conditions. It is notable that in this group of experimental disease models (which includes allergic encephalomyelitis, experimental thyroiditis, and experimental aspermatogenesis) the pathologic lesions appear to be the result of delayed rather than primary hypersensitivity to the autologous antigen. H. S. Lawrence has proposed that certain autoimmune disorders may arise after a foreign agent (X) produces an alteration of the host's tissue so that the host's immune mechanism is directed against itself plus the exogenous agent (self + X). According to Lawrence's postulate, delayed hypersensitivity can then be looked upon as a reaction against "self + X." He suggests that the self + X reaction constitutes a type of homograft rejection and that autoimmune phenomena represent a similar sequence of events. Other theories of autoimmunity propose (1) proliferation of "forbidden clones" of immunologically competent cells, (2) release of sequestered antigens, and (3) loss of suppressor activity by subpopulations of circulating T lymphocytes.

Despite these interesting concepts, it must be pointed out that none of the connective tissue diseases has yet been proved to be autoimmune in origin. Criteria that must be fulfilled before any human disease is considered an autoimmune disorder include not only positive identification of free circulating or cell-

bound autoantibodies, but also successful direct transfer of the disease from host to recipient by antibody-
containing serum or by immunologically stimulated
lymphoid cells.

GENETIC FACTORS
It is known that certain connective tissue diseases have
a greater than expected familial incidence. However,
no simple mendelian patterns of inheritance are discernible, and genetic studies on the various connective
tissue diseases have been limited to twins, families,
and occasionally populations. The studies of leukocyte antigen groups (HL-A) in transplantation immunology have been extended to a variety of connective
tissue diseases, and several striking correlations have
been found. The most dramatic has been the association of the HL-A group B-27 with ankylosing spondylitis in 95 percent of cases, and its further association with a wide variety of diseases characterized by
sacroiliitis.

LYSOSOMES
Abnormal lysosomal function and increased proteolytic enzyme activity (e.g., collagenase) probably play
a major role in the pathogenesis of certain connective
tissue diseases. Lysosomes are a heterogeneous group
of cytoplasmic inclusions that contain a number of
acid hydrolases such as acid phosphatase. It is known
that when cells are injured, these enzymes are released
into the surrounding fluids and act upon appropriate
substrates. The lysosomes can be seen in electron
micrographs as discrete inclusion bodies and can be
stained by means of electron histochemical techniques. Their high content of destructive enzymes
has led some to call them "suicide bags." Since these
enzymes damage connective tissue components, and
since SLE can be clinically activated by sunlight and
symptomatically relieved by adrenocortical steroids,
several investigators have studied the effects of ultraviolet irradiation on lysosomes. They postulate that
in the pathogenesis of lupus, lysosomes are released
locally, causing tissue destruction. It is possible that
these lysosomes are activated by sunlight and that one
of the major pharmacologic effects of cortisone is the
protection of lysosomes against injury, thus retarding
release of their potentially harmful enzymes.

**Nomenclature and Classification of Diseases
of Joints and Connective Tissue**
Despite the generalizations made above, there are a
great many specific disorders affecting joints and
connective tissue. A tentative classification has
recently been provided by a Committee of the
American Rheumatism Association:

I. Polyarthritis of unknown etiology
  A. Rheumatoid arthritis
  B. Juvenile rheumatoid arthritis (including Still's disease)
  C. Ankylosing spondylitis
  D. Psoriatic arthritis
  E. Reiter's syndrome
  F. Others
II. "Connective tissue" disorders (acquired)
  A. Systemic lupus erythematosus
  B. Progressive systemic sclerosis (scleroderma)
  C. Polymyositis and dermatomyositis
  D. Necrotizing arteritis and other forms of vasculitis
    1. Polyarteritis nodosa
    2. Hypersensitivity angiitis
    3. Wegener's granulomatosis
    4. Takayashu's (pulseless) disease
    5. Cogan's syndrome
    6. Giant cell arteritis (including polymyalgia rheumatica)
  E. Amyloidosis
  F. Others
    (See also Rheumatoid arthritis, I, A; Sjögren's syndrome, VI, G)
III. Rheumatic fever
IV. Degenerative joint disease (osteoarthritis, osteoarthrosis)
  A. Primary
  B. Secondary
V. Nonarticular rheumatism
  A. Fibrositis
  B. Intervertebral disk and low back syndromes
  C. Myositis and myalgia
  D. Tendinitis and peritendinitis (bursitis)
  E. Tenosynovitis
  F. Fasciitis
  G. Carpal tunnel syndrome

H. Others
(See also Shoulder-hand syndrome, VIII, C)
VI. Diseases with which arthritis is frequently associated
   A. Sarcoidosis
   B. Relapsing polychondritis
   C. Schönlein-Henoch purpura
   D. Ulcerative colitis
   E. Regional enteritis
   F. Whipple's disease
   G. Sjögren's syndrome
   H. Familial Mediterranean fever
   I. Others
   (See also Psoriatic arthritis, I, D)
VII. Diseases associated with known infectious agents
   A. Bacterial
      1. Gonococcus
      2. Meningococcus
      3. Pneumococcus
      4. *Streptococcus*
      5. *Staphylococcus*
      6. *Salmonella*
      7. *Brucella*
      8. *Streptobacillus moniliformis* (Haverhill fever)
      9. *Mycobacterium tuberculosis*
      10. *Treponema pallidum* (syphilis)
      11. *Treponema pertenue* (yaws)
      12. Others
      (See also Rheumatic fever, III)
   B. Rickettsial
   C. Viral
      1. Rubella
      2. Mumps
      3. Viral hepatitis
      4. Others
   D. Fungal
   E. Parasitic
VIII. Traumatic and/or neurogenic disorders
   A. Traumatic arthritis (the result of direct trauma)
   B. Neuropathic arthropathy (Charcot's joint)
      1. Syphilis (tabes dorsalis)
      2. Diabetes mellitus (diabetic neuropathy)
      3. Syringomyelia

4. Myelomeningocele
5. Congenital insensitivity to pain (including familial dysautonomia)
6. Others
C. Shoulder-hand syndrome
D. Mechanical derangement of joints
E. Others
(See also Degenerative joint disease, IV; Carpal tunnel syndrome, V, G)
IX. Disorders associated with known or strongly suspected biochemical or endocrine abnormalities
   A. Gout
   B. Chondrocalcinosis articularis ("pseudogout")
   C. Alkaptonuria (ochronosis)
   D. Hemophilia
   E. Sickle cell disease and other hemoglobinopathies
   F. Agammaglobulinemia (hypogammaglobulinemia)
   G. Gaucher's disease
   H. Hyperparathyroidism
   I. Acromegaly
   J. Thyroid acropachy
   K. Hypothyroidism
   L. Scurvy (hypovitaminosis C)
   M. Hyperlipoproteinemia type II (xanthoma tuberosum and tendinosum)
   N. Fabry's disease (angiokeratoma corporis diffusum or glycolipid lipidosis)
   O. Hemochromatosis
   P. Others
   (See also Inherited and congenital disorders, XII)
X. Neoplasms
   A. Synovioma
   B. Primary juxtaarticular bone tumors
   C. Metastatic malignant tumors
   D. Leukemia
   E. Multiple myeloma
   F. Benign tumors of articular tissue
   G. Others
   (See also Hypertrophic osteoarthropathy, XIII, I)
XI. Allergy and drug reactions
   A. Arthritis due to specific allergens (e.g.,

serum sickness)
B. Arthritis due to drugs
C. Others
 (See also Systemic lupus erythematosus, II,
 A, for drug-induced lupus-like syndromes,
 e.g., hydralazine and procainamide syn-
 dromes; Hypersensitivity angiitis, II, D, 2)
XII. Inherited and congenital disorders
A. Marfan's syndrome
B. Homocystinuria
C. Ehlers-Danlos syndrome
D. Osteogenesis imperfecta
E. Pseudoxanthoma elasticum
F. Cutis laxa
G. Mucopolysaccharidoses (including Hurler's
 syndrome)
H. Arthrogryposis multiplex congenita
I. Hypermobility syndromes
J. Myositis (or fibrodysplasia) ossificans
 progressiva
K. Tumoral calcinosis
L. Werner's syndrome
M. Congenital dysplasia of the hip
N. Others
 (See also Disorders associated with
 known or strongly suspected biochem-
 ical or endocrine abnormalities, IX)
XIII. Miscellaneous disorders
A. Pigmented villonodular synovitis and
 tenosynovitis
B. Behçet's syndrome
C. Erythema nodosum
D. Relapsing panniculitis (Weber-Christian
 disease)
E. Avascular necrosis of bone
F. Juvenile osteochondritis
G. Osteochondritis dissecans
H. Erythema multiforme (Stevens-Johnson
 syndrome)
I. Hypertrophic osteoarthropathy
J. Multicentric reticulohistiocytosis
K. Disseminated lipogranulomatosis (Farber's
 disease)
L. Familial lipochrome pigmentary arthritis
M. Tietze's syndrome
N. Thrombotic thrombocytopenic purpura
O. Others

Polyarthritis of Unknown Etiology

RHEUMATOID ARTHRITIS
Rheumatoid arthritis is a chronic systemic inflammatory disease of unknown etiology. It is characterized
by symmetrical involvement of the small peripheral
joints, the presence of rheumatoid factors and, in
some patients, rheumatoid nodules.

Classification of Diagnostic Criteria
Most difficulties in diagnosis concern not patients
with classic rheumatoid arthritis but those who have
signs or symptoms placing them in categories that
have variously been described as possible, probable,
early, mild, borderline, overlapping, or the like. To
ensure some degree of uniformity in classification
among different observers, the American Rheumatism
Association has proposed a number of diagnostic criteria consisting of eleven possible requirements and
twenty possible exclusions.

Requirements. According to these criteria, a patient
cannot be considered to have definite rheumatoid
arthritis unless he has had at least five of the following eleven findings:

1. Morning stiffness
2. Joint tenderness or pain on motion (observed by
 a physician) in at least one joint
3. Swelling (soft tissue thickening or fluid, not bony
 overgrowth alone, observed by a physician)
4. Swelling of at least one other joint (interval of
 not more than 3 months, free of joint symptoms
 between the two joint involvements, observed
 by a physician)
5. Symmetrical simultaneous joint swelling (observed
 by a physician)
6. Subcutaneous nodules (observed by a physician)
 over bony prominences, on extensor surfaces, or
 in juxtaarticular areas
7. X-ray changes typical of rheumatoid arthritis
 (must include at least juxtaarticular osteoporosis)
8. Synovial fluid analysis that demonstrates a poor
 mucin precipitate (with shreds and cloudy
 solution)
9. Positive result of agglutination test (demonstration of rheumatoid factors by any method that

in any laboratory has been positive in not over 5 percent of normal controls)

10. Characteristic histologic changes in synovial membrane, with three or more of the following findings:
    a. Marked villous hypertrophy
    b. Proliferation of superficial synovial cells, often palisaded
    c. Marked infiltration of chronic inflammatory cells with a tendency to form lymphoid nodules
    d. Deposition of compact fibrin either on surface or interstitially
    e. Foci of cell necrosis
11. Characteristic histologic changes in nodules, showing granulomatous foci with:
    a. A central zone of cell necrosis
    b. A concentric area containing proliferative fixed cells, often palisaded
    c. Peripheral fibrosis and chronic inflammatory cell infiltration, predominantly perivascular

An awareness of these criteria is mandatory if one is to assess adequately the patient who presents with joint involvement. Since patients may have disease of varying severity, not all are classifiable as having definite rheumatoid arthritis. For this reason, it is considered acceptable to label certain patients as having "probable" (when three or four criteria are present) or even "possible" (when two criteria are present) rheumatoid arthritis.

Exclusions. Since findings in rheumatoid arthritis are known to overlap those of related connective tissue disorders and a variety of other diseases, a number of exclusions have arbitrarily been added to the criteria. If any exclusion is present, a classification of rheumatoid arthritis should not be made. These exclusions actually delineate disorders which in practice should always be considered in the differential diagnosis of any patient who presents with joint symptoms. The exclusions are listed below:

1. The typical butterfly rash of systemic lupus erythematosus
2. A high concentration of LE cells

3. Histologic evidence of polyarteritis nodosa
4. Weakness of neck, trunk, or pharyngeal muscles or persistent muscle swelling of dermatomyositis
5. Scleroderma
6. A clinical picture characteristic of rheumatic fever
7. A clinical picture characteristic of acute gouty arthritis
8. Tophi
9. A clinical picture consistent with infectious arthritis
10. Tubercle bacilli in the joints or histologic evidence of joint tuberculosis
11. A clinical picture characteristic of Reiter's syndrome
12. A clinical picture consistent with the shoulder-hand syndrome
13. A clinical picture characteristic of hypertrophic pulmonary osteoarthropathy
14. A clinical picture characteristic of neuropathy (Charcot's joint)
15. Homogentisic acid in the urine detectable by alkalization
16. Histologic evidence of sarcoid
17. Multiple myeloma
18. Characteristic skin lesions of erythema nodosum
19. Leukemia or lymphoma
20. Agammaglobulinemia

In reviewing these exclusions, it becomes apparent that in each of the syndromes specifically mentioned a synovitis may occur that mimics the typical joint manifestations of rheumatoid arthritis. This list also includes some entities that could be considered as variants of rheumatoid arthritis (for example, in agammaglobulinemia a clinical picture entirely consistent with rheumatoid arthritis occurs in approximately one-third of reported cases). Other more widely accepted variants of rheumatoid arthritis are considered to be:

1. Juvenile rheumatoid arthritis
2. Felty's syndrome
3. Ankylosing (rheumatoid) spondylitis
4. Psoriatic arthritis
5. Arthritis associated with inflammatory intestinal disease
6. Intermittent hydrarthrosis
7. Palindromic rheumatism

Etiology

The cause of rheumatoid arthritis is unknown. Although it possesses many of the features of an infectious disease, there is to date no evidence to support the theory that organisms actually invade joints, despite recent direct efforts to isolate infectious agents (viruses or mycoplasmas). The observations of a number of investigators did much to advance the theory that rheumatoid arthritis and other related diseases might be due to hypersensitivity, in that typical pathologic lesions revealed vasculitis, fibrinoid deposition, granulomas and, often, lymphoid hyperplasia.

More recently, attention has been focused on the role of rheumatoid factors in the pathogenesis of rheumatoid arthritis. Though possessing properties of autoantibodies (against immunoglobulin G), they do not themselves appear to be harmful, as evidenced by experiments in which rheumatoid factors have been transfused into the circulation of normal volunteers without untoward effects. In addition, asymptomatic relatives of patients with rheumatoid arthritis may have high titers of rheumatoid factors in their serum, whereas agammaglobulinemic patients, though prone to develop rheumatoid arthritis, lack rheumatoid factors along with other types of immunoglobulins. In addition to the abnormalities in humoral immunity, there is now abundant evidence for the importance of cell-mediated immunity in rheumatoid arthritis, including (1) the presence of a polyarthritis similar to rheumatoid arthritis in children with agammaglobulinemia; (2) reports of striking clinical improvement in patients with rheumatoid arthritis following removal of lymphocytes by thoracic duct drainage; (3) the finding of T cell predominance in the rheumatoid synovium; (4) impaired lymphocyte transformation in the presence of plant lectins such as concanavallin A and phytohemagglutinin; and (5) the discovery that adjuvant-induced chronic inflammatory arthritis in experimental animals can be passively transferred by viable lymphoid cells but not by sera and is dependent on intact T cell function.

Pathologic Changes

The lesions in rheumatoid arthritis may be proliferative (synovitis, serositis, uveitis), necrotizing (nodule), or vascular (vasculitis in blood vessels of any size). The earliest joint change is swelling and congestion of the synovial membrane and the underlying connective tissue, which become infiltrated with polymorphonuclear leukocytes, lymphocytes, and macrophages. There is usually a concomitant increase in volume of the synovial fluid. At this stage the pathologic process is still reversible, and no permanent change in the joint has yet taken place.

If the disease progresses past this stage, hypertrophy of the synovial membrane, with proliferation of villi, develops. The external capsular layer becomes thickened, pannus is formed, and the cartilage disappears (seen by x-ray as narrowing of the joint space). By means of the pannus, firm fibrous adhesions form across the joint space, and small subchondral bone cysts situated just under the subchondral plate break through to form erosions. Owing to irregular "scarring" of the fibrous tissue in the capsule, and the patient's adoption of the position of flexion for relief of pain, deformities and subluxations occur. Periarticular muscle atrophy and synovial sheath effusions are also frequent at this time. Finally, the joint space may be completely obliterated as fibrous and bony ankyloses develop.

In addition to lesions of the synovial membrane and the formation of the rheumatoid nodule (for histologic appearance see requirement No. 11), involvement of other connective tissue such as tendons, bursae, muscles, and sclera is not uncommon in rheumatoid arthritis. Hyperplasia of lymph nodes may occur, and when it is associated with splenomegaly, the condition is called Felty's syndrome. Pericarditis is found at autopsy in more than one-third of patients studied; other cardiac abnormalities found in rheumatoid arthritis include focal areas of nonspecific myocarditis, granulomatous valvulitis, and coronary arteritis. Vasculitis may be widespread, and it has been suggested that severe vascular changes occur more frequently in patients treated with large doses of corticosteroids. Amyloidosis is found in approximately 25 percent of the patients examined at autopsy.

Epidemiology

The prevalence (that is, the number of people with a

disease at any given moment) of rheumatoid arthritis has been estimated from several population studies to be between 2 and 4 percent, but a more realistic prevalence of "definite" rheumatoid arthritis is probably closer to 5 cases per 1,000 normal population. The incidence (the number of cases of a disease becoming clinically evident within a specified period of time) is not known. There may be large numbers of mild cases of polyarthritis which occur and then remit quickly without coming to a physician's attention. If this is so, then rheumatoid arthritis may be a common disease, often of subclinical nature, with only the more severe cases being brought to attention. The average age at onset is about 40, but the disease can occur at all ages. About 5 percent of cases occur before the age of 5. No reason for this low frequency in early childhood has yet been established, although it may be relevant that this is not characteristic of diseases known to be solely infectious in origin. The available data, drawn from hospital and population studies, suggest that there is an increased incidence of rheumatoid arthritis in women at and following the menopause. Women appear to be affected three times more commonly than men. Some studies have shown a slight familial aggregation of rheumatoid arthritis, but recently other studies have failed to confirm these findings and have shown that the distribution of the disease in families does not fit any single genetic hypothesis. Rheumatoid arthritis is sometimes precipitated by and often aggravated in emotional disturbances. Few detailed psychological and psychiatric studies have been reported.

Clinical Features

Constitutional. Patients with rheumatoid arthritis may have manifestations of the disease prior to the onset of actual joint pain or swelling. This prodromal phase is characterized by fatigue, malaise, anorexia, paresthesia, or low-grade fever. The fatigue associated with rheumatoid arthritis is often very noticeable, usually coming on in early afternoon or, in severe cases, in late morning. Joint stiffness is a major source of complaint, being most pronounced in the morning immediately on waking. The duration of morning stiffness and the degree of fatigability are often directly proportional to the activity of the joint dis-

ease as indicated by the number of swollen or painful peripheral joints.

Joints. Initially the small joints of the hands and feet tend to be involved more frequently than the large joints (elbows, shoulders, knees, and hips). Sometimes the onset is monoarticular, and a period of months may elapse before other joints are affected. The disease tends to be symmetrical, affecting the same joints on each side, but every diarthrodial joint of the body, including the temporomandibular, the sternoclavicular, the cricoarytenoid, and the apophyseal, may be involved at some stage. The affected joints are usually enlarged (due to soft tissue swelling or effusions), tender, and painful on motion, and they may be red and warm. Periarticular muscle atrophy may develop with surprising rapidity, and weakening of capsules and ligaments may lead to subluxations and deformities. Spontaneous rupture of an inflamed Baker's cyst into the popliteal space and hence to the posterior calf frequently mimics the clinical features of acute thrombophlebitis of the lower leg.

Other Systems. Despite its predilection for the joints, tendon sheaths, and muscles, rheumatoid arthritis frequently produces symptoms and signs indicative of involvement in other systems. Although usually clinically silent throughout life, cardiac lesions of various types can be shown by autopsy to occur in at least half of the patients with rheumatoid arthritis. Vasculitis may be widespread, and involvement of coronary arteries may lead to death in some cases. Valvular heart disease, myocardial conduction defects, arrhythmias, and pericarditis may occur more commonly than was previously thought. Vasomotor abnormalities are also common, and many patients exhibit sweaty, cold, clammy, and often cyanotic extremities, Raynaud's phenomenon, and paresthesia. Neuropathy occurs occasionally in rheumatoid arthritis and is also probably secondary to vasculitis.

Rheumatoid arthritis is perhaps the most common cause, excluding pregnancy, of palmar erythema. Other skin manifestations include erythematous morbilliform eruptions and an increased incidence of psoriasis in association with rheumatoid arthritis. The eye may be the site of extensive involvement and may show uveitis, keratoconjunctivitis (part of Sjögren's syndrome), scleromalacia perforans, or band keratopathy. Pulmonary diffusion defects may be more common in rheumatoid arthritis than was previously suspected, and extensive nonspecific fibrous lesions occur in the lungs of patients with rheumatoid arthritis who are exposed to dust, for example, in coal miners (Caplan's syndrome). Except for amyloidosis, no specific renal lesion has been identified. Secondary amyloidosis is a complication of rheumatoid arthritis in 5 to 15 percent of patients. Its appearance does not clearly relate to the severity, duration, or any other definable aspect of the disease.

Laboratory Findings
In rheumatoid arthritis, laboratory data will often mirror the degree of constitutional involvement as evidenced by hypochromic anemia, mild polymorphonuclear leukocytosis, elevated erythrocyte sedimentation rate, and change in plasma proteins. In the acute phases of the disease there may be a rise in the alpha globulins (hence the C-reactive protein elevation), but as the disease becomes more chronic there is almost always a hyperglobulinemia reflecting increases in both the 7S and 19S immunoglobulins.

Rheumatoid Factors (Antiimmunoglobulins). Rheumatoid factors have been shown to be serum proteins of relatively high molecular weight (approximately 900,000), which by ultracentrifugation possess a sedimentation constant of 19 Svedberg units. In vivo, rheumatoid factors circulate as a complex with autologous immunoglobulin G (IgG) to form a soluble 22S macromolecule (Fig. 46-1A). There are other anti-IgG factors belonging primarily to the IgG and IgA classes that have serologic properties different from those of classic rheumatoid factors. In vitro, rheumatoid factors react with homologous and autologous immunoglobulin as well as with immunoglobulin from other species. The nature of this reaction suggests that rheumatoid factors represent antibodies to the host's own antigen-antibody complexes, with cross reactivity to immunoglobulin from other humans and from other species.

Rheumatoid factors can be demonstrated in the serum of most patients with progressive and severe rheumatoid arthritis. They are detected by means of several specific tests: the latex fixation test, the bentonite flocculation test, and the sensitized sheep red blood cell agglutination test. In the two former tests (Fig. 46-1B), the serum to be tested is added to inert carrier particles that have been coated with pooled Cohn fraction II human gamma globulin. If the test is positive, visible flocculation of the carrier particles will occur. In the sensitized sheep red cell agglutination test (Fig. 46-1C), the sheep cells are sensitized by a subagglutinating dose of rabbit amboceptor (incomplete rabbit antibody), and agglutination occurs when serum containing significant titers of rheumatoid factors is added.

Unfortunately for diagnostic purposes, rheumatoid factors are not present exclusively in the serum of patients with rheumatoid arthritis; they occur in a number of disorders, including the remaining connective tissue diseases (especially SLE), hepatitis, leprosy, syphilis, subacute bacterial endocarditis, and chronic tuberculosis. All these conditions are associated with sustained tissue inflammation and necrosis. It is of interest that rheumatoid factors can be produced experimentally in animals by repeated antigenic stimulation with immunoglobulin or even with globulin. The characteristics of rheumatoid factors are summarized below:

1. They are immunoglobulins with S value of 19 (IgM).
2. They represent antibodies to human IgG in either native, denatured, or aggregated form, and they cross react with immunoglobulins of other species.
3. They can be produced experimentally in animals by sustained antigenic stimulation.
4. They originate in plasma cells of synovial membrane, spleen, lymph nodes, and rheumatoid nodules.
5. They occur in 70 to 95 percent of patients with rheumatoid arthritis; they are more common in patients with nodules, vasculitis, and destructive bony changes seen on x-ray.
6. They have a low incidence in the variants of rheumatoid arthritis (ankylosing spondylitis, psoriatic arthritis, juvenile rheumatoid arthritis).
7. They have a high incidence in other connective

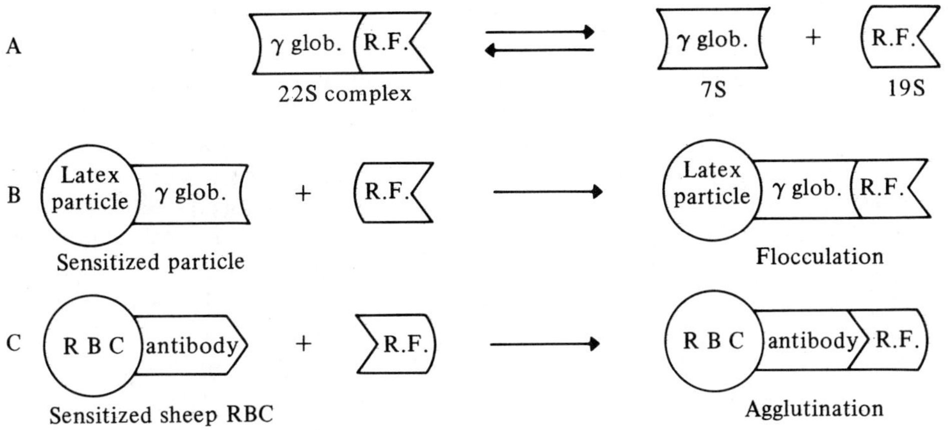

Figure 46-1. Mechanism of the latex fixation and sheep red cell agglutination tests. A. Rheumatoid factors (RF) circulate as soluble complexes formed by interaction of 19S macroglobulin and autologous 7S gamma globulin (γ glob.). B. Latex particles coated with heterologous 7S gamma globulin combine with rheumatoid factors as demonstrated by visible flocculation. C. Sheep red blood cells (RBC) coated with incomplete antibody (rabbit 7S gamma globulin) combine with rheumatoid factors to form visible agglutinates.

tissue diseases and in chronic inflammatory disorders (syphilis, leprosy, hepatitis).

8. They may antedate clinical disease; they may vary with the severity of disease and treatment; and they are not incompatible with good health.

Joint Fluid. Changes in the joint fluid of patients with rheumatoid arthritis reflect the degree of inflammation in the synovial membrane. The fluid is usually nonviscous and cloudy, and the mucin clot forms poorly in dilute acetic acid. Its white cell count is usually moderately elevated (generally about 19,000 cells per cubic millimeter), but it can vary between 1,000 and 100,000. The cells are predominantly polymorphonuclear, and many cells contain inclusions, some of which have been shown by immunofluorescent techniques to consist of rheumatoid factors. Because it represents an inflammatory exudate, synovial fluid in rheumatoid arthritis contains increased amounts of plasma proteins — for example, 7S and 19S immunoglobulins, fibrinogen, and hapto-

globin. IgG-anti-IgG "intermediate complexes" are particularly conspicuous in certain rheumatoid arthritis synovial fluids and correlate well with a marked depression in total hemolytic complement activity. Decreased levels of C4 and C2 suggest that the "classic" as well as "alternate" complement pathways may be activated in the synovial fluid of patients with rheumatoid arthritis. Increased levels of lysosomal enzymes (acid hydrolysates) and collagenase may contribute to the pannus formation and the destruction of articular cartilage. Synovial fluid sugar may be moderately decreased (20 mg per 100 ml) when compared simultaneously with the fasting blood sugar level.

Prognosis
The prognosis is impossible to predict in any one patient who develops rheumatoid arthritis. There is evidence that the future course is worse if rheumatoid factors are present in the patient's serum, if he has rheumatoid nodules, or if he delays going to a physician at the onset of the disease. Following appropriate treatment, about 25 percent of patients can return to their former occupations, and some of these may never have further evidence of the disease. About half the patients experience remissions alternating with exacerbations, with varying degrees of discomfort, disability, and joint damage over a period of years. In the remaining 25 percent, periods of remission are less pronounced and less prolonged, and patients in this group often become severely debilitated and disabled.

Treatment

The successful treatment of rheumatoid arthritis depends on the coordinated efforts of the physician, orthopedic surgeon, physiatrist, physiotherapist, occupational therapist, nurse, and social worker. The program of therapy must be carefully coordinated to meet the needs of each individual patient. In the absence of a specific cure, treatment of rheumatoid arthritis is aimed at suppressing inflammation, relieving pain, and preventing deformities. It is vital to institute treatment promptly, since there is good evidence that patients who are treated adequately during the first year of the disease stand the best chance of remission.

Bed Rest. It is recommended that during the acute phase the patient be hospitalized with complete bed rest until there are definite signs of improvement. How long this period of complete rest should last is a matter of some controversy, but recent studies indicate that prolonged hospitalization comparable to sanatorium therapy for acute tuberculosis some years ago may prove to be best for the patient in the long run.

Physiotherapy. The objective of physical therapy is to maintain proper posture and to achieve full power and range of motion in the joints. Beds should have firm mattresses, cages should be provided to remove heavy bedclothes from painful areas, and on no account should pillows be used to flex painful knees. Active exercises are designed to preserve normal muscle tone. Affected joints should also be passively exercised daily in order to prevent permanent contractures or limitation of motion. The application of heat prior to these exercises is often useful in relieving stiffness, diminishing muscle spasm, and improving the local circulation. As the patient improves, he should be taught to exercise his own joints and should continue these exercises as long as arthritis persists. Temporary splinting may be necessary to immobilize an acutely inflamed joint, to correct contractures, or to preserve a position of optimum efficiency.

Salicylates. Aspirin (0.6 to 1.0 gm 4 to 5 times per day) is still the mainstay of conservative management of rheumatoid arthritis and should be prescribed for every patient with the disease. Experimental studies in animals have demonstrated that aspirin acts as an antiinflammatory agent as well as an analgesic and antipyretic, and its antiinflammatory effects may explain how it relieves morning stiffness, reduces joint swelling and erythema, and lowers the sedimentation rate. Absorption of aspirin from the gastrointestinal tract may vary in different patients; for this reason, as well as to prevent toxic effects, serum salicylate levels should be determined at least initially in every patient who takes more than 3.0 gm of aspirin per day. Most patients can tolerate a serum level of 20 mg per 100 ml without troublesome symptoms of tinnitus, deafness, nausea, epigastric distress, or vomiting. Aspirin is a gastrointestinal irritant and should be prescribed with caution for patients who have a peptic ulcer diathesis. It also produces a reversible hepatotoxicity in certain patients, and allergic reactions in others, infrequently leading to urticaria (see Chap. 45). In patients who are unable to tolerate salicylates, a trial with other nonsteroid antiinflammatory drugs is indicated.

Chrysotherapy. Gold salts are advocated by some authorities for patients whose joints are red, hot, and tender, and who have failed to respond markedly to salicylate therapy. The compounds most frequently used, gold thiomalate and gold thioglucose, are water-soluble, contain 50 percent metallic gold, and are given intramuscularly.

The principal objections to chrysotherapy for rheumatoid arthritis are its considerable risk of toxicity and its limited long-term beneficial effects. The toxic manifestations include dermatitis, stomatitis, proctitis, albuminuria, hematuria, jaundice, purpura, aplastic anemia, agranulocytosis, and occasionally death. Gold accumulates in the body, and more than 80 percent of that given in the course of a 6-week period is retained in the tissues. If toxic effects develop, treatment with dimercaprol will result in prompt excretion of the metallic gold.

Antimalarials. Several controlled therapeutic trials have shown that certain antimalarial compounds have a moderate, but significant, beneficial effect in patients with rheumatoid arthritis. Hydroxychloroquine sulfate (200 mg daily) can be administered orally to most patients without undue upper gastrointestinal tract distress. Antimalarials, like gold salts, are poorly excreted and accumulate in the body, with an affinity for pigmented tissues. Toxic side effects are less serious than those with gold but include skin eruptions, alopecia and blanching of hair, headache, mental confusion, gastrointestinal distress, and most important, visual disturbance. Because of their predilection for pigmented areas, the antimalarials accumulate with time in the retina and iris. Early symptoms include reversible blurring of vision; a long-term hazard is the accumulation of the drug in the retina and potential visual impairment. Detailed ophthalmologic examination is now recommended at 6-month intervals for all patients receiving antimalarial therapy.

Steroids. During the initial and often acute phase of rheumatoid arthritis, steroid derivatives are rarely indicated, despite their dramatic antiinflammatory effects. It now is generally accepted that in spite of maximally tolerable, symptom-suppressing doses (e.g., 10 to 20 mg prednisone per day), joint destruction and deformity progress relentlessly.

The indications for steroids in rheumatoid arthritis include eye complications such as iritis, and the chronic inanition or the progressive downhill course seen in rare patients with apparent widespread rheumatoid vasculitis. Unfortunately, patients are all too often started on this treatment without due regard to the severity of the disease or the unfortunate consequences that may ensue from the therapy. The side effects of cortisol and related compounds are legion and include peptic ulcers; weight gain with redistribution of adipose tissue, producing moon facies and central obesity; acne; ecchymoses; hirsutism; diabetes mellitus; secondary infection; osteoporosis; psychoses; cataracts; myopathy; arteritis; and aseptic necrosis of bone.

The intraarticular injection of corticosteroids has been advocated by some in the treatment of acute inflammation that is confined to only one or two joints. Although this maneuver is occasionally useful, the benefit is usually temporary, and chronic injection of corticosteroids into the joint space may actually lead to development of a neuropathic joint, presumably due to excessive trauma resulting from interference with pain-sensitive defense mechanisms.

Nonsteroid Antiinflammatory Drugs. The major nonsteroid antiinflammatory drugs (NSAID) are the salicylates (e.g., aspirin or acetylsalicylic acid, sodium salicylate, choline salicylate), phenylbutazone, indomethacin, and a whole series of newer drugs, including ibuprofen, fenoprofen, naproxen, and tolmetin. These drugs are also analgesics and antipyretics, but their principal mode of action in rheumatoid arthritis probably depends on their ability to inhibit the synthesis of prostaglandin E2 and F2d. These two prostaglandins are mediators of inflammation and are found in measurable amounts in the synovial fluid of patients with rheumatoid arthritis. Aspirin and indomethacin also inhibit platelet aggregation, and it is conceivable that a decrease in thrombin-platelet interaction may decrease prostaglandin synthesis in some other way.

Other Therapeutic Agents. Other antirheumatic drugs, including penicillamine, have been used in the treatment of rheumatoid arthritis and appear to be of value for selected patients, particularly those unable to tolerate gold salts. Recently the use of immunosuppressives and antimetabolites has been advocated, but further study is needed because of the possibility of an increased tendency to neoplasia following prolonged administration of these agents.

JUVENILE RHEUMATOID ARTHRITIS
The concept that a distinct form of arthritis exists in childhood was advanced by Still in 1896. At present it is generally agreed that it would be wiser to drop the term *Still's disease* and to regard juvenile rheumatoid arthritis as a variant of rheumatoid arthritis. Although rheumatoid arthritis occurring before the age of 6 differs from the adult variety in several respects, careful studies have not revealed any differences between the two types that cannot be accounted for by the age of the patient.

Clinical Picture
Approximately 50 percent of patients with juvenile rheumatoid arthritis have a polyarthritis indistin-

guishable from that in adults. The onset is insidious, the small peripheral joints are commonly involved, and rheumatoid factors and subcutaneous nodules may be present. The cervical spine — and notably the apophyseal joints between C2 and C3 — is affected in many cases, and bony fusion may ultimately result in these areas. Disruption of the ossification centers and premature closure of the epiphyses alter bone growth near the affected joints (most strikingly at the temporomandibular joint), producing the receding chin and birdlike appearance of children with chronic juvenile rheumatoid arthritis.

In approximately 25 percent of juvenile patients the onset of arthritis may be explosive, characterized by a high fever that is often out of proportion to the severity of the arthritis. Skin rashes are common, the most characteristic being an evanescent, salmon-colored, morbilliform or maculopapular rash on the trunk and forearms. Nonarticular lesions occur in a sizable proportion of cases and include pleurisy and enlargement of the spleen, lymph nodes, and liver. Clinical laboratory abnormalities, which may be pronounced, include a profound anemia and a high white blood cell count (15,000 to 50,000 cells per cubic millimeter). Rheumatoid factors are usually absent, although they have been reported by workers using special inhibition tests or methods for detecting IgG-anti-IgG antibodies.

A third group of patients (about 25 percent) with juvenile rheumatoid arthritis have large joint involvement more than small joint involvement, with the knee presenting the initial symptoms in more than one-third of the patients. In these patients, four joints or less eventually develop pain and swelling (oligoarthritis), and there are only minimal systemic manifestations. On the other hand, one of the most dreaded complications of juvenile arthritis, band keratitis and uveitis, not infrequently accompanies oligoarthritis, and there is a significant (though unexplained) correlation with positive serologic tests for antinuclear antibodies in this form of arthritis.

Prognosis and Treatment
The prognosis for arthritis with an onset before puberty is somewhat better than for arthritis that develops after puberty. About half the juvenile

patients appear to have a complete remission, with no evidence of further disease activity. Less than one-sixth of the patients seen in hospitals or clinics progress to severe disability, although the remainder have disease that continues into adult life. Recent studies indicate that the development of amyloidosis is a problem in juvenile arthritis. Treatment is similar to that for the adult form of the disease, although orthopedic intervention may be required more often to prevent permanent deformities or contractures.

ANKYLOSING SPONDYLITIS
Ankylosing spondylitis (rheumatoid spondylitis; Marie-Strümpell disease) is a chronic arthritis of the spine, involving primarily the sacroiliac and apophyseal joints and adjacent soft tissues. Since more than 25 percent of patients with this disease ultimately acquire peripheral joint disease that is pathologically indistinguishable from rheumatoid arthritis, the disease had been considered by some to be a variant of rheumatoid arthritis. Most patients note the onset of symptoms before age of 30. Males are affected ten times more frequently than females. From 2 to 5 percent of relatives of patients with ankylosing spondylitis have been found to suffer from the same condition, indicating a greater familial aggregation than is found in rheumatoid arthritis.

A significant recent observation regarding ankylosing spondylitis is its association with the histocompatibility antigen, HL-A B27. Not only do more than 95 percent of patients with ankylosing spondylitis possess this genetic marker, but also approximately one-quarter of unselected "normal" blood donors who are HL-A B27 positive have signs and symptoms of chronic sacroiliac disease. A high association of this histocompatibility antigen has also been made with a variety of disorders characterized by sacroiliitis (e.g., Reiter's syndrome, granulomatous ileitis, uveitis).

With the exception of the predilection for bony ankylosis, the morphologic features of the proliferative chronic synovitis involving the diarthrodial joints of the spine are indistinguishable from those seen in rheumatoid arthritis. Inflammatory changes also occur in the intervertebral ligaments, as well as in cartilaginous joints such as the manubriosternal joint, the symphysis pubis, and the intervertebral disk.

Clinical Picture

In contrast to rheumatoid arthritis, constitutional symptoms in ankylosing spondylitis are usually mild. The first symptom is often back pain, which is unrelieved by rest and is often lessened by standing or walking. About 10 percent of patients may appear at first to have sciatica, but objective neurologic signs are rare. There is usually well-defined morning stiffness localized to the back. If the disease progresses, limitation of motion may become apparent not only in the lumbar area but also in the thoracic and cervical spine. Diminished chest expansion may lead to restrictive lung disease and increased susceptibility to pulmonary infections.

In at least half the patients with ankylosing spondylitis, peripheral joint disease never develops, but approximately one-quarter of the patients are said to manifest root joint disease (hips and shoulders) and another quarter have characteristic rheumatoid arthritis of the peripheral joints. Subcutaneous nodules rarely, if ever, complicate ankylosing spondylitis, but uveitis and urethritis occur with greater frequency than in rheumatoid arthritis. Aortic valvular lesions are found in from 1 to 4 percent of patients; if aortic incompetence ensues, it may result in cardiac enlargement, coronary insufficiency, and ultimately congestive heart failure.

Laboratory and X-ray Findings

The laboratory findings are nonspecific in ankylosing spondylitis. Elevation of the erythrocyte sedimentation rate is found in more than 80 percent of cases, and moderate elevation of proteins in the cerebrospinal fluid has been reported. There is a striking absence of rheumatoid factors in the serum. Proteinuria heralds the onset of a nephrotic syndrome resulting from amyloidosis in as many as 10 percent of patients with prolonged disease. The HL-A B27 histocompatibility antigen is present in 95 percent of patients (see earlier in this section).

The earliest articular lesions in ankylosing spondylitis are almost invariably detected by x-ray at the sacroiliac joints bilaterally. Osteoporosis is followed by erosions of the joint margin. Later, bone adjacent to the joint space becomes more dense, and finally complete ossification of the joint may occur. Similar changes are seen at the apophyseal joints, with involvement usually commencing in the lumbar spine and spreading cephalad to the cervical joints. All the interspinous ligaments tend to ossify, and erosions may appear on the symphysis pubis, ischial tuberosities, iliac margins, and sites of tendon insertions on the calcaneus, frequently in association with reactive sclerosis and fluffy proliferation of bone in adjacent areas.

Prognosis and Treatment

The overall prognosis for relief of pain and maintenance of function is generally good. About three-quarters of the patients are able to work full time, especially if they stay in light occupations.

Response to therapy is somewhat different in ankylosing spondylitis from that in rheumatoid arthritis. Gold salts, which provide symptomatic relief in many patients with peripheral arthritis, are not effective in the treatment of spondylitis. Radiotherapy, phenylbutazone (Butazolidin), and indomethacin, which are less useful in the treatment of rheumatoid arthritis, often provide dramatic relief for those patients with acute spondylitis. Radiotherapy, however, is rarely used except in the most refractory cases because of its potential to induce leukemia years later. Arthroplasty of the hip, often a useful corrective surgical procedure in rheumatoid arthritis, is rarely successful in ankylosing spondylitis because of rapid evolution of postoperative contractures and finally complete immobilization of the joint.

PSORIATIC ARTHRITIS

A small proportion of patients with psoriasis who acquire peripheral joint disease manifest a clinical picture that is classic for rheumatoid arthritis. Most cases are atypical, however, in that there is an unusual distribution of joint involvement, absence of rheumatoid factors in the serum, and often a distinctive radiologic appearance of the joints themselves.

Clinical Picture

In contrast to rheumatoid arthritis, in which the distal interphalangeal joints are not commonly involved, inflammatory changes in these joints may be the predominant or presenting features in psoriatic arthritis.

There tends to be a relatively asymmetrical distribution of arthritis in other peripheral joints, and changes in the hands and feet are remarkable for lack of ulnar deviation despite often gross resorptive changes at the metacarpal and metatarsal heads (arthritis mutilans). Ankylosis of the interphalangeal joints is more common in psoriatic than in rheumatoid arthritis, and a significant proportion of patients with arthritis and psoriasis exhibit changes at the sacroiliac joints that are indistinguishable from those observed in ankylosing spondylitis.

Laboratory and X-ray Findings
The laboratory abnormalities in patients with psoriatic arthritis do not differ significantly from those observed in other forms of inflammatory arthritis, except for the absence of rheumatoid factors in psoriatic patients. Recent studies have shown a multiple relationship of psoriatic arthropathy with HL-A antigens, and in patients with psoriasis alone, an increase of HL-A 13 as compared to controls. There is also a significant association with the HL-A B27 allele in psoriatic arthritis, especially in patients with sacroiliitis. Radiologically the association between psoriasis and arthritis can be suspected when any or all of the following abnormalities are seen: (1) absence of juxtaarticular osteoporosis despite marked erosive changes at the distal and proximal interphalangeal joints; (2) "penciling" of the metacarpal and metatarsal heads caused by severe bone resorption; (3) paradoxical widening of the joint space in the presence of erosions; (4) resorption of the distal phalangeal tuft; and (5) ankylosis of the interphalangeal joints.

Treatment
The therapy of arthritis associated with psoriasis is basically similar to that of rheumatoid arthritis. Drug reactions involving the skin are more frequent, however, and the use of gold salts and antimalarials is particularly limited. Systemic administration of corticosteroids is not advised because of the difficulties encountered when one attempts to reduce or discontinue maintenance therapy.

REITER'S SYNDROME
A clinical triad of arthritis, conjunctivitis, and urethritis constitutes Reiter's syndrome. Monoarticular arthritis occasionally occurs, but an asymmetrical polyarthritis with a predilection for the knees, ankles, and small joints of the feet is more frequent. The onset is often sudden, and the involved joints are red, hot, painful, and tender. Joint effusions are common, and synovial fluid analyses reveal turbid fluid, average white cell counts of 20,000 cells per cubic millimeter (60 percent polymorphonuclear leukocytes), and a poor mucin test.

Of the various polyarthritides of unknown etiology, the Reiter syndrome has the most features suggestive of an infectious origin. In addition to the striking relationship of the Reiter syndrome to postvenereal urethritis, outbreaks of the disease have been observed to follow epidemics of dysentery. Mycoplasmas have been isolated from the urogenital tract of patients with Reiter's syndrome, and in several instances these organisms were cultured from the joint fluid. Recently, the *Chlamydia* group of agents has been implicated in this condition. Arguments against an infectious etiology include the fact that the disease is confined almost entirely to males and that antibiotic therapy has proved to have little effect on it.

The conjunctivitis is of short duration and usually without sequelae; the discharge is either mucoid or purulent. Occasionally other eye complications including iritis, keratitis, or iridocyclitis may develop in association with the joint and genitourinary symptoms. The urethral discharge can be mucoid, purulent, or watery and contains many polymorphonuclear cells, but on Gram's stain it is negative for organisms. The finding of gonococci in the urethral smear does not rule out the possibility that the associated arthritis is of the Reiter type instead of being gonococcal in origin. Diarrhea may precede the clinical triad by several weeks; it is usually mild and nonbloody, lasts from 3 to 5 days, and is thought by some to be an integral part of the syndrome. Cutaneous lesions are frequently associated with the Reiter syndrome and may include keratodermia blennorrhagica, secondary purulent infection of the subungual keratoses, buccal or palatal plaques or ulcers, and balanitis circinata.

Although symptoms of the triad may develop

asynchronously over a period of months or years, the full syndrome usually develops within 10 to 14 days of onset. The disease is usually self-limited and subsides in 4 to 10 weeks, although it recurs in about 20 percent of patients. Occasionally it becomes chronic, in which case spinal involvement with sacroiliac changes is common. In this regard one should note that approximately 80 percent of patients with Reiter's syndrome have the HL-A B27 gene. Treatment is primarily symptomatic, although corticosteroids or phenylbutazone and other nonsteroid anti-inflammatory drugs may reverse the inflammatory articular signs in some cases. Other cases progress to a chronic arthritis despite all modes of therapy.

ARTHRITIS ASSOCIATED WITH INFLAMMATORY INTESTINAL DISEASE

Approximately 20 percent of patients with ulcerative colitis and 5 percent of patients with granulomatous enteritis develop polyarthritis. The clinical joint manifestations appear to be comparable in the two groups. Patients with Whipple's disease may also present with articular changes, and the characteristic rodlike PAS-positive forms have been found in the synovium.

Peripheral joint disease in patients with inflammatory intestinal disease is usually acute and migratory in nature, often involving the large joints and only rarely associated with residual joint damage. The arthritis usually appears after, but sometimes simultaneously with, the onset of colitis or enteritis, and then exacerbations of the underlying disorders and of the arthritis often, but not always, parallel one another. Erythema nodosum, uveitis, and pyoderma gangrenosum all seem to occur more frequently in arthritic patients with inflammatory bowel disease than in those without such disease.

There is good clinical evidence of an association between ulcerative colitis and ankylosing spondylitis. Genetic factors appear to be clustered in these two conditions and also in regional enteritis, and HL-A B27 is now established as a common ground among the three diseases.

SJÖGREN'S SYNDROME

Sjögren's syndrome is also a clinical triad consisting of rheumatoid arthritis, keratoconjunctivitis sicca (dry eyes), and xerostomia (dry mouth), all of which need not necessarily be present at one time. In a recent survey it was demonstrated that keratoconjunctivitis sicca and xerostomia may also be associated with SLE, polyarteritis nodosa, scleroderma, and polymyositis. Although the Sjögren syndrome is generally considered to be a benign disorder, the development of reticulum cell sarcomas has been noted in several patients with the syndrome. Histologic examination of the parotid and lacrimal glands (indistinguishable from the findings in Mikulicz's disease) demonstrates metaplasia of the epithelium of the ducts, forming a so-called myoepithelial island. Round cell infiltrations of lymphocytes and plasma cells are also seen.

Clinically, enlargement of the lacrimal glands and diminished tear production cause dry, irritated eyes. Both the Schirmer test (measurement of lacrimal gland secretion with filter paper) and rose bengal staining of the cornea and conjunctiva are used as diagnostic aids. Involvement of the salivary glands can be detected by a history of dryness of the lips and mouth, by hypertrophy of the salivary glands, and by a sialogram. Biopsy of the buccal or nasal mucosal membranes is used to confirm the diagnosis of Sjögren's syndrome. Widespread connective tissue involvement is common, with arthritis and myositis being the most prominent features. Involvement of the kidneys has recently been described.

High titers of rheumatoid factors are demonstrable in the serum of almost every patient with the syndrome, whether or not signs and symptoms of rheumatoid arthritis are present. Other serologic abnormalities that are frequently noted include increased immunoglobulin levels, a 70 percent incidence of antinuclear factors, and a 30 percent incidence of antithyroid antibodies.

The etiology of the Sjögren syndrome is unknown. Because of evidence of serologic abnormalities in relatives of patients with the syndrome as well as in the patients themselves, and because of the broad overlap of the disorder with other connective tissue diseases, it has been suggested that there is an abnormality in the development of the immunologic apparatus in these patients.

Connective Tissue Disorders

SYSTEMIC LUPUS ERYTHEMATOSUS

Systemic lupus erythematosus (SLE), also known as disseminated lupus erythematosus (DLE), is a chronic inflammatory disorder of unknown etiology, with naturally occurring remissions and exacerbations. It involves multiple body systems and is characterized by the presence of the lupus erythematosus (LE) cell, antinuclear antibodies, and circulating immune complexes in the serum. Systemic lupus erythematosus usually involves the skin (classically with a butterfly eruption over the malar eminences) and is often characterized by arthritis, serositis, vasculitis, and central nervous system disease. Renal involvement is a common, significant, and often ominous component of the disease.

Diagnostic Criteria

As in many other chronic multisystemic disorders of unknown etiology, precise diagnostic criteria for SLE are not available. The criteria listed below are more useful for purposes of classification than for bedside diagnosis; they will be most helpful in studies of the natural history of the disease, in epidemiologic surveys, and in drug trials. The approach to establishing criteria for SLE was different from the empiric method used with acute rheumatic fever. Approximately 250 patients with unequivocal SLE diagnosed by experienced rheumatologists were compared in regard to 74 specific items with similar numbers of patients with either possible SLE, definite rheumatoid arthritis, or other medical disorders. The 74 items were then analyzed individually and in selected combinations for sensitivity and specificity. According to these 74 criteria, a patient should not be classified as having definite SLE unless he has at least four of the following findings:

1. Facial erythema (butterfly rash)
2. Discoid lupus
3. Raynaud's phenomenon
4. Alopecia
5. Photosensitivity
6. Oral or nasopharyngeal ulceration
7. Arthritis without deformity
8. LE cells
9. Chronic false-positive serologic test for syphilis
10. Profuse proteinuria: greater than 3.5 gm per day
11. Cellular casts (in urine): may be red cell, hemoglobin, granular, tubular, or mixed
12. Pleuritis and/or pericarditis
13. Psychosis and/or convulsions
14. Hemolytic anemia and/or leukopenia and/or thrombocytopenia

At the time of the original data collection, sufficient data were not available to include items that recent advances suggest might be very helpful (e.g., antinuclear antibody testing, especially for anti-DNA antibodies; serum complement levels).

Etiology

Although an etiologic agent has not been identified in patients with SLE, a naturally occurring experimental model of SLE is found in the NZB/NZW hybrid mouse; this condition is most interesting because of its close resemblance to the human disease. Chronic viral infection has been demonstrated in these animals, and there is impressive, though inconclusive, evidence that murine oncogenic type C virus is a causative agent of this lupuslike syndrome. A naturally occurring multisystemic disease resembling human SLE has also been recognized in several breeds of dogs, and there is preliminary evidence that C type RNA viruses may be present in filtrates from affected tissues in these animals. Independent evidence obtained by different techniques in different laboratories shows that C type RNA virus antigens are present on the peripheral blood lymphocytes of certain patients with SLE and, as noted subsequently, cytoplasmic inclusions resembling the nucleocapsid of paramyxovirus have been seen in the kidney and skin of patients with SLE.

Perhaps the most striking pathogenic abnormality in SLE is the patient's propensity to form autoantibodies to cell nuclei, cell membranes, cytoplasmic ingredients, and plasma proteins. It can be argued that all the clinical and pathologic abnormalities in SLE are directly related to autoimmune phenomena: For example, the proliferative renal and skin lesions correlate well with the presence of circulating immune complexes and anti-DNA antibodies; the pronounced T cell and B cell impairment may be caused by the action of cell membrane lymphotoxins; and the hematologic complications are the result of unusually high titers of circulating anticoagulants, antiplatelet antibodies, and Coombs-positive hemolysins. The recent demonstration that T lymphocytes and brain tissue share common antigenic determinants also raises the intriguing possibility that many of the central nervous system abnormalities in SLE have an immunologic basis.

Pathology

On histologic examination of tissue sections, no specific abnormalities may be present. However, the most characteristic and possibly pathognomonic finding is the *hematoxylin body* — that is, the tissue equivalent of the LE cell — which is a round, smudgy, eosinophilic body that is larger than a nucleus, usually occurs in clusters, and is found in synovial membrane, heart, kidney, and almost any tissue of the body. Another well-known pathologic lesion is *fibrinoid,* a homogeneous eosinophilic material in the ground substance that resembles fibrin but that immunochemically has been shown to contain a variety of substances, including fibrin and gamma globulin; it is nonspecific in nature. Vasculitis, including necrotizing arteritis, is also occasionally found in SLE.

Renal lesions are common in SLE, and a wide spectrum of glomerular changes may occur. Mild involvement may be manifest by focal hypercellularity or by thickening of the basement membrane. With more severe involvement, generalized proliferative or membranous changes with focal fibrinoid, necrosis, and "wire loops" occur. Hematoxylin bodies, often associated with necrosis, are sometimes seen at autopsy, but rarely in biopsy specimens.

In recent years, increasing numbers of lupus kidney biopsy specimens have been studied by light and electron microscopy. The latter technique has demonstrated a number of electron-dense deposits both in the basement membrane and on each side of it, as well as other nonspecific pathologic changes. The presence of the dense deposits, together with the evidence obtained by immunofluorescent and elution techniques that immunoglobulins G and M, complement, DNA, and anti-DNA antibodies are present in

glomeruli in lupus nephritis, has led to the important hypothesis that the renal lesion is immunologically mediated and is related to antigen-antibody complexes. It has also been suggested that the dense deposits may be related to fibrin and its degradation products, and that intravascular coagulation abnormalities may be in part responsible for the lesions.

The characteristic finding in the spleen is the "onionskin" lesion, consisting of concentric rings of collagen laid down around the arterioles; this periarteriolar fibrosis is common but is not specific. The cardiac lesion is the sterile or nonbacterial verrucous endocarditis first noted by Libman and Sacks and known by their names. It consists of small endocardial vegetations, which may occur on several valves and in any chamber. The vegetations are made up of fibrin, platelets, and hematoxylin bodies. There may also be a valvulitis in SLE, and the interstitial connective tissue of the myocardium may show fibrinoid degeneration and occasionally inflammatory cells, although myocardial lesions are not extensive. Evidence of pericarditis is present in approximately 50 percent of patients.

The lungs in patients with lupus may show pleural lesions, basilar pneumonitis with atelectasis, or a mucinous edema. The liver rarely shows any specific lesion. The classic skin lesion is characterized by hyperkeratosis, keratotic plugging of the hair follicles, degeneration of the basal cell layer, edema of the cutis, dilatation of superficial capillaries, and a lymphocytic cellular infiltrate. The synovial membrane may show a layer of eosinophilic fibrinlike material on its surface without a significant synovial cell proliferation. The degree of inflammation varies. Blood vessels may have a wide variety of acute and chronic inflammatory lesions.

Epidemiology

Recent investigations show that SLE is a rather prevalent disorder with, in the majority of cases, a more benign outcome than previous studies had indicated. It is now thought that the overall prevalence of SLE is approximately one case per 1,000, and that women between the ages of 15 and 64 are at higher risk, with a prevalence of approximately one in 700. Blacks have SLE, whether systemic or chronic discoid, three times as frequently as the general population, and black women between the ages of 15 and 64 may have the condition as commonly as rheumatoid arthritis.

Clinical Features

Because of its very widespread manifestations, SLE may present findings in any organ system. One of the most classic features is a skin rash characterized by a diffuse, erythematous, butterfly-like eruption over the malar eminences of the face and the bridge of the nose. This rash usually blanches on pressure and is to be distinguished from the classic rash of discoid lupus, which is a raised, red, scaly eruption that may occur anywhere on the body, including the face. (There is increasing evidence that a small but definite proportion of patients with discoid lupus evolve into the classic picture of the disseminated disease. The supposition that discoid lupus usually represents the benign end of the spectrum of systemic lupus erythematosus is supported by the serologic findings of significant plasma protein and immunologic abnormalities in patients with the discoid variety.) Other skin lesions seen in patients with SLE include upper eyelid capillary telangiectasia, periungual erythema, red spots on the hands, capillary dilatation over the fingertips, and palmar erythema. Patients may report sensitivity to either sunlight or drugs.

The disease is characterized by spontaneous exacerbations and remissions. There may be constitutional manifestations such as fever, fatigue, generalized weakness, or weight loss. There is no characteristic pattern as the disease unfolds, and it may initially involve one or many organ systems. The arthritis is classically described as transient, and the joint pains and inflammation are said to leave few residua. However, the arthritis on rare occasions may be as severe and deforming as that of classic rheumatoid arthritis, although radiologically joint erosions are rare. There is no one clinical criterion for differentiating the arthritis of SLE from that of rheumatoid arthritis. Serositis, including pericarditis, is not uncommon in SLE and in a few cases may be accompanied by pericardial effusion, a serious complication that must be carefully watched for. Pleurisy with or without effusions is also common, as are a variety of focal or diffuse

(though usually transient) pulmonary infiltrates. Basilar pneumonitis with atelectasis is not unusual. One has to diagnose such lesions with care because SLE is very often complicated by bacterial infection, especially if the patient is taking corticosteroids. Acute sterile peritonitis as well as perisplenitis and perihepatitis have been noted; these conditions may be confused with an acute "surgical" abdomen.

Myocarditis occurs but is not a common clinical lesion. It is caused by a diffuse vasculitis involving the coronary arteries and is characterized by tachycardia out of proportion to the fever. Cardiac dilatation, systolic murmurs at the base, and arrhythmias may also occur. The lesions of Libman-Sacks verrucous endocarditis may cause a variety of murmurs but usually do not in themselves produce severe functional abnormalities; these lesions may, however, be complicated by superimposed bacterial endocarditis. Hypertension does occur but is not common in SLE unless there is severe and long-standing renal involvement; on rare occasions, it may be a severe and early manifestation.

Gastrointestinal symptoms may include nausea, vomiting, oral mucous membrane ulcers, ulcers lower in the alimentary tract, and symptoms of peritoneal inflammation. Several years ago when LE cells were demonstrated in a number of young women with severe liver disease and hypergammaglobulinemia, a syndrome called lupoid hepatitis was described. Careful postmortem examinations have demonstrated that hepatic involvement is rarely an accompaniment of SLE; it is likely that the so-called lupoid hepatitis syndrome represents subacute hepatitis (chronic active hepatitis) with marked immunologic abnormalities (including LE cells) and is not necessarily related to lupus.

Central and peripheral nervous system involvement occurs in at least 20 to 30 percent of the patients with SLE. The disease may present as a seizure, as a psychotic episode, as aseptic meningitis, or in rare instances as hemiparesis. More subtle neuroophthalmic changes caused by aberrations of the postchiasmal visual pathways have recently been described in a large proportion of patients with active SLE. In association with the central nervous system findings, cytoid bodies may be observed on funduscopy. These bodies appear as soft, white, fluffy exudates in the absence of uremia; they are transient, may last up to 1 or 2 weeks, and in some series are said to occur in over half the patients. Polyneuritis or focal neuropathy is also observed. Progressive central nervous system involvement resulting from vasculitis is now believed to be a major cause of mortality in SLE.

Renal disease in SLE is the other important determinant of prognosis. It is present in 75 percent of the autopsy cases, but it is clinically apparent in a lesser number of patients studied during life. Biopsy material examined by electron microscopy suggests, however, that some abnormalities in glomerular structure occur in virtually all patients with systemic lupus. The early lesion is focal mesangial and may present only as albuminuria, although white blood cells, red blood cells, and casts may also be found in the urine. The early cases may be indistinguishable from acute glomerulonephritis. The disorder may also present with a nephrotic syndrome that is indistinguishable from idiopathic nephrosis unless other manifestations of lupus are present. Hypertension is not common unless the renal lesion is advanced. There are very few studies of the natural course of the untreated renal disease. Although diffuse proliferative lupus nephritis has been considered to be invariably fatal, evidence is accumulating that this is not necessarily so and that a reassessment of the prognosis of this syndrome is in order (see Chap. 53).

Laboratory Findings

Anemia is a common abnormality; in most cases it is normocytic and normochromic, although a small percentage of patients have a definite hemolytic anemia with reticulocytosis, a positive Coombs test, and hyperbilirubinemia. It is thought that the coating of the red cells with an abnormal protein, which leads to their destruction, is the best explanation for the hemolytic anemia. Leukopenia (a white cell count lower than 4,000 cells) is a characteristic finding, and there is frequently a marked reduction in the percentages and absolute numbers of B and T lymphocytes in the peripheral blood.

Despite having leukopenia, patients with SLE may respond with a leukocytosis to nonspecific inflammatory lesions or specific infections. Thrombocytopenia is seen in a small number of patients and represents a serious complication. The serum complement level is depressed, especially in the presence of active disease and more specifically in association with active nephritis. The erythrocyte sedimentation rate is usually increased during the acute phase of the disease and may remain elevated even during remission.

Urinary abnormalities may vary from simple proteinuria to proteinuria with red blood cells, red cell casts, granular casts, or the presence of a "telescoped" urinary sediment with elements of acute nephritis, chronic nephritis, and the nephrotic syndrome all present in the same urine specimen.

Plasma protein abnormalities are remarkably common and are so fundamental to the understanding of SLE that they have led some investigators to regard SLE as one of the major diseases in which autoimmune phenomena take place. In general, there is usually an elevation in the serum gamma globulin and some diminution in the serum albumin. Alpha$_2$ globulin may be increased. Cryoglobulins have been demonstrated in many instances, and cryoproteinemia has been related to disease activity. There is an excellent correlation between the presence of increased titers of fibrin split-products and lupus glomerulonephritis, although the pathogenic role of intravascular coagulation in progressive renal disease remains unknown.

Antinuclear factors are found in the serum of most patients with SLE. The LE or lupus factor reacts with nuclear material, which is then ingested by a phagocytic cell to form the inclusion body of the typical LE cell. Although the LE factor was originally considered to belong to the 7S IgG class, it has been shown that the antinuclear antibodies may belong to the IgM, IgA, or IgD classes. The essential consituents of a positive LE cell reaction are viable white cells, altered nuclear material, a phagocytosis factor, and the LE factor in the serum. In addition to the LE factor, which is an antinucleoprotein antibody, a whole series of antinuclear and anticytoplasmic factors have been demonstrated in the blood of patients with lupus. Complement fixation and hemagglutination tests have shown the presence of antibodies to nucleohistone (LE factor), extractable nuclear antigens (ENA), and desoxyribonucleic acid (DNA). These and other immunologic abnormalities in SLE are listed below:

1. Antinuclear antibodies
   Antinucleoprotein (LE factor)
   Anti-DNA (both native and denatured)
   Anti-ENA (both RNase sensitive and RNase insensitive [Sm antigen])
2. Anticytoplasmic antibodies
   Anti-RNA (ribonucleic acid and ribosomes)
   Antikeratohyalin
   False-positive serologic test for syphilis
3. Anti—cell membrane antibodies
   Antierythrocyte antibodies
   Antileukocyte antibodies
   Antilymphocyte antibodies (both T cells and B cells)
   Antiplatelet antibodies
4. Anti—plasma protein antibodies
   Antiimmunoglobulins (rheumatoid factors)
   Anticoagulants

A wide variety of methods for the demonstration of antinuclear factors have been devised:

1. Observe morphologic changes in cells
   LE cell only
2. Coat inert particles with antigen and observe agglutination on exposure to antibody
   Red blood cells
   Latex
   Bentonite
3. Identify antigen-antibody directly
   Complement fixation
   Precipitation
   Passive cutaneous anaphylaxis
4. Observe fluorescence of isolated nuclear constituents or cell nuclei in tissue slides after exposure to SLE serum (see patterns of fluorescence below)

The development of the fluorescent antibody technique and the recognition of patterns have provided a fairly simple system which may be useful in carrying out various clinical correlations and in following the course of the disease:

Pattern of Nuclear Fluorescence	Significance
Homogeneous	LE factor (antinucleoprotein antibody)
Shaggy	Anti-DNA antibody (acute SLE with nephritis)
Speckled	Antibody to soluble nuclear proteins (often seen in rheumatoid arthritis; Sjögren's syndrome; ulcerative colitis; scleroderma; mixed connective tissue disease)
Nucleolar	Not known; seen in scleroderma
Perinuclear	Antiperinuclear antibody (? directed against keratohyalin; found in buccal mucosa in rheumatoid arthritis)

Other antibodies occur frequently in SLE. Rheumatoid factors have also been found in approximately one-third of the patients. Occasionally patients with lupus will also show the presence of antithyroid antibodies. Another abnormal finding is the chronic biologic false-positive test for syphilis; a chronic false-positive reactor is a person with no clinical or epidemiologic evidence of syphilis who has a repeatedly positive serologic test for 6 months or more and negative treponemal antibody tests. Large numbers of these patients have been followed over a period of years, and it has been found that SLE develops in a significant percentage of them. Conversely, a small percentage of patients with known lupus are found to have false-positive serologic tests for syphilis. These reactions have served as indices for determining the epidemiology and the course of this disorder and already have indicated that in many cases lupus is present for a much longer time than had been suspected.

The role of the many unusual circulating antibodies found in SLE is difficult to ascertain. Certainly some are pathologic, in that they are associated with hemolytic anemia, leukopenia, and thrombocytopenia; others, such as the LE factor, lack cytotoxicity in tissue culture, have been transferred transplacentally without damaging the fetus, and have been transfused to normal subjects without producing any abnormality. Some antinuclear antibodies are not specific, in that they can be found in patients with rheumatoid arthritis, scleroderma, and liver disease. They also occur in normal relatives of patients with systemic lupus.

Drug-induced Lupuslike Syndromes

During the past 20 years a steady accumulation of reports has described lupuslike syndromes induced by various drugs. The list of agents includes the following: procainamide, hydralazine hydrochloride, isoniazid, phenytoin, trimethadione, penicillin, penicillamine, sulfonamides, tetracycline, propylthiouracil, alpha-methyldopa, and the oral contraceptives. Of patients taking procainamide, antinuclear antibodies develop in approximately 75 percent. Only a small number of these patients, however, develop a lupuslike clinical reaction, characterized by polyarthralgia, myalgia, fever, pleurisy, and pericarditis. As in other forms of drug-induced lupuslike syndromes, renal disease is notably absent in patients taking procainamide, and both the clinical and laboratory abnormalities disappear after the drug is discontinued.

Treatment

There is no specific treatment for SLE. A number of nonspecific measures, however, are exceedingly helpful in attaining remissions, and some are occasionally lifesaving. In general, the patients with active disease should have complete bed rest, an adequate diet, and should avoid stressful situations such as elective surgery, emotional stress, or nonessential drugs. These patients should also avoid direct sunlight and drugs known to sensitize (especially sulfa drugs, hydralazine hydrochloride, trimethadione, and other anticonvulsant agents). The patients with articular disease should have a conservative program of heat and exercises as outlined in the section on rheumatoid arthritis. Patients with active SLE should be given antiinflammatory medication, starting with the most benign agents (salicylates). Aspirin should be used as

it is in rheumatoid arthritis — that is, to tolerance. If the patients do not respond to salicylates, they may show a good response to antimalarial agents. The one most commonly used now is hydroxychloroquine sulfate (200-mg tablets), one tablet twice a day for 1 week, then one tablet per day thereafter. One must be cautious in utilizing antimalarial agents, however, because of ocular toxicity. Although minor side effects (transient leukopenia, gastrointestinal irritation) may be avoided by changing the dosage schedule, the ocular toxicity, owing to the affinity of hydroxychloroquine sulfate and chloroquine for pigment epithelium, may lead to scotomata and increasing loss of vision. This complication is probably related to the dose and duration of treatment. Patients receiving these agents must have a careful ophthalmologic examination at least every 3 months.

Steroids are indicated for acute hemolytic episodes, for severe leukopenia, and for thrombocytopenia. The other indications for steroids in SLE are not as clear-cut. Steroids should not be used routinely in all patients, many of whom (with mild or moderate disease) can be maintained on salicylates and antimalarial drugs alone. Patients who have more severe and occasionally life-threatening complications (that is, pericardial effusion, myocarditis, severe inanition) in addition to the hematologic complications already mentioned may often benefit from steroids given for short periods. Since steroids are difficult to withdraw, since they have many severe side effects, and since SLE is not always life-threatening, these drugs should always be used with caution.

The role of corticosteroids in lupus nephritis is more controversial. It is generally agreed that the usual doses (that is, about 20 mg of prednisone or its equivalent daily) will not affect the course of the nephritis. There are some who believe that larger doses (50 to 60 mg of prednisone daily for periods of up to 6 months) will favorably influence renal disease. There are, however, no controlled studies to support this view, whereas there are accumulating data indicating both that a number of patients with apparently severe renal disease will do well even without steroids and that the serious complications of steroid therapy often outweigh its possible beneficial effects.

Antimetabolites such as 6-mercaptopurine and azathioprine (Imuran) have also been used in lupus nephritis, usually together with systemic steroids. Although this form of therapy has many advocates and may be beneficial in individual cases, the overall results are disappointing, and there is mounting evidence that the prolonged use of immunosuppressive agents may lead to a more serious complication, namely, neoplasia.

NECROTIZING ARTERITIS AND
OTHER FORMS OF VASCULITIS

Polyarteritis Nodosa

Polyarteritis or periarteritis nodosa (PAN) was first described by Kussmaul and Maier more than a hundred years ago. The classic disease is a systemic disorder characterized by nodules and inflammatory lesions along the course of medium-sized muscular arteries. The lesions are segmental in distribution, involve arteries in almost any part of the body, and thereby may cause a wide variety of symptoms in any organ system. Clinical studies of this disorder have become somewhat complicated by numerous attempts to subdivide the types of vasculitis according to either the precipitating or sensitizing events or the type of blood vessel involved.

Numerous investigators have related the various kinds of arteritis to a variety of hypersensitivity phenomena. The classic work of Rich and Gregory demonstrated that lesions similar to those seen in periarteritis nodosa occur in patients dying from serum sickness and allergic reactions to sulfonamides. Similar lesions have been produced experimentally in rabbits on a hypersensitivity basis and are comparable to the lesions seen in human beings. Zeek termed this group of disorders *necrotizing angiitis* and subdivided them as follows: polyarteritis nodosa; hypersensitivity angiitis; rheumatic arteritis; allergic granulomatous angiitis; and temporal or cranial arteritis. One group of workers has classified polyarteritis on the basis of whether lung or renal disease predominates. In short, there are a number of overlapping syndromes, probably related to hypersensitivity phenomena, which are widespread in distribution and which may be of multiple etiologies. The vascular lesion is classically in the medium-sized artery, in which necrosis, fibrinoid change, acute leukocytic involvement, and nodule formation occur.

Clinical Picture. The clinical manifestations of polyarteritis nodosa are caused by acute or chronic occlusion of the vessels. The disease can begin at any age (peak incidence, ages 20 to 50), predominates in males (male-to-female ratio of 3:1), and is characterized by remissions and exacerbations. The patients may present simply with undiagnosed fever and tachycardia or with generalized aching in the joints or occasionally in the muscles. Symptoms may be primarily related to the lungs, in which sudden onset of asthma and an associated eosinophilia may be present. Almost any type of lesion may be seen on chest x-ray, but focal pulmonary infiltrates (often evanescent) are the most common.

Renal disease characterized by progressive azotemia is frequent and is the most common cause of death. On urinalysis, these patients have albuminuria, hematuria, red cell casts, and granular casts — that is, findings often indistinguishable from those of acute poststreptococcal glomerulonephritis. Hypertension commonly follows the initial renal disease. Multiple arteriolar thromboses or hemorrhages may occur throughout the body and lead to peripheral gangrene, myocardial infarction, or cerebral vessel thrombosis or hemorrhage. Neurologic abnormalities include symmetrical or asymmetrical peripheral neuropathy with both motor and sensory changes. Central nervous system disease may occur in almost any form; cerebral vascular disease may be the first evidence of periarteritis nodosa. Acute abdominal pain and abdominal emergencies resulting from mesenteric vessel occlusion, as well as gangrene in parts of the liver or spleen, are also part of this syndrome. These patients may also have erythema nodosum, urticaria, ecchymoses, and purpura. Acute polyarthritis and occasionally chronic polyarthritis can occur.

Laboratory Findings. Polymorphonuclear leukocytosis occurs in most patients, and eosinophilia may be marked when pulmonary lesions are present. Normocytic, normochromic anemia, an elevated erythrocyte sedimentation rate, and hyperglobulinemia are often present. Urinalysis reveals a variety of abnormalities including a "telescoped urine" — that is, a combination of red cells, white cells, red cell casts, fatty casts, and oval fat bodies. As in other connective tissue diseases, rheumatoid factors and LE factors are occasionally found in the serum. Diagnosis depends on histologic evidence and judicious biopsy of an affected site (usually skin, subcutaneous tissue, muscle, kidney, or testis).

Treatment. Therapy consists of supportive measures, relief of pain, transfusion, and the use of antiinflammatory medication, particularly corticosteroids. Doses of 40 to 60 mg of prednisone per day may be lifesaving, although their influence on long-term survival is not known.

Serum Sickness and Hypersensitivity Angiitis
Serum sickness was the name given by von Pirquet and Schick to a systemic disorder caused by the administration of foreign serum or serum products (see Chap. 45). It is characterized by fever, rash, lymphadenopathy, edema, arthralgia and arthritis, and myalgia, often with eosinophilia. In severe cases there may be renal, gastrointestinal, pulmonary, and nervous system manifestations. A similar disorder may be seen in drug hypersensitivity. The disease is caused by the interaction of the antigen with circulating antibody and the formation of soluble antigen-antibody complexes. The onset of symptoms in serum sickness coincides with the appearance of antibody and the disappearance of antigen at the time that antigen-antibody complexes are usually increasing. Pathologically, vascular lesions similar to those of polyarteritis nodosa are found. These lesions can be produced experimentally in animals or injection of foreign protein and have led to the concept that hypersensitivity plays an important role in polyarteritis nodosa and related disorders. Experimental studies by Dixon and co-workers have led to a greater understanding of the role of circulating complexes in these disorders, and through the use of fluorescent antibody and electron microscopic techniques, patterns of glomerular involvement have been defined.

The disorder usually is self-limited and lasts no longer than 1 to 3 weeks. Treatment with antihistamines may be adequate, but in severe cases cortico-steroids give excellent results.

Wegener's Granulomatosis
Wegener's granulomatosis is a generalized vasculitis of unknown etiology characterized by widespread necrotizing granulomatous lesions involving primarily the respiratory tract and kidneys. It affects young and middle-aged persons of either sex, and it may begin insidiously or acutely. The lesions commonly occur in the upper respiratory tract and progress from a severe sinusitis and rhinitis to ulcerating lesions of the face called midline granulomas, which are accompanied by nodular pulmonary infiltrates and an acute glomerulitis. Fever, skin eruption, leukocytosis, musculoskeletal complaints, eosinophilia, and hyperglobulinemia are present, and most patients develop progressive uremia. Although the outcome of this disease is usually fatal, some recent evidence indicates that isolated lesions of Wegener's granulomatosis may occur in the lungs and remain localized for long periods. Corticosteroid therapy may help to prolong life in this illness, and recently it has been shown that immunosuppressive treatments, especially with cyclophosphamides, may halt the disease.

Giant Cell Arteritis
Giant cell arteritis, also known as cranial arteritis, is an acute inflammatory disorder affecting large arteries, especially the temporal and occipital, but occasionally involving other vessels, including the aorta. The incidence is equal between sexes, and the disorder usually comes on late in life. The temporal vessels become red, tender, and thickened, which may cause severe headaches. Ocular complaints such as diplopia and loss of vision are among the more important complications. Patients may have fever, anemia, and vague articular aches and pains.

There is some discussion in the literature as to whether giant cell arteritis is strictly a local lesion or whether it has systemic manifestations. Many consider it to be part of a generalized granulomatous inflammation and have divided it into several stages: headache, ocular complications, and systemic complications. Involvement of the aortic arch and the branches may lead to a syndrome that is clinically and pathologically indistinguishable from brachiocephalic arteritis or pulseless disease. Symptomatic treatment and the use of systemic steroids (40 to 100 mg prednisone per day) are indicated in proved cases of giant cell arteritis because of the potential severity of the ocular complications.

Polymyalgia Rheumatica
Polymyalgia rheumatica is a clinical syndrome characterized by proximal girdle (especially shoulder) pain and stiffness, nonspecific generalized symptoms (fatigue, aching, weight loss), an unremarkable physical examination, and benign laboratory findings except for a significantly elevated sedimentation rate (at least over 50 mm per hour, usually more than 100 mm per hour). Arteritis is often present in these patients, and biopsy (deltoid muscle; temporal artery) is usually indicated. The disease usually responds to low-dose (10 to 20 mg), long-term steroid therapy, unless temporal arteritis is present, in which case higher doses are indicated.

SCLERODERMA
Scleroderma, or progressive systemic sclerosis, is a connective tissue disorder of unknown etiology. It affects primarily the skin but also involves synovial membranes, the gastrointestinal tract (especially the esophagus), and the heart, lungs, and kidneys. The dermatologic lesion is generally a severe, leathery induration of the skin, followed by atrophy and pigmentation. Scleroderma is more common in women than in men, may occur at any age, and is characterized by remissions and exacerbations. The course may be rapidly progressive, but local lesions may remain indolent for long periods. The skin lesion may be localized to small patches, in which case it is called *morphea;* rarely, it may be a sharply defined lesion, termed *linear scleroderma.* The lesion occasionally spreads widely through the skin and is called *generalized morphea* (see Chap. 5). The generalized form of scleroderma may itself be present for years as a disorder characterized by Raynaud's phenomenon (see Chap. 25) and by thickening of the skin of the fingers, in which case it has been referred to as *acrosclerosis.*

The pathology of scleroderma is that of replacement of the normal connective tissue with apparently increased amounts of collagen, and atrophy of dermal appendages. To date, no specific abnormalities in the collagen have been defined by histologic, immunofluorescent, or electron microscopic studies. However, more subtle alterations in the collagen molecule may be revealed as better understanding of the macromolecular biology of collagen is achieved. Recent data (on smaller collagen fibrils) suggest the presence of newly synthesized collagen and are consistent with other information indicating that there is an increased collagen synthesis in sclerodermatous skin (that is, increased activity of protocollagen proline hydroxylase; increased neutral-salt-soluble collagen). Other in vitro studies have demonstrated an increased collagen synthesis by the normal-appearing fibroblasts of sclerodermatous skin. Some investigators have tried to relate the abnormality in collagen to a microvascular abnormality (increased vasoconstriction), leading to hypoxia and to increased collagen synthesis.

As the disease develops, there is atrophy of the epidermis and its appendages, and subcutaneous calcification may subsequently occur. Similarly, replacement of submucosal connective tissue by collagen occurs in the gastrointestinal tract and elsewhere in the body. A thick rim of collagen may be laid down on the surface of the synovial membrane. Focal lesions may be found in the heart. In the kidney an unusual renal arteriolar lesion has been found and is associated with a rapidly fatal outcome. The renal interlobular arteries display a mucoid thickening and cellular proliferation of the intima. Fibrinoid alteration may also be seen in interlobular arteries and in arterioles.

In recent years, serologic studies of patients with this disease have demonstrated abnormalities (the occasional presence of antinuclear antibodies and rheumatoid factors) and a further overlap with rheumatoid arthritis and SLE. Sharp and co-workers have pointed out that many of the patients with mixed connective tissue disease have a peculiar "speckled" pattern seen on fluorescent antinuclear antibody testing, and a relatively benign clinical course (absence of renal and central nervous system manifestations).

Clinical Picture
Patients may first present with Raynaud's phenomenon, increasing stiffness of hands and arms, and non-

pitting edema followed by tightening of skin about the face and neck. The skin may become atrophic, lose its elasticity, and develop local ulcers. Normal body folds are lost, muscles become atrophic, and joint contractures may occur secondary to the skin lesion or resulting from primary sclerodermatous changes within the synovial membrane. When affected joints are moved, a characteristic leathery crepitus may be elicited. Patients may also complain of difficulty in swallowing if esophageal lesions are present. With more diffuse involvement a variety of intestinal symptoms may develop, including diarrhea and malabsorption, particularly when widespread small intestinal lesions are present. A multitude of symptoms may occur, often dominated by dyspnea resulting from pulmonary fibrosis and diffusion defects. Pulmonary hypertension and cor pulmonale may also result. X-ray study of the chest usually reveals diffuse pulmonary fibrosis. Lesions in the heart may result in pericarditis with effusion, symptoms of heart failure, or arrhythmias. Renal involvement is not common; if it occurs, the prognosis is very poor. The renal symptoms are usually those of rapid onset of hypertension and progressive azotemia. When there is no laboratory evidence of renal disease, the scleroderma may stabilize for years with little change.

Laboratory Findings
Laboratory studies reveal no unusual hematologic findings, although the erythrocyte sedimentation rate may be increased and there may be a mild anemia. Recently, hypergammaglobulinemia has been demonstrated in a number of patients, as well as the presence of antinuclear antibodies (including LE factor), and occasionally rheumatoid factors. It has been suggested that in scleroderma the fluorescent antinuclear antibody test shows a "speckled" pattern more often than the other patterns. With renal disease the urine may contain albumin, red cells, white cells, and casts. Synovial fluid of involved joints shows mild inflammation. X-rays of bones and joints demonstrate diffuse osteoporosis and areas of soft tissue calcification, particularly in the extremities. Chest films show diffuse pulmonary infiltrates, while a barium swallow will demonstrate dilatation of the esophagus and loss of peristalsis. Electrocardiography may reveal rhythm changes, T wave alterations, or other nonspecific changes of myocardial involvement.

Treatment
There is no specific treatment for scleroderma. Measures that have been tried include the use of corticosteroids, para-aminobenzoic acid, relaxin, and chelating agents. Some believe that the use of corticosteroids may lead to the appearance of or acceleration of renal disease. Penicillamine and other agents that decrease intramolecular cross linking of collagen are under trial, but to date they have not demonstrated striking results. Symptomatic treatment includes bed rest, local care of the skin, joint and muscle exercise, and salicylates in high doses when there are articular manifestations. The use of physiotherapy to prevent contractures, not only during the active phase of the disease but when the disorder is quiescent, is an important part of the overall treatment. Symptoms of malabsorption may respond to antibiotic therapy when they are caused by bacterial overgrowth in an atonic bowel.

POLYMYOSITIS
Polymyositis (dermatomyositis) is an acute, subacute, or chronic disease of unknown etiology characterized by edema, dermatitis, and muscle inflammation. The essential clinical feature is muscle weakness and tenderness. The primary lesion is a noninfectious, inflammatory, and degenerative process of muscle fibers and the connective tissue about them. The disorder is more common in females than in males and may occur at any age. In recent attempts at classification, some authors arbitrarily divide the cases into five types: (1) acute idiopathic polymyositis with disease confined primarily to muscles; (2) classic dermatomyositis with a characteristic skin eruption; (3) polymyositis (or dermatomyositis) associated with malignancy; (4) childhood dermatomyositis and polymyositis with vasculitis; and (5) mixed cases with muscle, skin, and other connective tissue manifestations. In practice it is not always easy to separate these types, or indeed to distinguish some cases of dermatomyositis that appear to overlap scleroderma or SLE in their manifestations.

Criteria

No official diagnostic or classifying criteria for polymyositis have been either accepted or scientifically tested. The following items, however, have been suggested as useful in establishing a clinical diagnosis:

1. Progressive symmetrical weakness of the limb-girdle muscles and anterior neck flexors
2. Muscle biopsy evidence of fiber necrosis with phagocytosis, regeneration, and basophilia
3. Elevation of skeletal muscle enzymes, especially CPK, and including SGOT, LDH, and SGPT
4. Electromyographic triad of (a) short and polyphasic motor-unit fibrillations, (b) positive sharp waves and insertional irritability, and (c) bizarre, high-frequency, repetitive discharges
5. Rash (heliotrope discoloration of eyelids, with peripheral edema and erythematous dermatitis over dorsum of hands, other joints, and torso)

Pathologic Changes

Histologically, skeletal muscle fibers show both degeneration (with varying amounts of vacuolization, necrosis, phagocytosis, and cellular infiltration) and regeneration. Of these changes, the most specific for dermatomyositis is regeneration, recognized by loss of striation, variation in size, and basophilic staining. Examination of involved skin may show changes comparable to those in scleroderma. Extensive or localized calcifications may occur in skin, subcutaneous tissues, tendons, and muscles. Vascular inflammatory infiltrates in other parts of the body may also be seen. In one detailed study of dermatomyositis of childhood it was suggested that the primary lesions were vascular, with perivascular collections of inflammatory cells as well as arteritis and phlebitis, and that this particular disorder was a distinct clinicopathologic entity.

Clinical Picture

The cardinal feature of all cases of polymyositis is muscular weakness, with particular involvement of the muscles of the pelvic and shoulder girdles, anterior neck, thighs, and arms. If the disease is progressive, the patient may experience difficulties in speech and swallowing and may lose voluntary control of breathing due to paralysis of the intercostal and accessory muscles. Muscular pain and tenderness may occur, especially in patients with skin rash and subcutaneous edema. The typical skin eruption consists of edema and dusky erythema of the face, periorbital regions, neck, shoulders, upper thorax, and proximal portions of the arms. A heliotrope (lilac) suffusion of the upper eyelids is characteristic. Constitutional symptoms include fever, malaise, and weight loss. Periarticular discomfort and frank polyarthritis may occur, and Raynaud's phenomenon may be present.

When the acute phase — which may last many months — passes, the patient may be left with muscle atrophy and contractures. Calcinosis is not an unusual complication. Some patients, especially children, who pass through the acute phase may do exceedingly well thereafter. In other patients the disease may have a very prolonged subacute or chronic course. The association of the disorder with neoplasms such as carcinoma of the breast, lung, stomach, ovary, or kidney is important, and occasionally the dermatomyositis will subside when such a primary focus is removed. The differential diagnosis includes other connective tissue disorders, myasthenia gravis, trichinosis, thyrotoxic myopathy, muscular dystrophy, and polyneuritis.

Laboratory Findings

The laboratory findings include a polymorphonuclear leukocytosis and often anemia. The erythrocyte sedimentation rate is elevated, creatinuria is usually present, and myoglobinuria may occur. In some cases antinuclear antibodies (including LE cells) or rheumatoid factors are found in the blood. Serum globulins may be elevated. Serum glutamic-oxaloacetic transaminase (SGOT), serum glutamic-pyruvic transaminase (SGPT), lactic acid dehydrogenase (LDH), and creatine phosphokinase (CPK) are usually elevated. The last noted (CPK) is possibly the most useful, but in some cases of active myositis all enzymes may be normal. Serum aldolase is usually elevated. Serial estimates of SGOT, SGPT, and serum aldolase probably provide the best laboratory guides to the course of the illness. These enzyme studies are also helpful in diagnosis, particularly in differentiating myopathy from weakness and wasting of muscles resulting from primary neurologic disease. Electromyography, although not specific, will suggest the presence of myopathic (as opposed to a normal or neuromyopathic) response. The usual findings on electromyography are short, small, polyphasic motor-unit fibrillations; positive sharp waves and insertional irritability; and bizarre, high-frequency, repetitive discharges. Muscle biopsy is indicated whenever the disease is suspected.

Treatment

Therapy is symptomatic only in the mildest cases and includes bed rest and physiotherapy. In most cases, corticosteroids in high doses must be used (20 to 40 mg of prednisone per day); this treatment will often result in lessening of the symptoms and slow but steady improvement in muscle strength. During the acute phases of the disease, 40 to 60 mg of prednisone may be needed. The dose should be lowered slowly to avoid exacerbations. Maintenance doses of prednisone (5 to 20 mg per day) may be needed for long periods. The role of immunosuppressive drugs in polymyositis is not clear, although wide-ranging claims have been made for them. On occasion, they seem to be very effective in steroid-resistant cases. Tumors should be searched for, and if a malignancy is found, its surgical removal may cause remission of the polymyositis.

Other Diseases Affecting Joints

DEGENERATIVE JOINT DISEASE

Degenerative joint disease (osteoarthritis, osteoarthrosis, hypertrophic arthritis) is a chronic disorder of joints without systemic manifestations, characterized by articular cartilage degeneration, bone remodeling, pain on joint motion that subsides with rest, and certain x-ray changes. It is the most common form of arthritis seen in clinical practice. It may occur in an idiopathic, primary form, or it may be secondary to previous joint damage (e.g., trauma, rheumatoid arthritis, dysplasia). When it involves many sites, particularly the weight-bearing joints, the apophyseal joints of the cervical spine, and the small joints of the hands (distal interphalangeal, proximal interphalangeal, and the first carpometacarpal joint), it is classified as *primary generalized degenerative joint disease.* Osteo-

phytosis of the spine should probably be distinguished from degenerative joint disease of the apophyseal joints. In the former condition, the osteophytes are formed most commonly at the anterior margins of the ends of the vertebral bodies and result from degenerative changes in the intervertebral disks. Various degrees of spinal rigidity may result from localized osseous bridging between vertebrae.

Pathogenesis

Aging appears to be the single most important factor in the pathogenesis of degenerative joint disease. The relationship is a complex one, however, in that certain elderly persons may show little evidence of the disease, whereas relatively young persons may have widely disseminated disease. Progressive joint remodeling occurs with age as a response to normal physical stresses. It has been suggested that "unbalanced" remodeling might lead to chondromalacia by interfering with the normal nutrition and metabolism of cartilage.

The hypothesis that the primary lesion in degenerative joint disease is an increased loss of proteoglycans from the cartilage matrix is supported by studies demonstrating that most of the chondrocytes in the morphologically involved areas show evidence of active sulfate uptake, thus indicating normal or increased chondroitin sulfate synthesis. The basis for the loss of proteoglycans in degenerative arthritis is not yet known. Proteoglycans exist in cartilage in very large (60–70 S) aggregates, in which many proteoglycans are noncovalently linked to a highly polymerized chainlike molecule of hyaluronic acid. In addition, tissue glycoprotein is present in the aggregates and appears to stabilize the proteoglycan-hyaluronate interaction. Recent evidence indicates an "aggregation defect" in osteoarthritic cartilage, that is, a smaller than normal proportion of aggregated to nonaggregated proteoglycans. In addition, the aggregates in osteoarthritic cartilage tend to be smaller than normal. Whether the abnormality is caused by the proteoglycans themselves or by other components of the aggregates remains to be determined, as does the relationship of these changes in proteoglycan organization to the aging process. Proteolytic enzymes, which have the capacity to degrade proteoglycans, exist in articular cartilage and may relate to the changes described.

Genetic and systemic factors may also be important in degenerative joint disease, judging by familial incidence of the disease (particularly Heberden's nodes) and the increased incidence and severity of the process in metabolic diseases such as acromegaly, diabetes, and alkaptonuria. An inherent relationship between obesity and degenerative joint disease has not been proved, and studies in mice reveal that obesity per se does not influence degenerative joint disease. Several other types of degenerative joint disease have inherited or acquired biologic bases but must be regarded as belonging to the secondary type. The so-called epidemic generalized degenerative joint disease (Kashin-Beck disease) found commonly in parts of eastern Siberia and Manchuria appears to be nutritional in origin. The articular changes closely simulate degenerative joint disease but develop only in children having a special metaphyseal defect associated with abnormal bone formation.

Pathology

In contrast to rheumatoid arthritis, the primary lesion in degenerative joint disease appears to reside in the articular cartilage rather than in the synovial membrane. First, the normally smooth, translucent articular cartilage becomes dull, focally opaque, and softened. Later, the altered cartilage becomes frayed and fibrillated, leading to denudation of the underlying bone. Reactive fibroblastic and osseous proliferation at the subchondral plate produces bony sclerosis, while periosteal bone formation at the joint margins leads to the appearance of osteophytes. Histologically these lesions show a loss of metachromatic material in the matrix and an increase in the proportion of cells relative to interstitial tissue. Multicellular chondrocyte clusters appear, probably as a result of cellular proliferation.

Clinical Features

Only a small proportion of patients with pathologic lesions of degenerative joint disease have symptoms. The presenting complaint is usually persistent pain in one or more joints. Constitutional symptoms are rare.

The pain is characteristically aggravated by motion and weight bearing but is relieved by rest. Tenderness, redness, and heat are usually negligible except during episodes of acute trauma to affected joints. Crepitation on motion, spasm or atrophy of surrounding muscles, limitation of motion, and hypertrophic bone changes may be detectable on physical examination.

Although the typical hypertrophic lesions of the distal interphalangeal joints (Heberden's nodes) and proximal interphalangeal joints (Bouchard's nodes) usually develop without symptoms, they may occasionally be preceded by acute inflammatory changes at these sites. Involvement of the first carpometacarpal joint is not uncommon, but other joints of the upper extremity, particularly the wrist and shoulder, are spared in primary osteoarthritis. The knees are frequently affected and may present with large synovial effusions; the synovial fluid, in contrast to exudates of inflammatory origin, contains few cells and demonstrates good mucin. Degenerative joint disease of the hip (malum coxae senilis) is the most disabling form of the disease and often requires surgical intervention. Degenerative joint disease of the cervical spine frequently involves the lateral intervertebral joints and the posterior facets. The close proximity of these joints to the cervical nerve roots renders the latter vulnerable to compression, which may be expressed clinically as neck, shoulder, or arm pain. In more advanced stages, cervical spondylosis leads to severe neuropathic changes, including atrophy of shoulder and hand muscles and loss of sensation and motor power.

Diagnosis of degenerative joint disease depends on the persistence of joint pain, on normal blood and serologic findings, and on a typical x-ray appearance. Radiologic findings in degenerative joint disease include narrowing of the joint space, subchondral sclerosis of bone, osteophytes and, less commonly, juxtaarticular bone cysts.

Any patient over age 50 who presents with a history of joint pain or swelling without constitutional symptoms should immediately be suspected of having degenerative joint disease. The main differential points between rheumatoid arthritis and degenerative joint disease are listed in Table 46-2.

Table 46-2. Major Differences Between Rheumatoid Arthritis and Degenerative Joint Disease

	Rheumatoid arthritis	Degenerative joint disease
Age at onset	Third and fourth decades	Fifth and sixth decades
Weight	Normal or underweight	Usually overweight
Constitutional manifestations	Present	Absent
Joints involved	Any joint (classically bilateral symmetrical proximal interphalangeal and metacarpophalangeal joints)	Mainly knees, hips, spine, and distal interphalangeal joints
Appearance of joints	Soft-tissue swelling	Bony swelling
Special deformities	Fusiform finger joints; ulnar deviation	Heberden's and Bouchard's nodes
Subcutaneous nodules	Present in 20%	Never present
X-ray	Osteoporosis and erosions	Osteosclerosis and osteophytes
Joint fluid	Increased cells; poor mucin	Few cells; good mucin
Rheumatoid factors	Usually present	Usually absent
Blood count	Anemia and leukocytosis	Normal
Erythrocyte sedimentation rate	Markedly elevated	Normal
Course	Often progressive	Slow or stationary
Termination	Ankylosis and deformity; amyloidosis	No ankylosis and no amyloidosis

Treatment

There are no specific forms of therapy for degenerative joint disease. The chief treatments are given below.

Analgesics and Antiinflammatory Agents. Aspirin given to tolerance is by far the most useful method of relieving joint pain. It must be recognized that older persons have less tolerance for large doses of aspirin and that their serum salicylate levels should not be allowed to exceed 20 mg per 100 ml. Phenylbutazone (Butazolidin) and indomethacin may help some patients, especially those with hip involvement; gold salts and systemic corticosteroids, however, are not indicated in degenerative joint disease. In an occasional patient infrequent intraarticular instillation of a long-acting corticosteroid may be a useful adjunct to other measures. Recently several additional nonsteroidal antiinflammatory drugs, such as ibuprofen, have been shown to give some symptomatic benefits.

Physiotherapy. As performed in rheumatoid arthritis, physiotherapy should be used primarily to aid in preventing permanent limitation of motion in an involved joint. Intermittent traction to the neck may relieve mild cervical neurologic symptoms. Heat treatments often offer symptomatic relief, although they do not affect the underlying process. In an acute exacerbation, the affected weight-bearing joint should be rested. Obese patients should be encouraged to lose weight. If the joint disability is severe, the patient may have to change his job or mode of life. Crutches may be necessary to reduce stress on severely affected hip or knee joints.

Orthopedic Management. When normal functioning of a joint is likely to be permanently impaired by progressive degenerative joint disease, orthopedic advice should be sought. Reconstructive surgery is often indicated when there is intractable pain or marked limitation of motion in a weight-bearing joint.

NONARTICULAR RHEUMATISM

The term *nonarticular rheumatism* is applied to a heterogeneous group of conditions producing pain and stiffness in connective tissue adjacent to and supporting the joints, but not affecting the actual articulation. The group includes such disorders as tendinitis and peritendinitis (bursitis), fasciitis, the carpal tunnel syndrome, the shoulder-hand syndrome, and prolapsed intervertebral disk. Although the general physician may see only a relatively small proportion of such cases, their socioeconomic implications can be great.

Tendinitis and Peritendinitis (Bursitis)

Altogether there are some 140 bursae in the body where acute, subacute, or chronic irritation may occur in association with inflammation of the surrounding tendons. When tendon sheaths or bursae become acutely inflamed, they cause severe pain, with resultant loss of motion in adjacent joints. Later, calcium deposits may appear. The most common site for calcium deposition is probably the tendon of the supraspinatus muscle; in older persons this is often associated with degenerative changes of the tendon secondary to constant trauma as it slides beneath the acromial spine. At its height, pain in this area can be excruciating but is often relieved spontaneously when the bulk of the calcium deposit is discharged into the underlying subacromial bursa. Some persons show a predisposition to calcium deposits in multiple tendon sites, and it has been postulated that these individuals may be suffering from a systemic disease (periarthritis calcarea). *Adhesive tendinitis* and *frozen shoulder* are the terms used to designate the results of muscle atrophy and prolonged immobilization of the shoulder secondary to supraspinatus or biceps tendinitis. No treatment of tendinitis is universally effective, but most patients respond promptly to a variety of measures including the oral administration of aspirin, corticosteroids, or phenylbutazone, or the direct percutaneous injection of procaine or hydrocortisone.

Shoulder-Hand Syndrome

The shoulder-hand syndrome is a potentially disabling condition characterized by shoulder pain, limitation of wrist motion, diffuse soft-tissue swelling of the hand, and vasomotor changes in the affected fingers. The pathogenesis of this syndrome is still obscure. It was first thought to represent varying degrees of reflex neurovascular response to a variety of disorders, the most common of which is acute myocardial infarction. In most patients with this condition gradual reduction of the shoulder disability and decrease in swelling of the hand occur over a period of weeks. Flexion deformities of the fingers, along with atrophy of the palmar soft tissues, may develop and result in Dupuytren's contractures. The skin of the affected hand may become chronically tight, smooth, shiny, and atrophic. In later stages, x-rays may reveal a spotty osteoporosis of underlying bone. Fortunately this progressive pattern does not always ensue and, except for the late irreversible changes, recovery may occur at any point. The condition is usually unilateral, but in one-third of the cases it affects both upper limbs simultaneously. Treatment consists of anti-inflammatory medication, intensive physiotherapy, and occasionally stellate ganglion block.

Gout

Primary gout is a hereditary disease, predominantly of males, that is characterized by recurrent attacks of acute arthritis, by elevation of the serum uric acid, by a therapeutic response to colchicine, and by the presence of urate crystals in the synovial fluid. *Secondary gout* is acute arthritis and hyperuricemia associated with diseases in which there is either an accelerated nucleoprotein turnover, or an interference with the renal handling of uric acid by drugs or intrinsic renal disease.

The term *gout* was derived from the Latin *gutta* (a drop) and refers to the belief that a poisonous substance was deposited in the joints in a drop-by-drop fashion. Gout and gouty arthritis have been known to physicians and other men of letters almost as long as recorded history. Its apparent predilection for famous people in diverse fields has given a unique historical record of its clinical aspects and social significance. Hippocrates, who is generally credited with the first clear-cut clinical description of gout in about 500 B.C., recognized its high incidence among males as well as its other clinical features. The drug colchicine (the extract of the meadow saffron) was introduced in the sixth century by Alexander of Tralles, but it was abandoned in many areas after centuries of use when fear of purgation became prominent. Benjamin Franklin, a famous sufferer from gout, introduced colchicine into the United States.

Uric acid was isolated from a urinary stone by Scheele in 1776. Subsequently, it was shown that the gouty tophus itself contained uric acid. In one of the earliest demonstrations of a serum abnormality in a clinical disorder, Garrod the elder, in the nineteenth century, demonstrated that there was increased uric acid in the blood of persons with gout. The younger Garrod, in 1931, classified gout as one of the first inborn errors of metabolism because of the known chemical abnormality and the familial incidence.

GENETICS AND HEREDITY OF GOUT

Some 20 percent of the relatives of patients with gout have asymptomatic hyperuricemia. There is an increased incidence of hyperuricemia and gout among Filipinos in North America and the Maoris. Although primary gout was once regarded as an inherited disorder of metabolism caused by a single genetic defect and characterized by the overproduction of uric acid, a complete reevaluation of this concept has taken place as the many factors involved in the hyperuricemia of gout have become apparent. It is unlikely that one genetic defect could cause an abnormality in the renal secretion of uric acid, an overproduction of uric acid, and also a combination of these two. Although some early work had led investigators to believe that primary gout was inherited as an autosomal dominant with incomplete penetrance, at least one study pointed out that multiple gene action was a more likely explanation for the genetics of primary gout. This polymorphic type of inheritance fits better with the biochemical and clinical picture as understood at this time.

Because of the high incidence of gout among famous people, it was formerly suggested that only the more intelligent in the population had gout, but certainly it is now clear that it can occur in all walks of life.

ACUTE GOUTY ARTHRITIS

The acute attack of gout is characterized classically by painful joint swelling. The first metatarsophalangeal joint is involved in over 50 percent of the initial episodes of gouty arthritis (podagra). The area becomes red, hot, and so exquisitely tender that even the slightest touch may be unbearable. No joint is exempt, and the attack may begin with involvement of the tarsus, the ankle, occasionally other large joints, or even small joints of the hand. Severe attacks may be accompanied by fever and leukocytosis. The acute attack will subside spontaneously in 1 or 2 weeks (occasionally longer), and the patient is then completely free of symptoms (this symptom-free interval has been called the intercritical period). In a review of 614 cases of gout, Gutman found that 62 percent

of the patients had a second attack within the first year, 16 percent after 1 to 2 years, 6 percent after 2 to 3 years, 5 percent after 3 to 5 years, and 4 percent after 6 to more than 10 years; 7 percent of the patients in this series had had only one attack of acute gout. When the condition is untreated, increasing numbers of acute attacks of gouty arthritis occur. These attacks become more and more closely spaced until, in the later, more severe cases, the patients are rarely free of pain. Approximately 50 percent of untreated patients develop chronic tophaceous gout in 10 years (see later in this section). A positive family history of gout may be obtained in some 20 or 25 percent of the patients with primary gout. The sex incidence is nine male patients for every female patient with primary gout.

During the acute gouty attack any joint in the body, and on occasion multiple joints, may be involved. For unknown reasons various types of trauma, especially surgical procedures, minor direct trauma to a joint or, occasionally, emotional disturbances, will trigger acute attacks of gout. A variety of drugs such as uricosuric agents and thiazide diuretics, which elevate serum uric acid, may also precipitate acute attacks of gouty arthritis. It has been recently shown that the starvation diet used in the treatment of obesity also leads to hyperuricemia and occasionally to acute gout.

In the acute gouty joint an effusion may be present that is characterized by an inflammatory synovial fluid. The white cell count in this fluid is usually elevated (a mean count of 21,000 cells, with counts higher than 100,000 cells per cubic millimeter being recorded), and the percentage of polymorphonuclear cells is also increased. Joint mucin is generally poor. The uric acid level of the synovial fluid is comparable to that of the serum. Urate crystals are found in the majority of the effusions, and during the acute phase about 90 percent of these crystals are intracellular. The crystals have a needlelike form and demonstrate negative birefringence when viewed in a polarizing microscope.

PATHOGENESIS OF GOUT

Until recently evidence suggested that the level of uric acid in itself was not related to the acute attack of gout — for example, many patients had hyperuricemia without having acute gout; probenecid (Benemid) could decrease the serum uric acid and not abort the acute attack, while colchicine did not affect the serum uric acid and did cure the acute attack; and experiments carried out in the past to increase the serum uric acid apparently did not cause acute gout. In the 1960s, however, a direct relationship of urate to gout was proved. By polarization microscopy it was found that urate crystals in needlelike form were present in the synovial fluid, that during acute attacks of gout they were usually intracellular, and that they decreased as the inflammation subsided. It was also demonstrated that an acute attack of gout could be precipitated by the intrasynovial injection of needlelike urate crystals in normal persons as well as in those subject to gout. It is well known that in patients with no family history of gout, any event that can cause hyperuricemia can ultimately cause attacks of acute gouty arthritis, thereby implicating the level of uric acid.

It has been proposed, therefore, that the development of acute gouty arthritis depends on the deposition of sodium urate in a needlelike form from hyperuricemic body fluids. The basic cause of the crystal deposition is not known, but it may reflect an alteration in the normal binding of urate to serum protein (albumin) or to connective tissue proteoglycans. A prime requirement may be a serum urate concentration above the point of saturation (6.4 mg per 100 ml). The appearance of these crystals evokes an acute inflammatory reaction with phagocytosis of the crystals; as a consequence of urate phagocytosis, a factor that is chemotactic for polymorphonuclear leukocytes is released from the cells. When the white cells ingest these crystals, there is a rise in their metabolic activity and an increased lactate production, which causes a decrease in the pH locally. The local decrease in pH may cause further urate crystal precipitation, and a self-sustaining propagation of the inflammation takes place. As a proton donor, urate interacts with the lipid membrane of the phagolysosome, resulting in its destruction and in the intracellular and extracellular release of its content of acid hydrolases. A possible explanation of the therapeutic efficacy of colchicine has come from the work on the crystal deposition

cycle; data now indicate that colchicine may interrupt this cycle by stabilizing the membranes of white cell lysosomes. This interruption would indeed prevent the release of acid hydrolases and thus alter leukocyte metabolism. In addition, colchicine may prevent release of the chemotactic factor mentioned above.

CHRONIC TOPHACEOUS GOUT

As the equilibrium between the production of uric acid and its excretion through the kidney and the gastrointestinal tract becomes disproportionate, urate is retained within the body (see Fig. 46-2). Slow accumulation of urates takes place and causes the production of tophi, most commonly in relatively avascular areas including cartilage, portions of synovial membrane, tendons, subcutaneous tissue, and kidney. Clinically, tophi may be seen about the joint or in the helix or anthelix of the ear of the patient. Occasionally they may spontaneously drain a white, chalky material. From a pathologic standpoint, the tophaceous nodule consists of a deposit of urate crystals plus a matrix and the foreign body granuloma evoked locally. The crystals are sodium acid urate and are generally arranged radially into small compact clusters. They are best preserved when the material has been fixed in absolute alcohol, since they are water soluble. In the joint afflicted by chronic gout there may be a chronic, nonspecific, tophaceous synovitis or degenerative joint disease resulting from disintegration of the articular cartilage. The classic punched-out cystic lesion seen by x-ray is caused by a tophaceous deposit in the bone marrow but is present in only a third of the cases. The clinical picture may occasionally resemble that of advanced and crippling rheumatoid arthritis, and there are several recorded instances in which chronic tophaceous gout has masqueraded as rheumatoid arthritis.

COMPLICATIONS OF GOUT
AND ASSOCIATED DISEASES

Renal functional impairment is frequent in gout. The most common pathologic findings are nephrosclerosis and pyelonephritis. Because of the relative insolubility of uric acid, microtophaceous deposits can occur in the renal tubules. Renal obstruction, inflammation, and secondary infection may follow.

Uric acid is the major constituent of approximately

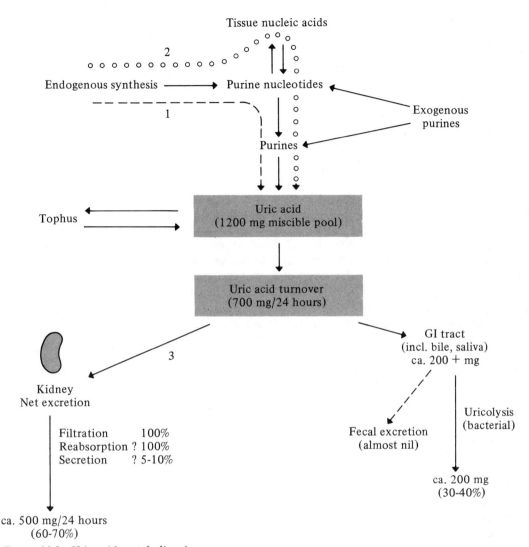

Figure 46-2. *Uric acid metabolism in man.*

5 to 10 percent of renal stones in the United States. Such stones occur in roughly 20 percent of the patients with primary gout and in almost double that number of patients with secondary gout (due to conditions such as polycythemia vera, leukemia, or myeloid metaplasia). In some patients gout is first discovered with the appearance of a uric acid stone. Uric acid is less soluble in urine than is its sodium salt, and at acid pH there is an increase in the uric acid available for local precipitation. Uric acid stones usually contain some calcium salts and are radiopaque on that basis.

An early onset and an increased incidence of hypertension have also been associated with gout. Other reported disease associations are generalized arteriosclerosis and diabetes mellitus.

URIC ACID METABOLISM
Uric acid is the final product of purine metabolism in man and is formed by the action of the enzyme xan-

thine oxidase on xanthine and hypoxanthine. The handling of uric acid by the body is outlined in Figure 46-2. The miscible pool of uric acid, as determined by radioactive isotopes, is approximately 1,200 mg; it is formed from exogenous dietary purines and from endogenous sources. There is only a slight reduction in the pool and in the serum uric acid if no purine is taken exogenously, and it has been amply demonstrated that uric acid is primarily formed from glycine and other simple precursors in the body. Although the biosynthetic pathways for purines have been elaborately worked out, the specific metabolic abnormality or abnormalities in primary gout are still to be determined.

The normal turnover of uric acid in 24 hours is roughly 700 mg. In the kidney, uric acid is thought to be filtered completely, and under normal circumstances it is completely reabsorbed. Evidence suggests that tabular secretion of uric acid by the kidney also takes place. The urinary output in the normal person is usually under 500 mg in 24 hours. The remainder of the uric acid is excreted into the gastrointestinal tract, where it is degraded by uricolysis by the bacterial flora. Fecal excretion of uric acid is practically nonexistent.

Metabolism in Primary Gout
Radioisotopic studies carried out in a small group of patients, utilizing first glycine-^{15}N and subsequently glycine-1-^{14}C, demonstrated two things: (1) an increased incorporation of the label into uric acid in patients with primary gout over a period of time; and (2) a rapid incorporation of the label in the gouty patient, with a peak in the urinary label within 1 day as opposed to 3 days in the normal person. These results indicated that at least a proportion of the patients with gout had an overproduction of uric acid, and that a shunt mechanism was probably utilized to account for the rapid incorporation of the label into the uric acid. It was found that all patients with an increased urinary excretion of uric acid (usually more than 600 mg per day) demonstrated the defect of overincorporation; these patients represented roughly 30 percent of the patients with gout. In the second group of patients — that is, those in whom the uric acid level was increased in the plasma but normal in

the urine — a proportion were also demonstrated to have overincorporation. This left a group in whom the uric acid level was elevated in the plasma but normal in the urine, and in whom no overincorporation was demonstrable. A relative renal defect in these patients (that is, lack of the tubular secretion of uric acid) has been proposed as the mechanism of the hyperuricemia. Finally, there is evidence that these several defects may be present in varying degrees — that is, overincorporation in some hyperuricemic patients, a renal defect in others, and the combination in a third group of patients who are not only overproducers of uric acid but also have a decreased urate clearance. Among the patients with overincorporation, abnormalities in feedback inhibition along with surpluses of substrates have been postulated to result from possible biochemical lesions.

Recent data indicate the presence of multiple potential and several demonstrated enzymatic abnormalities leading to purine overproduction. These abnormalities have been classified into three groups: (1) those leading to an increase in the availability of PP-ribose-P; (2) those that lead to a decrease in the intracellular pool of purine nucleotides; and (3) those that lead to an increase in glutamine concentration. The enzymes that lead to the first phenomenon (increased PP-ribose-P) are divided into those that cause an increase in the rate of its synthesis and those that cause a decrease in the rate of its utilization. Glucose 6-phosphatase deficiency and increased activity of glutathione reductase or of PP-ribose-P synthetase, or both, fall in the former category, while hypoxanthine-guanine phosphoribosyltransferase (HG-PRT) deficiency is classified in the second group.

The best characterized abnormalities are the HG-PRT deficiency, an X-linked disorder with two phenotypes: the first, the Lesch-Nyhan syndrome in males, with an almost complete enzyme deficiency, and the second, a group of individuals with only partial deficiency and minimal neurologic findings. The other well-characterized group has a deficiency in PP-ribose-P synthetase activity and also has considerable genetic heterogeneity. The potential enzyme defects are listed in tabular form.

I. ↑ PPRP available (causing purine overproduction)
   A. ↑ Rate of synthesis of PPRP

— Glucose 6-phosphatase deficiency
— Glutathione reductase increase
— PPRP synthetase increase (genetic heterogeneity) (proved)
B. ↓ Rate of utilization
— HG-PRTase deficiency (2 phenotypes: juvenile and adult) (proved)
— Xanthine oxidase deficiency
II. ↓ Intracellular purine nucleotides (causing purine overproduction)
A. ↓ Production of purine nucleotides
— HG-PRTase deficiency (see above)
— Adenosine kinase deficiency (mammalian cell line in culture only)
— ↑ Xanthine oxidase (? in gout)
B. ↑ Catabolism of purine nucleotides
— No evidence as yet
III. ↑ Glutamine concentration
↓ Renal glutaminase I (not proved)
↓ Glutamate dehydrogenase (not proved)

Metabolism in Secondary Gout

The mechanism of the hyperuricemia in patients who have polycythemia vera, myeloid metaplasia, leukemia, lymphoma, psoriasis, and other disorders associated with secondary gout seems to be reasonably straightforward. In these patients there is an increased breakdown of tissue or of white cell or red cell nucleic acids (see Fig. 46-2), with the release of increased amounts of purine and the subsequent appearance of increased amounts of uric acid. The mechanism of the hyperuricemia associated with the administration of a number of drugs such as the thiazides, pyrazinamide, or low doses of aspirin is explained by their interference with the renal tubular handling of uric acid. Uricosuric drugs such as probenecid, phenylbutazone, high doses of salicylate, and sulfinpyrazone have the opposite effect: They interfere with tubular reabsorption and cause increased uric acid excretion.

Juvenile Gout with Central Nervous System Dysfunction (Lesch-Nyhan Syndrome)

A syndrome of mental retardation, spastic cerebral palsy, choreoathetosis, and self-mutilating behavior associated with elevated levels of serum uric acid has been described in children. Inheritance follows an X-linked recessive transmission. These patients have marked overincorporation of simple precursors into uric acid and develop the stigmata of acute and chronic gout and its complications. Studies of HG-PRTase in these patients have shown the enzyme to be completely absent from their tissues. It is not yet known what the cause of the neurologic lesion is, but it is possible that it is more closely related to the oxypurine levels than to the uric acid levels in the cerebrospinal fluid.

TREATMENT

Acute Gout

One form of treatment for acute gouty arthritis is colchicine given orally in doses of 0.5 mg (or 0.65 mg) every hour until pain is relieved or until nausea or diarrhea occurs. Not more than 5 to 10 mg should normally be given in the treatment of any one acute attack. Paregoric should be administered immediately with the onset of diarrhea. On this regimen the majority of patients with acute gout will experience at least a 50 percent improvement in 24 to 48 hours. The earlier the treatment with colchicine is instituted, the more successful will be the therapeutic result. In some cases when colchicine cannot be easily administered orally, 1 to 3 mg may be given intravenously, again with relief occurring in the majority of cases in about 24 hours. An alternative treatment is phenylbutazone (Butazolidin), 400 mg immediately, followed by 200 mg in 4 to 8 hours and 200 mg 4 hours later — that is, a total of 800 mg on the first day. This dosage is usually followed by 600 mg in divided doses on the second day and 400 mg in divided doses on the third day. This regimen will abort the majority of the attacks of acute gout. Maintenance doses of colchicine (0.5 mg two or three times a day) should also be started at the same time to prevent recurrence of acute gout. The undesirable side effects of phenylbutazone include bone marrow depression, peptic ulcers, and sodium retention; this medication should therefore be used with caution. A third effective course of treatment is intramuscular corticotropin (ACTH), 100 units given intramuscularly and repeated on 3 consecutive days, again with maintenance doses of colchicine. Finally, indomethacin in doses varying from 100 to 400 mg per day for 3 days has been successfully used in the treatment of acute attacks.

Chronic Tophaceous Gout

In the treatment of chronic tophaceous gout the aim is to induce negative urate balance. Probenecid (Benemid), which causes a selective inhibition of the reabsorption of urates from the renal tubule, is commonly used. This drug has a very low toxicity. It should be given in doses of 1 to 2 gm per day, although occasionally up to 3 gm per day may be used. One can demonstrate in time a decrease in the miscible urate pool, an increased urate excretion, and a fall in the serum uric acid level toward normal. Tophi can be observed to decrease in size, although this may take well over a year. A second effective uricosuric agent is sulfinpyrazone (Anturane), which is a phenylbutazone analogue without antirheumatic properties; 50 mg of this potent uricosuric agent is given two to four times per day. A third uricosuric agent is aspirin in high doses (usually 5 to 6 gm per day). If a patient can tolerate this amount, an effective uricosuric result is obtained. It is important to be aware of the fact that low doses of aspirin (1 to 2 gm per day) cause hyperuricemia and that aspirin interferes with the action of probenecid and sulfinpyrazone, and so should not be used simultaneously with these drugs.

Whatever uricosuric agent is used, there are two potential hazards other than those due to the individual drug itself. The first of these, the provocation of an attack of acute gout, can usually be avoided by using colchicine prophylactically for several days before the uricosuric agent. The second problem is the appearance of renal colic resulting from the mobilization and excretion of large amounts of uric acid. It is important, therefore, to encourage a generous fluid intake whenever uricosuric treatment is undertaken.

A completely different approach to the treatment of tophaceous gout was made possible by the introduction of the drug allopurinol, which inhibits the enzyme xanthine oxidase. When this inhibition occurs, the production of uric acid is decreased. Although the decrease in uric acid is accompanied by an increase in xanthine and hypoxanthine, significant side effects (xanthine stones) have been reported only rarely. This drug is particularly valuable in treating patients who have urate stones, renal disease, or massive hyperuricemia due to tissue destruction (for example, associated with therapy of myeloproliferative diseases). The dose ranges from 200 to 600 mg per day and averages 400 mg per day. Differences in the responses of patients to allopurinol have recently been related to HC-PRTase activity, since allopurinol has a secondary effect as an inhibitor of purine synthesis de novo, and presence of the enzyme HG-PRTase may be necessary for this effect.

SUMMARY

Primary gout is a disorder characterized by hyperuricemia, acute arthritis, response to colchicine, and urate crystals in the synovial fluid. The mechanisms involved are an overproduction of urate and abnormalities in the renal handling of uric acid as well as enzyme abnormalities in some patients. Secondary gout is characterized by acute arthritis and hyperuricemia associated with diseases in which there is an accelerated nucleoprotein turnover, or interference with the renal handling of uric acid by drugs or intrinsic renal disease. The diagnosis of gout is dependent on the clinical appearance of acute episodic arthritis, associated with an increased serum uric acid level, adequate response to colchicine, and the appearance of urate crystals in the synovial fluid.

Ochronotic Arthropathy

Ochronosis and ochronotic arthropathy are the sequelae of alkaptonuria, an asymptomatic inborn error of metabolism that is characterized by an absence of the enzyme homogentisic acid oxidase. This disorder is transmitted by a single autosomal recessive gene and has been estimated to affect one person per 100,000. As a consequence of the enzyme defect, the body pool of homogentisic acid is greatly increased, and the urine contains large amounts of this compound. Though normal in color when passed, the urine darkens upon standing several hours, as a result of oxidation of the homogentisic acid. As a useful screening test, addition of a few drops of alkali ($10N$ NaOH) to the urine, by accelerating the oxidation of homogentisic acid, will produce immediate darkening of the sample. The polymerized oxidation products of homogentisic acid in vivo have a marked affinity for connective tissue and are responsible for the blue-black pigmentation which, by the third decade, becomes clinically evident in the sclerae, ear cartilage, and skin of alkaptonuric patients. The ochre color of this pigment in tissues viewed under the light microscope is responsible for the name given to the disorder, which is an inevitable consequence of the enzyme defect.

The pigment resembles melanin and accumulates especially in intervertebral disks and articular cartilage. Some 50 percent of patients with alkaptonuria ultimately develop progressive ochronotic arthropathy, which often leads to their total incapacitation by the sixth decade. Articular involvement is considerably more common in males than in females. The most common clinical presentation is stiffness and pain in the low back, caused by ochronotic spondylosis. Patients present with many of the features of ankylosing spondylitis. X-ray films are distinctive and show calcification of intervertebral disks, most advanced in the lumbar spine, with disk degeneration and narrowing of the intervertebral spaces. Osteophytes may be present but usually are not prominent. In contrast to ankylosing spondylitis, sacroiliac joints are uninvolved, syndesmophytes are absent, and ossification of paraspinous ligaments does not occur. In approximately 20 percent of males with ochronotic spondylopathy, the disease presents initially in the second or third decade with acute rupture of an intervertebral disk.

In peripheral joints, ochronotic arthropathy is marked by cartilage degeneration that resembles primary osteoarthritis. Knees, hips, and shoulders are most commonly involved. In sharp contrast to osteoarthritis, however, the small joints of the hands are spared. Pathologically, pigment deposits are seen in the articular cartilage, which becomes brittle and then fibrillates and fragments. As a result, osteochondral loose bodies may be seen within the joint. Fragments of cartilage may float free and become embedded in the synovial membrane, resulting in synovial effusions. Small fragments of pigmented cartilage may be numerous in the joint fluid, resembling a sprinkling of ground pepper. Chondrocalcinosis is occasionally associated with the peripheral joint disease, and the joint effusions may contain crystals of calcium pyrophosphate dihydrate. Treatment of ochronotic arthropathy should be aimed at relief of pain and prevention of deformities. Loose joint bodies may require surgical removal. Recent experimental evidence has indicated that ascorbic acid may inhibit the binding of homogentisic acid to connective tissue, suggesting that in the early stages of the disease, this drug may be of benefit.

Tumors and Tumorlike Conditions in Joints

Either benign or malignant primary or metastatic tumors of joint structures are rare. Diagnosis is established by biopsy, but difficulties may be encountered in distinguishing these tumors from certain nonneoplastic lesions. Synoviomas have the malignant character of sarcomas in other sites of the body. Pigmented villonodular synovitis has certain characteristics both of a benign neoplasm and of an inflammatory reaction. In this condition hemosiderin is deposited in the synovial tissues which, in addition, are infiltrated with giant cells and xanthoma cells. Most lesions occur in the knee, and the diagnosis may be suspected on obtaining a bloody tap from a nontraumatic effusion. Related to villonodular synovitis is a relatively common tendon-sheath tumor, giant cell tumor, or xanthoma, which most commonly occurs on the flexor tendons of the fingers. Synovial osteochondromatosis is a rare benign condition in which small nodules of bone and cartilage form within synovial villi. In leukemia, articular symptoms may result from direct leukemic infiltration of the synovial or paraarticular tissues. Articular symptoms associated with multiple myeloma may be caused either by direct invasion by plasma cells or by synovial deposits of amyloid (see later in this chapter).

Heritable Disorders of Connective Tissue

It is difficult to conceive of simple biochemical and biophysical techniques as directly solving the problem of the etiology of the many inflammatory connective tissue diseases already mentioned. There is a group of disorders, however, in which noninflammatory abnormalities are present, and which are related to connective tissue elements themselves (that is, fibroblasts, collagen, elastic tissue, mucopolysaccharides), and in which there is reason to believe that modern macromolecular biology offers the best hope for the elucidation of pathogenesis. These disorders — namely, Marfan's syndrome, the Ehlers-Danlos syndrome, pseudoxanthoma elasticum, osteogenesis imperfecta, and the mucopolysaccharidoses — are inherited diseases of connective tissue and have been ably reviewed by McKusick.

THE MARFAN SYNDROME

The classic triad known as the Marfan syndrome consists of dolichomorphism, aortic dilatation or dissection or both, and subluxation of the ocular lenses. The basic cause of this disorder is not known; it is inherited as an autosomal dominant. A large proportion of affected persons represent sporadic de novo, rather than inherited, mutations. A minimal prevalence figure of 1.5 : 100,000 of the population has been cited. Patients with the disorder have long, thin extremities, their arm span is greater than their height, and their lower body segment length (pubis to heels) is greater than the upper (pubis to vertex). Arachnodactyly is a hallmark of the syndrome. Funnel chest, kyphoscoliosis, and other skeletal deformities are common. The skeletal ligaments are often lax, leading to hyperextensible joints. In most patients the suspensory ligaments of the lens are also lax, resulting in ectopia lentis and associated iridodonesis (tremor of the iris), which may be the presenting sign. Abdominal hernias are not uncommon. Several patients have been described who suffered repeated spontaneous pneumothorax.

A wide variety of congenital defects in the heart, lungs, and skeleton (e.g., coarctation of the aorta, patent ductus arteriosus, cystic disease of the lungs, spina bifida occulta), and also in other areas, occur with greater than usual incidence in the Marfan syndrome. Although these defects are not part of the classic syndrome, they may be due to the influence of the connective tissue defect on embryogenesis. Fibromyxomatous degeneration of the mitral valve, with systolic prolapse of the posterior leaflet into the left atrium, is seen frequently and produces the syndrome of mid-late systolic clicks with late systolic murmurs. Endocarditis may develop on the abnormal valve. The classic aortic lesion is caused by cystic medionecrosis, resulting in progressive dilatation with aneurysm formation, aortic regurgitation and, ultimately, dissection or rupture (or both). The average age of death in a series of 72 patients with the Marfan syndrome was 32 years, with the aortopathy and its complications accounting for about 80 percent of the deaths.

HOMOCYSTINURIA

Homocystinuria is an autosomal recessive disorder with a prevalence of 5 per 1,000,000 population, in which the enzyme cystathionine synthetase is deficient. The disease must be distinguished from the Marfan syndrome, since patients with homocystinuria also exhibit arachnodactyly and other evidence of dolichomorphism, skeletal deformities, and ectopic lenses. Mental retardation may occur. Cardiovascular disease is a major problem in patients with homocystinuria and is signalled by multiple arterial and venous thromboses, resulting in renovascular hypertension, pulmonary embolism, myocardial infarction, and premature death. Cystic medionecrosis with aortic dilatation and dissection, as seen in the Marfan syndrome, is not a feature of homocystinuria. The specific diagnosis is made by demonstration of homocystine in the urine, for which the silver nitroprusside test serves as a useful screening procedure. The test is performed by saturating 6 or 7 ml of urine with solid sodium chloride, following which 0.25 ml of 1% sodium nitroprusside and 0.25 ml of 0.7% sodium cyanide are added. If homocystine is present, a pink or purple color develops immediately. Although the etiology of the disorder is unknown, recent evidence has suggested that a primitive collagen cross-link (derived from hydroxylysine and the hydroxylysine-derived aldehyde, hydroxylysino-hydroxynorleucine) is "trapped" in homocystinuria, preventing formation of more complex cross-links.

THE EHLERS-DANLOS SYNDROME

The Ehlers-Danlos syndrome is characterized by hyperextensible joints together with fragility and hyperelasticity of the skin. A variety of other abnormalities, including diaphragmatic hernia, respiratory and gastrointestinal tract ectasia, and congenital cardiac abnormalities, have also been reported. Characteristically, the stretched skin returns easily to its original shape, although with the passage of time, dermal elasticity may also be lost. The skin may be fragile, may bruise easily, and may develop calcified spherules or molluscoid pseudotumors. "Cigarette paper" scars develop over points of trauma, such as shins and knees. The articular laxity may result in genu recurvatum and recurrent joint dislocations. The disorder is usually inherited as an autosomal dominant; however, it has become apparent that patients with the Ehlers-Danlos syndrome constitute a clinically and genetically heterogeneous group. The basic defect is thought to affect the organization of collagen bundles into their normal meshwork. In certain instances, specific biochemical abnormalities of collagen have been elucidated (Table 46-3).

PSEUDOXANTHOMA ELASTICUM
Pseudoxanthoma elasticum is an inherited connective tissue disorder involving the skin, eyes, and arteries. Its prevalence has been stated to be at least 1 : 160,000. The areas of integument that are subject to the greatest amounts of wear and tear (the flexural areas of the neck, axilla, and groin) undergo deterioration, develop yellowish papules, and take on a redundant appearance. Histologically, the affected skin shows fragmentation of elastic fibers, which have a granular, irregular appearance and show a strong affinity for calcium. In 85 percent of patients, examination of the optic fundus reveals angioid streaks, which appear as irregular, pigmented, brownish peripapillary lines that radiate outward. Although the presence of these lesions is not pathognomonic of pseudoxanthoma elasticum (they have been reported in Paget's disease and in sickle cell anemia), they are indicative of a systemic disease and represent a breakdown in Bruch's membrane behind the retina. In some patients, retinal hemorrhage or central chorioretinitis and subsequent chorioretinal fibrosis develop and may lead to blindness.

The arteries undergo premature degeneration and calcification; the extent of the latter, as seen on x-rays, is often striking. The arterial disease results in diminished peripheral pulses with vascular insufficiency, intermittent claudication, angina pectoris, renovascular hypertension, and a striking predilection for gastrointestinal hemorrhage. The hemorrhagic

features of the disease are attributable to degeneration of the elastic media of small and medium-sized arteries. All the aforementioned vascular complications may occur at a very early age. Sudden death is not uncommon, and approximately 50 percent of patients with this disorder do not survive beyond age 50. The disorder is genetically heterogeneous. Although in most instances it is transmitted as a autosomal recessive, autosomal dominant forms also exist. The pathogenesis of pseudoxanthoma elasticum is not known, although many authorities believe that it represents an abiotrophy of the elastic fiber in the connective tissue.

OSTEOGENESIS IMPERFECTA (FRAGILITAS OSSIUM)
Osteogenesis imperfecta is an inherited connective tissue disease affecting the skeletal system, the eye (blue sclerae), the joints (loose jointedness), the ear (progressive deafness), and the teeth (dentinogenesis imperfecta). It may be the disease that afflicted the artist Toulouse-Lautrec.

Clinically, the bones are exceedingly weak and prone to develop multiple fractures (including intrauterine fractures). Although this tendency lessens with puberty, patients with the disorder are usually short, with bowed, osteoporotic bones, platybasia, "codfish" vertebrae, and a bulging calvaria. The blue appearance of the sclera, the otosclerosis, the dental abnormalities, and the loose jointedness, as well as the skeletal abnormality, are believed to be caused by a defect in the maturation of collagen, which is deficient throughout the body. Plasma calcium, inorganic phosphate, and alkaline phosphatase levels are usually normal. The disorder seems to be inherited as an autosomal dominant; its frequency has been estimated to be 1 in 40,000 births.

THE MUCOPOLYSACCHARIDOSES
A number of heritable syndromes resulting from abnormalities in mucopolysaccharide metabolism are recognized. The associated phenotypic features differ in severity in these syndromes, which have in common an abnormal urinary excretion of mucopolysaccharides. In some cases, the basic metabolic abnormality has been demonstrated in fibroblast cultures (see Table 46-4).

Table 46-3. Heterogeneity of Ehlers-Danlos Syndrome

Type	Transmission	Skin hyperextensibility	Joint hypermobility	Other	Biochemical defect
I	Autosomal dominant	++++	++++	Skin fragility ++++	?
II	Autosomal dominant	+ to ++	+ to ++	....	?
III	Autosomal dominant	+	++++	....	?
IV	Autosomal dominant	0 to +	+ (usually only digits)	Bruisability ++++ Rupture of bowel ++++ Rupture of arteries ++++	Absence of type III collagen
V	X-linked recessive	++++	+	Bruisability ++	?
VI	Autosomal recessive	++++	++++	Fragilitas oculi	Lysyl hydroxylase deficiency
VII	Autosomal recessive (?)	++	+++	Bruisability ++	Procollagen peptidase deficiency

0 to ++++ = estimated ranges of severity of clinical findings.

Table 46-4. The Mucopolysaccharidoses

Type	Syndrome eponym	Inheritance	Clinical features	Urine	Enzyme deficiency
I	Hurler's	Autosomal recessive	Gargoylism, mental retardation, hepatosplenomegaly, corneal clouding, stiff joints, vertebral abnormalities, early demise	Dermatan sulfate Heparan sulfate	α-L-iduronidase
II	Hunter's	X-linked recessive	Gargoylism less severe than in type I, normal intellect, no corneal clouding	Dermatan sulfate Heparan sulfate	. . . .
III	Sanfilippo A	Autosomal recessive	Severe CNS abnormalities, mild somatic changes	Heparan sulfate	Heparan sulfate sulfatase
	Sanfilippo B	Autosomal recessive	Same as IIIA	Heparan sulfate	N-acetyl-hexosaminidase
IV	Morquio's	Autosomal recessive	Dwarfism, kyphosis, flat vertebrae with wedging, diffuse epiphyseal osteo-dystrophy, aortic regurgitation	Keratan sulfate	. . . .
V	Scheie's	Autosomal recessive	Corneal clouding, aortic regurgitation, normal intellect, coarse facies, claw hands	Dermatan sulfate Heparan sulfate	α-L-iduronidase
VI	Maroteaux-Lamy	Autosomal recessive	Severe vertebral and epiphyseal abnor-malities, corneal clouding, normal intellect	Dermatan sulfate	. . . .
VII	. . . .	Autosomal recessive	Hepatosplenomegaly, dysostosis, mental retardation, leukocyte inclusions	Dermatan sulfate	β-glucuronidase

Miscellaneous Disorders

AMYLOIDOSIS

Systemic amyloidosis is a pathologic condition characterized by the accumulation of a fibrous glycoprotein, called amyloid, in the extracellular connective tissue. It occurs in association with rheumatoid arthritis, chronic osteomyelitis, tuberculosis, bronchiectasis, and a great variety of other inflammatory conditions *(secondary amyloidosis)*. In addition, amyloidosis appears de novo with no other disease association *(primary amyloidosis)*. Several heredofamilial forms of systemic amyloidosis have also been recognized. Amyloidosis has been found in frequent association with familial Mediterranean fever; it is also present in 10 to 15 percent of patients with multiple myeloma. Amyloid may also accumulate in local deposits (that is, nonsystemically), either diffusely within an organ or as a tumoral mass. Localized amyloid tumors are most commonly observed in the respiratory and urinary tracts. Amyloid deposition is also related to aging, and amyloid may be found in the hearts of elderly persons, in the "senile" plaques within the brain of patients with Alzheimer's disease, and in the pancreas of patients with diabetes mellitus.

Clinical Features

Since any organ system may be involved, the clinical manifestations of amyloidosis are truly protean. In patients with rheumatoid arthritis or other predisposing conditions, the development of systemic amyloidosis should be suspected if either albuminuria or hepatosplenomegaly develops. In primary systemic amyloidosis or in amyloidosis associated with plasma cell dyscrasias (e.g., multiple myeloma, Waldenstrom's macroglobulinemia, heavy-chain disease), peripheral neuropathy may occur as a result of pressure on a nerve (as in the carpal tunnel syndrome) or of direct infiltration of a nerve. In such cases the neuropathy is often the presenting feature. Serum M-components (monoclonal immunoglobulin abnormalities) are also uniformly observed. As with the neuropathy, the arthropathy and, perhaps, also the macroglossia (due to infiltration of the nerves, joints, and tongue, respectively, with amyloid) appear only in patients with *primary* systemic amyloidosis, or with amyloidosis associated with plasma cell dyscrasias (that is, these symptoms have not been reported in patients with true *secondary* amyloidosis). Primary amyloid nephrosis is being seen with increasing frequency as greater numbers of renal biopsies are carried out. In other respects, however, a marked overlap is found in organ distribution and tinctorial characteristics of the deposits obtained from patients with primary and secondary systemic amyloidosis, those with amyloidosis associated with plasma cell dyscrasias, or those with localized amyloidosis. The only valid *clinical* separation of the various types of amyloidosis currently appears to be based on the associated disease, if any, and on the heredofamilial aspects. Biochemical differences between primary, myeloma-related, and secondary amyloidosis have been demonstrated (see the next section).

Etiology

The cause of amyloidosis is not known. Many possibilities, especially immunologic factors, have been studied. Recent evidence suggests that amyloid may be formed locally by reticuloendothelial cells, but the primary stimulus of its formation is not known. Under the electron microscope, all types of amyloid have an ultrastructure consisting of fine fibrils that are approximately 75 Å in diameter. Biochemically, however, the fibrils from patients with primary amyloidosis and those with multiple myeloma consist of fragments or complete portions of immunoglobulin light chains, especially the variable segments, whereas the fibrils from patients with secondary amyloidosis are comprised of a nonimmunoglobulin protein (AA). In the sera of normal persons, as well as that of patients with secondary amyloidosis, a circulating alpha globulin (SAA) is present that is immunologically related to the secondary amyloid fibril and may represent a precursor of the fibril protein.

Diagnosis and Treatment

The diagnosis of amyloidosis can be firmly established only by tissue examination. Rectal biopsies produce a high incidence of positive results in proved cases. In selected patients, skin, gingival, renal, and liver biopsies are of value. All biopsy specimens must be stained with Congo red and viewed in the polarizing micro-scope for green birefringence. There is no known treatment for amyloidosis. Following removal of a source of chronic infection such as a focus of osteo-myelitis, however, regression of amyloid has occasion-ally been observed. When amyloidosis of the kidneys is the predominant clinical problem, renal transplan-tation may be of benefit. There is also great interest in the therapeutic potential of colchicine, since this agent is capable of preventing acute attacks of familial Mediterranean fever as well as suppressing amyloid formation in casein-treated mice.

FAMILIAL MEDITERRANEAN FEVER

Familial Mediterranean fever (familial paroxysmal polyserositis) is an autosomal recessively inherited disease of unknown etiology that is most frequently encountered in ethnic groups of Mediterranean an-cestry, particularly Sephardic Jews, Armenians, Turks, and Arabs. The diagnosis is based entirely on a his-tory of recurrent, self-limited attacks of fever, rash, and pain in the abdomen, chest, and joints; the last symptom represents inflammation of the peritoneal, pleural, and synovial membranes. Amyloidosis has been reported in 40 percent of Sephardic Jews with familial Mediterranean fever, but this complication appears to be less common in North American pa-tients of Armenian origin. The attacks can be fre-quent, painful, and often disabling. Recent studies from both the United States and Israel indicate that colchicine, 0.5 mg twice a day, seems to reduce the incidence and severity of attacks of familial Medi-terranean fever.

CALCIUM PYROPHOSPHATE CRYSTAL DEPOSITION DISEASE

This disorder, originally named *pseudogout* (or *chon-drocalcinosis* in the European literature), is a syn-drome characterized by acute attacks of monoarticular arthritis that usually involves large joints, especially the knee. It is seen in both males and females, usually those over age 50, and it commonly has a self-limited course of 2 to 4 weeks. The patients have radiologic-ally demonstrable articular cartilage calcification and often have degenerative joint disease. Synovial fluid analysis shows an inflammatory joint fluid containing crystals that have weakly positive birefringence (urate

crystals exhibit negative birefringence); x-ray diffrac-tion and biochemical studies have characterized the crystals as calcium pyrophosphate dihydrate. The disorder may be seen in association with hyperpara-thyroidism, ochronosis, neuropathic arthropathy, and hemochromatosis. Diabetes mellitus is also a common associated disease. Treatment is symptom-atic since the attacks are short-lived, and joint aspira-tion alone affords considerable relief. The use of colchicine and other drugs has generally not proved to be effective in this disorder.

The pathogenesis of the crystal deposition is not known. The pyrophosphate (PPi) concentrations have not been found to be elevated in plasma or urine, and the synovial fluid alkaline phosphate levels are generally normal. On the other hand, synovial fluid levels of PPi are consistently increased in pseudogout, suggesting a local abnormality in pyrophosphatase. This abnormality is not specific for pseudogout, how-ever, and occurs also in osteoarthritis.

HYPERTROPHIC OSTEOARTHROPATHY

Hypertrophic osteoarthropathy is a syndrome charac-terized by clubbing of the fingers and toes, periostitis with new bone formation at the distal ends of the long bones, and swelling and pain of the peripheral joints. Idiopathic and hereditary forms have been described, but the disorder usually occurs secondary to lesions in the intrathoracic cavity. These lesions include lung tumors (either benign or malignant), aortic aneurysms, congenital cyanotic heart disease, pulmonary tuberculosis, bronchiectasis, and others. Hypertrophic osteoarthropathy occurs in 5 to 10 per-cent of patients with intrathoracic neoplasms and may be the presenting feature of bronchogenic carcinoma. Occasionally the syndrome is observed in association with chronic extrathoracic conditions such as cirrhosis or chronic diarrheal states (for example, inflammatory bowel disease).

The primary anatomic change appears to be over-growth of connective tissue, secondary to increased blood flow. Measures that normalize blood flow in the limbs may cause prompt regression of the osteo-arthropathy. Reversal of signs and symptoms after vagotomy suggests that the pathogenesis may be mediated by a neurogenic reflex in which the afferent fibers run in the vagus nerve.

Clinically, the onset may be insidious or acute. Patients often fail to note clubbing of the fingers until bone deformities or joint pain and swelling supervene. Uncommonly, bone or joint symptoms may antedate clubbing by weeks or months. Bouts of profuse sweating of the hands and feet may occur, as well as Raynaud's phenomenon. Gynecomastia appears in about one-fifth of the patients. Thickening of the skin, especially on the forehead and extremities (pachydermoperiostosis) may occur and is characteristic of the hereditary form of the disease. Therapy is directed against the primary cause. Surgical removal of an intrathoracic lesion or vagotomy often leads within days to regression of the bone and soft tissue lesions. Supportive analgesic drugs or corticosteroids may be useful for the bone and joint pain.

ACUTE BACTERIAL ARTHRITIS

Acute bacterial joint infection is a remediable form of arthritis, but one that demands prompt diagnosis and treatment. Although the incidence has lessened with the use of antibiotics, acute joint infections are not uncommon, particularly in the very young, the elderly, and in persons with already damaged joints (especially those with rheumatoid arthritis). Infections may reach joints by hematogenous spread, by local direct implantation (e.g., following trauma), or by spread from contiguous bone infection (osteomyelitis). Common infecting organisms include *Staphylococcus aureus, Neisseria gonorrhoeae,* and *Streptococcus pyogenes.* In infants, *Hemophilus influenzae* is commonly implicated in acute bacterial joint infections. Infections with gram-negative enteric bacilli occur most often in elderly or debilitated persons with compromised host defenses or with established extra-articular infections with the same organism.

Clinical Features

The disorder usually presents as an acute monoarticular arthritis of a large joint, although any joint may become infected. Polyarthritis occurs in 10 to 20 percent of cases and is especially notable as a prodromal feature in gonococcal arthritis. The infected joint is usually red, hot, tender, and painful on motion. In patients who are severely debilitated or who are receiving cytotoxic drugs, however, these classic signs of inflammation may be less prominent. One-third of patients with acute bacterial arthritis may not be febrile, and in many leukocytosis is absent in the peripheral blood.

Laboratory Findings

In any patient in whom an infectious arthritis is suspected, prompt joint aspiration is mandatory. Smears of the joint fluid should be examined by Gram's stain. Aerobic and anaerobic cultures with appropriate antibiotic sensitivity studies should be carried out. White cell counts in infected fluids may range from a few thousand to 250,000 cells per cubic millimeter. Counts higher than 50,000 cells per cubic millimeter are typical, and if the white cell count in the synovial fluid is higher than 100,000 cells per cubic millimeter, infection should be considered present until proved otherwise. However, in rare cases of noninfectious synovitis (e.g., acute rheumatoid arthritis or gout) counts of this magnitude may be encountered. The percentage of polymorphonuclear leukocytes in the synovial fluid in infectious arthritis is usually over 90 percent. Glucose in the synovial fluid falls precipitously after infection, often to less than 30 mg per 100 ml, and the difference between the synovial fluid and blood sugar concentrations is usually over 50 mg per 100 ml. The synovial fluid mucin is generally of poor quality. X-ray examinations of affected joints in the first 7 to 10 days may show effusion and periarticular swelling but little else. Subsequently, generalized demineralization, destruction of cartilage, and loss of detail of subchondral bone occur; if the disease is untreated, further destructive changes may ensue.

Treatment

Successful treatment depends on appropriate antibiotic therapy and adequate drainage of the joint. Choice of antibiotics is determined by the sensitivities of the organisms cultured from (or presumed to be present in) the joint space. If a joint infection is discovered and appropriately treated within 1 week of its onset, results are almost always excellent. Delay in therapy often leads to complications, for example, joint contracture, chronic synovitis, secondary osteomyelitis, or ankylosis. Infected joints should be completely aspirated daily, or as frequently as the effusion reaccumulates. The response to therapy can be assessed by sequential analyses of the fluid (outlined above). Serial measurements of antibiotic concentrations or of the bacteriocidal capacity of the fluid may be of great value in monitoring the adequacy of treatment. In most cases, parenteral administration of antibiotics results in adequate synovial fluid concentrations of the drug, obviating the need for intraarticular administration of the antibiotic. With infections produced by relatively resistant organisms, however, such as some gram-negative bacilli, the difference between the minimal inhibitory concentration of the antibiotic and the concentration achieved in the synovial fluid with systemic antibiotic administration may be small. In such instances, if a prompt response to systemic therapy is not apparent, consideration should be given to supplementary intraarticular injection of the antibiotic. For some antibiotics (e.g., polymyxin, gentamycin, carbenicillin) data are not yet available to indicate whether or not adequate synovial fluid levels can be achieved by systemic administration. The infected joint should be immobilized with splints during the acute phase. Passive and active motion are instituted when signs of acute inflammation have subsided. In severe and in antibiotic-resistant infections, open drainage may be necessary.

Bibliography

ACUTE SUPPURATIVE ARTHRITIS

Brandt, K. D., Cathcart, E. S., and Cohen, A. S. Gonococcal arthritis. *Arthritis Rheum.* 17:503, 1974.

Goldenberg, D. L., and Cohen, A. S. Acute infectious arthritis: A review of patients with nongonococcal joint infections (with emphasis on therapy and prognosis). *Am. J. Med.* 60:369, 1976.

AMYLOIDOSIS

Cohen, A. S. Amyloidosis. *N. Engl. J. Med.* 277:522, 574, 628, 1967.

ANKYLOSING SPONDYLITIS

Blumberg, B., and Ragan, C. The natural history of rheumatoid spondylitis. *Medicine* 35:1, 1956.

McEwen, C., DiTata, D., Lingg, C., Porini, A., Good, A., and Rankin, T. Ankylosing spondylitis and spondylitis accompanying ulcerative colitis, regional enteritis, psoriasis and Reiter's disease: A comparative study. *Arthritis Rheum.* 14:291, 1971.

Schlosstein, L., Terasaki, P. I., Bluestone, R., and Pearson, C. M. High association of an HL-A antigen, W27, with ankylosing spondylitis. *N. Engl. J. Med.* 288:704, 1973.

CALCIUM PYROPHOSPHATE CRYSTAL DEPOSITION DISEASE (PSEUDOGOUT)

McCarty, D. J., Jr. Calcium pyrophosphate dihydrate crystal deposition disease—1975. *Arthritis Rheum.* 19:275, 1976.

Skinner, M., and Cohen, A. S. Calcium pyrophosphate dihydrate crystal deposition disease. *Arch. Intern. Med.* 123:636, 1969.

DEGENERATIVE JOINT DISEASE

Bollet, A. J. An essay on the biology of osteoarthritis. *Arthritis Rheum.* 12:152, 1969.

Mankin, H. J. Reaction of articular cartilage to injury and osteoarthritis. *N. Engl. J. Med.* 291:1285, 1335, 1974.

Sokoloff, L. *The Biology of Degenerative Joint Disease.* Chicago: The University of Chicago Press, 1969.

ETIOLOGY, CLASSIFICATION, AND GENERAL REFERENCES ON ARTHRITIS AND CONNECTIVE TISSUE DISEASES

Cohen, A. S. *Laboratory Diagnostic Procedures in the Rheumatic Diseases* (2nd ed.). Boston: Little, Brown, 1975.

Hollander, J. E., and McCarty, D. J., Jr. *Arthritis and Allied Conditions* (8th ed.). Philadelphia: Lea & Febiger, 1972.

Samter, M. *Immunological Diseases* (3rd ed.). Boston: Little, Brown, 1978.

GIANT CELL ARTERITIS

Fauchald, P., Rygvold, O., and Oystese, B. Temporal arteritis and polymyalgia rheumatica: Clinical and biopsy findings. *Ann. Intern. Med.* 77:845, 1972.

Hunder, G. G., Disney, T. F., and Ward, L. E. Polymyalgia rheumatica. *Mayo Clin. Proc.* 44:849,
1969.

GOUT

Holmes, E. W., Kelley, W. N., and Wyngaarden, J. B.
Control of purine biosynthesis in normal and
pathologic states. *Bull. Rheum. Dis.* 26:848,
1975–76.

Proceedings of the second conference in gout and
purine metabolism. *Arthritis Rheum.* 18:659,
1975.

Rundles, R. W., Wyngaarden, J. B., Hitchings, G. H.,
and Elion, G. H. Drugs and uric acid. *Annu.
Rev. Pharmacol.* 9:345, 1969.

Wyngaarden, J. B., and Kelley, W. N. *Gout and Hyperuricemia.* New York: Grune & Stratton, 1976.

HERITABLE DISORDERS OF CONNECTIVE TISSUE

Beighton, P., Price, A., Lord, J., and Dickson, E.
Variants of the Ehlers-Danlos syndrome. *Ann.
Rheum. Dis.* 28:228, 1969.

Carey, M. C., Donovan, D. E., Fitzgerald, O., and
McAuley, F. D. Homocystinuria: I. A clinical
and pathological study of nine subjects in six
families. *Am. J. Med.* 45:7, 1968.

Goodman, R. M., Smith, E. W., Paton, D., Bergman,
R. A., Siegel, C. L., Ottesen, O. E., Shelley,
W. M., Pusch, A. L., and McKusick, V. A.
Pseudoxanthoma elasticum: A clinical and
histopathological study. *Medicine* 42:297,
1963.

McKusick, V. A. *Heritable Disorders of Connective
Tissue* (4th ed.). St. Louis: Mosby, 1972.

HYPERTROPHIC OSTEOARTHROPATHY

Mendlowitz, M. Clubbing and hypertrophic osteoarthropathy. *Medicine* 21:269, 1942.

JUVENILE RHEUMATOID ARTHRITIS

Ansell, B. M. (ed.). Rheumatic Diseases in Childhood.
In *Clinics in Rheumatic Diseases.* Philadelphia:
Saunders, 1976.

Bujak, J. J., Aptekar, R. G., Decker, J. L., and Wolff,
S. M. Juvenile rheumatoid arthritis presenting
in the adult as fever of unknown origin.
Medicine 52:431, 1973.

Calabro, J. J., Katz, R. M., and Malty, B. A. A critical
reappraisal of juvenile rheumatoid arthritis.
Clin. Orthop. 74:101, 1971.

NONARTICULAR RHEUMATISM

Mattingly, S. The Painful Shoulder. In A. S. J. Dixon
(ed.), *Progress in Clinical Rheumatology.*
Boston: Little, Brown, 1965.

Steinbrocker, D., and Argyros, T. G. Shoulder-hand
syndrome: Present status as diagnostic and
therapeutic entity. *Med. Clin. North Am.*
42:1533, 1958.

PERIARTERITIS NODOSA

Frohner, P. P., and Sheps, S. G. Long-term follow-up
study of periarteritis nodosa. *Am. J. Med.* 43:8,
1967.

Rose, G. A., and Spencer, H. Periarteritis nodosa.
Q. J. Med. 26:43, 1957.

POLYMYOSITIS

Bohan, A., and Peter, J. B. Polymyositis and dermatomyositis. *N. Engl. J. Med.* 292:344, 1975.

Walton, J. N., and Adams, R. D. *Polymyositis.*
Baltimore: Williams & Wilkins, 1958.

PSORIATIC ARTHRITIS

Wright, V. Psoriatic arthritis. *Bull. Rheum. Dis.*
21:627, 1971.

REITER'S SYNDROME

Morris, R., Metzger, A. L., Bluestone, R., and Terasaki, P. I. HL-A W27: A clue to the diagnosis
and pathogenesis of Reiter's syndrome. *N. Engl.
J. Med.* 290:554, 1974.

Weinberger, H. W., Ropes, M. W., Kulka, J. P., and
Bauer, W. Reiter's syndrome, clinical and
pathologic observations. *Medicine* 41:35, 1962.

RHEUMATOID ARTHRITIS

Goldie, I. F. Synovectomy in rheumatoid arthritis:
A general review and an 8 year follow-up of
synovectomy in 50 rheumatoid joints. *Semin.
Arthritis Rheum.* 3:219, 1974.

Gordon, D. A., Stein, J. L., and Broder, I. The extra-
articular features of rheumatoid arthritis. *Am.
J. Med.* 54:445, 1973.

Johnson, J. S., Vaughn, J. H., Hench, P. K., and
Blomgren, S. E. Rheumatoid arthritis, 1970–
1972. *Ann. Intern. Med.* 78:937, 1973.

O'Sullivan, J. B., and Cathcart, E. S. The prevalence of rheumatoid arthritis. *Ann. Intern. Med.* 76:573, 1972.

Ropes, M. W., Bennett, G. A., Cobb, S., Jacox, R., and Jessar, R. A. 1958 revision of diagnostic criteria for rheumatoid arthritis. *Bull. Rheum. Dis.* 9:175, 1958.

Short, C. L., Bauer, W., and Reynolds, W. E. *Rheumatoid Arthritis.* Cambridge, Mass.: Harvard University Press, 1957.

Stage, D., and Mannik, M. Rheumatoid factors in rheumatoid arthritis. *Bull. Rheum. Dis.* 23:720, 1973.

Williams, R. C. *Rheumatoid Arthritis as a Systemic Disease.* Philadelphia: Saunders, 1974.

Ziff, M. Pathophysiology of rheumatoid arthritis. *Fed. Proc.* 32:131, 1973.

SCLERODERMA

Campbell, P. M., and LeRoy, E. C. Pathogenesis of systemic sclerosis: A vascular hypothesis. *Semin. Arthritis Rheum.* 4:351, 1975.

D'Angelo, W. A., Freis, J. F., Masi, A. T., and Shulman, L. E. Pathologic observations in systemic sclerosis (scleroderma). *Am. J. Med.* 46:428, 1969.

Medsger, T. A., Jr., Masi, A. T., Rodman, G. P., Benedek, T. G., and Robinson, H. Survival with systemic sclerosis (scleroderma): A life table analysis of clinical and dermographic factors in 309 patients. *Ann. Intern. Med.* 75:369, 1971.

Rodnan, G. P. Progressive Systemic Sclerosis (Diffuse Scleroderma). In M. Samter (ed.), *Immunological Diseases* (3rd ed.). Boston: Little, Brown, 1978.

SJÖGREN'S SYNDROME

Shearn, M. A. *Sjögren's Syndrome.* Philadelphia: Saunders, 1971.

SYSTEMIC LUPUS ERYTHEMATOSUS

Blomgren, S. E., Condemi, J. J., and Vaughan, J. H. Procainamide-induced lupus erythematosus. *Am. J. Med.* 53:338, 1972.

Cohen, A. S., Reynolds, W. E., Franklin, E. C., Kulka, J. P., Ropes, M. W., Shulman, L. E., and

Wallace, S. L. Preliminary criteria for the classification of systemic lupus erythematosus. *Bull. Rheum. Dis.* 21:643, 1971.

Dubois, E. L. *Lupus Erythematosus* (2nd ed.). Los Angeles: University of Southern California Press, 1974.

Estes, D., and Christian, C. L. The natural history of systemic lupus erythematosus by prospective analysis. *Medicine* 50:85, 1971.

Fessel, W. J. Systemic lupus erythematosus in the community: Incidence, prevalence, outcome, first symptoms; the high prevalence in black women. *Arch. Intern. Med.* 134:1027, 1974.

Rothfield, N. F. (ed.). Systemic Lupus Erythematosus. *Clinics in Rheumatic Diseases.* Philadelphia: Saunders, 1975.

Sergent, J. S., Lockshin, M. D., Klempner, M. S., and Lipsky, B. A. Central nervous system disease in systemic lupus erythematosus. *Am. J. Med.* 58:644, 1975.

Sharp, G. C. Mixed connective tissue disease. *Bull. Rheum. Dis.* 25:828, 1975.

WEGENER'S GRANULOMATOSIS

Byrd, L. J., Shern, M. A., and Tu, W. H. Relationship of lethal midline granuloma to Wegener's granulomatosis. *Arthritis Rheum.* 12:247, 1969.

Carrington, C. B., and Liebow, A. A. Limited forms of angiitis and granulomatosis of Wegener's type. *Am. J. Med.* 41:497, 1966.

Wolff, S. M., Fauci, A. S., Horn, R. G., and Dale, D. C. Wegener's granulomatosis. *Ann. Intern. Med.* 81:513, 1974.

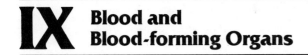

IX Blood and Blood-forming Organs

47

The Anemias

Lewis R. Weintraub

Normal hematopoiesis occurs in the sternum, vertebrae, ribs, skull, and proximal end of the humerus and femur. Approximately 40 percent of the marrow cavity in these areas is comprised of hematopoietic cells; the rest is fat. A pluripotential cell exists within this marrow and under the stimulus of the renal hormone erythropoietin (or of other unknown factors) gives rise through mitotic division to a daughter cell that differentiates into a proerythroblast. The proerythroblast matures through a series of three to four mitotic divisions. The nucleus is then unable to carry out DNA synthesis; it becomes pyknotic and eventually is extruded from the cell. However, the remaining erythrocyte still contains some RNA in ribosomes and is capable of synthesizing hemoglobin, although it is no longer able to divide. Such a cell is called a reticulocyte and is delivered into the peripheral circulation. The total maturation from proerythroblast to reticulocyte takes 4 to 6 days. The reticulocyte loses its ribosomes during its first 24 hours in the peripheral circulation and then becomes a mature erythrocyte.

The mature red cell remains in the peripheral circulation for approximately 120 days. Aging gradually takes place during this time and is characterized by (1) progressive decrease in enzymes necessary to maintain the integrity of the cell wall and protect the hemoglobin from oxidative degradation and (2) loss of cell surface area with decrease in mean corpuscular volume and increased rigidity of the cell wall. These changes eventually lead to the sequestration of the cell in the reticuloendothelial cells throughout the body and to the catabolism of the cell and its contents. The iron liberated by the degradation of the hemoglobin is released from the reticuloendothelial cell and picked up by the plasma protein transferrin (a beta globulin). Transferrin is carried through the circulation back to the bone marrow and the developing erythroid cells. The transferrin molecule delivers its iron to the erythroblasts and then returns to the circulation to pick up additional iron from the reticu-

loendothelial cells. It may also carry iron recently absorbed from the intestinal epithelial cells.

Bilirubin is formed from the degradation of the heme ring, and it enters the plasma in an unconjugated form. It is subsequently conjugated by the hepatic parenchymal cells and excreted in the bile. When free hemoglobin enters the plasma it is bound by the plasma protein haptoglobin (an alpha globulin). This complex is rapidly cleared and completely degraded by the reticuloendothial system. If the plasma hemoglobin level exceeds the haptoglobin-binding capacity, the hemoglobin is filtered in a dimeric form by the renal glomeruli and appears in the urine. Some of the hemoglobin may be reabsorbed by the renal tubules and become catabolized. The iron from this hemoglobin is incorporated into ferritin within the renal tubules and subsequently appears in the urine as hemosiderin.

Anemia is defined as a decrease in the red cell or hemoglobin mass. Such a decrease can result from either impaired production or increased destruction of red blood cells. The physician considers the hemoglobin concentration, hematocrit, and red cell count to determine the degree of an anemia. One must remember that these are all concentration measurements, not direct measurements of either red cell or hemoglobin mass. A direct relationship between the red cell and hemoglobin mass and the three laboratory tests just mentioned exists only if reciprocal changes in the plasma volume occur, maintaining a constant blood volume.

Anemia Secondary to Decreased or Ineffective Red Cell Production

IRON DEFICIENCY

The total body iron in the normal adult is between 3 and 4 gm. Approximately 70 percent of this iron is incorporated in hemoglobin within the circulating red cell mass. Of the iron from senescent red cells, 90 to 95 percent is reused for new hemoglobin synthesis. The remaining 5 to 10 percent of the iron circulating through the plasma is exchanged between the other body iron pools: (1) storage iron (ferritin) in the liver and spleen, (2) enzymes (heme and nonheme iron proteins) in all cells capable of carrying out oxidative metabolism, and (3) myoglobin. Each day approximately 1 mg of iron is lost from the body by desquamation of iron-containing epithelial cells from the skin and gut and by the 0.5 to 1.0 ml of blood lost in the stools. Women may lose an additional 50 ml of blood per month with each menstrual period, bringing their average daily iron loss up to 1.5 to 2.0 mg. There is no active mechanism for iron excretion.

The normal dietary intake of iron is 10 to 15 mg per day. The body retains only 1 mg to compensate for the amount lost; thus body iron balance is solely regulated by the ability of the small intestinal epithelial cell to accept or reject dietary iron. Although iron absorption in the normal individual is maximal in the duodenum, iron may be absorbed efficiently throughout the small intestine; hence exclusion of the duodenum per se will not result in iron deficiency. The major form of dietary iron is organic in the form of heme from myoglobin and hemoglobin. Heme is insoluble in the acid environment of the stomach. It becomes soluble in the alkaline pH of the duodenum and becomes available for absorption. The heme ring is taken up into the epithelial cell intact; within the cell the heme ring is oxidized, and the iron is then released and subsequently taken up by transferrin in the plasma.

Clinical Features. Iron deficiency is the commonest cause of anemia. In the adult this is due, with limited exceptions, to blood loss. Bleeding may be due to peptic ulcer disease, hiatus hernia, gastrointestinal malignancies, menorrhagia, or severe and prolonged epistaxis. Hemorrhoidal bleeding is another frequently overlooked cause of iron loss. Less obvious sites of iron loss include vascular anomalies of the intestinal mucosa, which may be associated with skin telangiectasias, and bleeding ectopic gastric ulcers in a Meckel's diverticulum. In all instances bleeding may be intermittent and may not be obvious to the physician at the time of his examination.

Malabsorption or dietary deficiency as a primary cause of iron deficiency is a very rare phenomenon in the United States. In children a relative dietary deficiency may occur because of the increased requirements for iron necessary for growth and an increasing red cell mass. A similar relative deficiency occurs in pregnant women due to the increased requirements of the fetus.

The anemic patient may complain of fatigue, exertional dyspnea, irritability, and difficulty in concentrating. In addition, the patient with iron deficiency may develop pica, a craving to ingest certain items such as ice (pagophagia), salty crackers, celery, or other foods. These desires immediately disappear when the iron deficiency is corrected. Indeed some of the food cravings experienced during pregnancy may be related to iron deficiency.

Findings on physical examination in iron deficiency anemia may be pallor, atrophy of the tongue, brittle hair, and koilonychia. The last two changes represent epithelial cell abnormalities secondary to depletion of essential iron-containing enzymes within skin cells. Splenomegaly may also be noted, reflecting an alteration in red cell plasticity and increased splenic phagocytosis.

Laboratory Features. With excessive iron loss, the gastrointestinal tract will increase its absorption of dietary iron to a maximum of 5 to 8 mg per day and so maintain body iron balance. If iron loss exceeds this amount, then iron is mobilized from the liver to compensate for the deficit. Thus with the increased delivery of iron to the bone marrow, red cell production can increase and the individual does not become anemic. However, each day that blood loss continues, the iron stores diminish. In stage I of iron deficiency, a normal hemoglobin mass persists along with normochromic and normocytic red cells, but total reserve iron stores are diminished. The serum iron may be low, and the serum ferritin value is decreased.

If blood loss continues at the same rate, the iron stores will eventually become seriously depleted and stage II of the iron deficiency ensues, in which the bone marrow can no longer maintain its increased production. The individual becomes anemic, and his red cells become microcytic. The mean corpuscular hemoglobin decreases, but the mean corpuscular concentration remains normal; therefore the cells remain normochromic. The serum iron is low, and total iron-binding capacity is increased. No stainable iron is present in the bone marrow, and the serum ferritin level is very low. As the iron deficiency becomes still greater and hemoglobin production decreases, the mean corpuscular hemoglobin falls at a faster rate than the mean cell volume. The mean corpuscular hemoglobin concentration now is decreased, and this is stage III of iron deficiency. The red cells are hypochromic and microcytic. Stage IV of iron deficiency occurs when the red cells become fragmented and exhibit severe poikilocytosis in addition to hypochromasia and microcytosis. The red cell membrane loses its plasticity, and its survival is decreased. Sequestration of the rigid cells in the spleen leads to splenomegaly. Recent studies suggest that in iron deficiency a decrease in glutathione peroxidase, the red cell enzyme, leads to oxidative damage of the red cell membrane, decreasing its plasticity and increasing the rate of membrane loss.

Treatment. The most important factor in the therapy of iron deficiency is to search for the site of blood loss. If bleeding can be stopped, the patient will regenerate his hemoglobin mass without any other specific therapy. The rate of recovery may be enhanced by the addition of pharmacologic doses of iron. Ferrous sulfate is the most effective and least expensive form of oral iron. The ingestion of 0.3 gm ferrous sulfate three times per day by the iron-deficient individual results in the retention of 20 to 25 mg of elemental iron by the body. Further increases in the total dose of ferrous sulfate result in only a negligible increase in total body retention. Gastric intolerance of oral iron is best dealt with by reducing the dose to 0.3 gm once or twice per day. This dose will only slightly prolong the period of repair of the anemia. Failure to respond to oral iron in almost every instance points to continued blood loss at a rate faster than the body can assimilate the pharmacologic iron. The use of parenteral iron in the form of iron dextran or iron sorbitol complexes should be limited to rare patients who cannot tolerate any oral dose of iron or to the patient in whom continued bleeding defies any type of correction (i.e., a patient with hereditary telangiectasia of the intestines or nasal mucous membranes). Greater amounts of iron can be administered parenterally in a shorter time than can be administered orally in treating patients with persistent blood loss, but it should be remembered that anaphylaxis can occur with parenteral iron, and hence there should be a very strong indication for its use.

SIDEROBLASTIC OR IRON-LOADING ANEMIAS
The sideroblastic anemias are commonly misdiagnosed as iron-deficiency anemias. The red cells are hypochromic and microcytic, but in contrast to iron deficiency, the serum iron is elevated. In the bone marrow stainable iron is increased, and pathologic sideroblasts are present. The sideroblast is a normoblast with perinuclear Prussian blue-staining granules; these represent nonheme iron that has been delivered to the normoblast but has not yet been utilized for heme synthesis. Since the perinuclear region is the normal location of the mitochondria and the site of heme synthesis, any abnormality in the cell that results in a block in heme synthesis may be associated with an excess accumulation of such nonheme iron granules around the nucleus; this is the pathologic, or "ringed," sideroblast. There are at least seven different enzymatic reactions in the synthesis of heme from the initial union of glycine and succinic acid to form delta-aminolevulinic acid, to the final incorporation of iron into the porphyrin ring to form heme. An abnormality anywhere along this synthetic pathway can result in such a sideroblastic anemia. The defect may be hereditary, acquired, or neoplastic.

Hereditary. The familial or sex-linked sideroblastic anemias characteristically appear in young men. Despite the fact that this is a genetic abnormality, the anemia does not become apparent until the third or fourth decade of life. In addition to the abnormality in heme synthesis, these patients have a defect in their gastrointestinal cells that allows them to absorb more iron than is needed. The overabsorption leads to an excess accumulation of iron in the liver, heart, pancreas, and other organs throughout the body. A clinical picture similar to familial hemochromatosis may develop. In many instances the patients may die of liver or heart failure caused by iron storage disease.

The exact defect has not been elucidated in familial sideroblastic anemia, and the syndrome may represent more than one enzymatic deficiency. Some patients demonstrate partial improvement in heme synthesis following the administration of pharmacologic doses of pyridoxine (200 mg per day). This coenzyme is essential in the initial step of heme synthesis, the union of glycine and succinic acid to form delta-aminolevulinic acid. Despite their response to treatment, patients with familial sideroblastic anemia do not demonstrate any other clinical features of pyridoxine deficiency. Thalassemia major is also a sideroblastic anemia. The inheritance pattern and associated elevation of A_2 or fetal hemoglobin distinguish it from the familial sex-linked sideroblastic anemias. Thalassemia will be discussed in more detail later in this chapter, under Hemoglobinopathies.

Acquired. Lead poisoning results in a sideroblastic anemia. Lead has been demonstrated to interfere with three different enzymes in the heme synthetic pathway: delta-aminolevulinic acid synthetase, delta-aminolevulinic acid dehydrase, and heme synthetase. Lead poisoning should be considered whenever there is a history of paint pica, industrial exposure, use of improperly glazed pottery, or potential contamination of water by lead pipes. The diagnosis can be easily excluded by determining the lead level in the blood. Alcoholism may also be associated with a sideroblastic anemia. In this instance blood levels of pyridoxal 5-phosphate, the active enzymatic form of pyridoxine, have been demonstrated to be low. Alcohol may inhibit the enzymatic phosphorylation of pyridoxine, or it may increase the rate of dephosphorylation. Clinically, acquired sideroblastic anemia secondary to alcoholism does not respond to pharmacologic doses of pyridoxine, but it will respond to pyridoxal 5-phosphate.

Isoniazid (INH) and cycloserine have been incriminated as the cause of sideroblastic anemia in several instances. These drugs are antagonists of pyridoxine, and the anemia will improve with the addition of pharmacologic doses of pyridoxine despite continuation of the INH or cycloserine. Chloramphenicol has also been incriminated with significant frequency as a cause of sideroblastic anemia. It is known that chloramphenicol interferes with mitochondrial membrane metabolism. Since this organelle is the site of heme synthesis, it is understandable that a sideroblastic anemia might develop if it is disturbed. The anemia is reversible when the drug is discontinued. This process does not appear to be directly related to the idiosyncratic fatal aplastic anemia associated with chloramphenicol. Isolated cases of sideroblastic anemias have also been described in association with an assorted group of diseases, including lupus erythematosis, rheumatoid arthritis, infectious mononucleosis, and multiple myeloma. The exact relationship of the anemia to the primary diseases remains to be elucidated.

Idiopathic. Elderly patients often develop a refractory sideroblastic anemia that does not fall into any of the preceding categories. Not infrequently the anemia may be associated with an unexplained leukopenia, monocytosis, or thrombocytopenia. Pelger-Huët nuclear anomaly may be seen in the peripheral leukocytes. Megaloblastic or megaloblastoid abnormalities of erythroid maturation may also be present with normal serum folate and B_{12} levels. The abnormalities suggest that the idiopathic variety of sideroblastic anemia may be a form of myeloproliferative disorder. Indeed, many who initially manifest idiopathic sideroblastic anemia eventually develop acute myelogenous leukemia, which unfortunately proves to be extremely refractory to most forms of chemotherapy.

ANEMIA OF CHRONIC INFLAMMATORY DISEASES
Chronic inflammatory disease is the second most common cause of anemia, following iron deficiency. The red cells are usually microcytic and at times slightly hypochromic; in addition, the serum iron is low. These findings are similar to those in early iron deficiency. However, certain other features distinguish the anemia of chronic inflammatory disease from iron deficiency: (1) the total iron-binding capacity is decreased and (2) abundant stainable iron is present in the bone marrow reticuloendothelial cells.

Following the intravenous injection of radioactive iron (^{59}Fe) bound to transferrin in a patient with the anemia of chronic disease, there is almost 80 to 90 percent uptake of the isotope into the hemoglobin in the circulating red cell mass. In contrast, if hemoglobin in the form of denatured red cells is tagged with ^{59}Fe and is introduced into the same patient, less than 50 percent of the initial radioactivity finds its way into the peripheral red cell mass. It must be remembered that iron bound to transferrin is delivered directly to the normoblasts for heme synthesis. When denatured red cells or senescent red cells are cleared from the circulation by the reticuloendothelial cells, the hemoglobin is catabolized and the iron is then released to the plasma transferrin, which brings the iron to the erythroblasts. Thus the laboratory features of the anemia of chronic inflammatory disease suggest that there is a major defect in the release of iron from reticuloendothelial cells following the catabolism of senescent red cells. This is a form of internal iron deficiency. The exact reason for this defect as well as for the decrease in transferrin levels remains to be elucidated.

Recently, levels of plasma erythropoietin have been measured in patients with the anemia of chronic inflammatory disease and compared to plasma erythropoietin levels in other patients with a comparable degree of anemia. Although elevated, the erythropoietin level in chronic inflammatory disease is not as great as it is in other anemias. Hence an inadequate release of erythropoietin in response to anemia may be a second defect impairing red cell production in infection.

In addition to the above abnormalities, cross transfusion experiments have established that there is a mild decrease in red cell survival due to unknown extracorpuscular factors in patients with chronic inflammatory disease. The magnitude of the decrease in the life span of the red cell would not be great enough to produce anemia if red cell production were not impaired. The normal bone marrow can increase its production and maintain a normal red cell mass when the red cell life span is decreased to one-sixth to one-eighth of normal. Unfortunately the mechanisms responsible for the abnormalities of hematopoiesis in the anemia of chronic disease are not known. Correction of this anemia can be achieved only by correction of the basic inflammatory disease (Table 47-1).

FOLIC ACID DEFICIENCY

Folic acid (pteroylmonoglutamic acid) is a nutrient essential for several biochemical reactions within the human body. In its reduced form, tetrahydrofolic acid, it serves as a carrier of single-carbon atom units of several types. Perhaps one of the most important forms of folic acid is $N^5 N^{10}$ methylene tetrahydrofolate. This coenzyme serves as a donor of a one-carbon atom unit as well as two hydrogen atoms required for the conversion of desoxyuridylate to thymidylate, one of the preliminary steps in DNA synthesis. As a result of this reaction the folate is changed to dihydrofolate. Through a series of reactions the dihydrofolate is regenerated to its active coenzymatic form.

Folic acid is an ingredient of many foods, such as leafy vegetables, fruits, grains, eggs, milk, liver, yeast, and meats. It exists as a polyglutamate due to the

Table 47-1. Differential Diagnosis of Hypochromic Anemias

Type of anemia	Serum Fe/total iron-binding capacity ratio	Bone marrow iron	Hemoglobin electrophoresis
Iron deficiency	Decreased/increased	Absent	Normal
Sideroblastic anemias — familial, acquired, idiopathic	Increased/normal or decreased	Increased + sideroblasts	Normal
Thalassemia	Increased/normal or decreased	Increased + sideroblasts	Increased A_2 and/or fetal hemoglobin
Anemia of chronic inflammatory disease	Decreased/decreased	Increased, no sideroblasts	Normal

conjugation of the glutamic acid residue of the folic acid molecule. Folic acid is water soluble and heat labile, and following ingestion its polyglutamates must be deconjugated. This may take place within the intestinal lumen and may also occur in the brush border of the small intestinal epithelial cells. Absorption of the monoglutamate form of the folic acid takes place primarily in the jejunum, where the folic acid is transferred across the epithelial cell to the plasma. Subsequent methylation and reduction of the folate takes place in the liver.

The total body store of folic acid is in the range of 5 mg. The minimal daily requirement to compensate for losses is 50 μg. Since folic acid may be partially destroyed by cooking and may not be completely deconjugated and absorbed, the minimal total food folate content should be in the range of 600 μg.

Clinical and Laboratory Features. In addition to the general symptoms of anemia, both glossitis and diarrhea are common features of folic acid deficiency. The glossitis and diarrhea are due to the decreased DNA synthesis and cellular turnover in the epithelial cells of the tongue and small intestine, respectively. The peripheral blood displays a macrocytic normochromic anemia associated with hypersegmented polymorphonuclear cells. Mild leukopenia and thrombocytopenia may also be present. The bone marrow examination reveals an asynchrony between nuclear and cytoplasmic maturation. The cell is large, and nuclear maturation lags behind cytoplasmic development, a pattern termed *megaloblastic maturation.* Abnormal leukocyte and megakaryocyte maturation is also evident. Serum lactic dehydrogenase and bilirubin are usually elevated secondary to an increase in the intramarrow destruction of the abnormal hematopoietic precursors. If an individual were to go on a diet free of folic acid, reduced levels of serum folate would be noted within 3 to 4 weeks, hypersegmentation of the polymorphonuclear cells in 12 weeks, macro-ovalocytes in peripheral blood in 18 weeks and, finally, a megaloblastic marrow and anemia in 19 to 20 weeks.

Dietary deficiency of folic acid may be seen in patients who (1) are anorexic due to any cause and whose total food intake is reduced, (2) selectively avoid foods rich in folic acid – the "tea and toast" diet, or (3) excessively cook or boil all their food, thus destroying folic acid. Folic acid deficiency is commonly associated with alcoholism. Although the alcoholic may maintain his caloric intake with alcohol, the ingestion of foods containing essential nutrients is usually diminished. In addition to a decrease in folate intake in these individuals, the alcohol itself may also interfere with the enzymatic reduction of folic acid to the active tetrahydrofolate form. The occurrence of folate deficiency may be less common in the beer-drinking alcoholic because of the folic acid in yeast used to make beer. Malabsorption syndromes secondary to tropical sprue, celiac disease (nontropical sprue), and jejunal granulomatous disease may all be associated with folic acid deficiency.

Many drugs have been incriminated as causing folate deficiency. Prolonged use of the anticonvulsants, phenytoin (Dilantin) or phenobarbital, or of estrogen-containing birth-control pills has been associated with low serum folates and at times with a megaloblastic anemia. The anemia may be corrected with pharmacologic doses of folic acid despite continuation of the incriminating agents. The drugs that cause folate deficiency may do so by inhibiting the intestinal deconjugating enzyme and thereby interfering with the absorption of dietary folates. Methotrexate, a cancer chemotherapeutic agent, irreversibly combines with dihydrofolate reductase, thereby blocking the formation of the active coenzyme and producing a megaloblastic anemia. Such an anemia can be overcome by giving the patient folinic acid (tetrahydrofolate), thus eliminating the need for the reductase enzyme. A relative deficiency in folic acid may develop in pregnant women and in infants due to the increased requirements of fetal and infant growth. Increased requirements for folic acid are also reported in the hypermetabolism of malignant tumors and with erythroid hyperplasia in chronic hemolytic diseases.

Treatment. Every attempt should be made to delineate and correct the cause of the folate deficiency. While this is in progress, or if the cause is not correctable, one may institute therapy with pharmacologic doses of folic acid. One milligram per day is more than adequate to correct megaloblastic anemia. This dose is also adequate in malabsorption syndromes, since absorption of the free monoglutamate is less impaired than the absorption of the polyglutamates.

VITAMIN B_{12} DEFICIENCY

Vitamin B_{12} (cyanocobalamin) is a coenzyme essential for several metabolic processes, including the conversion of methylmalonate to succinate and of homocysteine to methionine. The initial steps in DNA synthesis also require vitamin B_{12}, reflecting its role in folic acid metabolism. Vitamin B_{12} is necessary for the regeneration of N^5-methyltetrahydrofolate to tetrahydrofolic acid, the precursor of N^5N^{10} methylene tetrahydrofolate, a compound essential for the transformation of desoxyuridylate to thymidylate. In patients with B_{12} deficiency, N^5-methyltetrahydrofolate accumulates, causing elevated serum folate levels even though there is actually an internal metabolic folate deficiency.

Vitamin B_{12} is found in liver, beef, seafoods, and to a lesser degree in dairy products. It is not present in significant amounts in vegetables. The normal diet may contain from 5 to 30 μg of the vitamin, and the daily requirement is approximately 2 to 5 μg. In contrast to folic acid, B_{12} resists destruction by cooking. Within the stomach, B_{12} binds to intrinsic factor (IF), a glycoprotein secreted by the gastric parietal cells. The IF-B_{12} complex is subsequently taken up in the intestinal epithelial cells of the terminal ileum, and the B_{12} is transferred to a plasma carrier protein (transcobalamin). The total body store of B_{12} ranges between 2 and 5 mg, mostly in the liver.

Clinical and Laboratory Features. Vitamin B_{12} deficiency produces a megaloblastic anemia with clinical features and laboratory findings in the peripheral blood and bone marrow similar to those found in folate deficiency. In addition, neurologic abnormalities due to inadequate myelin synthesis are also present; these may be manifested by paresthesias, disturbances in position and vibratory sense, abnormal gait, difficulties in concentration, and even an organic psychosis. The exact metabolic defect in the neurologic system responsible for these changes is unknown. Dietary deficiency of B_{12} is a rather rare phenomenon because of the widespread distribution of the vitamin in foods. It is occasionally seen in a strict vegetarian who eats no dairy products. Malabsorption of B_{12} can occur as a result of (1) lack of intrinsic factor, (2) competitive utilization of B_{12} by intestinal bacteria or parasites, (3) diseases of the small intestine causing malabsorption, or (4) surgical removal of the terminal ileum.

Pernicious anemia is an example of B_{12} deficiency secondary to a lack of intrinsic factor production by the gastric parietal cells and associated with gastric mucosal atrophy and histamine-fast achlorhydria. Patients with impaired intrinsic factor production also have circulating antibodies against both gastric parietal cells and intrinsic factor. This association has prompted the speculation that pernicious anemia may be an autoimmune disorder. The disease is more common in the older age groups, but occasionally it may be seen in young adults and children. A familial incidence is not uncommon. Surgical removal of the stomach also eliminates the site of intrinsic factor production. Since the body stores of vitamin B_{12} are large and daily loss is minimal, clinically symptomatic megaloblastic anemia may not occur for 5 to 6 years following surgery. The clinical manifestations of acquired B_{12} deficiency are similar to those of pernicious anemia with the exception of the associated circulating antibodies. Abnormal bacterial growth in a small intestinal diverticulum or intestinal parasites like the fish tapeworm may consume all the available intestinal B_{12} and lead to a deficiency state. Tropical sprue, celiac disease, regional enteritis, and terminal resection of the ileum all may result in a megaloblastic anemia due to the failure to absorb the IF-B_{12} complex.

A reduction in the serum B_{12} level (normal is under 175 pg per milliliter) is common to all the disorders described above. The Schilling test, which measures the urinary excretion of radioactive B_{12} following an oral dose of radioactive B_{12}, is of help in determining the specific cause of the B_{12} deficiency. Renal function must be normal in order to validate the results. In normal individuals more than 7 to 10 percent of an oral dose of 0.5 μg of radioactive B_{12} is excreted in the urine in 24 hours. In malabsorption syndromes one may see 3 to 5 percent of the test dose excreted, and in pernicious anemia less than 2 percent is excreted. Repeating the study after giving either hog intrinsic factor or oral antibiotics to suppress abnormal bacterial growth will help to elucidate the specific defect (Table 47-2).

Treatment. Treatment of B_{12} deficiency consists in the parenteral administration of B_{12}. The initial dose is 100 μg intramuscularly daily for 3 to 5 days followed by monthly injections of 100 μg. The belief expressed in the literature that larger initial doses are effective in the treatment of the neurologic complications is without proof. Since the vitamin has no potential side effects, some physicians advocate doses of 1,000 μg per day for 2 weeks followed by 100 μg biweekly in the presence of severe neurologic disease. As in folate deficiency, a brisk reticulocytosis is seen in 5 to 7 days following initial therapy.

Table 47-2. Schilling Test in B_{12}-Deficient Megaloblastic Anemias

Cause of anemia	Without intrinsic factor	With intrinsic factor	Postoral antibiotic without intrinsic factor
Postgastrectomy pernicious anemia	Abnormal	Normal	Abnormal
Small intestinal diverticulum (bacterial overgrowth)	Abnormal	Abnormal	Normal
Primary diseases or resection of the terminal ileum	Abnormal	Abnormal	Abnormal
Dietary deficiency	Normal	Normal	Normal

APLASTIC ANEMIA

Either an abnormality in the microcirculation of the bone marrow or damage to the marrow pluripotential cells could result in reduced marrow cell populations and cause anemia, leukopenia, and thrombocytopenia. Such marrow failure is termed an *aplastic* or *hypoplastic* anemia and is characterized by a marrow with an increased fat-to-cell ratio. A number of agents, given in a sufficient dosage, are toxic to the bone marrow and may produce an aplastic anemia. These include ionizing radiation, benzene, alkylating agents, and antimetabolites employed in cancer chemotherapy. Other common drugs have also been incriminated; in these cases the process may not be dose-related and appears to represent an idiosyncratic reaction of the host to the drug. Such agents include chloramphenicol, phenytoin, sulfa drugs, tolbutamide, and phenylbutazone. In some instances viral illnesses have also been associated with marrow aplasia. In a great number of cases of aplastic anemia no cause can be found.

Clinical and Laboratory Features. Aplastic anemia is usually normochromic and normocytic. The reticulocyte count is low and the serum iron is elevated because of the lack of erythroid precursors and the underutilization of iron for hemoglobin synthesis. Treatment consists in removal of the incriminating agent, if any can be found, and supportive therapy with transfusions of red cells, platelets, and leukocytes as indicated by the clinical situation. In some instances recovery may occur in weeks to months. Hemorrhage and infection are the major causes of death in this condition. Androgens in large pharmacologic doses have been beneficial in improving erythroid production in a few patients. The mechanism of action may be through direct stimulation of the stem cell to differentiate. Androgens may also potentiate the action of erythropoietin.

Sustained pure red cell aplasia is a rather rare disorder in which granulocyte and platelet production remain normal. Approximately one-third of the reported cases have been associated with a thymoma. Antibodies against erythropoietin and erythroblasts have also been demonstrated in some cases. These observations have led to the speculation that pure red cell aplasia is an autoimmune disease. In some instances improvement has been noted after surgical thymectomy or after therapy with corticosteroids or immunosuppressive antimetabolites and alkylating agents.

Anemia Secondary to Decreased Red Cell Survival

HEMOGLOBINOPATHIES

Sickle Cell Anemia

The normal adult hemoglobin molecule is composed of two pairs of polypeptide chains ($\alpha_2^A \beta_2^A$) and four heme rings. Normal adult hemoglobin is termed hemoglobin A. Hereditary abnormalities in the synthesis of hemoglobin may cause a molecule to be made with altered physiochemical properties that result in premature destruction of the cell and a hemolytic anemia. Sickle cell hemoglobin (hemoglobin S) represents a single amino acid substitution of valine for glutamic acid in the beta chain of the hemoglobin molecule. As a result of this change, the hemoglobin S molecule ($\alpha_2 \beta_2^S$) will polymerize and form rigid tactoids under the following conditions: (1) decreasing oxygen tension, (2) decreasing pH, (3) increased osmolarity, and (4) decreasing temperature. The cell becomes distorted and assumes a classic sickle shape. The rigid cell becomes easily trapped in the microcirculation, resulting both in its premature destruction and in vasoocclusive phenomena.

Clinical and Laboratory Features. Sickle cell *trait* (hemoglobin AS) occurs in 8 to 10 percent of black Americans, 3 to 6 percent of Americans of Puerto Rican descent, and to a lesser extent in Americans of Italian, Sicilian, Greek, and Syrian descent. Approximately 25 to 45 percent of the hemoglobin on electrophoresis is S. The affected individual is not anemic, red cell survival is normal, and life expectancy is normal. Rarely morbidity or mortality can occur due to in vivo sickling under conditions leading to severe hypoxia, such as high-altitude mountain climbing, high-altitude flying in nonpressurized airplanes, or deep anesthesia without adequate oxygenation. Hyposthenuria and hematuria of renal origin may also be seen in individuals with sickle cell trait. The conditions of low oxygen tension, acid pH, and high tonicity may predispose to microinfarctions in the renal medulla.

Sickle cell *disease* (hemoglobin SS) occurs in approximately 1:400 births in the black population of the United States. The sickle hemoglobin comprises 70 to 99 percent of the total hemoglobin mass; the remainder is fetal hemoglobin (hemoglobin F, or $\alpha_2^A \gamma_2^F$). The classic laboratory features of hemolytic anemia are present: reticulocytosis, bone marrow erythroid hyperplasia, and indirect bilirubinemia. Sickle cells are present on the peripheral blood smear made in the routine fashion. Initially the spleen is enlarged due to sequestration of the rigid sickle cells. However, with time autoinfarction occurs; the spleen becomes atrophic, and functional hyposplenism occurs. Howell-Jolly bodies (remnants of the nucleus) appear in the peripheral red cells since they no longer are "pitted," that is, removed from the cell in the spleen. Recurrent painful abdominal crises that occur may mimic an acute abdomen. Painful crises in the extremities are also common. Such crises are thought to be secondary to impairment of blood flow to various parts of the body. Infections may predispose the affected individual to these episodes, although crises may occur without any known cause. Treatment consists in administering pain medication, maintaining hydration, and ensuring adequate oxygenation. Unfortunately the only treatment for the anemia to date is transfusion. Multiple transfusions eventually lead to the complications of iron storage disease with cardiac and hepatic decompensation. The anemia may increase acutely secondary to transient bone marrow aplasia associated with viral illnesses. Such aplastic crises are more common than hemolytic crises. Some individuals with hemoglobin SS appear to have a mild anemia with hemoglobin levels in the range of 10 to 11 gm per 100 ml. They suffer few crises and fortunately reach adult life. In these patients the concentration of hemoglobin F is in the range of 20 to 25 percent, and in vivo sickling is less than in individuals with lower concentrations of hemoglobin F. A combination of sickle trait and other genetic hemoglobin abnormalities, such as hemoglobin C or thalassemia, results in a syndrome with clinical severity intermediate between that found with hemoglobin SS and that found with hemoglobin SA.

Hemoglobin C Disease

Hemoglobin C represents a genetic substitution of lysine for glutamic acid in the sixth position from the N-terminal of the beta chain ($\alpha_2^A \beta_2^C$). Hemoglobin

C is less soluble than hemoglobin A within the red cell. When such hemoglobin precipitates within the red cell, it adheres to the plasma membranes and reduces the plasticity of the cell. If the cell rigidity is great enough, the cell will be sequestered in the microchannels of the splenic cords.

Clinical and Laboratory Features. Hemoglobin C is present in 2 to 3 percent of the black population in America. Individuals with hemoglobin C trait have no anemia and are asymptomatic. The peripheral blood smear reveals increased target cells. Homozygous C disease is characterized by a hemolytic anemia with hemoglobin levels in the range of 8 to 12 gm per 100 ml. There is a marked increase in target cells. Affected patients have the generalized symptoms of anemia and, occasionally, fleeting arthralgias and abdominal pain.

Thalassemia

Thalassemia, in contrast to sickle cell anemia, represents a genetic quantitative rather than qualitative abnormality in hemoglobin production. The basic defect appears to be a disturbance in messenger RNA activity, resulting in a decreased rate of alpha-chain or beta-chain synthesis. In beta thalassemia, the most frequent form of the disease, beta-chain synthesis is decreased but alpha-chain synthesis remains normal. There are concomitant increases in the production of gamma and delta chains that combine with alpha chains to form fetal and A_2 hemoglobin, respectively. Unfortunately the increases cannot match the decrease in beta-chain synthesis; hence, the net total hemoglobin production is decreased and the red cell is hypochromic. The excess free alpha chains are unstable and precipitate within the red cell, binding to the inner surface of the cell membrane. These rigid inclusions impair the passage of the red cell through the microcirculation of the spleen and other organs. In the early stages the precipitated alpha chains are removed from the cell in the spleen. This process further distorts the membrane and increases its rigidity. Eventually there is premature sequestration and destruction of the red cells in the spleen and other organs. Thus thalassemia is a disease of decreased survival as well as of decreased production of red cells.

Clinical and Laboratory Features. Beta thalassemia minor represents the genetic heterozygote state. It is characterized by a mild anemia with the mean corpuscular volume, mean corpuscular hemoglobin, and mean corpuscular hemoglobin concentration all reduced. In addition, numerous target cells are seen. Hemoglobin electrophoresis reveals an elevation in A_2 hemoglobin. Hemoglobin F as measured chemically (resistance to alkaline denaturation) is normal or slightly elevated. Symptoms of anemia are absent in these patients, and life expectancy is normal. The spleen is usually not palpable. Frequently the anemia is misdiagnosed as due to iron deficiency and the patient is mistakenly maintained on oral iron.

Beta thalassemia major represents the homozygous form of the disease. The anemia is quite severe (less than 7 gm per 100 ml) and requires transfusion therapy for the relief of symptoms. The liver and spleen are enlarged. The peripheral red cells are hypochromic, microcytic, and poikilocytic. Nucleated red blood cells are also seen. The hemoglobin F level is markedly increased, usually in the range of 30 to 90 percent. In contrast to thalassemia minor, the A_2 level may be low or normal. Due to the severe anemia, growth and development are retarded. In addition to the complications of severe anemia, the patients develop iron storage disease secondary to the multiple transfusions. Restrictive myocardiopathy and cirrhosis similar to that seen in patients with familial hemochromatosis develop and may lead to the early death of the patient, often in childhood.

Alpha thalassemia is less common. In the homozygous form no significant amount of hemoglobin A, A_2, or F can be synthesized since there is little alpha-chain production. In utero, gamma-chain synthesis occurs and hemoglobin Bart (γ_4) is formed. Unfortunately this hemoglobin exhibits no Bohr effect and is an inefficient carrier of oxygen. In addition, it is unstable and will cause red cells to sickle. Intrauterine death of the affected fetus usually occurs. In the heterozygous form of alpha thalassemia a significant rate of alpha-chain synthesis does occur so that A, A_2, and F hemoglobin can be made. During the first 3 months of life a small amount of hemoglobin Bart (γ_4) may be found. After this early period, trace amounts of hemoglobin H ($delta_4$) may be seen.

Minimal anemia and hypochromic cells are noted in the laboratory. Hemoglobin H is unstable and will denature to form hemoglobin inclusions, which may be visualized with a supravital stain.

RED CELL ENZYME DEFICIENCIES
The mature normal red cell, lacking mitochondria, is dependent on only two pathways for the generation of compounds necessary for its survival. Both of these pathways are glucose dependent. Approximately 90 percent of the glucose entering the cell undergoes anaerobic glycolysis (Embden-Meyerhof pathway), in which glucose is broken down to lactate through a series of eleven enzymatic reactions. During this process three important products are generated: (1) reduced nicotinamide-adenine dinucleotide (NADH, DPNH), a compound essential for the maintenance of the reduced state of the ferrous iron in the hemoglobin molecule; (2) 2,3-diphosphoglycerate (2, 3-DPG), which binds to hemoglobin and enhances oxygen delivery to tissues; and (3) ATP, which is essential for the maintenance of the red cell membrane. Extracellular sodium ions will normally diffuse across the semipermeable red cell membrane and bring water into the cell. The red cell has an ATP-dependent sodium pump mechanism that will transport the sodium ions and water out of the cell against a concentration gradient. If ATP levels are reduced, the pump will not function efficiently; sodium ions and water will enter the cell, cell size will increase, and eventually the red cell will rupture, causing intravascular hemolysis. Adenosine triphosphate also binds calcium ions; if ATP is not available, the calcium will bind to the lipids of the red cell membrane. Such binding has been demonstrated to cause an increase in membrane rigidity, a decrease in red cell plasticity, and hence an increase in the sequestration and destruction of red cells in the microcirculation.

Pyruvate Kinase Deficiency

Clinical and Laboratory Features. Pyruvate kinase (PK) deficiency is the most common enzymatic deficiency in the Embden-Meyerhof pathway. Genetic deficiencies of the other enzymes are quite rare, and their clinical manifestations may be similar to PK deficiency. Erythrocyte PK deficiency is inherited as an autosomal recessive trait, and only the red cells appear to be affected. Only individuals homozygous for the defect manifest clinical anemia. In most affected individuals the anemia is detected in childhood; occasionally milder forms of the disease may go undiagnosed until adult life.

The magnitude of the anemia varies from case to case. Hemoglobin levels are usually in the range of 6 to 11.5 gm per 100 ml. In general, symptoms of anemia will correlate with the degree of anemia. As in all chronic congenital hemolytic disorders there is an increased incidence of cholelithiasis due to the increased bile pigment turnover. Physical examination may reveal scleral icterus and a variable degree of splenomegaly. The red cell indices are normal or may reveal a slight increase in the mean corpuscular volume, reflecting the degree of reticulocytosis associated with the hemolytic disorder. The peripheral blood smear will show mild anisocytosis and poikilocytosis with some polychromatophilia. Elevation of the indirect bilirubin and decreased or absent haptoglobins are seen as a result of the increased rate of hemoglobin catabolism. If the patient's red cells are incubated under sterile conditions for 48 hours, free hemoglobin rises due to an accelerated rate of autohemolysis. The addition of ATP (but not glucose) to the initial incubation medium corrects the abnormality in the PK cells. This test system is known as the autohemolysis test. The diagnosis of PK deficiency is confirmed by direct assay of PK activity in red cell hemolysates. Unfortunately no specific therapy is available. Splenectomy may result in a partial improvement, but in some cases the improvement is only transient.

Glucose 6-Phosphate Dehydrogenase Deficiency
The aerobic hexose monophosphate shunt or pentose phosphate pathway is responsible for the metabolism of the remaining 10 percent of the glucose in the mature red cell. Through a series of enzymatic reactions initiated by glucose 6-phosphate dehydrogenase (G-6-PD), reduced nicotinamide-adenine dinucleotide phosphate (NADPH, TPNH), a high-energy compound, is generated. This in turn supplies an electron via the enzyme glutathione reductase to maintain glutathione in a reduced form. Glutathione protects the hemo-

globin molecule and red cell membrane from oxidative damage, because when confronted with an oxidant drug or peroxide, the reduced glutathione will be oxidized preferentially. The oxidized form of glutathione consists of two glutathione molecules joined by a disulfide linkage. If adequate levels of reduced glutathione cannot be maintained, the oxidants will then use hemoglobin or the red cell membrane as a substrate. Oxidation of ferrous to ferric iron impairs the ability of the hemoglobin molecule to bind oxygen. Oxidation of the sulfhydryl group of the amino acids in hemoglobin results in denaturation and subsequent precipitation of the hemoglobin molecule. The precipitated hemoglobin is the Heinz body that is visible with supravital stains of the peripheral blood. The precipitated hemoglobin adheres to the internal surface of the red cell membrane and causes an increase in membrane rigidity. Some of the Heinz bodies are removed from the cell by the splenic macrophages. However, the increase in membrane rigidity secondary to the Heinz body formation eventually leads to the premature sequestration and destruction of the red cell.

The structural gene responsible for G-6-PD is located on the X chromosome. Therefore the abnormality is fully expressed in affected males and only rarely in homozygous females. Since only one X chromosome is randomly expressed in each erythroid stem line, the female heterozygote for G-6-PD deficiency will have an average enzyme activity about half that found in normal individuals; however, this varies considerably from case to case. There are many genetic variants of G-6-PD deficiency. Functional reduction in enzyme activity may be the result of (1) decreased rate of synthesis of the enzyme, (2) decreased stability of the enzyme, or (3) production of an abnormal enzyme variant with decreased functional activity under physiologic conditions.

Clinical and Laboratory Features. Approximately 11 percent of American black males have G-6-PD deficiency. This genetic variant (A−) of the enzyme has been shown to have a decreased stability in vivo. Enzyme activity in a sample of red cells from affected patients is approximately 5 to 15 percent of normal. The young red cells have nearly normal activity, but as they age, their activity falls to zero. Under normal conditions the affected individuals have normal hemoglobin concentrations and reticulocyte counts; however, when exposed to oxidant drugs they are hemolyzed. These oxidant drugs include the following:

1. Primaquine and related antimalarials
2. Sulfonamides
3. Sulfones
4. Nitrofurans
5. Acetanilid
6. Aminophenazone
7. Aspirin
8. Vitamin K
9. Quinidine
10. Chloramphenicol

Viral infections may also precipitate a hemolytic crisis; the responsible mechanism is unknown. With hemolysis the hemoglobin falls, and subsequently reticulocytosis appears. First spherocytosis and then fragmentation of the red cells occur as a result of membrane loss when the spleen removes the precipitated hemoglobin. Heinz bodies are demonstrable on supravital stains. The diagnosis is confirmed by specific enzyme screening tests or assays for G-6-PD activity. As the reticulocyte count increases, the mean red cell activity of G-6-PD will return toward normal, since there is now a greater population of younger red cells with higher enzyme activity. As a result, a compensated hemolytic state may develop in which the patient's hemoglobin may return to normal despite continuation of the oxidant drug. If the reticulocyte count is elevated, then the enzyme assay may be falsely normal.

A variant of the G-6-PD enzyme exists in Caucasians of Mediterranean origin and Sephardic Jews. Enzyme activity in the peripheral red cells of affected individuals is usually less than 1 percent. Hemolysis occurs upon exposure to oxidant drugs. Since enzyme activity is virtually absent, even in young cells, the anemia is quite severe and is *not* self-limited, as in the A− variety. In some individuals hemolytic anemia is a constant finding throughout life, even in the absence of any oxidant drug or other stress. The defect that separates these individuals from those with periodic oxidant-related hemolysis remains to be defined.

RED CELL MEMBRANE ABNORMALITIES

Hereditary Spherocytosis

Hereditary spherocytosis is a hereditary hemolytic anemia transmitted as an autosomal dominant trait with varying penetrance. The characteristic feature in the peripheral blood is the appearance of the spheroidal cell completely filled with hemoglobin and lacking the normal central pallor. The exact metabolic defect or defects within the cell causing spherocytosis have not been elucidated.

The spherocytes demonstrate (1) a marked deficiency of total surface area while red cell volume is only slightly reduced (the change in the ratio of the surface area to volume is responsible for the spheroidal shape of the cell as well as for the characteristic increase in the mean corpuscular hemoglobin concentration to more than 36 percent); (2) decreased membrane plasticity; (3) increased permeability to sodium necessitating an increased rate of sodium extrusion by the ATP pump and hence an increased rate of glucose utilization; (4) reduced total lipid content while the relative distribution of the various lipids remains normal; (5) an increased susceptibility to lipid membrane oxidation.

The spherocyte has a shortened survival and is preferentially destroyed in the spleen. The rigid membrane impedes the passage of the red cell through the spleen, causing stasis in the splenic cords and relatively vacant sinuses. Under such conditions of stasis, the glucose supply of the cell becomes depleted and more sodium and water leak through the abnormal membrane and accumulate within the cell. In addition, glucose deprivation also leads to increased lipid membrane oxidation and instability. All of these features cause the ultimate death of the cell and splenic enlargement.

Clinical and Laboratory Features. The magnitude of the anemia in individuals affected by hereditary spherocytosis is variable and depends on the penetrance of the dominant genetic abnormality. As in other hereditary hemolytic anemias there is an increased incidence of cholelithiasis secondary to the increased rate of bilirubin excretion. Gallbladder disease may be present, even in the patient whose bone marrow is capable of increasing production enough to compensate for the decreased survival. In addition, patients with compensated anemia may be troubled by episodes of severe anemia during viral-induced aplastic crises. Splenomegaly is a characteristic clinical feature. Examination of the peripheral blood reveals the classic spherocytes, an increased mean corpuscular hemoglobin concentration, a normal mean corpuscular hemoglobin, and a slightly reduced mean corpuscular volume. The spherocyte is more susceptible to osmotic lysis, and thus the osmotic fragility curve (the magnitude of red cell lysis in varying concentrations of sodium chloride) is abnormal. However, in some individuals the defect in the red cell is not severe enough to cause an abnormal osmotic fragility curve. If their cells are incubated in plasma under sterile conditions, glucose deprivation occurs, and after 24 hours the metabolic defect in the affected red cells is accentuated. The osmotic fragility curve then becomes abnormal as compared to that of normal cells incubated under similar conditions.

Once the diagnosis of hereditary spherocytosis is confirmed, the patient should have a splenectomy. Removal of the organ that preferentially destroys red cells allows their survival to approach 90 to 95 percent of normal. The anemia is easily corrected, even though the defect in the cell persists. Patients with compensated hereditary spherocytosis should also have their spleen removed to prevent the complications of cholelithiasis and aplastic crisis. Splenectomy is usually not performed during the first decade of life, since there may be an increased incidence of severe infections in the postsplenectomy state in children. In this age group splenectomy should be limited to patients with significant symptomatic anemia.

Hereditary Elliptocytosis

Hereditary elliptocytosis is a genetic abnormality transmitted as an autosomal dominant trait in which the affected individual's red cells are elliptical or ovoid in shape. Red cell survival is usually normal, but in 10 to 15 percent of patients with this trait, the red cell survival is decreased and hence hemolytic anemia may occur. The defects responsible for the abnormal shape of the cell as well as the shortened life span are not known. There is no correlation between the number of elliptocytes in the peripheral blood and the degree of hemolysis. On sterile incubation, these cells show a greater fall in ATP and a greater rise in sodium efflux than normal incubated cells. These abnormalities are similar to those demonstrated in hereditary spherocytosis. However, there is no correlation between the magnitude of these defects and the decreased survival of the cell. When hemolytic disease is present, it can be corrected by splenectomy, as is done in hereditary spherocytosis.

Paroxysmal Nocturnal Hemoglobinuria
Paroxysmal nocturnal hemoglobinuria (PNH) is an acquired red cell abnormality in which fixation of complement to the membrane occurs in the absence of any demonstrable antibody and the amount of complement activation necessary to produce hemolysis is considerably less than for normal cells. An in vitro increased susceptibility to complement lysis can be demonstrated by activating the alternative properdin-dependent pathway, which bypasses complement components C1, C4, and C2. The activation is accomplished in vitro by (1) acidifying the plasma, (2) adding insulin, or (3) decreasing the ionic strength of the solution in which the red cells are suspended. The mechanism by which complement is activated in vivo in this condition has not been elucidated. The activation of the terminal components of the complement cascade (C5 $\longrightarrow$ C9) leads to the destruction of the red cell membrane and to intravascular lysis of the cell. Free hemoglobin produced in excess of the serum haptoglobin-binding capacity is filtered by the kidneys and appears in the urine. For some unknown reason the accelerated hemolysis occurs at a greater rate during sleep, giving rise to the name paroxysmal nocturnal hemoglobinuria.

The disease is relatively rare and usually occurs in the third or fourth decade of life. The patient will present with a normochromic normocytic hemolytic anemia. Less than a third of the patients will have gross hemoglobinuria. In these individuals iron loss may be great enough to cause iron deficiency and thus increase the severity of their anemia. Patients with this disorder also have an increased incidence of severe intravascular thrombotic episodes, the cause of which is not known. A small but significant number of patients with paroxysmal nocturnal hemoglobinuria

will subsequently develop aplastic anemia or acute leukemia, suggesting that the disease may be a myeloproliferative disorder of which the first manifestation is the production of an abnormal clone of red cells with increased susceptibility to complement lysis.

The diagnosis of paroxysmal nocturnal hemoglobinuria is confirmed in the laboratory by performing the acid hemolysis test, the inulin hemolysis test, or the so-called sugar water test (low ionic strength solution). All three tests potentiate the activation of complement sufficiently to cause in vitro lysis of diseased cells but not of normal cells. There is no specific treatment.

Traumatic Intravascular Hemolytic Syndrome
(Microangiopathic Hemolytic Anemia)
Traumatic intravascular hemolytic syndrome is an acquired hemolytic disorder characterized by distorted and fragmented red cells (schistocytes), increased plasma hemoglobin, hemosiderinuria, and decreased haptoglobin levels. Traumatic injury to the red cell membranes can occur because of prosthetic cardiac valves, diseased aortic valves, abnormal endothelium in small vessels such as is seen in diffuse vasculitis, or intravascular fibrin strands deposited in disseminated intravascular coagulation. The red cells may undergo complete intravascular lysis, and the freed hemoglobin and hemosiderin may appear in the urine. If partial red cell destruction occurs from trauma, the fragmented cells have decreased membrane plasticity, causing them to sequestrate and be destroyed in the spleen. Hemolysis is greatest in this disorder when the patient is active and cardiac output is increased. Hence this disorder may be called paroxysmal daytime hemoglobinuria. Correction of the primary abnormality, if possible, will cure the anemia.

IMMUNE HEMOLYTIC ANEMIAS

Drug Induced
The ingestion of several drugs may result in the production of an immune hemolytic anemia. In each instance the presence of an antibody on the surface of the red cell is responsible for the ultimate destruction of the cell. The mechanism by which the antibody fixes to the membrane varies with the incriminating drug; there are three such mechanisms known.

(1) The drug may adhere to the surface of the red cell through a physiochemical interaction. Antibody produced against the drug is then combined with the drug-red cell complex. This mechanism may be seen in individuals receiving high doses of intravenous penicillin (in excess of 20 million units per day). The antibody involved is an IgG immunoglobulin. (2) The drug may stimulate specific antibody production and form an immune complex within the plasma. The complex in turn may adhere to the surface of the red cell. This mechanism is seen in individuals with quinidine-induced immune hemolysis. The antibody is usually an IgM immunoglobulin. (3) The drug may alter the immune surveillance mechanism of the individual and result in the production of an autoantibody directed against a normal antigenic structure on the red cell membrane. This mechanism occurs following the ingestion of alpha methyldopa (Aldomet). The antibody here is an IgG immunoglobulin and is directed against the Rh locus on the surface of the red cell. The production of the autoantibody occurs in approximately 10 percent of patients receiving alpha methyldopa for periods longer than 6 months. Of those patients that develop the antibody, only 10 percent will show evidence of a hemolytic anemia. Thus only 1 percent of patients receiving methyldopa will evidence a drug-induced hemolysis.

In all of the examples given above, an antibody, either IgG or IgM, is present on the surface of the red cell. As a result, the Coombs test, which detects such antibodies, will be positive in each instance. The Coombs reagent is rabbit immune serum raised against human globulins. The reagent will cause human red cells coated with immunoglobulins to agglutinate in vitro by cross-linking any globulin on the surface of the cell by the polyvalent antibody. In the first two examples given above, the drug must be present in the patient's plasma for the Coombs test to be positive. If the immunoglobulin is an autoantibody, a drug is not a necessary part of the antigen-antibody complex; therefore, the Coombs test may remain positive for months after levels of the initiating drug have become undetectable.

Because reticuloendothelial cells possess receptors for IgG, an IgG-coated red cell will adhere to their membranes. The cells engulf part of the phagocytic reticuloendothelial red cell membrane adjacent to the receptor, and the remainder of the cell is set free. Through this process the ratio of red cell surface area to volume decreases and an acquired spherocytosis occurs. Eventually the whole cell is sequestered and destroyed. Immune IgM complexes on the red cell surface enhance the binding and the subsequent activation of complement that will lead to membrane destruction and intravascular hemolysis. In addition, the phagocytic reticuloendothelial cells have receptors for complement (C3). Hence phagocytosis and extravascular destruction of cells coated with IgM also occur.

Once the diagnosis of drug-induced hemolytic anemia is made or suspected in the presence of a positive Coombs test, the drug should be immediately discontinued. In the first and second mechanisms described above, the Coombs test and the hemolysis will persist only for as long as it takes the body to catabolize or excrete the drug. The antibody may persist for a longer period but is of no hazard to the red cell in the absence of the antigen. In the third mechanism described, hemolysis may persist for up to 6 weeks after the drug has been discontinued, even though there is no detectable methyldopa left in the body. The use of steroids does not appear to enhance the rate of recovery. During the recovery period, the Coombs test will also remain positive. Indeed, the positive Coombs test may persist for up to a year without evidence of hemolysis. Perhaps the concentration of autoantibody on the surface of the red cell either is not great enough to induce hemolysis or its nature changes and does not allow attachment and sequestration of the red cell by the reticuloendothelial cells.

Autoimmune IgG-7S Warm-Reacting Antibody Hemolytic Anemia

The spontaneous production of an IgG antibody directed against an individual's own red cells can occur and cause a significant hemolytic anemia. In many instances the antibody has been demonstrated to have specificity against one of the Rh antigens on the red cell membrane, for example, the c, e, or the Rh loci. In approximately one-half of the cases, the antibody has no apparent specificity and will agglutinate all human red cells. If the production of the autoantibody is great enough, free antibody will be present in the patient's plasma as well as on the red cells, giving rise to a positive indirect as well as direct Coombs test. Some of the red cell IgG autoantibodies will fix sublytic amounts of complement to the membrane of the cell. If these antibodies are highly dissociable, then at any one time there may not be a large enough concentration of the IgG molecules on the surface of the cell to give a positive conventional Coombs test. However, if a specific anticomplementary immune rabbit serum (nongamma Coombs reagent) is used, a positive test may be seen, since the complement is not freely dissociable. The IgG antibody reactivity is greatest at $37°C$ ($98.6°F$); hence this entity has been referred to as warm autoimmune hemolytic anemia. The mechanism of destruction of the IgG-coated red cell is similar to that described in IgG drug-induced hemolytic anemias.

The severity of the anemia varies considerably from patient to patient. Splenic enlargement on physical examination is a common finding. Examination of the peripheral blood reveals spherocytosis and polychromatophilia, the latter being a manifestation of the increased population of reticulocytes. Elevation of the indirect bilirubin supports the diagnosis of hemolysis. The direct Coombs test and the nongamma Coombs test should be positive. If the number of IgG molecules on the cell surface is less than 500, the Coombs test will be negative, and more sensitive research techniques will be required to confirm the autoimmune process. In approximately 40 percent of patients with an autoimmune hemolytic anemia, some associated disease is present; these diseases include (1) lymphomas and chronic lymphatic leukemia, (2) systemic autoimmune or connective tissue disorders such as lupus erythematosus, and (3) nonlymphoid malignancies (ovarian and breast cancers). In many instances the hemolytic anemia will precede the clinical appearance of the related disorder.

The initial treatment of choice is the administration of corticosteroids. In many instances hemolysis may be decreased within 48 hours, but the Coombs test remains positive. These changes suggest that the mechanism of action of the steroids may be to suppress recognition of the antibody-coated red cells as well as to inhibit phagocytosis, rather than to suppress antibody production. If steroid therapy does not alter the rate of hemolysis within 2 to 4 weeks or if continued high doses of steroids are necessary to suppress hemolysis, splenectomy should be performed. The operation will correct the hemolytic process in approximately 60 percent of the patients, but the Coombs test will remain positive. These findings suggest that improvement is due to removal of the organ that preferentially sequesters the antibody-coated red cells and that ending the role of the spleen as a major source of antibody production is of secondary importance. Recently immunosuppressive therapy has been tried in patients who have failed to respond to steroids and splenectomy. Azathioprine, cyclophosphamide, and 6-mercaptopurine have all been used with limited success. However, these drugs have the potential of increasing the severity of the anemia by suppressing the bone marrow's ability to maintain an increased rate of erythroid production.

Autoimmune IgM-19S Cold-Reacting Antibody Hemolytic Anemia

Cold-agglutinin hemolytic disease is characterized by the presence of an IgM antibody, most commonly directed against the I antigen on the red cell surface. This antigen is absent on fetal red cells but appears on the membrane during the first year of life in practically all individuals. In rare instances the cold antibody may be directed against the i antigen. In contrast to I, i is present in significant numbers on the surface of fetal cells but decreases during the first year of life.

The IgM cold antibody will bind to the antigenic site on the red cell as the temperature is reduced from $37°C$ ($98.6°F$). Maximal binding occurs at $4°C$ ($39.1°F$), causing gross agglutination of the cells. The extent of the reaction at higher temperatures varies with each case and is referred to as the thermal amplitude of the antibody. Under conditions that promote IgM antibody binding, complement is also fixed to the membrane. The IgM antibody is dissociable, and when the temperature returns to $37°C$, the antibody will leave the red cell surface. However, complement remains fixed to the membrane, and its subsequent activation leads either to lysis or to sequestration of the cell.

In vivo binding of the cryoantibody to the red cell may occur in the blood vessels of the skin and distal parts of the body, where the temperature may fall below 32°C (87.8°F). Clinical hemolytic anemia is usually not seen unless either the titer of cold agglutinins is over 1:1,000 or the antibody has a high thermal amplitude. In addition to symptoms of anemia, the patient may complain of Raynaud's phenomenon. Cold-agglutinin hemolytic anemia may be an idiopathic entity or it may be associated with a systemic disease. In the idiopathic variety and in that associated with mycoplasmal pneumonia or lymphoid malignancy, the antibody is an anti I. In cold-agglutinin hemolysis associated with infectious mononucleosis, the antibody is directed against i. Unfortunately steroids and splenectomy are of little value in the treatment of cold-agglutinin hemolytic anemia. Alkylating agents (chlorambucil and cyclophosphamide) have been of some value in the treatment of cold-agglutinin hemolysis in patients with lymphoid malignancies or the idiopathic type. Cold-agglutinin hemolysis associated with mycoplasmal pneumonia and infectious mononucleosis is usually self-limited.

Autoimmune IgG-7S Cold-Reacting Antibody Type (Paroxysmal Cold Hemoglobinuria)

Paroxysmal cold hemoglobinuria is a very rare disorder that may be associated with syphilis or may represent an idiopathic phenomenon. The IgG antibody in this disorder is directed against the red cell antigen P. The antibody has increased affinity for the red cell at lower temperatures, and the red cell-antibody complex fixes complement to the membrane. When the temperature returns to 37°C, the severity of the complement activation is greater than that associated with the IgM cryoantibody. As a result, acute, severe hemolysis occurs and free hemoglobin passes into the urine. The Donath-Landsteiner test reproduces these conditions in vitro and is diagnostic for paroxysmal cold hemoglobinuria. There is no specific therapy for this disorder. The idiopathic variety is usually self-limited, and the condition will usually disappear if the patient with syphilis is treated with penicillin.

Bibliography

Chanarin, I. *The Megaloblastic Anemias.* Oxford, Eng.: Blackwell, 1969.

Fairbanks, V., Fahey, J., and Beutler, E. *Clinical Disorders of Iron Metabolism.* New York: Grune & Stratton, 1971.

Surgeoner, D. (ed.). *The Red Blood Cell* (2nd ed.). Vols. 1 and 2. New York: Academic, 1975.

Valentine, W., et al. Hereditary enzymatic deficiencies of erythrocytes. *Semin. Hematol.* 4:307, 1971.

Weed, R., et al. The red cell membrane. *Semin. Hematol.* 7:249, 1970.

Williams, W. J. (ed.). *Hematology.* New York: McGraw-Hill, 1972.

Wintrobe, M. (ed.). *Clinical Hematology* (7th ed.). Philadelphia: Lea & Febiger, 1974.

48

Polycythemic Syndromes

Aaron Miller

The term *polycythemia* is commonly used to refer to an abnormal increase in the number of red blood cells. This is usually, but not always, associated with an increase in red cell mass. Normally, erythropoiesis and consequently red cell mass are controlled by the renal production and the release of erythropoietin. The etiologic relationship of erythropoietin to the polycythemias constitutes a reasonable basis for their classification.

Primary Polycythemia

Polycythemia vera is an intrinsic disorder of the bone marrow that is characterized by the excessive production of erythrocytes, leukocytes, and platelets. Erythropoiesis is not under normal regulatory control. Thus erythropoietin levels in both plasma and urine are low.

Clinical Features. Polycythemia vera affects the middle-aged and elderly. Initial symptoms are variable, nonspecific, and may involve any organ system. They can be ascribed to circulatory disturbances caused by an increased red cell mass with its resultant hypervolemia and hyperviscosity. Common symptoms include headache; dizziness; pruritus, especially after a warm bath; abnormal auditory and visual sensations; paresthesias; and epistaxis. Because of the hyperuricemia resulting from the increased breakdown of nucleoprotein, attacks of gouty arthritis are not uncommon. Physical findings include plethora and suffusion of the skin and mucous membranes and engorged retinal veins. Splenomegaly is the most important physical sign and is found in about 80 percent of patients.

Laboratory Findings. The red cell count, hemoglobin, and hematocrit are characteristically increased in polycythemia vera. Leukocyte and platelet count are also moderately elevated. An increase in basophils and a shift to the left in the neutrophil series are commonly found. The platelets may be functionally defective.

Bone marrow aspiration reveals a hypercellular marrow with an increased number of megakaryocytes; storage iron is frequently absent. An increase in reticulin fibers may also be seen in a biopsied specimen. Red cell mass is increased with plasma volume unaffected or slightly decreased. Other relevant abnormalities include elevations of leukocyte alkaline phosphatase, blood histamine, serum vitamin B_{12} and B_{12}-binding capacity, and serum uric acid.

Complications. Polycythemia vera runs a chronic course. With time, the hematocrit falls to normal or subnormal levels while the leukocyte and the platelet count remains elevated. The bone marrow is then diffusely or patchily fibrotic, and splenic and hepatic enlargement may be considerable. The hematologic picture may simulate that of chronic granulocytic leukemia but can be distinguished from this disease by histochemical and chromosome studies. In other patients the picture is identical to that of agnogenic myeloid metaplasia. In about 10 percent of patients a terminal, acute, leukemialike illness develops. It is unclear whether this is a sequel of the disease or a consequence of ^{32}P therapy.

Treatment. Decreasing the red cell mass by venesection (phlebotomy) is an effective and rapid means of controlling symptoms of polycythemia vera. Some patients can be effectively treated for years with phlebotomy alone plus agents to control the pruritus and the hyperuricemia. However, myelosuppressive therapy may also be required in patients with very active erythropoiesis or with problems arising from excessive thrombocytosis and marked splenic enlargement. Commonly used agents have been ^{32}P and various alkylating compounds. The median survival for patients treated with myelosuppressive drugs is on the order of 13 years.

Secondary Polycythemias

Most cases of secondary polycythemia can be shown to be due to an excessive release of erythropoietin produced as a physiologic response to tissue hypoxia. More rarely, erythropoietin-induced polycythemia is inappropriate since tissue hypoxia is absent. Hypoxic polycythemia may accompany diseases associated with impaired ventilation or perfusion of the lung, or it may follow cardiac shunts that permit venous blood to bypass the pulmonary capillary bed. It occurs in high-altitude dwellers and may also result from interference with the transport and release of oxygen, such as occurs in smokers or patients with a variety of abnormal hemoglobins. Nonhypoxic polycythemias are found in patients with intrarenal disease and in association with certain tumors of the liver, cerebellum, or endocrine organs.

Clinical Features. In secondary polycythemia the symptoms of the primary disorder usually predominate, but those secondary to the polycythemia can also occur. The physical signs are again those of the primary disorder. Splenomegaly is not found.

Laboratory Findings. Red cell count, hemoglobin, and hematocrit are elevated in secondary polycythemia. Unlike the case in polycythemia vera, the leukocyte and platelet count, the number of basophils and bone marrow megakaryocytes, and the levels of leukocyte alkaline phosphatase and blood histamine are not increased. In the hypoxic group, arterial oxygen saturation is below 90 percent or the affinity of hemoglobin for oxygen is increased.

Treatment. Venesection to lower the hematocrit in secondary polycythemia should be considered when the physiologic gain accruing from the increase in red cell and total blood volume have been negated by the hyperviscosity of the blood. However, it is usually difficult to document this clinical situation. Since the wisdom of the body may be superior to that of the attending physician, it seems wise to avoid phlebotomy in such circumstances.

Relative Polycythemia
Any condition in which the venous hematocrit is elevated in the presence of a normal red cell mass is referred to as *relative polycythemia*. Relative polycythemias can be found transiently in sick and obviously dehydrated patients with a reduced plasma volume. However, another group of subjects maintain chronically elevated hematocrits in the absence of a dehydrating primary disorder. This relatively common condition has been called stress, spurious, or pseudopolycythemia. The patients usually have a

normal to high normal red cell mass and a plasma volume at the lower limits of normality. It is unclear whether the syndrome constitutes a distinct disease entity. A large number of these patients are smokers. The relation between smoking and the red cell mass findings has not been adequately explored.

Clinical Features. Patients with relative polycythemia are usually white, middle-aged, mildly overweight, and anxious. Symptoms are nonspecific and include headache, fatigue, weakness, and nervousness. Moderate hypertension and evidence of coronary artery disease by ECG or the history are common. Splenomegaly is not found.

Laboratory Findings. The hemogram in relative polycythemia is normal except for the elevated red cell parameters. Leukocyte alkaline phosphatase, bone marrow megakaryocytes, arterial oxygen saturation, and the hemoglobin affinity for oxygen are all normal. Serum uric acid, cholesterol, and triglycerides are often elevated.

Treatment. Myelosuppressive treatment is contraindicated in relative polycythemia. Phlebotomy is also not indicated, since it seems unlikely that the modestly elevated hematocrit is responsible for the symptoms. Therapy should be directed toward the associated hypertension and coronary artery disease.

Bibliography
Balcerzak, S. P., and Bromberg, P. A. The secondary polycythemias. *Semin. Hematol.* 12:353, 1975.
Berlin, N. I. Diagnosis and classification of the polycythemias. *Semin. Hematol.* 12:339, 1975.
Weinreb, N. J., and Shih, C. F. Spurious polycythemias. *Semin. Hematol.* 12:397, 1975.

49

Principles of
Blood Transfusion and
Blood Component Therapy

Charles P. Emerson

Safe and maximally effective blood replacement requires the close collaboration of those responsible for the clinical care of the patient with those responsible for a competently operated and suitably equipped blood bank. The physicians in charge of both should agree on the patient's therapeutic requirements; what suitable materials are available to meet these requirements — whole blood, washed and unwashed red cell concentrates, platelet concentrates, fresh frozen plasma, or serum albumin; the manner and quantity in which these materials should be administered; and the risks entailed in their use. They must also be familiar with the early and late complications of replacement therapy and the steps that are indicated for the avoidance of these complications and in their treatment. Certain precepts and precautions must be observed:

1. Whenever indicated and feasible, blood components should be used instead of whole blood, which might burden the patient unnecessarily with excess fluid volume, acid, electrolytes, or other unneeded or potentially hazardous substances including antibodies.
2. Whenever possible the physician should avoid emergency or stat transfusions that curtail the standard, officially prescribed, and rather lengthy (1- to 2-hour) compatibility testing.
3. Extreme precautions should be taken to ensure that the correct blood is given to the right patients; misidentification of either the recipient or the blood label at the bedside is responsible for most transfusion disasters.
4. Every transfused patient should be checked at frequent intervals during and after the procedure for the earliest clinical signs of reaction so that the transfusion may be halted or the problem identified and the damage minimized.

5. All unnecessary transfusions should be avoided and as little blood used as possible. The incidence of complications, infectious and otherwise, is directly proportional to the number of units transfused.

Almost all donor blood is currently collected in plastic bags containing a preservative-diluent solution, either citrate-phosphate-dextrose (CPD) or acid-citrate-dextrose (ACD). The red cells in CPD-preserved blood are suitable for transfusion as long as 4 weeks after collection, at which time approximately 70 percent may be expected to persist in the recipient after infusion and then be eliminated at a rate of 1 to 2 percent per day. An official dating period of 3 weeks has been established for both ACD and CPD blood stored continuously at 1 to 6°C; at the end of that time 75 to 80 percent of CPD and 65 to 75 percent of ACD red cells are viable. Certain plasma components remain essentially intact during that period of storage and even longer; thus outdated plasma is perfectly suitable for the salvage, fractionation, and preparation of stable, injectable concentrates of albumin, fibrinogen, and gamma globulin.

Platelets and granulocytes, on the other hand, lose their viability in a matter of hours after collection; and certain important labile ingredients of the plasma, including clotting factors V and VIII, lose their coagulant properties at an exponential rate of approximately 50 percent per week of storage. The immediate separation and prompt freezing of plasma following blood collection effectively prevents deterioration of these labile factors, and almost every hospital blood bank has a depot of single-unit donations of such freshly frozen plasma.

The general availability of multiple interconnected plastic bag collection devices has made it possible to prepare with ease and safety red cell concentrates by the immediate separation of plasma from freshly collected whole blood and also to sequester from the plasma a cryoprecipitate in which factor VIII is concentrated. Single-unit platelet concentrates, if desired, can also be prepared, and the residual plasma may be frozen again and stored indefinitely as a source of all clotting factors or as a blood volume expander in cases of oligemia. Red cell concentrates thus prepared, with a hematocrit value of 60 to 80 percent, have a 3-week shelf life in storage; and they may be administered to anemic patients with therapeutic benefits equal to or surpassing those of whole blood. Such red cell concentrates frozen in a glycerol medium and stored at $-85°C$ in a mechanical refrigerator or at $-196°C$ in liquid nitrogen maintain their viability for many years, and after thawing and removal of the cryoprotective glycerol, the cells are as effective therapeutically as on the day of their freezing. Red cells preserved by freezing are increasingly in demand, especially for patients with rare blood types. Furthermore, the manner in which glycerol is removed from thawed blood produces red cells of exceptional quality, that is, the cells are essentially free of irregular isoantibodies, white cells (hence histocompatibility antigens), potentially antigenic plasma proteins, and viral contaminants.

Blood Component Therapy

Red cell replacement should be regarded as the therapy of choice whenever a transfusion is indicated for correction of anemia, especially an anemia severe enough to produce symptoms related to inadequate oxygen-carrying capacity; an anemia unresponsive to specific antianemic therapy; an anemia not otherwise correctable within the time available; or an anemia associated with circulatory impairment or renal or hepatic disease. In most patients requiring intraoperative transfusions and in elderly or debilitated patients or young children susceptible to volume overload, red cell concentrates alone or supplemented as needed with fresh or frozen plasma and/or serum albumin are effective and desirable.

Leukocyte-poor (leukocyte-free) red cells prepared by continuous-flow centrifugation of donor blood or by filtration of the blood through nylon filters are employed for the transfusion of sensitized patients who have developed leukocyte antibodies in response to earlier transfusions. Because of their circulating leukoagglutinins, such patients are highly liable to have febrile reactions and, occasionally, transient pulmonary infiltrates if they are given blood that has not been so processed. Leukocyte-free red cell transfusion is also considered mandatory for patients who are candidates for renal transplantation, the success of which depends on the avoidance of immunization against tissue antigens shared by donor leukocytes and donor kidneys.

Donor Platelets. Properly collected and processed, donor platelets are capable of functioning for primary hemostasis (see Chap. 52) and accordingly may play an important role in the management of severe thrombocytopenic purpura. The platelets in freshly collected whole blood (or in platelet concentrates) are viable and hemostatically effective for 8 to 11 days in a recipient lacking incompatible platelet antibodies. However, 1 unit of donor platelets, which is the amount collected in a single donation of 500 ml blood, would raise the platelet count of a 70-kg adult at most only about 5,000 per cubic millimeter and hence would be totally inadequate for an acutely thrombocytopenic patient, for whom no less than 8 to 12 units might be required. Platelets in such quantities have to be pooled from multiple units of fresh donor blood or, preferably, extracted from a single donor by plateletpheresis, a process involving continuous flow centrifugation. The yield from plateletpheresis may be 10^{11} platelets contained in 400 to 500 ml. The material may be given by rapid intravenous injection without preliminary crossmatching. Donor platelets preferably should be given promptly after collection, but they will retain their viability for as long as 48 hours when kept at room temperature (22 to 26°C). If they are stored at 4°C for more than 24 hours, their survival in the recipient's circulation is relatively brief. However, there is evidence that such refrigerated platelets are hemostatically more effective immediately after transfusion than those previously maintained at room temperature; their quick disappearance after injection may more reflect their prompt utilization than their nonviability. Patients rarely bleed spontaneously with platelet counts above 10,000. Therefore, platelet transfusions should be reserved for more severely thrombocytopenic patients and patients with active or imminent bleeding. The effect of a platelet transfusion is limited to a few days at best, and in patients with autologous platelet antibodies (e.g., patients with idiopathic thrombocytopenic purpura) or homologous antibodies stimulated by prior transfusions, such transfusions will almost certainly be ineffective.

Leukocyte Concentrates. Prepared by leukapheresis from single donors, which involves continuous-flow centrifugation or a filtration-flow process, leukocyte concentrates are under investigation in many centers for the treatment of patients with life-threatening agranulocytosis. The life span of neutrophils in the circulating blood is no more than 8 to 10 hours. However, injections of 10^{11} granulocytes, repeated daily for 3 to 5 days, have reportedly improved the survival of patients with sepsis who have had temporary myelosuppression by anticancer chemotherapy, as compared with patients who have been treated similarly except for granulocyte transfusions. Obviously granulocytic transfusions are at best of temporary benefit and are potentially useful only in patients in whom granulopoiesis is destined to resume spontaneously and imminently.

Human Albumin. This blood component is available as a purified homogenous plasma fraction in both 5 and 25 percent solutions, with or without sodium; and in a plasma protein fraction containing 5 percent albumin and a mixture of other low-molecular-weight plasma proteins. Both types of fractions, in contrast to all other therapeutic blood components, are completely safe from the standpoint of viral contamination, including hepatitis infectivity, since they are capable of heat sterilization and have been exposed to 60°C for 10 hours before packaging. Moreover, these human albumin fractions are free of isoantibodies, are nonantigenic and nonpyrogenic, and are stable at room temperature for extended periods of time. Their principal use is in restoring or maintaining blood volume in patients with acute blood loss (given in conjunction with red cell concentrates) and in patients with burns, intestinal obstruction, mesenteric thrombosis, peritonitis, and other plasma-losing conditions. Salt-poor albumin solution is indicated in oligemic patients with heart, liver, lung, or renal disease or in patients who are otherwise susceptible to fluid overload.

Clotting Factors
Ten plasma proteins are known to be involved in the clotting reaction and hemostasis (see Chap. 52). All are present in freshly collected blood and retain their original activity for at least a year in freshly separated, frozen plasma stored continuously at −30°C. Three factors, namely V (proaccelerin), VIII (antihemophilic factor), and XI (plasma thromboplastin antecedent, or PTA), deteriorate at a rate of 50 percent per week in whole blood or plasma stored at 4°C; the others remain unchanged for 3 weeks at this temperature. The turnover rate of these factors, that is, their half-lives in vivo following injection, are: factor I (fibrinogen), 4 days; factor II (prothrombin), 2 to 5 days; factor V, 24 hours; factor VII (proconvertin), 5 to 7 hours; factor VIII, 8 to 12 hours; factor IX (plasma thromboplastin component, or Christmas factor), 24 to 48 hours; factor X (Stuart factor), 30 to 50 hours; and factor XI, 40 to 84 hours. Factor concentrates are also available but, except for the treatment of hemophilia, these preparations are little used at present because they are prepared from large pools of donor plasma and carry unacceptably high risks of hepatitis. Preparations of factor VIII (antihemophilic globulin) are indispensable in the treatment of patients with hemophilia A; the cryoprecipitate provides in 10-ml quantities half of the activity present in 200 ml of fresh or freshly frozen plasma. High-potency factor VIII and factor IX concentrates (for hemophilia B) are also available with up to thirty times the activity contained in normal plasma (see Chap. 52).

Immune and Hyperimmune Gamma Globulins
Fractionated plasma from immunized donors containing high concentrations of antibodies against certain infections such as tetanus, pertussis, or hepatitis or against specific blood group antigens may be of great value in many conditions. Immune plasma is harvested from these donors by a process known as plasmapheresis, using a constant-flow centrifugation device that separates and removes the plasma and reinfuses the formed elements. The gamma-globulin fraction of this plasma, in which the high-potency immunoglobulins are concentrated, is suitable for intramuscular but not for intravenous injection.

One important hematologic application of hyperimmune gamma globulin is the injection of hyperimmune anti-Rh_O (D) into Rh-negative mothers immediately following the delivery of Rh-positive infants in order to destroy promptly any Rh-positive fetal cells that have entered the maternal circulation at the time of delivery, before these fetal cells have had time to produce Rh sensitization of the mother. Such Rh sensitization would almost certainly produce erythroblastosis fetalis in subsequent Rh-positive offspring. Hyperimmune anti-Rh_O (D) gamma globulin (RhoGAM) is also given in large quantity to any Rh-negative woman who at any time prior to her menopause has inadvertently received a transfusion of Rh-positive blood.

Special Transfusion Problems

OLIGEMIC SHOCK

One of the major applications of blood transfusions is the treatment or prevention of shock (forward failure) due to blood volume loss from spontaneous or traumatic (including surgical) hemorrhage or from burns, peritonitis, or other plasma-losing conditions. The therapeutic objective is to maintain sufficient blood volume to sustain arterial pressure and support the circulation sufficiently to deliver an adequate supply of oxygen to the tissues. If blood is required at all, the amount used should be judged on the amount and rate of loss; changes in vital signs, especially pulse and arterial pressure; and the likelihood of continued losses. Postural signs, that is, rises in pulse and falls in blood pressure when the patient is rapidly shifted from a prone to a sitting or upright position, are particularly helpful indications of the need for blood transfusion. A systolic pressure below 100 mm Hg in the supine position suggests that the blood volume has been reduced to less than 70 percent of normal. Hematocrit readings may not drop significantly for several hours after an acute hemorrhage, but progressive falls are highly significant. A decrease in the hourly urine output occurs from oligemia, even without a drop in blood pressure, and therefore diminished urinary output may be a sensitive indication of oligemia. The central venous pressure may or may not fall significantly; on the other hand, a rising venous pressure during transfusion indicates an adequate volume return to the right heart and suggests the need for caution with respect to further transfusions.

Selection of Therapeutic Agents

Balanced salt solutions, involving as they do fewer hazards than blood transfusions, should be used to restore blood volume when the blood loss has been small and the hemoglobin concentration is normal. A previously healthy patient after severe injury can tolerate massive saline infusions; he eliminates the excess fluid and salt over the next few days by dint of massive diuresis. Elderly patients and others with diminished cardiac reserve, impaired renal function, or both should not be exposed to excessive salt loads. In general, acute, severe blood loss is to be replaced with whole blood or red cell concentrates in amounts equivalent to the estimated volume deficit. In addition, balanced salt solutions in up to 3- and 4-liter amounts per 24 hours may be given to normal adult men and half this amount to normal adult women. In the treatment of severe burns, intestinal obstruction, mesenteric thrombosis, pancreatitis, and other plasma-losing conditions, appropriate replacement is provided in the form of 25 or 5% human albumin, "plasma protein fraction," or whole plasma, again supplemented by large volumes of balanced salt solution and with due precautions as mentioned above.

MASSIVE TRANSFUSIONS

One of the problems encountered in massive blood replacement results from the marked decrease in the buffering capacity of stored bank blood, caused in part by the highly acid preservative solutions. Each unit of bank blood has an acid load of approximately 8 mEq per unit, and in the course of rapid transfusion exogenous acids may accumulate in the patient. To avoid acidosis in massively transfused patients, sodium bicarbonate may be administered at the rate of 45 mEq per each 5 units of blood administered. The oxygen tension of stored blood may be reduced to between 9 and 19 mm Hg and the oxygen saturation to between 20 and 40 percent; in addition, the stored blood has been depleted of its organic polyphosphates, especially 2,3-diphosphoglycerate, with the result that its oxygen delivery is greatly reduced and may not be restored for several hours after transfusion. Hypothermia, which inevitably develops when a massive transfusion is given with refrigerated blood, should be prevented by the use of blood warmers set at 100°F

(38°C). Clotting defects caused by depletion of platelets or of factors V, VIII, and XI can be averted by interspersing blood transfusions with infusions of fresh whole blood or freshly frozen plasma in the ratio of 1 unit for every 5 to 10 units of stored blood. Significant thrombocytopenia is unlikely to develop in an individual not already deficient in platelets; these deficient individuals should receive platelet concentrates preoperatively and intraoperatively.

The sudden onset during surgery of generalized oozing requires immediate investigation of all possible causes, including hemolytic transfusion reaction or a consumption coagulopathy (see Chap. 52).

COMPLICATIONS OF TRANSFUSIONS

Immediate Hemolytic Reactions
Any unfavorable reaction occurring during a transfusion calls for immediate interruption of the procedure and a prompt, systematic search for the cause. The injection needle should be kept patent with a slow saline drip either to permit the administration of mannitol and other intravenous medications, if necessary, or to facilitate the resumption of the transfusion if incontrovertible evidence is obtained to indicate that the incident was not attributable to the transfusion in question. Hemolytic reactions are characterized by rapid destruction of red cells, often with hemoglobinemia and hemoglobinuria. These accidents are most often brought about by the introduction of red cell antigens into a recipient whose plasma contains antibodies specific for those antigens. The two most dangerous examples of such incompatibility reactions are those produced by (1) the transfusion of type A or type B blood into individuals lacking A or B antigens (hence possessing A or B antibodies, respectively); and (2) the transfusion of D+ (Rh-positive) red cells into a patient who has been isoimmunized against the Rh_O (D) factor as the result of an earlier Rh-positive transfusion or an Rh-positive pregnancy (not treated postpartum with prophylactic anti-Rh_O [D] hyperimmune globulin).

Hemolytic transfusion reactions are usually manifested by chills, fever, and back pain or, in the case of anesthetized patients, by the onset of oozing from surgical wounds or venipuncture sites. Hemoglobinuria succeeded by oliguria, even a complete anuria, may be anticipated if hemolysis has been severe, for example, in patients who have received more than 100 or 200 ml of ABO-incompatible red cells.

Investigation of a Transfusion Reaction. As already stated, the transfusion must be stopped immediately and the needle kept open with a saline drip. A fresh specimen of the patient's blood is sent immediately to the blood bank together with what is left of the donor blood. The fresh blood specimen is centrifuged immediately, and the supernatant plasma is examined visually for free hemoglobin, which is detectable as a pink or reddish discoloration. The blood bank staff will retest the fresh blood specimen, the residual donor blood, and the pilot samples for ABO and Rh types, for serologic evidence of incompatibility (or compatibility), and for agglutininability by antiglobulin serum (i.e., the direct Coombs test). The urine should be examined for hemoglobin after centrifugation, and the urine output should be carefully monitored and recorded. The residual donor blood should be examined by a Gram stain for evidence of bacterial contamination, and the blood should be cultured using at least two incubator temperatures (20 and 37°C). Finally, a careful clerical check should be made to confirm the identity of the patient and the accuracy of both the clinical and the blood bank records.

Treatment of Hemolytic Reactions. The following steps are to be carried out without delay, simultaneously with the investigations specified above.

1. Inject mannitol intravenously (25 gm to an adult), infusing a 20 or 25 percent solution over a 5-minute period in an attempt to establish a diuresis. Subsequently mannitol should be administered in a 2.5 to 5 percent solution in saline in volumes equivalent to the urine output. A maximum of about 150 gm of mannitol can be given safely within 24 hours to a patient whose urine output exceeds 100 ml per hour. Intravenous diuretics (furosemide, 20 to 40 mg, or ethacrynic acid, 50 mg) are indicated for overhydrated patients.

2. Obtain baseline levels of blood urea nitrogen, creatinine, and electrolytes.

3. If there is no evidence of circulatory overload, hydrate the patient with intravenous normal saline, 1,500 to 2,000 ml plus 44 mEq of sodium bicarbonate during the first 2 hours. If urine flow is not adequate in response to these measures, salt and fluid must thereafter be restricted.

4. If the patient still requires blood, concentrated red cells may be administered, providing the compatibility test with a fresh specimen of blood from the patient is completely satisfactory and assuming also that the mechanism of the hemolytic reaction itself has been explained and its recurrence accordingly forestalled. If ABO incompatibility was the cause, type O blood cell concentrates should be selected for subsequent transfusion.

5. If the patient bleeds profusely after a febrile transfusion reaction there is a good possibility that defibrination is occurring; in this case laboratory screening for disseminated intravascular coagulation is indicated (see Chap. 52). Heparin should be administered intravenously at once in a dose of 7,500 to 10,000 units and continued at the rate of 1,000 units per hour until the partial thromboplastin, prothrombin, and thrombin times and the platelet counts are satisfactory. Transfusions of platelets and fresh frozen plasma may be required.

Circulatory Overload

Circulatory overload, a transfusion complication that is most common in infants and elderly patients, is manifested by tachypnea, cyanosis, and auscultatory signs of pulmonary congestion. Treatment consists in interrupting the transfusion, placing the patient in an orthopneic position, and applying measures appropriate for congestive heart failure, including oxygen inhalation and the administration of intravenous diuretics. In severe cases a phlebotomy may be advisable (to reduce the blood volume) while concentrated red cells are simultaneously administered in a different vein, if the need for donor red cells remains urgent. The risk of circulatory overload is minimized if red cell concentrates are used rather than whole blood and if transfusions are administered with the patient in a sitting, rather than supine, position.

Allergic Reactions

Urticarial lesions, with slight or no fever, develop in about 3 percent of all transfusions. Such reactions are seldom serious. The inciting agent may be antigenic material associated with the donor leukocytes, platelets, or plasma, or, conversely, an antibody in the donor blood with specificity for an antigen in the recipient. Allergic reactions rarely occur with transfusions of thoroughly washed red cells. Treatment consists in the parenteral administration of an antihistamine or epinephrine. The routine administration of an antihistaminic drug prior to a transfusion as a prophylactic against allergic reactions is not advised, and on no account should an antihistaminic drug or, for that matter, any medication be added directly to the donor blood.

Bacterial Contamination

Contaminated donor blood is likely to produce profound circulatory collapse, a dangerous situation calling for emergency measures. Clinical symptoms and signs developing almost immediately following the start of the infusion include severe chills, fever, severe abdominal cramps, vomiting, diarrhea, tachypnea, hypotension, and the hemorrhagic manifestations of disseminated intravascular coagulation. Initial leukopenia is followed by leukocytosis.

Confirmation of bacterial contamination may be obtained rapidly by performing a Gram stain on the donor blood obtained from the container or tubing. The donor blood and blood from the patient should be cultured aerobically and anaerobically at 4, 20, and 37°C, since some cryophilic (cold-growing) organisms will not grow well at 37°C. Gram-negative organisms capable of growing at 4°C are the most common bacterial contaminants. The contaminating organisms may no longer be viable at the time of transfusion, but the endotoxins responsible for the transfusion reaction may be demonstrated by means of pyrogen tests in rabbits. Treatment is designed to combat shock and includes the parenteral administration of corticosteroids, norepinephrine, and appropriate antibiotics (see Chap. 6).

Leukoagglutinin Reactions

Many multitransfused patients develop antibodies specific for leukocyte antigens and thereafter exhibit febrile reactions, sometimes severe, in response to transfusions of blood containing these antigens. Alternatively, donor blood, especially blood from multiparous donors previously sensitized to specific leukocyte antigens that are possessed by their offspring but not by them, may produce reactions in recipients whose blood contains those antigens. Such reactions are manifested primarily by fever and, depending on the relative quantities of leukocyte antigen and antibody, by dyspnea and cough, with pulmonary infiltrates visible on x-ray. Treatment includes measures to control the fever and alleviate respiratory distress.

IgA-Induced Transfusion Reactions

Severe anaphylactic reactions caused by antibodies to immunoglobulin A, in recipients who lack IgA on a congenital basis, constitute a rare but important type of immediate transfusion complication. Selective absence of IgA has been found in approximately 1 per 900 individuals, so it may be assumed that the risk of such reactions is in the order of 0.1 percent of transfusions involving the injection of material containing plasma. Symptoms appear almost immediately after the start of such transfusions and in almost all instances include severe pain in the chest, epigastric pain, nausea, dyspnea, diaphoresis, hypotension, and cyanosis. Treatment involves immediate cessation of the transfusion and maintenance of arterial pressure with vasopressors and, in certain cases, corticosteroids.

The presence of IgA antibodies in most but not all of the patients who have had a severe anaphylactic reaction to transfusion has been explainable on the basis of isoimmunization through earlier transfusions or pregnancies. In the absence of such stimuli the assumption has been that the patient has been immunized in utero by exposure to maternal IgA. Prevention of IgA reactions in vulnerable patients depends on the exclusive use of donors lacking IgA (rosters of such individuals are being compiled throughout the country) and on the use of thoroughly washed red cells plus albumin in lieu of whole blood or plasma in the event further transfusions are required.

DELAYED COMPLICATIONS OF TRANSFUSION

Late Hemolysis of Donor Red Cells

Several days to a few weeks after a transfusion, a primary or an anamnestic immune reaction may develop in response to the donor red cells if enough incompatible donor red cells are still present at that time. The hematologic picture is that of idiopathic autoimmune hemolytic anemia (see Chap. 47) with manifestations of hyperbilirubinemia, reticulocytosis, and anemia, and the appearance of a positive direct Coombs test. The severity of the process depends on the relative proportions of donor and the patient's own cells in the circulation at the time. The process is self-limited, and as soon as the sensitized donor cells have been cleared from the circulation, the only residual manifestations are the presence of blood group isoantibody in the patient's circulation and anemia. The anemia can be corrected if necessary by transfusions of compatible red cells, that is, red cells for which the patient possesses no antibodies.

Posttransfusion Thrombocytopenia

A situation analogous to the late hemolysis of red cells occurs from time to time as the result of the antigenicity of donor platelets and is responsible for the syndrome of posttransfusion purpura (see Chap. 52). Almost all such patients have been women, and almost all of them have been found to possess an isoantibody directed against the platelet antigen Pl^{A1}, which they themselves lack. Thrombocytopenia in patients so afflicted develops about a week after transfusion. The platelet count usually drops to 10,000 or less and may persist for 3 to 6 weeks or longer before spontaneous recovery occurs and the count rises to baseline levels. No therapy is available to hasten recovery except for removal of the offending antibody by exchange transfusion, a procedure that may be undertaken in severe cases. A 60 percent exchange has sufficed to control previously intractable bleeding. Any patient who has experienced posttransfusion purpura must be considered disqualified as a recipient of whole blood or red cell concentrates containing platelets, since the platelet antigen Pl^{A1} is possessed by 98 percent of the donor population.

TRANSMISSION OF INFECTION

A number of infections are transmissible by transfusion of blood or blood components donated by asymptomatic carriers. Among these infections are syphilis, hepatitis, malaria, and the so-called postpump syndrome. These are discussed in detail elsewhere in this textbook (Chaps. 30, 41).

Hepatitis
Hepatitis may be induced by a variety of viral agents, predominantly but not exclusively by hepatitis A and hepatitis B viruses. Hepatitis A has a relatively short incubation period (e.g., 3 weeks), and hepatitis B has a long incubation period (3 to 6 months). Susceptible recipients respond with signs and symptoms ranging from asymptomatic abnormal liver function tests only to the rapid development of acute hepatic necrosis. The mortality of posttransfusion hepatitis in adults approaches 5 to 10 percent; children tend to have milder disease. All blood components may transmit hepatitis with the exception of serum albumin and Plasma Protein Fraction, both of which are heat sterilized in the course of processing, and immune (and hyperimmune) serum globulin. With respect to all other blood products including, of course, whole blood, the risk of hepatitis is proportional to the number of units administered and the number of donors who have contributed to the pool from which the components have been derived. The greatest risk is incurred with the use of pooled plasma, fibrinogen, and commercial preparations containing mixtures of clotting factors II, VII, IX, and X. The prophylactic value of hyperimmune gamma globulin in patients known to have received blood from hepatitis B carriers has been reported favorably. Universal screening of donors for the presence of hepatitis surface antigen by a radioimmunoassay technique promises to eliminate at least three-fourths of the infectious donors who carry this particular virus, but a substantial number of posttransfusion hepatitis infections are due to viruses other than A or B, still unidentified.

Malaria
Viable malarial parasites persist in stored blood and pose, even in the United States, a risk that is more than negligible. About 20 cases have been recorded in the past decade. Malaria may manifest itself as early as 2 weeks following transfusion, but generally the latent period is longer, as long as 3 months in one recorded instance. The possibility of this complication should be considered in a patient with unexplained fever 2 weeks to 4 months following transfusion. Donors from endemic areas should be excluded for a period of 2 years after discontinuing suppressive antimalarial therapy and for 6 months after residence in such an area. Those with a history of malaria should be accepted only for plasma donation.

Syphilis
With venereal disease on the rise, the hazard of posttransfusion syphilis is of increasing concern. Fortunately the spirochete does not remain viable after several days of refrigerated storage, but transfusions of fresh blood, fresh blood components, or components of plasma freshly frozen at temperatures below $-20°C$ can transmit the disease. A negative serologic test for syphilis of the donor is no absolute guarantee that he does not have spirochetemia (seronegative primary disease). As with malaria, the danger is that the cause of symptoms, which may not appear for 1 to 4 months following transfusion, may go unrecognized and the disease may go untreated.

Postpump Syndrome
A clinical picture suggesting infectious mononucleosis has been described in individuals who have received freshly collected whole blood, especially in patients who have had open heart surgery under cardiopulmonary bypass in the recent past, when strictly fresh blood transfusions were considered mandatory. Major clinical features include fever and splenomegaly and the presence of atypical lymphocytes in the peripheral blood, all developing about a month postoperatively. Other features of this illness have been hepatomegaly, cervical lymphadenopathy, and a rubellalike rash. In most cases the illness has lasted several weeks but has proved relatively benign. The major proportion of these cases have probably not been instances of infectious mononucleosis, since the majority have had negative heterophil antibody tests and have lacked antibodies to the Epstein-Barr virus. The most frequent cause is cytomegalovirus infection transmitted by the fresh blood or due to reactivation of latent cytomegalovirus in the recipient. In many instances

the virus has been recovered in the recipient's urine and in his circulating leukocytes. Complement-fixing antibody levels have been shown to increase, and the course of the illness has been consistent with the clinical picture of megalovirus infection.

A third possible cause of the postpump syndrome has been a host-versus-graft or graft-versus-host reaction. Such transfusions could well provide a graft of living lymphocytes, and both electron microscopic and tritiated thymidine autoradiography studies have demonstrated that the atypical cells characteristic of the postpump syndrome are actively dividing lymphocytes somewhat similar to the lymphoblasts seen in mixed lymphocyte cultures.

Bibliography

Boggs, D. R. Transfusion of neutrophils as prevention or treatment of infection in patients with neutropenia. *N. Engl. J. Med.* 290:1055, 1974.

Huestis, D. W., Bove, J. R., and Busch, B. *Practical Blood Transfusion.* Boston: Little, Brown, 1969.

Mollison, P. L. *Blood Transfusion in Clinical Medicine* (5th ed.). Philadelphia: Davis, 1972.

National Research Council Panel (H. Chaplin, Jr., Chairman). Current status of red cell preservation and availability in relation to the developing national blood policy. *N. Engl. J. Med.* 291:68, 1974.

Valeri, C. R. *Blood Banking and the Use of Frozen Blood Products.* Cleveland: CRC Press, 1976.

50

Disorders of
the Granulocyte

Mark J. Brauer

This chapter considers disorders of granulocytes, or
mature polymorphonuclear white cells, the major
phagocytes in the blood. Increases in the number of
these cells both in the peripheral circulation and in
the bone marrow may be either appropriate or exaggerated in response to infection or inflammation and,
in fact, may occur in the absence of any obvious
stimulus. Abnormal decreases in either the number
or the phagocytic function of granulocytes may result
in clinical disorders characterized by chronic, recurrent bacterial or fungal infections. Finally, neoplastic
proliferations of leukocytes may occur with predictably dire effects. Before considering these various
disorders, it is necessary first to review the normal
morphology and physiology of granulocytes.

Morphology and Function

Myeloblasts are the most primitive identifiable cells
of the granulocytic series. These cells, comprising less
than 5 percent of all bone marrow cells, proliferate
into the promyelocytes, which are large cells with
prominent nucleoli and large azurophilic granules
containing myeloperoxidase, hydrolytic enzymes, and
mucopolysaccharides. Promyelocytes, in turn, give
rise to myelocytes, which develop specific staining
granules identifying them as neutrophils, eosinophils,
or basophils. The next cell of the series is the metamyelocyte, a product of myelocyte maturation that
is smaller than the myelocyte and has an indented
nucleus and many specifically staining granules. The
metamyelocyte does not divide, but matures to a
band form and then to a polymorphonuclear leukocyte over a 6- to 7-day period. Phagocytic efficiency
is not reached until the band and polymorphonuclear
stages of cell development.

Circulating blood monocytes are derived from the
promonocytes present in limited numbers in the bone
marrow. The circulating monocyte ingests and
destroys bacteria and particulate material less efficiently than the mature polymorphonuclear leuko-

cyte. In addition, human monocytes have a surface
receptor that is specific for the Fc portion of IgG
immunoglobulin, and they can bind particles coated
with such a globulin. When Rh antibodies, for example, are fixed to human red cells, monocytes bind
the cells, leading to their sequestration and death,
a process referred to as immune hemolysis.

Granulopoiesis

The average postmetamyelocytic granulocyte spends
from 6 to 7 days maturing in the bone marrow before
it is released into the peripheral circulation. The
marrow is estimated to contain about 25 times more
cells than the number circulating in the blood. Once
in the peripheral circulation, about half the granulocytes move centrally in the axial stream of the blood
vessels, while the other half are marginated along the
walls of the venules and arterioles. These marginated
cells are ready either to leave the circulation in response to an appropriate chemotactic stimulus or to
reenter the central circulation in response to exercise
or epinephrine (demargination). Polymorphonuclear
leukocytes spend 6 to 12 hours in the peripheral circulation, but once they enter the tissues, they survive
only 2 or 3 days and never reenter the bloodstream.
Thus only worn-out granulocytes are regularly found
in body secretions or excretions.

Granulocyte production appears to be homeostat-
ically regulated to maintain a total neutrophil count
in the range of 1.8 to 7.25×10^3 cells per cubic millimeter in the peripheral blood. In man, a production
rate of 1.6×10^9 cells/kg/day has been estimated to
be necessary to maintain this level in the face of the
aforementioned short half-life. The system must also
be able to respond rapidly to the demands of micro-
bial invasion or heightened cell loss.

All blood cells are derived from stem cells, most of
which are committed to one or another line of differentiation. For example, stem cells responsive to the
hormone erythropoietin appear capable of making
only cells of the erythroid line (see Chap. 47). Pluripotent stem cells, which are capable of giving rise to
mixed colonies of erythroid, granulocytic, and megakaryocytic cells, have been demonstrated experimentally using the technique of spleen colony assay.
Other experimental studies suggest that a stem cell

exists with the capacity for differentiation along both the lymphoid and myeloid pathway. In any case, regulatory factors appear to operate at the stem cell level (as already mentioned, erythropoietin clearly regulates erythropoiesis). Stem cells committed to the megakaryocytic or granulocytic cell lines are thought to respond to thrombopoietin and granulopoietin, respectively. One theory holds that the pluripotent stem cells can sense depletion of the committed cell compartments and can feed in more of the specifically depleted components. Thus granulopoietin acting on the target-committed precursor cell causes a loss of cells in that granulocyte compartment, thereby initiating recruitment of additional granulocyte-committed stem cells from the pluripotent stem cells.

In vitro bone marrow culture systems have shown that colonies of granulocytic (or monocytic) cells are stimulated to develop from their stem cells by colony-stimulating activity substances. Such substances include (1) a glycoprotein purified from human urine with a molecular weight of 45,000 daltons; (2) human peripheral leukocytes, especially monocytes; (3) human tissue macrophages; (4) bacterial endotoxins; and (5) immunologically stimulated lymphocytes. There is evidence that several kinds of colony-stimulating activity substances may be involved in the regulation of granulopoiesis. For homeostasis a system of inhibition (negative feedback) must also exist, lest granulopoiesis get out of control. Recently evidence for an inhibitor of granulopoiesis, granulocyte chalone, has been obtained; this substance, extractable from intact neutrophils, appears to be a polypeptide with a chain length of 20 to 30 amino acids. It is known to inhibit DNA synthesis of granulocytic precursor cells and is cell-specific. Figure 50-1 shows a scheme for the regulation of granulopoiesis based on both stimulation and negative feedback action on stem cells.

Figure 50-1. Scheme for the regulation of granulopoiesis.

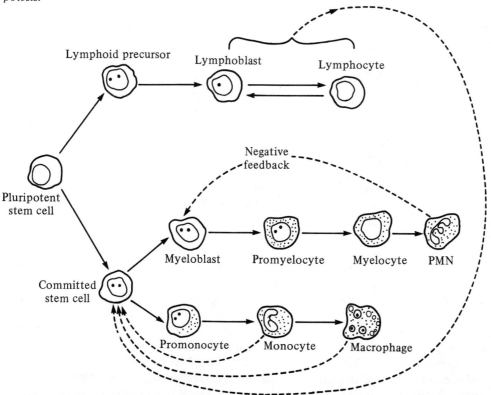

Leukocytosis and Leukemoid Reactions

Leukocytosis is defined as a peripheral leukocyte count above 10,000 per cubic millimeter (the normal average is 7,000, and the normal range is 5,000 to 10,000) (Table 50-1). Fluctuations as great as 3,000 to 4,000 cells can occur in the leukocyte count during a normal day's activities. With complete rest a low-normal white blood cell count is seen; ordinary activity produces a rise in the count; and a high-normal white cell count is commonly found in the afternoon. Physiologic variations greater than this normal range have been described without demonstrable disease. In such varied and unique situations as a quarter-mile run, parturition, an epileptic seizure, an episode of pain, or an emotional disturbance, a transient leukocytosis to 20,000 to 30,000 cells per cubic millimeter may be found, the predominant cells being mature granulocytes.

Granulocytosis is a predominantly granulocytic leukocytosis with a shift to less mature forms as indicated by an increased percentage of bands and the appearance of metamyelocytes and myelocytes in the blood. Frequently these cells also exhibit toxic granulation; that is, a tinctorial change in which the granules stain more deeply and appear larger. While a specific list of all the diseases causing granulocytosis is too long to detail, the general types of disorders are acute infections, usually bacterial; intoxication due to physical or chemical agents; acute hemorrhage; and disorders associated with rapid destruction of tissue.

Eosinophilic granulocytosis (defined as an eosinophil blood count above 200 per cubic millimeter) is frequent in patients with allergic disorders such as bronchial asthma, hay fever, or angioneurotic edema. In respiratory allergies a helpful diagnostic finding is the presence of large numbers of eosinophils in nasal and bronchial secretions. Parasitic infestations, especially those in which tissue invasion occurs, such as trichinosis, can produce marked elevations of eosinophils. On occasion, eosinophilia may be seen in patients with Hodgkin's disease. Rarely, eosinophilia has been found with chronic pyogenic infections such as osteomyelitis.

Lymphocytosis occurs when the absolute lymphocyte count in the blood is above the normal maximum of about 2,000 per cubic millimeter. This is characteristic in pertussis, in which leukocyte counts of 20,000 to 30,000 and higher, with up to 60 percent lymphocytes, are found. Many viral infections produce a lymphocytosis of varying degrees. They may also cause plasmacytosis. The most striking example of benign plasmacytosis is that found in serum sickness.

A *leukemoid reaction* is a leukocytic response in the peripheral blood of such magnitude or abnormal cell morphology or both as to be out of the ordinary and raise a suspicion of leukemia. The term *leukemoid reaction* is not a diagnosis; rather, it only implies the recognition of an abnormal laboratory finding, similar to that implied by the terms *anemia* and *low platelet count*. Leukemoid reactions are often found in association with nonspecific systemic disturbances such as fever, weight loss, and malaise; they may also be associated with localized processes. The course of a leukemoid reaction usually follows that of the underlying disorder.

Leukemoid reactions may involve various cell types. Associations observed between individual cell types and certain conditions include:

Table 50-1. Normal Laboratory
Values for Leukocytes

Site of blood sampling and test	Value
Peripheral blood	
Total leukocytes (per cu mm $\times 10^3$)	5–10
Leukocyte differential count (percent)	
Segmented neutrophils	55–70
Juvenile (band) forms	2–5
Eosinophils	1–3
Basophils	0.5–1.5
Lymphocytes	20–35
Monocytes	3–7
Bone marrow differential distribution (percent)	
Blast forms	3
Promyelocytes	6
Myelocytes (neutrophilic)	16
Metamyelocytes and band forms	24
Segmented neutrophils	20
Eosinophils (all stages)	3
Basophils (all stages)	1
Lymphocytes	20
Plasma cells	3
Erythroblasts and normoblasts	25
Leukocyte alkaline phosphatase	13–130

1. Neutrophilic reactions
   a. Acute: pyogenic infections, drug reactions, liver necrosis, fulminating tuberculosis
   b. Chronic: infection (fungal, bacterial), neoplasms (Hodgkin's disease, carcinoma), bone marrow hyperactivity (hemolytic anemia)
2. Lymphocytic reactions
   a. Acute: infectious mononucleosis, pertussis
   b. Chronic: tuberculosis
3. Eosinophilic: collagen vascular disease, Hodgkin's disease, allergy, parasitic infestation
4. Monocytic: tuberculosis, fungal infection, bacterial endocarditis

Diagnosis. Diagnostic efforts in leukemoid reactions should always be made to exclude leukemia; the peripheral blood smear will often do this, but a bone marrow examination may be necessary. Peripheral blood findings in acute neutrophilic leukemoid reactions may mimic acute leukemia, but a more typical picture is a definite leukocytosis with a modest increase in immature forms. Chronic leukemoid neutrophilic reactions may attain blood counts seen in chronic myelogenous leukemia, but usually they are lower. Nucleated red blood cells with marked anisocytosis and poikilocytosis suggest either myelofibrosis or bone marrow invasion by tumor or granuloma. A leukemoid reaction in association with a high hematocrit and high platelet count suggests polycythemia vera. The diagnosis of leukemia is generally established by bone marrow analysis. A bone marrow biopsy may reveal tumor involvement, granuloma, or myelofibrosis. Most often in leukemoid reactions, the marrow shows only increased cellularity without specific abnormalities.

Laboratory Tests. Certain laboratory tests are very helpful in distinguishing leukemoid reactions from leukemia or other disorders associated with leukocytosis.

1. The leukocyte alkaline phosphatase level is low in chronic myelogenous leukemia but elevated in myeloid leukemoid reactions.
2. The heterophil or monospot tests are often positive in infectious mononucleosis, never in malignant lymphocytosis.
3. The presence of the Philadelphia chromosome is strong support for the diagnosis of chronic myelogenous leukemia.

No treatment is indicated for leukemoid reactions other than therapy of the underlying disease. It should be emphasized that every effort should be made to attain a definitive diagnosis, since antileukemic therapy may produce fatal bone marrow depression if erroneously given.

Leukopenia and Agranulocytosis
Leukopenia exists when the white blood cell count drops below the lower limit of normal, 5,000 cells per cubic millimeter. In some instances the reduction in total leukocytes is balanced and the differential count remains essentially normal. Much more often, the neutrophils are disportionately low, in which case the term *neutropenia* or *granulocytopenia* is more descriptive. Generally, leukopenia will not cause difficulty if the white cell count is above 2,500 and the neutrophils are over 20 percent. With total counts below this level and more severe neutropenia, invasion of the mucous membranes, skin, and blood by microorganisms becomes increasingly frequent and severe. There is, however, considerable variability from individual to individual, and no precisely critical level can accurately be assumed. Leukopenia may be a secondary finding in many disorders, or it can be the result of significant primary disease. Thus a reduced number of circulating neutrophils may result from the impaired production of neutrophils, their accelerated destruction, or less commonly from their abnormal marginal cell distribution.

A large number of defects in neutrophil production has been described as leading to neutropenia. Aplasia or hypoplasia of the bone marrow may be either idiopathic or related to ionizing radiation; toxic agents such as benzene or alcohol; cytotoxics (antimetabolites, alkylating agents) or drugs that interfere with cell maturation such as antibiotics (chloramphenicol, sulfonamides); thiazide diuretics; anticonvulsants (phenytoin); antithyroid medications (propylthiouracil); and phenothiazines (chlorpromazine). Bone marrow infiltration and replacement by either neoplastic cells or lipid storage cells (Gaucher's disease) may compromise granulocyte production. Megaloblastic anemia due to deficiency of vitamin B_{12} or folic acid not infrequently is associated with significant leukopenia. Certain disseminated bacterial infections such as salmonella and viral disorders including influenza, infectious hepatitis, and mononucleosis may lead to significant but often transient neutropenia. Finally, paroxysmal nocturnal hemoglobinuria, an acquired disorder, and certain congenital or hereditary disturbances of neutrophil production may lead to reduced circulating granulocytes. Cyclic changes in the leukocyte count have been observed in the congenital-hereditary group.

Neutrophil destructive disorders include hypersplenism, an entity associated with hepatic cirrhosis (Banti syndrome), portal vein thrombosis, chronic infections of the reticuloendothelial system, and rheumatoid arthritis (Felty's syndrome). Leukocyte antibodies may develop following the administration of certain drugs such as aminophenazone, mercurial diuretics, and phenylbutazone and lead to destruction of mature granulocytes. Isoimmune antileukocyte antibodies may develop during pregnancy and may be transmitted transplacentally, while autoimmune antileukocyte sensitization may occur in adults with collagen vascular disorders such as systemic lupus erythematosus and cause moderate granulocytopenia.

Acute infections may cause transient, severe neutropenia due to shifts of granulocytes from the central axial circulation into other body compartments; this may result from increased neutrophil margination along capillaries or arteriolar walls. In some instances increased movement of neutrophils into inflammatory exudates temporarily outstrips marrow reserve.

Granulocytopenias due to cytotoxic agents or drugs usually revert within 7 to 14 days after discontinuing the responsible agent. During this time the severity of the illness is related to the presence and extent of infection and the promptness with which appropriate antibiotic therapy is instituted. Neutropenias associated with other reversible disorders such as megaloblastic anemias usually respond within 3 to 4 days of appropriate therapy. In contrast, irreversible infiltrative processes of the bone marrow such as acute leukemia or myelofibrosis may lead to progressive diminution in mature cell production and ultimately cause death from septicemia.

The degree and duration of granulocytopenia predict the prognosis. Brief episodes of drug-induced agranulocytosis may be tolerated with a favorable outcome. However, severe depression of granulocyte production for a period longer than 10 to 14 days is ordinarily associated with severe, uncontrollable sepsis. Certain chronic neutropenic states, such as may occur with paroxysmal nocturnal hemoglobinuria or idiopathic or drug-induced bone marrow aplasia, may occasionally terminate in acute myeloblastic leukemia.

AGRANULOCYTOSIS

Agranulocytosis is a disease characterized by an acute course with high fever, sore throat, prostration, and, in severe cases, death. There is marked leukopenia with decreased or even totally absent neutrophils. Membranous ulcerations with little surrounding tissue reaction may be found in the mouth and pharynx. In some cases, fatigue, weakness, and malaise precede the acute onset by several days. Initially, infection occurs in body areas such as the pharynx or rectum, where bacteria are normally present in large numbers but are kept under control by the neutrophils. These local infections become generalized as the disease progresses; septicemia is to be anticipated; pneumonia is the commonest cause of death.

The peripheral blood smear in agranulocytosis is usually unremarkable except for the decreased or absent neutrophils. The bone marrow is usually hypocellular with a decrease both in the myeloid-erythroid (M/E) ratio and in all myeloid elements. The megakaryocyte and erythroid series are usually normal, as compared to the situation in aplastic anemia, in which the erythroid, megakaryocyte, and myeloid series are all greatly decreased. In some cases of leukemia, a leukopenic picture may be found in the peripheral smear but the bone marrow will contain a great number of younger cells, especially blast forms. Monocytosis has been noted in the peripheral blood early in the recovery phase of acute agranulocytosis.

It should be noted that neutropenia alone is not an indication for treatment (other than for the primary disease) except when there is evidence of neutrophilic dysfunction. For example, patients with chronic idiopathic neutropenia may be completely well despite a profound neutropenia of many years' duration, and they need no treatment. However, patients with other types of neutropenia (e.g., acute leukemia or aplastic anemia) have potentially life-threatening diseases. Thus knowledge of both the basic disease and the patient's susceptibility to infections in the past figure importantly in the therapeutic approach. In managing the patient with agranulocytosis, specific antibiotics are employed pending results of bacterial cultures and sensitivity tests. Reverse isolation procedures are of dubious benefit, since the patient may readily become autoinfected. If a particular agent or drug is suspected as being at fault, it should be immediately discontinued. Compatible leukocyte transfusions are available at special centers throughout the country but still are viewed as experimental in nature. The most important therapeutic maneuver involves detecting the cause of the neutropenia and, if possible, removing it. The use of steroid compounds is not usually beneficial. Splenectomy has proved helpful only in some patients with congestive splenomegaly or Felty's syndrome; otherwise, it is of little value.

Phagocytic Dysfunctional Syndromes

Phagocytosis in vivo is determined by both serum and cellular factors, and it occurs primarily in tissue sites beyond the limits of the vascular tree. There are six steps involved in phagocytosis as performed by polymorphonuclear leukocytes and monocytes.

1. *Chemotaxis.* This is a process responsible for the migration of phagocytes from the circulation to inflammatory sites in tissue. Polymorphonuclear leukocytes appear to be attracted by chemotactic factors in the exudate; complement components constitute one type of chemotactic factor.
2. *Opsonization.* This is a process in which bacteria are coated with opsonins that make them more susceptible to ingestion by phagocytes; IgG, IgM antibody, and complement have been shown to act as opsonins.
3. *Ingestion.* This is the process in which the phagocytic cell invaginates its membrane attached to

bacteria and sweeps in the bacteria by pinocytosis. Energy derived from ATP is essential for this reaction to proceed.

4. *Phagosome formation.* A portion of the cell wall with attached bacteria invaginates and then pinches itself off, forming a phagosome. Complex alterations in lipid metabolism accompany this process.
5. *Degranulation.* The phagosome containing entrapped bacteria becomes the focal point for the collection and degranulation of lysosomal and peroxidative enzymes; the contents of the lysosomal granules are transferred to the phagosome.
6. *Bacterial killing.* This process, which leads to bacterial death, is the least well understood; one important aspect involves the generation of hydrogen peroxide, which interacts with myeloperoxidase and halide ions in the phagosome to iodinate and kill bacteria. Lack of either H_2O_2 or myeloperoxidase leads to chronic and recurrent infections. A recently described form of molecular oxygen, designated superoxide O_2^-, a product of conversion of oxygen to hydrogen peroxide, has been postulated to be a potent bactericidal factor generated during phagocytosis and responsible for the death of microbes within phagocytic vacuoles.

Decreased chemotaxis may result either from cellular defects, in which leukocytes fail to respond appropriately to chemotactic factors, or from a serum deficiency in chemotactic factors. Serum inhibitors of chemotaxis have also been demonstrated. The lazy leukocyte syndrome, described first in children and characterized by a fever, neutropenia, gingivitis, and otitis media, appears to be the result of the patient's neutrophils failing to respond appropriately to chemotactic stimuli; the production of chemotactic factors in the patient's serum seems normal. Impaired chemotaxis has also been described in patients with diabetes mellitus, rheumatoid arthritis, and uremia. A rare entity, Job's syndrome, is characterized by cold staphylococcal abscesses, high IgE levels, and eczematous dermatitis and is most likely explained by defective cellular (neutrophil) chemotaxis.

Defective opsonization is characteristic of the sera of patients with little or no gamma globulin, and it results in an increased susceptibility to infection by encapsulated bacteria. Complement (C3) deficiency seen in systemic lupus erythomatosus and in glomerulonephritis may result in pyogenic infections. The serum in sickle cell anemia has been shown to be deficient in levels of a heat-labile opsonin, 5-6S pseudoglobulin, which may, in consort with splenic shutdown due to recurrent microinfarctions, contribute to the decreased resistance to pneumococci seen in sickle cell anemia.

Chronic granulomatous disease (CGD) is a rare inherited entity that is transmitted by the X chromosome. It is characterized by recurrent, severe infections of the skin, lung, lymph nodes, liver, and many other tissues. *Staphylococcus aureus,* enteric bacilli *(Klebsiella-Aerobacter, Escherichia coli, Serratia marcescens),* and certain fungi *(Candida* and *Aspergillus)* are the organisms most commonly found in the lesions. Notable by their absence from the infected areas are beta-hemolytic streptococci, pneumococci, and *Haemophilus influenzae.* The polymorphonuclear leukocytes of these patients fail to kill certain ingested bacteria and fungi normally, and this is associated with demonstrable impairment of leukocyte metabolism. Any patient with a history of severe staphylococcal or gram-negative infection since childhood with a normal or elevated immunoglobulin level, leukocytosis, and normal delayed hypersensitivity should be suspected of having CGD.

Chemotaxis and phagocytosis are normal in CGD. However, the neutrophils do not kill certain bacteria; they readily kill certain other organisms (e.g., streptococci, pneumococci). In the leukocytes of patients with CGD there is a marked decrease in the metabolic activity normally induced by phagocytosis. Hydrogen peroxide is deficient in these leukocytes. Of note is the fact that the streptococcal and pneumococcal organisms generate their own H_2O_2, which may account for the destruction of these organisms in CGD patients. Nitroblue tetrazolium dye can be used in a histochemical test to identify leukocytic oxidative activity during phagocytosis. Oxidized nitroblue tetrazolium is colorless, but when reduced, it precipitates in the cytoplasm as blue formazan. Approximately 80 to 90 percent of normal leukocytes reduce nitroblue tetrazolium during phagocytosis; in contrast, less than 10 percent of the neutrophils from patients

with CGD do so. This test has become highly useful in screening patients for possible CGD. In some patients the disease is apparent early in life and progresses relentlessly to death before age 10. In others the onset appears later and the course is more benign. Therapy includes appropriate antibiotics and surgical drainage of the lesions when indicated.

Myeloperoxidase deficiency has been described as associated with a corresponding decrease in the leukocyte peroxidase granule content. The disease may be either hereditary or acquired (preleukemic) and is characterized by bouts of severe disseminated candidiasis. In the Chédiak-Higashi syndrome, a rare autosomal recessive disease, one finds giant lysosomelike granules in all granule-containing white cells. The main clinical features of this syndrome are (1) oculocutaneous albinism with rotatory nystagmus, (2) recurrent staphylococcal infections, and (3) a lymphomalike accelerated phase. Neutropenia is common. Giant granule degranulation with release of contents is delayed or absent, causing a marked decline in bacterial killing. Treatment with antibiotics and supportive measures is initially effective, but death in the second decade is frequent.

Granulocytic Leukemias

ACUTE LEUKEMIA
Acute leukemia may be defined as a neoplastic proliferation of abnormal, undifferentiated, or poorly differentiated leukocytes within the bone marrow, which can lead to replacement or repression of normal functioning tissue with subsequent marrow failure and death. Neoplastic cells themselves are often individually indistinguishable by light microscopy from normal immature hematopoietic cells. Acute leukemia occurs in all races and may develop at any age. In the untreated state, leukemic cells enter the blood, where they usually become the predominant leukocyte. Organ invasion also occurs not infrequently. The untreated disease often leads to death after a brief and stormy illness.

PRELEUKEMIA
Preleukemia is the term used when symptoms and laboratory findings (or both) are suggestive of acute myelocytic leukemia, but the diagnosis cannot be

established on the basis of available evidence. Cryptic cytopenias, refractory anemias, and abnormalities in leukocyte morphology such as the Pelger-Huët anomaly may be some features found in the peripheral blood. The marrow may have a low-normal cell count or may be hypercellular, with or without shift to the left and with or without megaloblastoid changes in the erythroid series. The changeover from preleukemia to overt acute leukemia may be either gradual or abrupt; no certain method of predicting the course of preleukemia is yet available.

ACUTE MYELOBLASTIC LEUKEMIA

Acute myeloblastic leukemia is a hematopoietic neoplasm in which the normal bone marrow elements are replaced by a population of immature myeloid precursors. Cytogenic studies suggest that the leukemic cells are clonal in origin. Investigations of cell kinetics in patients have shown that the leukemic cells do not proliferate more rapidly than normal myeloid precursors and that they frequently have extended generation times. It would appear that in acute granulocytic leukemia there is a deficit in cellular maturation and that the increased cell accumulation relates to decreased cell death and removal. Since cell maturation and ultimately cell death are normal means of granulocyte disposal, the defect in cell maturation permits the leukemic cell population to expand steadily and unceasingly, despite the fact that neoplastic cells are actually growing at a lower rate than normal.

Several subtypes of acute myeloblastic leukemia have been defined: typical myeloblastic, promyelocytic, myelomonocytic, monocytic (Schilling), and erythroleukemia. Acute forms of leukemia derived from eosinophils, basophils, and megakaryocytes, although quite rare, display unique characteristics as well as some features in common with the other acute leukemias.

In the majority of patients with acute leukemia no cause can be found; the possible etiologic role of viruses is still uncertain. However, there is an increased incidence of leukemia in patients with genetic defects (Down's syndrome) and hereditary conditions (Fanconi aplastic anemia, ataxia-telangiectasia) and a high concordance rate among identical twins. In addition, frequency rates of leukemia are higher following exposure to excessive radiation, chemicals such as benzene and chloramphenicol, and in patients with aplastic anemia. Acute lymphoblastic leukemia has not been associated with any of the aforementioned factors; 80 to 90 percent of patients with acute lymphoblastic leukemia are children, whereas 80 to 90 percent of patients with acute myeloblastic leukemia are adults.

Diagnosis. Presenting complaints in acute myeloblastic leukemia are often general, consisting of weakness, malaise, anorexia, fever, and unexplained purpura. Joint pain, lymph node swelling, and excessive bleeding may all be initial symptoms. Sternal tenderness is common, as well as gingival hyperplasia with periodontal infiltration. Spleen and liver enlargement may be detected but are less prominent than that in the chronic leukemias. Pallor is almost invariably present, and evidence of a bleeding diathesis with purpuric spots, ecchymosis, and retinal hemorrhages is frequent. Unusual physical findings in acute myeloblastic leukemia associated with high white cell counts include priapism due to vascular engorgement and evidence of peripheral or central nervous system involvement due to focal infiltrates.

Laboratory Tests. Laboratory findings in acute leukemia are of great diagnostic and clinical significance. The total white cell count is variable, ranging from low (5,000 per cubic millimeter) to elevated (20,000 to 100,000 per cubic millimeter) to very high (greater than 100,000 per cubic millimeter). The total polymorphonuclear leukocyte count is depressed, sometimes to zero. Normochromic, normocytic anemia occurs early. The platelet count is much below normal (below 50,000 per cubic millimeter). The blood smear shows immature and abnormal cells, and Auer bodies (red-staining rods in the cytoplasm of myeloblasts) occur in 10 to 20 percent of the cases and are pathognomonic of acute myeloblastic leukemia. The presence of peroxidase-staining granules in the cytoplasm suggests myeloblastic leukemia rather than lymphoblastic leukemia. In the bone marrow there is massive proliferation of immature blast cells (even when there is leukopenia in the peripheral blood), while red cell and megakaryocyte precursors are reduced or absent. In one variant, acute promyelocytic leukemia, disseminated intravascular coagulation is regularly observed. Hyperuricemia is the most frequent biochemical abnormality in acute leukemia.

Treatment and Prognosis. Untreated patients with acute leukemia die within a few months as a result of anemia, infection, hemorrhage, and tissue infiltration. With the more efficacious therapy now available, remission rates of more than 50 percent have been achieved in adults with acute myeloblastic leukemia, and remission rates of more than 90 percent have been obtained in patients under 15 years of age with acute lymphoblastic leukemia.

During the initial phase of chemotherapy, referred to as induction, patients receiving antileukemic agents are at great risk from the effects of pancytopenia. With supportive therapy in the form of platelet transfusions, bleeding has become a less significant problem. Most leukemic deaths now result from bacterial, fungal, or bizarre opportunistic infections (toxoplasmosis, cytomegalic inclusion disease, *Pneumocystis* pneumonia). Finally, as survival has increased in acute leukemia, especially the childhood form, leukemic meningitis has increased in frequency. Since the chemotherapeutic agents currently in use do not cross the blood-brain barrier, this complication might be expected. Attempts to eradicate central nervous system lesions with irradiation and intrathecal agents are strongly recommended.

CHRONIC MYELOGENOUS LEUKEMIA
Chronic myelogenous leukemia is a myeloproliferative disorder characterized by a prominent overproduction of granulocytes. Its most characteristic feature is the presence in 90 percent of the patients of a marker, the Philadelphia chromosome, which has shortened long arms on the G22 chromosome. Recent studies using fluorescein labeling techniques have indicated that the abnormality represents a translocation between G22 and C6 chromosome with the deleted portion of the former being situated on the latter. This marker persists throughout the disease, even when there is transformation to an acute blast crisis or when the patient goes into remission following therapy. In patients who do not have the Philadelphia chromosome the disease has a different course, with survival shortened to 8 to 12 months as compared with 30 to 40 months in patients who do have the Philadelphia chromosome.

Another characteristic feature in patients with chronic granulocytic leukemia is the finding of a low leukocyte alkaline phosphatase level. During remission, the leukocyte alkaline phosphatase can rise to normal in some patients. Of note is normal or high leukocyte alkaline phosphatase in patients with leukocytosis due to polycythemia vera, myelofibrosis, or leukemoid reactions.

An increased incidence of chronic granulocytic leukemia has been reported in persons exposed to radiation, for example, atomic bomb survivors and patients who have had unprotected irradiation for diseases such as ankylosing spondylitis. Benzene exposure on a chronic basis has also been incriminated.

Diagnosis. The onset of chronic granulocytic leukemia may be insidious and the course prolonged. There are no symptoms early in the disease, and it may be discovered only when a routine examination discloses a leukocytosis. The initial white cell count may be 12,000 to 15,000 and continue so for years. As the disease progresses, the neutrophil count rises and increasing numbers of metamyelocytes and myelocytes appear in the peripheral blood. The neutrophil count may be as high as 500,000 per cubic millimeter or higher, with segmented forms about equal in number to the metamyelocytes and myelocytes. Eosinophils and basophils are increased, as often are the blood platelets. Bone marrow aspiration reveals marked cellularity, with an increased myeloid-erythroid ratio and a preponderance of myelocytes and metamyelocytes. The disease may terminate in a blast crisis in which (see below) the myeloblast is the predominant cell in the bone marrow and peripheral blood.

Physical findings disclose moderate to massive splenomegaly; at times the spleen fills the left side of the abdomen. Infarction pain and early satiety are associated with such massive splenic enlargement. Weakness, nervousness, and weight loss due to the increased metabolic rate are common in the fully developed state. Fever, if present, may be related to the malignancy itself or, more likely, to infection. The cause of the fever should be searched for and treated accordingly.

Treatment and Prognosis. While there is no cure for chronic granulocytic leukemia, remissions can be rather easily achieved by a number of treatments. Busulfan (Myleran), which behaves as an alkylating agent, is the chemotherapeutic agent of choice, since it is more selective than other drugs in its action on the myeloid series. Up to 80 percent of patients treated with busulfan achieve remission. Unfortunately, within 5 years of diagnosis from 40 to 80 percent of patients with chronic granulocytic leukemia develop the blast crisis phase, which has proved to be almost totally refractory to therapy and rapidly fatal. Blast crisis closely resembles acute myeloblastic leukemia; cytogenetic studies suggest that it occurs by clonal transformation within the Philadelphia-chromosome positive population of leukemic cells.

Myeloproliferative Syndromes

Because of its diverse cell population, the bone marrow can respond in a variety of ways to various stimuli. Pyogenic infection leads to leukocytosis; hemorrhage leads to elevated platelet and reticulocyte counts. These reactions are self-limited, and there is a reversion to normal once the evocative stimulus abates.

Myeloproliferative disorders are examples of proliferation with apparently no stimulation. The proliferation is partially or totally self-perpetuating and resembles neoplastic diseases with similar clinical and hematologic characteristics. The spectrum of such diseases includes chronic myelogenous leukemia, polycythemia vera, myelofibrosis with myeloid metaplasia, and essential thrombocythemia. Initially one cell line usually predominates, but all cells seem to be overactive; for example, in polycythemia the leukocyte count and platelet count are often elevated. Fibrosis of the bone marrow is another common feature, suggesting that connective tissue proliferation may also be common to all myeloproliferative disorders. Splenic enlargement is often seen. Terminal blast transformation occurs with variable frequency

in all conditions. The only unique finding, the Philadelphia chromosome, is seen exclusively in chronic granulocytic leukemia. Of note is the fact that leukocytosis is a feature common to the various myeloproliferative syndromes. The term *myeloproliferative syndrome* should be used with caution so as not to generalize too greatly.

Bibliography

Regulation of Granulopoiesis
Barr, R. D., Whang-Peng, J., and Perry, S. Hemopoietic stem cells in human peripheral blood. *Science* 190:284, 1975.
Boggs, D. R. The kinetics of neutrophilic leukocytes in health and disease. *Semin. Hematol.* 4:359, 1967.
Golde, D. W., and Cline, M. J. Regulation of granulopoiesis. *N. Engl. J. Med.* 291:1387, 1974.
Stohlman, F., Jr., Quesenberry, P., and Tyler, W. S. The regulation of myelopoiesis as approached with in vivo and in vitro techniques. *Progr. Hematol.* 8:259, 1973.

Leukopenia and Agranulocytosis
Greenberg, P. L., and Shriver, S. L. Granulopoiesis in neutropenic disorders. *Blood* 41:753, 1973.
Pisciotta, A. V. Immune and toxic mechanisms in drug-induced agranulocytosis. *Semin. Hematol.* 10:299, 1973.
Quie, P. G. Pathology of bactericidal power of neutrophils. *Semin. Hematol.* 12:143, 1975.
Yunis, A. A., and Bloomberg, G. R. Chloramphenicol Toxicity: Clinical Features and Pathogenesis. In C. V. Moore and E. B. Brown (eds.), *Progress in Hematology*. Vol. 4. New York: Grune & Stratton, 1966. P. 138.

Phagocytic Dysfunction Syndromes
Karnovsky, M. L. Chronic granulomatous disease — pieces of a cellular and molecular puzzle. *Fed. Proc.* 32:1526, 1973.
Klebanoff, S. J., and Hamon, L. B. Role of myeloperoxidase-mediated antimicrobial systems in intact leukocytes. *J. Reticuloendothel. Soc.* 12:170, 1972.

Miller, M. E. Pathology of chemotaxis and random mobility. *Semin. Hematol.* 12:59, 1975.

Quie, P. G. Infections due to neutrophil malfunction. *Medicine* 52:411, 1973.

Stossel, T. P. Phagocytosis. *N. Engl. J. Med.* 291: 717, 774, 833, 1974.

Ward, P. A. Leukotactic factors in health and disease. *Am. J. Pathol.* 64:521, 1971.

Granulocytic Leukemias

Beard, M. E. J., and Fairley, G. H. Acute leukemia in adults. *Semin. Hematol.* 11:5, 1975.

Bierman, H. R. The leukemias — proliferative or accumulative. *Blood* 30:238, 1967.

Gunz, F., and Baikie, A. G. *Leukemia* (3rd ed.). New York: Grune & Stratton, 1974.

Stryckmans, P. A. Current concepts in chronic myelogenous leukemia. *Semin. Hematol.* 11:101, 1974.

Tjio, J. H., Carbene, P. P., Whang, J., and Frei, E., III. The Philadelphia chromosome and chronic myelogenous leukemia. *J. Natl. Cancer Inst.* 36:567, 1966.

Ward, H. P., and Block, M. H. The natural history of agnogenic myeloid metaplasia (AMM) and a critical evaluation of its relationship with the myeloproliferative syndrome. *Medicine* 50:357, 1971.

51

The Lymphoproliferative Disorders

Albert L. Sullivan

Classification

The lymphoproliferative disorders are characterized by either an abnormal decrease or an increase in the cells involved in immune responses, namely lymphocytes and macrophages (or histiocytes). These diseases are presently classified by descriptive histologic or serologic criteria, since with few exceptions their etiology and pathogenesis are unknown. The criteria used include (1) morphology of individual proliferating cells (e.g., plasma cells in multiple myeloma, Sternberg-Reed cells in Hodgkin's disease); (2) distribution of the proliferating cells (e.g., capsular invasion of the lymph nodes in malignant lymphoma); and (3) associated antibody response (e.g., heterophil antibody in infectious mononucleosis and monoclonal immunoglobulin in multiple myeloma).

The lymphoproliferative diseases are further divided into benign and malignant categories. Certain ones are considered benign because they are self-limited (e.g., infectious mononucleosis), because they have a defined etiology, as in the graft-versus-host reaction, or because of their localized behavior, as in the Sjögren syndrome. Other lymphoproliferative dis-

orders clearly involve unregulated proliferation and are known as malignant lymphomas. Hodgkin's disease has been considered a form of malignant lymphoma by most observers for years, but some now doubt its malignancy, whereas others consider it totally separate from other malignant lymphomas because of its different natural course and response to therapy. Multiple myeloma and macroglobulinemia are usually distinguished from the malignant lymphomas because of their special secretory product, monoclonal immunoglobulin.

Recent advances in the identification of the cells involved in the normal immune responses permit further classification of the lymphoproliferative disorders. Two clearly separate lymphoid systems and also the reticuloendothelial system normally take part in immune responses. The cells mediating the functions of these three separate systems are the B-lymphocyte, T-lymphocyte, and macrophage (Table 51-1).

A decreased proliferation of either of the lymphoid systems leads to characteristic anatomic and clinical changes. A pure B-lymphocyte deficiency, as in sex-linked agammaglobulinemia, leads to loss of lymphoid follicles in lymph nodes and agammaglobulinemia and results in an increased incidence of the common bacterial infections, but not increased fungal, viral, or myobacterial infections. A pure T-lymphocyte depletion, as occurs in hereditary thymic aplasia, leads to

Table 51-1. Cells Mediating the Immune Response

	B-lymphocyte	T-lymphocyte	Macrophage[a]
Origin	? Gut (bursa in chickens)	Thymus gland	Bone marrow
Major function	Protection against extracellular infection (common gram-positive and gram-negative bacteria)	1. Protection against intracellular infection (tuberculosis, fungus, virus) 2. Tumor surveillance	1. Antigen processing for lymphocyte recognition 2. Scavenger for foreign antigens opsinized with immunoglobin or complement
Mediated by	Antibodies	Cells	? RNA adjuvant
Identifying cellular markers	1. Surface membrane immunoglobulin 2. Complement receptor 3. IgG receptor	1. Sheep erythrocyte receptor 2. Transforms with phytohemagglutinin	1. IgG receptor 2. Complement receptor

[a]Or histiocyte.

loss of parafollicular lymphocytes in lymph nodes and results in an inability to develop delayed hypersensitivity skin reactions and in an increased occurrence of viral, fungal, and protozoal infections.

Diseases involving increased lymphoid proliferation may also be assigned to either the B- or T-lymphoid systems. Assignment can be certain when the abnormally proliferating lymphoid cells have been typed as B or T as defined by their surface membrane markers or their responses to mitogens (Tables 51-1 and 51-2). Other lymphoproliferative disorders in which cell typing has not yet been performed have been classified as either B- or T-lymphocyte disorders by assuming that the abnormally proliferating cells ablate normal function of that arm (B or T) of the immune systems from which they are derived. For example, chronic lymphocytic leukemia cells have been typed as B-lymphocytes in most cases because there is immunoglobulin on their surface membranes as well as receptor for complement (both of which are characteristic B-lymphocyte properties). Chronic lymphocytic leukemia cells neither transform under the influence of phytohemagglutinin nor bear receptors for sheep red blood cells (both T-lymphocyte properties). On the other hand, no such studies have been performed on abnormal cells from patients with Hodgkin's disease, which is presumed to be a disease involving abnormal T-lymphocyte proliferation because normal T-lymphocyte function (delayed cutaneous hypersensitivity, ability to reject foreign skin grafts) is frequently depressed, whereas B-lymphocyte function (antibody production) remains unimpaired.

Manifestations

The clinical manifestations of lymphoproliferative disorders generally depend on the location of the proliferating cells. Most commonly, proliferation occurs within the lymph nodes, spleen, or bone marrow, leading to lymphadenopathy, splenomegaly, or bone pain. In certain cases the disorder is detected only by laboratory tests revealing either cellular proliferation (peripheral blood lymphocytosis in chronic lymphocytic leukemia) or accumulation of secretory products of the proliferating cells (a monoclonal gamma globulin band on protein electrophoresis in multiple myeloma). Less commonly, overt immunologic manifestations occur, such as deficiency states (hypogammaglobulinemia in chronic lymphocytic leukemia, delayed skin test unresponsiveness in Hodgkin's disease) or autoimmune phenomena (antibody-mediated thrombocytopenia or hemolytic anemia in chronic lymphocytic leukemia). In addition, nonspecific generalized symptoms may occur such as pruritus, night sweats, fever, or weight loss.

Diagnosis

The initial diagnosis of lymphoproliferative disorders is not generally made by either history or physical examination, which are nevertheless extremely important in defining the laboratory tests and procedures that might be helpful. Determination of serum antibodies frequently leads to a diagnosis in benign lymphoproliferative disorders. Detection of a specific antibody, particularly if the titer is rising, or

Table 51-2. Classification of Malignant Lymphoproliferative Disorders by Cell Surface Markers

B-lymphocytes	T-lymphocytes	Macrophages	Undefined
1. Chronic lymphocytic leukemia[a] 2. Lymphocytic lymphoma[a] (nodular, diffuse, poorly or well differentiated) 3. Burkitt's lymphoma 4. Leukemic reticuloendotheliosis[b] ("hairy cell" leukemia)	1. Sézary syndrome (erythroderma with peripheral blood lymphocytosis) 2. Mycosis fungoides 3. Mediastinal lymphoma (frequent in children with a leukemic phase indistinguishable morphologically from acute lymphoblastic leukemia)	1. Leukemic reticuloendotheliosis[b] ("hairy cell" leukemia) 2. Malignant histiocytosis (histiocytic medullary reticulosis)	1. Histiocytic lymphoma 2. Hodgkin's disease

[a]Majority of cases in adults. T-lymphocyte origin more common in children with lymphocytic lymphoma.
[b]Features of both a B-lymphocyte and macrophage.

finding a nonspecific antibody frequently establishes the appropriate diagnosis. Examples of specific antibodies are those directed against Epstein-Barr virus or against *Toxoplasma* organisms. Anti-DNA and heterophil antibodies are examples of nonspecific antibodies. However, biopsy of the bone marrow or removal of an enlarged lymph node or an enlarged spleen is frequently necessary to make the initial diagnosis, particularly if the history and physical examination do not suggest one of the benign lymphoproliferative disorders.

Electrophoresis of serum or urine proteins is diagnostic in lymphoproliferative disorders associated with the secretion of a monoclonal immunoglobulin. The abnormal immunoglobulin appears as a narrow band of protein (M spike), usually in the gamma or beta region. Definitive proof that a suspect immunoglobulin band arises from a single clone of cells requires demonstration that it consists of a single type of heavy chain (one of the five possible — alpha, delta, gamma, epsilon, or mu) and a single type of light chain (one of the two possible — kappa or lambda). Separation of the protein in question by electrophoresis in agar followed by precipitation with specific antisera against heavy and light chains (immunoelectrophoresis), respectively, is used to establish its monoclonal or polyclonal origin.

The most recent diagnostic advance is the typing of lymphoid cells by surface markers or by their response to mitogens (see Table 51-1). The procedure is readily performed with peripheral blood cells and recently has been applied to tissue cells such as those of spleen and lymph nodes (see Table 51-2). The use of these techniques should allow a more rational classification of the lymphoproliferative disorders to evolve than has morphology alone and may provide insight into the pathophysiology of these disorders.

Benign Lymphoproliferative Disorders

The nonneoplastic lymphoproliferative disorders are outlined in Table 51-3. Many disorders produce the clinical manifestations of lymphadenopathy and splenomegaly, with or without lymphocytosis. In certain cases the underlying cause of the increased lymphoid proliferation is evident when the patient is first seen; in others the proliferation is the presenting manifestation of an unknown disease that may be diagnosed either by specific laboratory tests or by its natural course as the disease evolves. In either case, biopsy of lymphoid tissue may be advisable to exclude a malignant lymphoproliferative process.

Only the syndrome of infectious mononucleosis will be considered at length, since the other causes of benign lymphoproliferation are considered elsewhere in this text. Infectious mononucleosis is a self-limited disorder caused by the Epstein-Barr virus. The disease is characterized by fever, pharyngitis, malaise, lymphadenopathy, splenomegaly, and atypical lymphocytosis in the peripheral blood. The peak incidence occurs between the ages of 17 and 25 years; the disease is uncommon beyond the age of 30 and very rare after the age of 40. The estimated incidence in the general population is 50 per 100,000.

Conclusive data derived from serologic surveys and from viral cultures have implicated the Epstein-Barr virus as the cause of infectious mononucleosis. The virus is able to infect B-lymphocytes and change them in a manner that allows them to be established in long-term culture in vitro. The morphologically and functionally atypical peripheral blood lymphocyte is a T-lymphocyte. The cause of its transformation is unclear, but it does not result from direct infection with Epstein-Barr virus.

The prodromal stage of infectious mononucleosis lasts several days, with nonspecific symptoms such as mild fever and malaise. The midstage lasts several days to several weeks and is characterized by fever, lymphadenopathy involving all groups of nodes, and severe exudative pharyngitis. Petechiae on the palate are frequent. Splenomegaly, with the spleen tip extended 2 to 4 cm below the costal margin, is present in the majority of patients. Liver dysfunction as evidenced by elevated transaminase and alkaline phosphatase levels occurs in most cases. Jaundice and a palpable liver occur less frequently. Transient skin rashes include urticarial lesions, macular eruptions, and petechiae. The appearance of petechiae suggests the possibility of an immune-based thrombocytopenia, a rare but dangerous complication of infectious mononucleosis. Only minimal neurologic symptoms such as headache or photophobia may be present; however, severe complications, including meningitis,

Table 51-3. Benign Lymphoproliferative Disorders

Etiology	Clinical findings	Laboratory findings
1. Infectious		
Infectious mononucleosis (IM)	Pharyngitis, fever, malaise, lymphadenopathy, splenomegaly	Atypical lymphocytes, + heterophil antibody, + EB virus antibody
Cytomegalovirus IM	Fever, malaise, splenomegaly	Atypical lymphocytes, + cytomegalovirus antibody
Toxoplasma IM	Fever, malaise, lymphadenopathy, splenomegaly	Atypical lymphocytes, + *Toxoplasma* antibody
Bacterial Viral Spirochetal Myobacterial Fungal	May present with or manifest lymphadenopathy and/or splenomegaly	Specific skin test; antibody or culture evidence of etiology
2. Immunologic		
Hypersensitivity states[a] Serum sickness	History of drug or foreign protein; lymphadenopathy/splenomegaly	Atypical lymphocytes, + heterophil antibody, specific antibody
Graft versus host disease	History of bone marrow transplant; lymphadenopathy/splenomegaly; rash	
3. Unknown		
Sarcoidosis	Lymphadenopathy/splenomegaly	+ Kveim test

Collagen vascular diseases
  Systemic lupus erythematosus
  Polyarteritis nodosa
  Rheumatoid arthritis
	May manifest lymphadenopathy or splenomegaly	+ Antinuclear antibody, + rheumatoid factor

Sjögren syndrome[a]	Parotid gland swelling; dry eyes and mouth	+ Rheumatoid factor
4. Storage diseases		
Gaucher's[b]	Hepatosplenomegaly	Thrombocytopenia, anemia, leukopenia, increased acid phosphatase (non-prostatic)

[a]Certain cases of phenytoin sensitivity and Sjögren syndrome have progressed to malignant lymphoma.
[b]Not due to lymphoid or histiocytic proliferation but to accumulation of glucocerebroside in histiocytes leading to massive hepatosplenomegaly and hypersplenism.

meningoencephalitis, and acute polyneuritis, occur in 1 percent of the cases. When neurologic complications appear, the mortality increases to 11 percent.

There is constant danger in infectious mononucleosis that the soft, enlarged spleen will rupture, and because of this, palpation of the spleen should be limited and not overly vigorous. Any person in whom splenic rupture occurs with minimal or no trauma should be investigated for the possibility of infectious mononucleosis.

When suspected clinically, the diagnosis is established by finding atypical lymphocytes in the peripheral blood and heterophil antibodies in the serum. In the acute stage, at least 20 percent of the lymphocytes are atypical. The atypical lymphocytes include cells that have (1) round, unstained areas in the cytoplasm, giving a foamy appearance; (2) large size with a variation in the blue stain of the cytoplasm (these cells appear wavy or rolled up at the edges); (3) resemblance to monocytes; (4) resemblance to plasma cells in staining qualities; (5) nucleoli resembling blast forms.

The heterophil antibody is a nonspecific agglutinin of certain mammalian erythrocytes. The classic test for heterophil antibody is based on the fact that sheep erythrocyte agglutinating activity can be absorbed from the sera of patients with infectious mononucleosis by beef erythrocytes but not by guinea pig kidney homogenate. The heterophil antibody is present in up to 90 percent of patients with infectious mononucleosis and may be detectable by a rapidly performed slide test using formalin-treated horse erythrocytes.

Antibodies to Epstein-Barr virus of the IgM class persist for a finite period following the illness. Less specific Epstein-Barr virus antibody titers persist indefinitely following infection; hence, a positive virus antibody test is not conclusive evidence of recent infection unless the antibody is demonstrated to be of the IgM class.

In the usual case of infectious mononucleosis, treatment is symptomatic and includes rest, analgesics, and antipyretics. In more severe cases, the morbidity may be reduced by using a short course of steroids.

Certain other infectious agents may cause an illness resembling infectious mononucleosis. Cytomegalovirus can produce malaise, fever, hepatosplenomegaly, and atypical lymphocytosis. Pharyngitis does not occur, and lymphadenopathy is unusual. *Toxoplasma* infection may produce a clinical picture identical to infectious mononucleosis with the exception of pharyngitis. These entities may be suspected when the clinical findings and peripheral blood picture resemble those found in infectious mononucleosis but the heterophil antibody is not present. Specific serologic tests confirm the diagnosis.

Malignant Lymphoproliferative Disorders

The malignant lymphoproliferative disorders have been identified and classified by histologic criteria that are changing with increasing experience. The presently accepted pathologic classification of malignant lymphomas is presented along with persisting clinically accepted synonyms in Table 51-4.

The chronic lymphocytic leukemias, the lymphocytic lymphomas of adults, and Burkitt's lymphoma have all been shown to involve primarily a B-lymphocyte proliferation (see Table 51-2). The lymphocytic lymphomas of children more commonly involve T-lymphocyte proliferation.

Undifferentiated malignant lymphoma (Burkitt's), a relatively common tumor in certain parts of Africa, has been suspected to be due to the Epstein-Barr virus. This lymphoma is uncommon in this country, and it occurs at a younger age than the other types of malignant lymphoma. The American tumor does not appear to be related to the Epstein-Barr virus. Burkitt's lymphoma usually involves extranodal sites, has a high proliferative rate, and is dramatically responsive to chemotherapy. Certain patients in

Table 51-4. Classification of Malignant Lymphomas

Pathologic classification	Popular clinical synonym
Malignant lymphoma, undifferentiated	Burkitt's lymphoma
Malignant lymphoma, histiocytic ⎫ Malignant lymphoma, mixed ⎭	Reticulum cell sarcoma
Malignant lymphoma, poorly differentiated lymphocytic ⎫ Malignant lymphoma, well-differentiated lymphocytic	Lymphoblastic lymphoma ⎫ Lymphocytic lymphoma ⎬ Lymphosarcoma Chronic lymphocytic leukemia ⎭ Follicular = nodular

Nodular or Diffuse

Africa and in this country have experienced long, disease-free survivals following chemotherapy.

The other malignant lymphomas are rare in individuals under the age of 40. After the age of 50, the annual incidence increases to 30 to 45 per 100,000. The etiology is unknown. Individuals with these disorders usually are first seen because of enlarged lymph nodes; systemic symptoms are unusual. An elevated leukocyte count with 50 percent or more mature lymphocytes may be the only finding in chronic lymphocytic leukemia for as long as 5 years before the onset of symptoms. Occasionally histiocytic or lymphocytic lymphomas present in extranodular sites (tonsils, intestine, bone) as apparently isolated lesions. Radiotherapy frequently results in long disease-free intervals (and possibly cure) in such patients. The malignant lymphomas lead to morbidity and mortality by expanding into large, symptomatic tumor masses; by infiltrating vital organs (such as liver, bone marrow); or by altering normal immune function, thus increasing the patient's susceptibility to infection, autoimmune hemolytic anemia, or thrombocytopenia.

A third of the patients with chronic lymphocytic leukemia and certain patients with other malignant lymphomas have hypogammaglobulinemia. Delayed skin hypersensitivity to previously experienced antigens remains intact. Patients with these B-lymphocyte malignancies may frequently have extracellular bacterial infections because of their inability to produce antibodies against invasive organisms.

In general, the less differentiated malignant lymphomas have a worse prognosis than those having a more differentiated histologic picture, and in any category, histologically nodular forms generally have a better prognosis than histologically diffuse forms. The mean survival periods are diffuse histiocytic — 1 year; diffuse, poorly differentiated lymphocytic — 2 years; nodular, poorly differentiated lymphocytic — 8 years; well-differentiated lymphocytic — 9 or more years. These lymphomas are not generally staged to determine the extent of spread, as is done in Hodgkin's disease, since the majority are widespread (stage IV); even those that appear to be localized frequently reappear following apparently curative therapy.

Therapy may be withheld initially in newly diagnosed patients who do not have potentially curable lesions in order to allow the rate of progression of the disease to be determined. It is not uncommon, especially for patients with more histologically differentiated or with nodular lesions (or both), to have long intervals in which the disease is quiescent and no therapy is required. As with the other malignant lymphoproliferative disorders, two forms of therapy are currently available — radiotherapy and chemotherapy. In patients with apparently localized disease without systemic symptoms (fever, night sweats, weight loss), radiotherapy is commonly used. In patients with obviously widespread disease or systemic symptoms, chemotherapy is usually given. Recently combination chemotherapy has been employed in patients with widespread disease, and an increased percentage of responders and longer disease-free intervals were obtained in these patients compared to patients treated with any single agent.

Two uncommon malignant lymphomas that involve the skin have recently been demonstrated to be due to T-lymphocyte proliferation. In mycosis fungoides, the skin abnormalities represent the most prominent, and in many cases the sole, manifestation of the disease for a number of years. The skin lesions may vary from erythema multiforme to ulcerating tumors of the skin. In the Sézary syndrome, generalized erythroderma is coupled with peripheral blood lymphocytosis that is indistinguishable from that in chronic lymphocytic leukemia.

The leukemic cells of about 20 percent of the patients with acute lymphoblastic leukemia bear T-lymphocyte markers. Leukemic cells from the other 80 percent have neither B- nor T-lymphocyte markers, and there is no evidence that these cells are lymphoid in origin. Of interest is the fact that patients with acute lymphoblastic anemia of T-lymphocyte origin have clinical features (lymphadenopathy, splenomegaly, thymic masses, high blast count) that are associated with a poor prognosis.

HODGKIN'S DISEASE

The binucleate Sternberg-Reed cell is the characteristic cell of Hodgkin's disease, which, like the other malignant lymphoproliferative disorders, is a disease recognized by histologic criteria. There are two peak age incidences, one in the third decade and the other in the seventh decade of life. The overall incidence is 2 to 3 per 100,000. The etiology is unknown, but Hodgkin's disease is frequently associated with depressed, delayed hypersensitivity and may be associated with T-lymphocyte depletion in the peripheral blood. Even those individuals with minimal disease (stage I) demonstrate impaired peripheral blood lymphocyte transformation with phytohcmagglutinin (a lymphocyte mitogen). The humoral arm of the immune response (antibody production) remains intact until late in the disease. These findings suggest that Hodgkin's disease is an abnormality of the T-lymphocyte system, but no formal proof of this exists.

Asymptomatic lymphadenopathy is the most common presenting sign of Hodgkin's disease, although in the elderly, severe prostration and fever of unknown origin may be the first evidence of the disease. Patients with Hodgkin's disease are always classified according to the histologic type and extent of disease (clinical stage), since it has been clearly shown that both of these factors indicate the prognosis and the therapy to be used in the individual patient (Tables 51-5 and 51-6).

Patients with nodular sclerosis (40 percent) and patients with mixed cellularity (40 percent) comprise most of the cases of Hodgkin's disease. About 90 percent of the patients with lymphocyte predominance and 70 percent of those with nodular sclerosis are in clinical stage I or II at the time of diagnosis. In contrast, about half the patients with mixed cellularity and one-third of those with lymphocyte-depleted disease are in clinical stage I or II. Although Hodgkin's disease has an overall male predominance, nodular sclerosis presenting with cervical and mediastinal lymph node enlargement is more common in young women.

In addition to the above symptoms, pain at the sites of involvement following ethanol ingestion and generalized pruritus may occur in patients with Hodgkin's disease, although they are not considered prognostically significant. Proper evaluation of patients with histologically proved Hodgkin's disease for purposes of staging should include history, physical

Table 51-5. Classification and Staging of Hodgkin's Disease

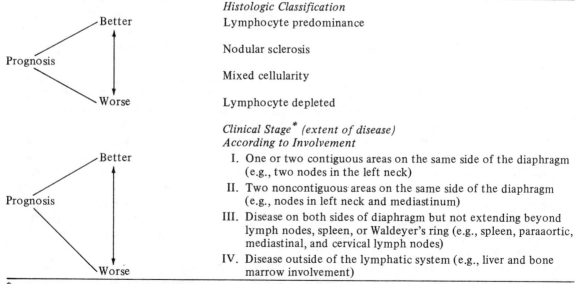

Histologic Classification

Lymphocyte predominance

Nodular sclerosis

Mixed cellularity

Lymphocyte depleted

Clinical Stage* (extent of disease)
According to Involvement

I. One or two contiguous areas on the same side of the diaphragm (e.g., two nodes in the left neck)

II. Two noncontiguous areas on the same side of the diaphragm (e.g., nodes in left neck and mediastinum)

III. Disease on both sides of diaphragm but not extending beyond lymph nodes, spleen, or Waldeyer's ring (e.g., spleen, paraaortic, mediastinal, and cervical lymph nodes)

IV. Disease outside of the lymphatic system (e.g., liver and bone marrow involvement)

*Each stage is subclassified according to the presence or absence of symptoms:
A = no symptoms
B = fever, night sweats, unexplained weight loss (greater than 10 percent of body weight in the 6 months prior to evaluation)

Table 51-6. Treatment of Hodgkin's
Disease as Determined by Stage

Stage of disease	Currently accepted treatment
Stage I-A or B Stage II-A or B Stage III-A	Radiotherapy
B Stage IV-A or B	Systemic combination chemotherapy

examination, hemogram, chest x-ray, bone marrow
biopsy, bone x-rays, liver function tests, and liver
scan and biopsy (if liver function tests are abnormal
or if hepatomegaly exists). In addition, lymphangiography is routinely performed to assess infradiaphragmatic nodal involvement. Recently, exploratory
laparotomy with splenectomy and multiple retroperitoneal lymph node biopsies has been advocated
as part of the clinical staging procedure in patients
with less than stage IV disease in order to confirm the
extent of infradiaphragmatic disease suggested by
other tests.

The currently accepted therapy of Hodgkin's disease is determined by the stage of the disease (Table
51-6). The efficacy of radiotherapy in patients with
stage II-B disease is questionable, since many of
these patients experience relapse following intensive
radiotherapy. The optimal extent of radiotherapy is
currently under investigation. In some centers, the
best results have been obtained when all central
lymph node areas have been treated regardless of the
initial extent of disease. Other studies suggest that
more limited radiotherapy may produce similar
results. In any case, radiotherapy has led to results
that, projected beyond 5 years, suggest that the
majority of patients with stage I or II disease can be
cured. As with the malignant lymphomas, treatment
with a combination of several chemotherapeutic
agents has markedly improved both the number of
Hodgkin's patients responding to therapy and the
length of the disease-free interval after therapy in
comparison to the results obtained with single-agent
therapy.

MONOCLONAL GAMMOPATHIES
The five classes of immunoglobulins (IgG, IgA, IgM,
IgD, IgE) are determined by the heavy chain type.

Two types of light chain (kappa and lambda) are associated with the five types of heavy chain. A monoclonal gammopathy may be suspected when a narrow-
based spike appears in the immunoglobulin region of
the electrophoretic pattern of serum or urine. Definitive proof that such a spike is composed of immunoglobulin derived from a single clone of cells would be
the demonstration of an identical amino acid sequence for all molecules composing the spike. In
practice, immunoelectrophoresis is employed to
determine that the immunoglobulin spike is composed
of a single heavy chain and/or single light chain and
is therefore monoclonal.

Monoclonal gammopathies are uncommon in
patients under the age of 30. The incidence increases
with age and reaches a peak in the sixth to seventh
decades. The incidence of a monoclonal serum component of 100 to 300 per 100,000 has been reported
in healthy blood donors, whereas the incidence of
frank multiple myeloma is 2 to 4 per 100,000.

The etiology is unknown, although monoclonal
gammopathies can be induced regularly in certain
strains of mice by various chemicals. The lymphoproliferative disorders associated with the production
of a monoclonal immunoglobulin may be classified
either by the type of immunoglobulin produced or
by the clinical presentation of the disorder. The
latter is more helpful with regard to prognosis and
choice of therapy. The various clinical presentations
of monoclonal gammopathy are outlined below.

1. *Presenting without evidence of disease.* Benign
   monoclonal gammopathy is characterized by a
   spike on serum protein electrophoresis, but abnormal protein is less than 2 gm per 100 ml. In addition, there is no anemia, no lytic bone lesions, and
   no excess urinary excretion of light chains; less
   than 25 percent of the marrow is involved with
   plasmacytosis; and there is no reduction in the
   serum concentration of other immunoglobulins.
2. *Presenting with lymphadenopathy and hepatosplenomegaly.*
   a. Waldenström's macroglobulinemia is character-
      ized by a monoclonal IgM in the serum. The
      disorder is frequently associated with a hyper-
      viscosity syndrome.

b. Gamma heavy chain disease is characterized by a monoclonal gamma chain in serum and urine. It is frequently associated with swelling of the palate and uvula.

3. *Presenting with destructive bone lesions (lytic lesions or osteoporosis).* Multiple myeloma is characterized by a monoclonal IgG, IgA, IgD, or IgE in serum or a monoclonal light chain in urine (Bence Jones protein). Multiple myeloma is further characterized by anemia, hypercalcemia, and recurrent bacterial infections secondary to a decrease in normal immunoglobulins.

4. *Presenting with malabsorption.* Alpha heavy chain disease is caused by an intestinal lymphoma that produces monoclonal alpha chains without a spike on electrophoresis because of polymeric heterogeneity. This condition most frequently occurs in Arabs and Sephardic Jews.

5. *Presenting as chronic lymphatic leukemia.* Mu-chain disease displays a clinical course which is similar to that of chronic lymphatic leukemia without mu chains.

The above malignancies are all derived from B-lymphocytes. They are frequently associated with a depression in the concentration of normal immunoglobulin. Patients affected by these disorders frequently have recurrent bacterial infections, particularly bacterial pneumonias.

No therapy is required for patients with benign monoclonal gammopathy. Certain patients with this condition, when observed over a number of years, progress to frank multiple myeloma. Chemotherapy is the major therapy used for the other monoclonal gammopathies. As in the other malignant lymphoproliferative disorders, chemotherapy with multiple agents has proved more effective in inducing remission and increasing disease-free intervals than therapy with any single agent. Radiotherapy is used in multiple myeloma when lytic lesions give rise to pain. Plasmapheresis is usually successful in reversing the hyperviscosity syndrome associated with Waldenström's macroglobulinemia, since the large IgM molecule is largely confined to the intravascular space.

Bibliography

Aisenberg, A. C. Malignant lymphoma. *N. Engl. J. Med.* 288:883, 1973.

Aisenberg, A. C., and Long, J. C. Lymphocyte surface characteristics in malignant lymphoma. *Am. J. Med.* 58:300, 1975.

Berard, C. W., Gallo, R. C., Jaffe, E. S., Green, I., and DeVita, V. T. Current concepts of leukemia and lymphoma: Etiology, pathogenesis, and therapy. *Ann. Intern. Med.* 85:351, 1976.

Carter, R. L. Infectious mononucleosis: Model for self-limiting lymphoproliferation. *Lancet* 1:846, 1975.

Cline, M. J., and Golde, D. W. A review and reevaluation of the histiocytic disorders. *Am. J. Med.* 55:49, 1973.

Gajl-Peczalska, K. J., Bloomfield, C. D., Coccia, P. F., Sosin, H., Brunning, R. D., and Kersey, J. H. B and T cell lymphomas: Analysis of blood and lymph nodes in 87 patients. *Am. J. Med.* 59:674, 1975.

Levin, W. C. (ed.). Symposium on myeloma. *Arch. Intern. Med.* 135:27, 1975.

Lukes, R. J., and Collins, R. D. New approaches to the classification of the lymphomata. *Br. J. Cancer* 31(Suppl. II):1, 1975.

52

Hemostasis and Thrombosis

Lilia Talarico and Daniel Deykin

Normal hemostasis involves an integrated series of reactions between blood vessels, blood platelets, and certain plasma constituents responsible for blood coagulation. The role played by each of these factors differs according to the size of the blood vessel and the severity of the vascular injury. Arrest of bleeding from small vessels depends mainly on primary hemostasis, which results from vasoconstriction and the formation of a platelet plug. When larger vessels are injured, primary hemostasis is inadequate, and the platelet plug must be reinforced by fibrin evolved through the activation of the coagulation mechanism.

Primary Hemostasis

Vasoconstriction
The most immediate effect of vascular trauma is vasoconstriction, which slows blood flow and facilitates interactions between the vascular component, platelets, and local coagulation mechanisms.

Formation of the Temporary Platelet Plug
Platelets are cytoplasmic structures derived from megakaryocytes in the bone marrow. In the peripheral blood they number 150,000 to 400,000 per microliter; their life span of about 10 days is probably determined by senescence. In conditions of increased demand on hemostasis, platelets may be used at random.

A platelet has no nucleus or DNA, but it has a plasma membrane surrounded by an amorphous coat containing sialic acid, adsorbed plasma proteins, and clotting factors. Its cytoplasm contains glycogen, microtubules, mitochondria, and two types of granules: the alpha granules and the dense bodies. Alpha granules contain fibrinogen, acid hydrolases, and cathepsins; dense bodies contain calcium, serotonin, adenosine triphosphate (ATP), and adenosine diphosphate (ADP). Platelets can synthesize fatty acids and phospholipids; their major source of energy derives from glucose.

When vascular damage or trauma disrupts the endothelium, the subendothelial structures are exposed to the flowing blood, initiating a series of events that lead to the formation of the platelet plug. The sequence of events may be summarized as follows: (1) Platelets adhere to the exposed subendothelial and perivascular structures (of which collagen is the most important), which change the platelets' configuration from disks to spiny spheres, probably because of contraction of the platelet marginal microtubules; (2) the platelet granules are forced to the center of the platelets, thereby releasing the granule contents into the canalicular system and thence out into the surrounding environment; (3) the substances released include ATP, ADP, serotonin, platelet factor 4, and catecholamines; released ADP derives from a granule-bound storage pool that is distinct and independent from the metabolic pool responsible for platelet metabolism.

Adenosine diphosphate is a powerful aggregating substance; therefore, more platelets now aggregate at the site of injury, building up over the layer of platelets already adhering to the collagen. In addition to ADP, serotonin, epinephrine, and thrombin can directly aggregate platelets and induce the release of endogenous ADP; this amplifies and sustains further aggregation of platelets with formation of the platelet plug (Fig. 52-1).

The changes in platelet structure associated with the release and aggregation phenomena allow platelet phospholipids (platelet factor 3) to become exposed and available for the reactions leading to the conversion of prothrombin to thrombin, thus mediating the platelet contribution to the coagulation mechanism (see under Coagulation Mechanism). Platelets contain and can release a cationic protein (platelet factor 4); this factor has antiheparin activity and also inhibits the anticoagulant action of fibrin and fibrinogen split products. Cofactors in plasma also appear necessary for normal platelet function in primary hemostasis; in addition to calcium these include at least two coagulation factors, fibrinogen and the von Willebrand factor.

The exact mechanisms responsible for the platelet aggregation and release reactions are not completely understood. Recent studies have shown that changes in platelet membranes induced either by the process

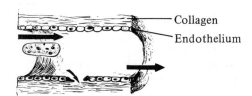

Collagen
Endothelium

1. Vessel disruption
   a. Construction
   b. Exposure of collagen

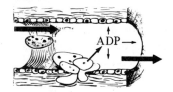

ADP→

2. Platelet reactions with collagen
   a. Swelling, degranulation
   b. Synthesis of prostaglandin
   c. Release of ADP and other contents

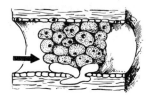

3. Platelet reactions with ADP
   a. Loose aggregation, morphology intact,
      reversible
   b. Secondary ADP release; self-
      perpetuating aggregation

Figure 52-1. Formation of temporary hemostatic plug. (From D. Deykin, Thrombogenesis. N. Engl. J. Med. 276:622, 1967. Reproduced by permission.)

of adhesion or by direct aggregating agents (or both) result in the production of arachidonic acid from membrane phospholipids. Arachidonic acid is converted by the enzyme cyclo-oxygenase into the cyclic endoperoxide prostaglandin G_2 from which unstable intermediates are formed. These intermediates, named thromboxanes, can induce both immediate aggregation and the release reaction.

The platelet plug is a permeable structure and must undergo consolidation for hemostatic effectiveness. Consolidation occurs through the activation of the coagulation mechanism with the formation of thrombin. Thrombin is an enzyme that induces both irreversible aggregation of the platelets available at the site of injury and local formation of fibrin, which is the final supporting structure of the permanent hemostatic plug.

Coagulation Mechanism

The coagulation mechanism involves various factors

in a sequence of reactions leading to the formation of a proteolytic enzyme, thrombin, which is capable of converting a soluble protein, fibrinogen, into insoluble fibrin (Fig. 52-2). The coagulation mechanism can be divided into three stages: activation of factor X, conversion of prothrombin to thrombin, and polymerization of fibrinogen to fibrin.

Activation of factor X can take place through two distinct pathways, intrinsic and extrinsic. The intrinsic pathway is initiated by the activation of a plasma protein, factor XII. In physiologic conditions, this factor is activated by contact with subendothelial structures, perhaps collagen, exposed at the site of vascular damage. Activation alters the factor XII molecule and unmasks an active serine protease, which in turn acts on the next factor, factor XI, activating it into its enzymatic form.

In addition to its role in coagulation, factor XII participates in the activation of kallikreinogen to kallikrein with subsequent release of kinins capable of producing pain, capillary permeability, and smooth muscle contraction. Factor XII also participates in the activation of the complement and fibrinolytic system.

Other factors (e.g., Fletcher, Flaujeac, or Fitzgerald

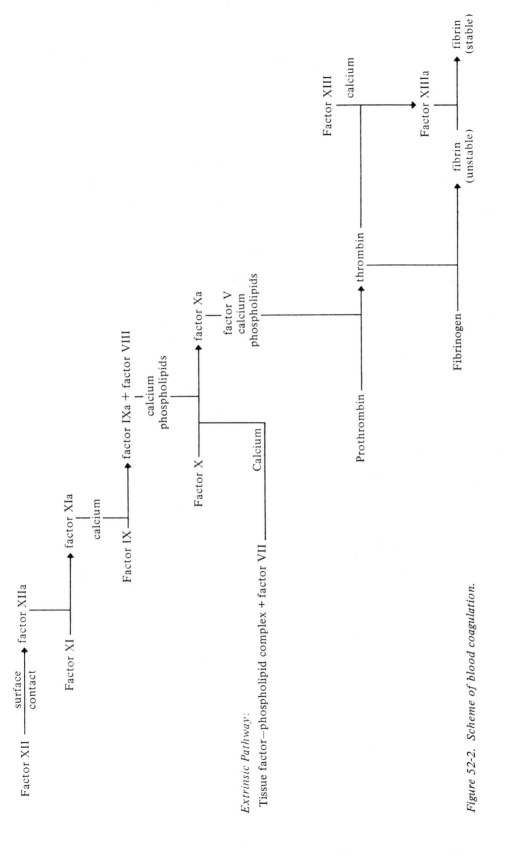

Intrinsic Pathway:

Extrinsic Pathway:

Figure 52-2. Scheme of blood coagulation.

factors) have been shown to participate, with factor XII, in the contact activation and kinin formation.

Calcium is not required for the reaction between factors XII and XI, but it is necessary for the next reaction, the activation of factor IX by activated factor XI. Here again factor IX is the substrate for activated factor XI, and in turn it is converted into activated factor IX, a serine protease. In the presence of calcium and phospholipid derived from platelets, activated factor IX combines with factor VIII to form a complex that activates factor X to its enzymatic form, again a serine protease.

The extrinsic pathway is initiated by the release of tissue factor, a protein found in endothelial cells and liberated by vascular injury. Tissue factor forms a complex with phospholipid, calcium, and coagulation factor VII. This complex activates factor X directly. Platelets play no role in the extrinsic system, which in effect can bypass the clotting reactions involved in the intrinsic pathway.

The conversion of prothrombin (a single chain molecule weighing approximately 73,000) to thrombin is produced by two segmental cleavages effected by factor Xa. In the first cleavage, factor Xa splits prothrombin into two portions: the amino terminal and the carboxyl terminal. The amino terminal portion has, in turn, two regions; one region binds calcium and phospholipids and the other region binds factor V. In the presence of the intact amino terminal portion the carboxyl terminal portion of prothrombin is cleaved by Xa between a disulfide bridge to form the two-chain active enzyme *thrombin.* The binding of calcium and phospholipids accelerates both the binding of factor V and the splitting of the carboxyl portion. If the amino terminal portion has an altered structure (as seen in vitamin K deficiency or in the presence of warfarin), then calcium is not bound properly and the second cleavage by Xa to form thrombin is greatly retarded.

The polymerization of fibrinogen into fibrin is mediated by the proteolytic action of thrombin. The fibrinogen molecule consists of two identical subunits each composed of three chains — alpha, beta, and gamma chains, joined by disulfide bonds. Thrombin cleaves the two alpha and the two beta chains releasing fibrinopeptides A and B from the N-terminal group of the chains. The remaining portion of the fibrinogen molecule is termed the *fibrin monomer.* The fibrin monomer can spontaneously polymerize by hydrogen bonding to form unstable fibrin. Stabilization of the fibrin is then achieved through the activation of factor XIII by thrombin in the presence of calcium. Activated factor XIII is a transamidase that catalyses the formation of covalent bonds between glutamyl and lysyl groups in adjacent molecules of fibrin. This reaction is the final step of blood coagulation and is responsible for the formation of stable, hemostatically effective fibrin.

The coagulation mechanism is an enzymatic process capable of amplification and autocatalysis. However, its activation must remain restricted to the site of local injury. Various mechanisms operate in this restriction: Spillage of thrombin into the systemic circulation is impeded by its adsorption at the site of fibrin formation; neutralization of thrombin is carried out by antithrombin (antithrombin III); and dilution of thrombin precursors is produced by the rapid blood flow. In addition, should activated procoagulants escape into the circulation, clearance mechanisms remove them; some activated factors are cleared by the liver cells, and larger molecules such as the tissue factor-lipoprotein complex or the fibrin monomers are cleared by the reticuloendothelial system.

FIBRINOLYTIC MECHANISM

Fibrin is not a permanent structure. Once it has fulfilled its hemostatic function, it is removed by the macrophages and by a process of lysis. Activation of the fibrinolytic system results in the formation of a proteolytic enzyme, plasmin. Plasmin is derived from an inactive precursor, plasminogen, by the action of various activator enzymes present in tissues, blood, and other body fluids. Vascular endothelium represents one important source of such activators. Another activator is urokinase, produced in the kidneys and excreted in the urine (see under Fibrinolytic Agents). The activation of factor XII also indirectly converts plasminogen to plasmin. Some bacterial enzymes such as streptokinase can activate plasminogen to plasmin.

Plasmin is a nonspecific enzyme that attacks complement components, fibrin, fibrinogen, factors V and

VIII, polypeptides such as ACTH (corticotropin), and growth hormone. Its action in plasma is opposed by several inhibitors of the fibrinolytic pathway. The proteolytic effect of plasmin on the molecule of fibrinogen consists first in the cleavage of small peptides from fibrinogen, leaving behind a large fragment designated as fragment X. This fragment is still clottable by thrombin, though at a slower rate, and it can also form complexes with fibrinogen or fibrin monomers, delaying their polymerization. Plasmin can split fragment X further into fragments Y and D; fragment Y eventually is split into fragments D and E. Fragment Y forms unclottable complexes with fibrin monomers and fibrinogen; fragments D and E inhibit fibrin polymerization, resulting in the formation of abnormal, fragile polymers. Both fragments X and Y interfere with platelet aggregation induced by thrombin and other aggregating agents. Similar inhibitory fragments are derived from the action of plasmin on fibrin. All these fragments together are known as fibrinogen-fibrin split products (FSP) or fibrin degradation products (FDP).

Clinical Evaluation of Hemorrhagic Disorders

A proper evaluation of any hemorrhagic disorder requires a carefully obtained history and a thorough physical examination of the patient. It is important to know the duration of the bleeding tendency, the frequency of the bleeding manifestations, the temporal relations of the bleeding to trauma, and whether the occurrence of bleeding was spontaneous. The family history can contribute to the diagnosis of inherited disorders and to the evaluation of their mode of inheritance. The presence of associated conditions must be investigated because acquired hemorrhagic disorders are common in many systemic diseases and may be induced by therapeutic agents. The type of bleeding is of limited help, since no type or site is strictly characteristic of any given hemorrhagic disorder.

In general, disorders of primary hemostasis are characterized by purpuric manifestations affecting particularly the skin and mucosal surfaces. Spontaneous bleeding is manifested by petechiae, ecchymoses, epistaxes, gastrointestinal and urinary tract bleeding, and menorrhagia. Posttraumatic bleeding

is usually immediate and, when superficial, may be arrested by local pressure. Petechiae are not common in disorders of coagulation, and superficial ecchymoses may occur, but they usually develop into hematomas. Bleeding into muscles is frequent; hemarthrosis is practically limited to severe coagulation disorders, particularly factor VIII or IX deficiencies. In coagulopathies posttraumatic bleeding is usually delayed in onset, because primary hemostasis is temporarily adequate.

Laboratory Tests of Hemostasis

LABORATORY TESTS OF PRIMARY HEMOSTASIS

Platelet Count. The exact platelet number can be determined either by counting them in a counting chamber with a phase microscope, or by using automated electronic counters. Examination of the peripheral blood smear permits a rapid estimate of platelet number and morphology; in addition, it may yield other diagnostic information.

Bleeding Time. This test evaluates primary hemostasis at the level of the small vessels. It reflects vasoconstriction, the number and functioning of the platelets and, in addition, the presence of von Willebrand factor. The bleeding time test is performed by making a small incision on the volar surface of the forearm after having inflated a blood pressure cuff around the upper arm to a pressure of 40 mm Hg. The accuracy of the test can be improved by using a template that allows standardized incisions of reproducible length and depth. The wound is gently blotted until the bleeding ceases. Prolongation of the bleeding time is very informative in nonthrombocytopenic patients. In severe thrombocytopenia, this test is superfluous; the bleeding time is expected to be prolonged.

Platelet Aggregation. This test is performed by measuring the optical density of a preparation of platelet-rich plasma in a spectrophotometer (platelet aggregometers are available). The addition of direct aggregating substances or of substances that induce the release of platelet ADP will be followed by the formation of platelet aggregates and a drop in optical density. The rate and degree of aggregation can be recorded in graphic patterns from which an estimation of either primary phase (direct) or secondary phase aggregation (due to released ADP) can be made.

Platelet Factor 3 Activity. This test measures the contributing effect of the platelet phospholipids to the coagulation mechanism.

Capillary Fragility. This is commonly evaluated by the tourniquet test, or Rumpel-Leede test. Intracapillary pressure is increased by applying a sphygmomanometer cuff around the patient's arm at a pressure of 80 mm Hg for 5 minutes. When the cuff is deflated, the forearm is examined for the presence of petechiae. Normally only a few petechiae appear; the test can be graded from 0 to 4+ according to the number of petechiae. This test may be positive in scurvy, vasculitis, and thrombocytopenia.

LABORATORY TESTS FOR BLOOD COAGULATION

Prothrombin Time. This is a widely used screening test for the evaluation of both the extrinsic pathway of factor X activation and the common pathway of thrombin formation. The prothrombin time refers to the time required for plasma to clot following the addition of tissue thromboplastin and calcium. This test is influenced by the activity of a number of factors beside prothrombin, including factors V, VII, and X and fibrinogen. Indeed, the prothrombin time test depends more on the concentration of factor VII and X than on that of prothrombin itself. Moreover, since the end point of the test is the formation of fibrin, either a deficiency of fibrinogen or the presence of anticoagulants such as heparin will prolong the time.

Partial Thromboplastin Time. This test measures the clotting time of recalcified platelet-poor plasma, to which a platelet lipid substitute has been added. It may be abnormal in any clotting defect except the one involving factor VII. The test is sensitive to clotting factor levels below 25 to 30 percent of normal. The test is also prolonged in the presence of interfering substances such as circulating anticoagulants or heparin.

Thrombin Time. The thrombin time test measures the clotting time of plasma upon addition of thrombin, thus evaluating the rate of conversion of fibrinogen to fibrin. The test is prolonged in hypofibrinogenemia, afibrinogenemia, dysfibrinogenemia, and in the presence of anticoagulants such as heparin or fibrin degradation products. Certain paraproteins can inhibit the conversion of fibrinogen to fibrin.

Specific Assays of Clotting Factors. Factors II, V, VII, and X are measured by a modification of the prothrombin time; factors VIII, IX, XI, and XII are measured by a modification of the partial thromboplastin time. The plasma concentration of the factor assayed is expressed as activity percent of normal. Fibrinogen can be measured directly by measuring the protein content of a fibrin clot. The normal fibrinogen level is 200 to 450 mg per 100 ml.

Fibrin Stability Test, or Screening Test for Factor XIII. Plasma clotted by recalcification is incubated in a solution of 5% urea or 1% monochloroacetic acid. These substances disrupt hydrophobic bonds between fibrin monomers; therefore, if fibrin has not been stabilized by factor XIII, the clot will dissolve.

Classification of the Disorders of Hemostasis
The disorders of hemostasis can be divided into three major groups: vascular defects, platelet abnormalities, and defects of coagulation factors. This separation is not absolute, since combined defects are not unusual. The groups are described in the list below.

I. Vascular defects
   A. Hereditary hemorrhagic telangiectasia
   B. Allergic purpuras
   C. Nonallergic purpuras
II. Platelet disorders
   A. Quantitative
      1. Thrombocytopenias
         a. Thrombocytopenia due to decreased production
         b. Thrombocytopenia due to increased destruction
            (1) Immune thrombocytopenia
            (2) Nonimmune thrombocytopenia

c. Thrombocytopenia due to sequestration of platelets

d. Thrombocytopenia due to loss of platelets

2. Thrombocytosis

a. Primary: thrombocythemia

b. Secondary: reactive thrombocytosis

B. Qualitative

1. Congenital or idiopathic

2. Acquired

III. Defects of blood coagulation

A. Inherited

1. Defects of coagulation factors XII, XI, X, IX, VIII, VII, V, II, I

2. von Willebrand disease

B. Acquired

1. Vitamin K deficiency

2. Liver disease

3. Acquired deficiency of factor X and of factor IX

4. Circulating anticoagulants

IV. Thrombosis

VASCULAR DEFECTS

Vascular defects may be due to anatomic or functional abnormalities involving capillaries, venules, or arterioles. They may be either hereditary or acquired.

Hereditary Hemorrhagic Telangiectasia

Also known as Rendu-Osler-Weber disease, hereditary hemorrhagic telangiectasia is transmitted as an autosomal dominant trait. The inherited vascular defect is anatomically characterized by defective development of the muscular and connective tissue elements, with formation of telangiectasias and, occasionally, arteriovenous aneurysms. Increased fragility and lack of constriction of the abnormal vessels are responsible for the bleeding in this disorder. The lesions are present on oral and nasal mucosal surfaces, lips, fingers, ears, and throughout the gastrointestinal tract. Pulmonary arteriovenous aneurysms may also be present. Epistaxis represents the most common symptom. Although the vascular disorder is present from birth, the typical lesions may not appear until adulthood. Laboratory tests reveal no coagulation

defects, and the bleeding time in noninvolved vessels is normal.

There is no treatment for hereditary hemorrhagic telangiectasia; cauterization of the bleeding vessels and application of nasal packs can be employed for epistaxes, but their effect is only temporary. Administration of estrogen preparations has been beneficial in reducing nosebleeds by producing stratitication of nasal epithelium with better protection to the underlying capillaries. Septal dermoplasty has been of help in some cases of intractable epistaxis. Chronic iron deficiency and anemia due to the frequent bleeding episodes are common complications of this disorder.

Allergic Purpuras

Among the acquired defects are the allergic purpuras, the most common of which is Henoch-Schönlein purpura. This disorder is seen most often in children following infections, especially beta-hemolytic streptococcal infection. It is characterized by the combination of purpura, joint and abdominal pain, and glomerulonephritis. This disorder may occur as a single episode lasting only a few weeks, but such episodes may recur. In addition to infections, many other causative agents including drugs, foods, vaccines, and chemicals have been described.

The purpuric lesions are usually symmetrical and involve mostly the lower extremities, the buttocks, and the dorsal areas of the upper extremities. The lesions vary in size and are often preceded by urticarial eruptions. Therapy with steroids is beneficial.

Autoerythrocyte and DNA sensitization are rare conditions characterized by painful ecchymoses. The lesions can be reproduced by intradermal injection of erythrocyte stroma or DNA respectively. These disorders may represent psycogenic conditions.

Hyperglobulinemic purpura is a vasculitis that can occur with a variety of disorders or it may be idiopathic. In the latter form, complexes of IgG-anti IgG immunoglobulins have been demonstrated.

Nonallergic Purpuras

The nonallergic purpuras include a variety of noninflammatory vascular abnormalities. The etiology is variable, and the pathogenesis is not always understood. In mechanical and orthostatic purpura the vascular damage is produced by increased intravascular pressure due to strenuous muscular activity (e.g., weight lifting or paroxysms of cough) or to stasis. Chronic stasis purpura can induce pigmentation on the lower extremities due to deposition of hemosiderin. In inherited disorders of connective tissue (Ehlers-Danlos syndrome, pseudoxanthoma elasticum, osteogenesis imperfecta, the Marfan syndrome), the increased vascular fragility is due to the abnormal structure of collagen and loss of perivascular support. Occasionally affected patients may also exhibit abnormalities of platelet function. Elderly individuals, patients with Cushing's disease, and patients on long-term steroid therapy often exhibit easy bruising (senile and steroid purpura). The ecchymoses are usually more frequent on the forearms and dorsum of the hands. The lesions tend to have a reddish color, persist for long periods of time, and fail to undergo the discoloration changes of the usual ecchymosis. Degeneration of dermal connective tissue, lack of support of the vasculature, and inadequate inflammatory response are responsible for this type of purpura.

Increased viscosity and sludging of red cells in the microcirculation, as it may occur in polycythemia, macroglobulinemia, and cryoglobulinemia, can induce capillary anoxia and increased vascular fragility. Deposition of amyloid in the skin and small blood vessels may result in increased vascular fragility and purpura.

Vitamin C is necessary for the synthetic formation of subendothelial collagen tissue. Characteristic manifestations of scurvy are gingival and perifollicular hemorrhage; in young children subperiosteal hemorrhage can occur. The hemorrhagic manifestations respond to vitamin C therapy.

PLATELET DISORDERS

Thrombocytopenias Due to Decreased Production of Thrombocytes

Thrombocytopenias due to decreased production of thrombocytes include rare familial, congenital forms; these are usually associated with other abnormalities such as errors of development (congenital malformations), errors of metabolism (aminoaciduria), and overall marrow failure (Fanconi syndrome). Among other genetically determined forms are the Wiskott-Aldrich syndrome and the May-Hegglin anomaly. The Wiskott-Aldrich syndrome is a sex-linked trait affecting only males, and it is characterized by thrombocytopenia, eczema, and recurrent infections. The megakaryocytes are abnormal; platelet production is defective; and the platelets have decreased storage pools of ADP and an abnormally short survival. The May-Hegglin anomaly is transmitted as an autosomal dominant trait and involves the granulocytic series as well as the platelets. It is characterized by both thrombocytopenia and the presence of basophilic inclusions (Döhle bodies) in the leukocytes. A rare form of isolated thrombocytopenia is characterized by the presence of immature megakaryocytes in the bone marrow and by the stimulation of platelet production in response to transfusions of plasma, suggesting a deficiency of thrombopoietin, the humoral factor necessary for normal megakaryocytic maturation and platelet production.

Acquired thrombocytopenias are common manifestations of many toxic, nutritional, or anatomic disturbances of stem-cell proliferation and differentiation. Neonatal rubella can induce megakaryocyte damage, and similar damage has been described after prenatal maternal ingestion of thiazide drugs. Acquired aplastic anemia, either idiopathic or secondary to exposure to ionizing radiations, myelosuppressive drugs, or chemicals, is a pancytopenic condition due to failure of all hematopoietic series including megakaryocytes. Decrease in megakaryocytes also can result from bone marrow infiltration by metastatic neoplastic cells, leukemic cells, or granulomas. In nutritional megaloblastic anemia due to either folate or B_{12} deficiency the arrest in DNA synthesis can affect the megakaryocytic series, causing decreased or ineffective thrombopoiesis. Depression of megakaryocyte maturation and thrombocytopenia is a frequent complication of severe alcoholism. Thrombocytopenia is a common manifestation of paroxysmal nocturnal hemoglobinuria; in contrast to the anemia, the decrease in platelets is not due to accelerated destruction, but rather to decreased production.

Thrombocytopenias Due to Increased Peripheral Destruction of Thrombocytes

Thrombocytopenias due to increased peripheral

destruction of thrombocytes can be caused by various immune mechanisms; by increased platelet consumption, either through disseminated intravascular clotting or generalized vascular damage; or by direct platelet injury from bacterial toxins. As a rule, all these conditions are characterized by peripheral thrombocytopenia, normal or increased megakaryocytes in the bone marrow, and shortened platelet survival. The accelerated turnover of platelets is also manifested by the presence of large young circulating platelets (megathrombocytes).

Drug-induced Immune Thrombocytopenia. Immune platelet destruction can be induced by drugs to which patients have become sensitized. A large number of pharmacologic agents have been associated with immune thrombocytopenia, but definite etiologic relationship has not always been established. In some cases, degradation products of the drug appear responsible for the sensitization. The pathogenetic mechanism of the thrombocytopenia is not completely defined; numerous studies suggest that either the drug or its metabolite combines with a plasma protein, forming an antigenic complex against which the patient produces an antibody. The antigen-antibody complex coats the platelets, and as a consequence immune damage results in agglutination and lysis. The antibody itself is harmless to platelets; the drug must be present for the immune reaction to occur. Indeed, improvement of thrombocytopenia follows discontinuation of the drug, despite the persistence of the antibody for a much longer period of time.

The clinical features of drug-induced thrombocytopenia are similar to those of any thrombocytopenia. The severity of bleeding depends on the degree of thrombocytopenia. A very careful history is of the utmost importance in identifying the drug responsible for the thrombocytopenia.

Treatment of drug-induced thrombocytopenia consists in withdrawing the offending agent. Although therapy with steroids may improve the clinical manifestations of thrombocytopenia, it does not seem to accelerate recovery, which rather is related to the rate at which the drug is metabolized, excreted, or both. Discontinuation of some drugs like quinine and quinidine is followed by recovery within a few days.

Recovery after discontinuing other drugs that remain in the tissues for a long time, such as gold, may be quite delayed.

Posttransfusion Purpura. This is a very rare form of immune thrombocytopenia that develops about 1 week following a blood transfusion. In addition to antigens common to all leukocytes, platelets have specific antigens; the most common is the Pl A1 antigen, which is present in 98 percent of all people. Posttransfusion thrombocytopenia and purpura have been described in Pl A1-negative individuals following transfusion of Pl A1-positive platelets. Theoretically, development of antibodies against Pl A1 antigen should not induce thrombocytopenia in the Pl A1-negative recipient. A satisfactory explanation is that the antibody induced by the initial exposure to the Pl A1 antigen combines with transfused soluble Pl A1 antigens to form soluble immune complexes which then can coat the recipient's Pl A1-negative platelets, causing their destruction.

Almost all posttransfusion purpura patients who have been described have been women with a history of one or more pregnancies, suggesting a previous sensitization to fetal platelet Pl A1 antigens. Other factors may play a role in the development of posttransfusion purpura, since its occurrence is much rarer than 2 percent, as would be statistically expected. The diagnosis should be suspected in patients who become severely thrombocytopenic shortly after a blood transfusion. In most cases the antibody can be demonstrated by complement fixation and platelet agglutination or lysis. The thrombocytopenia is self-limited, but it may persist for 3 to 6 weeks. Steroids are of no value, and splenectomy is not indicated. The most satisfactory therapy consists in plasmapheresis with removal, or at least reduction, of the antibodies.

Idiopathic Thrombocytopenic Purpura (ITP). This disease is also mediated by an immune mechanism. It can occur in acute and chronic forms. Acute ITP is seen most often in children following a viral infection after an interval of a few days to a few weeks. The mechanism of the immune damage is not clear, but it is somehow related to the preceding infection.

It is possible that viral antigen-antiviral antibody complexes form and adsorb onto the platelets or that transient aberrations of the immunocytes or changes in platelet antigenic structure are caused by the virus and result in the formation of antibodies to autologous platelets. The thrombocytopenia persists for a week or a few months; in the majority of cases it subsides spontaneously. Steroid therapy is of no value in hastening the recovery, but it may be clinically beneficial in severe cases. Occasional patients fail to recover after several months and progress into chronic forms of ITP requiring protracted therapy with steroids and, eventually, splenectomy.

Chronic ITP is predominantly a disorder of young adults, and it affects women more often than men. The thrombocytopenia and the hemorrhagic manifestations usually are less abrupt in onset than in acute ITP, and unlike acute ITP, chronic ITP does not remit spontaneously. The pathogenesis of the thrombocytopenia is related to the development of an antiplatelet antibody. The antibody is a 7S IgG that reacts with both autologous and homologous platelets independently of specific antigens. The antibody is specific for platelets, since the other blood elements are unaffected by it.

The clinical manifestations of chronic ITP do not have any specific features other than the hemorrhagic manifestations related to the degree of thrombocytopenia. Bruising, menorrhagia, petechiae, and bleeding with minimal trauma are common.

The diagnosis of ITP should be limited to cases in which all the possible etiologic factors have been considered and satisfactorily excluded. Laboratory findings include a decreased platelet count, which can vary from extremely low values to 75,000 to 100,000 per cubic millimeter; other blood elements are normal. If anemia is present, it is usually due to blood loss. The bone marrow aspirate shows no abnormalities; the megakaryocytes are increased and the young forms are increased. Bleeding time and capillary fragility are abnormal; platelet survival is consistently decreased. Antiplatelet antibodies can be detected in the serum of about 70 percent of patients with chronic ITP.

The therapy of ITP is mainly with steroids, for example, prednisone, 0.5 to 2.0 mg/kg/day depending on the severity of the condition. The response to this therapy may occur after a few days or a few weeks, and its effectiveness presumably is due to suppression both of phagocytic activity in the reticuloendothelial system and of immune mechanisms. Either the recurrence of thrombocytopenia or the long-term need for steroid therapy represents a sufficient indication for splenectomy, which will induce a more satisfactory and prolonged remission in the majority of cases. The spleen represents the organ of major platelet destruction, but if the platelets are heavily coated by antibody, destruction may also take place in the liver. About 10 percent of the patients fail to respond either to steroids or to splenectomy; some of these refractory cases may eventually benefit from therapy with immunosuppressive agents such as cyclophosphamide, vincristine, or azathioprine. Transfusions of platelets are of little value because the platelets have a very short survival; such transfusions should be limited to episodes of life-threatening or central nervous system bleeding.

Secondary symptomatic immune thrombocytopenia, a form indistinguishable from ITP, may complicate various conditions known to be associated with abnormal immune responses, including systemic lupus erythematosus, lymphoproliferative disorders, sarcoid, and autoimmune hemolytic anemia (Evans syndrome). The thrombocytopenia of infectious mononucleosis is due to the development of a cold agglutinin specific for the i antigen that is present on platelet membranes. The therapy of all these disorders includes specific treatment of the underlying disease, steroid therapy, and occasionally splenectomy.

Neonatal Immune Thrombocytopenia. This platelet disorder occurs in newborns of mothers with idiopathic or secondary immune thrombocytopenia, owing to the transplacental passage of maternal antiplatelet antibody to the fetus. As the antibody is only passively transferred, the duration of the thrombocytopenia is limited to the life span of the antibody. Occasionally the degree of thrombocytopenia is so severe that it requires steroids and platelet transfusion; exchange transfusion may be needed in some cases to accelerate the removal of the antibodies.

Isoimmune Neonatal Thrombocytopenia. This is due to maternal isoimmunization to fetal platelet antigens and transplacental passage of the antibody back to the fetus. The mother's platelets lack the specific antigen, and therefore they are not affected by the antibody. This syndrome is similar to erythroblastosis fetalis but with the fetal platelet as antigenic stimulus and target cell for the antibody rather than the erythrocyte. Steroid therapy, exchange transfusion, and transfusion with washed maternal platelets may be required in severe cases.

Nonimmune Thrombocytopenias. These include thrombohemolytic thrombocytopenic purpura (TTP), a rare condition of unknown etiology that is characterized by hemolytic anemia, thrombocytopenia, variable and fluctuating neurologic abnormalities, and renal dysfunction. Its onset is usually abrupt, its course acute, and its outcome often fatal. Rare chronic forms have been described.

The pathogenesis of TTP is a primary, widespread vascular lesion characterized by hyaline fibrinoid deposition within the lumina of arterioles and capillaries, without inflammatory reaction. Thrombi containing platelet aggregates and fibrin have been shown in the microcirculation. The vasculature of any organ or system may be involved in TTP, producing complex clinical features. Trauma and fragmentation of the erythrocytes as they circulate through the impaired blood vessels are responsible for the hemolytic anemia and for the invariable presence of schistocytes on examination of the peripheral blood smear (microangiopathic hemolytic anemia). The thrombocytopenia is due to excessive consumption of platelets at the sites of the vascular lesions; some patients also demonstrate evidence of disseminated intravascular coagulation (DIC) and consumption coagulopathy. The bone marrow shows marked erythroid activity and increased megakaryocytes.

The therapy of TTP includes steroids and splenectomy; in addition, administration of anticoagulants, dextran, and other drugs that inhibit platelet aggregation has been effective in some cases. Satisfactory results have also been reported with plasmapheresis.

The hemolytic uremic syndrome is a disease of infants and children. It is similar to TTP except that it lacks neurologic involvement. A viral etiology has been suggested, but no specific infectious agent has yet been isolated. The vascular lesions of hemolytic uremic syndrome are similar to those in TTP but are mostly limited to the kidneys. The mechanisms of hemolysis and thrombocytopenia are identical to those in TTP; occasionally DIC may be present. Therapy with steroids, anticoagulants, and dialysis has reduced the mortality rate in hemolytic uremic syndrome, but often some degree of renal failure persists.

In the Kasabach-Merritt syndrome, thrombocytopenia is due to consumption of platelets in a vascular tumor (giant cavernous hemangioma). Other coagulation abnormalities consistent with DIC and microangiopathic hemolysis are usually present. Anticoagulation therapy can control the coagulopathy; more effective therapy consists in surgical excision or irradiation of the tumor.

Various bacterial infections, particularly gram-negative sepsis, are often complicated by thrombocytopenia which can be due to direct platelet injury, endothelial damage or to DIC. Purpura fulminans is a severe postinfectious complication characterized by thrombosis, hemorrhagic necrosis of the skin and DIC. Heparin and dextran have been used successfully.

Thrombocytopenia Due to Sequestration of Platelets Normally about one-third of the peripheral platelet mass is pooled in the spleen at any one time; this pooled fraction is in exchange with the circulating fraction. Marked enlargement of the spleen or hypersplenism such as may occur in liver disease with congestive splenomegaly can delay the splenic transit of platelets and produce splenic sequestration of platelets and peripheral thrombocytopenia. Studies with transfused platelets labeled with isotopes have demonstrated decreased recovery but normal survival of the infused platelets. The thrombocytopenia of hypersplenism is usually moderate, in the range of 50,000 to 100,000 per cubic millimeter. More severe reductions may be encountered in splenomegaly associated with other diseases such as Gaucher's disease, lymphoma, or sarcoidosis, in which increased platelet destruction as well as sequestration within the spleen can occur. Hypothermia can produce aggregation and sequestration of platelets in various organs. The resulting thrombocytopenia is usually reversed by rewarming of the body temperature.

Thrombocytopenia Due to Loss of Platelets
Thrombocytopenia may be due to actual loss of platelets, for example, in an exchange transfusion or if excessive blood loss is replaced with multiple transfusions of stored blood. Loss of viable platelets, dilution with platelet-poor transfused blood, and lack of an immediate compensatory increase in platelet production are responsible for the thrombocytopenia. Loss of platelets during extracorporeal circulation or hemodialysis is probably due to platelet damage by the apparatus, adhesion to foreign surfaces, or aggregation by the ADP released by damaged erythrocytes and platelets.

Excessive Platelets: Thrombocythemia and Thrombocytosis
Marked elevation of the platelet count due to increased production can be seen in various conditions. The term *thrombocythemia* applies to the elevated count associated with myeloproliferative diseases and in particular to essential thrombocythemia, a primary neoplastic proliferation of megakaryocytes. In this condition, the platelet count can rise in the order of millions. The manifestations include both thrombosis and hemorrhage, the former due to spontaneous clumping of platelets in the circulation and the latter to associated qualitative platelet defects and to interference by the high number of platelets with the clotting mechanism. Therapy consists in administration of myelosuppressive agents; anticoagulants or drugs which inhibit platelet function may be required in patients with thrombotic tendency.

Thrombocytosis usually refers to the elevated count secondary to a variety of conditions: acute and chronic inflammatory processes, cancer, Hodgkin's disease, iron deficiency, splenectomy, and so on. The platelet count usually is only moderately elevated, although it can approach 1 million. The elevation may be transient, and it can be corrected by effective therapy of the associated disease. The thrombocytosis following splenectomy can reach very high levels in the second week postoperatively,

but then it gradually decreases over the next few months to normal levels. Thrombotic complications are very rare in thrombocytosis; bleeding manifestations have not been described.

Qualitative Platelet Disorders
Various bleeding disorders due to functional platelet defects have been described; these may be either congenital or acquired. A satisfactory classification of the congenital forms is not available at present. For simplicity, they can all be designated with the terms *thrombopathia* or *thrombocytopathy* and can be divided into defects of adhesion, release reaction, or aggregation. Deficiency or abnormal release of platelet factor 3, at one time considered a specific defect, can occur with any type of thrombopathy.

A rare form of adhesion defect has been described in which there is impaired platelet adhesion to collagen in the absence of other abnormalities. Other bleeding disorders due to defective interaction between the subendothelial structures and platelets include von Willebrand disease and the Bernard-Soulier syndrome (giant platelet syndrome). In von Willebrand disease, the defect is not intrinsic to the platelets; rather, it is due to the deficiency of a plasma factor closely related to the factor VIII molecule, the von Willebrand factor. This disorder will be described later in this chapter, under Disorders of Blood Coagulation. The Bernard-Soulier syndrome is a rare bleeding disorder characterized by the presence of large, bizarre platelets. Contrary to von Willebrand disease, in this disorder the interaction mediated by factor VIII is impaired because of an intrinsic platelet defect: The platelet membrane lacks a glycoprotein needed for its binding of factor VIII and other clotting factors.

Defects of release reaction and second-phase aggregation represent the most common qualitative platelet abnormalities. They are characterized by failure of the platelets to release ADP from the granules and to aggregate at the site of injury. These disorders can be divided into two broad groups. In the first group, the defect is strictly in the release mechanism, since the ADP content of the granules is normal. The nature of the abnormality is not known; in one case, a defect of the enzyme cyclo-oxygenase that catalyzes the formation of prostaglandin G2 has been demonstrated. In the second group, the abnormality of release is due to a diminished amount of the granule pool of ADP (storage pool disease). In addition to idiopathic cases, defect of storage pool has been described in association with oculomotor albinism (Hermansky-Pudlak syndrome) and in Wiskott-Aldrich syndrome. Both defects of release may produce variable prolongation of the bleeding time and abnormal platelet aggregation tests. While the platelets can be aggregated by exogenous ADP and other direct aggregating agents, collagen-induced aggregation, which depends on released ADP, is abnormal or absent. The differential diagnosis between the two groups is based on the measurement of the pool of adenine nucleotides and serotonin.

Defect of primary aggregation (Glanzmann thrombasthenia) is due to failure of the platelet membrane to respond to ADP. The nature of this rare defect is not clear. Frequent but not constant biochemical abnormalities, including decreases of platelet actomyosin, platelet fibrinogen, or glycolytic enzymes, have been demonstrated. More recent studies have shown the absence of a membrane-specific glycoprotein. Glanzmann thrombasthenia is transmitted as an autosomal recessive trait and is manifested only in homozygous individuals. Bleeding manifestations are variable. Diagnostic laboratory features include prolonged bleeding time, abnormal clot retraction, lack of response to exogenous and endogenous ADP as shown by absence of primary and secondary aggregation, and impaired activity of platelet factor 3. Content and release of ADP and serotonin are normal. The only available therapy is platelet transfusion.

Acquired qualitative platelet disorders can develop in the course of many pathologic conditions. In uremia the platelet dysfunction is manifested by prolonged bleeding time, abnormal platelet adhesiveness and release reaction, and defective availability of platelet factor 3. The degree of the abnormalities, particularly the bleeding time, correlates with the frequency and the severity of the hemorrhagic manifestations. The defect is not intrinsic to the platelets but is due to interference by urea metabolites (guanidinosuccinic and phenolic acid); in fact, normal platelets acquire the defect when incubated in uremic plasma, and the

platelet abnormality in uremic patients is improved by dialysis.

Platelet function may be impaired by macroglobulins and other paraproteins as well as by antibodies. Thrombopathy is common in myeloproliferative diseases. In fibrinolysis and in liver disease the platelet abnormality may be due to the presence of fibrin and fibrinogen split products. Many drugs may inhibit platelet function; the most important is aspirin (acetylsalicylic acid, ASA) because of its widespread use. Other nonsteroidal antiinflammatory drugs (phenylbutazone, indomethacin), vasodilators (dipyridamole), and most antihistaminics may induce similar defects. The plasma expander dextran adsorbs onto the platelets, interfering with membrane function and surface charges. The effect of drugs on platelets can be of great clinical significance: in patients with associated coagulation abnormalities such as hemophilia, liver disease, or anticoagulation, concomitant impairment of primary hemostasis by these antiplatelet drugs may precipitate or aggravate bleeding.

DISORDERS OF BLOOD COAGULATION
Including calcium and phospholipids, 12 factors, 10 of which are proteins, are recognized as specific coagulation factors. By international agreement these factors are designated with Roman numerals I through XIII according to the order of their discovery; there is no factor VI. Additional coagulopathies due to deficiencies of previously unrecognized factors have been described recently. They include a variant form of hemophilia A designated as Heckathorn disease, an autosomal form of factor VIII deficiency, a variant form of hemophilia B, and the deficiency of an unknown factor designated as Passovoy factor.

The coagulation defects can be due to decreased synthesis of the factors (e.g., afibrinogenemia, factor XI deficiency) or to the synthesis of abnormal factors with deficient activity (e.g., factors VII, VIII, IX, X, and dysfibrinogenemia).

The inherited disorders of coagulation are usually limited to deficiency of a single factor; rare exceptions are those represented by a combined factors V and VIII deficiency and the deficiency of all the vitamin K-dependent factors. Factor VIII and factor IX deficiencies are inherited as sex-linked recessive traits and von Willebrand disease as an autosomal dominant trait; all the other inherited factor deficiencies are autosomal recessive. Often patients with a congenital, inheritable defect lack any family history of bleeding; their disease may represent spontaneous genetic mutations.

The acquired disorders of coagulation, in contrast to the inherited disorders, are rarely due to a single factor deficiency; more often they involve a group of factors that share some biologic or physicochemical properties. The acquired disorders can occur at any age and are usually induced by a concomitant pathologic condition.

Inherited Coagulation Disorders

Factor XII Deficiency. Also known as Hageman factor deficiency, factor XII deficiency is transmitted as an autosomal recessive trait. It is not associated with a bleeding tendency; actually some patients have shown a tendency to thrombosis, suggesting that in vivo the intrinsic pathway can be activated without the participation of factor XII. The diagnosis of factor XII deficiency is strictly a laboratory one, with findings of a prolonged clotting time, a prolonged partial thromboplastin time, but a normal prothrombin time, fibrinogen level, thrombin time, and bleeding time.

Factor XI Deficiency. Also known as PTA or plasma thromboplastin antecedent deficiency, factor XI deficiency is transmitted as an autosomal recessive trait. It has been described most frequently in individuals of Jewish ancestry. The clinical manifestations are usually mild; spontaneous bleeding is rare, and the defect is often detected because of postsurgical or posttraumatic bleeding. The screening laboratory tests are similar to those for factor XII deficiency; specific diagnosis requires assay of factor XI activity. Factor XI is stable on storage; its biologic life span is about 3 days. Satisfactory correction of this defect is easily obtained with transfusion of plasma.

Hemophilia A. Factor VIII deficiency (also known as classic hemophilia or hemophilia A) is a sex-linked recessive trait affecting males and transmitted through females. It is due to a genetic defect in the X chromosome. A male hemophiliac will transmit the defect to all his daughters, who will be carriers of the trait. A female carrier will transmit the trait to one-half of her daughters and the disease to one-half of her sons. Female carriers can be asymptomatic; their factor VIII level can be variable, because of variability of expression of one of the two X chromosomes (Lyon hypothesis). The incidence of hemophilia A is about 1 in 20,000. The characteristic family history is not present in all patients; these de novo cases probably arise from a spontaneous mutation in the patient's X chromosome or in one of the mother's.

Extensive research on the biochemical and physiologic properties of purified factor VIII indicates that it is a glycoprotein with molecular weight of 1.2×10^6 daltons which can be dissociated into high-molecular-weight and low-molecular-weight components. Three functionally distinct properties have been identified for this complex factor: the antigen, the procoagulant, and the von Willebrand factor (see later under von Willebrand Disease). The antigen can be detected by specific antibodies, the procoagulant corrects the coagulation abnormality in hemophilia A and in patients with von Willebrand disease, and the von Willebrand factor corrects the abnormality of platelet function and the bleeding time of patients with von Willebrand disease. The antigen and the von Willebrand factor activities are related to the high-molecular-weight fraction, which is produced by the endothelial cells and is genetically controlled by an autosomal chromosome. It is not certain whether the procoagulant activity, which is controlled by the X chromosome, is a separate molecule that attaches to the large molecule or whether it is the result of conversion of the large molecule to a clot-promoting factor. In normal individuals there is good correlation among the three activities.

In hemophiliacs, the antigen and the von Willebrand factor activities are normal, but the coagulant activity is decreased. In von Willebrand disease all three activities are decreased. Thus hemophilia A, which was at one time considered to be due to decreased synthesis of factor VIII, is in fact the result of the synthesis of a functionally defective factor VIII molecule.

The immunologic determination of the factor VIII antigenic activity has been applied to the detection of asymptomatic female carriers of hemophilia A. In female carriers, the affected X chromosome directs the synthesis of functionally inactive but antigenically normal factor VIII; the normal X chromosome directs the synthesis of functional and antigenically normal factor VIII. As expected, the antigenic level of factor VIII in female carriers is in excess of the factor VIII coagulant activity.

Hemophilia can be classified as severe, moderate, or mild, with a spectrum of manifestations ranging from frequent episodes of spontaneous bleeding to bleeding occurring only after trauma or surgery. The severity of the disease parallels the degree of the deficiency. Affected members of the same family usually exhibit similar degrees of severity. In severe hemophilia, bleeding can occur in any organ or tissue. Hemarthroses are frequent; hematomas can be extensive and can induce vascular or neurologic damage by compression. Subperiosteal bleeding can result in formation of pseudotumors. The laboratory tests show a prolonged partial thromboplastin time but normal prothrombin time, thrombin time, fibrinogen level, platelets, and bleeding time. Definite diagnosis is made by measuring factor VIII activity.

Therapy of bleeding consists in temporary replacement of factor VIII by transfusing fresh plasma or concentrated preparations to an adequate hemostatic level. Infusions of fresh or fresh-frozen plasma can be sufficient to control minor hemorrhages in which a low factor VIII level (5 to 10 percent) is adequate for hemostasis. Major trauma, surgery, or bleeding in dangerous sites requires higher levels (50 percent or more) of factor VIII and more prolonged correction of the defect. In these cases, concentrated preparations must be used to avoid the risk of circulatory overload, which would be inevitable if whole plasma were used.

Cryoprecipitate is an easily available form of factor VIII concentrate; unfortunately, the content of the factor in each preparation varies greatly. More concentrated forms containing 10- to 100-fold more factor VIII activity than plasma are commercially available. These preparations carry a high risk of hepatitis but are of great value in severe hemorrhage and for surgical procedures. Home therapy programs and self-administration of factor VIII concentrates at the earliest sign of bleeding have decreased the morbidity and have improved the therapy of hemophilia. The administration of antifibrinolytic drugs is effective in reducing the bleeding and in decreasing the transfusion requirement in dental extractions.

Occasionally, patients with hemophilia develop antibodies to factor VIII following transfusion therapy (see under Circulating Anticoagulants).

Hemophilia B. Factor IX deficiency (also known as hemophilia B, PTC, or plasma thromboplastin component deficiency, Christmas disease) is a bleeding disorder that is clinically indistinguishable from factor VIII deficiency and, like that disorder, is inherited as a sex-linked defect. The discovery of factor IX was prompted by the observation that the plasma of some hemophiliacs could correct the clotting abnormality of other hemophiliacs, suggesting the defect of a factor other than factor VIII. Factor IX is synthesized in the liver and is one of the vitamin K-dependent factors. Congenital factor IX deficiency, like factor VIII deficiency, is not the result of decreased factor synthesis. Immunologic studies have shown that patients with factor IX deficiency represent a heterogeneous group: The majority synthesize antigenically reactive protein similar to factor IX, but lack its coagulant activity; some have an abnormal form of factor IX with an inhibitory effect on the prothrombin time when this test is performed with ox thromboplastin. The incidence of hemophilia B is approximately 1 in 100,000, about five times less common than factor VIII deficiency, from which it can be differentiated only by laboratory assay of factor IX.

Treatment of the bleeding manifestations of hemophilia B consists in replacement therapy. Factor IX is stable in fresh-frozen plasma; its biologic half-life is approximately 24 hours. Concentrated preparations are available that contain an average of 15 times the factor IX activity of normal plasma. Postinfusion recovery of factor IX is lower than the recovery achieved with factor VIII because of the significant exchange of plasma factor IX with the extravascular space due to its small molecular size.

Factor V Deficiency. Also known as parahemophilia, this is a very rare disorder with an incidence of about 1 in 1 million. It is transmitted as an autosomal, incompletely recessive trait. The clinical manifestations can be severe, especially with trauma or surgery; spontaneous bleeding may also occur. The coagulation tests show prolonged prothrombin time and partial thromboplastin time; definite diagnosis is made by factor V assay. Factor V is labile on storage. Its biological half-life is about 24 hours, so daily infusions of fresh or fresh-frozen plasma must be given to achieve and maintain a satisfactory level of factor V.

Factor VII Deficiency. Also known as proconvertin or SPCA deficiency, factor VII deficiency is a very rare disorder that is transmitted as an autosomal recessive trait with a high degree of penetrance. The clinical manifestations depend on the degree of deficiency; in severe cases, spontaneous bleeding can occur. The laboratory tests show prolongation of the prothrombin time with normal partial thromboplastin time because factor VII is not required for the intrinsic pathway of clotting. Definite diagnosis requires factor VII assay. The abnormal prothrombin time is corrected by using Russell's viper venom (Stypven) instead of tissue extract because Stypven can activate factor X in the absence of factor VII. Although factor VII is stable in vitro, its biologic half-life is only 4 to 5 hours, and therefore plasma infusions for replacement therapy must be given three to four times per day. The level required for hemostasis is about 25 percent of normal.

Factor X Deficiency. Also known as Stuart-Prower factor deficiency, factor X deficiency is a rare disorder that is transmitted as an autosomal recessive trait with a high penetrance. Patients with factor X deficiency represent a heterogeneous group; some can synthesize a protein with the antigenic properties of normal factor X, and others show partial synthesis that does not correlate with the level of the coagulant activity. Factor X is stable in frozen plasma; the biologic half-life is about 48 hours, and a level of 20 to 25 percent is adequate for hemostasis. Therapy consists in transfusion of plasma.

Factor II Deficiency. Also known as prothrombin deficiency, factor II deficiency is an extremely rare disorder, and only a few cases have been studied. Little is known about its genetic transmission; most likely it is an autosomal recessive trait. Bleeding manifestations can occur in severe cases. The level adequate for hemostasis is low, about 10 to 15 percent, and its biologic half-life is rather long, about 50 to 60 hours, so that satisfactory correction can be accomplished with plasma transfusion.

Factor I Deficiency. This is a rare disorder caused by deficient synthesis of fibrinogen. It is transmitted as an autosomal recessive trait; the homozygous state results in almost complete absence of fibrinogen (afibrinogenemia) and severe bleeding manifestations. The heterozygous state shows mild reduction of fibrinogen (hypofibrinogenemia) without bleeding tendency. In afibrinogenemia, the level of fibrinogen is unmeasurable by all physicochemical techniques and immune techniques reveal only traces of fibrinogen. The bleeding manifestations can be present from birth, but for some unknown reason, patients with factor I deficiency usually are less affected than hemophiliacs. Some patients exhibit a defect of primary hemostasis with prolonged bleeding time. The laboratory tests show unclottable blood, even with the addition of thrombin. The therapy consists in replacement of fibrinogen by transfusion of either plasma or concentrated preparations (Cohn fraction I). A level of 80 to 100 mg per 100 ml is adequate for hemostasis.

The dysfibrinogenemias represent a heterogeneous group of disorders characterized by normal synthesis of an abnormal variant of the fibrinogen molecule. The majority of patients with a dysfibrinogenemia are asymptomatic; some have shown a mild bleeding tendency, abnormal healing of wounds, or tendency to thrombosis. Dysfibrinogenemias are probably transmitted as autosomal dominant traits.

Factor XIII Deficiency. This deficiency is also known as fibrinase or fibrin-stabilizing factor deficiency. Factor XIII is an enzyme activated by thrombin and calcium; it allows the covalent binding of the fibrin molecule. In the absence of factor XIII the coagulation mechanism proceeds normally but results in hemostatically unstable fibrin. In severe deficiency hemorrhages are frequent and can occur at any site. Bleeding is often delayed several hours following trauma; wound healing can be defective. This disorder is transmitted as an autosomal recessive trait.

The diagnosis of factor XIII deficiency is based on the demonstration of the solubility of the fibrin clot in a solution of 5% urea or 1% monochloroacetic acid; all other clotting tests are normal. Very small amounts of factor XIII are required for normal hemostasis, and therefore effective therapy can be achieved with plasma transfusion. The biologic half-life of factor XIII is 2 to 3 days.

Von Willebrand Disease. This is a complex bleeding disorder involving defects of both primary hemostasis and blood coagulation. It is characterized by a prolonged bleeding time, decreased factor VIII activity, abnormal platelet adhesiveness, and overresponse of factor VIII to transfusion. It is transmitted as an autosomal dominant trait. Although hemophilia A and von Willebrand's disease both have a deficiency of factor VIII, they differ in many respects, including their genetic transmission.

In von Willebrand disease the defect of factor VIII involves the coagulant activity and the activity responsible for the adhesion of platelets to the subendothelial structure known as von Willebrand factor. Deficiency of this activity is responsible for the prolonged bleeding time and for the defective adhesion of platelets to glass beads and defective aggregation by ristocetin. All the abnormalities of platelet function can be corrected in vivo and in vitro by normal plasma, by preparation containing factor VIII, and by hemophiliac plasma, indicating that such activity of factor VIII is independent of its coagulant activity. Immunologic studies have shown that in von Willebrand disease the factor VIII-related antigen is decreased as well. Recent immunofluorescent studies have shown that endothelial cells synthesize and

release the factor VIII portion that has the antigenic and the von Willebrand factor components but lacks the coagulant activity. It has been suggested that the component synthesized by the endothelium represents a precursor molecule which is then converted into a coagulant factor at a different site by an unknown mechanism controlled by the X chromosome. Endothelial cells of patients with von Willebrand disease have decreased amounts of factor VIII antigen and von Willebrand factor. It seems likely that in this disorder the synthesis of the precursor molecule is impaired, with the result that all three components of the factor VIII complex are reduced in parallel. In hemophilia A, on the other hand, the endothelial synthesis of the precursor molecule is normal but the conversion is impaired; therefore the coagulant activity is decreased while the factor VIII antigen and the von Willebrand factor are normal.

When patients with von Willebrand disease are transfused with normal plasma or factor VIII concentrate they exhibit the immediate increment in all the factor VIII components to the levels accounted for by the material infused. Following the infusion, the antigen and the von Willebrand factors gradually decrease over the next 12 and 24 hours respectively. The coagulant activity shows an additional increase (overresponse) over the following 8 to 12 hours; thereafter it decreases at a slower rate than in transfused hemophiliacs. This delayed increment in factor VIII coagulant activity is observed even when hemophiliac plasma, devoid of coagulant activity, is infused. The nature of the stimulus responsible for this transient synthesis of factor VIII coagulant activity is not known. Von Willebrand disease is heterogenous in its clinical presentation and laboratory manifestations; variability has been observed even among affected members of the same family. The typical cases exhibit prolongation of the bleeding time, decreased factor VIII coagulant activity and factor VIII-related antigen, decreased platelet adhesiveness, and aggregation by ristocetin.

The bleeding manifestations in von Willebrand disease are variable in severity, with bruising, epistaxis, and menorrhagia among the more common. Severe bleeding may occur when factor VIII deficiency is marked. The therapy consists in transfusion of either plasma or factor VIII concentrate. Since these patients can synthesize factor VIII after transfusion and since the biologic half-life of factor VIII is longer than in hemophilia A, a satisfactory level of factor VIII can be reached and maintained with smaller and less frequent transfusions. In surgical patients, factor VIII administration should begin 12 to 24 hours before surgery in order to make use of the maximal response (overresponse) to transfusion. Correction of the factor VIII level does not always correct the abnormality of the bleeding time, or does so only transiently; this accounts for the difficulties encountered in some cases.

Acquired Coagulation Disorders

Deficiency of Vitamin K-dependent Coagulation Factors. The synthesis of factors II, VII, IX, and X by the liver is dependent on the presence of vitamin K. In animals, this vitamin is derived both from its synthesis by the intestinal flora and from dietary intake; it is fat soluble and is absorbed in the small intestine in the presence of bile salts. The mechanism by which vitamin K promotes the synthesis of factors II, VII, IX, and X is not certain; recent studies have shown that when vitamin K is deficient or when its utilization is blocked, a defective form of prothrombin is produced. The defect is due to the lack of a peptide containing the gamma carboxyglutamic acid residue responsible for the calcium-dependent binding of prothrombin to phospholipids. A similar defect may involve all the vitamin K-dependent factors. A bleeding tendency due to the deficiency of factors II, VII, IX, and X can arise in any condition in which the synthesis, absorption, or utilization of vitamin K is reduced.

Reduced synthesis of vitamin K may occur after the administration of broad-spectrum antibiotics with sterilization of the intestinal flora. In this setting, the vitamin K deficiency can be further enhanced in severely ill patients by lack of dietary sources of vitamin. Normal newborns exhibit depressed levels of the vitamin K-dependent factors because of a combination of decreased synthesis of the vitamin, lack of body stores, and immaturity of the hepatic enzyme system for protein synthesis. Occasionally, particularly in premature newborns, this deficiency

state may be very severe, causing hemorrhagic complications. This condition is known as hemorrhagic disease of the newborn. Decreased absorption of vitamin K can occur in biliary tract obstruction or in bowel diseases such as steatorrhea, sprue, malabsorption, and intestinal lymphoma. Decreased utilization of vitamin K occurs after the administration of coumarin and coumarinlike drugs. These drugs act as indirect anticoagulants and are widely used for the therapy and prophylaxis of thromboembolic disorders (see under Thrombosis and Antithrombotic Therapy). Overdosage or the accidental or surreptitious ingestion of coumarin can result in severe coagulopathy and bleeding manifestations such as ecchymosis, epistaxis, and gastrointestinal and urinary tract bleeding.

The laboratory findings in all these forms of vitamin K deficiency show prolongation of the prothrombin time and partial thromboplastin time and decreased levels of factors II, VII, IX, and X. The therapy consists in administration of vitamin K. Various preparations are available, including water-soluble forms suitable for oral and parenteral use. Synthesis of the clotting factors with correction of the coagulopathy occurs 6 to 24 hours following administration of 5 to 10 mg of vitamin K_1; the dose for newborns is 100 to 200 μg. In cases of severe bleeding or emergency surgery, a more prompt correction of the defect can be achieved by transfusion of plasma or concentrated preparations containing factors II, VII, IX, and X. In patients on anticoagulants because of a high risk of thromboembolic complications, sudden complete reversal of anticoagulation by vitamin K administration may be followed by a recurrence of thromboembolic events and refractoriness to further anticoagulant therapy.

Liver Disease. The liver is the organ of synthesis of the vitamin K-dependent factors, of factor V, and, in addition, of fibrinogen. Therefore, abnormalities of clotting mechanisms are common complications of liver disease. In obstructive liver disease, the coagulopathy involves mainly the vitamin K-dependent factors because of malabsorption of this vitamin, with little or no impairment at the cellular site of synthesis. This defect can be easily corrected by parenteral administration of vitamin K. Hepatocellular disease, on the other hand, impairs the synthesis of all the liver-produced factors. In severe liver disease, additional defects may contribute to the severity of the hemorrhagic manifestations. Thrombocytopenia is a frequent occurrence in patients with portal hypertension and congestive splenomegaly; thrombopathy may be present as well. Increased fibrinolysis can develop because of either decreased synthesis of inhibitors or decreased clearance of activators. Impaired clearance of procoagulants can be responsible for DIC.

The laboratory tests in liver disease may show prolongation of prothrombin time and partial thromboplastin time; depression of factors II, V, VII, IX, X, variable platelet counts, bleeding times, fibrinogen levels, and fibrin and fibrinogen split products. The therapy is mainly of the replacement type, with transfusions of fresh-frozen plasma and platelets when indicated. Concentrated preparations of factors II, VII, IX, and X are available. They may contain activated forms which can be thrombogenic; their use in patients with liver disease is not without risk. Besides, they do not correct the deficiency of factor V. In patients with overt evidence of DIC or severe fibrinolysis, heparin and antifibrinolytic drugs have been used. In any event, the effectiveness of these therapeutic measures may be very transient and disappointing and often is limited by the irreversibility of the underlying liver damage.

Occasionally acquired coagulation defects can involve a single factor. For example, factor X deficiency has been described in a few cases of amyloidosis; it appears to be due to selective absorption of the factor to the amyloid tissue. Factor IX deficiency has been described in patients with nephrotic syndrome with massive proteinuria; the deficiency probably results from extensive loss of factor IX in the urine.

Circulating Anticoagulants (Inhibitors). Occasionally a bleeding disorder may arise following the appearance in the blood of an abnormal substance that inactivates a specific coagulation factor or inhibits a particular clotting reaction. The inhibitors most commonly encountered are those directed against the antihemophilic factors VIII and IX and the inhib-

itor of the reaction of prothrombin conversion. The latter is known as lupus anticoagulant from its initial description in SLE. Inhibitors to fibrinogen have developed following transfusion therapy in patients with afibrinogenemia. The use of some drugs has been associated with the development of inhibitors; for example, inhibitors against factor V have been observed to develop following streptomycin therapy, and inhibitors against factor XIII have been seen to develop during isoniazid therapy for tuberculosis.

A circulating anticoagulant against factor VIII has been encountered in three groups of patients: (1) patients with hemophilia A who have been transfused repeatedly; (2) women in the first year postpartum; and (3) previously healthy individuals of both sexes in whom the anticoagulant has appeared spontaneously in association with a great variety of diseases. In patients in the second and third groups a condition called hemophilialike syndrome develops and is indistinguishable from classic hemophilia. The inhibitor is generally considered to be an antibody, usually an IgG antibody of the kappa light-chain type. The type of bleeding and the laboratory findings are similar to those of factor VIII deficiency. The presence of the inhibitor is demonstrated by the observation that the plasma or serum of these patients mixed with normal plasma produces a decrease in activity of factor VIII in the normal plasma. The inactivation of factor VIII is usually enhanced by extending the time of incubation of the mixture. The inhibitor can be titrated and expressed in arbitrary units.

The treatment of patients with circulating anticoagulant against factor VIII is very difficult and unsatisfactory because factor VIII supplied by transfusion is destroyed rapidly. Effective modes of therapy have included highly concentrated preparations of factor VIII, plasmapheresis to decrease the level of the inhibitor, animal preparations of factor VIII because of the species specificity of the antibody, and immunosuppression therapy because of the immune nature of the inhibitor. Satisfactory control of hemostasis has been achieved by the administration of preparations containing factors II, VII, IX, and X. The effectiveness of such preparations may be due to the presence of an activated factor which bypasses factor VIII and the site of the anticoagulant. In patients with hemophilia A, the anticoagulant may reappear in response to subsequent transfusions of factor VIII.

A circulating anticoagulant of factor IX has appeared in about 5 percent of patients with severe factor IX deficiency following transfusions. The type of reaction between factor IX and its inhibitor and the physicochemical properties of the inhibitor appear to be similar to those for factor VIII inhibitor. The spontaneous occurrence of a factor IX inhibitor is very rare.

The lupus anticoagulants can be detected in about 10 percent of patients with systemic lupus erythematosus and occasionally in a variety of pathologic conditions. The significance of such inhibitor in relation to bleeding tendency is doubtful; other defects of hemostasis, notably thrombocytopenia, are often responsible for the bleeding. The in vitro coagulation defect is manifested by a slightly prolonged prothrombin time and an abnormal partial thromboplastin time. Interestingly, the plasma level of each of the individual clotting factors can be normal in some cases. Occasionally the inhibitor may be specific, directed against factor VIII, IX, XI, or XII. Effective therapy of the basic disease usually improves the coagulation abnormality.

THROMBOSIS AND ANTITHROMBOTIC THERAPY
Thrombosis is not a single pathologic process. Three forms are separable by their pathogenesis, by their gross and ultrastructural morphology, by the turnover of clotting constituents, and by response to antithrombotic therapy; they are the white thrombus, the red thrombus, and disseminated thrombosis.

Arterial Thrombus
The white (arterial) thrombus is initiated by vascular injury and endothelial denudation. The primary pathologic event is the reaction between platelets and exposed subendothelial tissue. In the forming arterial thrombus the platelet-fibrin mass grows along the wall of the injured vessel. As the thrombus becomes concentric, areas of red cells and fibrin are incorporated, reflecting local generation of thrombin. The continued disruption of the surface of the mural thrombus by axial blood flow and the redeposition of new platelet masses give the thrombus a laminar appear-

ance, distinguishing it from the uniformly distributed red cell-fibrin meshwork of a solid clot that forms in vitro. The crucial features of the arterial thrombus are its genesis from an injured vessel wall and its growth by extension along the injured vessel wall. Only when the lumen becomes almost totally occluded does the coagulation mechanism become dominant.

Venous Thrombus
In most red (venous) thrombi there is no evidence of prior vascular injury to the veins either at sites of recently formed thrombi or in the lining of valve pockets (without thrombi). It is likely that turbulent flow in proximity to the sites of thrombosis, such as the valve cusps, leads to selective deposition of platelets at those sites and that coagulation is then initiated by the turbulent, platelet-rich blood. Whatever its cause, the venous thrombus grows by extension of the thrombus into the vein lumen, and propagation occurs primarily through coagulation. The resultant thrombus is composed primarily of red cells and fibrin, but because it grows in slowly flowing blood, platelets become enmeshed in thrombus, giving it a laminar appearance also. The laminar structure of both the arterial and venous thrombi reflects their formation in flowing blood. Although both are distinct from a blood clot formed in vitro, their laminar similarity does not mean that they share a common pathogenesis.

Recent studies have provided kinetic data in support of fundamental differences between arterial and venous thrombi. Using radioactive tracers to label platelets and fibrinogen, it has been shown that there is increased turnover of both platelets and fibrinogen in patients with venous disease, reflecting activation of the coagulation mechanism. In patients with arterial disease (atherosclerosis) selective consumption of platelets has been demonstrated, reflecting the reaction between platelets and the vessel wall. Furthermore, in patients with venous thrombosis the accelerated turnover of platelets and fibrinogen was restored to normal by anticoagulants; antiplatelet drugs were ineffective. In patients with arterial disease the antiplatelet drug dipyridamole restored platelet turnover to normal, but anticoagulants were ineffective in doing so.

Disseminated Thrombus

Disseminated intravascular coagulation apparently results when there is a disturbance in the normal hemostatic response to local vascular injury, namely in the balance between the forces leading to the deposition of the hemostatic plug at the site of the injury and the forces preventing the extension of the plug beyond that site. A variety of diseases that lead either to widespread vascular injury or to the circulation of thromboplastic substances may evoke a widespread rather than a localized hemostatic response. Whether a bleeding diathesis or a microvascular thrombosis (or both) occurs depends on the generation of a preponderance of plasmin, thrombin, or fibrinogen degradation products in local areas. In contrast to other hemostatic disorders, these balances may shift rapidly and differ markedly in various parts of the vascular tree at the same time.

There are no generally available tests that by themselves are diagnostic of DIC. The most consistent findings are prolongation of the thrombin time, depression of fibrinogen, lowered platelet count, and the presence of fibrin and fibrinogen degradation products. In many cases, however, one or more of these abnormalities may not be present. It is difficult to make the diagnosis of DIC in the presence of a normal thrombin time. Clotting factor levels are quite variable. They may be elevated, depressed, or unchanged. Red cell fragmentation is helpful when present, but it must be distinguished from other causes of abnormal red cell morphology. The major challenge of the DIC syndrome lies not in the diagnosis or the therapy of the fulminant form but rather in the recognition of milder forms and in the selection of appropriate therapy for patients with laboratory evidence of DIC but not yet in serious hemostatic difficulty. There is an astonishing lack of controlled clinical data to assist in this decision.

Antithrombotic Therapy

Antithrombotic therapy is presently available in four classes of agents: antiplatelet, fibrinolytic, afibrinogenic, and anticoagulant. Each class of agents has a fundamentally different therapeutic premise and a different mode of action.

Antiplatelet Agents. Use of these agents is based on the premise that by interfering with the sequence initiated by the adhesion of platelets to exposed subendothelial tissue and the subsequent buildup of platelet fibrin masses, the formation and growth of arterial thrombi can be retarded. Agents now in use have been selected to interfere with the platelet sequence after, not before, platelet adherence to collagen has occurred, so as to minimize the risk of hemorrhage. For example, aspirin (ASA) acts by inhibiting prostaglandin synthetase, resulting in the blockage of production of cyclic endoperoxides and thromboxanes that participate in platelet aggregation. Adenosine diphosphate release is also impaired by ASA, but what link, if any, exists between platelet prostaglandin formation and ADP release is not known at present. The effect of ASA is related to its acetyl group and is permanent on all platelets once they are exposed to it. Aspirin is readily absorbed but is also rapidly hydrolyzed in plasma, having a biologic half-life of approximately 20 minutes; the salicylate moiety does not affect platelets. Therefore a single dose of ASA acts as a "pulse"; when exposed to platelets for a short period, it has effects lasting for the 10-day life span of the exposed platelets. The antihemostatic effect is apparent within 1 hour of ingestion and is detectable for at least 4 days.

The major toxicity of ASA is its tendency to induce gastrointestinal bleeding, which reflects both its local irritant action on the gastric mucosa and its systemic antiplatelet effect. In some patients with mild underlying disorders of hemostasis (which may have escaped prior detection), ASA ingestion may produce severe hemorrhage following a trauma or surgery. Large doses may cause severe metabolic abnormalities and other forms of salicylate toxicity (vertigo, tinnitus, nausea, fever, confusion) and may exacerbate or provoke hepatitis or asthma. These toxic effects ordinarily are not seen at the usual daily dose levels (600 to 1,200 mg) of aspirin administered for its antiplatelet action. The rare urticarial reaction provoked by aspirin can occur at any dose level.

Sulfinpyrazone is a mild antiinflammatory and uricosuric drug that also impairs the second phase of platelet aggregation, that is, the release reaction, but the mechanism is not firmly established. The drug is rapidly absorbed and has a plasma half-life of approximately 3 hours. Unlike ASA, sulfinpyrazone affects platelets only when the drug is present in the plasma. Toxic reactions are rare. Dipyridamole is a vasodilator drug that impairs the responsiveness of platelets to ADP, although it does not itself block the release reaction. The metabolism of dipyridamole has not been fully studied. Toxic reactions include nausea, vomiting, and headaches.

Available data have produced mixed and often contradictory assessments of the clinical usefulness of antiplatelet agents; they appear to have limited effectiveness at best, and different ones are not interchangeable in different clinical settings. Dipyridamole, given in addition to the oral anticoagulant warfarin, lowers the incidence of peripheral arterial embolism from artificial heart valves; ASA alone is not effective for this purpose, but its use allows the dose of dipyridamole to be reduced. Sulfinpyrazone reduces the incidence of thrombi in arteriovenous shunts placed for long-term hemodialysis. Mass trials of aspirin in the prevention of recurring myocardial infarction are now under way, but given the uncertainty of the role of thrombosis as the cause of myocardial infarction and the many factors that can cause death once infarction has occurred, prevention of primary occurrence may be a more valid test of the effectiveness of ASA.

Fibrinolytic Agents. Use of these agents is based on the premise that by activating endogenous plasminogen bound to fibrin within the interstices of a thrombus, local digestion of the thrombus (thrombolysis) can be induced without causing systemic fibrinogenolysis. A corollary of this premise is that fibrinolytic therapy has no prophylactic value but instead is intended only to attack an existing thrombus. Streptokinase, a bacterial enzyme, converts plasminogen to plasmin. Theoretically, within the general circulation both streptokinase and plasmin are inhibited by antiplasmin, but at the surface of a thrombus or within it, streptokinase will activate plasminogen locally. The enzyme must be given by continuous infusion; toxic effects include pyrogenic reactions and bleeding. Urokinase is a similar human enzyme excreted by the kidney. Urokinase has been isolated

and purified from urine; its action is similar to that of streptokinase except that it does not cause pyrogenic reactions. Although theoretically attractive, fibrinolytic therapy has been of limited value in practice. Contrary to theory, it may cause generalized activation of plasminogen and lead to a distinct bleeding tendency. To date, no convincing data have been collected to demonstrate that fibrinolytic therapy decreases mortality or morbidity from either pulmonary embolism or coronary thrombosis. Fibrinolytic therapy may enhance dissolution of peripheral venous thrombi, but the value of this effect (compared to its distinct toxicity) also remains to be proved.

Afibrinogenemic Therapy. The use of Ancrod (Malayan pit viper venom) is based on the premise that rendering the patients essentially free of fibrinogen will thereby prevent the deposition or extension of a venous thrombus. Ancrod cleaves the alpha chain of fibrinogen, releasing fibrinopeptide A, but it also partially degrades the remaining alpha chain of fibrin monomer. This abnormal fibrin will clot in the microcirculation, but the clots contain noncrosslinked fibrin. Activation of plasminogen, which occurs by a mechanism not yet established, dissolves these abnormal fibrin clots rapidly. The venom must be given by continuous infusion; occasional pyrogenic reactions and a mild bleeding tendency are the major toxic effects. Clinical trials of Ancrod have been limited but do show it to be effective in preventing the extension of venous thrombi. To date the superiority of Ancrod over conventional anticoagulant therapy has not been shown.

Anticoagulant Therapy. The premise of anticoagulant therapy is that either by retarding the synthesis of certain clotting factors or by accelerating the inactivation of certain clotting factors, one can prevent the deposition or extension of stasis or venous-type thrombi. A corollary of this premise is that anticoagulants have no effect on established thrombi and that all anticoagulant therapy is prophylactic. Heparin, a naturally occurring sulfated polysaccharide, consists of hexuronic acid, acetylated glucosamine, and many sulfuric acid ester groups. Its average molecular weight lies between 8,000 and 10,000; it is extremely acidic because of its high sulfuric acid content. Heparin binds to a plasma alpha globulin, variously known as the heparin cofactor or antithrombin III, and thereby strikingly potentiates the inhibitory effect of this protein on thrombin and on activated factors IX, X, XI, and XII. The effect on factor X outweighs the effect on thrombin. Heparin is active as an anticoagulant both in vitro and in vivo. Following an intravenous dose of heparin, 20 to 25 percent is recoverable unchanged in the urine; most of the remainder is degraded in the liver; and a small amount may be taken up by mast cells. The rate of clearance from plasma is variable, but the average half-life is approximately 1 hour. The major toxic effect of heparin is bleeding, usually from mucous membranes and open wounds. Other toxic effects of heparin include thrombocytopenia, alopecia and, on prolonged usage, metabolic bone disease. A specific antidote for heparin is protamine sulfate.

There is no standard dose of heparin. When heparin is given by intermittent intravenous injection, its usual dose is in the range of about 5,000 units every 4 hours. When given by continuous intravenous infusion, the dose must be controlled by clotting assays; after an initial loading dose, the usual dose is approximately 1,000 units per hour. Recent studies have shown continuous infusion to cause less bleeding than intermittent injection. In low-dose heparin therapy, the drug is given subcutaneously every 8 hours, theoretically to provide preferential inhibition of activated factor X, thereby affording antithrombotic protection but with less risk of bleeding.

The coumarins are a class of water-soluble derivatives of coumaric acid; the most commonly used is warfarin. The coumarins act by inhibiting the hepatic synthesis of factors II (prothrombin), VII, IX, and X. The precise mechanism of inhibition is unknown, but it is dependent on coumarin inhibition of vitamin K_1 oxide reductase, leading to impaired vitamin K action. Vitamin K is essential for the gamma carboxylation of glutamic acid residues in factors II, VII, IX, and X, which is required for the binding of calcium by those clotting factors. Warfarin is completely absorbed from the gut. It is transported in plasma bound to albumin, from which it can be displaced by more tightly binding drugs. Warfarin crosses the placenta and also appears in maternal milk. It is degraded in the liver by enzymes localized on the endoplasmic reticulum. The clearance of warfarin from the plasma varies widely from person to person, and therefore the dose must be individualized. The drug is effective only in vivo.

Warfarin therapy is monitored with the prothrombin time. If hemorrhage occurs, the drug is discontinued and plasma and vitamin K_1 are given. Drug interactions are a major cause of hemorrhage in patients receiving warfarin. Although bleeding is the major toxic reaction, rare instances of hemorrhagic platelike infarction of the skin occurs in patients receiving warfarin. There is clear evidence that either warfarin or full-dose heparin therapy prevents recurring pulmonary embolism, and thus it is mandatory in patients who have pulmonary embolism but no contraindication to anticoagulants. Warfarin also reduces the incidence of peripheral embolism in patients with cardiac valvular stenoses and atrial fibrillation and in patients with artificial heart valves. One recent large-scale trial of low-dose heparin has shown that it is effective in reducing fatalities from postoperative pulmonary embolism. The role of heparin in the treatment of DIC remains controversial.

Bibliography

Aledart, L. M. (ed.). Recent advances in hemophilia. *Ann. N.Y. Acad. Sci.* 240:1, 1975.

Baldini, M. Idiopathic thrombocytopenic purpura and the ITP syndromes. Symposium on Hemorrhagic Disorders, *Med. Clin. North Am.* 56:47, 1972.

Biggs, R. *Human Blood Coagulation, Hemostasis and Thrombosis.* Oxford, Eng.: Blackwell, 1976.

Blomback, B., and Blomback, M. Molecular structure of fibrinogen. *Ann. N.Y. Acad. Sci.* 202:77, 1972.

Bowie, E. J., Thompson, J. H., Didisheim, P., and Owen, C. A. *Laboratory Manual of Hemostasis.* Philadelphia: Saunders, 1971.

Deykin, D. Emerging concepts of platelet function. *N. Engl. J. Med.* 290:144, 1974.

Deykin, D. The clinical challenge of disseminated intravascular coagulation. *N. Engl. J. Med.* 283:636, 1970.

Deykin, D. Warfarin therapy. *N. Engl. J. Med.* 283: 801, 1970.

Feinstein, D. I., and Rapaport, S. I. Acquired inhibitors of blood coagulation. *Progr. Hemostasis Thromb.* 1:75, 1972.

Frantantoni, J. C., Ness, P., and Simon, T. L. Thrombolytic therapy. *N. Engl. J. Med.* 293:1073, 1975.

Gallus, A. S., and Hirsh, J. Treatment of venous thromboembolic disease. *Semin. Thromb. Hemostasis* 2:291, 1976.

Macfarlane, R. G. An enzyme cascade in the blood clotting mechanism and its function as a biochemical amplifier. *Nature* 202:498, 1964.

Ratnoff, O. Some relationships among hemostasis, fibrinolytic phenomena, immunity and inflammatory response. *Adv. Immunol.* 10:145, 1969.

Ratnoff, O. D., and Bennett, B. The genetics of hereditary disorders of blood coagulation. *Science* 179:1291, 1973.

Roberts, H. R., and Cederbaum, A. I. The liver and blood coagulation — physiology and pathology. *Gastroenterology* 63:297, 1972.

Rosenberg, R. D. Action and interaction of antithrombin and heparin. *N. Engl. J. Med.* 292: 146, 1975.

Sherry, S. Fibrinolysis. *Annu. Rev. Med.* 19:247, 1968.

Spaet, T. H. Hemostatic homeostasis. *Blood* 28:112, 1966.

Weiss, H. J. Platelet physiology and abnormalities of platelet function. *N. Engl. J. Med.* 293:531, 580, 1975.

Zimmerman, T. S., Ratnoff, O. D., and Powell, A. E. Immunological differentiation of classic hemophilia (factor VIII deficiency) and von Willebrand's disease. *J. Clin. Invest.* 50:244, 1971.

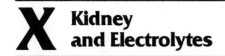

X Kidney
and Electrolytes

53

Diseases
of the Kidney

Norman G. Levinsky and William G. Couser

Tools of Renal Diagnosis

Accurate diagnosis of disorders of the kidney depends largely on the skillful and discriminating application of a variety of laboratory tests and other special diagnostic aids. A careful history and physical examination must, of course, be the starting point. These alone will often indicate the presence of renal disease and many times suggest the correct diagnosis. However, the existence, nature, and severity of kidney disease can rarely be definitively established without the use of at least some of the techniques listed here.

LABORATORY TESTS

Microscopic Examination of the Urinary Sediment. An essential part of the workup of every patient, the examination of the urinary sediment is without question the most valuable of all renal diagnostic procedures. Its usefulness depends on the care with which the urine specimen is obtained and the skill and experience of the analyst. The sediment examination, when properly done, provides a reliable screening test for the discovery of renal disease and is also an invaluable aid in differential diagnosis.

Bacteriologic Examination of the Urine. Bacterial infection of the urinary tract is recognized by the presence of bacteriuria. Bacteriuria is best diagnosed by the examination of a freshly voided, midstream urine specimen that has been collected with suitable precautions for avoiding contamination; catheterization is rarely needed to obtain a satisfactory specimen. The identification of bacteria on microscopic examination of the urine or the presence of a significant number of bacteria on quantitative culture usually indicates active infection. In clean, freshly voided specimens from male patients any bacterial count of 5,000 organisms per milliliter or greater is suspicious, and counts of 100,000 per milliliter or higher are usually considered diagnostic of infection. In female patients contamination of voided specimens is more

likely, and the criterion of significance is generally considered to be counts of 100,000 per milliliter or more. This subject is considered in more detail in the section dealing with urinary tract infections.

Measurement of Urinary Protein. Proteinuria (excretion of more than 0.150 gm of protein per day) is not always a feature of renal disease, nor is it necessarily pathognomonic of a kidney disorder, but the quantitative measurement of the total daily protein excretion is nevertheless of considerable help in diagnosis. Qualitative determination of the protein content of a single specimen on a scale of 0 to 4+ is of more limited value because of the dominant effect of urine flow rate on the results.

In general, heavy, continuous proteinuria (more than 4 gm per day) indicates a disease that diffusely increases glomerular permeability (e.g., glomerulonephritis, idiopathic nephrotic syndrome, or intercapillary glomerulosclerosis), although it should be remembered that these conditions may also produce more moderate degrees of proteinuria. Diseases that primarily involve the tubules or interstitial tissue (e.g., pyelonephritis or the nephropathies of hypercalcemia and potassium depletion) and those that do not primarily damage renal parenchyma (e.g., hydronephrosis) characteristically cause only minimal proteinuria (less than 0.5 gm per day) or may not increase protein excretion at all. Arteriosclerotic and hypertensive vascular disease of the kidney usually resemble this group of diseases in this respect, but in accelerated hypertension, ischemic damage of glomeruli may be severe and diffuse enough to produce heavy proteinuria. Intermittent proteinuria caused by emotional stress, physical exertion, or the assumption of the upright position is a common and usually benign phenomenon in healthy adolescents and young adults. However, intermittent excretion of protein — not necessarily related to posture — may also be seen during the course of those diseases that characteristically cause only slight proteinuria, and it sometimes also occurs in the healing or latent stages of glomerulonephritis.

Kidney Function Tests. Tests of kidney function are chiefly of use in the evaluation of the severity of renal disease and in following its progress. Although certain general patterns of dysfunction are sometimes associated with specific types of disease, functional tests are rarely of great help in differential diagnosis.

Glomerular filtration rate is best estimated in clinical practice by the endogenous creatinine clearance. Blood levels of creatinine are inversely related to the creatinine clearance and hence are a useful index of changes in glomerular filtration. Blood urea (or urea nitrogen) is not as reliable in this respect because it is significantly influenced by variations in the rate of urea production and by the state of hydration. The function of the countercurrent mechanisms in the renal medulla as well as the integrity of the collecting ducts is measured by the various tests of concentrating ability, but maximum urine concentration is also influenced by glomerular filtration rate, by diet, and, of course, by the integrity of the hypothalamic-neurohypophyseal system that regulates the synthesis and release of antidiuretic hormone.

In certain disorders initially limited to the medulla or the tubules (e.g., pyelonephritis or the nephropathies of hypercalcemia or potassium depletion), concentrating ability may be significantly impaired before there is any definite fall in creatinine clearance. Conversely, certain diseases that are at first largely confined to the glomeruli (e.g., acute glomerulonephritis) may cause a significant fall in creatinine clearance when concentrating ability is still relatively well preserved. However, the intimate anatomic and functional relation between glomeruli and tubules inevitably results in a nearly uniform reduction in all clinical function tests when renal disease advances, and even in the early stages of most diseases the functional tests are at best of limited diagnostic help.

ROENTGENOGRAPHIC EXAMINATION

Various roentgenographic techniques are available for the examination of the urinary system and are of great help in the recognition of certain types of renal disease. A plain film of the abdomen is useful in assessing the size and shape of the renal shadows and in identifying stones or nephrocalcinosis. Intravenous pyelography can give a more definitive picture of renal size and shape; provided renal function is not too

severely impaired, it also furnishes information about the anatomy of the pelvocalyceal system and the lower urinary tract. Even with moderate to advanced chronic renal insufficiency, the renal collecting system will usually be visualized adequately by the use of larger doses of intravenously administered contrast media and of nephrotomography. When intravenous urography is useless and x-ray films of the urinary tract are essential, the ureters may be catheterized and retrograde pyelography carried out. Cinefluoroscopic examination of the lower urinary tract during micturition (voiding cystourethrogram) is often valuable in diagnosing disorders of ureteral or bladder function that may be the cause of renal disease.

Renal angiography permits visualization of the arterial tree in the kidney and is particularly useful in identifying obstruction or narrowing of a major vessel. It is also helpful in the diagnosis of space-occupying lesions in the kidney, particularly in the differentiation of tumors and benign cysts.

The length of the normal kidney is between three and three and one-half times the distance between the upper ends of the second and third lumbar vertebral bodies. Slight symmetrical enlargement of the kidneys is seen in acute glomerulonephritis, the nephrotic syndrome, renal vein thrombosis, and in infiltrative diseases like leukemia or myeloma. More marked, often asymmetrical, enlargement is caused by hydronephrosis, polycystic disease, tumors, and cysts; also these latter conditions usually cause characteristic changes of the pelvocalyceal collecting system in the pyelogram. Slight and equal reduction in renal size is common in almost any diffuse bilateral disease leading to renal failure. Severe symmetrical contraction usually means chronic glomerulonephritis, bilateral hypoplasia, or chronic pyelonephritis. However, the hallmark of chronic pyelonephritis is irregular, bilaterally unequal, or unilateral contraction of the kidneys, with characteristic distortion of the pelvocalyceal system seen on pyelography. When renal disease is purely unilateral, contraction of one kidney is usually accompanied by enlargement of the contralateral healthy one.

RENAL BIOPSY

Percutaneous needle biopsy of the kidney often provides valuable diagnostic, prognostic, or therapeutic information at minimal risk to the patient. In most cases, the data from the history, physical examination, and the various diagnostic methods mentioned above are adequate for practical purposes. Since biopsy is not entirely free of the risk of hemorrhage and other complications, it cannot be recommended as a routine procedure. However, classification of glomerular diseases by histologic, immunofluorescent, and ultrastructural techniques has proved increasingly valuable for precise diagnosis and for determination of prognosis and treatment. Biopsies may also be of value in selected patients in whom the cause of renal insufficiency cannot be established by other means.

Renal Diseases
In the following pages the major medical diseases of the kidney are discussed briefly, with emphasis on their natural history and pathophysiology. An effort is also made to show how the tools of renal diagnosis just described can be used in differential diagnosis. Only the basic principles of treatment are considered. For a more detailed discussion the reader should consult the references at the end of this chapter.

ACUTE RENAL FAILURE
Acute renal failure is a general term for the sudden development of renal insufficiency due to any of a number of causes. Although in most cases oliguria (conventionally defined as the excretion of less than 300 to 400 ml of urine per day) or anuria is present, azotemia may sometimes develop rapidly despite normal urinary output.

Pathogenesis. The major causes of acute renal failure are listed below.

1. Renal circulatory failure (prerenal azotemia) due to factors such as fluid and electrolyte depletion, hemorrhage, myocardial failure, sepsis
2. Acute nonspecific renal failure (acute tubular necrosis or cortical necrosis)
   a. Subsequent to renal circulatory failure
   b. Toxins (carbon tetrachloride, heavy metals, certain antibiotics, and anesthetics)
   c. Intravascular hemolysis (mismatched trans-

fusion, etc.)
   d. Myoglobinuria (crush injuries, prolonged seizures, etc.)
   e. Burns
   f. Premature separation of the placenta
3. Other causes of primary renal injury
   a. Acute glomerulitis and vasculitis (glomerulonephritis, lupus erythematosus nephritis, periarteritis, etc.)
   b. Acute interstitial nephritis (severe diffuse pyelonephritis, papillary necrosis, drug-induced nephritis, etc.)
   c. Severe hypercalcemia
   d. Intratubular obstruction (sulfonamides, urates after cytotoxic drug therapy, myeloma protein after urogram)
4. Arterial or venous obstruction (embolism, thrombosis, aneurysm)
5. Obstruction (prostatism, bladder or cervical neoplasms, renal calculi, ureteral swelling after instrumentation, etc.)
6. Hepatorenal syndrome

Except as required for the discussion of differential diagnosis, this section will be limited to the first two categories listed above, renal circulatory failure (prerenal azotemia) and acute nonspecific renal failure. Some of the specific entities listed under primary renal injury are discussed elsewhere in this chapter. The hepatorenal syndrome is discussed in Chapter 41.

Reduced renal circulation due to fluid depletion, cardiovascular failure, and hypotension (prerenal azotemia) is a common cause of acute renal failure. Renal parenchymal integrity is preserved for a variable period of time, and restoration of normal circulation during this interval will return renal function to normal. At some point, renal damage may become self-perpetuating and renal insufficiency will persist despite restoration of the circulation. This type of acute renal failure is often called acute tubular necrosis, a term also applied to acute renal insufficiency induced by toxins, heme pigments, and a variety of other causes. In many cases, no definite cause can be determined. These types of acute renal failure are linked by the common clinical features described below. They probably also share pathogenic pathways to some extent. Although the cause of persistent renal insufficiency is unknown, current evidence indicates that persistent arteriolar vasoconstriction; tubular obstruction by epithelial cells, pigment, and proteinaceous casts; and back-leak of filtrate through damaged tubular epithelium all are important factors.

Pathologic Changes. In many cases of acute renal failure no definite changes are found in the kidneys; in others there are varying degrees of tubular necrosis characterized by disrupted, necrotic, or regenerating tubular epithelium; tubular casts; interstitial edema; and leukocytic infiltration. In postischemic renal failure, there is often a striking disparity between the severity of the functional loss and a relative paucity of anatomic changes. In tubular necrosis due to toxins, uniform destruction of a single segment, most often the proximal convoluted tubule, is usually noted. When tubular necrosis occurs after shock, hemolysis, trauma, and so forth, a spectrum of lesions may be seen. These may range from patchy focal necrosis of the tubular epithelium alone to cortical necrosis, in which the cortex is partially or totally infarcted and thrombosis of arterioles is noted.

Clinical Features. Acute renal failure (with or without the histologic changes of tubular necrosis) often develops in a setting of hypotension or extensive tissue trauma. This is particularly common postoperatively, after traumatic injuries and accidents, or after obstetrical hemorrhage. In some patients, especially in the elderly, transient hypotension of apparently minimal severity may be sufficient to cause acute renal failure. Increasingly, acute renal failure is due to drugs such as antibiotics, radiologic contrast media, and anesthetics prescribed by physicians. In many cases the precipitating event cannot be determined. Cortical necrosis is found in similar clinical circumstances but is especially frequent in pregnancy that has been complicated by toxemia, septic abortion, or uterine hemorrhage.

The clinical course of acute renal failure is usually divided into an oliguric and a diuretic phase. The oliguric phase may last from 2 days to 3 or 4 weeks. During this period, azotemia gradually increases, and

the clinical features of uremia, including nausea, vomiting, stupor, twitching, and so forth, gradually develop (see later in this chapter, under Uremia). In uncomplicated cases, blood urea nitrogen increases by about 10 to 20 mg per 100 ml per day, plasma potassium rises less than 0.5 mEq per day, and acidosis develops slowly. The rate at which azotemia, hyperkalemia, and acidosis progress is increased markedly if traumatized tissue, fever, infection, or other causes of increased catabolism are present. If water and sodium are not restricted, disturbances of water and sodium metabolism such as edema and hyponatremia may arise. Anemia develops gradually, and leukocytosis is frequently present. Moderate hypertension may occur, especially if fluid overloading is present. Congestive heart failure and pulmonary edema may develop; they are the result of excessive fluid intake and not of intrinsic myocardial disease. Infections are frequent and are the commonest cause of death in the oliguric phase of acute tubular necrosis.

Urine volume usually increases stepwise after the variable period of maximal oliguria; it may increase only to normal levels or to a diuretic phase. As urine volume rises, azotemia may continue to increase for a short time, but within a few days after the daily output exceeds 800 to 1,000 ml, the blood urea and creatinine levels begin to fall. In the diuretic state, urine volume may reach a maximum of several liters a day, especially if there has been significant positive fluid balance during the oliguric phase. In a minority of patients, a true polyuric phase may occur in which marked polyuria and sodium and potassium wasting require vigorous replacement therapy. The diuretic phase gradually wanes after days or weeks. Thereafter the kidney is completely healed, and for practical purposes, renal function may be considered normal.

It should be emphasized that although the foregoing is a description of the so-called typical clinical course of acute tubular necrosis, there is great variation in the duration and severity of the features described. Thus quite often azotemia may develop in the absence of definite oliguria (nonoliguric acute tubular necrosis). Furthermore, in several conditions such as cortical necrosis and acute glomerulonephritis with prolonged anuria, recovery of renal function is not to be expected, and the diuretic phase may never appear.

Diagnosis. The first step in the diagnosis of acute renal failure is to look for reversible or specifically treatable causes of acute renal failure, such as urinary tract obstruction, acute pyelonephritis, circulatory failure, or hypercalcemia. The urinary volume may be helpful in differential diagnosis. Most conditions causing acute renal failure result in oliguria, but not anuria; complete anuria suggests urinary tract obstruction, arterial infarction, or cortical necrosis, but it also occasionally occurs in acute glomerulitis. In most of the renal parenchymal causes of acute renal failure, daily urine output is either low but relatively constant or else gradually and progressively rising; relatively large and irregular variations in output suggest variable degrees of obstruction. It should be remembered, however, that partial urinary-tract obstruction may cause progressive azotemia despite normal or even increased urine volumes.

The examination of the urinary sediment is extremely valuable in establishing the cause of renal failure. In urinary tract obstruction, the sediment is scanty; occasional red cells, white cells, and hyaline or granular casts may be the only elements seen. Proteinuria is minimal. In the initial phases of acute renal failure due to shock and circulatory insufficiency, hyaline and granular casts in moderate numbers are present. If acute tubular necrosis or cortical necrosis develops, the sediment characteristically contains numerous renal epithelial cells, epithelial cell casts, and coarsely granular casts; occasionally, hemoglobin and red cell casts are seen, especially when intravascular hemolysis has occurred. Proteinuria is minimal or moderate. In acute glomerulonephritis and vasculitis, hematuria and red cell casts are the characteristic features. Protein excretion is usually moderate or heavy.

The urinary specific gravity and sodium concentration are especially helpful in distinguishing prerenal failure from acute tubular necrosis. In the former, specific gravity is usually over 1.020 and sodium concentration is less than 15 mEq per liter; in tubular necrosis, specific gravity is less than 1.018 and sodium more than 20 mEq per liter. (Lower sodium concen-

trations may occur in nonoliguric tubular necrosis.)

When the history, clinical features, and urinary findings are not sufficient to establish the diagnosis, renal biopsy may be indicated. Sometimes a plain x-ray film of the abdomen may be helpful by revealing kidney size or the presence of an obstructing stone. Retrograde ureteral catheterization should be performed without delay if the clinical circumstances suggest the possibility of obstruction.

Prognosis. Acute tubular necrosis is potentially completely reversible, whereas total cortical necrosis is irreversible. There is no clear demarcation between these conditions, but rather a spectrum from minimal tubular necrosis with transient oliguria through full-blown tubular necrosis with prolonged oliguria, through patchy cortical necrosis intermixed with areas of tubular necrosis, to complete, irreversible cortical necrosis. Since the clinical circumstances in which these conditions occur are similar and since even biopsy may be misleading in patchy disease, the prognosis must be determined on clinical grounds. Oliguria continuing for more than 4 weeks suggests irreversible disease such as cortical necrosis, but occasional instances of tubular necrosis with recovery after even longer periods of oliguria have been reported. In acute glomerulonephritis in adults, anuria or severe oliguria persisting for more than a few days usually indicates severe disease with an acute or subacute irreversible course.

Treatment. Patients with brief, uncomplicated acute renal failure can often be managed by conservative therapy alone. Fluid intake should be restricted to a volume equivalent to urine output plus extrarenal losses, including an allowance of 300 to 400 ml per day for basal insensible loss.

To avoid overhydration, it is usually advisable to adjust intake so that the patient will lose 100 to 200 gm of weight per day. The use of sodium, potassium, and protein is not permitted. Caloric requirements are met by giving at least 150 gm of carbohydrate in the daily allotment of fluid. This can be given orally or as an intravenous hypertonic glucose solution if nausea or vomiting interferes with oral intake. Infections can be prevented by avoiding inlying venous or urethral catheters. Hyperkalemia can be controlled by infusions of glucose and ion-exchange resins. Although conservative measures may suffice for a few days, patients with persistent renal failure are best managed with peritoneal dialysis or hemodialysis. Early dialysis is also beneficial in patients with increased catabolism and rapidly developing uremia. Dialysis increases the patient's well-being by controlling uremic symptoms and permitting liberalized food and fluid intake. With appropriate management, death from fluid overloading and electrolyte imbalance should not occur. However, about half the patients with acute renal failure do die, largely from superimposed infections or from complications of their underlying diseases.

Prevention. Acute renal failure can be prevented in many cases, for example, by maintaining normal fluid balance and blood pressure during and after surgery, by supporting plasma volume in burned patients with infusions, and by avoiding nephrotoxic antibiotics. It has been suggested that infusion of mannitol or of potent diuretics such as furosemide may prevent or even reverse acute renal failure, if administered soon after oliguria develops. Although some support for this view is available in uncontrolled clinical studies, evidence for the efficacy of these agents in treating acute tubular necrosis is not conclusive.

Glomerular Diseases

Despite the availability of hemodialysis and renal transplantation, chronic renal failure still represents a major cause of death and disability in the young adult. Sixty to seventy percent of patients with chronic renal failure have some form of glomerular disease. The past two decades have witnessed significant advances in understanding the pathogenesis of glomerular diseases due in large part to three developments: the widespread application of percutaneous renal biopsy as a diagnostic tool in the evaluation of renal diseases, the development of experimental animal models that resemble the diseases seen in man, and the routine application of immunofluorescent and electron microscopic techniques to study human biopsy material in the light of known mechanisms defined in animal models. With these techniques

glomerular diseases can now be classified more precisely in terms of etiology, pathogenesis, and prognosis than was ever possible in the past using clinical and light microscopic features alone. As the understanding of glomerular diseases has rapidly expanded, some confusion in terminology has inevitably resulted. Several classifications are in use based on clinical features, pathogenic mechanisms, or histopathology. This discussion will concentrate on the clinical features and pathogenesis of the major currently recognized glomerular diseases. The renal manifestations of certain systemic diseases with glomerular lesions mediated by similar mechanisms will be discussed as well. Rare diseases and lesions reflecting renal involvement by systemic hereditary or metabolic disorders (e.g., diabetes, amyloid) are mentioned for completeness but are dealt with in more detail elsewhere in the text.

PATHOGENESIS OF GLOMERULAR DISEASES
Most glomerular diseases are now believed to be mediated by deposition within the glomerulus either of antibody directed against antigenic constituents of the glomerular basement membrane itself *(anti-GBM nephritis),* or of circulating soluble immune complexes *(immune complex nephritis).*

Anti-GBM Nephritis. Four to eight percent of cases of glomerulonephritis in man are mediated by anti-GBM antibody. Most such cases present as a severe, acute rapidly progressive glomerulonephritis (RPGN). Anti-GBM nephritis associated with hemorrhagic pneumonitis is called Goodpasture's syndrome (see later). Anti-GBM antibody-mediated lesions are usually characterized by extensive epithelial cell crescent formation as seen under light microscopy and by the presence of IgG anti-GBM antibody and sometimes complement deposited in a linear pattern along the glomerular basement membrane as seen under immunofluorescence microscopy. What causes a patient to initiate production of antibody to his own glomerular basement membrane is not known.

Immune Complex Nephritis. Most cases of human glomerulonephritis now appear to be consequent to deposition within the glomerulus of immunoglobulin in the form of immune complexes. Immune complex

Date_____

TO: _____

FROM: Peg N. Kruk/Hoop

/ / For your information.

/ / For your information - Please comment.

/ / Please xerox _____copies, and
      return to me.

/ / Please make _____copies, and
      mail out original.

/ / Please mail out - NO COPIES.

/ / Please make _____copies, forward
      copies to those designated, and
      mail out original.

/ / Please type envelope and mail out.

/ / Send to:_____

      _____

      _____

COMMENTS:_____

_____

_____

Thank you.

nephritis is recognized immunopathologically by the presence of discrete deposits of immunoglobulin and usually of complement in a granular, "lumpy-bumpy" pattern as seen by fluorescence microscopy. The localization of these deposits can be more precisely defined by electron microscopy. Although the antigenic component of such complexes, that is, the agent inciting the disease, is usually not identifiable in a particular patient, both exogenous antigens (bacterial, viral, protozoal, foreign proteins, drugs) and endogenous "self" antigens (DNA, tumor antigens) have been found to induce formation of pathogenic immune complexes. Glomerular immune complex deposition leads to a spectrum of clinical and pathologic findings ranging from acute crescentic glomerulonephritis to chronic membranous nephropathy with nephrotic syndrome. The type of lesion produced depends on several factors, the predominant ones being the intraglomerular site of complex deposition and the quantity of deposited complexes. Low-molecular-weight immune complexes formed in slight antigen excess tend to deposit on the basement membrane and cause more severe disease than complexes of higher molecular weight formed in antibody excess, which deposit predominantly in the glomerular mesangium and cause less capillary wall damage. Understanding of these concepts may become relevant to the therapy of immunologically mediated glomerular diseases, since treatment that reduces antibody production may alter complex size and localization in ways that increase rather than diminish the severity of the disease.

Mediation of Immunologic Renal Injury. Deposition of immunoglobulins within the glomerulus results in tissue injury by activation of mediator mechanisms. Identification of these mechanisms provides additional points for potential therapeutic intervention. In addition to immunoglobulins, the best defined mechanism involved in the mediation of glomerular injury is the complement system. Activation of the complement system by immunoglobulin, either directly, starting with the C1 components, or through the alternate complement pathway starting at C3, generates leukotactic factors that attract polymorphonuclear leukocytes to the site of immune reaction. Interaction of the polymorphs with immunoglobulin

deposits within the glomerulus results in local release of proteolytic lysosomal enzymes that directly damage the capillary basement membrane and lead to proteinuria, hematuria, and the clinical features of acute glomerulonephritis. In other cases, the immunoglobulin deposits may not be functionally capable of complement activation and polymorphs are not part of the glomerular pathology, which suggests that antibody may also mediate tissue damage by mechanisms currently undefined that are independent of complement and polymorphonuclear leukocytes.

Severe glomerular injury is usually associated with epithelial cell proliferation and so-called crescent formation within the glomerulus. The formation of crescents has been shown to result from leakage of fibrin from the capillary into the Bowman capsule.

An association has been noted between the presence of cold-precipitable globulins (cryoglobulins) and some glomerular diseases. The disease mixed essential cryoglobulinemia is often associated with vasculitis and severe glomerulonephritis with glomerular deposits of the immune complex type. Cryoglobulins are also frequently present in other immunologically mediated diseases such as poststreptococcal nephritis and the nephritis of systemic lupus erythematosus (SLE), and the levels may correlate with the activity and severity of renal disease.

Prior release of vasoactive amines (histamine, serotonin) mediated by interaction of antigen with sensitized cells coated with specific IgE antibodies apparently facilitates the deposition of immune complexes in glomerular capillary walls. No role for cell-mediated immunity (delayed hypersensitivity) in the pathogenesis of glomerular diseases has yet been established.

PRINCIPAL DISEASES CAUSING
ACUTE GLOMERULONEPHRITIS
The diseases most commonly presenting as acute glomerulonephritis and their most frequent clinical and pathologic features are summarized in Table 53-1 and described in more detail below.

Poststreptococcal Glomerulonephritis
(Postinfectious Glomerulonephritis)
Although glomerulonephritis may follow exposure to several infectious agents, the nephritis that develops after a 1- to 3-week latent period following group A beta-hemolytic streptococcal infection represents the

Table 53-1. Summary of Diseases Causing Acute Glomerulonephritis[a]

Glomerular disease	Common clinical and laboratory findings	Renal pathology[b]
Poststreptococcal glomerulonephritis (GN)	2:1 male-female; 1- to 3-week latent period; ↑ BP; proteinuria, hematuria, edema; ↑ ASO titer; ↓ C3-C9, ± C1, 4, 2; usually ↑ BUN and creatinine; 95% resolve, 5% progress rapidly	LM: diffuse proliferation, poly-morphs IF: coarsely granular IgG and C3 EM: subepithelial "humps"
Rapidly progressive glomerulonephritis (RPGN)		
Idiopathic	Acute, oliguric, azotemic GN; male-female; ± BP, C3, ASO, ANA; no lung disease; irreversible renal failure	LM: over 50 percent crescents IF: IgG linear (1/3), granular (1/3), negative (1/3) EM: no deposits if linear IF
Goodpasture's syndrome	As in RPGN, but 4:1 young male-female; hemorrhagic pneumonitis, iron deficiency anemia	LM: changes may be focal early IF: linear IgG in 100%, C3 in 50% EM: no deposits
Focal glomerulonephritis		
IgG-IgA nephropathy	Recurrent macroscopic hematuria 1 to 3 days after upper respiratory infection; ± BP, C3, ASO, BUN; ↑ IgA; 10 to 20% progress to renal failure	LM: focal proliferation IF: mesangial IgA, IgG, C3 EM: mesangial deposits
Henoch-Schönlein purpura	As above, with skin, joint, and gastrointestinal involvement; 10 to 20% RPGN; focal form rarely progresses	As above, fibrin deposits prominent
Chronic glomerulonephritis	Chronic renal failure, small kidneys, ↑ BP	End-stage kidney

[a]Excludes nephritis of systemic lupus erythematosus.
[b]LM, IF, and EM = light, immunofluorescent, and electron microscopy.

prototype of acute glomerulonephritis. It generally presents with hypertension, mild edema, either dark urine or gross hematuria, proteinuria, and red cell casts. The disease is commonest in older children with an almost 2:1 predominance in males, but it can occur in any age group. The severity ranges from attacks presenting with all the above features and also oliguric renal failure and hypertensive encephalopathy, to subclinical cases detectable only by careful urinalysis. The latter form is especially common in epidemics. Malaise and abdominal pain are other commonly associated symptoms. About 20 percent of patients with severe, acute disease and azotemia manifest a transient nephrotic syndrome.

Associated laboratory features in poststreptococcal nephritis include a marked lowering in total serum complement, reflecting a reduction in C3 and late-reacting complement components, with C1, C4, and C2 usually remaining normal; elevations in titers of antibodies to antistreptolysin O and other streptococcal antigens (hyaluronidase, streptokinase); and usually a reduction in renal function with mild anemia.

In contrast to acute rheumatic fever, the infection preceding glomerulonephritis must be with a nephritogenic strain of streptococcus, most commonly M type 12, although several other types have also been associated with this disease. The attack rate for glomerulonephritis in patients with streptococcal infection varies widely from about 5 percent in sporadic cases to over 50 percent in some epidemics. In contrast to rheumatic fever, early penicillin therapy probably does not reduce the incidence of glomerulonephritis, whereas the risks of subsequent prophylaxis generally exceed the risks of a second infection with a nephritogenic strain of streptococcus.

Pathology and Pathogenesis. Streptococcal nephritis produces a diffuse proliferative glomerulonephritis by light microscopy with an increase in mesangial cells, a polymorphonuclear leukocytic exudate and, depending on the severity, variable numbers of epithelial cell crescents. Immunofluorescence microscopy shows coarsely granular deposits of IgG and C3 along the basement membrane, and electron microscopy reveals characteristic subepithelial, electron-dense "humps."

The disease is believed to be mediated by deposition of immune complexes containing some antigenic component of the streptococcus and specific antibody to it. It is thus presumably analogous to acute serum sickness, in which a brief antigenic exposure leads to antibody production, resulting in immune elimination of circulating antigen as well as glomerular immune complex deposition.

Edema is believed to reflect the renal retention of salt and water due to an acute decrease in filtration rate with well-preserved tubular function, while hypertension reflects fluid volume overload, possibly exacerbated by activation of the renin-angiotensin system.

Course and Prognosis. The prognosis of poststreptococcal glomerulonephritis is a subject of continuing controversy. About 5 percent of patients sustain glomerular damage so severe that renal function does not recover following the acute episode, and they have a course similar to that of rapidly progressive glomerulonephritis, developing end-stage renal failure in a few months to 1 to 2 years. This course is most frequent in older patients and in those with severe loss of renal function, persistent reductions in serum complement, the nephrotic syndrome, and extensive crescent formation on initial biopsy. No specific therapy has been shown to reduce the incidence or to alter the course of the disease; hence only symptomatic therapy is indicated.

It is generally accepted that 95 percent or more of patients recover spontaneously from the acute episode and have a return of renal function and serum complement to normal within 3 to 6 weeks without specific therapy. Long-term follow-up studies reveal some evidence of renal dysfunction in up to 50 percent of such patients, including slight proteinuria, decreased inulin clearance, mild hypertension, and morphologic changes on biopsy. Whether these abnormalities represent early stages of progressive renal disease or are simply persistent residua of the previous acute nephritis is not yet clear. At the present time, it appears that the development of chronic renal failure several years after recovery from acute poststreptococcal glomerulonephritis is a rare, though possible, event.

*Rapidly Progressive Glomerulonephritis
(Crescentic Glomerulonephritis)*

The term *rapidly progressive glomerulonephritis* (RPGN) may be applied to severe nephritis associated with several diseases, including streptococcal nephritis, Henoch-Schönlein purpura, SLE, Wegener's granulomatosis, polyarteritis nodosa, and Goodpasture's syndrome (see later). In many cases the disease is idiopathic and involves only the kidney. In all cases biopsies reveal crescent formation in more than 50 percent of the glomeruli. The idiopathic variety of RPGN affects adult men and women with equal frequency. The clinical abnormalities are insidious in onset, as the disease is not preceded by any identifiable inciting event. The patient's complaints are nonspecific ones of malaise, nausea, loin pain, and often a decrease in urine output. Urinalysis is consistent with severe glomerular inflammation, showing proteinuria, red cells, and red cell casts. Oliguria or anuria may be established at the time of presentation, and mild anemia and eosinophilia are common features. Serum complement levels, antistreptolysin O titers, antinuclear antibodies, and lupus erythematosus cell preparations are normal (or negative). Hypertension and edema are usually absent, and proteinuria in the nephrotic range is uncommon. Kidney size as seen by intravenous pyelogram is normal. The natural history of RPGN from the onset of clinical symptoms to end-stage renal failure is usually one of days to weeks, although occasional spontaneous recoveries occur.

Pathology and Pathogenesis. The hallmark of RPGN is the presence of cellular crescent formation in more than 50 percent of the glomeruli. Glomerular involvement is usually diffuse, with necrosis, fibrin deposits, and a prominent polymorphonuclear leukocytic exudate. Immunofluorescence microscopy reveals linear staining for IgG anti-GBM antibody deposits in the glomeruli of about one-third of the patients, usually accompanied by complement. Circulating antibodies reactive with glomerular basement membrane can usually be demonstrated in such cases by immunofluorescence or radioimmunoassay. Electron microscopic changes are nonspecific, since anti-GBM antibody deposits cannot be seen ultrastructurally.

Another one-third of patients exhibit granular staining for presumed immune complexes, while the remainder have nonspecific or negative immunofluorescence.

Course, Prognosis, and Therapy. In contrast to the high incidence of recovery in oliguric poststreptococcal nephritis with renal failure, most patients with RPGN pursue an inexorable course to irreversible renal failure irrespective of the underlying pathogenic mechanism. At present, no form of therapy, including steroids, immunosuppressive agents, and anticoagulants, has been shown to be of consistent benefit (see Goodpasture's Syndrome, below).

Renal transplantation carried out in the presence of circulating anti-GBM antibody may result in an immediate, severe recurrent nephritis in the transplant.

Goodpasture's Syndrome

Goodpasture's syndrome is a relatively uncommon disease affecting predominantly young men (3 to 4:1) usually between 15 and 40 years of age. The characteristic clinical picture of hemoptysis with pulmonary infiltrates, iron deficiency anemia, and severe glomerulonephritis may develop slowly. Patients often present with hemoptysis, cough, and shortness of breath before significant renal involvement is apparent. Initial urinalysis may reveal only hematuria, but rapid progression of the renal lesion with proteinuria, casts, and renal failure is invariable. The course of the renal disease is indistinguishable from that described for RPGN, and the glomerular lesion is mediated by anti-GBM antibody deposition. The anemia reflects intraalveolar pulmonary hemorrhage, which may wax and wane. Up to one-third of patients with Goodpasture's syndrome die of severe pulmonary disease. As in RPGN, hypertension is usually not prominent, nephrotic syndrome is uncommon, and serum complement levels and other serologic studies are normal. Renal biopsy in the early stages may reveal a focal proliferative glomerulonephritis, but usually this progresses to diffuse involvement with extensive crescent formation.

Immunofluorescence reveals linear staining for IgG in all glomeruli accompanied by complement deposits in about 50 percent of patients. Anti-GBM antibodies are demonstrable in the serum of most patients with Goodpasture's syndrome.

Although no specific therapy has been consistently shown to benefit the renal disease, the pulmonary lesions on occasion may respond to steroids. Plasma exchange combined with steroids and cytotoxic drug therapy has reduced circulating antibody levels and has been of benefit to the renal and pulmonary lesions in a few patients.

Focal Glomerulonephritis

In focal glomerulonephritis histologic inflammatory changes are present in some glomeruli, while others are entirely spared; often only some segments of a given glomerulus are involved while the adjacent capillary loops are normal. All the following diseases may produce the histologic picture of focal nephritis:

1. Systemic lupus erythematosus
2. Polyarteritis nodosa
3. Goodpasture's syndrome
4. Wegener's granulomatosis
5. Subacute bacterial endocarditis
6. Henoch-Schönlein purpura
7. IgG-IgA nephropathy (Berger's disease)

Although focal changes in some diseases represent early lesions that progress to diffuse nephritis (Goodpasture's syndrome), the focal lesion itself is generally associated with a favorable prognosis. Lupus (SLE) nephritis is often focal and will be discussed later in this chapter. Two diseases commonly causing focal nephritis and exhibiting similar clinical and renal immunopathologic features are described below.

IgG-IgA Nephropathy ("Benign" Recurrent Hematuria, Berger's Disease)

IgG-IgA nephropathy accounts for up to 20 percent of cases of acute glomerulonephritis in adults, affecting predominantly men between ages 16 and 35. Such patients present with gross hematuria, usually associated with an upper respiratory tract infection. In contrast to poststreptococcal nephritis, the hematuria appears the day of, or 1 or 2 days after, the infection. Hypertension and edema are usually absent, proteinuria is generally minimal (less than 1 gm per day), and renal function and serum complement are normal. Serum IgA levels may be elevated. There is no associated systemic disease. Although the preceding respiratory infection can be streptococcal, it is usually viral. Forty percent of patients have only one episode of gross hematuria, which generally lasts 2 to 5 days, but another 30 percent have hematuria that recurs several times per year. Microscopic hematuria with red cell casts often persists between attacks.

Pathology and Pathogenesis. Renal biopsy in patients with IgG-IgA nephropathy reveals focal nephritis by light microscopy in more than 80 percent of cases. A characteristic finding by immunofluorescence is the glomerular deposition of immunoglobulin, predominantly IgA, within the mesangium rather than on the basement membrane and involving all glomeruli including those that appear normal by light microscopy. Although the pathogenesis of this disease is not understood, it is believed to represent a consequence of mesangial deposition of immune complexes containing IgA as either the antigen or the antibody along with complement.

Course. Most patients with IgG-IgA nephropathy maintain normal renal function for years, although recurrent hematuria may persist. About 25 percent of patients suffer a progressive loss of renal function over several years, often associated with the appearance of hypertension. At present, no clinical or pathologic criteria allow accurate prediction of which patients will experience progressive disease, but significant proteinuria and diffuse proliferative changes on biopsy are regarded as poor prognostic signs. No form of therapy has been shown to be of benefit. Recognition of this disease is of some clinical importance, since it has been shown to recur frequently when such patients undergo renal transplantation.

Henoch-Schönlein (Anaphylactoid) Purpura

The nephritis associated with Henoch-Schönlein purpura reflects renal involvement by a generalized vasculitis with other clinical manifestations in the skin (purpura, 100 percent), joints (arthritis and edema, 80 percent), and gastrointestinal tract (abdominal pain, melena, 40 to 50 percent). Although the syndrome is more common in the pediatric age group, its occurrence in adults is well documented. The incidence of significant clinical renal involvement is about 50 percent, with histologic abnormalities present in over 75 percent of cases. About 10 percent of children and up to 25 percent of adults have a diffuse proliferative glomerulonephritis with crescents and a course similar to that described above for RPGN. The remaining patients manifest a more benign form of acute nephritis, with hematuria and mild proteinuria as the major clinical findings. Hypertension and edema are less common, and serologies and complement levels are normal. The acute nephritis usually develops within a month of the onset of the syndrome and resolves within 4 to 6 weeks. The persistence of microscopic hematuria and a recurrence of urinary abnormalities over a period of years without significant loss of renal function, as well as the finding of focal nephritis with mesangial deposition of IgA, are clinical and pathologic features common to both Henoch-Schönlein and IgG-IgA nephropathies and suggest that the renal lesions in these two diseases may be mediated by similar mechanisms.

Steroid therapy may benefit other systems involved in this disease, but it has little demonstrable beneficial effect on the nephritis.

Idiopathic Hematuria
Although the frequency of recurrent macroscopic hematuria as a clinical manifestation of focal or mesangial immune complex nephritis has been noted above, it should be stressed that not all patients with recurrent hematuria will have this type of lesion. Hematuria may be the presenting sign of various lesions of the kidneys and urinary tract, including infection, papillary necrosis, polycystic and medullary sponge kidneys, renal stones, atheroembolic disease, malignancies, blood dyscrasias, and hemoglobinopathies, all of which should be carefully excluded by appropriate laboratory and radiologic procedures. Up to one-third of all patients with idiopathic hematuria determined to be of renal parenchymal origin by the presence of red cell casts will have biopsies that are entirely normal by light, fluorescence, and electron microscopy. These patients generally have minimal or no proteinuria and a benign course. Another 10 percent will have more severe glomerular lesions, including diffuse proliferative and membranoproliferative glomerulonephritis and focal glomerular sclerosis (see below). The remainder have some form of focal nephritis. After careful general medical and urologic evaluations have excluded other nonglomerular sources of the hematuria, renal biopsy for diagnostic and prognostic purposes is indicated, particularly in patients with additional clinical findings such as casts in the urine sediment, proteinuria, hypertension, or a decrease in renal function.

Chronic Glomerulonephritis
Chronic glomerulonephritis is the term applied to end-stage kidney disease resulting from glomerular lesions that have progressed to the point at which currently available clinical, laboratory, and pathologic techniques cannot classify the original disease. The possibility that in rare cases chronic glomerulonephritis may evolve in patients whose initial disease was acute poststreptococcal glomerulonephritis has been discussed above. It is clear that most patients with other glomerular lesions, including rapidly progressive glomerulonephritis, membranous nephropathy, focal glomerular sclerosis, and membranoproliferative glomerulonephritis, as well as some patients with focal glomerulonephritis, regularly progress to chronic glomerulonephritis with renal failure. However, most patients with chronic glomerulonephritis present with end-stage kidney disease without any past history of acute nephritis or other renal disease. Such patients are usually hypertensive with bilaterally small kidneys, variable degrees of proteinuria, and urinary sediment abnormalities, including red cells; white cells; hyaline casts; granular casts; and numerous broad, waxy casts (renal failure casts). Although in each patient potentially reversible causes of decreased renal function such as salt and fluid volume depletion and urinary tract obstruction and infection must be excluded, no specific therapy is available for the renal disease itself. These patients are managed conservatively for chronic renal failure and are usually candidates for long-term hemodialysis and renal transplantation.

NEPHROTIC SYNDROME

The nephrotic syndrome is a clinical condition caused by several different diseases whose major renal manifestation is an increase in glomerular permeability to serum proteins. The classification of glomerular diseases into those causing nephritis and those causing nephrotic syndrome is an arbitrary one, since proteinuria is a feature of all glomerular diseases. Among the diseases discussed above, however, nephrotic syndrome is relatively uncommon, less severe, and signs of glomerular inflammation predominate over those of altered permeability. In the nephropathies discussed in this section the nephrotic syndrome is the usual presenting feature and major clinical manifestation.

The causes of nephrotic syndrome are multiple and include immunologic mechanisms such as immune complex deposition (SLE nephritis), biochemical abnormalities of the basement membrane (diabetic nephropathy), infiltrative diseases (amyloid), congenital and hereditary defects in glomerular function (congenital and hereditary nephrosis), direct toxic effects (heavy metals, various drugs), and mechanisms that remain undefined (lipoid nephrosis). About one-third of American adults with nephrotic syndrome have some underlying systemic disease, the most common being diabetes, SLE, and amyloidosis. Two-thirds of adults (and 80 to 90 percent of children) have an idiopathic nephrotic syndrome due to a primary renal lesion. Clinical features alone cannot differentiate the diseases causing idiopathic nephrotic syndrome, and renal biopsy is routinely employed to provide a specific diagnosis. Although prognosis and response to therapy are clearly dependent on the underlying cause of the nephrotic syndrome, the pathophysiology is much the same in all patients.

Definition and Pathophysiology. The hallmark of nephrotic syndrome is heavy proteinuria, usually greater than 3.5 gm/1.73 square meter/day in adults and 40 mg/square meter/hour in overnight collections in children. These figures are obviously arbitrary, since either early or resolving states of diseases causing the nephrotic syndrome may result in lesser degrees of proteinuria. The other clinical signs of nephrotic syndrome are consequent to the proteinuria and include a lowered serum albumin (less than 3.0 gm

per 100 ml), edema, hyperlipidemia (serum cholesterol greater than 300 mg per 100 ml) and lipiduria. The presence of these associated features of the nephrotic syndrome depends largely on the severity and duration of proteinuria.

Proteinuria, which can reach levels of 30 to 40 gm per day, reflects an increase in the permeability of the glomerular capillary wall to serum proteins. Glomerular capillary permeability is determined by several factors, including the integrity of the capillary wall itself, glomerular hemodynamic factors, and the net negative charge on the capillary wall that is conferred largely by the sialoprotein coating of epithelial cells and slit pore regions. In some noninflammatory diseases of the glomerular capillary wall (lipoid nephrosis) the urine protein is composed largely of albumin, and thus proteinuria is said to be selective. Diseases associated with inflammatory changes of the basement membrane itself are accompanied by urinary excretion of all classes of serum protein, or nonselective proteinuria.

Hypoalbuminemia, which may be as low as 0.5 gm per 100 ml in patients with severe nephrotic syndrome, reflects primarily the loss of albumin in the urine. Edema ranges from mild peripheral edema to generalized anasarca and results from reduced plasma oncotic pressure due to the lowered albumin concentration. This in turn leads to contraction of plasma volume and renal retention of salt and water through activation of the renin-angiotensin-aldosterone system and probably other as yet undefined mechanisms. Plasma volume contraction can be clinically significant in the nephrotic patient, who may exhibit postural hypotension and even circulatory collapse with oliguric renal failure. Mild elevations in blood urea nitrogen and serum creatinine in nephrotic patients often reflect decreased renal perfusion due to hypovolemia rather than progression of the underlying renal disease, and this must be kept in mind in the management of these patients.

Hyperlipidemia is due to an increase in all major lipid fractions, including triglycerides, free and esterified cholesterol, and phospholipids, and it is believed to reflect an increase in hepatic lipoprotein synthesis that accompanies the increase in synthesis of albumin. The degree of hyperlipidemia is quite variable, but it may be sufficient to give fasting plasma a milky appearance. Nephrotic patients with persistent hyperlipidemia have been shown to have an increased incidence of atherosclerotic disease. Lipiduria parallels more closely urine protein excretion than serum lipid levels and includes fat droplets, either free or incorporated into fatty casts that have a characteristic Maltese cross pattern under polarized light, and oval fat bodies, which are degenerating renal epithelial cells swollen with fat globules.

Serum levels of immunoglobulins, particularly IgG and IgA, tend to be low in the nephrotic syndrome, probably contributing to the significantly increased risk of infection. Nephrotic syndrome is also a hypercoagulable state, in part reflecting increased levels of platelets and some clotting factors resulting from mechanisms similar to those causing hyperlipidemia. Thromboembolic phenomena are common both as complications and as causes of death in patients with uncontrolled nephrosis.

The use of steroid and immunosuppressive therapy in patients with nephrotic syndrome is covered in the discussions of specific diseases below. Symptomatic therapy includes judicious use of diuretics and salt restriction for edema and increased protein and calorie intake to compensate for urinary losses if there is no concurrent renal failure. Because of its rapid and virtually quantitative excretion in the urine, intravenous albumin is of little benefit in severe nephrosis except for the short-term restoration of intravascular volume prior to surgical procedures, including renal biopsy.

PRINCIPAL DISEASES CAUSING NEPHROTIC SYNDROME

The major clinical and pathologic features and the approximate frequency of the diseases causing idiopathic nephrotic syndrome in children and adults are summarized in Table 53-2.

Lipoid Nephrosis (Minimal Change Disease)

Lipoid nephrosis is most common in children and accounts for about 80 percent of the cases of childhood nephrosis, as compared with 15 to 20 percent of the cases of idiopathic nephrotic syndrome in adults. Proteinuria is often severe and may be either insidious or abrupt in onset, usually without any definable inciting event. Blood pressure is either normal or low, and the clinical and laboratory findings are those described for nephrotic syndrome in general. Serum complement levels and serologies are usually normal, and IgM and IgE levels may be elevated. The kidneys are either normal in size or somewhat enlarged.

Pathology. Light microscopy of renal biopsy material reveals no significant changes and no immune deposits in lipoid nephrosis. Diffuse fusion of the epithelial cell foot processes with a normal basement membrane is seen by electron microscopy.

Course and Treatment. The pathogenesis of lipoid nephrosis is not known. There is no evidence that it is mediated by currently recognized immune mechanisms. Since there is no glomerular destruction, the disease does not progress to renal failure. Prognosis relates entirely to the course and complications of the nephrotic syndrome. Death, when it occurs, is usually a consequence of either infection or thromboembolic phenomena. Spontaneous remissions have been reported in up to 40 percent of patients and have been noted to follow some viral infections, especially measles.

Of all renal lesions, lipoid nephrosis is the most responsive to therapy with corticosteroids. About 90 percent of patients with lipoid nephrosis will respond within 2 months to adequate steroid therapy, and their proteinuria will disappear. Nonresponders have usually been those with focal sclerotic changes as seen on biopsy, and they may have a different disease (see below). Although over half of steroid-responsive patients later relapse or become steroid-dependent, long-term remissions can be induced in more than 75 percent of younger patients by appropriate use of steroid therapy alone. The addition of cytotoxic agents, including cyclophosphamide or chlorambucil, reduces the frequency of relapses and effects longer remissions in selected patients, but these potential benefits must be carefully weighed against the gonadal toxicity and mutagenic potential of these drugs.

Table 53-2. Summary of Principal Causes of Idiopathic Nephrotic Syndrome[a]

| Glomerular disease | Approximate frequency (percent) | | Clinical and laboratory findings | Renal pathology[b] |
	Children	Adults		
Lipoid nephrosis	75	20	Heavy proteinuria, ↓ albumin, ↑ cholesterol, edema, ↓ IgG, ↑ IgM; normal ASO, C3, ANA, BP; steroid-sensitive, nonprogressive	LM: normal IF: negative EM: diffuse foot process fusion
Focal glomerular sclerosis	10	10	As above with hematuria, early ↑ BP, steroid-resistant, progressive	LM: juxta-medullary sclerotic lesions IF: IgM plus C3 in sclerotic lesions EM: diffuse foot process fusion
Membranous nephropathy	2	50	Nephrotic syndrome as above; BP, ASO, C3, ANA normal; slowly progressive; renal vein thrombosis and cancer associated	LM: early normal, late GBM thickening and "spikes" IF: granular IgG and C3 on GBM EM: diffuse subepithelial electron-dense deposits
Membranoproliferative glomerulonephritis	10	10	Nephrotic syndrome, young females, ↓ C3–C9, 1/3 nephritic, ↑ BP, slowly progressive	LM: ↑ GBM and mesangial cells, lobulation, "tram-tracks" IF: granular C3 EM: subendothelial deposits or "dense-deposit disease"
Proliferative glomerulonephritis	3	10	See Table 53-1	See Table 53-1

[a]Excludes nephritis of systemic lupus erythematosus, diabetes, and amyloid.
[b]LM, IF, and EM = light, immunofluorescent, and electron microscopy.

Focal Sclerosing Glomerulopathy

In contrast to the steroid-responsive and nonprogressive nature of lipoid nephrosis, another apparently identical clinical syndrome responds poorly to steroids and goes on to progressive renal failure. The pathologic correlate of this clinical course is the development of focal sclerotic lesions in one or more lobules of some glomeruli near the juxtamedullary junction. These sclerotic lesions contain deposits of IgM and C3 as seen by fluorescence microscopy, but in all other respects the pathologic findings in noninvolved capillary loops and glomeruli are identical to those in lipoid nephrosis. Because the focal sclerosing glomerulopathy lesion initially involves only juxtamedullary glomeruli, deep in the renal cortex, it is easily missed on needle biopsy. There is much controversy about whether focal sclerosis is a progressive lesion that develops in some patients with lipoid nephrosis or is an entirely separate disease. Because of its unique clinical and histologic features, the disease is treated here as a separate entity.

Although the exact prevalence is difficult to determine because the diagnosis rests heavily on the site from which the biopsy specimen was obtained and how extensively it is examined, focal sclerosis is probably present in about 10 percent of children and up to 50 percent of adults with the idiopathic nephrotic syndrome and the biopsy findings of minimal change disease in most glomeruli. Most cases of focal sclerosing glomerulopathy are resistant to steroids. Progression to renal failure accompanies the extension of sclerotic changes to involve more superficial glomeruli and may take place within a few months or slowly over several years. In addition to steroid resistance, the presence of an unusual amount of hematuria and early hypertension are additional clinical features suggesting focal sclerosis in a patient with idiopathic nephrosis. Early recognition of focal sclerosis is important because of its poor response to steroid therapy, its unfavorable prognosis, and its tendency to recur promptly in some patients receiving renal transplants. Although the pathogenesis of this disease, like that of lipoid nephrosis, is entirely unknown, the observations in patients with renal transplants suggest the presence of some as yet unidentified circulating factor, probably not an immunoglobulin, that mediates the marked increase in glomerular basement membrane permeability seen after transplantation.

Membranous Glomerulonephropathy (Membranous Nephropathy)

Membranous nephropathy is the most common cause of idiopathic nephrotic syndrome in adults (30 to 40 percent of all cases and over 50 percent of nephrotic adult patients with relatively normal renal function). The clinical features are those of the nephrotic syndrome in general and are usually insidious in onset, without an acute phase or any antecedent event. The ratio of men to women is about 2:1. Early in the disease, blood pressure and kidney size are normal and complement levels and serologies (except in SLE) are unremarkable. Urinary protein excretion is usually sufficient to cause nephrotic syndrome before any significant impairment in renal function is apparent.

Pathology and Pathogenesis. By light microscopy, the glomeruli in membranous nephropathy show progressive, diffuse thickening of the glomerular capillary wall without increased cellularity. In the early stages, the disease cannot be differentiated from lipoid nephrosis (or focal sclerosis) by light microscopy alone. In more advanced stages, the thickened basement membrane is easily seen projecting between subepithelial deposits to give the characteristic spikes seen on silver stain. Immunofluorescence reveals bright, finely granular deposits of IgG and, usually, complement distributed uniformly along the basement membranes of all gomeruli. Electron microscopy reveals uniformly distributed electron-dense deposits on the subepithelial surface of the basement membrane which become intramembranous as the disease progresses.

Membranous nephropathy is now believed to be mediated by chronic deposition of immunoglobulin, probably as immune complexes containing antigens that may persist in the circulation for prolonged periods of time. In selected patients, epimembranous basement membrane deposits have been shown to contain exogenous antigens derived from bacteria or viruses (hepatitis B antigen) as well as endogenous antigens including DNA and components of several tumors. In most cases, however, the inciting antigens have not been identified.

Course and Prognosis. Spontaneous remissions of membranous nephropathy have been reported in up to 25 percent of patients, and such remissions usually occur early in the disease. More commonly the nephrotic syndrome is persistent, and renal function is lost gradually. About half the patients develop renal failure in 10 years, but some survive up to 20 years before requiring dialysis. Several cases of sudden decreases in renal function resulting from a superimposed acute, crescentic anti-GBM nephritis have been reported.

Renal vein thrombosis is a particularly common complication of membranous nephropathy and is present by venography in 30 to 40 percent of the patients, usually without any apparent adverse effect on either renal function or progression of the disease. Anticoagulant therapy to prevent embolic episodes may be indicated in such patients. Membranous nephropathy mediated by tumor antigen-antibody complexes may sometimes be the presenting sign of an otherwise occult neoplasm. Older patients presenting with membranous nephropathy should be carefully evaluated for malignancy.

Numerous trials of steroids and immunosuppressive agents have produced no immediate effect on the proteinuria in membranous nephropathy. However, patients treated with steroids appear to have less proteinuria and better preservation of renal function when compared to untreated controls several years later.

Membranoproliferative Glomerulonephritis

This disorder, which is also called mesangiocapillary glomerulonephritis, lobular glomerulonephritis, or chronic hypocomplementemic glomerulonephritis, is responsible for about 10 percent of cases of idiopathic nephrotic syndrome. In its classic form, membranoproliferative glomerulonephritis presents as nephrotic syndrome in adolescent girls (the female-male ratio is about 3 : 1) with a mean age of 16. Seventy percent of patients have persistently low levels of complement components C3 through C9 and normal levels of C1, C4, and C2, and virtually all patients will manifest hypocomplementemia at some time during their course. Although nephrotic syndrome is usually the major clinical feature of this disease, up to one-third of patients present with signs of acute glomerulonephritis. Such presentations may on occasion follow streptococcal infections and may mimic poststreptococcal glomerulonephritis. Persistent hematuria, sometimes macroscopic, and hypertension early in the disease, are common clinical features. The course is an indolent one, with slow progression to renal failure, although 50 percent of patients survive for over 10 years and a 15-year survival is not unusual. There appears to be no correlation between the serum complement levels and the prognosis.

Pathology. Light microscopy in membranoproliferative glomerulonephritis reveals diffuse changes with both basement membrane thickening (membranous change) and cellular proliferation, usually involving mesangial cells. The glomeruli may have a characteristic lobular appearance and show splitting of the basement membrane by special stains. Immunofluorescence is usually positive for C3, often without IgG, in a granular pattern in the periphery of capillary loops.

Electron microscopy reveals two distinct patterns. About two-thirds of the patients have subendothelial deposits and prominent mesangial changes, and one-third exhibit diffuse, homogenous, nonimmune, dense intramembranous deposits (so-called dense-deposit disease). To date, the subendothelial and dense-deposit varieties of this disease have not been well correlated with any specific clinical characteristics except for the frequent recurrence of dense-deposit disease in renal transplants.

Pathogenesis and Treatment. A circulating factor capable of activating C3 in vitro (C3-nephritic factor) has been demonstrated in patients with the dense-deposit form of membranoproliferative glomerulonephritis, but the role of the abnormalities in complement metabolism in the pathogenesis of the nephritis is unclear. The disease may represent a chronic immune complex nephropathy that develops in a setting of immune deficiency. Steroids have little immediate effect on the proteinuria, but longer-term therapy may contribute to improvement in renal pathologic changes and preservation of renal function in selected patients.

Other Causes of Proteinuria

Although the glomerular diseases described above are those to which the physician must be most attuned in evaluating the patient with significant proteinuria, it is important to remember that abnormal quantities of protein can appear in the urine as a result of a variety of other disturbances. Any process affecting renal hemodynamics and either increasing the filtered load of protein or decreasing its tubular reabsorption, or both, including fever, hypertension, exercise, dysproteinemias, chronic pericarditis, and severe right heart failure, as well as a variety of vascular and interstitial diseases, can increase urinary protein excretion. In the absence of significant glomerular pathology, however, the amount of protein excreted daily in these conditions rarely exceeds 2 gm. It is worth noting that renal vein thrombosis, once regarded as a cause of nephrotic syndrome, is now generally believed to be a consequence of several proteinuric states, particularly membranous nephropathy.

It is also known that assumption of the upright posture increases urine protein excretion severalfold in everybody (orthostatic proteinuria). A common clinical problem is that of the patient who persistently exhibits qualitative proteinuria in the upright posture alone. Although up to 50 percent of such patients will demonstrate some glomerular abnormalities on biopsy, these abnormalities are usually minimal. Follow-up studies have shown that although proteinuria persists in about half of these patients 10 years later, there is no apparent progression of renal disease. Further evaluation by renal biopsy is unnecessary in a patient with orthostatic proteinuria alone, but it should be considered when protein excretion exceeds 1 gm per day, when proteinuria persists in the recumbent position, or when certain other clinical findings are present, including abnormalities of the urine sediment, decreased renal function, or hypertension.

RENAL INVOLVEMENT IN CONNECTIVE TISSUE DISEASES

Although the clinical features of the major connective tissue diseases are covered in detail elsewhere (see Chap. 46), the renal aspects of those with prominent kidney manifestations will be reviewed here.

Systemic Lupus Erythematosus

Nephritis secondary to systemic lupus erythematosus (SLE) is the most common type of acute glomerulonephritis seen in the adult population and represents a major cause of death in SLE. Clinical manifestations of nephritis are present in 60 to 70 percent, and some kind of renal pathology is found in over 90 percent of SLE patients. The renal lesions as well as the clinical manifestations are widely variable and presumably reflect glomerular deposition of immune complexes containing DNA, viral, and other antigens as well as components of the complement system. Ten to fifteen percent of patients have only mild proteinuria or hematuria, essentially normal glomeruli by light microscopy, and only mesangial deposition of immunoglobulin by immunofluorescence and electron microscopy. Such patients generally have mild systemic disease, normal complement levels, and a favorable prognosis. With greater amounts of mesangial immunoglobulin deposition, a focal proliferative nephritis is seen by light microscopy (30 to 40 percent of patients); this type of lesion also has a relatively good prognosis (70 percent of the patients have a 5-year survival), although some patients, particularly those with subendothelial electron-dense deposits, may progress to diffuse proliferative lesions. Another 10 to 20 percent of patients with SLE nephritis will manifest heavy proteinuria and membranous glomerular lesions with clinical characteristics and prognosis similar to those of idiopathic membranous nephropathy. Diffuse proliferative glomerulonephritis develops in 40 to 50 percent of patients and is largely responsible for renal failure in SLE. Women predominate 3 : 1, and such patients generally exhibit extensive immune deposits on the basement membrane, active urine sediments, proteinuria in the nephrotic range in over 50 percent, significant systemic disease, low levels of serum complement, and declining renal function. The 2-year survival rate of patients with diffuse proliferative SLE nephritis is about 10 percent, although early high-dose steroid therapy has improved this figure to 20 to 25 percent at 5 years. The role of additional immunosuppressive agents in the treatment of diffuse proliferative SLE nephritis remains controversial, but when carefully used in selected patients such agents appear to further improve these figures. Because of the apparent benefit of early therapy in some patients with progressive lesions and because of the difficulty in predicting the type of glomerular involvement from the clinical characteristics alone, renal biopsy has achieved widespread acceptance as a routine part of the early diagnostic evaluation of patients with SLE.

Polyarteritis (Periarteritis) Nodosa

The renal manifestations of polyarteritis include those of the classic form, in which involvement of medium-sized arteries leads to renal ischemia and infarction with loin pain, hematuria, and severe hypertension, as well as the signs of multisystem involvement discussed elsewhere (Chap. 46). The diagnosis of polyarteritis involving the kidney is probably best confirmed by abdominal angiography, which demonstrates multiple small aneurysms of involved vessels including those in the kidney. Early steroid therapy may halt or reverse the progression of the renal lesions. A systemic vasculitis with similar lesions has also been described in association with some forms of drug abuse and Australia antigenemia.

In the microscopic form of polyarteritis, which involves capillaries including those in glomeruli, an acute glomerulonephritis may develop that is initially focal but often becomes rapidly progressive, with crescent formation and renal failure. Such acute disease responds poorly to therapy. Although polyarteritis is widely believed to be an immunologically mediated disease, the renal immunopathologic findings in the microscopic form of polyarteritis are not characteristic of either immune-complex or anti-GBM antibody-induced nephritis, and the underlying pathogenic mechanisms are not clear.

Wegener's Granulomatosis

Necrotizing granulomatous vasculitis in Wegener's granulomatosis may produce an acute glomerulonephritis with proteinuria, hematuria, normal blood pressure, and normal or high serum complement in association with midline lesions in the upper and lower respiratory tracts. The renal lesion is a severe, focal proliferative one that is characterized by necrosis, a rapidly progressive course, and 90 percent mortality in 2 years. Early treatment with steroids and cytotoxic drugs, particularly cyclophosphamide, may be of considerable benefit. Renal biopsy is of particular importance in order to identify early the potentially fatal renal involvement in patients who

may appear clinically to have more limited forms of Wegener's granulomatosis as well as to differentiate it from other diseases such as Goodpasture's syndrome, which produces a clinically similar picture. The pathogenesis is not known.

Scleroderma

Clinical renal involvement in scleroderma can be quite severe and can result in death. In patients with so-called scleroderma kidney, the principal clinical manifestations are severe hypertension and renal failure. The renal lesions are primarily vascular and are not unlike those in other renovascular diseases, including malignant hypertension, thrombotic thrombocytopenic purpura, and hemolytic uremic syndrome. There is little evidence of an immunologic basis for the renal involvement.

Urinary Tract Infections
William R. McCabe, M.D.

Infections of the urinary tract are second in frequency only to bacterial infections of the respiratory tract. Clinical studies have demonstrated that asymptomatic bacteriuria occurs in 1.2 percent of all schoolgirls aged 5 to 14, and that each year acute symptomatic urinary infections occur in 5 percent of all adult women aged 20 to 40.

Etiology and Pathogenesis. The most frequent etiologic agents of urinary tract infection are *Escherichia coli* and species of *Klebsiella, Enterobacter, Proteus,* and *Pseudomonas,* although enterococci, staphylococci, and other species may occasionally be responsible. Of the *E. coli* that cause urinary infections, 40 percent belong to six serogroups – O1, O2, O4, O6, O18, and O75 – out of the more than 140 O serotypes. Spontaneously occurring initial infections are caused by *E. coli* almost exclusively. It is believed that the fecal flora serve as the source, since strains of *E. coli* of the same serologic type as those isolated from the urine may be found in the feces prior to or at the onset of urinary infection. Bacteria other than *E. coli* are more frequent in patients with recurrent infections or in those who have been catheterized or undergone other urinary tract manipulations. Adenoviruses have been implicated as a cause of hemorrhagic cystitis, but there is no evidence that viral infections produce pyelonephritis.

Bacteria usually enter the bladder by the ascending route. This probably accounts for the greater incidence of spontaneous infections in females, the frequent onset of symptomatic infections after sexual intercourse, and the frequency with which bladder catheterization is followed by infection in both sexes. Once bacteria reach the bladder, the urine provides an excellent culture medium, but this does not assure establishment of infection, because there are host defense mechanisms. Micturition is one important defense mechanism, since it effectively rids the bladder of large numbers of bacteria; in contrast, incomplete emptying provides a continuous medium for bacterial multiplication. Once bacteria become established in the bladder, they tend to persist for prolonged periods, and a change in the infecting organism or superinfection with other species is rare except after therapy.

In approximately 50 percent of urinary infections, involvement of the upper tract has been demonstrated, while in the other 50 percent only the bladder is affected. Ascent of bacteria from the bladder to the kidney through the ureteral lumen, periureteral lymphatics, or the bloodstream has been proposed. Most evidence indicates that ascent through the ureteral lumen is most important. Reflux of bladder urine also has been emphasized as an important cause of extension of infection to the kidney, but recent studies have demonstrated that urinary infection itself results in reflux. Obviously bladder infection is a prerequisite if reflux is to lead to the development of renal infection.

Urinary infections tend to differ from infections in other sites caused by the same bacteria. Other gram-negative bacillary infections are usually acute and produce severe symptoms, but urinary infections may be asymptomatic. The chronicity of many urinary tract infections and their refractoriness to treatment are puzzling, since the bacteria are susceptible to antibiotics and a brisk antibody response is usually present in renal infection.

A variety of factors are associated with an increased frequency of urinary tract infections, including (1) the shorter urethra in the female; (2) pregnancy; (3) obstruction, especially of the bladder neck; (4) diabetes mellitus; (5) hypertension; and (6) catheterization or instrumentation of the bladder. The last is an extremely important predisposing factor, and the greater frequency of catheterization in patients with factors 2, 3, 4, and 5 may be responsible for the higher incidence of urinary infections in these patients. Renal calculi, previous renal scarring, and vesicoureteral flux are also thought to predispose to renal infection.

Pathologic Changes. Both acute and chronic inflammatory changes occur in response to bladder infection. In acute pyelonephritis, the renal lesions may be focal or diffuse, unilateral or bilateral. The pelvic and calyceal mucosae are acutely inflamed, and areas of leukocytic infiltration are scattered throughout the renal parenchyma. The inflammatory reaction primarily involves the tubules and renal interstitium, extending into the glomeruli only infrequently. Involvement is most marked in the renal medulla, probably because its milieu of high ammonia concentration, high tissue fluid osmolality, and relatively low blood supply inhibits host defense mechanisms. Multiple small abscesses may form in severe infections. Ischemic infarction and necrosis of renal papillae (papillary necrosis) may occur in diabetics, in alcoholics, or in patients with urinary obstruction.

The pathologic changes in chronic pyelonephritis are similar to those seen in interstitial nephritis except for the almost uniform occurrence of either focal or diffuse chronic inflammatory changes of the mucosa of the renal pelvis or calyces. The renal lesion is characterized by interstitial infiltration with lymphocytes and plasma cells, atrophic and dilated tubules filled with colloid casts, and fibrosis. In extensively involved kidneys, a specialized type of periglomerular fibrosis is present. These changes are often termed *thyroidization* of the kidney. The entire kidney may be diffusely involved, but these changes are more often seen in a segment of the kidney drained by a distorted pelvocalyceal collecting system. The presence of granulocytes suggests active infection. Grossly there are coarse, irregular depressions (scarred areas) of the kidney surface resulting from variable thinning of the renal cortex.

Clinical Features. The clinical manifestations of urinary tract infection are quite protean. Some patients may have periods of asymptomatic infection (asymptomatic bacteriuria) interrupted by acute symptomatic episodes, but many others may be entirely asymptomatic. Bladder involvement is generally marked by urinary frequency, nocturia, dysuria or burning on urination, and urgency. Renal infection may be associated with pain in the flank or costovertebral angle that may radiate to the groin or external genitalia and with tenderness to palpation of the costovertebral angle. Chills, fever, and cloudy or malodorous urine may also be present. Symptoms are notoriously unreliable in the diagnosis of urinary tract infection and may be entirely absent despite significant infection. This makes diagnosis particularly difficult in patients with renal infection who may be asymptomatic, in patients who have symptoms of bladder infection only, or in patients with symptoms of both bladder and renal involvement. Rarely, patients with chronic pyelonephritis may present with symptoms and findings of renal insufficiency without any history of a preceding symptomatic renal infection.

Diagnosis. Urinary tract infection can be recognized with certainty only by culture and microscopic examination of the urine. White blood cells, five or more per high power field, are found on microscopic examination of the urinary sediment in most patients with urinary tract infection, but they may be absent in asymptomatic bacteriuria. Clumps of leukocytes are frequent in severe, acute infections. Leukocyte casts also may be found, and these provide evidence of renal involvement. The finding of erythrocytes in the urine is unusual except in hemorrhagic cystitis. Proteinuria may occur with renal infections, but it rarely exceeds the 2+ level (2.0 gm per day).

Bacteriologic culture of the urine is necessary to establish the presence of infection. Normally the urinary tract is sterile except for the distal 1 to 2 cm of the urethra, which may contain small numbers of gram-positive and gram-negative bacteria. Therefore, even bladder catheterization does not exclude urethral contamination, because urethral inhabitants may be introduced by the catheter into the bladder. Differ-

entiation between urinary tract infection and urethral contamination can be achieved by quantitation of the number of bacteria in clean-voided urine specimens that have been carefully collected and promptly cultured. Urine is an excellent culture medium that allows bacterial multiplication to occur even during the period the urine resides in the bladder. Bacterial counts usually exceed 100,000 per milliliter of urine in active infections, whereas bacteria swept into clean urine from the urethra never attain such numbers. In males, bacterial counts as low as 5,000 to 10,000 per milliliter should be regarded as suspicious and should be repeated.

A valuable indication of the degree of bacteriuria may be obtained from a Gram stain of the urine. The visualization of 1 bacteria per oil immersion field in a simple smear made of one loopful of uncentrifuged urine, dried and stained, is adequate evidence of the presence of at least 100,000 bacteria per milliliter and therefore is a useful method of diagnosing infection promptly. Abnormalities of renal function may result from renal infection. Diminution of maximal concentrating ability is almost uniformly found with renal infection and is the earliest detectable functional change. Glomerular filtration usually remains preserved, despite impairment of tubular functions.

Excretory urography is usually normal in acute pyelonephritis, whereas diminution in renal size may be seen in chronic pyelonephritis. The most characteristic abnormality is calyceal dilatation or blunting that is contiguous with an area of scarring or diminution in renal substance. Obstructing lesions, congenital anomalies, or calculi also may be seen.

Definition of whether infection is limited to the bladder or also involves the upper urinary tract may be difficult and is not required for adequate management. The methods used to distinguish upper from solely lower tract involvement include measurement of antibacterial antibody in serum and quantitative urine cultures obtained by bladder and ureteral catheterization after a bladder washout. These techniques are more suitable for research studies than for routine clinical use. Most investigations have indicated that approximately 50 percent of urinary tract infections, including asymptomatic bacteriuria, are associated with upper urinary tract involvement.

Principles of Treatment. Quantitative cultures and antibiotic sensitivity testing should be routine in all patients with suspected urinary tract infection, but therapy need not be withheld until such results become available. Bacteria isolated from patients with spontaneous initial attacks of uncomplicated infection are usually sensitive to the broad-spectrum antibiotics and often to the sulfonamides. Therapy may be started with full doses of one of these agents if the patient is acutely ill. There is no particular merit of one antibiotic over another if the infecting organism is equally sensitive to both. The object of therapy is not only the relief of symptoms but also, and of greater importance, the permanent eradication of bacteriuria. Defervescence and disappearance of other symptoms may occur without antibiotic therapy but without disappearance of bacteriuria. For this reason it is essential that quantitative urine cultures be obtained during and after therapy to ensure the effectiveness of therapy. Persistent fever or other symptoms after 2 or 3 days of therapy indicate ineffectiveness of therapy and also suggest the possibility of structural genitourinary tract abnormalities.

In the absence of such abnormalities, failure of therapy may be due to (1) the presence or development of bacterial resistance to the antibiotic employed, (2) recurrence of infection with the original infecting organism after cessation of therapy, or (3) reinfection with a different bacterial species or serotype. Although reinfection with a different organism may occur during therapy, especially when indwelling catheters are present, it usually occurs weeks or months after treatment. In contrast, recurrence of infection with the original infecting organism can occur very rapidly.

Patients with nosocomial or chronic infections are often infected with bacteria that are resistant to the sulfonamides and are often resistant to several other antibiotics as well. The more nephrotoxic agents such as gentamicin, kanamycin, and the polymyxins are usually reserved for treatment of such organisms, but these agents must be used with caution because of their nephrotoxicity and ototoxicity.

Since recurrences of infection are frequent and often asymptomatic, patients should be followed with quantitative urine cultures at 3-month intervals for a year after treatment.

Course and Prognosis. Most urinary tract infections are self-limited in that the symptoms usually subside within a few days, even in the absence of treatment, although bacteriuria may persist. Thus disappearance of symptoms does not correlate with resolution of infection. In contrast, persistence of fever and symptoms despite adequate antibiotic therapy is often indicative of structural anomalies of the urinary tract. Progression to renal damage severe enough to produce renal insufficiency is infrequent, despite the prevalence of urinary tract infections. Inability to identify patients who may progress to significant renal injury necessitates vigorous efforts to ensure eradication of bacteriuria in all cases.

Interstitial Nephritis

An interstitial infiltrate is the most prominent histologic feature in a number of acute and chronic conditions. Usually there is associated morphologic and functional evidence of damage to tubules, while glomeruli are relatively spared. Infection of the kidney is the cause of tubular interstitial disease in many patients. This condition, termed *acute* or *chronic pyelonephritis,* has already been described in the preceding section. However, there is increasing evidence that many cases of acute and most cases of chronic interstitial nephritis are not due to direct bacterial invasion of the kidney. A number of other causes of interstitial nephritis are now well recognized, as shown in the list below. In many patients the cause of interstitial nephritis cannot be determined.

1. Causes of acute interstitial nephritis
   a. Hypersensitivity to drugs (methicillin, penicillin, phenindione, sulfonamides, etc.)
   b. Infection (pyelonephritis)
   c. Radiation nephritis
   d. Idiopathic
2. Causes of chronic interstitial nephritis
   a. Analgesic abuse (phenacetin, usually combined with aspirin)
   b. Hyperuricemic nephropathy (gouty nephropathy)
   c. Hypercalcemia, hypokalemia
   d. Obstructive uropathy
   e. Associated with nephrolithiasis
   f. Hereditary nephritis

g. Arteriolar nephrosclerosis

h. Neoplastic infiltrates: lymphoma, leukemia, myeloma

i. Nephrotoxins: lead, cadmium

j. Radiation nephritis

k. Infection (pyelonephritis)

l. Idiopathic

Acute interstitial nephritis is characterized by a cellular infiltrate in which lymphocytes, plasma cells, eosinophils, and leukocytes are present in variable proportions, together with interstitial edema and tubular degenerative changes. Clinically the picture is usually that of nonoliguric acute renal failure, in that rapidly progressive azotemia is the most prominent feature. Skin rash and eosinophilia are common in drug-related disease. Hypertension is not noted except in radiation nephritis, in which the renal microvasculature is prominently involved. Urinalysis typically reveals only minimal proteinuria and a scanty sediment in which occasional leukocytes and finely granular casts are present. Roentgenographic studies reveal the kidneys to be bilaterally normal in size or enlarged. Diagnosis depends on recognition of the possible causes (such as drugs) in patients with progressive azotemia and typical urinary findings. In obscure cases, renal biopsy may be required to establish the diagnosis. Treatment varies with the cause. In drug hypersensitivity reactions, corticosteroid therapy may be helpful if withdrawal of the offending agent does not suffice.

Chronic interstitial nephritis is characterized by an interstitial infiltrate in which lymphocytes and plasma cells predominate. Interstitial fibrosis and tubular degeneration and atrophy are usually prominent, and periglomerular fibrosis is typical in advanced cases. Histologic features vary somewhat according to the causative agent. Clinically, renal failure usually progresses slowly. There is early evidence of tubular functional damage, such as decreased urinary concentrating ability, hyperchloremic acidosis, or salt-wasting. The urinalysis typically reveals minimal proteinuria and a scanty sediment in which leukocytes, occasional leukocyte clumps, and rare leukocytic and degenerating cell casts are the key elements. Patients are usually asymptomatic, and the condition is often discovered in the evaluation of hypertension, proteinuria,

or azotemia noted on routine screening studies. In some cases, bacterial infection is superimposed and the symptoms of pyelonephritis may be prominent (see preceding section). In analgesic nephropathy, papillary necrosis is frequent and the key symptom may be recurrent attacks of renal colic as sloughed papillae are passed. Hypertension is often a prominent feature, but some patients may remain normotensive throughout the course of the disease. In other patients, severe or even accelerated hypertension may develop; in such instances, renal failure may progress more rapidly than is otherwise typical of chronic interstitial nephritis. The intravenous urogram may be especially helpful in diagnosis. In the early stages of chronic interstitial nephritis the kidneys may be of normal size, but more typically they are contracted, often asymmetrically. Calyces are blunted and distorted, and overlying cortical scars may be prominent.

Diagnosis of chronic interstitial nephritis depends on recognition of possible causative factors together with typical urinalysis, functional pattern, and roentgenographic changes. Renal biopsy may be nondiagnostic, since the condition is characteristically patchy in distribution within the kidney and is most prominent in the renal medulla.

Treatment of chronic interstitial nephritis consists in the removal of offending agents such as analgesics, specific treatment of underlying causes where possible (e.g., therapy of hyperuricemia with allopurinol), and appropriate therapy of superimposed infection and hypertension. In analgesic nephropathy, removal of the inciting drug has usually prevented further deterioration of renal function and often has resulted in progressive functional improvement; hence recognition of this relatively frequent cause of interstitial nephritis is especially important. It is also important to remember that many patients who abuse analgesics deny ingesting them.

Other Diseases of the Kidney

OBSTRUCTIVE UROPATHY

<u>Definition and Pathogenesis.</u> Obstruction to the flow of urine often leads to anatomic and functional damage to the kidneys and is one of the common causes of acute and chronic renal failure. Obstruction in the urinary tract may occur at any level from the renal

pelvis to the urethral meatus. Among the causes of urinary obstruction are prostatic enlargement, strictures, congenital valves, pressure from extrinsic structures such as tumors or blood vessels, periureteral fibrosis, stones, blood clots, and neuromuscular dysfunction that interferes with normal voiding. Congenital obstructions of the urethra, bladder neck, and ureteropelvic junctions, though common, may be missed until adult life.

Clinical Features. Acute ureteral obstruction usually causes colic, whereas acute bladder neck obstruction causes local symptoms due to distention of the bladder. On the other hand, gradually developing chronic obstruction may be asymptomatic when the obstruction is located above the bladder, although it may be associated with abnormal voiding patterns (hesitancy, multiple voiding, enuresis, dysuria, dribbling, etc.) when the obstruction is at the level of the bladder neck or the urethra. Urinary tract infections are frequent when the obstruction is at the bladder neck or below but are less common when the obstruction is above the bladder unless pathogenic organisms have been introduced by retrograde catheterization. Because urinary concentrating ability is often decreased in obstructive uropathy, polyuria may be a feature of chronic partial obstruction. Oliguria, it should be stressed, is not a feature of chronic partial obstruction.

Eventually azotemia develops, and uremic symptoms may be the first manifestations of chronic obstructive uropathy. The urine contains little or no protein, and the sediment is sparse. Azotemia in the presence of minimal proteinuria or sediment abnormalities should always alert the physician to the possibility of obstructive uropathy, especially if kidney size is normal or increased.

Diagnosis and Treatment. Definitive diagnosis of obstructive uropathy usually requires roentgenographic evaluation by intravenous pyelography or cystoscopic and retrograde urologic study, which should be performed without delay if obstruction is suspected. Surgical relief of acute or even chronic obstruction may restore renal function nearly to normal. However, parenchymal damage from pressure, ischemia, and infection eventually may become

irreversible. A temporary phase of diuresis and electrolyte-wasting, which occasionally may be severe, may follow the relief of severe obstruction. This phase requires careful attention to the adequate replacement of fluid and electrolyte losses.

NEPHROLITHIASIS

Definition and Pathogenesis. Approximately 90 percent of kidney stones are composed of calcium salts; nearly all the rest are urate stones. Cystine stones are formed in patients with the rare hereditary metabolic disorder, cystinuria, and xanthine stones in the still rarer condition, xanthinuria. In perhaps one-third to one-half of cases, stone formation is related either to increased excretion of calcium or uric acid or to persistent alterations in urinary acidity favoring precipitation of the normally dissolved amounts of these materials. In the remaining cases, alterations in the physicochemical characteristics of urine that favor crystallization presumably occur, but the nature of such changes and the identity of the factors concerned are as yet unknown.

Calcium Stones
Calcium stones may be composed of calcium oxalate, calcium phosphate, or mixtures of the two. Such stones are often associated with hypercalciuria, as in hyperparathyroidism, idiopathic hypercalciuria, ingestion of excessive vitamin D, sarcoidosis, acute osteoporosis due to immobilization, Cushing's syndrome, or renal tubular acidosis. Calcium oxalate stones may also be formed in the rare condition known as primary hyperoxaluria, in which oxalate excretion is increased. Calcium oxalate and phosphate stones are formed at any urine pH. Mixed calcium, magnesium, and ammonium phosphate stones are formed in urine that is persistently alkaline due to infection with urea-splitting organisms. In many cases no specific cause for calcium stone formation can be discovered.

Uric Acid Stones
The solubility of uric acid is markedly affected by urine pH, and uric acid stones are formed only in acid urine. In many patients, increased uric acid excretion due to gout or to hematologic disorders such as lymphoma or leukemia is present. In other

patients, the formation of uric acid stones is related to the secretion of persistently acid urine (pH less than 5.5), which favors the precipitation of the normal amounts of uric acid present in the urine. The mechanism responsible for the persistent aciduria is not yet fully defined.

Cystine Stones

In cystinuria, a rare hereditary disorder, the urine contains increased amounts of cystine and of the common diamino acids: arginine, lysine, ornithine. The exact mechanisms responsible for the increased excretion of the amino acids have not been clarified. Cystine is relatively insoluble at acid or neutral pH, and cystine stones tend to form if more than 300 mg of cystine is excreted in the average daily urine volume. Except for recurrent lithiasis and the renal damage that may ensue, patients with cystinuria are in good health.

Clinical Features and Diagnosis. Stones in the renal pelvis are often asymptomatic, although hematuria, crystalluria, proteinuria, and vague flank pain may occur. Large staghorn (triple-phosphate) calculi are commonly associated with recurrent pyelonephritis. Renal colic, that is, severe, spasmodic pain in the flank, usually radiating along the course of the ureter to the genitalia, indicates that a stone has moved from the pelvis into the ureter. Hematuria is almost always found. Colic abruptly disappears when the stone is passed into the bladder, usually to be voided per urethra shortly thereafter. Some patients may pass only a single stone in a lifetime; others may be subject to repeated episodes of renal colic.

Even in the absence of colic, the diagnosis of lithiasis is usually made easily from the urinary findings and roentgenographic examination. Calcium and cystine stones are radiopaque, whereas uric acid stones are radiolucent and can be identified only by pyelography. Stones may be single or multiple, and they vary greatly in size. Mixed calcium, magnesium, and ammonium phosphate stones sometimes grow to a large size, filling many branches of the intrarenal collecting system (staghorn calculi). In many patients with hypercalciuria and calcium stones, nephrocalci-nosis, or calcifications of the renal parenchyma, also may be noted.

Treatment and Prevention. The treatment of stones already formed is usually limited to the symptomatic relief of renal colic, although sometimes surgery or retrograde catheterization is needed to remove an impacted stone that may be obstructing urine flow. Attempts at dissolving stones through lavage of the renal pelvis have not been notably successful.

Of greatest importance is a systemic search for a specific cause of the stone formation, because once recognized, many of these causes can be eliminated. Chemical analysis of stones is essential. Every patient should also have multiple examinations of blood and urine for disorders of calcium metabolism; stones are frequently the sole clinical manifestation of hyperparathyroidism. Several causes of hypercalciuria, such as hyperparathyroidism, vitamin D excess, and Cushing's syndrome, are amenable to specific treatment, and thereby further stone formation can be prevented. Control of urinary tract infection may decrease the formation of mixed phosphate stones. When no specific cause for calcium stones can be discovered, decreased calcium ingestion and increased water intake may lessen the frequency of stone formation. Relatively small amounts of sodium phosphate taken orally may decrease the formation of idiopathic calcium stones. Administration of thiazide diuretics decreases urinary calcium excretion, and clinical studies suggest that it may reduce calcium stone formation.

The formation of uric acid stones can almost always be prevented by increased water intake and alkalinization of the urine. The latter can be accomplished by alkali ingestion (sodium bicarbonate or citrate) in the daytime and administration of a carbonic anhydrase inhibitor such as acetazolamide at bedtime. Allopurinol, an inhibitor of urate production, is also useful in the treatment of urate lithiasis.

The frequency of cystine stone formation is decreased by restricting the intake of methionine, by increasing water intake, and by alkalinization of the urine to above pH 7.5. D-penicillamine (β, β-dimethylcysteine), which converts cystine in the urine to the soluble disulfide of cysteine and penicillamine, has proved successful in reducing stone formation and may even result in dissolution of existing stones. However, a relatively high incidence of hypersensitivity reactions limits the use of this drug to patients in whom more conservative measures have failed.

TOXEMIA OF PREGNANCY

Definition and Pathogenesis. Much confusion in the past has resulted from including all cases of proteinuria, hypertension, and edema during pregnancy within the term *toxemia of pregnancy*. This diagnosis should be reserved for a specific syndrome of pregnancy in which the clinical findings appear after the fifth month of gestation and are not related to other known renal disease or preexisting hypertension. When convulsions and other manifestations of encephalopathy are absent, the condition is called preeclampsia; if these signs occur, eclampsia is said to have developed. The cause of toxemia of pregnancy is unknown. It seems to be closely associated with the presence of placental tissue, because toxemic symptoms usually subside promptly after delivery of the placenta.

Pathologic Changes. The characteristic changes in the kidney in toxemia are swelling of endothelial and mesangial cells and the presence in glomerular capillaries of subendothelial deposits that appear to be made up of fibrin or related materials. These changes usually disappear promptly after delivery. In eclampsia vascular lesions may also be found in the liver and central nervous system.

Clinical Features and Course. Toxemia is most frequent in older women and primigravidae. Hypertension and edema usually precede proteinuria, but occasionally the order is reversed. Often these findings are not progressive; they usually respond partially to treatment and disappear after delivery. Rarely, hypertension becomes severe, azotemia supervenes, or severe headaches, visual disturbances, and vomiting may signal the development of the full syndrome of eclampsia, with convulsions and coma. In such cases, maternal death may occur, due to cerebral hemorrhage, congestive heart failure, or acute renal failure. Fetal mortality is high in eclampsia or in severe, un-

controlled preeclampsia. Some evidence suggests that toxemia of pregnancy may predispose to hypertension in later life, but this point is controversial. In any event, the risk of permanent damage in a woman who was free of renal and vascular disease prior to pregnancy is clearly not great. Unrecognized preexisting disease that is exacerbated by pregnancy may account for many cases in which some of the manifestations of toxemia continue in the postpartum period.

Treatment. The use of low-sodium diets, diuretics, and antihypertensive drugs has greatly improved the prognosis of toxemia. In those patients in whom a prompt response to these measures does not occur, the addition of sedation and bed rest may be helpful. If azotemia, intractable hypertension, or signs of eclampsia develop, it is often necessary to empty the uterus in order to avoid serious maternal consequences.

Other Forms of Renal Disease in Pregnancy
Asymptomatic urinary tract infection (bacteriuria) and acute pyelonephritis are especially common in pregnant women, perhaps in relation to the physiologic stasis in the urinary tract during this period. Postpartum urinary tract infection in many cases is probably related to catheterization at delivery; catheterization should be avoided whenever possible. Preexisting pyelonephritis often becomes active during pregnancy. Some observers believe that pyelonephritis predisposes to the development of toxemia, but this relation has not been clearly established. Prophylactic treatment of asymptomatic bacteriuria reduces the incidence of subsequent acute pyelonephritis and to this extent probably improves the prognosis of the pregnancy.

Acute renal failure is an important complication of pregnancy. It usually occurs in relation to uterine hemorrhage (premature placental separation), septic abortion, or eclampsia. The pathologic and clinical features are those of acute tubular necrosis or cortical necrosis.

Preexisting chronic renal disease or hypertension may undergo exacerbation during pregnancy, with the appearance of clinical features of toxemia. If the patient is not seen early in pregnancy and the history is uncertain, the clinical picture may be indistinguishable from true toxemia of pregnancy. In general, the prognosis for mother and fetus is fairly good in latent chronic renal disease and in benign early essential hypertension. On the other hand, chronic asymptomatic pyelonephritis, if untreated, is likely to flare up. The presence of any degree of azotemia or of significant hypertensive vascular disease makes pregnancy hazardous for both mother and fetus.

Recently a new entity of postpartum renal failure has been recognized clinically as an acute, severe, and usually irreversible renal failure beginning 1 day to several months postpartum. A few of the patients have had toxemia, but in the majority pregnancy and delivery were normal. A microangiopathic hemolytic anemia is found in all patients and thrombocytopenia in most patients with postpartum renal failure. Slowly developing hypertension, unexplained fever, congestive heart failure, and seizures are frequently associated. Pathologically, glomerular capillaries and the smaller arteries in the kidney show thrombi, endothelial hyperplasia, subendothelial deposits of fibrin, and fibrinoid necrosis. The renal lesions are similar to those found in an experimental Shwartzman reaction. Postpartum renal failure can be considered a form of hemolytic uremic syndrome occurring in the postpartum period. Treatment of postpartum renal failure with anticoagulants has been of uncertain benefit. Renal failure is usually irreversible in women with the fully developed syndrome, but sometimes a milder, transient renal failure may occur.

POLYCYSTIC DISEASE OF THE KIDNEYS

Definition and Pathogenesis. Polycystic disease is the commonest inherited disorder of the kidneys. It is believed due to a defect in the fetal development of the renal tubular system, which deforms a variable fraction of the nephrons and causes them to develop cystlike dilatations at some point along their course. These cysts tend to increase slowly and thereby to enlarge the kidneys, sometimes to an enormous extent. Interstitial fibrosis, ischemia due to internal distortion of renal architecture, and frequent superimposition of chronic infection contribute to the progressive loss of renal function. Cysts also occur in the liver in about a third of the cases, but they are of no functional significance.

The overall incidence of the disease has been estimated at somewhat less than 1 per 1,000, but the autopsy frequency is slightly greater. The pattern of inheritance appears to be that of an autosomal dominant, with a high degree of penetrance and no sex linkage. The disease described here is related pathogenically to other less common forms of polycystic disease, but the latter are not always hereditary, and they often lead to severe dysgenesis and neonatal renal failure.

Clinical Features. Polycystic disease is present from birth, but it does not usually cause any signs or symptoms until the cysts have expanded enough to cause significant distortion of renal architecture and function. The usual time of onset is in middle-age, but sometimes the disease is not discovered until later in life. The first manifestation may be episodic flank pain or hematuria. Pyelonephritis is a common complication, and often the early symptoms are those ascribable to recurrent, acute renal infection. In some patients, a visible or palpable irregular mass in the flanks is the first sign of the disease; in still others nothing is apparent until uremia and hypertension supervene.

More than half the patients reach end-stage renal failure within 10 years of the onset of symptoms, but the course is variable, and approximately 10 percent survive more than 20 years without developing chronic uremia.

Diagnosis. When the kidneys are grossly enlarged and nodular and masses are palpable bilaterally in the flanks, the diagnosis of polycystic disease is usually obvious. At earlier stages of the disease the diagnosis can often be made from the intravenous pyelogram, which characteristically reveals the calyces to be stretched and distorted by the multiple intrarenal cysts. Examination of the urine is helpful but not diagnostic. There is usually little or no proteinuria or cylindruria. The number of red cells and white cells in the urine is usually slightly increased; sometimes the urine is grossly bloody. If infection is active, there may be white cell casts and gross pyuria.

Treatment. There is no treatment for the underlying polycytic disease. However, meticulous management of urinary tract infection and secondary hypertensive disease may delay the development of terminal cardio-renal failure and thereby prolong life. The management of renal failure in these patients is essentially the same as that in other patients with uremia; this subject is discussed under Uremia.

Other Cystic Diseases

Solitary and Multiple Cysts. Cysts are thin-walled structures 1 to 10 cm in size that are apparently congenital in origin and that may occur singly or occasionally at multiple sites in the kidneys. Usually cysts are asymptomatic and are discovered incidentally when urograms are performed. Rarely, they may achieve such large size as to cause backache or a dragging sensation, obstruct the ureter, or even compress the renal artery, leading to hypertension. The main importance of cysts is in their differential diagnosis from neoplasms of the kidney, as described under Kidney Tumors.

Medullary Cystic Disease. This disease (also called juvenile nephrophthisis) may be inherited in variable genetic patterns or may occur without familial inheritance. It manifests itself as progressive renal failure in children and young adults. The usual findings of chronic uremia gradually develop and, in addition, profound salt-wasting is usually present. Growth retardation and uremic bone disease are prominent. Pathologically, small cysts crowd the medulla, and there are tubular dilatation and atrophy.

Medullary Sponge Kidney. This entirely different condition does not lead to renal failure. It is recognized in intravenous urograms as linear or cystic dilatation of collecting ducts near the calyces. It is usually asymptomatic; however, small stones may form in the dilated structures, and occasionally these may lead to bleeding, obstruction, or infection.

KIDNEY TUMORS
The most common malignant tumor of the kidney in adults is hypernephroma or renal cell carcinoma. This tumor presents clinically in most patients as flank pain, abdominal mass, or hematuria. In other patients the first manifestations may be those of metastases to lung, brain, bone, or liver. Patients may present with or develop a variety of metabolic disorders, including fever, hypercalcemia, leukocytosis, polycythemia, neuropathy, and myopathy. This tumor often grows as a solid mass into the vena cava and may cause venous obstruction or even progress into the right atrium.

Diagnosis can be made roentgenographically by infusion urograms and by angiography, which can differentiate cysts and malignant tumors with great accuracy. Cysts tend to be avascular, smooth, regular, and sharply separated from the parenchyma, and are not calcified. Neoplasms are irregular, extend into neighboring tissues, have prominent and irregular vasculature, and are sometimes calcified. About 20 percent of patients survive 5 years after surgical excision alone. Various combinations of chemotherapy now under trial show some promise of improved survival.

UREMIA
Uremia is the clinical condition that results from marked reduction in overall renal function. This state is characterized chemically by severe azotemia, which is an increase in plasma nonprotein nitrogenous compounds such as urea, uric acid, and creatinine. However, the increased plasma levels of these and other nitrogenous compounds have at most a limited part in the pathogenesis of uremia, the symptoms of which are not predictably related to the concentration of any of these substances. The uremic syndrome is compounded of numerous pathophysiologic and biochemical changes reflecting decreased excretory, tubular, metabolic, and regulatory activities of the kidneys.

Pathophysiologic Changes. Regulation of body fluids and electrolytes is a principal function of the kidneys. Uremic patients therefore suffer from a variety of disturbances of fluid and electrolyte balance. Sodium depletion may result from inability of the diseased kidneys to reduce sodium excretion appropriately when sodium intake is restricted by anorexia, nausea, or the prescription of a low-salt diet. Renal salt-wasting in the sense of inability to excrete a sodium-free urine is common in uremia, but profound salt-wasting, sufficient by itself to produce salt depletion on a normal sodium intake, is rare. Dehydration usually accompanies sodium depletion. Inability to excrete concentrated urine is routinely a feature of severe renal insufficiency. The deficiency of both sodium and water in uremia is most often the result of gastrointestinal losses from vomiting or diarrhea, compounded by an inadequate renal regulatory response. Salt and water depletion results in circulatory insufficiency, which may further compromise renal function.

Sodium excess and edema formation may result from renal retention of sodium and water due to glomerular tubular imbalance or from congestive heart failure due to hypertension and anemia. Water intoxication may arise from rapid oral or intravenous administration of fluids to uremic patients, in whom water diuresis characteristically is deficient because of defective renal diluting mechanisms.

In acute, oliguric renal failure, hyperkalemia is often prominent and may be life-threatening because of its cardiotoxic effects. Potassium excretory capacity in chronic renal failure remains relatively normal, although minor nonprogressive elevation of serum potassium is common. Severe hyperkalemia does not occur until the terminal oliguric stage unless severe acidosis or sodium depletion develops. Conversely, potassium depletion and hypokalemia may develop in relation to malnutrition and gastrointestinal losses. Renal potassium-wasting is a relatively uncommon disorder that occurs in renal tubular diseases without uremia and is not a feature of uremia per se.

In the initial phases of chronic renal failure, plasma phosphate is normal, probably because progressive secondary hyperparathyroidism maintains normal phosphate excretion despite decreasing renal function. When the glomerular filtration rate falls to 25 percent or less of normal, hyperphosphatemia develops. Gastrointestinal absorption of calcium is progressively impaired, probably because of decreased renal conversion of vitamin D to 1,25-dihydroxycholecalciferol, the form of the vitamin most potent in stimulating intestinal absorption. Despite the decrease in absorption, plasma calcium is normal in most patients with moderate renal failure, presumably because of

the skeletal effects of secondary hyperparathyroidism. In late renal failure, hypocalcemia is common. Although hypocalcemia rarely causes tetany in uremia because of the opposing neuromuscular effects of acidosis, tetany may occur if alkali is administered too rapidly. The common neuromuscular manifestations of uremia — muscle cramps, twitching, paresthesias — are not related to hypocalcemia and rarely respond to calcium infusions.

Bone disease is present histologically in nearly all patients with advanced renal failure but is only rarely symptomatic in adults. It may become more significant in patients maintained on chronic dialysis. Osteitis fibrosa cystica due to secondary hyperparathyroidism is most prominent, but osteomalacia is often present and osteosclerosis is sometimes a feature of uremic osteodystrophy. Metastatic calcification may occur, especially in patients whose calcium-phosphorus concentration product exceeds 70. Such deposits may be noted on physical examination as corneal band keratopathy and conjunctival deposits, and roentgenographically as deposits in skin and blood vessels. Parenchymal deposits in vital organs (heart, lungs, etc.) may lead to clinically significant impairment of function.

Metabolic acidosis is regularly a feature of the uremic state; the degree of acidosis is approximately proportional to the level of azotemia. Acidosis results from defective tubular excretion of acid, especially that fraction excreted as ammonium. Acidosis causes hyperpnea and may be a factor in the fatigue and nausea common in patients with uremia. Chronic acidosis may also play a role in the pathogenesis of bone disease.

Reduced glomerular filtration results in azotemia. Most of the increase in nonprotein nitrogen is due to urea, but the plasma concentrations of creatinine, uric acid, and a number of other nitrogenous compounds also increase. Elevated urea concentrations may contribute to anorexia, nausea, and fatigue. Some investigators believe that ammonia liberated from urea in the gastrointestinal tract is significant in the genesis of uremic stomatitis, vomiting, and diarrhea. Prolonged hyperuricemia in uremia may lead to secondary gout.

Plasma concentrations of compounds such as organic acids, phenols, and indicans have been found to be abnormally elevated, and others undoubtedly remain to be identified. Thus far, no direct relations between specific metabolites and individual clinical features of uremia have been discovered.

Clinical Features. Although the essential features are the same regardless of cause, the clinical picture of uremia varies greatly, depending on the rate at which it develops, the age of the patient, the nature of any underlying disease, and the particular response of the individual. Occasional patients with severe renal insufficiency may remain virtually asymptomatic. However, in the great majority of patients with marked impairment of renal function some of the following clinical manifestations develop.

Fatigue, lassitude, and decreased mental and physical vigor are prominent symptoms. Terminally, confusion, stupor, and coma usually develop. Restlessness and insomnia may be noted. Bizarre, psychotic behavior may occur episodically in severe uremia. Neuromuscular manifestations include coarse muscle twitches, muscle cramps, peripheral neuropathies with sensory and motor phenomena, and convulsions (most commonly related to hypertensive encephalopathy).

Gastrointestinal manifestations are almost uniformly present. Anorexia, nausea, vomiting, an unpleasant taste in the mouth, stomatitis, parotitis, and diarrhea may all be noted at one time or another. Ulceration and bleeding may occur in any part of the gastrointestinal tract, and clinically significant gastrointestinal hemorrhage occasionally may develop.

Malnutrition is a feature of chronic uremia, due both to the gastrointestinal manifestations described above and to unknown metabolic factors. A yellow brown discoloration of the skin may result from the deposition of unknown pigments. Occasionally, urea from sweat crystallizes on the skin as so-called uremic frost. Pruritus is common.

Hematologic findings in uremia include anemia and an abnormal bleeding tendency. The anemia is usually normochromic and normocytic and results from depression of erythropoiesis by decreased erythropoietin formation and possibly by uremic poisons. In severe uremia an increased rate of red cell destruction may occur. Malnutrition and bleeding may also contribute to the anemia. Qualitative defects in platelet

function appear to be the principal cause of the abnormal bleeding tendency; depression of plasma coagulation factors and increased capillary fragility may also play a role.

Circulatory disorders in uremia include hypertension, which may on occasion be severe enough to cause encephalopathy. Congestive heart failure is often present, due to hypertension and anemia. Pericarditis is usually a late event in chronic uremia, but it may also occur in severe acute uremia that is potentially reversible. A friction rub is often heard, and in occasional patients, precordial pain may be severe. "Uremic pneumonitis," a roentgenographic picture of central pulmonary congestion, is due to fibrinous alveolar exudation and pulmonary edema.

Treatment. The first step in the management of the patient with uremia is to establish the cause of renal failure. Uremia by itself is not an acceptable diagnosis, for it may reflect ignorance of a specific, potentially reversible cause. Uremia may result from renal disease, from inadequate circulatory supply to the kidney (prerenal), or from obstruction to urine flow. A search must be made for correctable causes of renal failure: Circulatory inadequacy, salt and water depletion, infection, hypercalcemia, and obstruction should all be considered. If careful diagnostic study reveals only irreversible renal disease, proper management, although only palliative, can often prolong useful, comfortable life considerably. A brief summary of general principles follows.

Modifications of the low protein diet devised by Giovannetti have gained wide acceptance as a means for ameliorating symptoms in advanced uremia. Daily protein intake is restricted to 20 to 40 gm, but care is taken to provide all essential amino acids. Although the underlying renal disease is not affected, many uremic symptoms such as fatigue, confusion, nausea, vomiting, and muscle twitching are frequently dramatically improved. By this means, patients with uremia may be given additional months of useful and relatively comfortable life.

Often food intake is restricted by anorexia, and the physician's problem is to encourage intake in order to prevent severe malnutrition. Ad libitum water intake should be allowed; either forcing or restricting fluids may overtax limited renal concentrating and diluting capacity. Signs of salt and water depletion should be treated vigorously with added salts and fluids by mouth or by vein, but the dangers of congestive failure and severe hypertension due to sodium overloading in these patients must be borne in mind.

Activity, except for the most strenuous types, need not be restricted in uremia. In any case, the activity of uremic patients is usually self-limited by fatigue and lassitude.

Acidosis need not be treated if it is mild. When the plasma carbon dioxide content is less than 15 mEq per liter, judicious alkali therapy may reduce symptoms such as hyperpnea, anorexia, or lassitude. Sodium bicarbonate or citrate is given by mouth until symptomatic benefit is obtained, with due caution to avoid sodium overload or a sudden change in blood pH that might precipitate tetany. The use of alkaline potassium rather than sodium salts runs the risk of hyperkalemia.

Hypocalcemia and hyperphosphatemia are usually asymptomatic and require no treatment. Rarely, hypocalcemia may cause tetany, especially after alkali therapy, and this may require treatment with intravenous administration of calcium gluconate. Uremic bone disease has been treated experimentally with 1,25-dihydrotachysterol and related compounds. In patients on chronic dialysis, normalization of plasma calcium by use of increased calcium concentration in dialysis fluids and reduction of plasma phosphate by ingestion of phosphate-binding gels has had some success experimentally. However, no well-established regimens are available, so treatment of uremic bone disease is best left to experts.

Uremic anemia responds only to transfusions. These should be reserved for severe, symptomatic anemia and should be carried out slowly and cautiously.

Congestive heart failure due to excessive fluid retention responds to sodium and water restriction. Large doses of potent diuretics such as furosemide and ethacrynic acid are usually effective except in far-advanced renal failure. If myocardial failure is due largely to hypertensive heart disease, administration of digoxin should be tried cautiously, remembering that both excretion of digoxin and clinical tolerance to the drug are impaired in uremia. Hypertension, when moderate or severe, should be treated because of its deleterious effect on cardiac and kidney function. However, too strenuous or rapid reduction of blood pressure in severe uremia may further compromise renal function.

Drug therapy of any kind requires a thorough understanding of the role of the kidney in excreting the particular drug chosen. Long-acting barbiturates, narcotics, sulfonamides, anticoagulants, and several antibiotics (e.g., kanamycin, gentamycin) are examples of drugs that must be used in reduced dosage or avoided altogether in patients with uremia.

Long-term Dialysis and Transplantation. During the past decade, maintenance dialysis and transplantation have become firmly established as reasonably successful means for prolongation of life and rehabilitation of many patients with terminal renal failure. However, many medical problems remain. Moreover, the high cost of these types of treatment has posed difficult economic problems for patients and for society as a whole.

Long-term hemodialysis is performed for 5- to 6-hour periods, two or three times weekly, using one of a number of commercially available dialyzers or artificial kidneys. Repeated access to the patient's circulation is obtained by creation of a permanent arteriovenous fistula. Adequate dialysis relieves most of the symptoms of uremia, and the majority of patients properly selected for this therapy are rehabilitated and able to return to part-time or full-time work. Hepatitis has been a serious problem among both patients and staff of dialysis centers. Despite dialysis, the intake of oral sodium, water, and protein must still be limited. Excess intake of sodium and water is especially troublesome and may lead to repeated episodes of pulmonary congestion, edema, and severe hypertension. In a minority of patients, hypertension may remain severe despite adequate control of sodium and water intake. Renin levels are regularly high in such patients, and nephrectomy may be required to relieve the hypertension. Anemia persists despite frequent dialysis. Transfusions are given only for acute blood loss or for major symptoms in order to avoid hepatitis and hemosiderosis. Progressive peripheral neuropathy, prominent in early reports of chronic dialysis, appears to be related to inadequate dialysis time, and it should not occur with present techniques. Renal osteodystrophy and metastatic calcification have been prominent problems in some patients.

Major psychological problems often develop in patients on prolonged dialysis. The cost of long-term dialysis in treatment centers is on the order of $8,000 to $15,000 per year. Considerable savings can be achieved by training psychologically suitable patients with adequate family assistance and home environments to perform dialysis themselves at home. Because of the numerous medical and economic problems, maintenance dialysis is usually reserved for selected patients unsuitable for transplantation. About 10 to 15 percent of patients on indefinite dialysis die each year of various causes, especially cardiovascular disease, which occurs with increased frequency in these patients.

For most patients with terminal renal failure, transplantation is now considered to be the treatment of choice. However, dialysis and transplantation are complementary modes of treatment, and patients in transplantation programs must be maintained on dialysis while awaiting suitable kidneys or when rejection occurs. The major determinants of success in transplantation are the severity of the rejection reaction and the complications of the immunosuppressive agents used to suppress rejection. Isografts between identical twins are usually successful, since rejection does not occur, and the transplanted kidney functions well indefinitely unless the original disease in the recipient affects it. Allografts from related living donors or from cadavers are rejected unless immunosuppressive agents are employed. Those currently in use are corticosteroids, azathioprine, and antilymphocyte globulin. Among the serious complications due to these agents are infections both by pathogens and by organisms not normally pathogenic and an increased incidence of certain neoplasms. When the transplanted kidney functions normally, all elements of the uremic syndrome are corrected and the patient is rehabilitated to a normal life. With current techniques of immunosuppression, kidney survival rates are about 70 to 80 percent for 2 years in patients who receive transplants from living related donors with whom they are well matched by histocompatibility testing. With cadaver transplants, in which close histocompatibility matching is impossible, somewhat lower kidney survival rates generally have been reported (about 50 percent in 2 years). Although information is less complete after the first 2 years, the rate of loss of kidneys appears to be slower. Late loss of function may be due to chronic rejection or to damage to the transplanted kidney by the recipient's original kidney disease.

The clinical course of a patient who receives an allograft depends largely on the severity of the rejection reaction. Acute rejection usually occurs in the first few weeks after transplantation. It is detected by various clinical tests, of which the most important is acute deterioration of renal function, and it is treated with increased doses of steroids. Patients in whom rejection does not occur are usually able to return to ordinary activity within 2 months after transplantation. Thereafter immunosuppressive therapy is slowly tapered down with careful monitoring for evidence of delayed rejection. Repeated or persistent rejection may call for removal of the transplant to avoid the potentially lethal complications of high doses of steroids and azathioprine.

Bibliography

Brenner, B. M., and Rector, F. C. (eds.). *The Kidney.* Philadelphia: Saunders, 1976.

Fairly, K. F., Carson, N. E., Gutch, R. C., Leighton, P., Grounds, A. D., and O'Keefe, C. M. Site of infection in acute urinary tract infection in general practice. *Lancet* 2:616, 1971.

Germuth, F. G., Jr., and Rodriguez, E. *Immunopathology of the Renal Glomerulus.* Boston: Little, Brown, 1973.

Habib, R. Focal glomerular sclerosis. *Kidney Int.* 4:355, 1973.

Hayslett, J. P., Kashgarian, M., Bensch, L. C., Spargo, B. H., Freedman, L. R., and Epstein, F. H. Clinicopathological correlations in the nephrotic syndrome, due to primary renal disease. *Medicine* 52:93, 1973.

Heptinstall, R. H. *Pathology of the Kidney* (2nd ed.).
Boston: Little, Brown, 1974.

Kincaid-Smith, P., Mathew, T. H., and Becker, E. L.
(eds.). *Glomerulonephritis: Morphology,
Natural History and Treatment.* New York:
Wiley, 1973.

Kunin, C. M., Deutscher, R., and Paquin, A., Jr.
Urinary tract infection in school children: An
epidemiologic, clinical, and laboratory study.
Medicine 49:91, 1964.

McCabe, W. R., and Jackson, G. G. Treatment of
pyelonephritis: Bacterial, drug, and host factors in success or failure among 252 patients.
N. Engl. J. Med. 272:1037, 1965.

Papper, S. *Clinical Nephrology.* Boston: Little,
Brown, 1971.

Stamey, T. A., and Pfau, A. Urinary infections:
A selective review and some observations.
Calif. Med. 113:16, 1970.

Strauss, M. B., and Welt, L. G. (eds.). *Diseases of the
Kidney* (2nd ed.). Boston: Little, Brown, 1971.

Thompson, A. L., Durrett, R. R., and Robinson, R. R.
Fixed and reproducible orthostatic proteinuria:
VI. Results of a 10-year follow-up evaluation.
Ann. Intern. Med. 73:235, 1970.

Wilson, C. B., and Dixon, F. J. Anti-glomerular basement membrane antibody-induced glomerulonephritis. *Kidney Int.* 3:74, 1973.

54

Fluid and Electrolyte Balance

Norman G. Levinsky

Acid-Base Balance

Disorders of acid-base balance are common complications of a great variety of disease states. Often the acid-base disturbance is a relatively minor aspect of the patient's general problem, but occasionally it is so severe that it threatens the patient's survival and demands direct action by the physician. Under any circumstances, however, it is always important to recognize the existence of an acid-base imbalance and to identify its pathogenesis, for this provides valuable insight into the physiologic state of the patient and the nature and seriousness of his disease.

EVALUATION OF ACID-BASE DISORDERS

Classification of acid-base disorders is based on the biochemical changes in extracellular fluid, but it must be remembered that the latter do not always parallel the conditions inside cells; indeed, sometimes intracellular and extracellular acid-base changes are in opposite directions. *Acidosis* refers to any physiologic disturbance that tends to add acid to the extracellular fluid or to remove base from it. Compensatory mechanisms may minimize or prevent any fall in pH of the blood, but if the pH is significantly depressed the biochemical change is referred to as acidemia. There are two types of acidosis: respiratory and metabolic. Respiratory acidosis is the result of an increase in the CO_2 tension of the alveolar gas — that is, the acid being added to the blood in this instance is carbonic (H_2CO_3). As a result of the buffering of the carbonic acid and as a result also of the increased production and reabsorption of bicarbonate by renal tubules, the extracellular concentration of bicarbonate* tends to rise in respiratory acidosis, even as the pH tends to fall. In *metabolic acidosis,* on the other hand, acids other than H_2CO_3 accumulate in the extracellular fluid and combine with bicarbonate or else there is a direct loss of bicarbonate from the body; in either case, the result is a fall in bicarbonate concentration.

Alkalosis is defined as a physiologic disturbance that tends to remove acid from or add base to the extracellular fluid. Alkalemia — that is, a significant increase in blood pH — occurs in alkalosis only when compensatory mechanisms are inadequate. As with acidosis, there are two types of alkalosis: respiratory and metabolic. Respiratory alkalosis is the result of a decrease in the CO_2 tension of the alveolar gas — that is, removal of H_2CO_3 from extracellular fluid. Tissue buffering (sometimes accompanied by increased production of lactic acid) and renal adjustments cause a reduction in extracellular bicarbonate concentration. Metabolic alkalosis is due to the addition of base to the extracellular fluid or to loss of acid other than carbonic acid. In this condition, extracellular bicarbonate concentration rises.

Compensatory responses by the lungs and kidneys create major problems in the clinical assessment of acid-base disorders. Primary changes in PCO_2 lead to renal compensatory responses that produce parallel changes in bicarbonate. Respiratory compensation for a primary alteration in plasma bicarbonate changes carbon dioxide concentration in the same direction. Consider the following values in a patient with chronic respiratory failure: PCO_2, 60 mm Hg; HCO_3, 33 m*M* per liter; pH, 7.36. The physician must know whether the elevated plasma bicarbonate is due to renal compensation alone or to a superimposed metabolic acid-base disorder. Such information can be obtained only from clinical observations, not by calculation or a priori reasoning. Observations have been made in each primary disorder in man, and the results are best visualized by a "confidence band" presentation, as shown in Figure 54-1. Each band for a primary disorder represents the mean ± 2 standard deviations, that is, 95 percent of the observations that would be expected from the compensatory responses to that

---

*Throughout this discussion *bicarbonate concentration* is used instead of *CO_2 content,* but it should be understood that for practical clinical purposes the two terms are synonymous. Actually, of course, CO_2 content as measured in the laboratory includes dissolved CO_2 gas and H_2CO_3 as well as bicarbonate ions, but the former two moieties are usually negligibly small when compared to bicarbonate. The term *CO_2 combining power* is not mentioned because it is an anachronism without any physiologic meaning. Neither are the terms *whole blood buffer base, base excess, base deficit,* and *standard bicarbonate* used. The disadvantages of this latter terminology are discussed in detail by Schwartz and Relman elsewhere (see Bibliography).

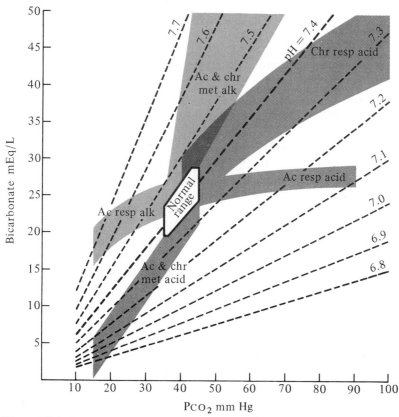

Figure 54-1. In-vivo nomogram showing bands for uncomplicated respiratory or metabolic acid-base disturbances. Each "confidence band" represents the mean ± 2 SD for the compensatory response to a given primary disorder. Ac = *acute;* Chr = *chronic;* Met = *metabolic;* Resp = *respiratory;* Acid = *acidosis;* Alk = *alkalosis. (Reprinted by permission from G. S. Arbus, An in vivo acid-base nomogram for clinical use.* Can. Med. Assoc. J. *109:291, 1973.)*

disturbance. In our example, inspection of the band for chronic respiratory acidosis indicates that 95 percent of patients with a chronic elevation of PCO_2 to 60 will have bicarbonate between 32 and 40 mM per liter resulting mainly from renal compensation. Therefore, the bicarbonate of 33 in the example is compatible with a compensated chronic respiratory acidosis alone. Obviously the use of this scheme does not eliminate the need for clinical judgment. If a patient had only recently developed hypercapnia, the same bicarbonate of 33 mM per liter would indicate superimposed metabolic alkalosis, since this value is well above the curve for acute respiratory acidosis.

METABOLIC ACIDOSIS

Pathogenesis. Metabolic acidosis is perhaps the most frequently encountered type of acid-base disturbance.

The major causes of metabolic acidosis are:

1. Renal insufficiency
   a. Primary tubular disease: hyperchloremic acidosis
   b. Azotemic renal failure: uremic acidosis
2. Ketoacidosis
   a. Diabetic acidosis
   b. Starvation ketosis
   c. Alcoholic ketoacidosis
3. Lactic acidosis
   a. Secondary to inadequate circulation
   b. Primary
   c. Drug-induced: phenformin
   d. Total fasting in obesity
4. Poisoning
   a. With increased anion gap: salicylates, methanol, ethylene glycol

b. With normal anion gap: ammonium chloride, acetazolamide, lysine/arginine chloride

Renal insufficiency is the commonest cause of chronic metabolic acidosis. The essential defect in all cases of renal acidosis is the inability of renal tubules to excrete endogenous acids at a rate equal to that at which they arise from intermediary metabolism. In some cases this defect includes a deficiency in the renal reabsorption of bicarbonate, so that the acidosis is due not only to retention of acid but also to loss of alkali. When the tubular defect occurs in the absence of a marked reduction of the glomerular filtration rate (and this is the case in the rare disease called renal tubular acidosis as well as in many cases of early chronic pyelonephritis), the reduction of plasma bicarbonate is associated with an equivalent rise in plasma chloride, causing a so-called hyperchloremic acidosis. On the other hand, when the glomerular filtration rate is very low and azotemia supervenes, metabolic anions such as phosphate and sulfate are retained in the plasma. In this condition, often referred to as uremic acidosis, there is usually little or no increase in plasma chloride concentration and the reduction in bicarbonate is approximately balanced by a rise in metabolic anions (unmeasured anions, anion gap).

Acidosis develops sooner or later in almost all patients with chronic progressive renal disease. When it is mild, it is of no particular consequence except in renal tubular acidosis, in which apparently even mild degrees of acidosis lead to hypercalciuria, osteomalacia, nephrocalcinosis, and lithiasis. In chronic renal failure, acidosis can become severe and may cause symptoms and signs that play an important role in the clinical picture of uremia.

Diabetic ketosis is probably the commonest cause of acute metabolic acidosis. Increased hepatic production of acetoacetic acid and beta-hydroxybutyric acid results from the defect in utilization of carbohydrate, and these acids accumulate in the extracellular fluid at the expense of bicarbonate. Despite the usual intense hyperventilation and a vigorous compensatory excretion of acid in the urine, blood pH is often reduced to very low levels.

Ketoacidosis may be associated with alcoholism. The typical patient gives a history of a recent high intake of alcohol, prolonged abstention from food, and often of protracted vomiting. Ketone bodies and lactate both accumulate in the plasma. Because the ratio of hydroxybutyrate to acetoacetate is unusually high, ketosis may be missed by the nitroprusside tests commonly in use; these tests respond only to acetoacetate. Blood glucose is usually normal or mildly elevated. The mechanism of this type of ketosis is unknown.

Starvation depletes carbohydrate stores and leads to overproduction of ketone bodies as a result of increased combustion of fat. This may produce a mild degree of chronic acidosis.

Another significant cause of metabolic acidosis is severe diarrhea, or intestinal malabsorption, as may occur in cholera, ileitis, sprue, severe ulcerative colitis, or in patients with a poorly controlled ileostomy. Liquid stool contains high concentrations of bicarbonate, typically 40 to 60 mEq per liter.

Pooling of urine in the colon of patients who have had a cystectomy and ureterosigmoidostomy sometimes causes hyperchloremic acidosis. This results from the intestinal secretion of bicarbonate into the urine in exchange for chloride and the subsequent excretion of alkali. Associated renal tubular insufficiency caused by ureteral obstruction and ascending pyelonephritis may further contribute to the development of acidosis. The use of ureterosigmoidostomy as a bladder substitute has now been largely superseded by the use of isolated ileal loops. This prevents stasis of urine and has virtually eliminated the problem of acidosis.

Lactic acidosis may be due to a number of causes. Most commonly it is secondary to circulatory failure, as in shock or sepsis. In these circumstances, lactic acid production is accelerated by the Pasteur effect, that is, tissue hypoxia stimulates glycolysis. The acidosis is usually moderate and the plasma lactate is less than 10 mM per liter, although severe acidosis may occur in shock or cardiopulmonary arrest. Primary or idiopathic lactic acidosis occurs either spontaneously or in association with a variety of conditions such as leukemia or cirrhosis. Its cause is obscure. Lactic acidosis has also appeared in some obese patients undergoing total starvation for weight reduction.

There are various types of acute acidosis due to

drug intoxication. Important among these are poisoning due to aspirin, methyl alcohol, and ethylene glycol. In each case the acidosis apparently is due to excessive production of a mixture of endogenous organic acids arising from a metabolic block caused either by the drug or by some degradation product of it. The quantities of endogenous acid released are greater than can be directly accounted for on a stoichiometric basis by the amount of ingested drug. In aspirin poisoning, the acid-base picture is complicated by the fact that the initial abnormality (and, in adults, often the only acid-base disturbance) is respiratory alkalosis due to direct stimulation of the respiratory center by the drug. In acidosis due to these agents, unmeasured anions are increased.

Acidosis of the hyperchloremic type results from the ingestion of ammonium chloride or other acidifying agents such as arginine hydrochloride. Ordinarily this acidosis is mild when the agents are used in therapeutic dosage, but some patients with latent or overt renal tubular impairment may become severely acidotic during the prolonged administration of even relatively small doses. The acidosis produced by the carbonic anhydrase inhibitor acetazolamide results from inhibition of bicarbonate reabsorption by the kidney. It is a self-limited acidosis that rarely becomes severe, because the drug becomes progressively less effective in producing a bicarbonate diuresis as plasma bicarbonate concentration is lowered.

Clinical Features. The symptoms and signs of metabolic acidosis are highly variable, depending on the severity and suddenness of the onset as well as on the clinical setting. The severer the acidosis and the more suddenly it occurs, the more evident its clinical manifestations will be. The symptoms and signs range from minimal fatigue, anorexia, malaise, and exertional dyspnea, to stupor or coma and intense hyperpnea (Kussmaul respiration). In extreme cases there is vascular collapse with hypotension.

Laboratory Findings. In metabolic acidosis, the characteristic findings in the blood are a reduced or low normal blood pH. The CO_2 tension (PCO_2) is also reduced, usually by about 1 mm Hg for each 1 mM per liter reduction in bicarbonate due to compensatory hyperventilation (see Fig. 54-1). In maxi-

mally severe cases, plasma bicarbonate may be less than 5 mEq per liter and pH may be below 7.0. (The lowest blood pH values compatible with life are in the range of 6.8 to 6.9; the most intense hyperventilation can lower PCO_2 only to approximately 10 mm Hg.) Acidosis tends to elevate plasma potassium by shifting potassium ions from cells to the extracellular space. In severe cases there may be marked hyperkalemia, but regardless of its initial level, plasma potassium always tends to fall as acidosis is corrected.

The reduction in plasma bicarbonate, which is the hallmark of metabolic acidosis, is associated with an increase either in the relative concentration of chloride (hyperchloremic acidosis) or in the concentration of the anions of the exogenous or endogenous acids responsible for the acidosis. Hyperchloremic acidosis is characteristic of renal tubular acidosis, early pyelonephritis, intestinal malabsorption, ureterocolostomy, or administration of ammonium chloride or acetazolamide. High anion acidosis is found in uremia, lactic acidosis, diabetic ketosis, or aspirin or methanol poisoning.

Other effects of severe acidosis on blood constituents include polymorphonuclear leukocytosis and hyperglycemia. The explanation for the former is not known, but hyperglycemia (and impaired glucose tolerance) is thought to be due to a direct inhibitory effect of lowered pH on one or more enzymes in the glycolytic pathway.

Treatment. When metabolic acidosis is relatively mild, no special treatment is usually required beyond that of the underlying disease. The only generally recognized exception to this rule is renal tubular acidosis, in which it is important to correct acidosis fully in order to avoid hypercalciuria and osteomalacia. Acidosis that becomes symptomatic or extremely severe ought to be corrected.

Chronic acidosis in renal failure probably should be corrected whenever the plasma bicarbonate level persists below 15 mEq per liter, because at such levels symptomatic deterioration may occur. Oral treatment is preferred to intravenous therapy whenever possible. Palatable solutions of sodium and potassium citrate are particularly useful in the management of chronic acidosis.

For acute or very severe cases, intravenous administration of alkali is necessary. Sodium bicarbonate is the agent of choice. A detailed discussion of the intravenous therapy of acidosis is beyond the scope of this chapter, but the essential principles can be summarized quite simply. The concentration of bicarbonate used intravenously is ordinarily between 44 and 132 mEq per liter (1 to 3 ampules per liter). Undiluted solutions (880 mEq per liter) should not be used to treat acidosis, since they may precipitate cardiac arrhythmias. The amount of alkali needed to correct an acidosis can be calculated on the assumption that the alkali will buffer equal amounts of extracellular plus intracellular acid. Hence an apparent distribution space of 40 percent of body weight (twice the extracellular volume) should be used. The rate at which the alkali is infused should be determined by the severity of the acidosis and by the patient's capacity to tolerate expansion of the extracellular space with sodium salts. Too rapid an administration of alkali not only risks circulatory overload, but also in some cases may cause troublesome hypokalemia or calcium deficiency tetany.

RESPIRATORY ACIDOSIS

Pathogenesis. Acute respiratory acidosis is usually the result of failure of ventilation due to (1) depression of the respiratory center by cerebral disease or drugs, (2) neuromuscular disorders, or (3) cardiopulmonary insufficiency. Chronic respiratory acidosis most often is due to chronic emphysema and bronchitis, in which effective alveolar ventilation is decreased and ventilation and perfusion are mismatched. Primary alveolar hypoventilation and the pickwickian syndrome (hypoventilation due to obesity) may also cause chronic hypercapnia. Diseases in which interference with alveolar gas exchange is the major abnormality, such as pulmonary fibrosis, pneumonia, and pulmonary edema, usually cause hypocapnia rather than elevated PCO_2. Hypoxia stimulates increased ventilation and, since CO_2 diffuses much more rapidly than O_2, PCO_2 is lowered unless the disease is extremely severe or respiratory fatigue supervenes.

Acute hypercapnia leads to an almost immediate rise in plasma bicarbonate owing to the buffering of H_2CO_3 by hemoglobin and other tissue buffers. This rise is modest (approximately 0.8 mEq per liter for each acute 10 mm Hg rise in PCO_2) and not sufficient to prevent a reduction in blood pH. With continued hypercapnia, renal excretion of acid gradually increases and results in further elevation of plasma bicarbonate. Simultaneously the renal threshold for bicarbonate increases, so that the newly generated bicarbonate is retained in the plasma. The final adjustment of plasma bicarbonate (the total rise is approximately 3 mEq per liter for each 10 mm Hg rise in PCO_2) brings the blood pH closer to the normal range.

Clinical Features. Patients with significant degrees of respiratory acidosis are usually cyanotic and have other obvious signs of pulmonary insufficiency. The relationship between the level of CO_2 tension and the clinical manifestations is variable, and it depends in part upon the speed with which hypercapnia develops. As a rule, hypercapnia per se has no important clinical effects until it reaches levels of 65 to 75 mm Hg and above. At that level mental processes become obtunded. At CO_2 tensions much above 90 mm Hg, patients are usually confused, stuporous, or comatose; and tremors, including asterixis and other neurologic signs, are common. Hypercapnia causes cerebral vasodilatation; this sometimes leads to increased intracranial pressure and papilledema. Occasionally generalized convulsions may occur. A common finding is dilatation of conjunctival vessels and chemosis, presumably due to the same cause.

Laboratory Findings. Analysis of blood reveals an elevated PCO_2, a low PO_2, a reduced pH, and usually an elevated bicarbonate concentration. Plasma chloride is usually reduced in inverse relation to the bicarbonate. In chronic steady states, blood pH is rarely below 7.20, but in acute conditions it may be much lower, particularly if severe anoxia and consequent lactic acidosis are superimposed on the hypercapnia. Serum potassium is often elevated if the respiratory acidosis is severe or acute.

Treatment. The only effective approach to the treatment of respiratory acidosis is to attempt to lower PCO_2 through the correction or amelioration of the underlying respiratory problem. The principles of management of pulmonary insufficiency are discussed elsewhere (see Chap. 23). Suffice it to say here that little or no lasting benefit accrues from attempts to correct blood pH by the administration of alkali.

METABOLIC ALKALOSIS

Pathogenesis. Metabolic alkalosis results from the loss of fixed acid or the accession of alkali by the extracellular fluid, or from the contraction of extracellular volume due to selective loss of sodium and chloride. The important clinical mechanisms leading to metabolic alkalosis are:

1. Volume (chloride) depletion due to
   a. Vomiting or gastric drainage
   b. Diuretic therapy (all agents in common use except acetazolamide, spironolactone, triamterene, amiloride)
   c. Posthypercapneic alkalosis
2. Hyperadrenocorticism in
   a. Cushing's syndrome
   b. Primary aldosteronism
   c. Bartter syndrome
3. Severe potassium depletion
4. Excessive alkali intake
   a. Acute excess
   b. Milk-alkali syndrome

Metabolic alkalosis is initiated by increased loss of acid, but excretion of excess bicarbonate is normally so rapid that alkalosis is not sustained unless bicarbonate resorption is stimulated or alkali is rapidly and continuously generated. Maintenance of metabolic alkalosis is commonly due to stimulation of bicarbonate reabsorption by a volume (chloride) deficit. During volume depletion, renal sodium conservation takes precedence over other homeostatic needs, including correction of alkalosis. In alkalosis, complete reabsorption of filtered sodium requires reabsorption of the excess bicarbonate. Alkalosis will be sustained until volume depletion is corrected by sodium chloride. This diminishes the avid tubular reabsorption of sodium and provides chloride as an alternative anion; excess bicarbonate can then be excreted with sodium.

Mineralocorticoids stimulate renal hydrogen ion secretion; elevation of plasma bicarbonate presumably is initiated by increased excretion of ammonium and titratable acid. Bicarbonate reabsorption is also enhanced thereby and sustains the metabolic alkalosis. Patients with hyperadrenalism are neither volume nor chloride deficient, and this type of alkalosis does not respond to sodium chloride. Most patients with Cushing's syndrome or primary aldosteronism have only minimal or moderate alkalosis. More marked alkalosis may occur in the extreme adrenal gland hyperfunction associated with tumors secreting corticotropin (ACTH) such as bronchogenic carcinoma. Moderate alkalosis is typical of patients with the Bartter syndrome.

Although alkalosis and potassium depletion are regularly associated, mild or moderate potassium depletion alone is rarely the cause of sustained metabolic alkalosis. However, when potassium depletion is extreme (serum potassium usually 2 mEq per liter or less), there may be an associated metabolic alkalosis that is resistant to correction with sodium chloride but does respond to potassium replacement.

As noted earlier, alkalosis due to alkali loads will not be maintained unless huge amounts are given. If renal function is compromised, alkalosis may be perpetuated by smaller amounts of alkali. This appears to be the mechanism of alkalosis in the milk-alkali syndrome, in which hypercalcemic nephropathy limits bicarbonate excretion, thus sustaining the alkalosis.

Clinical and Laboratory Features. Metabolic alkalosis, unless very severe, causes few clinical signs or symptoms. When severe, it may produce apathy, mental confusion, and slight depression of respiration. Occasionally signs of tetany may be apparent, particularly if the alkalosis develops rapidly and if serum calcium or potassium concentrations are reduced.

Laboratory findings include an increase in plasma or serum bicarbonate and an increase in blood pH. Respiratory compensation for metabolic alkalosis is clearly evident only in severe cases; the usual finding is only a very slight rise in CO_2 tension. Plasma chloride concentration is usually low, as is the concentration of potassium. The electrocardiogram, even when the potassium concentration is only slightly reduced, may show marked, so-called hypokalemic changes in the T and U waves. In most cases of chronic alkalosis the urine does not contain much bicarbonate and in fact may be neutral or even acid in reaction. This is sometimes referred to as paradoxical aciduria and is simply a reflection of the fact that the renal reabsorptive threshold for bicarbonate is increased.

Treatment. If possible, the specific factors responsible for the genesis and maintenance of the alkalosis should be identified and corrected. When potassium depletion is present, the administration of potassium chloride by mouth or vein is usually indicated. Alkaline salts of potassium may not be effective in correcting the alkalosis unless the intake also provides adequate amounts of chloride. In many cases, adequate amounts of sodium chloride will suffice to permit the kidneys to excrete bicarbonate and correct the alkalosis. The use of acidifying salts is not usually necessary and is best avoided unless the alkalosis is severe and intractable.

RESPIRATORY ALKALOSIS

Pathogenesis. Respiratory alkalosis results from alveolar hyperventilation, which reduces the CO_2 tension in the alveolar air and hence in the arterial blood. The hyperventilation in most cases is a reflection of increased activity of the respiratory center. The major clinical causes of hyperventilation that lead to respiratory alkalosis are

1. Psychoneurotic: the hyperventilation syndrome
2. Hyperventilation in anesthesia and artificial respiration
3. Secondary to hypoxia
   a. Pulmonary disease
   b. Cyanotic heart disease
   c. High altitude
4. Brain damage: encephalitis, vascular disease, etc.
5. Hyperpyrexia
6. Exercise
7. Bacteremia (especially when due to gram-negative organisms)
8. Hepatic coma
9. Salicylate intoxication
10. Pregnancy

Clinical Features. Depending on the severity and the acuteness of the hyperventilation, an overt increase in the respiratory rate and/or depth will be more or less apparent. In such mild states of chronic hyperventilation as those existing in pregnancy and at high altitudes, no change in respiration will be clinically detectable. In severe, acute cases, patients may complain of paresthesias, numbness, and tingling, and sometimes of twitching or frank tetany. Confusion or coma may supervene in extreme cases. These neurologic manifestations are probably due to reduced cerebral circulation as well as to the direct effects of low PCO_2 and high blood pH on neuromuscular excitability.

Analysis of blood reveals a decrease in CO_2 tension and a fall in serum bicarbonate concentration (see Fig. 54-1). Blood pH is usually only slightly increased but in severe cases may be markedly deviated in the alkaline direction. In acute, severe hyperventilation, serum lactate and pyruvate are significantly increased owing to stimulation of glycolysis by intracellular alkalosis; but in chronic conditions the change in plasma organic anions is negligible and there is a rise in chloride concentration that is approximately equal to the fall in bicarbonate. With the onset of hyperventilation the urine is usually alkaline, but with sustained hyperventilation it usually reverts to its usual reaction.

Treatment. As in other acid-base disturbances, treatment of respiratory alkalosis is sometimes unnecessary if the primary cause can be identified and eliminated, or in any event if the disturbance is mild and transient. When hypocapnia is very severe and the patient is symptomatic, it may become necessary to have him rebreathe into a bag or to have him breathe a mixture of 7 percent CO_2 and 93 percent O_2. Administration of acidifying salts is contraindicated.

"MIXED" ACID-BASE DISORDERS

Although the preceding discussion has considered each of the four primary types of acid-base disorder separately, it is not uncommon in clinical practice to find two types occurring simultaneously in the same patient. A frequent combination is respiratory alkalosis and metabolic acidosis, which is often seen in salicylate poisoning. The combination of respiratory acidosis with metabolic acidosis is also frequently encountered. This occurs acutely in asphyxia and in other acute clinical conditions with severe ventilatory and circulatory failure. In these situations, hypercapnia and hypoxic lactic acidemia may combine to cause very severe acidemia. In patients with chronic respiratory acidosis who are given ammonium chloride or acetazolamide, a combined disturbance will develop. In these cases the serum bicarbonate may be within normal limits, and yet blood pH may be dangerously low because of hypercapnia. These examples emphasize the need for careful and complete laboratory investigation of each patient with suspected acid-base disturbance. Although much can be deduced from the clinical background and the single determination of plasma bicarbonate, accurate diagnoses will not always be made unless pH and PCO_2 are also known, as well as the plasma electrolyte pattern.

Sodium and Water Metabolism

PATHOPHYSIOLOGY

The physiologic mechanisms that regulate sodium and water metabolism are closely interrelated. Sodium salts account for more than 90 percent of the total osmolality of the extracellular fluid; hence with only a single exception (which is discussed later), variations in plasma sodium concentration are always reflected in equivalent changes in plasma osmolality. Since water moves rapidly across cellular membranes to dissipate osmotic gradients, intracellular and extracellular fluids are always in osmotic equilibrium. The plasma sodium concentration, therefore, is an index not only of the relative proportions of sodium and water in extracellular fluid but also of the relation between total body solute and total body water. For example, a primary decrease in the concentration of solute within cells would cause intracellular water to shift out and dilute the plasma sodium.

Plasma osmolality is regulated by a receptor-effector system that involves the hypothalamus, the neurohypophysis, and the kidney. Hypothalamic osmoreceptors are able to detect changes of 2 percent or less in plasma osmolality. Small increases in osmo-

lality stimulate the secretion of antidiuretic hormone (ADH) from the neurohypophysis, while minimal decreases below the level set by the osmoreceptors suppress ADH secretion. The normal plasma osmolality is approximately 280 to 300 mOsm per kilogram of water, which is equivalent to a plasma sodium of 136 to 145 mEq per liter. When secretion of ADH is maximal, urine volume may be as little as 400 to 500 ml per day and urinary osmolality 800 to 1,400 mOsm per kilogram. Maximum water diuresis may exceed 20 liters per day; minimal urinary osmolality is 40 to 80 mOsm per kilogram. These efficient mechanisms can maintain plasma osmolality within narrow limits despite large variations in the volume and concentration of fluid intake.

Since regulation of plasma osmolality is equivalent to regulation of plasma sodium, it should be apparent that the primary determinant of plasma sodium concentration will be water metabolism rather than the total sodium content of the body. For example, primary excess of total sodium content could cause at most only a transient hypernatremia if water were available. Thirst would stimulate increased water intake, and the ingested fluid would be retained because ADH secretion would be stimulated. The result would be an expanded extracellular volume rather than hypernatremia. Conversely, loss of sodium without water would lead to decreased plasma sodium concentration only transiently if the osmoregulatory system were functioning normally. Decreased plasma osmolality would shut off ADH secretion, leading to a water diuresis. Plasma sodium concentration would be restored to normal, while extracellular volume would be decreased. Thus changes in total sodium content tend to result in changes in extracellular volume, whereas changes in plasma sodium concentration reflect changes in the regulation of water.

It is crucial to understand that the plasma sodium concentration per se gives no information about the amount of sodium present in the body. This amount is determined by the volume of the extracellular fluids as well as by the concentration of sodium in these fluids. Since changes in volume tend to be greater than changes in plasma sodium concentration, extracellular fluid volume is the dominant factor in determining the body sodium content. Plasma sodium concentration reflects merely the relative proportions of sodium and water, not the absolute amount of sodium in the body. Hyponatremia or hypernatremia indicates that the mechanisms controlling water metabolism are defective; either may occur whether total sodium content is decreased, normal, or increased.

The sodium content of the body, and hence the extracellular volume, depends on the balance between dietary intake and renal excretion of sodium. In normal subjects, extrarenal losses of sodium are negligible and renal excretion is closely regulated so as to be equal to dietary intake. About one-half of an administered sodium surfeit is excreted within the first day after its ingestion and the remainder over the next several days. If sodium intake stops, sodium excretion decreases to less than 5 to 10 mEq per day within 2 to 4 days. Thus extracellular volume can be maintained within normal limits despite wide variations in dietary sodium intake.

The mechanisms that regulate sodium excretion are incompletely understood. Changes in aldosterone secretion and in glomerular filtration rate are probably important. Recent evidence indicates that other very potent mechanisms regulate tubular sodium reabsorption; these include oncotic and hydrostatic forces in the peritubular circulation, which help determine proximal reabsorption, and possibly a hormonal inhibitor of tubular transport (natriuretic hormone). How these factors are integrated is unknown, but it is believed that receptor mechanisms respond to changes in plasma volume or some "effective" function thereof.

CLINICAL DISORDERS

Excesses and deficits of sodium and water occur in many clinical settings. The features of an underlying disease may overshadow those of the fluid and electrolyte disorder. A practical clinical classification of disorders of sodium and water metabolism is given in the facing outline, but it must be emphasized that mixed disturbances are much more common than isolated excesses or deficits.

Sodium and Water Depletion

Combinations of sodium and water deficits are much more common than isolated deficits of either constituent. The term *dehydration* is often used for combined deficits, but this usage is confusing. *Dehydration* should be used to describe relatively pure water depletion, and *volume depletion* or some similar term should be used for combined deficits. As already noted, elimination of sodium from the diet will not cause sodium depletion, since urinary sodium excretion will then decrease rapidly to negligible levels. Therefore sodium depletion must result either from extrarenal losses or from abnormal renal function. The principal causes of volume depletion are given in the outline below.

I. Combined sodium and water depletion (volume depletion)
  A. Extrarenal losses
    1. Gastrointestinal (vomiting, diarrhea, therapeutic gastrointestinal suction)
    2. Abdominal sequestration (rapid accumulation of ascites, peritonitis)
    3. Cutaneous (sweating)
  B. Renal
    1. Kidney disease (chronic renal failure; salt-wasting renal disease, e.g., medullary cystic disease, postoperative uropathy)
    2. Solute diuresis (diabetic glycosuria)
    3. Adrenal gland disease (Addison's disease, hypoaldosteronism)
II. Hyponatremia
  A. Associated with sodium depletion (volume depletion)
  B. Associated with sodium retention and edema (congestive heart failure, hepatic cirrhosis, nephrosis)
  C. Primary dilutional (excessive water administration, usually coupled with defective water diuresis, as in renal failure or after an operation)
  D. Adrenal gland insufficiency
  E. Syndrome of chronic inappropriate secretion of antidiuretic hormone (with pulmonary neoplasms or central nervous system diseases such as those due to neoplasms, meningitis, encephalitis, trauma; or after ingestion of drugs such as chlorpropamide)

F. Essential hyponatremia or sick-cell syndrome (chronic illness, e.g., pulmonary tuberculosis, hepatic cirrhosis, congestive heart failure)

G. Osmotic (hyperglycemic, mannitol-induced)

H. Artifactual (hyperlipemia, hyperproteinemia, laboratory error)

III. Hypernatremia

A. Extrarenal water loss
1. Skin and lungs (insensible losses, increased by fever)

B. Renal
1. Diabetes insipidus
2. Nephrogenic diabetes insipidus
3. Solute diuresis (urea diuresis due to high protein fed by stomach tube, glycosuria)

C. Grossly excessive salt intake with limited access to water (rare)

D. Adrenal excess (Cushing's disease, primary hyperaldosteronism)

Clinical Features and Diagnosis. Sodium and water depletion can usually be suspected from the history: Inadequate intake, vomiting, diarrhea, sweating, or symptoms of renal or adrenal disease may be noted. On physical examination, the principal signs are those of plasma and extracellular volume depletion. Skin turgor is decreased. Turgor can be estimated by noting the rate at which skin over the forehead or the sternum returns to position when it is raised between the examiner's fingers; in patients with volume depletion, it will settle slowly. With moderate volume depletion, blood pressure is usually normal when the patient is recumbent, but it may drop in the erect or sitting positions (postural hypotension). With more severe degrees of volume depletion, recumbent blood pressure may be reduced or even shock may occur. The patient is often lethargic, weak, and obtunded. Oliguria usually occurs when volume depletion is moderate or marked, even though recumbent blood pressure may be normal.

Laboratory Findings. The hematocrit and plasma protein concentration may be increased in sodium and water depletion. The plasma sodium concentration may be increased, normal, or decreased, depending on the proportionate deficits of sodium and water; usually plasma sodium is slightly to moderately reduced. The urinary sodium concentration will be less than 10 mEq per liter if extrarenal losses have caused the volume depletion, but it is usually more than 20 mEq per liter if renal or adrenal disorders are at fault. Thus determination of urinary sodium concentration may be helpful in differential diagnosis if the cause of volume depletion is not evident from the history. The plasma creatinine and urea nitrogen levels are almost always increased, since renal hemodynamics are compromised by volume depletion (prerenal azotemia).

Treatment. Moderate sodium and water deficits can often be corrected by increasing the oral intake of sodium and water. When depletion is more marked, or if gastrointestinal function is disturbed, isotonic (0.85 percent) saline should be infused. The hyponatremia found in patients with combined sodium and water depletion ordinarily does not of itself require treatment, and the plasma sodium concentration cannot be used to determine the degree of sodium deficit. The clinical features of sodium and water depletion are due to reduction of plasma and extracellular fluid volumes. Since there is no convenient clinical method for assessing these volumes, the amount of saline solution to be given must be determined by the clinical response as indicated by the blood pressure, urine output, and skin turgor.

Hyponatremia

Hyponatremia, defined as a decrease in plasma sodium concentration below the normal range (136 to 145 mEq per liter), is a sign of dilution of body fluids by an excess of water relative to total solute. Hyponatremia is not synonymous with sodium depletion, which is only one of several clinical settings in which it may occur (see the outline on p. 734).

Since the normal response to dilution of body fluids is a water diuresis, most types of hyponatremia can be considered to result from defective urinary dilution. Three factors are required for normal water diuresis: (1) ADH secretion must be suppressed; (2) adequate amounts of sodium and water must reach the ascending limb of Henle's loop and the distal convoluted tubule, the sites at which the urine is diluted; and (3) these nephron segments must actively reabsorb sodium and be impermeable to water. Thus defective water diuresis may be due to (1) inappropriate secretion of ADH despite extracellular fluid hypotonicity, which normally shuts off ADH secretion; (2) reduction in the amount of sodium reaching the diluting segments due to reduced glomerular filtration or enhanced proximal tubular absorption of sodium; or (3) defective sodium transport or excessive water permeability at the diluting sites due to renal disease or adrenal insufficiency. The mechanism of hyponatremia in most of the categories listed in the outline on page 734 can be interpreted within this framework.

The principal factor in the hyponatremia seen with sodium depletion and, paradoxically, that associated with edematous states, is probably a decreased delivery of sodium and water to the diluting segments. Glomerular filtration tends to be reduced and proximal tubular sodium and water reabsorption enhanced in both cases due to contraction of extracellular volume in sodium depletion and to inadequate "effective" extracellular volume in edematous states. Inappropriate secretion of ADH stimulated by volume contraction has also been postulated in these conditions, but direct evidence is lacking. In some edematous patients, essential hyponatremia may occur as well; this mechanism is discussed later.

Voluntary water intake is normally regulated by thirst and, in any case, the normal kidney can excrete more than 20 liters of dilute urine per day. Hence primary dilutional hyponatremia ordinarily occurs only when there is a combination of defective water diuresis and water intake unregulated by thirst. For example, primary dilutional hyponatremia is common postoperatively, and when fluids are administered parenterally, a number of mechanisms limit water diuresis. Primary dilutional hyponatremia may be induced in patients with renal failure by forcing of fluids. Very rarely, psychoneurotic ingestion of huge quantities of fluids may overwhelm normal water excretory capacity and produce symptomatic dilutional hyponatremia. The hyponatremia of adrenal insufficiency apparently results from multiple causes of defective urinary dilution. Because of sodium

depletion, glomerular filtration is reduced and proximal tubular sodium reabsorption is probably enhanced; therefore, delivery of sodium to the diluting sites falls. Glucocorticoids are needed to maintain normal glomerular filtration and may also be necessary to maintain the normal impermeability to water of the diluting sites in the absence of ADH. Aldosterone deficiency decreases sodium reabsorption at the diluting sites. Finally, some investigators believe that inappropriate secretion of ADH occurs.

In the syndrome of chronic inappropriate secretion of ADH, the cause of which is unknown, the hyponatremia is due not only to water retention but also to urinary losses of sodium. Renal sodium wasting is related to the volume expansion, which elevates glomerular filtration and depresses tubular sodium reabsorption.

Essential hyponatremia, also known as the sick-cell syndrome, is one of the very few types of hyponatremia that do not result from a defect in water diuresis. It is believed that changes in cellular metabolism lead to a primary reduction in cellular osmolality. A decrease in intracellular solute would cause water to shift out of cells, thereby diluting extracellular fluids and initiating hyponatremia. Osmoreceptor cells in the hypothalamus are thought to be "reset," maintaining the decreased plasma osmolality as though it were the normal level for the patient.

Clinical Features and Diagnosis. The plasma sodium concentration in sodium depletion is usually no more than moderately decreased. The hyponatremia itself is of little clinical significance; the prominent findings are those related to extracellular volume depletion, and these have been discussed previously.

In conditions such as congestive heart failure, cirrhosis, and the nephrotic syndrome, there is some correlation between the severity of the edema and the frequency and severity of hyponatremia. Some degree of hyponatremia is usually present in markedly edematous patients unless water intake is restricted. However, the hyponatremia itself is ordinarily of no clinical significance; the major clinical features are those of the underlying disease. Occasionally symptomatic hyponatremia with signs of water intoxication (see below) may result from excessive oral or parenteral intake of dilute fluids or from vigorous diuretic therapy.

As previously noted, primary dilutional hyponatremia occurs in a clinical setting in which water diuresis is defective. The clinical features of dilutional hyponatremia, sometimes known as water intoxication, are most marked in the central nervous and neuromuscular systems. Patients become lethargic, confused, stuporous, or even comatose; if water intoxication develops rapidly, signs of hyperexcitability may occur, such as increased reflexes, muscular twitches, or convulsions. Since extracellular fluid volume is increased, blood pressure and skin turgor are normal or increased. Laboratory studies may reveal the hematocrit and plasma protein concentration to be decreased, but plasma creatinine and urea are normal unless preexisting renal disease is present.

Inappropriate secretion of ADH is defined by certain unique clinical features: (1) The urine is never maximally dilute, even when hyponatremia is marked; usually, urine osmolality is higher than plasma osmolality (the elaboration of hypertonic urine is presumptive evidence of ADH secretion if glomerular filtration is not decreased); (2) the glomerular filtration rate is normal or increased (plasma creatinine and urea are normal or low); and (3) during fluid loading, hyponatremia increases due both to urinary sodium-wasting and to water retention. When fluid intake is restricted, the hyponatremia and urinary sodium-wasting are corrected. The syndrome has been found in association both with pulmonary neoplasms and with disorders of the central nervous system such as tumors, trauma, meningitis, and encephalitis. Isolated cases have been noted in a wide variety of apparently unrelated disorders such as acute porphyria and hypothyroidism. An increasing number of drugs are found to induce the syndrome, either by stimulating ADH secretion or by potentiating its tubular action or both. The principal drugs include the oral hypoglycemic agents chlorpropamide and tolbutamide; the antineoplastic agents vincristine and cyclophosphamide; and the psychoactive drugs amitriptyline and carbamazepine. Since extracellular volume is normal or expanded, blood pressure and skin turgor are normal. When hyponatremia is moderate, patients are usually asymptomatic. However, when the plasma sodium is reduced to less than 115 mEq per liter by fluid administration, the findings of water intoxication may develop.

Essential hyponatremia (sick-cell syndrome) occurs in patients with a variety of chronic illnesses such as pulmonary tuberculosis, congestive heart failure, and cirrhosis. This type of hyponatremia is asymptomatic; it is believed that the lack of symptoms is due to the absence of cellular swelling in the central nervous system, because the primary decrease in cell osmolality causes a shift of water out of cells. Skin turgor, blood pressure, and renal function are normal. Except when altered by the underlying disease, sodium metabolism and water metabolism are both normal in these patients. The urine becomes dilute in response to water loading but concentrated during dehydration; sodium loads are excreted, but urinary sodium excretion is reduced appropriately in response to sodium restriction.

Since the osmotic effect of glucose in plasma will cause water to move out of cells and dilute plasma sodium, hyponatremia is present whenever hyperglycemia is marked. Plasma sodium will decrease about 1.6 mEq per liter for each increase of 100 mg per 100 ml in plasma glucose above normal. This type of hyponatremia is the sole exception to the rule that hyponatremia means decreased plasma osmolality; the sum of the osmolalities due to glucose and to sodium salts does not fall as hyponatremia progresses. In severe hyperlipemia, part of any unit volume of plasma pipetted for analysis will be lipid, which is sodium free. Hyponatremia will then be reported by the laboratory, because the sodium concentration, in milliequivalents per liter of plasma, will be low. A similar explanation accounts for hyponatremia reported when extreme hyperproteinemia is present. Sodium concentration per liter of plasma water is normal, however, and these types of hyponatremia have no clinical significance.

Differential Diagnosis. In practice, differentiation of the various types of hyponatremia described above is sometimes difficult. The categories are somewhat artificial, because more than one type of hyponatremia may be present in a given patient and because knowledge of the pathophysiology of hyponatremia is inadequate. Nevertheless, the classification outlined is useful as a framework for diagnosis and treatment.

The history is usually the most important factor in diagnosis. For example, prolonged vomiting, diarrhea, or nasogastric suction will indicate sodium depletion. Hyponatremia in the postoperative period should suggest either primary dilutional hyponatremia or hyponatremia associated with unreplaced sodium losses. Critical items in the physical examination include the state of consciousness; neuromuscular function; skin turgor; and the blood pressure, especially in relation to postural changes. Hyponatremia associated with sodium depletion is not likely to occur in the presence of normal skin turgor and normal upright blood pressure. The hyponatremia associated with edematous states may be suggested by edema found on physical examination. Laboratory studies of importance are the plasma creatinine or urea, urinary osmolality or specific gravity, and urinary sodium. The hyponatremia of sodium depletion is rare if plasma creatinine is normal. If urinary specific gravity is much below 1.006 to 1.008 or if urinary sodium is less than 10 mEq per liter during fluid loading, inappropriate secretion of ADH is ruled out.

Treatment. Hyponatremia itself is rarely of clinical significance when the plasma sodium is above 125 mEq per liter, except that neuromuscular symptoms may occasionally occur at even higher levels of plasma sodium if there has been a rapid decrease in the sodium concentration. When hyponatremia is associated with sodium depletion, one should try to correct the volume deficits. Primary dilutional hyponatremia is best treated by water restriction. If severe neuromuscular symptoms such as convulsions are present, hypertonic saline solution should be infused. The amount of sodium to be given must be calculated by multiplying the deficit in concentration (milliequivalents per liter) by total body water (55 percent of weight in men, 50 percent in women), because the osmotic effect of administered hypertonic saline will cause water to shift out of cells. Hyponatremia associated with edema responds to correction of the underlying disease; moderate water restriction may be necessary. Since edematous subjects have excess total sodium, hypertonic saline solution should not be administered except in rare instances in which hyponatremia is marked and stupor or other extreme symptoms occur. Hyponatremia due to inappropriate secretion of ADH responds to water restriction.

Hypernatremia

Hypernatremia always means that there is a deficit in body water relative to sodium. In most patients, hypernatremia is due to an absolute deficit in water caused either by losses or by deficient intake. In rare instances, administration of large excesses of salt may lead to hypernatremia despite normal total body water. Since hypernatremia normally stimulates thirst, severe, persistent hypernatremia is seen only when water losses occur in patients whose fluid intake is limited (e.g., infants or unconscious patients). Minimal persistent hypernatremia occurs in Cushing's disease and hyperaldosteronism; the mechanism is unknown. The principal circumstances that result in hypernatremia are listed in the outline on page 735.

Clinical Features and Diagnosis. The most notable symptoms of hypernatremia are confusion, obtundation, stupor, and coma, depending on the severity of hyperosmolality. It is believed that these central nervous system findings are due to dehydration of the brain; the clinical features of hyperosmolality due to extreme hyperglycemia (more than 800 to 1,000 mg per 100 ml) are similar. Since only about one-third of a water deficit is lost from extracellular fluids, the clinical features of extracellular volume depletion such as poor skin turgor or lowered blood pressure are usually not prominent.

Treatment. The treatment of hypernatremia is the administration of water, either by mouth or by intravenous infusions of dextrose in water. Since water deficits are drawn from both intracellular and extracellular fluid, calculations of water requirements must be based on total body water.

Potassium Metabolism

Disorders of potassium metabolism occur frequently in medicine and sometimes are of major clinical importance. To understand these, one must know a few elementary facts about the metabolism of potassium.

NORMAL BODY CONTENT

The body of a normal man contains about 40 to 46 mEq of potassium per kilogram of body weight, most of it in the lean-tissue mass. Almost all body potassium is "exchangeable," and under normal conditions it appears to be osmotically active. The greatest proportion — approximately 97 percent — of body potassium is found within cells, where it exists at a mean concentration of about 150 to 160 mEq per liter of cell water. Since the normal potassium concentration of extracellular fluid is only 4 to 5 mEq per liter, it is apparent that a very steep concentration gradient is maintained across the cell membrane. This is thought to be the result of a balance between the active transport of potassium into cells and a slower rate of passive outward diffusion from cells. Distribution of potassium between the intracellular and extracellular spaces is also greatly influenced by the relative acidity of the two compartments; all other factors being equal, extracellular acidosis tends to drive potassium out of cells to elevate the plasma concentration, whereas extracellular alkalosis has the opposite effect.

PHYSIOLOGY

The physiologic functions of potassium are still not entirely understood. Inside cells, potassium seems to be an important cofactor for several enzymes of intermediary metabolism. This relationship is probably responsible for the diabetogenic effect of severe potassium depletion and for certain disturbances in renal tubular cell function that are characteristic of potassium deficiency. Extracellular potassium greatly influences neuromuscular function. The ratio of intracellular to extracellular potassium concentration is the major determinant of membrane potential in nerve and muscle. Since extracellular potassium is low, small deviations in its absolute concentration will greatly influence the ratio. Conversely, only large changes in intracellular potassium will affect the ratio

significantly. The practical significance of these relations is illustrated by the effectiveness of glucose infusion in hyperkalemic toxicity by inducing movement of potassium from plasma to cells.

The external turnover of potassium is quite variable, but in the normal adult it will usually vary between 40 and 100 mEq per day, which is equal to the potassium content of the average American diet. Potassium is excreted from the body by three routes:

1. Skin: In the sensible and insensible perspiration, usually less than 5 mEq is excreted per day. Even when there is excessive sweating, losses of potassium from the skin are rarely of clinical significance.
2. Stool: Normal, formed stools contain only 5 to 10 mEq per day. However, the concentration of potassium in stool water is high (40 to 60 mEq per liter); hence very large quantities of potassium may be lost from the body when there is diarrhea or any other change in intestinal absorption that results in the excretion of bulky stools.
3. Urine: The urine is ordinarily the major route of potassium excretion. The kidneys normally regulate the excretion of potassium and defend the net balance of this ion. However, they respond relatively slowly to the withdrawal of potassium from the diet and do not reduce urine potassium concentrations to very low levels until the total body deficit has reached 200 to 300 mEq and the serum concentration has decreased at least moderately.

RELATION BETWEEN PLASMA CONCENTRATION AND TOTAL BODY CONTENT OF POTASSIUM

In general, potassium depletion leads to hypokalemia, but the severity of the latter is determined not only by the extent of the body deficit but also by the acid-base balance of the blood and the state of renal function. These considerations are discussed in more detail below. In certain acute situations (e.g., familial periodic paralysis and following the administration of glucose and insulin), rapid shifts of potassium from the extracellular space into cells may lower serum potassium concentration without any external loss of potassium. Thus potassium deficiency and hypokalemia are not necessarily related, and the terms should not be used synonymously.

Hyperkalemia is even less directly related to the body content of potassium, since significant increases in the latter probably do not occur. Instead, hyperkalemia usually is the result either of an impairment in renal excretion of potassium or of a disturbance in the mechanisms that regulate the distribution of this ion between cells and extracellular space. Indeed, it is common to find hyperkalemia in patients whose tissue spaces are actually depleted of potassium. This point will also be further explained below.

CLINICAL DISORDERS

Potassium Depletion and Hypokalemia
By potassium depletion is meant a significant external loss of potassium from the body, regardless of the change in the serum concentration of potassium. Ordinarily adult patients show few if any clinical or physiologic effects, and their serum potassium concentration is not significantly reduced until their body deficit is at least 100 mEq.

Etiology. The clinical causes of potassium depletion and hypokalemia are

I. Low potassium intake
II. Gastrointestinal loss (vomiting, diarrhea, villous adenoma, fistulas, ureterosigmoidostomy)
III. Urinary loss of potassium
    A. Renal tubular disease (renal tubular acidosis, Fanconi syndrome, leukemia [usually with lysozymuria])
    B. Glycosuria
    C. Diuretics (mercurials, thiazides, furosemide, ethacrynic acid, acetazolamide, etc.)
    D. Excessive adrenal steroids
       1. Primary aldosteronism
       2. Secondary aldosteronism (malignant hypertension, Bartter syndrome, juxtaglomerular tumors)
       3. Glucocorticoid excess
IV. Hypokalemia due to shift into cells (no depletion)
    A. Periodic paralysis
    B. Insulin effect

Clinical Features. If it develops gradually, potassium depletion, even when severe in degree, may be virtually asymptomatic. However, patients frequently note at least some vague malaise, weakness, and fatigue. Very severe depletion may cause marked generalized motor weakness of muscles, especially in the lower extremities, often associated with considerable aching and stiffness. Abrupt development or sudden exacerbation of potassium depletion may result in virtual paralysis of all peripheral skeletal musculature, even including the muscles of respiration. Polyuria and polydipsia are very common symptoms.

On physical examination, potassium-deficient patients sometimes show slight peripheral edema. They may also demonstrate decreased motor power, diminished or absent deep tendon reflexes, and occasionally signs of tetany. The cardiovascular manifestations of potassium depletion include hypotension and cardiac arrhythmias, the latter especially in patients taking digitalis.

Laboratory Findings. Potassium deficiency should be suspected from the history, which often reveals the existence of one or more of the depleting mechanisms listed above. However, the diagnosis cannot be confirmed without laboratory evidence. Hypokalemia is usually present, though not invariably, and generally it is roughly proportional to the body deficit of potassium. As already noted, the plasma concentration at any given level of potassium balance will be considerably influenced by the acid-base state of the body and by renal function. Thus a very acidotic or azotemic patient may have a normal or even elevated plasma potassium concentration despite a significant body deficit of potassium. Conversely, a severe alkalosis will tend to lower plasma potassium beyond the extent to be expected from the potassium balance.

The electrocardiogram usually shows characteristic changes, particularly in T and U waves, which are illustrated in Figure 32-32, page 380. The T wave is flattened, diphasic, or inverted, whereas the U wave remains upright and becomes more prominent. These alterations are only roughly correlated with the severity of the disturbance in potassium metabolism and do not appear to be clearly related either to serum concentration or to total body deficit. Potassium depletion enhances the toxic effects of digitalis on the myocardium, so if such a patient is taking a glycoside preparation there may also be electrocardiographic signs of digitalis intoxication.

Potassium-Depletion Nephropathy. Severe potassium depletion produces pathognomonic vacuolar lesions in the cytoplasm of the proximal convoluted tubules and a characteristic pattern of renal tubular dysfunction. Ability to concentrate the urine is usually impaired, and sometimes there is polyuria with the excretion of a persistently hypotonic urine. Sodium excretion is reduced (hence the tendency to peripheral edema), and the excretion of ammonia is relatively high. Renal threshold for bicarbonate is high, and the urine does not contain much bicarbonate even when the plasma bicarbonate is greatly elevated. Filtration rate is only slightly reduced, so the blood urea nitrogen and serum creatinine concentrations are not significantly increased. Urinalysis usually discloses only a low specific gravity, a trace of protein, and a few hyaline and granular casts.

Potassium-depletion nephropathy does not interfere with the normal potassium-conserving responses of the kidney. Thus when significant loss of potassium has occurred through the gastrointestinal route it is to be expected that the urine will contain less than 20 mEq per day; the same is true if the deficiency has resulted largely from inadequate intake. On the other hand, if a severely depleted patient is excreting more than 20 mEq of potassium in the urine per day, it is likely that renal potassium-wasting is the cause. In that case, if a kaliuretic steroid or diuretic drug is not currently being administered, one may conclude either that there is potassium-wasting renal tubular disease or that the patient is suffering from hyperadrenalism of one sort or another.

Treatment. It is preferable, whenever possible, to repair potassium deficiency gradually with oral supplements of potassium given in divided doses over a period of at least several days. However, acute neuromuscular or cardiovascular manifestations may require prompt intravenous administration of at least

enough potassium to alleviate the acute signs of deficiency.

If there is concomitant alkalosis with hypochloremia, potassium chloride is required; if there is acidosis, an alkalizing salt such as potassium citrate or gluconate is preferable. Oral therapy is best administered in the form of solutions or uncoated tablets; some enteric-coated preparations have been responsible for intestinal ulceration due to release of high local concentrations of potassium. Special caution must also be exercised to avoid sudden or excessive elevation in serum potassium concentration, which may be dangerous. This is particularly likely with intravenous therapy if renal excretory function is impaired or if the rate of infusion is rapid. Good general rules are

1. Never give potassium intravenously to oliguric or anuric patients or to patients in whom severe renal disease is known or suspected.
2. Never give potassium intravenously at a concentration greater than 60 mEq per liter or at a rate faster than 30 mEq per hour.
3. Whether using the oral or intravenous route, never give more than 200 mEq per day unless it is clear that continuing losses are large enough to warrant more intensive therapy.

When hypokalemia occurs together with hypocalcemia (as is often the case in patients with the malabsorption syndrome), restoration of a normal potassium concentration without concurrent administration of calcium will often precipitate signs of tetany. Similarly, administration of calcium without potassium to such patients may exacerbate the neuromuscular and electrocardiographic manifestations of potassium deficiency. Even in the absence of any apparent calcium deficit, patients sometimes manifest mild tetany during the period their potassium deficiency is being treated.

Hyperkalemia and Potassium Intoxication
Hyperkalemia may be defined as any rise in plasma potassium concentration above normal, regardless of the total body content of potassium. Ordinarily serum levels below 6.5 mEq per liter have relatively

little clinical effect, and true intoxication due to hyperkalemia does not begin to appear until concentrations of 7 or 8 mEq per liter have been reached.

Etiology. The important clinical causes of hyperkalemia are

1. Renal insufficiency
   a. Acute renal failure with oliguria or anuria
   b. Severe chronic renal failure (especially with oliguria or acidosis)
2. Adrenocortical deficiency
   a. Addison's disease
   b. Hypoaldosteronism
3. Diuretics interfering with renal excretion of potassium (spironolactone, triamterene, amiloride)
4. Increased potassium delivery to plasma
   a. Excessive intravenous or (rarely) excessive oral intake
   b. Increased release of potassium from red cells or tissues (as in severe acidosis, intravascular hemolysis, crushing injuries, massive infarction, internal hemorrhage, etc.)
   c. Shift from muscle due to succinylcholine or digitalis poisoning
   d. Acidosis
   e. Hyperkalemic periodic paralysis
5. "Pseudohyperkalemia" (thrombocytosis, leukocytosis, in vitro hemolysis)

Impairment in renal excretion of potassium may be either a primary or a secondary factor in hyperkalemia. Acute renal failure, particularly when associated with oliguria or anuria, is a common primary cause of severe hyperkalemia. In chronic renal disease, on the other hand, the serum potassium does not usually rise to clinically significant levels (i.e., plasma concentrations above 6.5 mEq per liter) until the terminal, oliguric phase of the illness or unless some superimposed factor increases the load or shifts extra potassium from the cells to the extracellular space. Functional renal impairment is a contributing factor in most instances of severe hyperkalemia due to hypoadrenalism. In this circumstance, renal hypoperfusion due to sodium depletion and circulatory insufficiency often adds to an already existing defect

in tubular secretion of potassium that has resulted from lack of aldosterone. (Aldosterone deficiency probably also contributes to hyperkalemia by altering the distribution of potassium between intracellular and extracellular fluid.) Increased potassium loads rarely cause dangerous hyperkalemia unless there is at least a moderate impairment of renal capacity to excrete potassium. The latter defect may be due to sodium depletion; to renal hypoperfusion, as in shock; to congestive heart failure; or to cirrhosis of the liver; or it may be due to the action of a drug that interferes with the renal excretion of potassium.

"Pseudohyperkalemia" may result from the release of potassium by platelets or leukocytes during clotting, when great numbers of these formed elements are present. In such cases there is no true elevation of potassium concentration in vivo, and "hyperkalemia" will be apparent only in samples of serum but not of plasma.

Clinical Features. The physiologic effects of hyperkalemia are due chiefly to the depolarization of the membranes of the cardiac and skeletal musculature. Hence the major clinical manifestations are cardiac arrhythmias and occasionally peripheral muscle weakness or paralysis.

Laboratory Findings. The diagnosis of hyperkalemia may be suspected from the clinical situation, but it must be established by chemical and electrocardiographic means. The serum potassium concentration is, of course, always elevated. The electrocardiogram usually reveals diagnostic changes, some of which are illustrated in Figure 32-31, page 379. Peaking of the T wave is the earliest change; later the QRS segment widens, the P-R interval lengthens, and the P wave disappears. Finally ventricular arrhythmias appear, culminating in fatal fibrillation or arrest. The severity of these abnormalities is generally closely related to the serum concentration of potassium, although it will also be influenced by concomitant levels of sodium and calcium and by the state of acid-base balance.

Treatment. The urgency and vigor with which treatment is initiated should depend on the severity of the hyperkalemia and the degree of electrocardiographic aberration. When life is threatened by severe cardiac toxicity, therapy must be begun at once with procedures that will rapidly lower the serum potassium concentration by causing potassium to shift into cells, even if the effect is only transient. Such measures include the rapid intravenous infusion of hypertonic glucose solutions with insulin and the infusion of sodium bicarbonate. Even though they do not affect the potassium concentration in the blood, calcium salts are also useful in an emergency because they transiently counteract the toxic effects of potassium on the heart. More lasting benefit is achieved by efforts to eliminate the cause of the potassium intoxication and by measures that remove potassium from the body. For the latter purpose, oral or rectal administration of sodium- or calcium-cycle ion-exchange resins has been used successfully. The most effective techniques for the removal of potassium are hemodialysis and peritoneal dialysis, but these are relatively slow in their effect and are not primarily useful in an emergency. The role of dialysis in the treatment of hyperkalemia in acute renal failure is mainly preventive.

Bibliography

ACID-BASE BALANCE

Arbus, G. S. An in vivo acid-base nomogram for clinical use. *Can. Med. Assoc. J.* 109:291, 1973.

Brackett, N. C., Jr., Wingo, C. F., Muren, O., and Solano, J. T. Acid-base response to chronic hypercapnia in man. *N. Engl. J. Med.* 280:124, 1969.

Levy, L. J., Duga, J., Girgis, M., and Gordon, E. E. Ketoacidosis associated with alcoholism in non-diabetic subjects. *Ann. Intern. Med.* 78:213, 1973.

Oliva, P. B. Lactic acidosis. *Am. J. Med.* 48:209, 1970.

Relman, A. S. Renal acidosis and renal excretion of acid in health and disease. *Adv. Intern. Med.* 12:295, 1964.

Schwartz, W. B., and Relman, A. S. A critique of the parameters used in the evaluation of acid-base disorders. *N. Engl. J. Med.* 268:1382, 1963.

Seldin, D. W., and Rector, F. C. The generation and maintenance of metabolic alkalosis. *Kidney Int.* 1:306, 1972.

DISORDERS OF SODIUM, POTASSIUM, AND WATER METABOLISM

Bartter, F. E., and Schwartz, W. B. The syndrome of inappropriate secretion of antidiuretic hormone. *Am. J. Med.* 42:790, 1967.

Brenner, B. M., and Berliner, R. W. Transport of Potassium. In J. Orloff and R. W. Berliner (eds.), *Handbook of Physiology.* Washington, D.C.: American Physiological Society, 1973.

Cannon, P. J. Juxtaglomerular cell hyperplasia and secondary aldosteronism (Bartter's syndrome): A reevaluation of the pathophysiology. *Medicine* 47:107, 1968.

Levinsky, N. G. Management of emergencies. VI. Hyperkalemia. *N. Engl. J. Med.* 274:1076, 1966.

Michelis, M. F., and Murdaugh, H. V. Selective hypoaldosteronism. *Am. J. Med.* 59:1, 1975.

Moses, A. M., and Miller, M. Drug-induced dilutional hyponatremia. *N. Engl. J. Med.* 291:1234, 1974.

Ross, E. J., and Christie, S. B. M. Hypernatremia. *Medicine* 48:441, 1969.

Schwartz, W. B., and Relman, A. S. Effects of electrolyte disorders on renal structure and function. *N. Engl. J. Med.* 276:283, 1967.

Surawicz, B. Relationship between the ECG and electrolytes. *Am. Heart J.* 73:814, 1967.

Weiner, M., and Epstein, F. H. Signs and symptoms of electrolyte disorders. *Yale J. Biol. Med.* 43:76, 1970.

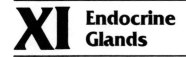

XI Endocrine Glands

55

The Pituitary Gland

Disorders of the Anterior Pituitary Gland
James C. Melby and Judith L. Vaitukaitis

The pituitary gland consists of three lobes, each differing in embryongenesis and histology. The anterior and intermediate lobes are derived from the embryonic pharynx of Rathke's pouch; the posterior lobe is a direct extension of neural tissue — axons of nerve cells that originate in the hypothalamus. The anterior pituitary secretes seven polypeptide or glycoprotein hormones, including growth hormone (GH); prolactin; thyroid-stimulating hormone (TSH); corticotropin (ACTH); melanocyte-stimulating hormone (β-MSH) or β-lipotropin (beta-LPH); luteinizing hormone (LH), and follicle-stimulating hormone (FSH). The various tropic hormones are elaborated by specialized cells distinguishable by their staining characteristics, and they are listed with their hormonal products in Table 55-1.

HYPOTHALAMIC REGULATION OF THE ANTERIOR PITUITARY

Hypothalamic Hypophysiotropic Peptides
The anterior pituitary communicates with the median eminence of the hypothalamus through the portal circulation, a network of blood vessels that supplies the median eminence and surrounds the infundibular stalk of the pituitary. Within the median eminence of the hypothalamus, small specialized secretory neurons (peptidergic neurons) elaborate the hypophysiotropic hormones, small polypeptides that are referred to as releasing and inhibitory factors. These releasing or inhibitory factors find their way through the portal vessel circulation to the anterior pituitary, where they exert their effects. The presently known hypothalamic hypophysiotropic peptides are also listed in Table 55-1.

Secretion of the releasing factors and the inhibitory factors by the hypothalamus involves both negative and positive feedback control systems. The negative feedback control systems are preeminent, and the positive feedback controls are less apparent. A variety of clinical conditions may be associated with disturbed long-loop negative feedback control; these will be discussed separately.

Monoaminergic Neurotransmitters Controlling the Hypothalamic Hypophysiotropic Peptidergic Neurons. Three monoamines function as neurotransmitters in the regulation of the secretion of the hypophysiotropic hormones. These neurotransmitters are dopamine, norepinephrine, and serotonin. Dopamine stimulates the hypophysiotropic peptidergic neurons to secrete both GH releasing factor and prolactin

Table 55-1. Adenohypophyseal Hormones: Sources and Hypothalamic Regulation

Cell type	Tropin	Molecular weight (daltons)	Hypothalamic hypophysiotropic peptides	
			Releasing factor (RF)	Inhibiting factor (IF)
Acidophils (35%)				
Somatotrophs	GH	21,700	GHRF	*SIF
Lactotrophs	Prolactin	22,500	Prolactin RF *TRF	Prolactin IF
Basophils (20%)				
Corticotrophs	ACTH	4,507	CRF	....
Melanotrophs	β-LPH	9,500	? MRF	MIF
Thyrotrophs	TSH	26,600 Glycoprotein	*TRF	....
Gonadotrophs	LH	30,000 Glycoprotein	*LRF	....
	FSH	30,000 Glycoprotein		

Note: * = known structure; ? = structure unknown; GH = growth hormone; C = corticotropin; β-LPH = beta-lipoprotein stimulating hormone; TSH = thyroid-stimulating hormone; LH = luteinizing hormone; FSH = follicle-stimulating hormone.

inhibiting factor. Pharmacologic agents that increase the synthesis and uptake of dopamine would thus be expected to induce a rise in growth hormone concentrations and a fall in prolactin levels in the serum. L-Dopa and apomorphine increase the pool of dopamine and markedly stimulate growth hormone secretion. These agents are used to test the ability of the anterior pituitary to secrete GH. Similarly, administration of the drug bromergocryptine results in increased dopamine activity with the elaboration of prolactin inhibiting factor and consequent suppression of prolactin secretion. For this reason, this agent is used in the treatment of galactorrhea. Chlorpromazine and reserpine block the uptake and storage of dopamine and norepinephrine in the hypothalamic neurons, and hence cause GH releasing factor and prolactin inhibiting factor levels to fall. Inhibition of prolactin inhibiting factor secretion leads to galactorrhea in some young women. Norepinephrine stimulates the hypophysiotropic peptidergic neurons to secrete LH releasing factor and TSH releasing factor. Serotonin activates corticotropin releasing factor and prolactin releasing factor secretion. The serotonin antagonist cyproheptadine has been used in the treatment of Cushing's syndrome due to the excessive production of pituitary ACTH (see Chap. 56). Pharmacologic agents that alter hypophysiotropic hormone secretion by disturbing the monoamine neurotransmitter control system are used both in a variety of tests of anterior pituitary function and in the treatment of neuroendocrine disorders.

A number of neuroendocrine syndromes may arise due to destruction of the hypothalamus and interruption of the hypothalamic-hypophyseal portal system, or both, as may occur, for example, with a tumor such as a craniopharyngioma. Several such syndromes are not accompanied by other demonstrable pathology, however. It is generally true that monotropic deficiencies of anterior pituitary hormones are rarely due to pathology within the pituitary but rather are associated with hypophysiotropic disturbances. In Table 55-2 are listed clinical syndromes that are associated with disturbed hypothalamic neuroendocrine secretion.

Table 55-2. Clinical Syndromes due to Altered Hypophysiotropic Hormone Secretion by the Hypothalamus

Clinical neuroendocrine syndrome	Hypophysiotropic hormone	Alteration
Cerebral gigantism	GHRF	Increased
	? SIF	Decreased
Acromegaly (acidophil hyperplasia)	GHRF	Increased
	? SIF	Decreased
Sexual ateliotic dwarfism (isolated GH deficiency)	GHRF	Decreased
	? SIF	Increased
Isolated TSH deficiency	TRF	Decreased
"Hypothalamic" hyperthyroidism	TRF	Increased
Isolated ACTH deficiency	CRF	Decreased
Cushing's syndrome	CRF	Increased
Wolff syndrome — tonic ACTH ↑	CRF	Increased
Isosexual precocious puberty	LRF	Increased
"Psychogenic" amenorrhea	LRF	Decreased
Olfactory-genital dysplasia (Kallman syndrome)	LRF	Decreased
Nonpuerperal galactorrhea (Chiari-Frommel syndrome)	PIF	Decreased

Note: GHRF = growth hormone releasing factor; SIF = somatostatin inhibiting factor; TSHRF = thyroid releasing factor; CRF = corticotropin releasing factor; LRF = luteinizing releasing factor; PIF = prolactin inhibiting factor.

THE ADENOHYPOPHYSEAL HORMONES AND DISORDERS OF SECRETION

Growth Hormone – Clinical Physiology and Disorders of Secretion

All of the actions of GH promote growth and maintenance of lean body mass. Growth hormone is anabolic and stimulates amino acid transport into cells and cell replication (number) but not hypertrophy. Further, GH stimulates the lipolysis of fat, promotes ketogenesis, and inhibits the action of insulin – the so-called diabetogenic effect. The actions of GH in promoting long bone and cartilage growth are mediated through somatomedin that GH stimulates the liver to synthesize (molecular weight, about 10,000). Somatomedin circulates in the plasma associated with macromolecules, and its biologic action is to stimulate the incorporation of the amino acids into mucoproteins of cartilage, uridine into RNA, and thymidine into DNA. Somatomedin may be the same substance as "nonsuppressible insulin-like activity-S" (NSILA-S). Both somatomedin and NSILA-S are increased after injections of GH, but both are markedly reduced by hypophysectomy. Somatomedin also may be responsible for the insulin resistance observed after GH administration.

Secretion of GH releasing factor is stimulated by dopaminergic activation of hypothalamic peptidergic neurons. Dopaminergic pharmacologic substances, including L-dopa and apomorphine, evoke intense acceleration of GH secretion and are used to test GH reserve. Release of GH releasing factor is also stimulated by hypoglycemia, hyperaminoacidemia, exercise, fasting, and fever. Somatostatin, which is composed of 14 amino acids, inhibits GH secretion. Inhibition of GH releasing factor, and perhaps also stimulation of somatostatin release (hence, inhibition of GH secretion) can be produced by the administration of dextrose. Somatostatin is a potent inhibitor of glucagon and insulin secretion. It also lowers plasma glucose levels independently of its effects on insulin and glucagon secretion.

Growth Hormone Deficiency

An acquired monotropic deficiency of GH in adults is without clinical manifestations. However, when GH deficiency occurs before puberty, dwarfism results. Growth hormone regulates somatic growth after 2 years of age, and its secretion increases sharply at 10 to 12 years of age. In the total absence of GH, one may attain a height of no more than 48 inches (120 cm). Isolated GH deficiency is rarer than GH deficiency associated with panhypopituitarism in children. Isolated or monotropic deficiency of GH results in proportionate dwarfism and delayed but normal puberty. This form of dwarfism is referred to as sexual ateliotic dwarfism, and it may be inherited as an autosomal recessive trait or it may be sporadic. Another type of sexual ateliotic dwarfism is the so-called Laron dwarfism, in which GH fails to stimulate the synthesis and elaboration of somatomedin. In these children, GH levels are measurable and respond normally to provocation. Laron dwarfism is not sporadic but is also inherited as an autosomal recessive trait. It is possible that the African pygmy has a similar form of dwarfism which is genetic, and normal GH responsiveness to provocative tests is preserved. In children with an isolated deficiency of GH it is possible to markedly stimulate growth with the administration of 2 to 5 mg of human GH twice per week for several months.

Growth Hormone Excess

Excessive secretion of GH by acidophilic adenomas or, more rarely, by a diffuse hyperplasia of the acidophils of the anterior pituitary (cerebral gigantism), results in overgrowth of long bones before epiphyseal closure and in enlargement of the acral parts of the skeleton (acromegaly) after epiphyseal closure. Acromegaly, a rare disorder that accounts for no more than 1 in 5,000 admissions to general hospitals, was described by Pierre Marie in 1886 and was attributed to acidophilic adenoma by Benda in 1900.

Clinical Features. The onset of symptoms and signs in acromegaly is insidious, beginning in the third or fourth decade with gradual enlargement of the hands and feet and coarsening of the facial features. Easy fatigability, muscle aching, heat intolerance, and excessive perspiration are generally noted. Acromegalic appearance results from prominence of the supraorbital ridges associated with overgrowth of the frontal sinuses; protrusion of the lower jaw (prognathism); enlargement of the nose and lips; and thickening, coarsening, and marked wrinkling of the skin of the face. Paresthesias of the ring and middle finger (carpal tunnel syndrome) due to median nerve compression may be observed early in the course of the disease. The basal metabolic rate is elevated in more than half of the reported cases. Menstrual irregularity and amenorrhea are common in women; progressive loss of libido occurs in men. Joint aches and pains are often present, and galactorrhea may occur (less than 5 percent of cases). Hypertension, present in 25 percent of the patients, is a serious complication that may lead to congestive heart failure. The voice is deep and hoarse because the volume of the larynx is increased. Visual field abnormalities may be demonstrable in half the patients; more than 50 percent complain of severe retroorbital, bitemporal, or frontal headache. Progressive thoracic kyphosis and genital regression occur in both men and women in the terminal phase.

Special Studies. X-ray study of the skull in acromegaly usually demonstrates an enlarged sella turcica exceeding 12 mm in depth and 15 mm in length. The distance between the anterior clinoid processes in the posteroanterior view is usually more than 22 mm. There may be marked enlargement of the frontal, ethmoidal, and mastoid sinuses. The bones of the spadelike hands demonstrate cortical thickening, with tufting of the tips of the distal phalanges. The serum phosphorus level may exceed 4.5 mg per 100 ml, but this is not a regular feature of acromegaly. The normal fasting recumbent plasma GH level is less than 5 ng per milliliter; in nearly all patients with acromegaly thus far studied, the hormone has exceeded this level. More importantly, ingestion of carbohydrate carried out in the standard glucose tolerance test, which normally results in a fall in the plasma GH level to less than 1 ng per milliliter within 60 minutes, usually fails to suppress GH levels below 5 ng per 100 ml; this finding is diagnostic. Results of this test in acromegalic patients are seen in Figure 55-1.

Treatment. The treatment of acromegaly and gigantism is controversial. Bragg-peak proton beam irradiation is most successful when the sella turcica is not

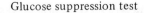

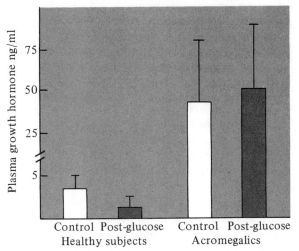

Figure 55-1. Plasma growth hormone levels 60 minutes after ingestion of 100 gm of glucose.

greatly enlarged and the pituitary tumor is entirely within the sella turcica. If suprasellar extension is demonstrated with or without visual impairment (bitemporal hemianopia), transsphenoidal hypophysectomy is required. If there is considerable suprasellar extension of the tumor, it may be necessary to use the transfrontal approach for hypophysectomy. Even with these measures it is difficult to reduce GH levels to within the normal range in a significant percentage of patients.

Thyroid-stimulating Hormone
Thyroid-stimulating hormone (TSH) is a glycoprotein composed of two dissimilar subunits, alpha and beta. The alpha subunit is common to LH, FSH, and human chorionic gonadotropin. Plasma concentrations of TSH are normally below 5 ng per milliliter. Thyroid-stimulating hormone stimulates the thyroidal trapping of iodine and the synthesis and release of thyroxin and triiodothyronine. Secretion of TSH is markedly accelerated in primary myxedema, in which there are low levels of thyroxin. The hypophysiotropic hormone from the hypothalamus, thyroid releasing factor, is a tripeptide amide that stimulates the secretion of TSH. Isolated TSH deficiency is the most common of the monotropic deficiencies of the anterior pituitary hormones, and it is probably due to failure of

elaboration of thyroid releasing factor. Synthetic thyroid releasing factor may be given intravenously and may distinguish between pituitary and hypothalamic disease when hypothyroidism is present. However, thyroid releasing factor can provoke a rise in TSH from pituitary tumors that secrete TSH poorly under physiologic circumstances. Thyroid releasing factor stimulation of TSH release in hypothyroidism is greatly augmented. No stimulation of TSH can be demonstrated in patients with hyperthyroidism. Thyroid releasing factor also stimulates prolactin secretion. Injections of 250 µg of thyroid releasing factor will induce a rise in both TSH and prolactin that is maximal within 30 minutes. Deficiency of TSH nearly always accompanies deficiencies of other anterior pituitary hormones when there is pathology such as is found in the Sheehan syndrome or in chromophobe adenoma.

Adrenocorticotropic Hormone (ACTH)

ACTH concentrations in plasma vary from 20 to 60 pg per 100 ml in the morning and fall below 10 pg per 100 ml late at night. ACTH stimulates adrenal steroidogenesis at a point between cholesterol and pregnenolone. Stimulation of ACTH secretion occurs through the action of corticotropin releasing factor. Corticotropin releasing factor, ACTH, and cortisol secretions all exhibit an endogenous circadian rhythm and also an ultradien periodicity of about 2 hours. Corticotropin releasing factor and ACTH secretions are controlled by a long-loop negative feedback control system.

A complete absence of ACTH secretion is incompatible with life. Partial ACTH deficiency occurs in panhypopituitarism, rarely as a selective or isolated monotropic deficiency, and in patients receiving long-term high-dose corticosteroid therapy for nonendocrine disorders.

Excessive ACTH secretion results in the Cushing's syndrome of cortisol excess. The cause of ACTH excess is unknown in patients with Cushing's disease, that is, in patients with the syndrome who have neither ACTH-producing pituitary chromophobe adenomas or ectopic ACTH production. Patients with Cushing's disease exhibit a loss of circadian rhythm of both ACTH and cortisol secretion and a loss of normal negative feedback sensitivity to administration of analogs of cortisol such as dexamethasone. Excessive ACTH secretion by a chromophobe adenoma of the pituitary is almost invariably associated with excessive secretion of beta-MSH or beta-LPH, and therefore hyperpigmentation is the hallmark of this type of Cushing's syndrome. Ectopic ACTH may be secreted by neoplastic tissue, particularly by an oat cell carcinoma of the lung, and this excessive ectopic production of ACTH may also be associated with excessive ectopic production of beta-MSH or beta-LPH or both. Five to ten percent of patients who undergo bilateral total adrenalectomy for Cushing's disease develop clinically significant pituitary tumors with hyperpigmentation, usually within several years after adrenalectomy (Nelson's syndrome). In these patients, ACTH, beta-MSH, and/or beta-LPH levels are extremely high.

Melanocyte-stimulating Hormone

It is likely that beta-LPH, a polypeptide more than four times the molecular weight of beta-MSH, may be the predominant melanocyte-stimulating substance in the human pituitary and human plasma. Beta-LPH exhibits biologic activity equal to that of beta-MSH. Beta-LPH secretory activity roughly parallels that of ACTH. Beta-LPH secretion can be suppressed by the administration of potent analogs of cortisol and stimulated by metyrapone, which inhibits cortisol biosynthesis.

Gonadotropins

The anterior pituitary synthesizes and secretes both FSH and LH. Another hormone, human chorionic gonadotropin, has biologic activity indistinguishable from that of LH and is normally secreted by the placenta. Human chorionic gonadotropin is used therapeutically and diagnostically in place of LH because it is more readily available and less expensive.

Gonadotropins are glycoprotein hormones (like TSH) weighing approximately 30,000 daltons and composed of two noncovalently linked subunits designated α and β. The α subunits of the different hormones are essentially identical in terms of their amino acid compositions, but the β subunits differ and confer on each hormone both its immunologic

Table 55-3. Normal Serum Levels of Hormones of Reproduction

Subject age and sex	LH (mIU/ml)	FSH (mIU/ml)	Prolactin (ng/ml)	Testosterone (ng/100 ml)	Estradiol (pg/ml)
Prepubertal	<10	<10	6	5–60	<10
Cycling women					
Follicular	5–20	5–15			Early follicular, 10–60;
Midcycle	30–150	15–100	<30*	20–100*	late follicular, 60–200;
Luteal	5–15	4–10			luteal, 60–200
Postmenopausal women	50–300	50–300	<30	20–100	<20
Men	5–20	5–20	6	350–1100	20–40

*No cyclic variation.

Note: LH = luteinizing hormone; FSH = follicle-stimulating hormone.

and its biologic specificity. Table 55-3 lists the normal levels of circulating FSH, LH, and other hormones of reproduction in prepubertal subjects and adults.

Controlling Factors. Both LH and FSH secretion are under the secretory control of a variety of hypothalamic factors, not all of which are known. Luteinizing hormone releasing factor is a decapeptide that stimulates the dose-related release of both LH and FSH. However, the LH response induced by LH releasing factor is usually considerably greater than FSH release so induced. Peak gonadotropin levels are observed 15 to 40 minutes after injection of an intravenous bolus of LH releasing factor, which acts directly on the pituitary cell membrane, binding to specific receptors with subsequent activation of the second messenger, adenosine $3':5'$-cyclic phosphate (cyclic AMP). A specific FSH releasing factor has not yet been identified, but its presence has been postulated to control pituitary FSH release directly. It is still not clear whether FSH and LH are both secreted by the same or by different pituitary cells, referred to as gonadotrophs.

Pituitary release of FSH may be modulated by a variety of substances. Estrogen exerts principally a negative feedback, primarily at the hypothalamic level, although a small number of pituitary estrogen receptors exist. Estrogen clearly exerts this effect in women and possibly in men. A hypothalamic enzyme that converts testosterone to estrogen has been identified in some animal species but not yet in man. *Inhibin,* a polypeptide not yet well characterized, is probably synthesized in the seminiferous tubules and may alter FSH secretion by negative feedback. Testosterone given in pharmacologic doses suppresses both LH and FSH levels in peripheral blood. Physiologic levels of testosterone do not appear to affect gonadotropin levels significantly.

Luteinizing hormone is the primary steroidogenic hormone of reproduction. Estrogen exerts variable effects on hypothalamic-pituitary LH release, depending on when in the menstrual cycle the estrogen is administered. If given from the first day of the menstrual cycle, tonic LH release is noted, consistent with the negative feedback of estrogen. However, if exog-enous estrogen is administered after the first day of the menstrual cycle, a positive feedback between estrogen and LH is noted, manifested by an increase in circulating LH levels. Progesterone exerts its anti-estrogenic action at the hypothalamic level and indirectly can cause a peripheral LH surge. Testosterone in pharmacologic doses can suppress plasma LH levels as well as urinary gonadotropin excretion, but it is less effective than estrogen. Most birth control pills contain both estrogen and progestins to suppress cyclic gonadotropin release and, consequently, ovulation. The latter will be discussed below.

Patterns of pubertal changes in boys and girls are discussed in Chapter 57, Disorders of the Male and Female Reproductive Systems. Both LH and FSH rise insidiously with the onset of puberty, FSH generally rising first. Starting with spontaneous menarche, LH and FSH undergo cyclic variation in peripheral blood in women.

Figure 55-2 depicts the mean daily plasma LH, FSH, estradiol. 17-hydroxyprogesterone, and progesterone concentrations during presumptively normal ovulatory cycles. Each menstrual cycle is characterized by a midcycle peak in plasma LH, usually accompanied by a concomitant FSH spike. The midcycle LH peak divides the menstrual cycle into two portions, the follicular phase, which precedes midcycle LH peak, and the luteal phase, which follows the midcycle preovulatory surge of LH and extends up to and includes the first day of menses.

The early follicular phase rise of FSH probably stimulates granulosa cell proliferation; the developing granulosa cells secrete estrogen, which circulates at highest levels in the latter part of the follicular phase. Estradiol levels decline just before or coincident with the preovulatory surge of LH. Both the height and the duration of elevated circulating estradiol may act to trigger the midcycle surges of both LH and FSH. In the late follicular phase, circulating 17-hydroxy-progesterone levels rise, probably reflecting granulosa cell maturation.

Twelve to thirty-six hours after the preovulatory surge of LH and FSH, ovulation occurs. The graafian follicle is transformed into a corpus luteum, which in the human secretes estradiol, 17-hydroxyprogesterone, and progesterone. The rising levels of these steroids

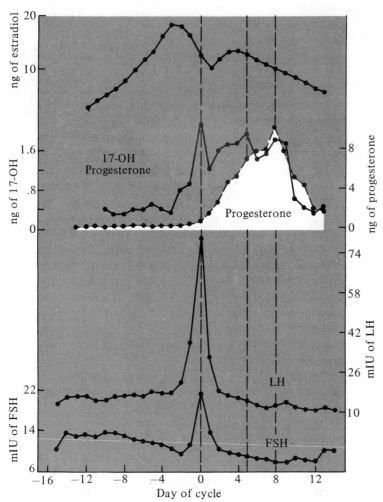

Figure 55-2. Mean daily plasma luteinizing hormone, follicle-stimulating hormone, estradiol, 17-hydroxy-progesterone, and progesterone concentrations during presumptively normal ovulatory cycles.

inhibit hypothalamic-pituitary secretion of LH and FSH. As a result, mean circulating LH and FSH levels of the luteal phase are lower than mean follicular phase levels of these hormones. The negative feedback effects of combined progestin and estrogen observed in the luteal phase are analogous to the pharmacologic effects of oral contraceptives containing the same agents. Since cyclic gonadotropin release is requisite for cyclic ovulation, the effect of oral contraceptives is to prevent ovulation.

Luteinizing hormone and FSH are secreted "circhorally" in men and women. This latter term was coined to describe spontaneous fluctuations occurring at hourly intervals in the circulating levels of LH and FSH. Generally, the higher the mean circulating gonadotropin level, the wider the absolute variation in plasma FSH or LH concentrations. There is no circadian rhythm of either FSH or LH release.

Starting with first stage of puberty (see Chap. 57), there is sleep-associated release of both LH and FSH. This pattern ceases with completion of puberty. Sleep-induced changes in LH are generally greater than those in FSH. This form of gonadotropin secretion probably requires maturation of higher centers in the central nervous system that have not yet been specifically identified.

In utero, the fetal circulating FSH levels in the female are in the castrate range in the late second trimester but steadily decline thereafter. LH levels are never in the castrate range in utero. During the neonatal period, circulating FSH levels in females are elevated for the first 2 years of life but do not exceed 15 to 20 mIU per milliliter. Luteinizing hormone levels are barely detectable. After the menopause, plasma gonadotropin levels are persistently elevated, signaling the loss of ovarian steroidogenic function; plasma LH and FSH levels range between 30 and 300 mIU per milliliter with mean concentrations of approximately 100 mIU per milliliter. Usually FSH levels exceed LH levels postmenopausally when one uses IRP2hMG (International Reference Preparation-2-human Menopausal Gonadotropin). Urinary gonadotropins by bioassay vary between 50 and 200 MUW (mouse uterine weight units) during menopause, which is the castrate range in either men or women. The MUW bioassay does not discriminate between LH and FSH biologic activities. Prepubertally, urinary gonadotropins are persistently less than 10 MUW units, and postpubertally urinary gonadotropin levels range between less than 10 to 50 MUW units, with most determinations being positive at 10 MUW units. In men there is a progressive small but significant rise of LH after the fifth decade with a concomitant fall of circulating testosterone levels, signaling relative Leydig cell failure.

Evaluation of Hypothalamic-Pituitary Function for FSH and LH Reserve. Clomiphene (Clomid) is a nonsteroidal compound that functions as an antiestrogen, competing with estrogen receptor sites in the hypothalamus. This interaction probably results in release of LH releasing factor, which will stimulate the pituitary to release both LH and FSH in men as well as women. However, minimal ovarian function, as reflected by peripheral estradiol levels greater than 10 pg per milliliter, is necessary for clomiphene to cause release of LH.

Clomiphene cannot evoke a hypothalamic-pituitary response either in normal prepubertal boys or in normal prepubertal girls. A normal female postpubertal response may be considered one in which at least a twofold elevation of basal LH and FSH levels is noted by the fifth day of clomiphene administration. Generally for this test 50 to 100 mg of clomiphene is given orally for 5 to 6 consecutive days, and circulating levels of FSH and LH are determined. Basal gonadotropin levels are usually tonically low in men and women with disorders of gonadotropin release at the hypothalamic-pituitary level.

In general, amenorrheic women who will respond to clomiphene have peripheral LH and FSH levels greater than 10 mIU per milliliter and plasma estradiol levels greater than 10 pg per milliliter. Progesterone acts as an antiestrogen at the hypothalamic level (like clomiphene) to induce transient rise of LH and FSH, which in turn stimulates ovarian steroidogenesis. For this test, either a single injection of 100 mg of progesterone in oil may be given intramuscularly, or 5 mg of a progestational agent may be given orally for 5 consecutive days. If withdrawal bleeding occurs (usually 3 to 7 days after administration ceases), then an intact hypothalamic-pituitary axis is implied. Approximately 80 percent of women who develop withdrawal bleeding after progesterone is given will respond to clomiphene with a significant rise in gonadotropin and possibly an ovulatory response.

After ovulation, the remaining follicle is transformed into a corpus luteum that secretes progesterone. Progesterone levels in excess of 3 ng per milliliter exert a direct effect on the thermoregulatory center in the hypothalamus to induce a basal body temperature shift, which is an indirect indicator of ovulation but is not diagnostic. Normal ovulatory cycles are usually associated with peripheral progesterone levels exceeding 10 ng per milliliter 5 to 8 days after the midcycle preovulatory LH surge. Table 55-4 summarizes a variety of hypothalamic-pituitary disorders in men and women, along with unique clinical features associated with those syndromes.

All the hypothalamic-pituitary syndromes are associated with low circulating gonadotropin levels and absent gonadal stimulation, as reflected by low estradiol levels (less than 10 pg/ml) in women and low testosterone levels in men (comparable to those found in women; less than 100 ng/100 ml). Patients affected

Table 55-4. Hypothalamic-Pituitary Disorders of Reproduction

Syndrome	Clinical signs and symptoms	Mode of inheritance	Comments
Kallman (men)	Congenital defects — hare lip, cleft palate, color blindness, nerve deafness, short fourth metacarpal, anosmia (secondary agenesis of olfactory nerve); small, unstimulated testes, <2 cm	X-linked	Some members of family may have congenital midline defects without hypogonadism
Olfactogenital dysplasia (women)	Same as Kallman	X-linked	Same as Kallman
Laurence-Moon-Biedl	Retinitis pigmentosa, obesity, mental retardation, congenital anomalies (e.g., congenital heart disease, ataxia, nystagmus, structural defects of kidneys and urogenital tract)	Autosomal recessive (?)	All signs and symptoms may not be present in all patients and relatives
Prader-Willi	Obesity, hypotonia, mental retardation, mild diabetes mellitus	Autosomal recessive (?)	. . . .
Delayed puberty	Retarded or absent secondary sexual development	May be familial or sporadic	This is a diagnosis of exclusion
Pituitary tumors and craniopharyngiomas	If developed prepubertally, markedly retarded or absent secondary sexual development. If onset postpubertally, regression of secondary sexual characteristics in both men and women, impotence in men and amenorrhea in women	None known except for those associated with multiple endocrine adenoma syndrome, type I, which is inherited as an autosomal dominant	Signs and symptoms reflext extent and anatomic position of tumor

with these syndromes usually lack development of secondary sexual characteristics, because the gonads have not been stimulated to secrete estrogen or testosterone necessary for inducing secondary sexual characteristics. Moreover, eunuchoid body proportions are usually encountered, such that the span exceeds the height and the lower body segment is greater than the upper body segment.

Pituitary tumors and craniopharyngiomas are also associated with hypogonadism and either absent or markedly retarded secondary sexual development, because there is interference with the hypothalamic-pituitary control of gonadotropin release. If the pituitary tumor is functional and is secreting an excess of a hormone, the patient may exhibit either Cushing's syndrome or gigantism.

Prolactin

Prolactin is a polypeptide hormone composed of 191 amino acids with a molecular weight of 16,000 to 18,000 daltons. In contrast to most other pituitary trophic hormones, prolactin acts directly on tissues and does not regulate a secondary endocrine gland. The only established function of prolactin in man is the initiation and maintenance of lactation, provided the tissue has been exposed to appropriate concentrations of estrogens, progestins, corticosteroids, and insulin. Prolactin is the only pituitary trophic hormone that is secreted by pituitary cells without direct hypothalamic stimulating factors intervening. Consequently, prolactin secretory control is under persistent inhibitory control by hypophysiotropic factors. Prolactin inhibitory factor is under dopaminergic control, resulting in decreased pituitary prolactin secretion. A prolactin releasing factor has not been identified. However, thyroid releasing factor stimulates the release of both pituitary prolactin and TSH. Prolactin levels are higher during sleep and fall insidiously as morning approaches. There appears to be a circadian rhythm of prolactin secretion. With daytime napping, prolactin levels tend to rise, but they usually do not exceed 30 ng per milliliter. Table 55-5 summarizes the various tests of pituitary-hypothalamic control of prolactin that may be used to assess patients presenting with apparent aberrations of prolactin secretory control. Table 55-6 summarizes a variety of clinical syndromes associated with aberrant prolactin secretion.

Anterior Pituitary Insufficiency

Childhood Type. Anterior pituitary insufficiency in the child leads to failure or retardation of growth (pituitary dwarfism). In more than a third of children having pituitary dwarfism, no discernible cause can be found, although GH deficiency is obvious and other pituitary tropic hormones are also demonstrably deficient in a high percentage of cases. Perhaps another third of the children with anterior pituitary insufficiency have craniopharyngiomas that directly invade the pituitary or interrupt its neural and vascular connections with the hypothalamus. Fifty percent of such children have symptoms before age 15, which may include diabetes insipidus (posterior pituitary), sexual infantilism, and growth failure. Pituitary dwarfism without an identifiable cause is never recognized before the second or third year of life. Growth retardation is a common manifestation of many childhood disorders, but further discussion of it is not within the scope of this section.

Adult Type. Anterior pituitary insufficiency in adults was described by Simmonds in 1914 (Simmonds disease). Because the onset of hypopituitarism is generally gradual and because deficiency of ACTH is usually the last feature to become clinically manifest, it is probable that Simmonds disease is more prevalent than recognized. The recorded incidence is in excess of 1 in 1,000 hospital admissions. The commonest cause of hypopituitarism in adult men is chromophobe adenoma, but in adult women it is postpartum hemorrhage and shock resulting in pituitary infarction and necrosis (the Sheehan syndrome). The primary vascular disturbance is presumably spasm of the arterioles supplying the anterior lobe and stalk, and its duration is the important determinant of tissue destruction. Also, thrombosis due to disseminated intravascular coagulation may play a role. Patients with diabetes mellitus may develop panhypopituitarism in a similar fashion following prolonged hypotensive episodes. Aneurysms of the carotid artery may compress the pituitary, causing severe headache preceded by transient blindness, but such symptoms may also result from hemorrhage into a chromophobe adenoma. Other causes of anterior pituitary failure in the adult include craniopharyngiomas, certain granulomas,

Table 55-5. Tests of Pituitary-Hypothalamic Control of Prolactin

Test substance	Mode of action	Sampling times
L-Dopa (3,4-dihydroxy-phenylalanine), 0.5 gm PO	Crosses blood-brain barrier, increases dopamine concentrations in hypothalamic neurons, and increases PIF. Increased PIF suppresses pituitary prolactin release. L-Dopa probably also has direct effect on cells secreting prolactin	−10, 0, +30, +60, +90, +120, +180 min; test should be carried out in afternoon
Chlorpromazine, 25 mg IM	Inhibits PIF secretion; consequently, circulating prolactin levels increase	−10, 0, +15, +30, +60, +90, +120 min
Thyrotropin releasing factor, 100−500 µg IV as bolus	Direct pituitary cell interaction; stimulates prolactin release	−10, 0, +15, +30, +60, +90 min

Note: PIF = prolactin inhibiting factor; PO = perorally; IM = intramuscularly; IV = intravenously.

Table 55-6. Syndromes or Diseases Associated with Altered Prolactin Secretion

Syndrome or disease	Comment
In women	
Chiari-Frommel	Postpartum amenorrhea and galactorrhea; most remit spontaneously and cyclic menses resume
Ahumada-del Castillo	Nonpuerperal amenorrhea and galactorrhea; patients should be followed closely for development of a pituitary tumor
Forbes-Albright	Amenorrhea and glactorrhea with a pituitary tumor. Tomography of sella turcica may be needed to discern small pituitary tumors, termed *microadenomas* (< 10 mm), usually located in inferolateral part of sella
Primary hypothyroidism	Amenorrhea and galactorrhea; all signs and symptoms remit with thyroid replacement therapy
In men or women	
Pituitary tumors	Galactorrhea may be present but need not be, even in presence of markedly elevated circulating prolactin levels. Tumor need not be prolactin-secreting to result in elevated circulating prolactin levels
Galactorrhea	1. Prolactin levels need not be elevated; some individuals manifest altered prolactin circadian rhythm 2. Result of neural stimulation from chest wall surgery or repeated breast manipulation 3. Drug-induced (phenothiazine, methyldopa, reserpine) 4. After pituitary stalk section; however, although prolactin levels may be elevated, galactorrhea need not be present

sarcoidosis, xanthomatosis, and metastatic replacement.

Therapeutic ablation of the pituitary has increased our understanding of hypopituitarism. Within 3 or 4 days after total hypophysectomy, the symptoms and signs of adrenocortical insufficiency appear, and circulatory failure results. Hypothyroidism generally is not evident for at least 4 weeks.

Clinical Features. The features of hypopituitarism depend on the cause, the degree of pituitary destruction, and the sex of the patient. Fully developed or severe panhypopituitarism is characterized by clinical manifestations of gonadal, thyroid, and adrenocortical insufficiency. Acute hypopituitarism can result from the Sheehan syndrome or from infarction of the anterior pituitary associated with head injury, especially when a fracture at the base of the skull involves hemorrhage into a pituitary tumor with ischemic necrosis (pituitary apoplexy). But hypopituitarism due to expansion of an intrasellar tumor or to the Sheehan syndrome often develops more gradually over a period of months to many years. The Sheehan syndrome is recognized in the majority of patients within 20 years after the postpartum hemorrhage; however, the clinical onset of this syndrome has been reported as long as 50 years after a postpartum hemorrhage. Cardinal features of the Sheehan syndrome are the absence of lactation in the postpartum period and the failure to resume menses. Acute anterior pituitary insufficiency, if severe, results in circulatory collapse and coma; death has been observed following hypophysectomy.

Gonadal hormones are usually the first to diminish and may be the sole hormones obviously deficient. Adult men have a loss of libido and potentia, with prostatic and testicular atrophy; the rate of beard growth is decreased, and there is a progressive loss of pubic and axillary hair. Adult women experience the cessation of menstrual periods without the occurrence of hot flashes, the nipples and areolae of the breasts become depigmented as they atrophy, and there is a paleness and thinning of the skin. Thyroid failure is variable. Many patients have only borderline abnormalities of thyroid function, whereas others are indistinguishable from patients with severe primary myxedema. In most patients cold intolerance, dry skin,

and a low basal body temperature develop. The majority of cases of hypopituitarism are recognized when the clinical manifestations of deficiency of both gonadotropin and thyroid stimulating hormone are obvious.

Blood pressure is usually not low before the development of other signs of secondary adrenal failure. Peripheral resistance rises, and left ventricular work increases so that the mean systemic arterial pressure may actually be elevated before the onset of adrenal insufficiency. When adrenocortical failure supervenes, it is limited to diminished cortisol and androgen production. In most patients the level of aldosterone seems to be adequate in that sodium deprivation will induce a rise in aldosterone secretion. Postural hypotension may be present, and infections and trauma may induce prostration. Weakness and fatigue are nearly always associated with the onset of cortisol deficiency, owing to lack of ACTH. One of the most serious features of hypopituitarism is the presence of hypoglycemia; insulin sensitivity is marked, and profound hypoglycemia may lead to death. The combination of hypothermia, the absence of the counterregulatory response of fatty acid mobilization normally induced by growth hormone, and the failure of hepatic gluconeogenesis because of the lack of cortisol explains the patients' tendency to develop severe hypoglycemia in response to an insulin challenge or to prolonged carbohydrate deprivation.

Patients with panhypopituitarism, even in the relatively severe phase, are usually not markedly cachectic, and they may even gain weight. In anorexia nervosa, a disease with cessation of menses in young adult women under the age of 40 years and usually in the second decade, cachexia is due solely to inadequate nutrition. In this condition, often confused with hypopituitarism, gonadotropin secretion ceases but the other tropic hormones are discharged normally. Anorectic patients rarely experience as severe weakness, fatigue, and impairment of ability to work as do patients with hypopituitarism.

Tests of Pituitary Function in Hypopituitarism

1. Growth hormone stimulation tests
   a. Apomorphine (0.75 mg) injected subcutaneously is the most effective stimulus of GH secretion.

Blood specimens should be obtained at 0, 45, 60, and 90 minutes after injection. Maximal GH level should be > 10 ng per milliliter of plasma. The results of this test appear in Figure 55-3.

   b. Insulin in a dose of 0.1 unit per kilogram body weight is injected intravenously, and GH levels are obtained at 0 and 60 minutes. If hypoglycemia has been induced, GH concentrations should exceed 10 ng per milliliter of plasma at 60 minutes.

2. Thyroid-stimulating hormone
   a. A basal serum TSH level is useful in patients suspected of hypopituitarism, provided hypothyroidism can be demonstrated. Thyroid-stimulating hormone levels are markedly elevated in primary hypothyroidism but are below 5 ng per milliliter of serum in secondary hypothyroidism.
   b. Thyroid releasing factor test for pituitary TSH reserve: 250 μg of synthetic thyroid releasing factor injected intravenously provokes maximal TSH levels in serum within 15 to 30 minutes. In some but not all patients with hypopituitarism due to pituitary disease, the response is nil. In patients with deficient thyroid releasing factor discharge by the hypothalamus, the response to thyroid releasing factor may be normal. Prolactin levels should also be obtained.

3. ACTH-metyrapone test
   Metyrapone, 750 mg, is given orally every 6 hours for 24 hours. Blood specimens are obtained at 8:00 A.M., just before the drug is given; and again at 8:00 A.M. 24 hours after the last dose. Metyrapone blocks the conversion of 11-deoxycortisol to cortisol; the consequent reduction of the circulating cortisol accelerates corticotropin releasing factor and in turn ACTH release, with a secondary increase in production of 11-deoxycortisol by the adrenals. The determination of 11-deoxycortisol levels in plasma in response to metyrapone administration tests the integrity of the negative feedback loop (hypothalamus to anterior pituitary to adrenal cortex). The level of 11-deoxycortisol in healthy subjects exceeds 10 μg per 100 ml of plasma after metyrapone, whereas in hypopituitaryism it is less

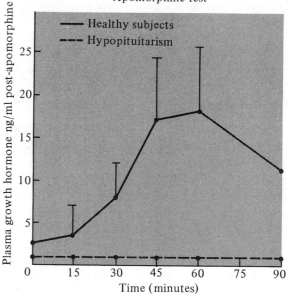

Apomorphine test

Figure 55-3. Plasma growth hormone levels after administration of 0.75 mg of apomorphine subcutaneously.

than 10. A comparison of patients with hypopituitarism and healthy subjects in the metyrapone test is seen in Figure 55-4.

4. Basal LH and FSH levels in plasma
   In postmenopausal and amenorrheic women these measurements are most useful, since they should be elevated in patients with primary gonadal failure and in postmenopausal patients.

Pituitary Tumors

Pituitary tumors account for 10 percent of all intracranial neoplasms. Chromophobe adenomas are the commonest, constituting 80 percent of all pituitary tumors. Chromophobe adenomas are rarely encountered before the third to fifth decade of life. Excessive secretion of prolactin can be demonstrated in nearly half of the patients with chromophobe adenoma, although the incidence of Forbes-Albright syndrome of galactorrhea and amenorrhea is seen in but a few. Rarely, chromophobe adenomas secrete excessive amounts of ACTH and beta-MSH, producing either Cushing's or Nelson's syndromes. Acidophilic adenomas account for 12 percent of pituitary tumors,

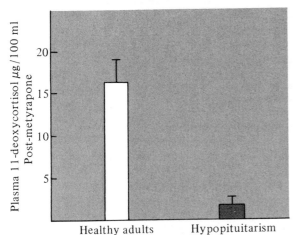

Metyrapone test

Figure 55-4. Plasma 11-deoxycortisol concentrations after administration of 750 mg of metyrapone every 6 hours for 24 hours.

and these may be the slowest growing. These tumors are usually associated with acromegaly or gigantism. Basophilic adenomas of extremely small size are relatively common in large autopsy series, but they are rarely clinically significant. Invasive chromophobe carcinoma is a rare tumor and may be associated with Cushing's syndrome. Craniopharyngiomas are not strictly pituitary tumors in that they arise from remnants of Rathke's pouch. They often appear early in life but also are recognized in adults. Craniopharyngiomas extend behind and above the sella turcica and often undergo a cystic degeneration so that they are referred to as suprasellar cysts. They may penetrate the hypothalamus and the floor of the third ventricle of the brain and may be associated with somnolence, delayed sexual maturation, and obesity.

Pituitary tumors, through local pressure and impingement on adjacent structures, cause roentgenographic abnormalities of the sella turcica, visual field defects, and headache. Erosion of the anterior clinoid process causes the sella turcica to have a flattened appearance, which is frequently seen with craniopharyngiomas. Chromophobe adenomas may simply erode the walls of the sella turcica uniformly until it appears to be enlarged or ballooned. Ordinarily the sella should not exceed 12 mm in depth or 15 mm in length. The adenoma first stretches the diaphragma

sellae, frequently causing retroorbital and bitemporal ("bursting" type) headaches; ultimately it may rupture the diaphragma sellae. As the tumor presses upward, it displaces the optic chiasm superiorly until it is finally limited by the anterior communicating arteries of the circle of Willis, which act as constricting bands on the inferior medial aspects of the optic nerves. It is thus common to have a visual defect in the superior temporal quadrant. Visual field loss may not be demonstrable with white test objects but may be clearly so with red ones. Classic bitemporal hemianopia often ensues. Palsies may occur in cranial nerves III, IV, and VI.

A pneumoencephalogram should be performed in all patients with enlargement of the sella turcica whether or not they have clinically manifested endocrine disorders. Enlargement of the sella turcica can be due to an anatomic variation that is referred to as the empty sella syndrome. Generally, this syndrome is without consequences and is easily distinguished by pneumoencephalography. Pneumoencephalography and computerized axial tomography scanning in patients with pituitary tumors may reveal suprasellar extension.

Ectopic Hormones
Ectopic hormonal syndromes were initially recognized because of the associated clinical signs and symptoms of excess circulating biologically active hormones found in some patients with tumors of nonendocrine origin. With the development of more sophisticated analytic techniques, it has become apparent that some varieties of excess circulating biologically active hormones may result in *no* clinical manifestations, and also that an excess of biologically *inactive* hormones may circulate. In some cases, ectopic hormones circulate in the form of prohormones but possess very little intrinsic biologic activity in that form. "Big" ACTH is an example (see Chap. 56). Table 55-7 summarizes the most commonly encountered ectopic hormonal syndromes, presenting the signs, symptoms, and type of tumor most likely to be associated with each.

A variety of hypotheses have been offered to explain the ectopic synthesis by nonendocrine tumor tissue of the wide variety of polypeptide hormones

Table 55-7. Ectopic Hormonal Syndromes

Ectopic hormone	Associated syndrome	Site and type of tumor most commonly associated
ACTH and/or MSH	Marked hypokalemic alkalosis, hypertension, edema, hyperglycemia, pigmentation, muscle weakness and wasting	*Lung, pancreas, thymus (thymoma), thyroid
Parathormone and parathormonelike substances	Increased calcium, low or normal phosphorus, anorexia, constipation, polyuria, drowsiness, coma	*Lung, kidney, liver (hepatoblastomas)
Human chorionic gonadotropin	Precocious puberty, gynecomastia; most have no signs or symptoms	*Gastrointestinal tract (liver and stomach), *pancreas, lung, breast, teratomas (gonadal or midline thoracic or intracranial)
Antidiuretic hormone	Hyponatremia, high urinary sodium excretion, lethargy, weakness, confusion, coma	*Lung, pancreas
Calcitonin	None known	*Lung, stomach
Prolactin	Galactorrhea (or no signs)	*Lung, kidney
Thyroid-stimulating hormone	Signs and symptoms of hyperthyroidism	*Lung, heart
Enteroglucagon	Malabsorption	*Kidney

*Most frequently associated tumor tissue associated with respective syndrome.
Note: ACTH = corticotropin; MSH = melanocyte-stimulating hormone.

that are encountered. The APUD (amine and precursor uptake in decarboxylation) cell concept cannot account for the ectopic production by tumors of the hormonal markers that are normally synthesized and secreted by the placenta (hCG and human chorionic somatomammotropin formerly named human placental lactogen). Tumors arising from APUD cells do produce serotonin and catecholamines as well as ACTH, parathormone, and antidiuretic hormone. Nonrandom derepression of the genome cannot explain these syndromes, since (1) the hormone or pieces of hormone identified from these syndromes has been identical to those found in endocrine tissue that normally synthesizes that hormone, and (2) specific hormones (e.g., ACTH or human chorionic gonadotropin) are more likely to be associated with specific tumor types (lung for the former and gastrointestinal tract for the latter). Cell hybridization has been postulated for genetic transfer of information found in cells capable of producing hormones. Whether cell hybridization occurs in vivo is unknown.

Disorders of the Posterior Pituitary
James C. Melby

Synthesis of the vasopressin and oxytocin octopeptides occurs in the neurons of the supraoptic and paraventricular nuclei of the hypothalamus. The octapeptides are bound to specific neurophysins and are transported as neurosecretory granules down the axons of the neurons to the posterior pituitary, where they are stored. The neurophysins are secreted with the active octapeptides in response to a variety of stimuli. Vasopressin acts to increase the permeability of epithelial membranes to water (the distal tubules of the kidney). Vasopressin secretion is stimulated by an acute increment in the osmolality of the extracellular fluid, an abrupt reduction in extracellular volume, or a nonspecific stress. Vasopressin secretion can be inhibited by significantly reducing plasma osmolality, increasing the volume of extracellular fluid, and by the administration of ethanol. The concentration of vasopressin in biological fluids is low, in the range of 1 to 2 pg per milliliter. This low level has made the radioimmunoassay of this octapeptide extremely difficult.

VASOPRESSIN EXCESS

The Schwartz-Bartter syndrome of inappropriate secretion of antidiuretic hormone (ADH) consists in plasma hypoosmolarity, renal sodium-wasting, and the excretion of a concentrated urine, all in the presence of normal hydration and normal renal and adrenal function. The syndrome may be associated either with the ectopic secretion of vasopressin by certain tumors (especially oat cell carcinoma of the lung) or with alterations in the secretion, metabolism, or antidiuretic action of ADH that can be caused by a variety of drugs or by diseases such as pulmonary tuberculosis, central nervous system disorders, acute intermittent porphyria, adrenal insufficiency, and myxedema. All the features of this syndrome can be reproduced by the administration of ADH and unlimited free water ingestion and can be reversed by the induction of negative water balance by fluid restriction. Even though it is not often possible to treat the underlying disease, fluid restriction and administration of sodium chloride effectively reverses the signs and symptoms of water intoxication observed in these patients (see Chap. 54).

VASOPRESSIN DEFICIENCY: DIABETES INSIPIDUS

Diabetes insipidus is a disorder of urinary concentration resulting from deficient secretion of ADH. It should be differentiated from other causes of polyuria such as psychogenic polydipsia, which results from abnormally excessive thirst, and nephrogenic diabetes insipidus, which results from renal refractoriness to the effects of vasopressin. In the majority of patients with diabetes insipidus, ADH secretion is markedly reduced but rarely totally absent. Better than 80 percent of patients with diabetes insipidus have very low but detectable concentrations of ADH in plasma. During water deprivation, plasma ADH may even be detected in a greater number of patients, approaching 95 percent or more. In diabetes insipidus, a limited capacity to secrete ADH is retained, and the secretion of ADH responds in the expected way to changes in hydration.

Diabetes insipidus is classified as either primary or secondary. In the primary group, the disease is divided between those individuals who have inherited the trait (familial diabetes insipidus) and those in whom no familial tendency can be demonstrated (idiopathic diabetes insipidus). The primary group represents about one-third of the total cases of this disease. In familial diabetes insipidus, the trait is an autosomal dominant. In patients with primary diabetes insipidus, the onset of the condition is often abrupt and memorable. Familial diabetes insipidus may also be associated with other congenital defects such as those in the Laurence-Moon-Biedl syndrome of obesity, hypogenitalism, retinitis pigmentosa, mental deficiency, and polydactyly.

Those with secondary diabetes insipidus are patients with metastatic cancer of the hypothalamus and pituitary, patients with posttraumatic diabetes insipidus after neurosurgery or a head injury, and patients with sarcoidosis, Hand-Schüller-Christian disease, histiocytosis, basal meningitis, or a variety of granulomas. Most often, patients excrete more than 5 liters of urine per day, and urinary volume has been recorded up to 25 liters per day. Patients exhibit hyposthenuria (specific gravity of 1.001 to 1.007), cold water thirst, and plasma osmolality after 8 hours of dehydration exceeding 310 mOsm per kilogram. The differential diagnosis includes psychogenic polydipsia, nephrogenic diabetes insipidus, and primary or secondary diabetes insipidus. Nephrogenic diabetes insipidus may be congenital or it may be acquired. Acquired nephrogenic diabetes insipidus is seen in patients with severe, prolonged hypokalemia, hypercalcemia, or after the long-term ingestion of lithium carbonate.

Water deprivation for 8 hours will distinguish between primary and secondary diabetes insipidus and psychogenic polydipsia. Plasma osmolality is obtained at the end of 8 hours, and in patients with psychogenic polydipsia, osmolality does not exceed 290 mOsm per kilogram, but in diabetes insipidus, plasma osmolality exceeds this amount. Subcutaneous injections of 5 units of aqueous vasopressin (Pitressin) will permit the patient with diabetes insipidus to concentrate his urine, whereas in patients with nephrogenic diabetes, urine concentration will be unaffected.

<u>Treatment.</u> Since nearly all patients with diabetes insipidus secrete some vasopressin, it is possible to treat their disease with chlorpropamide or clofibrate, singly or in combination with chlorothiazide, and to thereby ameliorate most of their clinical signs and symptoms. Although the effectiveness of these drugs varies, both chlorpropamide and clofibrate will reduce urine output significantly, increase urine osmolality, and restore plasma osmolality to normal. If chlorpropamide or clofibrate therapy does not relieve polyuria, chlorthiazide may be added to reduce urine volume by an additional 30 to 50 percent. In those patients without measurable vasopressin response to any stimulus, lysine vasopressin nasal spray may have to be used.

Bibliography

Anterior Pituitary Neuroendocrine

Boyar, R. M., Rosenfeld, R. S., Finkelstein, J. W., et al. Ontogeny of luteinizing hormone and testosterone secretion. *J. Steroid Biochem.* 6:803, 1975.

Crawford, J. D., and Osler, D. C. Body composition at menarche: The Frisch-Revelle hypothesis revisited. *Pediatrics* 56:449, 1975.

Daughaday, W. H. The Adenohypophysis. In R. H. Williams (ed.), *Textbook of Endocrinology* (5th ed.). Philadelphia: Saunders, 1974. P. 31.

Frohman, L. A., and Stuchura, M. E. Neuropharmacologic control of neuroendocrine function in man. *Metabolism* 24:211, 1975.

Malarkey, W. B., and Johnson, J. C. Pituitary tumors and hyperprolactinemia. *Arch. Intern. Med.* 136:40, 1976.

Melby, J. C. Assessment of adrenocortical function. *N. Engl. J. Med.* 185:735, 1971.

Rees, L. H., and Ratcliffe, J. G. Ectopic hormone production by nonendocrine tumors. *Clin. Endocrinol. (Oxford)* 3:263, 1974.

Root, A. Endocrinology of puberty: Normal sexual maturation. *J. Pediatr.* 83:1, 1973.

Rosen, S. W., Weintraub, B. D., Vaitukaitis, J. L., et al. Placental proteins and their subunits as tumor markers. *Ann. Intern. Med.* 82:71, 1975.

Ross, G. T., Cargille, C. M., et al. Pituitary and gonadal hormones in women during spontaneous and induced ovulatory cycles. *Recent Progr. Horm. Res.* 26:1, 1970.

Schwinn, G., von zur Muhlen, A., Kobberling, J., et al. Plasma prolactin levels after TRH and chlorpromazine in normal subjects and patients with impaired pituitary function. *Acta Endocrinol. (Kbh)* 79:663, 1975.

Sheehan, H. L., and Summers, V. K. The syndrome of hypopituitarism. *Q. J. Med.* 18:319, 1949.

Sparkes, R. S., Simpson, R. W., and Paulsen, C. A. Familial hypogonadotropic hypogonadism with anosmia. *Arch. Intern. Med.* 121:534, 1968.

Treloar, A. E., Boynton, R. E., and Behn, B. G. Variation of the human menstrual cycle through reproductive life. *Int. J. Fertil.* 12:77, 1967.

Vaitukaitis, J. L., Becker, R., Hansen, J., and Mecklenburg, R. Altered LRF responsiveness in amenorrheic women. *J. Clin. Endocrinol. Metab.* 39:1005, 1974.

Posterior Pituitary

Berndt, W. O., et al. Potentiation of the antidiuretic effect of vasopressin by chlorpropamide. *J. Clin. Endocrinol.* 86:1028, 1970.

Lant, A. F., et al. Long-term therapy of diabetes insipidus with oral benzothiadiazine and phyhalimidine diuretics. *Clin. Sci.* 40:497, 1971.

Miller, M., et al. Recognition of partial defects in antidiuretic hormone secretion. *Ann. Intern. Med.* 73:721, 1970.

Miller, M., and Moses, A. M. Urinary ADH in polyuric disorders and inappropriate ADH syndrome. *Ann. Intern. Med.* 77:715, 1972.

Robertson, G. L., Maheu, A., Athan, S., and Sinha, T. The development and clinical application of a new method for the radioimmunoassay of orgine vasopressin in human plasma. *J. Clin. Invest.* 52:2340, 1973.

56

Diseases of the Adrenal Gland

James C. Melby

Diseases of the Adrenal Medulla

PHEOCHROMOCYTOMA

Pheochromocytoma is a tumor of chromaffin tissue, usually in the adrenal medulla, but occasionally it presents as a paraganglioma originating in chromaffin tissues of the intrathoracic sympathetic chain or the organs of Zuckerkandl (associated with the abdominal aorta and in proximity to the origin of the inferior mesenteric artery). Ninety percent of pheochromocytomas occur in the abdomen. Sixty-five to seventy percent involve one adrenal gland, 15 percent both adrenals, and 20 to 30 percent are multicentric. Ten percent of pheochromocytomas are malignant. The incidence of pheochromocytoma is 0.2 percent in the hypertensive population. Eighty to ninety percent of pheochromocytomas are sporadic, and 10 to 20 percent are familial. Familial pheochromocytoma is bilateral, and 60 percent of the cases are inherited as an autosomal dominant trait. Familial pheochromocytoma is associated with other inherited disorders of neuroectodermal origin, such as von Recklinghausen's neurofibromatosis, von Hippel-Lindau disease, or Sturge-Weber syndrome (phakomatoses). The Sipple syndrome is the autosomal dominant inheritance of multiple bilateral adrenal pheochromocytomas, medullary carcinoma, amyloid deposits of the thyroid, and hyperparathyroidism. Occasionally ectopic corticotropin (ACTH) production is seen in the Sipple syndrome.

Clinical Features

Clinical manifestations of pheochromocytoma are often determined by the intermittence or constancy of secretion of the catecholamines (epinephrine and norepinephrine). Sixty percent of patients exhibit persistently elevated systemic arterial pressure. In over half of these patients there exists superimposed paroxysms of severe hypertension. Patients with persistently elevated blood pressure complain of headaches, sweating, palpitations, and weight loss, and they frequently exhibit fasting hyperglycemia. Patients with persistent elevations of blood pressure are more often younger (in the third and fourth decades). Forty percent of patients with pheochromocytoma exhibit only severe paroxysmal hypertension and have normotensive symptom-free intervals. Attacks are usually brief, lasting from 15 to 30 minutes, and they are accompanied by severe headache, sweating, tremor, and often back pain. The paroxysmal hypertensive form of pheochromocytoma occurs more often in the older age groups (fourth, fifth, and sixth decades).

Physical examination is rarely helpful except in the familial forms of pheochromocytoma, in which obvious neurofibromas, café au lait spots, or thyroid tumors are palpable. Excessive perspiration and orthostatic hypotension may be present. Deep subchondral or flank manipulation or palpation may elicit a hypertensive episode.

Diagnosis

The diagnosis of pheochromocytoma rests on the demonstration of excessive production of norepinephrine, epinephrine, or both (or their urinary metabolites), either spontaneously or after stimulation. These products can be detected in the urine as the catecholamines themselves, as their O-methylated metabolites (normetanephrine and metanephrine), and as the product of oxidative deamination, vanillylmandelic acid (3-methoxy-4-hydroxymandelic acid, or VMA). Of the three alternatives, the best for diagnosis are the urinary metanephrines. A rate of excretion in excess of 1.3 μg per 24 hours is diagnostic. In patients who have paroxysmal hypertension exclusively, the diagnosis is much more difficult because urinary excretion tests may be normal. Provocative tests to induce a paroxysm of hypertension are used only occasionally because of the dangers involved. Pressor tests with histamine, glucagon, or tyramine are positive in approximately 70 percent of cases, but both false-positive and false-negative tests may occur. Arteriography may be helpful in localizing pheochromocytomas.

Treatment

The treatment of pheochromocytoma is excision. Long-acting beta-adrenergic blocking agents such as phenoxybenzamine should be used to control blood pressure prior to surgery. Short-acting agents such as phentolamine are useful in controlling blood pressure during surgery.

Patients with malignant pheochromocytoma may survive many years with widespread metastases, and so they may require pharmacologic control of the humoral aspects of their disease. Most respond well to inhibition of synthesis of catecholamines by α-methyltyrosine, a drug that blocks the enzyme tyrosine hydroxylase, the rate-limiting step in catecholamine synthesis.

Disorders of the Adrenal Cortex

INTRODUCTION

Of the steroid hormones secreted by the human adrenal cortex into the adrenal venous effluent, only cortisol and aldosterone are essential to life processes, and together these account for most of the biologic activity. Both possess 21 carbon atoms and 4 or more oxygen atoms. In addition, dehydroepiandrosterone (DHEA) secreted as a sulfate ester (DHEA-S) is the principal adrenal androgen and has 19 carbon atoms. The adrenal cortex is functionally zoned, so that aldosterone is secreted entirely by the zona glomerulosa, cortisol exclusively by the zona fasciculata, and DHEA by the zona reticularis. Biosynthetic pathways for the production of these steroids are represented in Figure 56-1, in which the enzymes involved are listed below and their sites or action are depicted above. Deficiencies of all the individual enzymes involved in cortisol and aldosterone biosynthesis have been observed clinically and will be discussed below.

Cortisol Synthesis

Cortisol secretion is activated solely by adreno-corticotropic hormone (ACTH) acting on the zona fasciculata of the adrenal cortex. Corticotropin releasing factor, when elaborated by the hypothalamus, induces the discharge of ACTH and, indirectly, the discharge of cortisol. Cortisol concentrations in plasma have a cybernetic or negative feedback relationship with corticotropin releasing factor and hence, with ACTH. Advantage of this phenomenon is taken in the diagnostic inhibition test for Cushing's

syndrome, to be described later. Corticotropin and cortisol are secreted cyclically throughout a 24-hour period, and the secretions exhibit an endogenous circadian rhythm, having maximum concentrations from 8:00 to 9:00 A.M. and lowest concentrations after midnight. Cortisol and ACTH also have an ultradian rhythm with a period of about 1½ to 2 hours.

The basal secretion of cortisol varies from 10 to 28 mg per 24 hours, or approximately 5 to 10 μg per kilogram of body weight per hour. The basal cortisol plasma levels vary from 5 to 30 μg per 100 ml at 8:00 A.M. and fall to below 10 μg per 100 ml by 9:00 P.M. Infusions of ACTH will generally induce an increment in plasma cortisol levels by three to seven times within 2 to 4 hours. In plasma, cortisol circulates about 90 percent bound to a plasma α-globulin (transcortin or corticosteroid-binding globulin; it is metabolized by the liver, and 50 percent of its metabolites retain the dihydroxyacetone side chain at carbon 17. These metabolites are measured by a specific chromogen reaction and are referred to as 17-hydroxycorticosteroids (17-OHCS). Males excrete from 5 to 15 mg of 17-OHCS per 24 hours and females from 2 to 10 mg. Plasma cortisol is measured by the competitive protein-binding analysis, which is a specific technique and has the advantage of no interference by nonspecific substances. The cortisol secretion rate (CSR) is an accurate index of adrenal secretory activity (SA). Urine passed after the injection of a tracer dose of tritium (H^3)-labeled cortisol is collected, and the metabolites of cortisol are isolated by thin-layer chromatography. Specific activity of the isolated metabolites is determined by the counts per minute (CPM), and the secretion rate is then calculated as follows:

$$CSR = \frac{\text{injected dose of } ^3H \text{ (CPM)}}{\text{SA of urinary tetrahydrocortisone}}$$

Aldosterone Synthesis. Aldosterone is secreted by the zona glomerulosa, and its production is stimulated primarily by angiotensin II, potassium, and ACTH. Aldosterone in turn stimulates reabsorption of the sodium ion in the distal convoluted tubule and collecting ducts of the kidney, with concomitant loss of

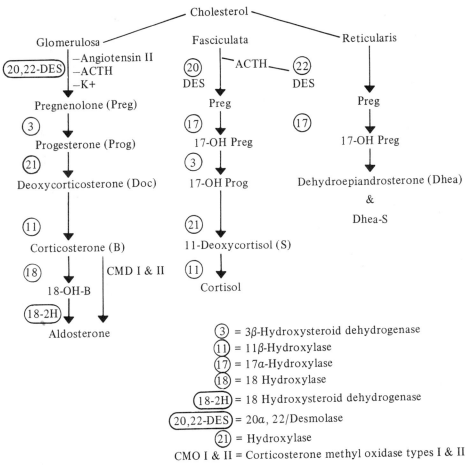

Figure 56-1. *Biosynthetic pathways for adrenal steroid hormones with functional zonation.*

potassium into the urine. Normally 30 to 150 µg of aldosterone is secreted daily; 30 to 50 percent of this amount is excreted as urinary tetrahydroaldosterone-3-glucuronide, while 5 to 10 percent is excreted as the 18-monoglucuronide of unreduced aldosterone. The aldosterone secretion rate (ASR) may be determined by injection of tritium-labeled aldosterone and isolation of one of its metabolites from the subsequent 24-hour urine specimen. The same calculation as for cortisol secretion is made for aldosterone:

$$ASR = \frac{\text{injected dose of }^{3}H\ (CPM)}{\text{SA urinary metabolite}}$$

Aldosterone circulates in low concentration in plasma (2 to 8 ng/100 ml), and it is measured by radioimmunoassay. Plasma aldosterone rises some twofold to threefold when the erect posture is assumed after recumbency.

Adrenal Androgens

The secretion of C-19 adrenal androgens — androstenedione, DHEA, and DHEA-S occurs in the cells of the zona reticularis. Dehydroepiandrosterone sulfate is produced in an amount of 10 to 20 mg per 24 hours. A small amount of secreted DHEA-S is converted to a more active androgen, testosterone, by the peripheral tissues. Urinary 17-ketosteroid excretion is a crude but reliable index of adrenal androgen secretion, although testicular androgens may contribute to a minor extent to the 17-ketosteroids. Males excrete

8 to 23 mg of ketosteroids per 24 hours in their urine, while females excrete 5 to 15 mg. All the adrenal virilizing syndromes are characterized by elevated excretion of 17-ketosteroids in urine.

INBORN ERRORS IN ADRENAL STEROID BIOSYNTHESIS

The inheritance of adrenal steroidogenic enzyme deficiencies occurs as a mendelian recessive characteristic. The incidence of the heterozygous state has been estimated to vary from 1 in 35 to 1 in 110, and the incidence of the homozygous state from 1 in 5,000 to 1 in 50,000 births.

Figure 56-1 depicted the enzymes involved in cortisol and aldosterone biosynthesis. The various inborn errors of cortisol and aldosterone biosynthesis are listed in Table 56-1, which lists diagnostic steroid profiles and includes data on the presence or absence of salt-losing states, hypertension, virilization, and disordered sex differentiation. It can be seen that virilism is regularly associated only with 21- and 11-β-hydroxylase deficiency and that hypertension accompanies only 17-α- and 11-β-hydroxylase deficiency. Salt-losing is a feature of 20-, 22-desmolase, 3-β-hydroxy steroid dehydrogenase, 18-oxydase, and 21-hydroxylase (involving glomerulosa and fasciculata) deficiencies. Hypertension in 17-α-hydroxylase deficiency is due to the excessive production of both deoxycorticosterone (DOC) and 18-hydroxy-11-deoxycorticosterone (18-OH-DOC), and hypertension in 11-β-hydroxylase deficiency is due to excessive secretion of DOC alone (see Chap. 25). Inborn errors of cortisol biosynthesis that have been encountered in adults include 17-α-hydroxylase, 11-β-hydroxylase, and 21-hydroxylase deficiencies. These will now be discussed briefly.

21-Hydroxylase Deficiency

This is the most common form of congenital adrenal hyperplasia, but in a few patients it may not be apparent until adult life. More than half the patients with 21-hydroxylase deficiency exhibit severe sodium loss in the neonatal period due to the inability to secrete aldosterone. In the salt-losing variety of this condition, it is likely that there is a 21-hydroxylase deficiency involving the cells of both the glomerulosa

and the fasciculata, whereas in the nonsalt-losing variety, 21-hydroxylase deficiency is limited to the zona fasciculata. It is interesting that patients who do not exhibit the salt-losing trait generally have, if anything, increased aldosterone secretion. Since the adrenal androgens are secreted without 21-hydroxylation, urinary 17-ketosteroid excretion is elevated. Normally, prepubertal children excrete no more than 2 mg of ketosteroids per 24 hours, and children under 2 years of age excrete much less. Children with congenital adrenal hyperplasia excrete from 3 to 40 mg of 17-ketosteroids per day. Adolescent and adult women excrete no more than 15 mg of 17-ketosteroids per 24 hours, whereas patients with virilizing hyperplasia of the adrenal cortex excrete from 16 to 80 mg of 17-ketosteroids per 24 hours. In virilizing hyperplasia an excess of the precursor 17-α-hydroxyprogesterone is secreted, and therefore large amounts of its metabolite, pregnanetriol, is excreted in urine (in excess of 4 mg per 24 hours). The rapid onset of virilism in the adult woman suggests a primary adrenocortical tumor more than a 21-hydroxylase deficiency, especially if urinary 17-ketosteroid excretion is markedly elevated (in excess of 100 mg per day). In congenital adrenal hyperplasia, 17-ketosteroid excretion can be suppressed by dexamethasone in a dose of 0.5 mg every 6 hours for 2 days, but it is not suppressed if an adrenocortical tumor is the source of the increased adrenal androgen production.

11-β-Hydroxylase Deficiency

This is the next most commonly observed form of congenital adrenocortical hyperplasia, and is occasionally encountered in adults. About 8 to 15 percent of patients with congenital adrenal hyperplasia have 11-β-hydroxylase deficiency. In addition to virilization, hypertension occurs in this condition. The hypertension results from excessive secretion of DOC in both the zona glomerulosa and the zona fasciculata. Urinary 17-ketosteroids are elevated. Plasma 11-deoxycortisol and urinary tetrahydro-11-deoxycortisol and dihydro-11-deoxycortisol are increased. Thus the urinary 17-hydroxycorticosteroids would be increased because of the marked increase in metabolites of 11-deoxycortisol (compound S) in urine.

Table 56-1. Inborn Errors of Cortisol and Aldosterone Biosynthesis

Enzyme deficiency	Salt-losing	Hyper-tension	Virilizing	Sex differentiation		Steroid profiles
				Male	Female	
20,22-Desmolase (lipoid hyperplasia)	+	0	0	Pseudohermaphroditism	No female sex maturation	No detectable steroids in urine
3-β-Hydroxysteroid dehyderogenase	+	0	0 to +	Hypospadius, incomp. development ambiguous genitalia	Virilization, variable ambiguous genitalia	Δ^5-Steroids: preg and 17-OH-preg ↑, DHEA and DHEA-S ↑, urinary 17-KS ↑; all other steroids ↓ or 0
17-α-Hydroxylase	0	+	0	Or male hypospadius, ambiguous genitalia	No female sex maturation	Plasma DOC ↑, 17-OHCS ↓, 17-KS ↓, aldosterone normal, plasma cortisol ↓, testosterone and E_2 ↓
11-β-Hydroxylase	0	+	+	Male macrogenitosomia	Male pseudohermaphroditism	Plasma DOC ↑, plasma 11-deoxycortisol ↑ (S), urinary 17-OHCS ↑ (THS, DHS), urinary 17-KS ↑
21-Hydroxylase — Glomerulosa and fasciculata (aldosterone deficiency)	...	0	+	Male macrogenitosomia	Male pseudohermaphroditism	Plasma 21-deoxycortisol ↑, urinary preg ↑, urinary 17-KS ↑, plasma cortisol low, 17-OHCS ↓
Fasciculata alone	+	...	...			...
8-Oxidase Corticosterone methyl oxidase — Type I	0	0	0	Normal male	Normal female	Type I ↓ aldosterone (plasma, urine), ↑ urinary 18-OH-THA
Type II	+	0	0			Type II ↓ aldosterone (plasma, urine), no increase in urinary 18-OH-THA

Note: preg = pregnanetriol; DHEA = dehydroepiandrosterone; DHEA-S = dehydroepiandrosterone sulfate; 17-KS = 17-ketosteroids; DOC = deoxycorticosterone; 17-OHCS = 17-hydroxycorticosteroids; E_2 = estradiol; THS = tetrahydrodeoxycortisol; DHS = dihydrodeoxycortisol; 18-OH-THA = 18-OH-tetrahydroaldosterone.

17-α-Hydroxylase Deficiency
This results in almost complete lack of steroidogenesis by the adrenals, ovaries, or testes except for the precursors of aldosterone in the adrenal. Enormous amounts of DOC and 18-OH-DOC are secreted, and these steroids induce sodium retention, hypertension, and greater or lesser degrees of hypokalemia. In these patients there is also an absence of development of secondary sex characteristics. Both urinary 17-hydroxy-corticosteroids and 17-ketosteroids are low. Aldosterone secretion is slightly decreased.

ADRENOCORTICAL HYPOFUNCTION

Primary Adrenocortical Insufficiency (Panhypo-corticalism – Underproduction of Cortisol, Aldosterone, and Androgens)
Bilateral destruction of the adrenal glands is followed within minutes to hours by a sharp reduction in cardiac output and by sodium depletion and dehydration that contract the blood volume. If salt and water are not replaced, profound shock and death ensue shortly. In acute adrenocortical failure, or addisonian crisis, hyperkalemia, hyponatremia, azotemia and, sometimes, hypoglycemia are observed. The electrolyte disturbance is due exclusively to aldosterone deficiency, while the hypoglycemia results from a lack of cortisol with a resultant diminished hepatic glucose output.

Acute adrenocortical insufficiency may occur in the course of chronic adrenocortical insufficiency (Addison's disease), or it may be the first manifestation of bilateral destruction of the adrenal glands or of anterior pituitary insufficiency. Symptoms of orthostatic hypotension, persistent tachycardia, and nausea suggest impending adrenal crisis. In a patient with known chronic adrenal insufficiency, a crisis is nearly always due to the precipitating stress of trauma, high environmental temperature, or acute febrile illness. Acute adrenocortical insufficiency is usually more severe in patients with untreated Addison's disease than it is in patients with secondary adrenal insufficiency or in patients who have previously received replacement therapy for Addison's disease. Heart size is reduced in the untreated patient, and the stroke volume cannot be increased. Approximately 3 percent

of patients who die in shock from gram-negative septicemia have demonstrable intraadrenal hemorrhage. In such cases, circulatory collapse has been attributed to adrenal insufficiency (Waterhouse-Friderichsen syndrome). However, studies have failed to demonstrate biochemical evidence of acute adrenal insufficiency during septic shock or permanently in survivors.

Chronic Adrenocortical Insufficiency (Addison's Disease)
In the early part of this century, the etiology of Addison's disease was thought to be tuberculosis involving the adrenal glands in more than 75 percent of the cases. In the last decade, tuberculous Addison's disease has accounted for no more than 20 to 25 percent of recognized cases, whereas idiopathic causes are now assigned in more than 70 percent of cases. Idiopathic Addison's disease is now thought to be mainly an autoimmune adrenalitis, because it is associated with a variety of conditions of autoimmune origin. It may be familial, and on histologic examination of the adrenal glands, there is a lymphocytic infiltration and fibrosis reminiscent of adenoid goiter. Two and one-half times as many women as men patients are affected with idiopathic Addison's disease, and in over half of these patients autoimmune disorders are clinically evident.

Hashimoto's thyroiditis affects more than half the women with idiopathic Addison's disease. Some 20 to 50 percent of patients with Addison's disease have diabetes mellitus, premature menopause, or both. Ten to 30 percent of Addisonian children have pernicious anemia, hypoparathyroidism, or alopecia totalis. Schilder's disease (spastic paraplegia) and hepatitis affect 6 percent. Organ-specific antibodies in Addison's disease include adrenal antibodies, demonstrable in 50 percent of the patients; gastric and thyroid cytoplasmic antibodies in 20 to 40 percent; and parathyroid antibodies in about 20 percent. Adrenal antibodies can also be demonstrated in about 10 percent of first-degree relatives of patients with idiopathic Addison's disease. Metastatic carcinomatosis, amyloidosis, or systemic mycoses occur in a small percentage of patients with Addison's disease.

<u>Clinical Manifestations.</u> Clinical manifestations of Addison's disease include pigmentation, muscle weakness, postural hypotension, and symptoms of fatigue, which may be present for years before the disease is recognized. Pigmentation results from oversecretion of β-lipotropin by the anterior pituitary, since its secretion is in a negative feedback relationship with cortisol. Postural hypotension is due in part to blood volume contraction resulting from aldosterone deficiency, but more importantly, the hypotension is due to reduced cardiac output because of cortisol deficiency. Cortisol is necessary for optimum contractility of the myocardium, on which it has a positive inotropic effect through its activation of a specific cardiac myosin. Serum sodium tends to be somewhat reduced and serum potassium slightly increased in about 40 percent of addisonian patients, but no obvious plasma electrolyte abnormality is present in the majority.

Renal function and water and electrolyte metabolism are all disturbed in Addison's disease. Renal plasma flow and glomerular filtration rate are reduced, resulting in moderate elevations of the blood urea nitrogen and serum creatinine. Proximal tubular reabsorption of sodium is elevated, whereas distal tubular reabsorption of sodium is nil in the absence of aldosterone. Total exchangeable sodium is decreased, due also to bone sequestration of sodium in the absence of aldosterone. There is defective exchange and excretion of potassium due to distal tubular sodium loss in the urine. Cortisol deficiency is exclusively responsible for abnormal water metabolism. Patients with Addison's disease are unable to excrete a water load, and administration of electrolyte-free solutions to patients with Addison's disease can precipitate a crisis of water intoxication and hyperpyrexia.

Special Investigations of Adrenocortical Failure

The diagnosis of primary adrenocortical insufficiency can be reliably established only by the demonstration of the failure of intravenous or intramuscular injections of ACTH to increase cortisol secretion. A single determination of the plasma cortisol or of the 24-hour excretion of 17-hydroxycorticorticosteroids in urine is not useful and may even be misleading. Any test employing ACTH with both control and test observations on plasma cortisol or urinary 17-hydroxycorticosteroids is satisfactory. Currently the most simple and convenient procedure is the rapid injection of 25 USP units of ACTH or 0.25 mg of α-1, 24-corticotropin intravenously. Blood samples for cortisol analysis are obtained both before injection of ACTH and 2 hours after. Figure 56-2 compares the results in patients so tested with responses in healthy subjects.

Secondary Adrenocortical Insufficiency

Secondary adrenocortical insufficiency may be due to panhypopituitarism, isolated ACTH deficiency, or suppression of the hypothalamic-pituitary-adrenal axis after exogenous corticosteroid therapy. Circulatory failure that does not respond to restoration of blood volume; that occurs during and after surgery or trauma; or that is found in patients with hypopituitarism having an acute febrile illness, in patients receiving maintenance corticosteroid therapy, or in patients whose corticosteroid therapy has been discontinued within 6 months, must be presumed to be due to secondary adrenocortical insufficiency. Practically all such failure is precipitated by an acute major physical insult such as surgery, trauma, or infection. Aldosterone deficiency is not a feature of either corticosteroid-induced adrenocortical hypofunction or pituitary hypofunction. Serum potassium is almost never elevated, even though hyponatremia may be seen due to dilution. It should be emphasized that patients with secondary adrenocortical insufficiency do not exhibit hyperpigmentation, since β-lipotropin secretion is reduced. Unfortunately clinicians often misdiagnose exacerbations of underlying disorders, for which corticosteroid treatment is being reduced or terminated, as representing episodes of adrenocortical insufficiency.

The metyrapone test should be used to determine the integrity of the negative feedback regulation of ACTH release in patients suspected of having secondary adrenocortical insufficiency. Metyrapone blocks the conversion of the precursor 11-deoxycortisol to cortisol. The consequent reduction in circulating cortisol causes acceleration of synthesis and release of ACTH, with increased production of 11-deoxycortisol by the adrenal glands; 11-deoxycortisol possesses the same side chain at carbon 17 as 17-

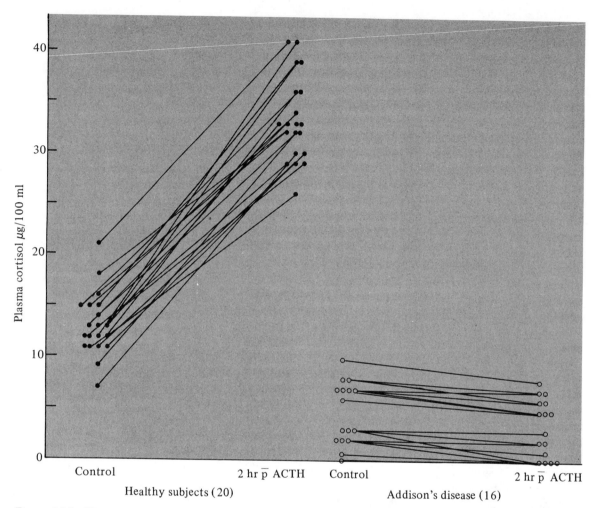

Figure 56-2. Plasma cortisol levels before and after 0.25 mg of α = 1,24 = corticotropin or 25 USP units of ACTH.

hydroxycorticosteroid and hence is measured as such in the urine. 17-Hydroxycorticosteroid is also measured by the competitive protein binding assay as the parent hormone, 11-deoxycortisol, in plasma. The test metyrapone is described in Chapter 55.

Treatment of Primary and Secondary Adrenocortical Insufficiency

Treatment of either acute primary or secondary adrenocortical insufficiency is nearly always successful if 100 mg of cortisol as a 21-succinate or 21-phosphate

ester is immediately injected intravenously and is followed by an intravenous infusion of cortisol phosphate or succinate in a dose of 15 to 20 mg per hour in saline over 24 hours. One should not use either hypotonic or potassium-containing fluids. Improvement can be expected within the first hour after the initial dose of cortisol, and restoration of the blood pressure should occur within 2 hours. Maintenance dosage of cortisol is approximately 20 mg by mouth daily. In chronic primary adrenocortical insufficiency it is necessary to replace aldosterone with 9-α-fluorocortisol (Florinef) in doses varying from 50 μg every other day to as much as 100 μg daily; the individual requirements for mineralocorticoid replacement vary enormously. Patients should be instructed to double their cortisol dosage if they have a severe upper respiratory infection or other febrile illness. They should be instructed also to contact their physician early in the course of any illness. They should be asked to wear a bracelet or identifying card describing their diagnosis and need for cortisol. It is wise to give patients water-soluble synthetic analogs of cortisol for immediate injection in case of emergency.

ADRENOCORTICAL HYPERFUNCTION – CUSHING'S SYNDROME OF CORTISOL EXCESS

Spontaneous Cushing's syndrome due to excessive secretion of cortisol results from either ACTH excess with adrenocortical hyperplasia (70 percent of cases) or from a primary adrenocortical tumor that autonomously secretes excessive amounts of cortisol (30 percent of cases). Alterations in the synthesis and/or discharge of ACTH with resultant adrenocortical hyperplasia are associated with disturbed neurohormonal secretion by the hypothalamus (abnormal or tonic discharge of corticotropin releasing factor) in half the cases of Cushing's syndrome. Ten to twelve percent of cases of Cushing's syndrome are due to an autonomous ACTH-secreting tumor of the pituitary that appears to be a chromophobe adenoma under light microscopy. These two forms of excessive secretion of ACTH by the pituitary resulting in Cushing's syndrome are referred to as pituitary Cushing's syndrome or, commonly, Cushing's disease. Nonendocrine tumors such as an oat cell carcinoma of the lung may produce ACTH not only in enormous quantities, but also ACTH of large molecular size and enhanced activity, referred to as "big" ACTH. When Cushing's syndrome arises from the hypersecretion of ACTH by such nonendocrine tumors, resulting in adrenocortical hyperplasia, it is referred to as ectopic Cushing's syndrome; approximately 10 percent of cases of Cushing's syndrome are of this type. Twenty-five to thirty percent of cases of Cushing's syndrome are due to primary adrenocortical neoplasm; adrenocortical carcinoma accounts for 10 to 15 percent, and benign solitary adrenocortical adenoma causes 15 to 20 percent. Corticotropin-producing tumors of the pituitary and ectopic ACTH production by nonendocrine tumors are frequently associated with excessive production of β-lipotropin, and patients with these neoplasms usually exhibit marked hyperpigmentation. Benign solitary adrenocortical adenomas secreting cortisol may produce a very mild form of Cushing's syndrome, but malignant adrenocortical tumors cause a very severe, rapidly progressive picture.

Clinical Features

An abnormal deposition of fat (centripetal obesity) that results in trunkal obesity, cervicodorsal and supraclavicular fat pads, facial mooning, a pouting appearance of the mouth, and muscle wasting of the extremities are common manifestations of Cushing's syndrome. Nearly all patients exhibit a proximal myopathy, some degree of osteoporosis, hypertension, plethora and, less commonly, purple abdominal striae. Some patients have generalized obesity. Further striking features such as easy bruisability and atrophy of the subcutaneous tissues may lead to the development of multiple ecchymoses in some patients. Most women have amenorrhea and reduced secretion of luteinizing and follicle-stimulating hormones. Frank diabetes may be precipitated by Cushing's syndrome, but an abnormal carbohydrate tolerance is demonstrated in most of the patients. Emotional lability and agitated depression are common manifestations; frequently patients complain that they cannot sleep. Hypokalemia and alkalosis are the hallmarks of Cushing's syndrome due to ectopic ACTH production by nonendocrine neoplasms. In these patients, ACTH stimulation of the adrenal zona fasciculata is so intense as to produce enormous quantities of DOC and 18-OH-DOC both of which are weak mineralocorticoids that if secreted in abundance can mimic a hypersecretion of aldosterone. Virilism in the female associated with cortisol excess is strongly suggestive of adrenocortical carcinoma as the cause of the Cushing's syndrome.

Screening Tests for Cushing's Syndrome

Diagnostic Inhibition Test (Rapid). This test is perhaps the most useful screening procedure for Cushing's syndrome. Patients with Cushing's syndrome fail to suppress their ACTH secretion and cortisol output with doses of cortisol (or its synthetic analo-

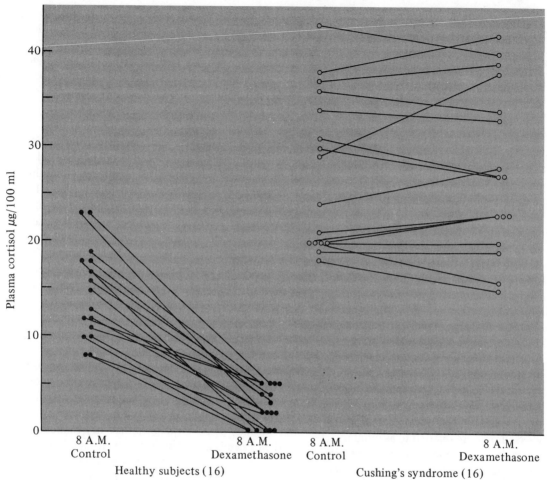

Figure 56-3. Plasma cortisol at 8 A.M. before and the morning after 1 mg of dexamethosone by mouth.

gues) that normally will just suppress adrenocortical function. One milligram of dexamethasone is given by mouth at 11:00 P.M. on the night before the measurement of the plasma cortisol. In normal subjects and in patients with nonendocrine disease, the plasma cortisol level will fall to below 5 μg per 100 ml, whereas in patients with Cushing's syndrome, it will remain above 10 μg per 100 ml. The results of this test are graphically represented in Figure 56-3.

Absence of Diurnal Variation in Plasma Cortisol.
Normal circadian variation is lost in Cushing's syn-

drome. Blood specimens are obtained at 8:00 A.M. and 9:00 P.M. for cortisol analysis. In healthy subjects and in hospitalized patients with nonendocrine disease, the plasma cortisol varies from 5 to 30 μg per 100 ml at 8:00 A.M. and always declines by more than 50 percent to less than 10 μg per 100 ml by 9:00 P.M. Patients with Cushing's syndrome may have normal or high normal plasma cortisol levels at 8:00 A.M., but they show no reduction of this level in the evening. The importance of this phenomenon cannot be overemphasized, since it explains the presence of florid Cushing's syndrome, even when the total cortisol production rate is only moderately increased. The value of this test is demonstrated in Figure 56-4.

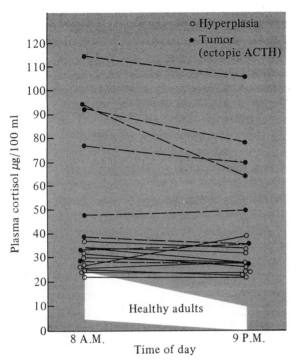

Figure 56-4. *Plasma cortisol levels at 8 A.M. and 9 P.M. in Cushing's syndrome.*

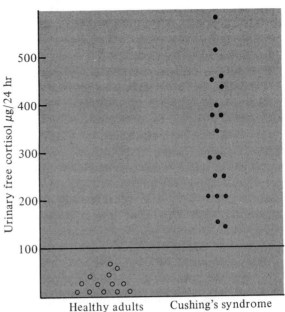

Figure 56-5. *Twenty-four-hour urinary free cortisol excretion.*

Urinary Free Cortisol Excretion. The excretion of free cortisol in urine is unaffected either by body weight or by conditions that modestly affect both plasma corticosteroid-binding globulin and plasma affinity for cortisol. Urinary free cortisol reflects the amount of cortisol unbound to transport plasma protein, and thus any increase in it would mirror an increment in nonprotein bound cortisol. Urinary free cortisol excretion is greater than 80 μg per 24 hours in patients with Cushing's syndrome, but it is not elevated in very obese patients. Urinary free cortisol is the preferred urinary measurement; 17-hydroxycorticosteroid excretion is not a very reliable screening test for Cushing's syndrome because it is dependent in part on the metabolic clearance rate of cortisol, which is increased in patients who are obese. The application of this test appears in Figure 56-5. Measurement of urinary 17-ketosteroids is not useful except in mixed Cushing's syndrome, in which virilism is also present.

Tests to Establish Etiology of Cushing's Syndrome
Once the diagnosis of Cushing's syndrome has been established by a failure to suppress plasma cortisol with dexamethasone, an absence of normal circadian variation of plasma cortisol, and an increased excretion of urinary free cortisol, certain test maneuvers may be carried out to determine whether the syndrome is due to abnormal regulation of ACTH secretion or to a primary adrenocortical neoplasm.

High-Dose Inhibition Test (Adrenocortical Tumor versus Cushing's Disease). Eight milligrams of dexamethasone are given by mouth every 6 hours for 2 days. Urine is collected the day before and on the second day of dexamethasone administration. The 17-hydroxycorticosteroid excretion of most patients with bilateral adrenocortical hyperplasia (Cushing's disease) is suppressed at this dose level to less than 50 percent of the basal amount on the second day of dexamethasone administration. In nearly all patients with adrenocortical tumors, urinary 17-hydroxycorticosteroid excretion is not appreciably suppressed by this dose of dexamethasone.

Metyrapone Test (Primary Adrenocortical Neoplasm versus Cushing's Disease). Metyrapone inhibition of cortisol biosynthesis induces a reciprocal rise in ACTH secretion in patients with Cushing's disease (disturbed regulation of ACTH secretion), but it does not affect ACTH secretion in patients with tumors. Thus patients with Cushing's disease exhibit a striking rise in plasma compound S (11-deoxycortisol) following the administration of 750 mg of metyrapone orally every 6 hours for 24 hours, using the measurement of compound S the morning after as compared with the morning just before the administration. In patients with adrenocortical tumors, there is a sharp fall in cortisol and no rise in plasma S after administration of metyrapone. Metyrapone binds partly to the mixed-function oxidase P-450 involved in 11-β-hydroxylation in the mitochondria; however, in the absence of ACTH drive, metyrapone will inhibit the other mixed-function oxidases in the microsomes and reduce all steroid hydroxylation, hence reducing the formation of steroids by a tumor that is ACTH dependent. Results of this test are shown in Figure 56-6.

Plasma ACTH Concentration. Plasma ACTH concentrations exceed 100 to 150 pg per milliliter at night, in patients with Cushing's disease, even after dexamethasone suppression. In patients who exhibit hyperpigmentation of the skin, with or without an enlarged sella turcica, ACTH concentrations in plasma exceed 300 pg per milliliter in the presence of a pituitary ACTH-producing tumor. Plasma ACTH concentrations may exceed 1,000 pg per milliliter in patients with Cushing's syndrome due to ectopic ACTH production. Hypokalemia and edema generally distinguish these patients from patients with other forms of Cushing's syndrome.

Adrenal Radioangiography. Elective adrenal arteriography is the most effective means of examining the adrenal glands in patients with Cushing's syndrome. It is not ordinarily safe to inject dye retrograde for adrenal venography because of the vulnerability of the corticomedullary vascular system of the adrenals in Cushing's syndrome. Selective adrenal arterio-

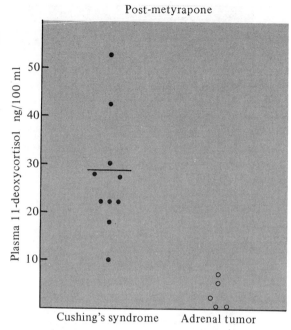

Figure 56-6. Plasma 11-deoxycortisol (compound S) in Cushing's syndrome of differing etiologies.

graphy will demonstrate either hyperplasia or unilateral neoplastic disease.

Radiocholesterol Scintiscanning. The noninvasive technique of administering ^{131}I iodocholesterol and observing its concentration permits the detection of an excessive concentration of isotope in adrenal glands with bilateral cortical hyperplasia. It is of interest that ^{131}I iodocholesterol may not be detected in highly malignant adrenal neoplasms, which are often associated with excessive production of androgens and a marked increment in urinary 17-ketosteroid excretion.

Treatment of Cushing's Syndrome
Treatment of Cushing's syndrome due to primary adrenocortical tumor is unilateral adrenalectomy, with chemotherapy for distant metastases if they exist. In patients with ectopic production of ACTH from nonendocrine tumor, treatment is directed at the primary tumor. In patients with chromophobe adenomas of the pituitary and Cushing's syndrome,

the treatment is either conventional supravoltage multiportal irradiation to the pituitary or proton-beam therapy. The majority of patients with Cushing's syndrome have Cushing's disease (altered ACTH secretion) but no other demonstrable pituitary abnormality. The treatment of the patients with Cushing's disease is more controversial. Conventional supravoltage multiportal irradiation of the pituitary is ineffective, with less than 20 percent of patients having permanent remissions. Proton-beam irradiation appears to produce remissions in up to 60 to 70 percent of patients so treated. In patients with less florid Cushing's disease, it appears to be safe to administer the adrenocytolytic agent, ortho-para'-DDD (Op'-DDD) (mitotane). This agent is given by mouth in a dose of 2.0 gm per day, as tolerated, for 6 months. Patients studied so far have experienced both clinical and biochemical remissions within 2 to 3 months. Approximately a third of the patients so treated have to be retreated because of relapse within 2 to 6 months after discontinuing therapy. Cyproheptadine (Periactin) is a serotonin antagonist that inhibits secretion of ACTH by inhibiting serotonin-mediated release of corticotropin releasing factor. Cyproheptadine in large doses (28 mg per day) can inhibit ACTH secretion in Cushing's disease and can induce remissions. Remission is maintained only by continuing therapy with cyproheptadine.

Hyperaldosteronism

SECONDARY ALDOSTERONISM (HYPERRENINEMIC HYPERALDOSTERONISM)

Secondary aldosteronism is the term used to describe excessive production of aldosterone by the adrenal glomerulosa under stimulation from outside the adrenal gland. Secondary aldosteronism, with the exception of a single entity — the rare syndrome of glucocorticoid-suppressible aldosteronism — results from excessive, prolonged stimulation by angiotensin II. In general, secondary aldosteronism is characterized by increased plasma renin activity, high plasma angiotensin II levels, and raised plasma aldosterone concentrations. The aldosterone hypersecretion is not inappropriate for the degree of activation of the renin-angiotensin system. The heightened activity of the renin-angiotensin system is most often due to

events reducing effective blood volume and extra-cellular fluid volume, with increasingly negative sodium balance. Secondary aldosteronism must be viewed as a physiologic counterregulatory response to these events, although the manifestations of aldosterone overproduction are predominant. Disorders associated with secondary aldosteronism are listed below.

I. Hyperaldosteronism associated with elevated plasma renin activity (hyperreninemic or secondary hyperaldosteronism)
   A. Without hypertension
      1. Edematous states
         a. Nephrotic syndrome
         b. Hepatic cirrhosis with ascites
         c. Localized edema
         d. Idiopathic edema
         e. Congestive cardiac failure
      2. Nonedematous states
         a. Salt-losing nephritis
         b. Bartter syndrome
         c. Renal tubular acidosis
   B. With hypertension
      1. Primary hyperreninism
         a. Juxtaglomerular cell tumor
         b. Wilms' tumor
      2. Secondary hyperreninism
         a. Accelerated hypertension
         b. Essential hypertension (10 percent)
         c. Hypertension treated with diuretics
         d. Oral contraceptive-induced hypertension
         e. Pregnancy

II. Hyperaldosteronism associated with suppressed plasma renin activity (hyporeninemic or primary hyperaldosteronism)
   A. Aldosterone-producing adenoma (primary aldosteronism, Conn syndrome)
   B. Idiopathic hyperaldosteronism — bilateral micronodular and/or macronodular adrenocortical hyperplasia
   C. Aldosterone-producing adrenocortical carcinoma
   D. Glucocorticoid-suppressible aldosteronism

Secondary aldosteronism is a concomitant of sodium depletion in pregnancy. With sodium depletion, there are increased circulating levels of angiotensin II and increased adrenocortical sensitivity to angiotensin II. Increased renin secretion results in part from negative sodium balance, and in pregnancy it is also accompanied by elevated levels of plasma renin substrate induced by the raised estrogen levels. In pathologic states, secondary aldosteronism leads to varying degrees of potassium depletion and, when edema is present, to positive sodium balance. When secondary aldosteronism accompanies hypertensive disorders in which volume contraction and negative sodium balance coexist, renin hypersecretion is reactive or secondary. On the other hand, the increased synthesis and release of renin by renin-producing tumors is primary and is unresponsive to alterations in either extracellular fluid volume or sodium balance. Hypertension precipitated by administration of estrogen-containing oral contraceptives is frequently hyperreninemic, though not necessarily renin dependent.

It is estimated that in over 15 percent of the adult hypertensive population elevated plasma renin activity and hyperaldosteronism can be demonstrated. A majority of these patients have moderately severe or accelerated hypertension, the level of which is determined more by elevated peripheral arteriolar resistance than by any other determinant of blood pressure. Using angiotensin II blockade by a specific competitive antagonist of the vascular action of angiotensin II (Saralasin acetate [P-113], or sar 1, ala^8 — angiotensin II) causes hypertensive patients with hyperreninemia to respond with a significant reduction in blood pressure (see Chap. 25).

PRIMARY ALDOSTERONISM
(HYPORENINEMIC HYPERALDOSTERONISM)
Aldosterone overproduction results in hypertension, potassium depletion, and feedback suppression of plasma renin activity. Primary aldosteronism may be due to an aldosterone-producing solitary adenoma (Conn syndrome), to bilateral micronodular or macronodular hyperplasia of the adrenal cortex (idiopathic hyperaldosteronism), to an aldosterone-producing adrenocortical carcinoma, or to congenital aldosteronism (bilateral adrenocortical hyperplasia). Hypersecretion of aldosterone is semiautonomous in primary aldosteronism with the exception of patients with hyperaldosteronism that can be treated with glucocorticoids. Aldosterone stimulates active renal sodium transport by the distal convoluted tubule and collecting duct cells. With enhanced sodium reabsorption, a reciprocal movement of potassium and hydrogen ions takes place into the urine, leading to potassium depletion. Increased sodium reabsorption by the kidney leads to expansion of extracellular fluid volume and elevated total body sodium content. The expansion of the extracellular fluid volume and intravascular volume often exceeds 2 liters and may be as great as 4 liters. However, the expansion of the extracellular fluid volume is limited by the renal counterregulatory mechanism of inhibition of proximal tubular sodium reabsorption. This phenomemon has been referred to as mineralocorticoid "escape." Expansion of intravascular blood volume also leads to the development of volume-dependent hypertension. Patients with primary aldosteronism exhibit hypervolemia, increased extracellular fluid volume, increased exchangeable sodium, and high cardiac output. Hypervolemia, increased extracellular fluid volume, and high exchangeable sodium act directly to suppress juxtaglomerular cell activity in the kidneys, with a low plasma renin activity resulting. Primary aldosteronism is a generic term for disorders in which chronic aldosterone excess is independent of the renin-angiotensin system and results in volume-dependent hypertension. Estimates of the incidence of primary aldosteronism vary from 0.5 to 2.0 percent of the hypertensive population, with a prevalence of 115,000 to 460,000 cases in the United States at present (see Chap. 25).

Clinical Features
The peak age distribution of primary aldosteronism is between the third and fifth decades, with women affected more than men in a preponderance of 3:1. All the complications of severe, long-standing hypertension have been observed in patients with primary aldosteronism; more than half the patients have a persistent frontal headache, and there is no feature of hypertension that is excluded. The most obvious

clinical manifestation of primary aldosteronism is excessive renal potassium wastage. Spontaneous hypokalemia is observed in 80 percent of the patients; however, 20 percent of the patients have persistently normal serum potassium levels. A substantial portion of patients with spontaneous hypokalemia admit to no symptoms. Nocturnal polyuria and polydipsia are common signs of potassium deficiency, and neuromuscular manifestations, including weakness, paresthesias, intermittent paralysis, visual disturbances, and frank tetany may wax and wane with variations in potassium balance. Sodium restriction leads to potassium retention and lessens the hypokalemic manifestations. Demonstrably abnormal glucose tolerance (in over half the patients associated with insulinopenia) is due to potassium deficiency. Sensitivity to the thiazide diuretics may be associated with the appearance of cardiac irregularity, paralyses, and tetany due to acute potassium depletion; if this occurs in the routine treatment of any hypertensive patient, one should think of the possibility of primary aldosteronism as the cause of the hypertension.

Types of Primary Aldosteronism
Two major types of primary aldosteronism, solitary adenoma and bilateral macronodular and micronodular hyperplasia, account for 85 to 98 percent of cases of this disorder. Rarer forms include aldosterone-producing carcinoma, congenital or juvenile aldosteronism, and glucocosteroid-remediable hyperaldosteronism (see the list earlier in this Chapter, under Aldosteronism). This discussion will be limited to the commoner forms of primary aldosteronism.

Solitary Aldosterone-producing Adenoma (Conn Syndrome). The most common adrenal lesion responsible for the syndrome of primary aldosteronism is a solitary adrenocortical adenoma (in 60 to 70 percent of patients). The biochemical manifestations are more pronounced in the Conn syndrome than in other forms of primary aldosteronism. The diagnosis of primary aldosteronism is made by the demonstration of inappropriately raised blood aldosterone concentrations in the presence of low plasma renin activity, both before and after acute induction of negative sodium balance. The adrenal lesion must

then be identified and, if unilateral, localized. Unilateral adrenalectomy for the removal of a solitary adenoma results in the disappearance of hypertension for 1 or more years in 70 percent and permanently in 50 percent of patients, whereas bilateral total adrenalectomy for micronodular or macronodular hyperplasia of the adrenals (idiopathic hyperaldosteronism) results in the disappearance of hypertension in only a third of the patients so treated. In the Conn syndrome, aldosterone biogenesis by the adenoma appears to be only partially autonomous in that plasma aldosterone concentrations still exhibit a circadian rhythm paralleling plasma cortisol and ACTH levels.

Bilateral Macronodular and/or Micronodular, or Both, Adrenocortical Hyperplasia (Idiopathic Hyperaldosteronism). In this form of primary aldosteronism, both adrenal glands are involved with diffuse micronodular or macronodular, or both, changes in the presence of hyperplasia of the zona glomerulosa. The nodules secrete excessive amounts of aldosterone with resultant arterial hypertension, potassium depletion, and suppression of plasma renin activity. Of all patients with primary aldosteronism, 15 to 30 percent have the idiopathic type. The biochemical abnormalities may not be as pronounced in these patients as they are in the Conn syndrome; hypokalemia may be less severe, and the suppression of plasma renin activity may be incomplete. Activation of aldosterone biogenesis by small increments in plasma renin activity occurs in these patients when they stand after prolonged recumbency, and no parallelism can be demonstrated between their plasma aldosterone and cortisol concentrations.

Diagnosis
Primary aldosteronism should be suspected in hypertensive patients who have spontaneous hypokalemia, who have become hypokalemic after initiation of diuretic therapy, or who may become hypokalemic after ingestion of large amounts of sodium chloride. The salt-loading maneuver may be used as a provocative test for aldosteronism in hypertensive patients who have persistently normal serum potassium levels. In primary aldosteronism, sodium loading intensifies potassium depletion, while sodium depriva-

tion permits potassium repletion. When aldosterone secretion is suppressed by salt ingestion in healthy subjects, the distal renal tubular stimulus for sodium reabsorption is quickly dissipated; whereas patients with autonomous aldosterone secretion exhibit continued distal tubular sodium reabsorptive activity in the face of a marked increase in the filtered sodium load. Ingestion of sodium in excess of 200 mEq per day (nine 1-gm sodium chloride tablets/day) for 4 days does not influence the serum potassium in the absence of aldosteronism, whereas in patients with aldosteronism, it causes a reduction of serum potassium to below 3.5 mEq per liter.

Confirmation of Diagnosis

Diagnosis of primary aldosteronism rests on the demonstration of increased aldosterone secretion or plasma aldosterone concentration in the presence of low or hyporesponsive plasma renin activity. The simplest and best method of diagnosis is to obtain blood specimens simultaneously for plasma aldosterone concentration and plasma renin activity after stimulation by acute volume depletion. The patient is given 80 mg of furosemide by mouth, and 3 hours later specimens for plasma renin activity and plasma aldosterone are obtained. The patient remains upright during the test. Elevation of plasma aldosterone inappropriate for the level of suppressed plasma renin activity is diagnostic (Fig. 56-7). This test should be performed in patients ingesting normal amounts of sodium in their diets (100 ± 30 mEq/day) and in whom diuretic therapy has been discontinued for 3 weeks and other antihypertensive medications for 1 week. Equally as reliable as measurements of the 18-monoglucuronide or tetrahydroaldosterone of aldosterone excreted in the urine over 24 hours is the measurement of the secretion rate of aldosterone by the radioisotope dilution method.

Distinction Between Unilateral and Bilateral Adrenal Disease and Localization of Unilateral Adlosterone-producing Adenomas: Adrenal Venous Aldosterone Levels. Adrenal angiography coupled with measurement of aldosterone in the adrenal venous effluent from both adrenal glands obtained by percutaneous adrenal vein catheterization has reliably distinguished solitary

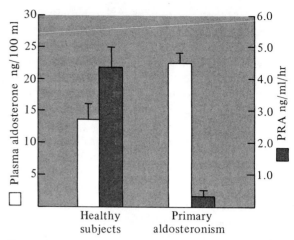

Figure 56-7. Plasma aldosterone and plasma renin activity (PRA) 3 hours after 80 mg of furosemide by mouth.

aldosterone-producing adenoma from the bilateral involvement of idiopathic aldosteronism. In idiopathic aldosteronism, concentrations of aldosterone in the venous effluent of the two adrenal glands may differ by 20 to 50 percent. In the Conn syndrome, concentration of aldosterone in the adrenal venous effluent from the tumor-bearing gland is 20 to 50 times that in the venous effluent of the contralateral gland.

Adrenal Imaging with Radioactive Iodocholesterol. Adrenal scintigraphy using ^{131}I-19-iodocholesterol is a noninvasive, painless technique in which scintiscans are performed following the intravenous administration of ^{131}I-19-iodocholesterol. Dexamethasone suppression is carried out concurrently with scintigraphy to differentiate idiopathic aldosteronism from the Conn syndrome. Asymmetric uptake between the two adrenal glands during suppression scintiscans is obvious 5 days after the tracer has been injected in patients with solitary aldosterone-producing adenomas. No lateralization is observed in patients with bilateral micronodular or macronodular hyperplasia. An even more useful and apparently superior agent is ^{131}I-6-iodomethyl-19-norcholesterol (NP-59) which accumulates in the adrenal glands more rapidly, permitting scintigraphy within 1 day of administration. Adrenal imaging with the latter agent should supplant adrenal vein catheterization for diagnosis and localization in primary aldosteronism. Adrenal venous aldosterone measurements can be obtained whenever the results of scintigraphy are ambiguous. Certain nonaldosterone mineralocorticoid hypertensive syndromes have been described in patients with hypertension and suppressed plasma renin activity and are listed below.

1. Pseudomineralcorticoid hypertensive syndromes
   a. Glycerrhizic acid derivative ingestion (licorice, carbonoxalone)
   b. Inappropriate excessive renal sodium conservation (Liddle's syndrome)
2. Deoxycorticosterone (DOC) excess
3. 18-hydroxy-11-deoxycorticosterone (18-OH-DOC) excess
4. 16, 18-dihydroxy-deoxycorticosterone (16- α-18-OH-DOC) excess
5. 16-β-hydroxy-dehydroepiandrosterone (16-β-OH-DHEA) excess
6. Dehydroepiandrosterone sulfate (DHEA-S) excess

ISOLATED HYPOALDOSTERONISM

Selective deficiency of aldosterone secretion without alterations in cortisol production results in persistent hyperkalemia, renal salt wastage, and postural hypotension in some patients. Hyperkalemia may be associated with profound muscle weakness and cardiac arrhythmias. Clinical manifestations are reversed by the administration of exogenous mineralocorticoids such as 9-α-fluorocortisol. Possible etiologies, including specific deficiencies of enzymes involved in aldosterone biosynthesis, selective destruction of the adrenal zona glomerulosa, and a variety of alterations in function of the renin-angiotensin system, are listed below.

1. Deficiencies of enzymes involved in aldosterone biosynthesis
   a. Corticosterone methyl oxidase type 1 deficiency — ? 18-hydroxylase deficiency
   b. Corticosterone methyl oxidase type 2 deficiency — ? 18-hydroxysteroid dehydrogenase deficiency
2. Failure of adrenal zona glomerulosa function
   a. Heparin and polysulfated glycosaminoglycan-induced adrenal glomerulosa failure

   b. ? Autoimmune glomerulosa insufficiency; isolated hypoaldosteronism associated with idiopathic hypoparathyroidism
3. Altered function of the renin-angiotensin system
   a. Following unilateral adrenalectomy for an aldosterone-producing adenoma
   b. Idiopathic hyporeninemic hypoaldosteronism
   c. "Big" renin hypersecretion, diabetes, renal disease, and hypoaldosteronism

In the disorders of aldosterone biosynthesis and in situations in which there appears to be failure of adrenal cortical zona glomerulosa function, plasma renin activity is usually elevated. In contrast, disorders in which alterations in the function of the renin-angiotensin system are observed generally are characterized by low or unmeasurable plasma renin activity.

Bibliography

Bongiovanni, A. M. Disorders of Adrenocortical Steroid Biogenesis. In J. B. Stanbrade, J. B. Olyngaarden, and D. S. Fredrickson (eds.), *The Metabolic Basis of Inherited Disease* (3rd ed.). New York: McGraw-Hill, 1972. P. 857.

Conn, J. W. Primary aldosteronism: A new clinical syndrome. *J. Lab. Clin. Med.* 45:3, 1955.

Conn, J. W., Cohen, E. L., and Rovner, D. R. Suppression of plasma renin activity in primary aldosteronism: Distinguishing primary from secondary aldosteronism in hypertensive disease. *J.A.M.A.* 190:213, 1964.

Dale, S. L., and Melby, J. C.: Altered adrenal steroidogenesis in "low-renin": Essential hypertension. *Trans. Assoc. Am. Physicians.* 87:248, 1974.

Lipsett, M. The differential diagnosis of hirsutism and virilism. *Arch. Intern. Med.* 132:616, 1973.

Melby, J. C.: Assessment of adrenocortical function. *N. Engl. J. Med.* 285:735, 1971.

Melby, J. C.: Systemic corticosteroid therapy: Pharmacologic and endocrinologic considerations. *Ann. Intern. Med.* 81:505, 1974.

Melby, J. C.: Therapeutic possibilities in Cushing's syndrome. *N. Engl. J. Med.* 285:288, 1971.

Melby, J. C.: Aldosterone Inhibitors (Adrenal Cortex). In E. B. Astwood and C. Cassidy (eds.), *Clinical Endocrinology.* Vol. 2. New York: Grune & Stratton, 1968. P. 477.

Melby, J. C.: Identifying the adrenal lesion in primary aldosteronism. *Ann. Intern. Med.* 76:1039, 1972.

Sapira, J. D., Altman, M., Vandyk, K., and Shapiro, A. P.: Bilateral adrenal pheochromocytoma and medullary thyroid carcinoma. *N. Engl. J. Med.* 273:140, 1965.

Spark, R. F., and Melby, J. C.: Aldosteronism in hypertension: A spironolactone response test. *Ann. Intern. Med.* 69:685, 1968.

57

Disorders of the Male and Female Reproductive Systems

Judith L. Vaitukaitis and Christopher Longcope

Developmental changes in the two sexes are indistinguishable for the initial 6 weeks of fetal life. However, in the seventh week the testis becomes distinguishable from an ovary and secretes at least two substances that exert local effects on ductal development as well as on differentiation of male external genitalia. Testosterone secreted by the normal fetal testis stimulates development of the wolffian ducts and their derivatives — vas deferens, epididymis, seminal vesicles — and stimulates differentiation of male external genitalia. In addition to testosterone, the testis secretes a second substance, müllerian regression factor, which is thought to be a polypeptide and which stimulates involution of the müllerian ducts. In contrast to male differentiation, which requires normally functioning testes to be present, female development will occur spontaneously in the absence of gonads; moreover, differentiation of müllerian ducts into a uterus, tubes, and upper portion of the vagina will also take place in the absence of any gonads.

Obviously if the testes fail to synthesize and secrete müllerian regression factor, the internal genitalia of both sexes will persist. If the testes cannot synthesize testosterone or if the target tissues of testosterone and dihydrotestosterone cannot utilize that steroid because of aberrations of intracellular metabolism or mediation of testosterone action, developmental defects ranging from ambiguous external genitalia to true hermaphroditism may result.

Puberty

Puberty encompasses a complex of ordered physiologic events that culminates in (1) the capacity to reproduce, and (2) the development of adult secondary sexual characteristics. The entire pubertal process requires 3 to 5 years for completion in both sexes. The staging of secondary sexual characteristics as outlined by Marshall and Tanner is a useful way to ascertain whether the pubertal process is normal, since the ordered set of physiologic events resulting in the development of secondary sexual characteristics and the capacity to reproduce requires an intact hypothalamic-pituitary-gonadal axis. The time prior to the development of pubic hair and breasts is referred to as Tanner stage I, while Tanner stage V alludes to full adult breast and pubic hair development. Table 57-1 summarizes these stages of puberty for both boys and girls.

In girls, in whom the onset of puberty may occur as early as 9½ years, progression of pubic hair and breast development parallel one another, and if there is any disparity between these events, a disturbance of reproduction reflecting an abnormality of the hypothalamic-pituitary-gonadal axis should be suspected. Most of these abnormalities are of a chromosomal nature and involve primary gonadal aberrations.

In contrast to girls, the first sign of pubertal development in boys is testicular enlargement, which starts approximately 6 months later than the first signs of puberty in girls. Moreover, the peak height velocity ("growth spurt") in boys usually occurs approximately 2 years later than in girls, starting approximately at the age of 14 to 15.

Precocious pseudopuberty is a pathophysiologic state in either a girl or a boy in which secondary sexual characteristics develop, but not the capacity to reproduce. Precocious pseudopuberty is termed *isosexual* if the secondary sexual characteristics are consistent with the sex of the individual, but *heterosexual* if the secondary sexual changes are contrary to the chromosomal sex of the individual. For example, a young girl undergoing precocious heterosexual pseudopuberty develops signs of excess circulating androgen, manifested by excessive and inappropriate hair growth, with or without clitoromegaly. Precocious isosexual pseudopuberty in girls usually results from secretion of estrogen from adrenal or ovarian tumors, or even from benign ovarian cysts.

Sex Steroids

The steroids responsible for secondary sexual characteristics are synthesized in the adrenal glands, gonads, and in a variety of peripheral tissues from precursors of biologically active steroids. The adrenals and

Table 57-1. Secondary Sexual Changes During Puberty

Tanner stage	Girls			Boys	
	Breast development	Pubic hair	Mean age (range)	Secondary sexual characteristics	Mean age (range)
1	No breast development; prepubertal	No pubic hair; prepubertal	< 9 yr	Prepubertal; testes < 2.4 cm in diameter, pubic hair absent	9.5
2	Glandular tissue coextends with areola	Few strands of hair	11 (9–13)	Early testicular enlargement with scrotal reddening; few strands of pubic or scrotal hair may be present	11.6 (10–14)
3	Glandular tissue extends beyond subareolar area	More pubic hair present	12 (10–14)	Further testicular enlargement, phallic enlargement, ± pubic and axillary hair	13 (11–15)
4	Progression of glandular tissue; plane of areola distinct from remainder of mammary tissue	Further progression so that mons pubis covered	13 (11–15)	Moderate amount of pubic, axillary, and facial hair; acne; voice change; adult body odor	14 (12–16)
5	Adult development; areola and remainder of breast tissue in same plane	Adult development with extension of hair growth to medial thighs	15 (12–18)	Adult testicular development (15 ml or > 4.5 cm in longest diameter); adult male body habitus; pubic hair extends to medial thigh	15 (13–17)

gonads can utilize acetate and cholesterol as precursors in the steroid synthetic pathway, which proceeds through the steps noted in Figure 57-1 to form the steroids with major biologic activity. The immediate precursors, which possess essentially no intrinsic biologic activity, are secreted by the adrenal glands and gonads and are carried in the blood to peripheral tissues, where they are converted to biologically active products. Target organs of sex steroids as well as muscle, adipose tissue, and skin can convert steroid precursors to biologically active forms of sex steroids and thus be exposed to high local concentrations of biologically active steroids.

In normal women 50 percent of circulating testosterone is synthesized in peripheral tissues, primarily from androstenedione, a steroid that is secreted by both the ovaries and the adrenals. Dehydroepiandrosterone and its sulfate, secreted in relatively large amounts from the adrenal gland, contribute only a small amount to circulating testosterone by peripheral conversion. In postmenopausal women, androstenedione is the precursor for peripheral tissue formation of testosterone as well as for most of the biologically active estrogens — estradiol and estrone. Moreover, in the adult man, peripheral conversion of testosterone and androstenedione accounts for between 60 and 80 percent of the biologically active

Figure 57-1. The major pathways for the synthesis of the androgens and estrogens secreted by the adrenal gland, ovary, and testis.

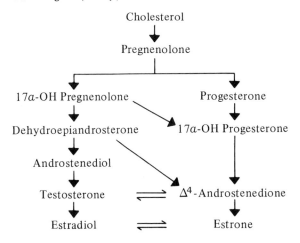

estrogens, estradiol and estrone. On the other hand, 5-α-reductase, an enzyme found in the cytosol of cells of the prostate and seminal vesicle, accounts for transformation of testosterone to dihydrotesterone.

In the blood, the biologically inactive precursor steroids circulate in an equilibrium between the free and the albumin-bound state. Since the binding affinity to albumin is weak, precursor steroids are potentially able to diffuse into cells and be transformed into biologically active steroids or be metabolized. In contrast to biologically active steroids, there are no specific intracellular binding proteins for inactive steroids.

The biologically active steroids circulate in the blood in an equilibrium between the free, albumin-bound, and globulin-bound states. While albumin binding is weak, globulin binding is strong with a slow dissociation rate; most of the biologically active steroids are bound to the globulins, referred to as TeBG or testosterone-estrogen binding globulin or sex-steroid—binding globulin. Consequently, only the small fraction of the total of biologically active steroid that exists in a free or an albumin-bound form is available for cell entry. The fraction that leaves the vascular bed and enters the cell does so by passive diffusion through cell membranes. It is this diffusible fraction of sex steroids that interacts with negative or positive feedback loops between the gonad and pituitary-hypothalamic axis.

Within the cytoplasm of the cell, however, the biologically active steroids become strongly bound to specific protein receptors. The initial steroid-receptor complex formed is apparently incapable of entering the nucleus. However, a transformation occurs in its structure to a complex with a smaller molecular weight protein, whereupon the steroid-receptor complex translocates into the nucleus, where it is bound to a portion of the chromatin. Following its binding to the chromatin, the genetic mechanism is activated, and through a series of steps, messenger RNA is formed and the specific effect(s) of the steroid are initiated. On the other hand, precursor steroids that enter the target cell can be acted upon by specific enzymes and can be transformed into active steroids, which then can bind to specific cytosol receptors and pass through the steps just described to initiate the specific effect(s). The mechanisms whereby steroids, having initiated their effects, leave the cell are uncertain at this time.

Thus there are various potential sites of steroid metabolism and action where abnormalities might occur, resulting in a variety of clinical syndromes. The sites are (1) altered steroidogenesis, resulting from enzymatic deficiencies and leading to altered sex steroid concentrations, (2) altered peripheral conversion of precursor steroids to biologically active forms, (3) aberrations of transport globulins, and (4) altered intracellular mediation of sex steroid action at the cytoplasmic or nuclear levels. Specific clinical syndromes have been identified with some of these four potential abnormalities. Altered steroidogenesis may result in an adrenogenital syndrome of varying severity due to deficiencies of 21-hydroxylase or 11-β-hydroxylase. As a result of excessive androgen production in utero, ambiguous genitalia of varying degrees result. In its severest form, female pseudo-hermaphroditism results (see Chap. 56).

In addition, as an example of (3) above, administration of either thyroxine or oral contraceptives that contain estrogen stimulates excessive synthesis of testosterone-estrogen binding globulin, resulting in a greater pool of bound sex steroid, even though the "free" pool may remain unchanged. However, the total circulating steroid, bound and free, will be increased.

An example of (4) above is the syndrome of testicular feminization, which occurs in genetic males as a result of altered cytoplasmic to nuclear translocation of the testosterone-receptor complex. Thus androgens, although present at normal male levels, are unable to bind to the nuclear chromatin. As a result, these patients have a female phenotype (male pseudo-hermaphrodite) but an XY karyotype. Patients with complete testicular feminization have Tanner V breast development but absence of both axillary and pubic hair. The disparity in breast development and pubic hair growth is a clinical sign that should cause this syndrome to be considered. Some patients have an incomplete form of the syndrome, probably reflecting an incomplete intracellular defect of testosterone metabolism. These patients may have inguinal or labial masses (testes) and male internal genitalia (vas deferens, epididymis). Circulating luteinizing hormone levels are usually elevated, whereas follicle-stimulating hormone concentrations may be normal or slightly elevated. The lower third of a vaginal pouch may be present, or only a dimple may be present at that anatomic site. The testes should be removed in these patients because of the higher incidence of tumors in intraabdominal testes or dysgenetic gonads containing a Y chromosome. Replacement estrogen therapy should then be instituted because the patients frequently have hot flashes after removing the testes, which secrete normal adult male levels of testosterone with a significant fraction of that androgen being converted to biologically active estrogens in peripheral tissues. The biologic effects of estrogen are unopposed by androgens and consequently exert a greater biologic affect.

Normal Male Physiology

The testis contains two sets of target tissues, namely the Leydig cells and the seminiferous tubules. The Leydig cells synthesize and release testosterone when stimulated by luteinizing hormone (LH), also known as interstitial cell stimulating hormone (ICSH). Normal male circulating levels of testosterone range between 350 and 1,100 ng per 100 ml. Levels below the lower limits of normal in the adult reflect either target organ (testicular) or hypothalamic-pituitary axis failure. Since the feedback between the target cell and the hypothalamic-pituitary axis is a negative feedback mechanism, high levels of circulating LH in the presence of low levels of circulating testosterone imply end-organ (Leydig cell) failure.

The second set of target tissues, the seminiferous tubules, is the site for spermatogenesis, which is dependent on follicle-stimulating hormone (FSH). The exact interaction of Leydig cell and seminiferous tubule functions is unknown. An androgen-binding protein with a high affinity for testosterone and dihydrotestosterone has been isolated from the fluid of seminiferous tubules and the epididymis. While the exact physiologic role of this androgen-binding protein has not been worked out, it is known to be regulated by FSH. The time required for maturation of sperm from the beginning of spermatogenesis to mature sperm has been estimated at 74 ± 4 to 5 days.

Sertoli cells line the basement membrane of the seminiferous tubule. When all the germinal elements are destroyed by some disease or chemical or physical process, only Sertoli cells are found within the seminiferous tubules. When testicular biopsies show this pattern, the patient is diagnosed as having Sertoli-cell-only syndrome, especially if a specific etiology cannot be discerned. When there is an aberration of seminiferous tubule function in the adult, elevated circulating FSH levels are usually encountered.

Obviously male hypogonadism can result because of a defect either at the target organ, namely the testis (hypergonadotropic), or at the pituitary-hypothalamic level (hypogonadotropic). The bases for differentiation of the site of abnormality are the circulating levels of testosterone and gonadotropin. In general, men with high levels of circulating gonadotropin who are hypogonadal have a defect at the target organ. The target organ defect may result from external or intrinsic aberrations of the testis.

HYPERGONADOTROPIC HYPOGONADISM IN MEN
The most common cause of hypergonadotropic hypogonadism is Klinefelter's syndrome, which occurs approximately once in every 500 male births. Clinically the syndrome is associated with small, firm testes and elevated circulating levels of FSH and LH. Characteristically the testes are firm because significant sclerosis has taken place, starting about the time of puberty. There are usually no physical stigmata of Klinefelter's syndrome at birth, and it is very difficult to make this diagnosis prior to puberty without doing routine buccal smears, which will usually reveal a percentage of Barr bodies in the normal female range. In normal men there should be fewer than 5 percent Barr bodies present in the cells of buccal mucosa. However, Klinefelter patients have an XXY karyotype that results in Barr bodies (two X chromosomes are necessary to make a Barr body).

The patient with Klinefelter's syndrome usually presents with arrested pubertal development. Phallic development and pubic hair may be normal, but axillary and beard hair are usually scant. Gynecomastia is frequently present. Because these patients have varying degrees of inadequate testicular testosterone synthesis, many have eunuchoid body propor-

tions. Testicular biopsies of patients with Klinefelter's syndrome will fail to show elastin around the basement membrane of seminiferous tubules with specific stains. This finding is sine qua non for the histologic diagnosis of Klinefelter's syndrome. The Leydig cells may appear clumped and hyperplastic. In addition, circulating testosterone levels may be in the low normal range, although they may be in the normal adult male range.

Hypergonadotropic hypogonadism may also be caused by infection or trauma. The testes are small and soft, in contrast to the small, firm testes of Klinefelter's syndrome. Since the seminiferous tubules are more susceptible than the Leydig cells to any type of injury, the patients will usually present with azoospermia or oligospermia, but they may have normal testosterone levels, reflecting the relative resistance of the Leydig cells to trauma or infection. If the infection and trauma are sufficiently severe, the patient will be permanently sterile. Testicular biopsies will show absent or arrested spermatogenesis. Some of the more common causes of postpubertal orchitis are trauma, gonococcal infection, and mumps. Interestingly, if a prepubertal male has mumps, the testes are usually spared. Unilateral involvement may be found in some patients, and the testicular damage may not be permanent in patients with milder infections. Usually the defects are progressive after these infections, so that early afterward, the patient may present with only mild oligospermia, but as years pass, the oligospermia may progress to azoospermia; in fact, Leydig cell function may dissipate completely.

In younger patients with hypergonadotropic hypogonadism due to trauma or infection, treatment consists in simply replacing natural testosterone with a long-acting testosterone preparation. It is better to start with a short-acting testosterone preparation (testosterone proprionate) in older men, in whom acute prostatic stimulation could lead to acute bladder retention and its sequelae. Patients presenting with oligospermia must be carefully evaluated over time, since febrile illnesses and other debilitating syndromes can cause oligospermia transiently. Therefore it may be necessary to evaluate the patient over several months, since the duration of the normal sperm cycle is on the order of 74 days.

In addition to trauma and infection, radiation damage and alkylating agents (as a result of their radiomimetic effects) can cause irreversible damage to the testis. Very small doses of radiation, as low as 50 rads, can cause significant changes in seminiferous tubules. When higher doses of radiation are given, small, soft testes that are indistinguishable from infected testes may result. With low levels of radiation on the order of 20 to 30 rads, FSH levels may be elevated, signifying seminiferous tubule damage, but LH and testosterone levels may be normal, reflecting the fact that Leydig cells are more resistant to damage.

The Sertoli-cell-only (or the del Castillo) syndrome is characterized by a lack of spermatogenesis but normal Leydig cell function. Consequently, LH and testosterone levels and the resulting secondary sexual characteristics are normal. However, plasma FSH levels are elevated, probably reflecting the fact that at an earlier time there had been direct damage to previously functioning seminiferous tubules in these patients. The seminiferous tubules contain only Sertoli cells, and the testes are usually smaller than normal in size. The testis may be of normal consistency, however, in the Sertoli-cell-only syndrome.

A rare cause of hypergonadotropic hypogonadism with isolated seminiferous tubule dysfunction is that of myotonic dystrophy. In patients presenting with myotonic dystrophy, lenticular opacities, and frontal baldness, approximately 80 percent have a primary testicular aberration characterized by complete hyalinization and fibrosis of the seminiferous tubules. The etiology of the latter is not known.

Hypogonadotrophic hypogonadal disorders are discussed in Chapter 55.

Normal Female Physiology

Primordial follicles first appear in the human fetal ovary around the fifth month of gestation. Initially they are found deep in the cortex at the corticomedullary junction. Starting with the sixth intrauterine month, the primordial follicles progressively increase in number and some become transformed into primary follicles containing growing oocytes. In the last 2 months of gestation, graafian follicles may actually be found in cross sections of the human fetal ovary and are normally found in ovarian cross sections from birth to the time of menopause.

At the time of menarche, cyclic gonadotropin release is initiated in women. As a result, cyclic ovulation occurs in the presence of continuing atresia of follicles. The first several menstrual cycles after menarche may be anovulatory. Luteinizing hormone usually interacts with the theca interna of the developing follicle and results in steroidogenesis. Specific receptors for FSH have been identified on granulosa cells. Prior to ovulation, granulosa cells secrete primarily estradiol. After ovulation the remaining granulosa cells of the graafian follicle are transformed into a corpus luteum that secretes estradiol, progesterone, and some 17-hydroxyprogesterone in the human.

OVARIAN DYSFUNCTION

Primary amenorrhea is defined as the absence of spontaneous menarche by age 16. *Secondary amenorrhea,* on the other hand, is defined as the cessation of spontaneous menses for at least 4 consecutive months. Primary gonadal disorders constitute between 30 and 50 percent of all causes of primary amenorrhea. Characteristically, circulating gonadotropin levels are elevated, with FSH being greater than LH when IRP2hMG (International Reference Preparation 2 of human Menopausal Gonadotropin) is used as the reference preparation. In addition, estradiol levels are usually less than 10 pg per milliliter and progesterone levels are less than 0.3 ng per milliliter.

The primary gonadal disorders include patients with Turner's syndrome, patients with dysgenetic gonads with XX or XY karyotype, the true hermphrodites with undifferentiated testes or ovotestes, and a few patients with polycystic ovary syndrome. Primary amenorrhea resulting from aberrations of the hypothalamic-pituitary axis constitutes only a small percentage of the cases, approximately 3 to 5 percent. The remainder of the patients have developmental abnormalities of the uterus or vagina such as dysgenesis or aplasia.

Patients with Turner's syndrome constitute approximately 30 percent of all cases of primary amenorrhea. These patients may have shield chest, webbed neck, short stature, short metatarsals, café au lait spots, black freckles, double-layered eyelashes, and various cardiac abnormalities. Classically these patients have an X0 karyotype and consequently have a lower than normal percentage of Barr bodies present in buccal smears when compared with their normal female counterparts.

A variety of ovarian tumors may result in primary or secondary amenorrhea. A small number of these tumors secrete biologically active substances, and these tumors are summarized in Table 57-2.

Secondary Amenorrhea

The differential diagnosis of secondary amenorrhea is somewhat complex. The most common cause is pregnancy and must be excluded before any patient undergoes further diagnostic evaluation. The second most common cause is that related to hypothalamic-pituitary dysfunction. However, the exact incidence is unknown in the United States, although it has been approximated in Sweden, where a 1-year rate of 4.4 percent was found for women with amenorrhea of at least 3 months' duration. Marked weight loss, commonly found among high school students and young women entering college, is frequently associated with secondary amenorrhea. The most extreme cases of marked weight loss are found among patients with anorexia nervosa. Both groups of patients, those undergoing voluntary weight loss and patients with bona fide anorexia nervosa, have gradations of the same aberrations of the hypothalamic-pituitary axis. In addition to weight loss, tumors or cysts in the areas of the hypothalamus may result in secondary amenorrhea by interfering with the hypothalamic-pituitary interaction of the various gonadotropin releasing factors.

In all the foregoing patients, plasma gonadotropins are tonically low, and consequently estradiol levels are low, usually ranging between 5 and 75 pg per milliliter. This reflects the absence of cyclic gonadal stimulation by FSH and LH. The precise pathophysiology for the hypothalamic-pituitary dysfunction is unknown.

Another cause of secondary amenorrhea is pituitary tumor. As a result of the tumor's presence, hypothalamic-pituitary interactions are again impeded, resulting in loss of cyclic gonadotropin release. Commonly, low circulating levels of gonadotropin are encountered, but in some cases in which the pituitary tumor is functioning, signs and symptoms of excessive circulating hormone may be present. For instance, if the tumor is secreting growth hormone, the patient will have signs and symptoms of acromegaly.

Patients with mosaic Turner's syndrome may undergo spontaneous puberty with normal sexual development. However, within a few years or so after spontaneous puberty, these patients may become amenorrheic. It may require careful analysis of several different tissues to demonstrate the chromosomal mosaicism. These patients may have a normal percentage of Barr bodies present on a buccal smear, or they may have a disparity between the percentage of Barr bodies present on buccal smears of the right and left cheeks. On the other hand, the number of Barr bodies may be totally within normal limits, and the chromosomal aberration may be limited to ovarian tissue. In essence, then, not only can a patient have mosaicism in terms of karyotype, but the mosaicism may be limited to a specific tissue. Ovarian biopsies of these patients will show absence of ova. Consequently, these patients have levels of circulating gonadotropin and estradiol indistinguishable from those in postmenopausal women.

Table 57-2. Ovarian Tumors Secreting Hormonally Active Substances

Steroid-producing		Nonsteroid producing	
Tumor	Steroid	Tumor	Nonsteroid hormone
Arrhenoblastoma	Testosterone	Dysgerminoma, teratoma, choriocarcinoma, adenoma	Human chorionic gonadotropin
Gonadoblastoma	Testosterone		
Granulosa-theca cell	Estrogen	Benign cystic teratoma, dermoid cyst	Serotonin
Lipoid cell tumors	Estrogen/testosterone	Teratoma, dermoid cyst	Thyroxine

Polycystic ovarian disease or Stein-Leventhal syndrome is commonly associated with secondary amenorrhea. Preceding the onset of amenorrhea, these patients will characteristically have a history of oligomenorrhea accompanied usually by varying degrees of hirsutism and acne, both reflecting excess androgen production. Although circulating testosterone levels may be in the normal female range, the production rates of testosterone are invariably elevated. Frequently the patients are overweight. In addition, these women may have inappropriately elevated plasma LH levels and tonically suppressed FSH levels, both of which are rather characteristic of polycystic ovarian disease. Studies carried out with exogenous estrogens suggest that there is an aberration of the feedback mechanism between ovarian steroids and pituitary-hypothalamic function, suggesting relative insensitivity of the hypothalamic-pituitary axis to the negative feedback effect of sex steroids. The ovaries may be of normal size or they may be markedly enlarged secondary to cyst formation. Perhaps a better name for this syndrome would be chronic anovulation.

Patients with polycystic ovarian disease will usually have an ovulatory response to clomiphene (Clomid), a fertility drug. Clomiphene functions as an antiestrogen agent primarily at the hypothalamic level, where it competes with estrogen for binding sites and indirectly stimulates pituitary gonadotropin release, which in turn stimulates the ovaries. Patients with polycystic ovarian disease on clomiphene may develop ovarian hyperstimulation, which is characterized by rapid, painful enlargement of the ovaries; consequently patients on clomiphene should be monitored closely while on the medication and for 1 to 2 weeks afterward. The dose of clomiphene should be tailored to the patient, who may require as little as 50 mg perorally daily for 3 days up to 200 mg perorally daily for 5 days. Ovarian wedge resection frequently restores cyclic menses in this group of patients, but unfortunately its effect is not long lasting and may persist for only a few months.

A variety of other factors may result in irreversible secondary amenorrhea. Among these are exposure to the alkylating effects of chemotherapy (most commonly busulfan [Myleran] and cyclophosphamide [Cytoxan]) or exposure to radiation per se. Less common causes of secondary amenorrhea are ovarian and adrenal tumors that actively secrete steroids that interfere with the normal feedback mechanisms between the ovarian-hypothalamic-pituitary axis.

Premature menopause is accompanied by high circulating FSH and LH levels comparable to those found in spontaneous menopause. The usual age for spontaneous menopause in the United States is 52 years of age. When the ovaries of patients with premature menopause are examined, they are essentially devoid of ova. No chromosomal aberrations have been described in these patients. The etiology of this syndrome is unknown, but commonly it is familial; consequently, a careful history should be obtained.

Treatment of Primary Gonadal Disorders

In men and women with primary gonadal failure, replacement sex steroid therapy is indicated. In young women, physiologic replacement of estrogen ranging between 15 and 30 μg of a synthetic estrogen per day is indicated to obviate severe osteoporosis from prolonged estrogen deprivation. Higher doses may be used to induce or restore secondary sexual characteristics more rapidly. Routine estrogen therapy for postmenopausal women is not recommended unless specific side effects dictate their use. Again, physiologic replacement doses should be used. In addition, a progestational agent, for example norethindrone acetate (Norlutate), 2.5 mg perorally daily for 5 consecutive days, should be added up to four times per year to attain adequate sloughing of endometrial tissue (which tends to slough partially with estrogen withdrawal alone). Obviously all patients with primary gonadal failure are sterile.

HIRSUTISM

Clinically, excessive circulating levels of biologically active androgens in women may result in acne, growth of excessive hair on the medial thighs, face, intermammary and periareolar areas, and in extreme cases may lead to virilization with clitoromegaly, frontal balding, and development of a male body habitus. Urinary 17-ketosteroid excretion has been traditionally used to screen for excessive androgen secretion. However, in normal women at least 80 percent of urinary 17-ketosteroids is derived from adrenocortical secretion of dehydroepiandrosterone and its sulfate ester, both of which are metabolized to androsterone and etiocholanolone. Only 10 percent of urinary 17-ketosteroid excretion results from metabolism of androstenedione secreted by the adrenal gland. Consequently, at least 90 percent of 17-ketosteroid excretion in women results from adrenal sources, and these are weakly androgenic at best. If, on screening, 17-ketosteroid excretion is clearly elevated (greater than 30 mg per day), the most likely source of androgen excess is the adrenal gland. If clinical signs of androgen excess are present but 17-ketosteroid excretion is normal, then the most likely site of excess androgen secretion is the ovary, testosterone being directly secreted by that gland. Ovarian tumors are usually associated with testosterone levels greater than 300 ng per 100 ml. There are exceptions to the foregoing generalizations, but they should enable the clinician to be correct approximately 90 percent of the time.

Most cases of hirsutism are idiopathic. However, idiopathic hirsutism is a diagnosis of exclusion. It is usually associated with normal female serum testosterone levels; however, testosterone production rates are usually elevated. Testosterone production rates result from the summation of direct testosterone secretion from the adrenal and ovarian glands plus peripheral conversion of precursor steroids to testosterone. After having excluded a tumor of the adrenal gland or ovary, idiopathic hirsutism is treated empirically with trials of one of the following: (1) combined estrogens and progestins to suppress gonadotropin-stimulated ovarian androgen secretion, (2) dexamethasone suppression of adrenal androgen secretion, or (3) a combination of both therapies, especially if neither is effective alone. Some physicians have used pharmacologic doses of thyroxine to increase sex steroid-binding globulins. Several months of clinical trial are generally needed before any therapeutic effect may be noted with any of the foregoing forms of therapy. Reversal of excessive hirsutism is rare, but in some cases the progression of hirsutism may be halted. Other adjunctive procedures such as electrolysis and depilatories may help cosmetically.

Bibliography

Anderson, D. C. Sex-hormone-binding globulin. *Clin. Endocrinol. (Oxford)* 3:69, 1974.

Baird, D., Horton, R., Longcope, C., and Tait, J. F. Steroid prehormones. *Perspect Biol. Med.* 11:384, 1968.

Baird, D. T., Horton, R., Longcope, C., and Tait, J. F. Steroid dynamics under steady-state conditions. *Recent Progr. Horm. Res.* 25:611, 1969.

Baird, P. A., and DeJong, B. P. Noonan's syndrome (XX and XY Turner phenotype) in three generations of a family. *J. Pediatr.* 80:110, 1972.

Bardin, C. W., and Lipsett, M. B. Testosterone and androstenedione blood production rates in normal women and women with idiopathic hirsutism or polycystic ovaries. *J. Clin. Invest.* 46:891, 1967.

DeVane, G. W., Czekala, N. M., Judd, H. L., and Yen, S. S. C. Circulating gonadotropins, estrogens, and androgens in polycystic ovarian disease. *Am. J. Obstet. Gynecol.* 121:496, 1975.

Faiman, C., and Winter, J. S. D. The control of gonadotropin secretion in complete testicular feminization. *J. Clin. Endocrinol. Metab.* 39:631, 1974.

Goldstein, J. L., and Wilson, J. D. Hereditary Disorders of Sexual Development in Man. In A. G. Motulsky and W. Lentz (eds.), *Birth Defects, Proceedings of the Fourth International Conference* (Vienna) (International Congress Series No. 310). Amsterdam: Excerpta Medica, 1974. P. 165.

Kirschner, M. A., and Jacobs, J. B. Combined ovarian and adrenal vein catheterization to determine the site(s) of androgen overproduction in hirsute women. *J. Clin. Endocrinol. Metab.* 33:199, 1971.

Liao, S. Cellular receptors and mechanisms of action of steroid hormones. *Int. Rev. Cytol.* 41:87, 1975.

Marshall, W. A., and Tanner, J. M. Variations in pattern of pubertal changes in girls. *Arch. Dis. Child.* 44:291, 1969.

Marshall, W. A., and Tanner, J. M. Variations in the pattern of pubertal changes in boys. *Arch. Dis. Child.* 45:13, 1970.

Paulsen, C. A., Gordon, D. L., Carpenter, R. W., Gandy, H. M., and Drucker, W. D. Klinefelter's syndrome and its variants: A hormonal and chromosomal study. *Recent Progr. Horm. Res.* 24:321, 1968.

Raynaud, J. P., Bouton, M. M., Gallet-Bourquin, D., Philbert, D., Tournemine, C., and Azadian-Boulanger, G. Comparative study of estrogen action. *Mol. Pharmacol.* 9:520, 1973.

Sherman, B. M., and Korenman, S. G. Hormonal characteristics of the human menstrual cycle throughout reproductive life. *J. Clin. Invest.* 55:699, 1975.

Siris, E. S., Leventhal, B. G., and Vaitukaitis, J. L. Effects of childhood leukemia and chemotherapy on puberty and reproductive function in girls. *N. Engl. J. Med.* 294:1143, 1976.

Teter, J. Prognosis, malignancy, and curability of the germ-cell tumor occurring in dysgenetic gonads. *Am. J. Obstet. Gynecol.* 108:894, 1970.

Walsh, P. C., Madden, J. D., Harrod, M. J., Goldstein, J. L., MacDonald, P. L., and Wilson, J. D. Familial incomplete male pseudohermaphroditism, type 2. *N. Engl. J. Med.* 291:944, 1974.

Wilson, J. D., and Gloyna, R. E. The intranuclear metabolism of testosterone in the accessory organs of reproduction. *Recent Progr. Horm. Res.* 26:309, 1970.

Wilson, J. D., Harrod, M. J., Goldstein, J. L., Hemsell, D. L., and MacDonald, P. C. Familial incomplete male pseudohermaphroditism, type 1. *N. Engl. J. Med.* 290:1097, 1974.

58

Thyroid Disease

Isadore N. Rosenberg

Physiology and Regulation of Thyroid Hormone Secretion

The thyroid gland synthesizes, stores, and secretes the iodine-containing amino acid thyroxine (T_4), 3, 5, 3'-triiodothyronine (T_3), and the peptide hormone calcitonin. The thyroid gland accumulates iodide from the circulation by an active transport mechanism that is sensitive to perchlorate and thiocyanate. The iodide so accumulated is organically bound to tyrosyl residues in thyroglobulin, a 19S glycoprotein of 660,000 daltons, to form monoiodotyrosyl and diiodotyrosyl residues. These residues then undergo "coupling", leading to the formation of thyroxyl and triiodothyronyl residues in thyroglobulin. Both the organic binding and coupling processes are mediated by a peroxidase, which can be inhibited by antithyroid drugs of the thiocarbonamide type, such as 6n-propylthiouracil and methimazole. Secretion of the thyroid hormones T_4 and T_3 into the circulation involves pinocytosis by the follicular cells of luminal colloid (colloid droplet formation), with formation of phagolysosomes and proteolytic release of the iodinated amino acids from thyroglobulin. The T_4 and T_3 are released from the gland, while the iodotyrosines undergo intracellular deiodination (mediated by an NADPH-dependent microsomal enzyme specific for free halogenated tyrosines); and the iodide so generated is reused for iodination of thyroglobulin.

Thyroid function is regulated by pituitary secretion of thyroid-stimulating hormone (TSH), a glycoprotein of 24,000 daltons composed of an alpha chain common to FSH, LH, and hCG (follicle-stimulating hormone, luteinizing hormone, and human chorionic gonadotropin) and a specific beta chain. Thyroid-stimulating hormone stimulates the thyroid by binding to receptors on the thyroid cell membrane, thus activating adenylate cyclase, and generating cyclic AMP (adenosine 3':5'-cyclic phosphate), which enhances colloid droplet formation, organic binding of iodine, synthesis of thyroglobulin, and trapping of iodide from the circulation. Secretion of TSH is governed by two opposing mechanisms: (1) hypothalamic drive mediated by thyrotropin-releasing hormone (TRH), a tripeptide that is produced in hypothalamic neurons, reaches the anterior pituitary by way of its portal venous plexus, and stimulates (by activating adenylate cyclase) the formation and secretion of TSH; and (2) feedback inhibition of TSH release, which is exerted by circulating thyroid hormones acting directly on the pituitary thyrotropic cell (the inhibition appears to involve DNA-dependent new protein synthesis).

The thyroid secretes both T_4 and T_3 in proportion to their relative concentrations in the thyroid. The thyroid T_4/T_3 ratio is 10 to 15:1 in iodine-replete regions; with dietary iodine deficiency, the proportion of T_3 increases. Studies of thyroid hormone secretion provide the data listed in Table 58-1. These data show that T_3 is bound only one-tenth as tightly to plasma proteins as T_4, is much more rapidly cleared from the blood, and is predominantly intracellular, whereas T_4 is mainly extracellular. Thyroxine arises only from thyroid secretion, while most of the extrathyroidal T_3 is derived from deiodination of secreted T_4. The sites and mechanisms of deiodination are not yet clear, but kidney and liver are known to catalyze this deiodination and there is some suggestion of impaired conversion of T_4 to T_3 in hepatic and renal disease. A normal T_3 level may sustain the euthyroid state even when T_4 is low (e.g., in severe iodine deficiency and after radioiodine therapy for hyperthyroidism); in these conditions of stimulated thyroid activity the production and secretion of T_3 are enhanced relative to T_4, a useful adaptive mechanism since the hormonal potency of T_3 is three to five times that of T_4. Increased plasma T_3 is characteristic of hyperthyroidism, and the plasma T_4/T_3 ratio is less than normal. Although plasma T_3 is subnormal in hypothyroidism, T_3 concentration is also low in starvation and in chronic illness and therefore is not per se a reliable index of hypothyroidism. A low T_3 in euthyroid individuals is often accompanied by a rise in plasma "reverse T_3" (3,3',5'-T_3); the curious reciprocal relationship between T_3 and reverse T_3 may indicate a shift of T_4 metabolism from the formation of a biologically active compound (T_3) to production of a noncalorigenic substance (reverse T_3). A possible biologic role of reverse T_3 is suggested by

Table 58-1. Plasma concentrations, pool sizes, and production rates of Thyroxine (T_4) and Triiodothyronine (T_3)

	T_4	T_3
a. Plasma concentration	4–11 μg/100 ml	60–180 ng/100 ml
b. Dialyzable fraction (%)	0.02	0.25
c. Plasma *free* hormone concentration (ng/100 ml) [a × b]	1–2	0.15–0.5
d. Metabolic clearance (L/day)	1	22
e. Volume of distribution (L)	10	40
f. Rate of turnover (%/day)	10	70
g. Half-time in circulation (days)	6.9	1.1
h. Extrathyroidal pool (μg) [a × e]	800	48
i. Disposal rate (μg/day) [a × d]	80	30
j. Secretion rate (μg/day)	80	6
k. Extrathyroidal production rate (μg/day)	0	24

Note: T_4 = thyroxine; T_3 = triiodothyronine.

recent reports that reverse T_3 both blocks the calorigenic action of T_4 and impairs the conversion of T_4 to T_3.

Approximately 80 percent of the T_3 produced daily is derived from metabolism of T_4; and since about 40 percent of the T_4 secreted daily is converted to T_3, which is three to five times as potent as T_4, the metabolic activity of T_4 can be largely accounted for by the T_3 formed from it. This has led to the suggestion that T_4 may be a metabolically inert prohormone, although some intrinsic biologic activity of T_4 is not excluded. This view is strengthened by the recent discovery, in the nuclei of cells of tissues responsive to thyroid hormone, of specific receptors of high affinity and low capacity that bind T_3 ten times more avidly than T_4. The nuclear receptor for thyroid hormone appears to be a nonhistone protein, and T_3-receptor DNA complexes have been characterized that may mediate the action of thyroid hormones in stimulating protein synthesis. The calorigenic effects of thyroid hormones may similarly be related to their enhancing the synthesis of cell-membrane Na^+-K^+-ATPase enzyme proteins, with consequent increased ATP hydrolysis and coupled oxygen utilization.

The circulating thyroid hormones are reversibly and noncovalently bound to plasma proteins. The major transport protein is thyroxine-binding globulin, an interalpha glycoprotein to which more than 75 percent of the circulating T_4 is bound; albumin

is a secondary carrier, while thyroxine-binding prealbumin is probably of minor significance under physiologic conditions. A reversible equilibrium exists between the concentrations of bound T_4, free T_4 (FT_4), and the unoccupied binding sites on the thyroxine-binding proteins (TBP_u), such that TBP_u + $FT_4 \rightleftharpoons$ bound T_4. Since 99.98 percent of the T_4 is bound, bound T_4 is essentially equivalent to total T_4, and the equilibrium constant, K, may be defined:

$$K = \frac{[\text{Total } T_4]}{[TBP_u]\,[FT_4]} \text{ , or } [FT_4] = \frac{[\text{Total } T_4]}{[TBP_u]} \times K$$

Hence FT_4 concentration is proportional to total T_4 concentration and inversely proportional to the TBP_u; FT_4 (and FT_3) are believed to be important determinants of thyroid hormone metabolism and action and correlate more closely than does the total T_4 (and T_3) with the thyroid hormone production rate, or thyroid state. Thus estrogen administration and pregnancy increase circulating thyroxine-binding globulin and are associated with high T_4 concentrations while FT_4 (and the thyroid state) remain normal; conversely, subnormal thyroxine-binding globulin is found in hypoproteinemic states and after androgen therapy, but again, free T_4 is normal and the individual remains euthyroid. Despite the importance of the free thyroid hormone concentrations as determinants of thyroid hormone metabolism and action and as indices of the thyroid state, they are not the sole determinants. Other factors, such as cellular metabolism of the hormone, including the conversion of T_4 to T_3, are probably important. Thus the FT_4 concentration is abnormally high in patients who are chronically ill and is subnormal in persons treated with phenytoin (dilantin), yet such individuals are euthyroid.

Evaluation of Thyroid Function

Determination of the production rates of T_4 and T_3 would provide the most useful information for assessing thyroid gland activity, but the necessary kinetic study is not feasible in the clinical setting. Clinical assessment of thyroid function may be considered under five headings: (1) measuring the concentration of the circulating hormones, T_4 and T_3; (2) assay of the reserve binding capacity of the thyroxine-binding proteins; (3) radioiodine studies of thyroid glandular activity; (4) assay of serum TSH and of TSH responses to TRH; (5) miscellaneous procedures.

CONCENTRATION OF CIRCULATING THYROID HORMONES

If the T_4 binding capacity is normal, the serum concentration of T_4 and T_3 (normal range, 4 to 11 and 0.06 to 0.18 μg/100 ml, respectively) as determined by competitive protein binding methods or radioimmunoassay will correlate well with the thyroid state, being high in hyperthyroidism and low in hypothyroidism. An important exception is the low T_3 found in euthyroid patients who are chronically ill or malnourished. Assays for T_4 and T_3 have virtually eliminated the need for chemical determination of protein-bound iodine and butanol-extractable iodine. Determination of FT_4 concentration (normally 1 to 3 ng/100 ml) from the product of the T_4 and the dialyzable fraction of T_4 (determined by equilibrium dialysis or ultrafiltration of serum containing highly purified radioactive tracer T_4) is technically difficult; similar information is more readily obtained from the free thyroxine index (see below).

RESERVE BINDING CAPACITY

The reserve binding capacity of the T_4 transport proteins is determined by equilibrating a trace quantity of labeled thyroid hormone (usually T_3) with serum in the presence of an adsorbent that binds the thyroid hormone and thus competes for the labeled material with the unoccupied sites on the transport proteins. An anion exchange resin is commonly used as the adsorbent (Sephadex, charcoal, and other materials have also been used), and the percentage of tracer bound to the resin is determined. The result is the resin T_3 uptake (RT_3U); in one commonly used procedure, normal RT_3U is 25 to 35 percent. The RT_3U is an inverse measure of unoccupied binding sites (TBP_u), and an increased or a decreased value indicates, respectively, a decrease or increase in TBP_u concentration. The increased saturation of serum protein binding sites in hyperthyroidism (with consequent reduction in unoccupied binding sites) and the decreased saturation in hypothyroidism explain the corresponding increases and decreases of RT_3U in these conditions. When the thyroid state is normal and there is a primary increase in thyroxine-binding globulin (as with estrogen administration, pregnancy, porphyria, or in idiopathic elevated thyroxine-binding globulinemia), RT_3U is low; when thyroxine-binding globulin is low (as in patients receiving androgens, anabolic steroids, salicylates, or phenytoin and in patients with acromegaly, hypoproteinemic states, or inherited deficiency of thyroxine-binding globulin), the RT_3U is high. It should be noted that alterations in thyroid hormone production rate show *concordance* of the abnormalities of serum T_4 and RT_3U (e.g., *both* values are high in hyperthyroidism and *both* are low in hypothyroidism), while *discordance* of the serum T_4 and RT_3U values is characteristic of primary abnormalities in thyroid hormone transport capacity. Thus pregnancy, in which circulating TBG capacity may increase twofold to threefold, is characterized by a high serum T_4 concentration and a low RT_3U, while persons given androgens show a low T_4 level and a high RT_3U. The numerical product of RT_3U and T_4, the free thyroxine index (FTI), tends to be normal in thyroxine-binding globulin abnormalities and abnormal in disturbances of thyroid function. These relationships are shown in Table 58-2.

RADIOACTIVE IODINE STUDIES OF THE THYROID

The thyroid radioactive iodine (RaI) uptake measures glandular avidity for accumulating and organically binding iodine; the uptake (expressed as a percent of the administered dose) usually is measured 24

Table 58-2. The Free Thyroxine Index and Its Relationship to Other Measurements of Thyroid Function

Condition	Thyroxine-binding capacity (μg T_4/100 ml)	T_4 (μg/100 ml)	T_3 (ng/100 ml)	RT_3U (%)	FT_4 (ng/100 ml)	FTI[*] μg/100 ml ($RT_3U \times T_4/30$)
Normal	15–25	4–11	60–180	25–35	1–3	3.3–13.0
Hyperthyroidism	↓	↑	↑	↑	↑	↑
Hypothyroidism	↑	↓	↓	↓	↓	↓
Pregnancy, estrogens	↑	↑	↑	↓	N	N
Androgens, hypoproteinemia	↓	↓	↓	↑	N	N

Note: T_4 = thyroxine; T_3 = triiodothyronine; RT_3U = resin triiodothyronine uptake; FT_4 = free thyroxine; FTI = free thyroxine index; N = normal; ↑ = increased; ↓ = decreased.
[*]In calculating FTI as the product of T_4 and RT_3U, the observed RT_3U is expressed as a fraction of normal (observed RT_3U divided by 30, the average normal value); in accordance with recent recommendations of the Committee on Nomenclature of the American Thyroid Association (*J. Clin. Endocrinol. Metab.* 42:595, 1976). FTI units (μg/100 ml), although formally correct, are usually omitted.

hours after administration of tracer ^{131}I, although shorter intervals are sometimes used. The RaI uptake is considerably dependent on the dietary intake of stable iodine. In iodine-deficient regions, euthyroid individuals may accumulate as much as 90 percent of the dose in 24 hours; in the United States the normal range of thyroid RaI uptake has declined from 15 to 45 percent a decade ago to 6 to 35 percent, paralleling the widespread increase in dietary iodide (possibly related to the use of iodate in bread processing). Large doses of iodide such as those used in radiologic contrast media dilute the tracer so extensively as to invalidate the thyroid RaI uptake as a clinical test of thyroid function. The contrast media used in intravenous pyelography lower the RaI uptake for 1 to 2 weeks, those used in cholecystography for 3 to 4 months, while agents used for myelography, bronchography, and lymphangiography may lower the RaI uptake for years. Thyroid clearance of plasma RaI determined from uptake of RaI over a 30-minute period and from the simultaneous plasma ^{131}I concentration averages 15 to 30 ml per minute; the product of thyroid RaI clearance and plasma stable iodide concentration yields the absolute iodine uptake, which, under steady-state conditions, is a reasonable approximation of the secretion rate of hormonal iodine. The absolute iodine uptake is normally about 2 μg per hour, with higher values, up to 50 μg per hour, being found in hyperthyroidism. The thyroid uptake of pertechnetate (TcO_4^-), an anion concentrated by the thyroid but not organically bound, has been used as a measure of glandular activity, the isotope uptake being measured 10 to 60 minutes after intravenous administration. Since pertechnetate and iodide compete for the same thyroid transport mechanism, administration of excess iodide, as well as perchlorate, or thiocyanate depresses pertechnetate as well as RaI uptake.

Thyroid scintiscans show the pattern of distribution of RaI in the thyroid and are therefore useful for (1) characterizing the functional activity of nodules as "cold," "warm," or "hot," that is, activity less than, equal to, or greater than the paranodular thyroid tissue; (2) for distinguishing diffuse toxic goiter, with its homogeneous pattern of RaI accumulation, from toxic nodular goiter, in which the pattern shows one or more hyperfunctioning areas; (3) for characterizing and localizing functioning thyroid tissue such as ectopic and sublingual thyroid and distant metastases of functioning thyroid cancer; and (4) for documenting changes in thyroid function (e.g., recovery from subacute thyroiditis) or thyroid size (e.g., after thyroid-suppressive therapy of nontoxic goiter). The isotope most used for thyroid scintigraphy has been ^{131}I, but equivalent resolution is achieved using pertechnetate and the scintillation camera technique.

The advantages of pertechnetate are its speed (imaging is done 20 to 30 minutes after intravenous injection of the isotope) and lower radiation exposure.*

SERUM TSH

Serum TSH as determined by radioimmunoassay normally ranges from undetectable (<0.5 μU/ml) to 5 μU per milliliter. Abnormally high values of TSH are characteristic of primary hypothyroidism, and modest elevations also occur in apparently euthyroid persons who may be in a prehypothyroid state, such as occurs in some cases of Hashimoto's thyroiditis and following RaI therapy of hyperthyroidism. Modest TSH elevations also occur in severe iodine deficiency. Serum TSH in hyperthyroidism is usually below the detection limit. The response of serum TSH to injected TRH is of considerable diagnostic usefulness. After pulse intravenous injection of 250 to 500 μg TRH in normal subjects, TSH rises, with a normal peak increment of 7 to 10 μU per milliliter at 15 to 30 minutes; this response is exaggerated in primary hypothyroidism and is absent in hyperthyroidism. Hypothyroidism secondary to pituitary TSH deficiency shows no response to TRH, while in hypothyroidism secondary to hypothalamic disease there is a response, although sometimes delayed or prolonged. The prolactin responses to TRH parallel those of TSH.

MISCELLANEOUS TESTS

Perchlorate Discharge Test. Sodium perchlorate, 1 gm given perorally 1 hour after tracer RaI, normally prevents further thyroid uptake of isotope; no efflux of RaI already accumulated occurs because iodide entering the thyroid is organically bound almost instantaneously. On the other hand, a prompt discharge of more than 10 percent of accumulated glandular RaI after perchlorate (positive perchlorate test) indicates the presence of appreciable amounts of unbound, diffusible inorganic iodide in the thyroid and hence impairment of organic binding capacity relative

---

*The radioactive isotope ^{123}I is becoming more widely used for thyroid uptake and imaging in preference to ^{131}I. The physical half-life of ^{123}I is much shorter (13 hours compared with 8 days for ^{131}I); it is a pure gamma ray emitter, and radiation dose to the thyroid is considerably less than with use of ^{131}I.

---

to iodide transport capacity. Positive perchlorate tests are seen in patients taking antithyroid drugs, in patients with dyshormonogenetic goiters due to peroxidase deficit, and in some patients with Hashimoto's thyroiditis and with Graves' disease previously treated with radioiodine. An iodide-perchlorate test, in which 500 μg of stable iodide is given with the tracer RaI, has been found to be even more sensitive for detecting the impaired capacity for organic binding in the above conditions.

Conversion Ratio. The fraction of the serum ^{131}I concentration present as protein-bound ^{131}I 48 to 72 hours after a tracer dose is normally 0.1 to 0.4. Higher values indicate a rapid turnover of thyroid organic iodine, such as in hyperthyroidism or in iodine-depleted thyroids.

TSH Stimulation Test. Bovine TSH, 5 to 10 units given intramuscularly for 1 to 3 days, the last injection 18 hours prior to tracer ^{131}I administration, normally increases the thyroid RaI uptake by 7 to 10 percent of the dose. The test distinguishes primary from secondary hypothyroidism; a response occurs only in the latter. Injection of TSH is also useful for demonstrating reversibly suppressed (i.e., unstimulated) thyroid tissue; thus TSH will increase the low thyroid RaI uptake of the euthyroid patient taking thyroid hormones, and scintigrams taken before and after TSH in patients with autonomously functioning nodules may reveal previously suppressed paranodular tissue.

Thyroid Suppression Tests. The function of the normal thyroid, unlike the hyperthyroid gland, is dependent on TSH; administration of a thyroid hormone such as triiodothyronine, 75 μg per day for 5 to 8 days, normally decreases thyroid RaI uptake to 60 percent or less of the control value, while the hyperthyroid gland is not suppressible. Nonsuppressibility, although characteristic of hyperthyroidism, is not specific for this condition; thus, nonsuppressible TSH-independent autonomous nodules may occur in euthyroid individuals and thyroid activity is nonsuppressible also in the majority of patients with euthyroid Graves' disease.

Hyperthyroidism

Hyperthyroidism is five times commoner among
women than men, as are most thyroid disorders. There
is a strong familial tendency, although the inheritance
pattern is not clear. Two major forms are recognized,
Graves' disease (toxic diffuse goiter) and the less
common Plummer's disease (toxic nodular goiter,
sometimes further subdivided into single toxic adenoma
and multinodular goiter with hyperthyroidism). The
manifestations of Plummer's disease are solely a consequence of the hypersecretion of thyroid hormones
by an enlarged thyroid gland functioning autonomously.
By contrast, in Graves' disease not only hyperthyroidism but also a characteristic dermopathy (pretibial
myxedema) and infiltrative ophthalmopathy may be
present, and the pathogenesis of the hyperthyroidism
may be abnormal circulating immunoglobulins with
thyroid-stimulating properties. In addition to
Graves' disease and Plummer's disease, hyperthyroidism
may occur in acromegaly and rarely with TSH-secreting
pituitary tumors; it may be associated with widely
metastatic functioning thyroid carcinoma; it may occur
after ingestion of large amounts of iodide by subjects
with either endemic or sporadic goiter (jodbasedow, or
Jod-Basedow); and it may be a manifestation of
hydatidiform mole and choriocarcinoma due to the
production by these tissues of large amounts of
chorionic gonadotrophin, which has intrinsic thyroid-
stimulating activity. Hyperthyroidism may also occur
as a manifestation of subacute and chronic thyroiditis,
and it may also result from excessive dosage of thyroid
hormones (thyrotoxicosis factitia).

PATHOGENESIS OF GRAVES' DISEASE

Hyperthyroidism

Many observations suggest the importance of immunologic factors in Graves' disease. Thus circulating antibodies to thyroid constituents are frequent and the
histology of the thyroid in Graves' disease often
resembles Hashimoto's (autoimmune) thyroiditis. In
several instances one member of a pair of identical
twins developed Hashimoto's disease and the other
Graves' disease. There is a correlation between Graves'
disease and the HL-A8 histocompatibility antigens
(the genes for which may be linked to immune response
genes). A possible pathogenetic role of antibody in
the hyperthyroidism of Graves' disease was suggested
by studies of the long-acting thyroid stimulator
(LATS). Long-acting thyroid stimulator is a polyclonal
7S IgG immunoglobulin with thyroid-stimulating
properties that are chemically and serologically
distinct from TSH, and it is present in the serum of
some patients with Graves' disease and is detected
by bioassay in mice and guinea pigs. The LATS activity
binds to and is neutralized by human thyroid microsomes. Although LATS has been detected in only
60 percent of Graves' disease patients, recent work
indicates a much higher prevalence of circulating
stimulators that are active on human, but not rodent,
thyroid tissue. Thus in many LATS-negative cases
of Graves' disease, a LATS protector is present in the
IgG fractions that prevents the neutralization of LATS
by human thyroid membranes; and infusions of LATS-
negative plasma containing LATS-protector in human
volunteers has stimulated thyroid glandular activity of
the recipients. Sera with LATS-protector activity have
been shown to stimulate colloid droplet formation and
cyclic AMP formation in human thyroid slices. Thyroid-
stimulating immunoglobulins, species-specific in their
ability to stimulate human but not mouse or guinea
pig thyroid, have been detected in over 90 percent of
patients with Graves' disease; they have been detected
in some patients with Hashimoto's thyroiditis, providing
another example of the similarities between Graves'
and Hashimoto's disease, but they are not reported in
Plummer's disease. The thyroid-stimulating immunoglobulins have been shown by radioreceptor assays to
displace TSH from specific binding sites on human
thyroid membranes. A current theory holds that
these thyroid-stimulating immunoglobulins are autoantibodies to thyroid cell receptors of TSH, and that
such antibodies, by interacting with the TSH receptor
on the plasma membrane of the follicular cell, activate
the thyroid and mimic TSH actions, such as stimulation of colloid droplet and cyclic AMP formation
and of thyroid secretion and hormone synthesis. The
transplacental passage of thyroid-stimulating immunoglobulins from mother to fetus may explain neonatal
hyperthyroidism, a self-limited disease of infants whose
mothers have or have had hyperthyroidism.

Cell-mediated immunity may also play a role in
Graves' disease. Lymphocytes of Graves' disease

patients, on exposure to thyroid antigen, inhibit leukocyte migration; such sensitized cells could infiltrate and possibly lead to stimulation or injury to the thyroid. Some hold the view that a heritable defect in immune surveillance (a T-lymphocyte function) with respect to forbidden clones of B-immunocytes is the prime disorder, permitting development of cells capable of synthesizing antibodies directed against thyroid antigens, including the TSH receptor.

Infiltrative Ophthalmopathy

The orbital pathology in Graves' disease includes edema and fatty infiltration of the ocular muscles and connective tissue, deposition of mucopolysaccharides, and lymphocytic infiltration. Circulating exophthalmos-producing substances bioassayed in fish have been detected in some cases, as well as substances that enhance radiosulfate uptake of mouse orbital tissues. Recent studies have emphasized the possible role of pituitary and of immunologic factors in the pathogenesis of ophthalmopathy. Thus a role of the pituitary is suggested by reports that TSH is exophthalmogenic. Pepsin treatment of TSH results in deletion of part of the alpha-chain, the altered molecule lacking thyrotropic activity but retaining exophthalmogenic activity and also retaining the capacity to bind to specific orbital receptors, such binding being potentiated by IgG present in serum of patients with Graves' disease.

Another hypothesis to explain infiltrative opthalmopathy holds that thyroglobulin may reach the orbit through a lymphatic pathway believed to connect the thyroid gland with the orbit, permitting the formation of soluble complexes of thyroglobulin with the antithyroglobulin antibodies present in most patients with Graves' disease. Such complexes may bind to orbital tissue and induce an inflammatory reaction, leading to edema, cellular infiltration, and stimulation of mast cell mucopolysaccharide synthesis. Whatever the pathogenesis may be, the edema of orbital contents and the inflammatory reaction may lead to exophthalmos, muscle weakness, diplopia, obstruction of orbital venous return, and serious disturbances of vision. Recent studies of the orbits using B-mode ultrasound, radionuclide, and computerized tomographic scanning techniques have led to better characterization of the orbital abnormalities in Graves' disease and permit improved discrimination between endocrine and non-endocrine exophthalmos.

CLINICAL MANIFESTATIONS

The signs and symptoms of hyperthyroidism include both those referable to hypermetabolism and others more specifically related to excessive thyroid hormone secretion. Symptoms include nervousness, tremulousness, irritability, heat intolerance, loss of weight and strength despite increased appetite and food consumption, polyuria and thirst, palpitation, exertional dyspnea, diarrhea, decreased libido, and menstrual instability generally in the direction of oligomenorrhia or amenorrhea, often with anovulation. In Graves' disease the ocular symptoms include photophobia, lacrimation, pain, and diplopia. Signs of hyperthyroidism include hyperkinetic behavior; moist, flushed, warm skin; fine tremor of hands, tongue, and body; goiter (often with bruit and thrill attesting to the vascularity of the enlarged thyroid); hyperdynamic circulatory signs such as tachycardia, forceful apical impulse, and widened pulse pressure; and arrhythmias such as atrial fibrillation and premature beats. Ocular signs, when present, vary from lid retraction signs, such as widening of the palpebral fissures, stare, and lid lag (these are classified as non-infiltrative ophthalmopathy, may occur in non-Graves' as well as Graves' hyperthyroidism, and are a result of excessive thyroid hormone secretion; they regress after treatment of the hyperthyroidism), to the more serious infiltrative ophthalmopathy, which includes edema of the lids, chemosis, exophthalmos, ophthalmoplegia, and papilledema. The infiltrative oculopathy, unlike the noninfiltrative variety, is not the consequence of hyperthyroidism and may precede, accompany, or follow the hyperthyroid stage of Graves' disease. It may be unilateral. Infiltrative ophthalmopathy is almost always present in patients showing dermopathy or pretibial myxedema. Pretibial myxedema typically occurs as large, indurated, non-pitting, confluent plaques that are often purplish and mainly are found on the extensor surfaces of the legs. The histologic picture is not distinguishable from myxedema.

Muscular weakness may occasionally be so severe

as to dominate the clinical presentation (thyrotoxic myopathy) and mimic primary neurologic disorders. There is profound atrophy and weakness, particularly of the proximal musculature of the pelvic and shoulder girdles; but the condition is completely reversible following treatment of the hyperthyroidism. Differentiation from myasthenia gravis (see Chap. 62) and hypokalemic paralysis, both of which may be associated with hyperthyroidism, is accomplished by the Tensilon test and serum electrolyte concentrations. The tremor of hyperthyroidism has been explained on the basis of accelerated rates of both tension development and of relaxation, which produces a briefer duration of the contractile period of skeletal muscle fibers.

Cardiac changes in hyperthyroidism include increased cardiac output (which is relatively greater than the increment in metabolic rate so that the arteriovenous oxygen difference is decreased), tachycardia, and increased contractility and oxygen consumption of myocardium. The enhanced contractility and rate are at least in part due to a direct cardiac action of thyroid hormones. Many of the features of hyperthyroidism, such as tremor, tachycardia, restlessness, and palpitation, resemble catecholamine excess. Although adrenergic blocking agents considerably ameliorate the hyperdynamic cardiovascular manifestations of hyperthyroidism (suggesting an adrenergic component in their pathogenesis), no abnormality of catecholamine production or metabolism has been documented, and the claim that the cardiovascular features of hyperthyroidism are mediated solely by catecholamines is unfounded. In so-called thyrocardiac cases, especially among older patients, cardiovascular manifestations predominate, and angina pectoris, congestive heart failure, and tachyarrhythmias (but, curiously, not myocardial infarction) are prominent.

DIAGNOSIS
Laboratory tests in hyperthyroidism show an abnormally high serum T_4, T_3, RT_3U, thyroid RaI uptake, FTI, and FT_4 concentration. The thyroid RaI uptake is nonsuppressible, and TRH injection produces no rise in serum TSH. Serum cholesterol is often low; serum calcium, phosphorus, and alkaline phosphatase may be high.

T_3 thyrotoxicosis. Serum T_3 is regularly increased in all forms of hyperthyroidism proportionately more than T_4, so the T_4/T_3 serum concentration ratio is less than normal. In a small group of hyperthyroid cases encompassing both diffuse and nodular toxic goiter, serum T_4 is normal (RT_3U, thyroid RaI uptake, and FT_4 may also be normal), but T_3 is high, and such cases are designated T_3 thyrotoxicosis. Thyroid glandular activity is not suppressed by exogenous hormone. Both hyperthyroidism early in its development and recurrent hyperthyroidism may show the increment in serum T_3 concentration before T_4 rises to abnormal values.

Euthyroid Graves' disease refers to cases in which infiltrative ophthalmopathy occurs without hyperthyroidism, which may appear later or never develop at all. The diagnosis is established by demonstrating nonsuppressibility of the thyroid (in three-fourths of cases), by nonresponse to TRH, by the presence of some of the immunologic abnormalities of Graves' disease, by ultrasound and computed tomographic X-ray scans of the orbit, and by eliminating other causes for the ocular signs.

TREATMENT
There are three general methods for treating hyperthyroidism: antithyroid drugs, surgery, and radioiodine therapy.

Antithyroid Drugs
The thiocarbonamide drugs 6n-propylthiouracil and methimazole inhibit thyroid organic binding of iodine and the synthesis of T_4 and T_3. Initial doses are 100 to 150 mg of propylthiouracil or 10 to 20 mg of methimazole every 8 hours, with lowering to maintenance dosage of approximately 50 mg propylthiouracil or 5 mg methimazole every 8 hours after 4 to 8 weeks, when the patient is euthyroid. Drug therapy for a 12- to 18-month period may be followed by a prolonged remission in 20 to 50 percent of patients with Graves' disease. Factors favoring prolonged remission after antithyroid drug therapy of Graves' disease are short duration of the hyperthyroidism, decrease of thyroid size during therapy, and return of normal thyroid suppressibility by exogenous thyroid hormones; low dietary iodine intake may also favor sustained remission. Sustained

remissions in Plummer's disease are unlikely. The most serious toxicity of these antithyroid drugs, fortunately rare (0.2 percent incidence), is agranulocytosis; fever, rash, and arthralgias are additional side effects with an incidence of about 3 percent. Perchlorate and thiocyanate, 1 to 2 gm daily, can control hyperthyroidism by their action on inhibiting glandular iodide transport and in effect creating thyroid iodine depletion; these agents are less well tolerated than the thiocarbonamide drugs, their effectiveness is compromised if dietary or other sources of iodide are excessive, and they are unsuitable for the preparation of patients for surgery, since pharmacologic doses of iodide are customarily given preoperatively to such patients to diminish the vascularity and friability of the gland.

Beta-adrenergic blockade by propranolol (10 to 40 mg four times per day) is often a helpful temporary adjunct to more specific antithyroid drug therapy until euthyroidism is achieved.

Surgical Therapy
The patient should be euthyroid at the time of operation, and this usually requires 4 to 6 weeks of therapy with an antithyroid drug (propylthiouracil or methimazole). During the last 2 weeks before surgery, iodide in the form of 5 drops of saturated solution of KI is coadministered three times per day. Surgical thyroidectomy for Graves' disease is rarely necessary. Possible complications of subtotal thyroidectomy include hypoparathyroidism, vocal cord palsy, hypothyroidism, and recurrence of hyperthyroidism. While surgical therapy is effective in Plummer's disease and eliminates the thyroid enlargement more completely than RaI therapy, it appears to have no substantial advantage over RaI therapy.

RaI Therapy
This is effective, simple therapy for Graves' disease. Usually a single 3- to 5-mCi dose of ^{131}I is sufficient to restore the euthyroid state in 8 to 12 weeks. The major complication of RaI therapy is hypothyroidism, which may occur within a few weeks or may occur insidiously years after the treatment; the incidence of hypothyroidism is at least 25 percent. Radioactive iodine therapy is probably the treatment of choice in patients over 40 and is often used in patients 20 to 40 years old, especially those with recurrent hyperthyroidism. It is contraindicated in pregnancy because of the potential radiation damage to the fetal thyroid and other tissues, and it should be used with cautious discrimination in juvenile hyperthyroidism. In toxic multinodular goiter much larger doses of RaI are required (20 to 40 mCi), and the risk of hypothyroidism is less. Propranolol is often prescribed for several weeks in conjunction with RaI therapy to provide symptomatic relief until the radiotherapeutic effect is achieved and also to minimize the very rare occurrence of thyroid storm following RaI therapy. The therapeutic usefulness of the ^{125}I isotope, which emits no beta radiation, is a much weaker gamma emitter, and thus is theoretically less likely to induce hypothyroidism, has not yet been established.

Treatment of Ophthalmopathy
Noninfiltrative eye changes usually respond to correction of the hyperthyroidism. Infiltrative ophthalmopathy may respond to high doses of corticosteroids (80 to 120 mg prednisone per day), especially when inflammatory changes are prominent and the disease is active and progressive. When steroids are ineffective, surgical decompression of the orbit through a temporal or maxillary approach may be necessary to save vision or ocular integrity. X-ray therapy directed at the orbits may be helpful in cases of progressive oculopathy, and some authorities have found radioablation (using ^{131}I) of all remaining thyroid tissue helpful in controlling progressive cases (malignant exophthalmos).

Thyroid Storm
This is a life-threatening exacerbation of untreated or poorly controlled hyperthyroidism characterized by fever, extreme tachycardia, and alarming deterioration of function of various body systems, especially the cardiovascular, central nervous, and gastrointestinal systems. There is usually a precipitating factor such as a surgical procedure, trauma, infection, pulmonary embolism, metabolic disturbance, or gastrointestinal bleeding. The mortality is high if the condition is untreated. Therapy includes the following measures:

1. An antithyroid drug — Propylthiouracil, 200 mg,

or methimazole, 20 mg – is given every 6 hours, by stomach tube if necessary. Propylthiouracil has some theoretical advantages over methimazole; although both block thyroid hormone synthesis, only propylthiouracil inhibits the peripheral conversion of T_4 to T_3.

2. Iodide is given, at least 10 mg daily, to decrease acutely the secretion of thyroid hormones.
3. Antiadrenergic therapy is instituted. Choices include propranolol, 20 to 60 mg every 4 hours by mouth; reserpine, 1 to 3 mg intramuscularly every 8 hours; or guanethidine, 80 to 120 mg per day orally.
4. Appropriate treatment of coexisting disorders that may have triggered the storm is provided.
5. Antipyretic measures are taken, such as application of cooling blankets and iced sheets, but salicylates are not given, since they may displace thyroid hormones from their plasma binding protein.
6. Intravenous corticosteroids equivalent to 300 mg cortisol daily are given for hyperthermia and possible relative adrenal insufficiency.
7. In desperately ill comatose patients, exchange transfusion and plasmapheresis have achieved rapid depletion of the extrathyroidal thyroid hormone pool.

Hypothyroidism

Hypothyroidism may be either primary (i.e., due to disease of the thyroid or to conditions that interfere with its function), or secondary (due to defective TSH secretion). A further rare cause is tissue unresponsiveness to thyroid hormones. Primary hypothyroidism may be classified as either nongoitrous or goitrous.

NONGOITROUS PRIMARY HYPOTHYROIDISM

Nongoitrous hypothyroidism may occur either spontaneously (idiopathic) or as a complication of RaI or surgical therapy of hyperthyroidism. Idiopathic hypothyroidism is a variant of Hashimoto's thyroiditis in which goiter has not appeared but in which the presumed autoimmune inflammatory process has resulted in a fibrotic, scarred gland lacking sufficient thyroid parenchyma to sustain normal thyroid secretion. Hypothyroidism following RaI therapy or thyroidectomy may occur weeks or many years after the

therapy. There is evidence that some hyperthyroid patients with Graves' disease, although never treated with ablative therapies, may develop hypothyroidism spontaneously.

GOITROUS PRIMARY HYPOTHYROIDISM

Goitrous hypothyroidism has three major causes: (1) excessive dosage of goitrogenic drugs, (2) dyshormonogenetic thyroid disorders, and (3) chronic thyroiditis.

Overdose of Goitrogenic Drugs

Drugs that interfere with thyroid hormone synthesis provoke an enhanced TSH secretion, and the resulting increase in thyroid size and function may sustain the euthyroid state; the goiter then represents an adaptive compensatory mechanism. If such compensation is inadequate, the goiter persists or increases, but hypothyroidism develops. Drugs that may cause goiter and hypothyroidism include the antithyroid drugs propylthiouracil and methimazole, perchlorate, and thiocyanate; iodides in pharmacologic doses (such as used in the treatment of bronchitis); lithium salts, as used in manic depressive disorders; resorcinol ointments applied to denuded skin; and aminoglutethimide, formerly used in treatment of epilepsy. In addition, certain plants (cabbage, rutabaga, turnip) contain thioglycoside precursors of goitrogens; thioglycosidases, enzymes which are present in uncooked plants as well as in the digestive tract of animals, can generate an active goitrogen (e.g., 5-vinyl, 2-thiooxazolidone, or goitrin), and ingestion of large amounts of the foodstuff may cause goiter and possibly hypothyroidism.

The antithyroid drugs propylthiouracil and methimazole used in treating hyperthyroidism do not produce goiter unless the dosage is excessive. Reduction of the dosage or coadministration of thyroid hormones results in lowering of the circulating TSH and regression of goiter. Awareness of the goitrogenic potential of antithyroid drugs is of particular importance in the treatment of hyperthyroidism in pregnancy; propylthiouracil and methimazole freely traverse the placenta, and excessive maternal doses may cause fetal goiter and hypothyroidism. Since transplacental passage of thyroid hormones is negligible, fetal goiter cannot be prevented by maternal administration of thyroid hormones. Prevention of fetal goiter therefore requires limiting the antithyroid drug dosage to the minimum required for control of the maternal hyperthyroidism.

The mechanism by which hypothyroidism and goiter are caused by pharmacologic amounts of iodide is not clear; both persistent impairment of hormone synthesis and prolonged inhibition of hormone release may result from excess iodide. Patients with chronic thyroiditis and persons previously treated with RaI for hyperthyroidism seem exceptionally sensitive to iodide-induced hypothyroidism, and fetal goiter may also result from maternal ingestion of excess iodide (100 to 200 mg daily). The goitrogenic effects of lithium seem to be due to its iodidelike effect of inhibiting thyroid hormone secretion as well as to some alteration in thyroxine metabolism; resorcinol and aminoglutethimide are weak inhibitors of thyroid organic binding and hence of hormone synthesis.

Dyshormonogenetic Goiter
Congenital defects have been described in the thyroid capacity to (1) concentrate iodide; (2) organically bind iodine; and (3) dehalogenate iodotyrosines. These defects are rare, familial, and inherited as autosomal recessive traits, and they may result in goiter and, in extreme cases, in hypothyroidism. The goiter and the hypothyroidism respond to thyroid hormone replacement therapy. The nature of the defect in (1) is unknown; in (2) and (3) the gland is deficient in peroxidase and iodotyrosine dehalogenase, respectively.

Patients whose thyroid glands cannot trap iodide are also unable to maintain iodide concentration gradients in salivary and gastric secretions. Such patients may therefore be recognized by finding that the salivary-plasma radioiodide ratio is close to unity after administration of tracer [131]I. The goiter and hypothyroidism have been shown to respond not only to replacement dosages of thyroid hormones but also to increasing the intake of dietary iodide (to 5 to 10 mg per day), which permits sufficient iodide to enter the gland to sustain normal thyroid hormone secretion. The combination of familial thyroid peroxidase deficiency and nerve deafness is called the Pendred syndrome. Patients with glandular peroxidase deficiency show an abnormal perchlorate test. Subjects with thyroid dehalogenase deficiency also lack this enzyme in other tissues, especially liver and kidney; such patients are unable to deiodinate injected monoiodotyrosine labeled with ^{131}I, and chromatograms of their urine show the unchanged labeled iodotyrosine as the major excretion product rather than inorganic ^{131}I-labeled iodide, as occurs in normal subjects. A variety of dyshormonogenetic goiters have been described, characterized by defective synthesis of thyroglobulin and glandular secretion of abnormal iodoproteins. Patients with these goiters comprise a heterogeneous group and are recognized by the presence of labeled iodoalbuminlike proteins on serum electrophoresis after ^{131}I administration; analysis of their thyroid biopsies reveals little thyroglobulin.

Chronic Thyroiditis
Chronic thyroiditis of the Hashimoto type is one of the most common causes of goiter with hypothyroidism. This is discussed later in this chapter, under Thyroiditis.

SECONDARY HYPOTHYROIDISM
Defective TSH secretion that is inadequate to sustain normal thyroid secretory function may result from either anterior pituitary or hypothalamic disorders (see Chap. 55). Thus hypothyroidism may result from pituitary tumors, granulomas, and metastatic lesions, as well as from postpartum ischemic necrosis of the anterior pituitary, surgical hypophysectomy (as in palliative therapy of breast cancer), irradiation of the pituitary, or pituitary stalk section. In most cases the TSH deficiency and hypothyroidism are part of a broad spectrum of panhypopituitarism with clinical evidence of either deficiency or impaired reserve secretory capacity of one or more of the hormones, including melanocyte-stimulating hormone, gonadotropins, growth hormone, corticotropin, as well as TSH. A type of TSH deficiency that results from failure of hypothalamic stimulation of presumably normal pituitary thyrotropic cells has been characterized and termed *hypothalamic* or *tertiary hypothyroidism;* the TSH deficiency results from

defective hypothalamic synthesis or delivery of TRH to the thyrotropic cells.

TISSUE UNRESPONSIVENESS TO THYROID HORMONES
A few cases have been described of familial congenital hypothyroidism characterized by stippled epiphyses, goiter, abnormally high circulating T_4, increased thyroid RaI uptake, and normal or slightly increased TSH values. Administered thyroid hormones produce neither a normal calorigenic response nor normal suppression of thyroid RaI uptake, making it likely that tissue unresponsiveness to the action of thyroid hormones underlies the disorder. The mechanism may be deficient nuclear receptors for iodothyronines. A variant of this disorder, in which the anterior pituitary alone appears unresponsive to thyroid hormones, has been described and is characterized by *hyper*thyroidism due to feedback failure — that is, inappropriate secretion of TSH results from the failure of elevated thyroid hormone levels to normally inhibit pituitary TSH release.

CLINICAL MANIFESTATIONS OF HYPOTHYROIDISM
The symptoms and signs of hypothyroidism are largely secondary to the hypometabolism, impaired growth, and decreased protein synthesis consequent to thyroid hormone deficiency. The mucinous, hydrophilic extracellular deposits present in skin, heart, and skeletal muscle give rise to the term *myxedema.* Characteristic symptoms include lethargy, cold intolerance, impaired hearing, constipation, muscle cramps, menstrual disturbances, and paresthesias. Physical findings include dry, cool skin; pallor, often with malar flush, giving a "strawberries and cream" appearance; hypothermia; puffiness of face and extremities (nonpitting edema); thinning of scalp, eyebrow, and body hair; large tongue; husky, croaking voice; hypertension; bradycardia; cardiomegaly (largely due to pericardial effusion without tamponade); abdominal distention; and prolongation of the contraction and especially the relaxation phases of the deep tendon reflexes, particularly the biceps and ankle jerks.

The functions of many organ systems are altered in hypothyroidism. Pituitary secretion of growth hormone, gonadotrophins, and corticotropin is diminished, and anovulation is the rule; cortisol secretion is subnormal (though appropriate for the depressed cortisol degradation rate), while plasma cortisol is normal. Anemia (microcytic, normocytic, or macrocytic) is common. Alveolar hypoventilation and a tendency to carbon dioxide retention may be present. Cardiac output is subnormal, although probably not disproportionate to the decreased metabolic requirements, and cerebral blood flow is reduced. The glomerular filtration rate is diminished, blood urea nitrogen and uric acid may rise, and there is impairment of urinary dilution (sometimes related to inappropriate secretion of vasopressin). Metabolism and excretion of many drugs is slowed, and unless smaller than average dosages of digoxin, opiates, and sedatives are prescribed, toxicity may result. Atherogenesis is accelerated, and myocardial contractility and electrocardiographic voltage are reduced. Variable degrees of malabsorption occur, and glucose tolerance test curves may be flat. The sella turcica may become enlarged in primary as well as secondary hypothyroidism.

Syndromes of amenorrhea with galactorrhea and of precocious puberty secondary to hypothyroidism have been described. When hypothyroidism begins prenatally or at birth (sporadic cretinism), defects in myelin formation and cerebral maturation occur, with impaired intellectual function that may be irreversible if treatment is delayed. Epiphyseal dysgenesis, short stature, umbilical hernia, and retarded skeletal maturation are characteristic findings in hypothyroid children; these changes emphatically underscore the important role of thyroid hormones in normal growth and development.

DIAGNOSIS
The serum T_4, RT_3U, and thyroid RaI uptake are usually subnormal in hypothyroidism, although in some cases of goitrous hypothyroidism, normal or even high thyroid RaI uptakes are seen. Circulating autoantibodies to thyroid constituents, including thyroglobulin, microsomal antigens, and colloid and cytoplasmic antigens, are detectable in 50 to 80 percent of patients with primary idiopathic hypothyroidism, attesting to the close relationship of hypothyroidism to autoimmune thyroiditis; but these autoantibodies are absent in secondary and tertiary

hypothyroidism. Assays of plasma TSH and of the TSH response to injected TRH are valuable in distinguishing primary from secondary hypothyroidism; in the former, TSH is high and the response to TRH is exaggerated; in the latter, TSH is low and the response to TRH is blunted or absent. Tertiary hypothyroidism shows a low serum TSH, but there is a response to TRH. Administration of bovine TSH enhances thyroid RaI uptake and serum T_4 and T_3 in secondary and tertiary but not in primary hypothyroidism.

TREATMENT

Replacement therapy with thyroxine, the major thyroid secretion product, most closely approximates physiologic thyroid hormone secretion, and T_4 is currently considered the agent of choice for treating hypothyroidism. Especially with older patients, in whom cardiac arrhythmias or angina might be provoked by too rapid an increase in metabolic rate, therapy is started at a low dosage, 0.05 mg T_4 once daily, with increments at weekly intervals until the average daily maintenance dosage of 0.15 to 0.30 (average, 0.20) mg, taken once daily, is achieved. Other preparations that are used include thyroid USP (desiccated thyroid), triiodothyronine, and commercially available mixtures of T_4 and T_3 in a 4:1 ratio. Thyroid USP is effective, although the possibly variable T_4/T_3 ratio in this product of natural origin is a conceivable drawback. There appears to be little to recommend the use of triiodothyronine or the proprietary T_4-T_3 mixtures in 4:1 ratio (liotrix) in the therapy of hypothyroidism; maintenance dosages of these agents produce undesirably and unnecessarily high serum T_3 concentrations. Approximate equivalent dosages of these various thyroid preparations are l-T_4, 0.1 mg; thyroid (USP), 60 mg; l-T_3, 25 μg; and liotrix, 50 to 60 μg T_4 plus 12.5 to 15 μg T_3. The adequacy of replacement therapy is judged on clinical grounds (regression of symptoms and signs of hypothyroidism) and, when l-T_4 is used in the treatment of primary hypothyroidism, restoration of serum T_4 and T_3, as well as TSH to normal.

In secondary hypothyroidism there is often a coexisting cortisol deficiency. Therefore, since cortisol degradation is enhanced by thyroid hormone administration, therapy with a physiologic replacement dosage of cortisol should precede institution of thyroid replacement therapy in order to avoid provoking adrenocortical insufficiency.

Myxedema coma is the end stage of severe hypothyroidism. It is characterized by stupor; hypothermia; exaggeration of the signs of hypothyroidism; and impaired cardiac, central nervous system, pulmonary, and renal function. Myxedema coma may be precipitated by stresses, exposure to low environmental temperature, coexisting diseases (such as gastrointestinal bleeding, myocardial infarction, stroke, infection), or overdosage of drugs, especially sedatives. The mortality is high, and therapy must be promptly instituted. Treatment includes (1) intravenous l-T_4, given as a pulse initial intravenous injection of 300 to 600 μg to quickly replenish the extrathyroidal thyroxine pool and followed by a daily parenteral maintenance dosage of 50 to 75 μg (although T_3 in this situation has its advocates, its use carries a considerable risk of cardiac arrhythmias); (2) corticosteroids in amounts equivalent to 150 to 250 mg cortisol daily; and (3) treatment of associated diseases and correction of physiologic derangements such as hyponatremia, carbon dioxide retention, hypovolemia, infections, hypoglycemia, or hypotension.

Nontoxic Goiter

Thyroid enlargement in euthyroid individuals is present in 4 to 5 percent of the population, even in areas where goiter is not endemic, and is by far the commonest thyroid disorder. Nontoxic goiter is generally classified as diffuse or nodular, and the latter group is subdivided into multinodular or solitary nodules. Single nodules often turn out to be a predominant nodule in a multinodular goiter. In some patients the goiter may be apparently compensating for some defect in thyroid hormone synthesis or secretion and be TSH dependent, although serum TSH is seldom abnormally high. Usually there are no symptoms; rarely, a large benign goiter may produce stridor from tracheal compression or a substernal goiter may cause the superior vena caval syndrome. Dysphagia and hoarseness with vocal cord paralysis secondary to recurrent laryngeal nerve involvement is almost never seen with a benign goiter.

Since nodular goiter may be the result of a variety of causes, including inflammatory, degenerative, fibrotic, calcific, cystic and adenomatous as well as malignant lesions, the major clinical issue in evaluating a case of nodular goiter is to determine whether it represents a benign or a malignant disorder. To make this assessment, reliance is placed on analysis of risk factors, the clinical characteristics of the goiter, and some laboratory procedures.

RISK FACTORS

Ionizing Radiation. The major risk factor to be considered is exposure of the head and neck to ionizing radiation (x-ray or radium therapy) in early life. Such exposure enhances the frequency of thyroid cancer in adult life manyfold. Study of such irradiated individuals 20 to 30 years after exposure has indicated a high incidence of thyroid nodules and a tenfold greater incidence of thyroid cancer than in control populations. It is claimed that 7 percent of persons irradiated in the first decade of life ultimately have histologic thyroid cancer. Radioiodine therapy of hyperthyroidism in children and adults has not been shown to be associated with thyroid carcinogenesis.

Family History. Thyroid cancer, like other thyroid disorders, tends to be familial. This is particularly true of the medullary carcinoma, which shows an autosomal dominant inheritance pattern.

Age and Sex. Analysis of the proportion of malignancies among nodular goiters in various age groups shows the highest ratios to be in childhood and among the elderly. Similarly, although thyroid disease is five times more common among females than in males, the female-male ratio for thyroid cancer is 2:1. Hence, a male, a child, or an elderly person with a thyroid nodule is statistically at higher risk of harboring a malignant lesion.

CLINICAL CHARACTERISTICS OF THE GOITER
Such features as the size, growth rate, consistency, and regularity of the goiter, as well as the presence of tenderness, fixation to surrounding structures, and presence of supraclavicular and cervical lymph nodes must be assessed. A rapidly enlarging, hard, irregular, nontender thyroid mass adhering to neighboring structures is suggestive of a malignant process.

LABORATORY PROCEDURES
A careful assessment of the clinical characteristics and risk factors permits a fairly reliable assignment of the goiter patient to either a high-risk or a low-risk group with respect to a malignant lesion. Laboratory procedures may then be very helpful in further characterizing the goiter. Thyroid scintiscans using RaI or pertechnetate permit nodules to be classified as hot, cold, or warm, reflecting their function relative to extranodular thyroid tissue. Although cold nodules are much likelier to be malignant than hot or warm nodules, even cold nodules are mostly benign. Ultrasound study (A- and B-mode scans) of the thyroid permits distinction between cystic (anechoic) and solid (echogenic) structures, cysts almost always being benign. Soft tissue x-ray study may reveal thyroid calcification; gross or annular patterns suggest a benign lesion (except in medullary carcinoma), while tiny, faint calcifications are typical of the psamomma bodies in a papillary tumor. A high titer of circulating antithyroid antibodies may suggest chronic thyroiditis as the explanation of a nodular goiter, while high circulating calcitonin suggests a medullary thyroid carcinoma (see below). Needle biopsies of thyroid nodules can be performed with little morbidity under local anesthesia and provide histologic diagnosis; increasing experience has lessened earlier concerns that the procedure might disseminate tumors and that the needle biopsy specimen might not prove representative of the thyroid pathology.

TREATMENT
If the clinical and laboratory assessment suggests the goiter is benign, replacement dosage thyroid hormone is prescribed to suppress TSH secretion. A decrease in the size of the goiter or at least prevention of further enlargement is achieved in a substantial proportion of such cases. If the evaluation has suggested a malignant lesion, or if on thyroid suppression a nodular goiter previously considered benign shows progressive enlargement, appropriate surgical therapy is indicated, followed by life-long thyroid suppression therapy.

Thyroid Cancer

Thyroid cancer is relatively infrequent (0.5 percent of all clinical cancer); 25 new cases occur per million population per year. The most widely used classification divides thyroid cancer into differentiated, medullary, and anaplastic varieties, which comprise 80, 5, and 15 percent, respectively, of the cases. Differentiated cancer includes papillary and follicular tumors, the former being three times as common as the latter but, in many tumors, elements of both may be found. Although the morphologic differences are striking, papillary and follicular carcinomas are generally similar in their biologic behavior.

Papillary carcinoma occurs in all age groups but is characteristically a tumor of children and young adults, with peak incidence being in the 20 to 30 age group. The prognosis is considerably better when the disease occurs before the age of 40; in patients under 40, survival statistics in treated subjects do not differ appreciably from those in appropriate nontumor control groups. The tumor may be confined to the neck for many years and tends to follow an indolent course. Distant metastases are mainly to lung and bone. The tumors are TSH dependent, and both neck masses and distant metastases may regress in response to a thyroid suppressive regimen. The tumors tend to be multicentric with microscopic foci in both lobes; nevertheless, recurrence in the contralateral lobe after surgical lobectomy is rare.

Surgical therapy for papillary tumors should be a thyroid lobectomy with removal of all nodes visibly involved by tumor, with subtotal lobectomy on the contralateral side. Total thyroidectomy and radical neck dissection carry a much higher morbidity, especially with regard to hypoparathyroidism and vocal cord paralysis, and they have not been shown to provide a higher cure rate. Following surgery a life-long thyroid suppressive regimen should be instituted. The adequacy of the suppressive therapy can be gauged by use of TRH; there should be no rise in serum TSH following TRH injection. The RaI uptake of papillary tumors is very limited, but it may be increased by administration of exogenous TSH or, more commonly, by radio therapeutic ablation of the thyroid (40 to 50 mCi ^{131}I) to produce hypothyroidism and enhanced endogenous TSH secretion.

Although such stimulation of the RaI uptake of metastatic lesions undoubtedly improves their response to therapeutic doses of ^{131}I (100 to 200 mCi), it sometimes has been associated with conversion of a differentiated, relatively indolent, slow-growing tumor to a much more invasive and anaplastic one. For this reason (and because ^{131}I in doses of 100 to 200 mCi may cause pulmonary fibrosis and gonadal change), RaI therapy of metastatic differentiated tumors should probably be reserved for cases in which progression occurs despite an adequate thyroid suppressive regimen.

Follicular cancer is most prevalent in an older age group (50 to 60) and tends to be somewhat more angioinvasive than the predominantly papillary tumors; well-differentiated follicular carcinoma also may accumulate RaI more avidly, facilitating radioiodine therapy of distant metastases. The same general principles of therapy apply as for papillary tumors, that is, resection followed by thyroid suppression, with ^{131}I therapy for treatment of aggressive distant metastases.

Medullary carcinoma arises from the parafollicular or C cells of the thyroid, which synthesize and secrete calcitonin. The unique morphologic feature of this tumor is the presence of amyloid in the stroma. Its biologic behavior is more aggressive than the differentiated cancers. The tumor tends to occur in the upper and middle thirds of the thyroid lobe and is often bilateral. In addition to thyroid enlargement, clinical manifestations include diarrhea and the carcinoid syndrome, attributed to production of prostaglandin and serotonin, respectively, by the tumor, and Cushing's syndrome secondary to the tumor's ectopic ACTH production. About 30 percent of the cases are familial and are inherited as an autosomal dominant trait. Familial cases are often associated with pheochromocytoma of the adrenal medulla (frequently bilateral) and sometimes with parathyroid adenoma or hyperplasia, the constellation being designated multiple endocrine adenomatosis, type 2a. Multiple mucosal neuromas and an appearance similar to that in the Marfan syndrome are sometimes associated findings.

The diagnosis of medullary thyroid carcinoma is confirmed by finding a high serum calcitonin concentration ($>$ 1 ng per milliliter). By using calcitonin tests, it has been possible to diagnose and treat the disease in asymptomatic family members of affected patients. Since many medullary thyroid carcinomas produce high serum histaminase levels, there may be no flare on intradermal test injection of histamine. Therapy is total thyroidectomy; thyroid replacement therapy is necessary because of the induced hypothyroidism. The tumors are neither TSH dependent, nor do they accumulate radioiodine. The prognosis, while variable, is distinctly poorer than that of differentiated tumors; the 10-year survival is approximately 40 percent in patients with positive lymph nodes.

Anaplastic carcinoma is a highly malignant tumor, with its peak incidence in the older age groups (50 to 70). The tumor grows rapidly, is independent of TSH, is very invasive locally, and may metastasize distantly as well. The tumor is nearly always inoperable; hence surgical therapy may be only palliative, for example, freeing of the airway. This type of carcinoma is highly lethal; almost all patients die within 3 years. External radiation therapy is sometimes helpful, and some beneficial effects with adriamycin have been reported.

Thyroiditis

The two major inflammatory disorders of the thyroid are subacute thyroiditis (also called granulomatous, giant cell, viral, and de Quervain thyroiditis) and chronic lymphocytic thyroiditis (also called lymphadenoid goiter, autoimmune thyroiditis, and Hashimoto's disease).

SUBACUTE THYROIDITIS

Subacute thyroiditis is believed to be due to a viral infection; Coxsackie, mumps, and echovirus have been implicated on the basis of serologic studies rather than viral isolation. The onset is often preceded by an upper respiratory infection and may be either insidious or fairly acute. Symptoms include local pain, swelling, and tenderness of one or both thyroid lobes; the pain typically radiates to the ear. Hoarseness and sore throat may be present. Fever (generally in the range of 99 to 101°F, or 37.2-38.5°C), malaise, and fatigue may be present, as well as signs of hyperthyroidism such as tachycardia, sweating, weight loss, and weakness. The hyper-

thyroid state is transient and results from extrusion of hormonally active substances from the inflamed gland. The thyroid is enlarged, very tender, and often indurated; the hard, wooden consistency may suggest malignancy, but there is no fixation to surrounding tissue and the tenderness would be very unusual for thyroid cancer. Laboratory findings include a low thyroid RaI uptake, though it may be normal in less severe cases, and elevated serum T_4, T_3RU, and erythrocyte sedimentation rate; leucocytosis is unusual. When thyroiditis affects only a part of the gland, the RaI scan shows the enlarged, involved portion as a cold nodule. Thyroid antibodies are not detectable in the blood or appear only transiently and in low titer. A tissue diagnosis is seldom necessary, but it can readily be made by needle biopsy of the thyroid, which shows disrupted acinar structure, polymorphonuclear leukocytic infiltration, and a granulomatous reaction containing multinucleated giant cells.

Subacute thyroiditis is self-limited, with recovery usually in 4 to 8 weeks; some cases follow a more protracted course with one or more relapses, and some are active for 6 to 24 months. Eventually the inflammatory process subsides, and there are no permanent sequelae with respect to thyroid structure or function. A transient hypothyroid phase (seldom longer than 2 weeks) may sometimes intervene before full recovery. In severe cases, treatment with corticosteroids provides dramatically prompt relief of fever, local pain, tenderness, and swelling and ameliorates the hyperthyroid symptoms. A regimen of prednisone, 40 mg daily, is prescribed for 1 to 3 weeks with a fairly rapid reduction of dosage to the level required to provide symptomatic relief. When the disease runs a protracted course and flare-ups occur repeatedly if steroids are withdrawn, thyroid RaI uptake and scan studies during steroid therapy are useful for recognizing the subsidence of the inflammatory process, as evidenced by restoration of glandular accumulation of RaI. Cases of subacute thyroiditis of only modest severity may be effectively treated with salicylates, and the mildest cases require no treatment at all.

CHRONIC THYROIDITIS

A much commoner disorder than subacute thyroiditis, chronic thyroiditis (Hashimoto's thyroiditis, struma lymphomatosa) occurs predominantly in women, mainly in middle life, but it is also a frequent cause of goiter in childhood. There is often a strong family history of some thyroid disorder, including nontoxic goiter, Graves' disease, or myxedema. The course of chronic thyroiditis is characterized by painless, insidious, progressive enlargement of the gland; and there is a pronounced tendency for the eventual development of hypothyroidism (indeed, primary idiopathic hypothyroidism may be a form of Hashimoto's thyroiditis, in which compensatory goitrogenesis fails to occur). The physical findings consist of the goiter, which may be diffuse or nodular, and signs of early hypothyroidism; constitutional and local signs of inflammation such as fever, pain, and tenderness are almost invariably absent.

Pathogenesis
The pathogenesis of Hashimoto's thyroiditis is believed to be autoimmune and perhaps to include a host defect in immune surveillance. Observations supporting an autoimmune mechanism include the following facts:

1. Chronic thyroiditis has been produced in several species of experimental animals by immunization procedures using autologous or homologous thyroglobulin (plus Freund's adjuvant). The immunized animals develop humoral and cell-mediated immunity, and in inbred strains of rats, transfer of the disease has been accomplished by transfusion of spleen cells from an immunized animal to a normal recipient.
2. Circulating antibodies to human thyroid constituents are demonstrable in more than 95 percent of patients with Hashimoto's disease. These include precipitating antibodies to thyroglobulin, complement-fixing antibody directed against thyroid microsomal antigens, antibodies cytotoxic to thyroid cell cultures, and antibodies directed against human thyroid cytoplasmic and colloid antigens as demonstrated by fluorescent antibody techniques. In addition to these humoral antibodies, there is evidence of cell-mediated immunity. Thus lymphocytes from patients with

Hashimoto's disease, when incubated with thyroid antigens, generate leukocyte migration-inhibition factors. Intradermal injection of human thyroglobulin in patients with Hashimoto's disease elicits skin reactions of the delayed hypersensitivity type. Cellular immune mechanisms are probably more directly related to the pathogenesis of the thyroid disease than are humoral antibodies, which are believed to be harmless byproducts of the immunologic process rather than the cause of the thyroid lesions.
3. There is an association between Hashimoto's thyroiditis and other diseases in which abnormalities of the immune mechanisms are believed to play a role, for example, pernicious anemia, Sjögren's syndrome, rheumatoid arthritis, and perhaps diabetes. In the Schmidt syndrome of coexisting primary myxedema and adrenal insufficiency, not only circulating thyroid antibodies but also antiadrenal (and sometimes antiovarian) antibodies have been found, the multiglandular end-organ failure of thyroid, adrenal cortex, and ovary being ascribed to multiple autoimmune mechanisms.

Graves' disease and Hashimoto's disease seem related. Family histories of patients with one of these diseases often include cases of the other, and paired occurrence of these two diseases in monozygotic twins has been documented several times. In Graves' disease as well as in Hashimoto's, the frequency of both circulating antibodies and of thyroid antigen-sensitized lymphocyte populations is high, although circulating antibody titers in Graves' disease tend to be considerably lower than in Hashimoto's disease. The histologic appearance of the thyroid in many cases of Graves' disease shows lymphoid involvement resembling Hashimoto's thyroiditis. The thyroid-stimulating immunoglobulins so characteristic of Graves' disease have also been identified in some cases of Hashimoto's disease; indeed, it is believed that in some cases of euthyroid Graves' disease the absence of hyperthyroidism may be explained on the basis of glandular lymphoid infiltration extensive enough to impair thyroid reserve, so that hypersecretion of thyroid hormones cannot be sustained even in the presence of the abnormal thyroid stimulators.

Laboratory Tests

Clinical diagnosis of Hashimoto's thyroiditis is facilitated by serologic tests. Antithyroglobulin antibody titer is determined by the sensitive tanned erthrocyte agglutination procedure, in which red cells coated with human thyroglobulin are agglutinated in diluted serum containing the antibody; extraordinarily high titers, up to 1×10^6 or more, are often found. Precipitin tests and commercially available latex agglutination tests are much less sensitive and are unlikely to detect antibody titers less than 1×10^4. A positive serologic test for antithyroid antibody cannot be equated with Hashimoto's thyroiditis, since 8 to 12 percent of normal subjects show such antibody in low titer. Conversely, absence of detectable antibody does not exclude chronic thyroiditis, particularly in children, in whom histologically documented lymphocytic thyroiditis is often not accompanied by any detectable circulating antibody.

Thyroid RaI uptake may be high, normal, or low in Hashimoto's thyroiditis, depending on the amount of residual functioning thyroid parenchyma and the degree of TSH stimulation and responsiveness. Perchlorate discharge tests are positive in many cases, attesting to the impaired organic binding capacity. Thyroid scans reveal a characteristically mottled pattern of RaI distribution in a diffusely enlarged gland. Serum T_4 and T_3RU may be normal or low. Serum TSH is elevated in 30 to 40 percent of the patients, even before clinical hypothyroidism is apparent, and such patients are considered to be in a prehypothyroid state. Histologic diagnoses are seldom needed, but in puzzling cases they can be made by needle biopsy.

Treatment

The administration of thyroid hormones, either 0.2 to 0.3 mg of l-T_4 or 120 to 180 mg of thyroid USP daily, often results in considerable reduction in size of the goiter in Hashimoto's thyroiditis, and, of course, it alleviates whatever features of hypothyroidism may be present. Life-long treatment is required, since recurrence of the goiter will result from discontinuing thyroid therapy. In case the inflammatory reaction has led to a predominantly fibrotic gland, the fibrosis may be largely irreversible and regression of gland size only partial. Although corticosteroid therapy of Hashimoto's disease has been shown to diminish gland size, the need for life-long therapy and the risk of complications from the high dosage of steroids make such therapy unwarranted. There is no indication for thyroidectomy in uncomplicated Hashimoto's thyroiditis; removal of thyroid tissue is promptly followed by the development of myxedema.

OTHER FORMS OF THYROIDITIS

Suppurative pyogenic thyroiditis of bacterial origin is rare. Chills, fever, and localizing signs of suppuration may suggest the diagnosis, and thyroid RaI scan study may help in making it. Therapy includes antibiotics and surgical drainage of the abscess.

Riedel's thyroiditis is very rare, of unknown etiology, and is characterized by moderate enlargement of the thyroid. The gland is stony-hard and involved in an extensive fibrotic process that may extend outside the gland capsule, producing fixation and suggesting cancer. The disease is benign, although pressure phenomena may occur. Therapy is surgical resection of involved tissue.

Bibliography

Burrow, G. N. (ed.). Current concepts of thyroid disease. *Med. Clin. North Am.* 59:1043, 1975.

Hershman, J. M. Clinical applications of TRH. *N. Engl. J. Med.* 290:886, 1974.

Ingbar, S. H. and Woeber, K. A. The Thyroid Gland. In R. H. Williams (ed.), *Textbook of Endocrinology* (5th ed.). Philadelphia: Saunders, 1974. Pp. 95–233.

Kendall-Taylor, P. LATS and human specific thyroid stimulator; their relation to Graves' disease. *Clin. Endocrinol. Metabol.* 4:319, 1975.

Rosenberg, I. N. Evaluation of thyroid function. *N. Engl. J. Med.* 286:924, 1972.

Werner, S. C., and Ingbar, S. H. (eds.). *The Thyroid* (3rd ed.). New York: Harper & Row, 1971.

59

Disorders of
Carbohydrate Metabolism

S. Edwin Fineberg and Stephen H. Schneider

Diabetes Mellitus

Insulin secretion in diabetic patients has been described as being both qualitatively and quantitatively deficient with regard to the prevailing level of blood glucose. Early insulin release after an intravenous glucose stimulus is regularly impaired in diabetes, whether or not exogenous insulin is required for therapy. Furthermore, when compared with appropriate controls matched with regard to body weight and age, all diabetics have a relative to severe impairment in insulin secretion.

Human and experimental diabetes is also characterized by inappropriate glucagon secretion in the face of hyperglycemia. Insulin deficiency per se may generate this abnormality. Studies using somatostatin as a pharmacologic probe have recently demonstrated that glucagon excess in states of insulin deficiency contributes to the metabolic abnormalities that one observes in diabetic ketoacidosis. Overall growth hormone secretion is regularly increased when diabetes is uncontrolled. Although there is no evidence that this hormone plays an etiologic role in diabetes, current observations suggest that growth hormone may be necessary for the full expression of diabetic complications.

Glucose Tolerance

Traditionally diabetes has been defined in terms of glucose tolerance testing (Table 59-1). For maximum reliability any glucose tolerance test should be carried out after proper dietary preparation and under standardized conditions. The oral glucose tolerance test is the most specific of all carbohydrate tolerance tests (having the fewest false positives).

Drugs affecting glucose tolerance should be omitted, and at least 2 weeks should be allowed to elapse following an acute illness. Proper test preparation consists of a diet containing at least 150 gm of carbohydrate and taken for 3 or more days prior to testing. After an overnight fast of 8 to 16 hours, 40 gm per

square meter of body surface area of glucose is administered orally in 300 ml of water over a 5-minute period. A test should not be begun after 12 o'clock noon. Blood samples should be obtained just prior to the glucose load and at 60, 120, and 180 minutes after the meal. Rapid separation of serum or plasma is advisable. Edetate (EDTA) and oxalate cannot be used as anticoagulants for some glucose oxidase determinations of plasma glucose.

Tables 59-2 and 59-3 present a number of criteria that can be used to interpret an oral glucose tolerance test. Fasting hyperglycemia is always indicative of severely disordered carbohydrate tolerance.

For the Wilkerson criteria (Table 59-2), one assigns points to a glucose level above the upper limit of normal, that is, 1 point to a fasting plasma level above 130 mg per 100 ml. Diabetic glucose tolerance by

Table 59-1. Classification of Diabetes
by Carbohydrate Tolerance

Type	Glucose tolerance	Therapy required
Overt	↑Fasting and post-prandial glucose	Diet or diet and hypoglycemic agent
Chemical	Normal fasting but ↑postprandial glucose	Diet, search for precipitating factors
Stress	Normal or abnormal fasting glucose; ↑post-prandial glucose	Removal of stress – i.e., drugs, pregnancy, obesity, illness, endo-crinopathy

Table 59-2. Plasma-Adjusted
Criteria for Glucose Tolerance

Author and test	Time (hr)	Glucose (mg/100 ml)	Evaluation
Wilkerson	Fasting	130 or more	1 point
	1	195 or more	½ point
	2	140 or more	½ point
	3	130 or more	½ point
Fajans-Conn	Fasting	130 or more	Diabetes
	1	185 or more	Diabetes
	1½	165 or more	Diabetes
	2	140 or more	Diabetes

Source: Adapted from C. L. Meinert, Standardization of the oral glucose tolerance test. *Diabetes* 21:1197, 1973.

Table 59-3. Glucose Tolerance Evaluation
by the Glucose Tolerance Sum Method

Category of glucose tolerance sum (GTS)	GTS*	Percent of population	Evaluation
GTS 0–2	< 585	98–100	Normal
(sum of 0, 30, 60,	585–913	....	Equivocal
120 min)	> 913	....	Diabetic
GTS 0–3	< 527	98–100	Normal
(sum of 0, 60, 120,	527–819	....	Equivocal
180 min)	> 819	....	Diabetic

*Glucose tolerance sum is the sum of plasma glucose concentrations (mg/100 ml) at fasting and 30-, 60-, 120-, and 180-minute intervals following the administration of 40 gm of glucose per square meter of body surface area.
Source: Adapted from T. S. Danowski, T. H. Aarons, and J. D. Hydovitz, Utility of equivocal glucose tolerances. *Diabetes* 19:524, 1970.

these criteria is diagnosed when the sum of points is 2 or greater. In the Fajans-Conn criteria (Table 59-2), any level of glucose outside the upper limits of normal is considered diagnostic of diabetic carbohydrate tolerance. For the glucose tolerance sum (GTS), (Table 59-3), the plasma glucose concentrations obtained at 0, 30, 60, and 120 minutes (GTS 0–2) are totaled; or in the GTS 0–3, the concentrations at 0, 60, 120, and 180 minutes are added together. Danowski has presented evidence that 98 to 100 percent of the population having normal tests by the GTS method will also be normal by all other criteria. A partial summary of factors influencing glucose tolerance is found in Table 59-4. Aging is associated with roughly a 10 mg per 100 ml increase in the 2-hour plasma glucose for every decade of age over 40. However, fasting glucose levels remain normal, whatever the age of an individual.

Genetic, Viral, and Autoimmune Theories of Etiology
The genetics of diabetes is obscure; the only really clear inheritance pattern reported is that found in individuals with a "maturity onset" type of diabetes occurring in youth. In these patients, diabetes is inherited as an autosomal dominant trait. At least 40 percent of new diabetics have no family history of the disease. Most juvenile-onset diabetics do not have a predictable incidence of diabetes in their

parents. An identical twin of such a diabetic has at least a 30 percent chance of escaping the disease. The prevalence of diabetes in the United States is 1 to 2 percent and probably would be twice that if extensive screening were carried out. Factors that predispose to the clinical appearance of diabetes include obesity, increasing age, and the use of drugs that inhibit insulin secretion or stimulate gluconeogenesis. Diabetes is a rare disease in undernourished populations but has a high prevalence in well-nourished, overfed populations.

Pathologists have long commented that children who die within 1 year of the onset of diabetes have pancreatic islets infiltrated with lymphocytes. Diabetic children have recently been shown to have a high incidence of antibodies directed against beta cells, suggesting that childhood diabetes may have an autoimmune etiology. Pancreatophilic viruses such as mumps, rubella, and the enteroviruses have been shown to produce transient diabetes in a small number of individuals. Peak periods of diabetes in children correspond to epidemics of such viruses. Titers of antibodies directed against these viruses are increased in children with a recent onset of diabetes.

From such fragments of evidence, it has been suggested that the etiology of diabetes may be either genetic, infectious, or autoimmune; however, the well-known influences of nutrition and age may be required to finally bring about clinical disease.

Clinical Diabetes Mellitus
Diabetes may present as an acute metabolic crisis or, more commonly, as a chronic illness. Individuals presenting with the latter have a mild to moderate impairment of insulin secretion and are usually diagnosed as having maturity-onset diabetes. They are usually obese and can often be treated with diet alone. Other associated symptoms may include polyuria, polydipsia, weight loss, and a number of nonspecific complaints and symptoms. On the other hand, some diabetics who have severe insulin deficiency and require insulin early in their disease present with an acute metabolic crisis. They are usually thin, and their diabetes may be "brittle" (swinging readily from hyperglycemia to hypoglycemia). They are usually known as juvenile-onset diabetics. However, the terms *maturity-onset*

Table 59-4. Factors Affecting Glucose Tolerance

Factor	Effect on tolerance	Comment
Obesity	↓	Decreased insulin binding
Age	↓	Normal fasting blood sugar
Pregnancy	↓	Postprandial ↑ blood sugar
Endocrinopathies	↓	Cushing's syndrome, hyperthyroidism, hyperaldosteronism, acromegaly
Inactivity	↓	↑ Muscular activity, ↑ insulin action; inactivity has the opposite effect
Time of day	↑ ↓	Maximum insulin sensitivity and release in the A.M., minimum in the P.M.
Drugs	↓	Sympathomimetic agents, diuretics, diazoxide, phenytoin, corticosteroids, nicotinic acid
Drugs	↑	Caffeine, theophylline, propranolol, aspirin, alcohol
Stress, illness	↓	Intolerance may be transient or permanent

and *juvenile-onset diabetes* are misnomers; they really describe noninsulin-requiring versus insulin-requiring diabetic states, respectively. With onset below age 20, approximately 85 percent of diabetic individuals require insulin; over age 20, 85 percent do not. Also, diabetes starting before age 20 is often characterized by a short period of remission, when no therapy is required.

METABOLIC DISTURBANCES OF DIABETES MELLITUS: KETOACIDOSIS AND NONKETOTIC HYPEROSMOLAR HYPERGLYCEMIC COMA

Pathophysiology and Biochemistry

The basic biochemical defect in both diabetic keto-acidosis (DKA) and nonketotic hyperosmolar hyper-glycemic coma (NKHHC) is lack of insulin action. In the former, the ability to secrete insulin is very severely impaired, whereas in the latter, considerable ability to secrete insulin is retained. Both disorders are characterized by a marked glucagon excess. With severe insulin deficiency, muscle is less able to oxidize ketoacids, which accumulate and lead to metabolic acidosis. Also glucose production increases and utili-zation decreases, which soon causes serum glucose to exceed the renal threshold. This in turn leads to an osmotic diuresis with concomitant water and electro-lyte losses that may cause hypotension.

Sodium depletion is masked in diabetic acidosis because water loss is usually greater than solute loss.

Body K^+ depletion may be poorly reflected by the plasma K^+, since in acidosis H^+ shifts into the intra-cellular space in exchange for K^+. Consequently, patients with a high plasma K^+ upon admission have a relative maintenance of K^+ stores, whereas those with normal or low K^+ have moderate to profound K^+ depletion. Often neglected in DKA are concomitant magnesium and phosphate deficits; the former may lead to neuromuscular irritability, alteration in con-sciousness, and seizures and the latter to a depletion of red blood cell 2,3-diphosphoglycerate, which increases the binding affinity of hemoglobin for oxygen.

Blood glucose concentrations will not exceed 600 mg per 100 ml in DKA unless there is a contraction of blood volume and some degree of prerenal azotemia. Since thirst is not impaired in DKA, extreme hyper-glycemia is seldom seen. Hyperosmolarity of mild to modest severity is a regular feature and has recently been invoked as a causative factor in neurologic dysfunction.

In NKHHC accumulation of glucose in the extra-cellular space becomes marked because of the de-creased fluid intake often seen in such patients and also because of preceding mild to moderate renal insufficiency. Hyperosmolarity becomes profound, along with losses of water and electrolytes (Table 59-5). Water shifts from the intracellular fluid space to the extracellular fluid space to maintain osmotic

Table 59-5. Fluid and Electrolyte Replacement for Diabetic Ketoacidosis and Nonketotic Hyperosmolar Hyperglycemic Coma

| Fluid, electrolyte | DKA | | NKHHC[c] | |
	Replacement[a]	Deficit[b]	Replacement	Deficit
H_2O	6 L (0–18)	80 ml/kg	12 ± 3.5 L (SD)	90 ml/kg
K^+	165 mEq (0–620)	5 mEq/kg	215 ± 83 mEq	4 mEq/kg
Na^+	530 mEq (0–1,460)	6 mEq/kg	512 ± 161 mEq	6 mEq/kg
PO_4	....	0.5 mEq/kg	....	....
Mg^+	....	0.6 mEq/kg	....	....

[a]From Beigelman [3]
[b]From Arrieff [2]
[c]From Butler [6]
Note: DKA = diabetic ketoacidosis; NKHHC = nonketotic hyperosmolar hyperglycemic coma; SD = standard deviation. Ranges noted in parentheses denote the range of fluid volume or ion replacement required.

equilibrium, lowering plasma Na^+ concentrations until dehydration becomes profound. Plasma K^+ is also decreased by this water shift. An estimate of effective osmolarity is obtained by the following:

$$2 (Na^+ + K^+) + \frac{glucose}{18} \ (mg/dl)$$

Such a calculation is useful in gauging whether hyperosmolarity is present.

Clinical Presentation, Differential Diagnosis, Complications, Prognosis

A diabetic may present with an acute metabolic or neurologic abnormality due to one or a number of disorders, including (1) hypoglycemia, (2) DKA, (3) NKHHC, (4) lactic acidosis, or (5) disorders unrelated to diabetes per se (i.e., uremia, cerebrovascular accident, hepatic coma). Clinical features of each of these disorders are summarized in Table 59-6. Hypoglycemia can be determined quickly from a measurement of blood glucose.

Neurologic abnormalities may persist for up to one week after a hypoglycemic episode. An immediate bolus injection of 25 to 50 gm of glucose as 50% dextrose in water is indicated in hypoglycemia, along with the infusion of a 10% dextrose in water solution to maintain normoglycemia; a helpful adjunct to such therapy is 1 mg of glucagon intramuscularly (IM).

Diabetic ketoacidosis often occurs in young adults (average age of 38) who have previously required insulin therapy but have either contracted an underlying infection (urinary tract, pulmonary, or skin) or omitted their diabetic therapy. Other conditions such as cancer, myocardial infarction, or pancreatitis may precipitate the illness and lead to death. Hypotension is present in 16 percent of the patients. Fruity (acetone) breath should be sought along with signs of dehydration, which are usually prominent. Since increased respiratory exchange and acute neurologic dysfunction are seen in other disorders, the differential diagnosis must be based on the biochemical features (Table 59-7). An atypical presentation can be seen in diabetics after alcohol ingestion, in whom glucose concentrations can be normal or low and serum ketones as measured by nitroprusside reaction decreased. Alcohol metabolism leads to an inhibition of glucose production and to increased conversion of acetoacetate to beta-hydroxybutyrate. Also in hypotension or prolonged acidosis of unusual severity, more acetoacetate may be converted to beta-hydroxybutyrate. Since nitroprusside tablets detect only acetoacetate, they do not reflect the serum ketone concentrations accurately in this situation.

Nonketoacidotic hyperosmolar hyperglycemic coma can usually be differentiated from DKA by its clinical and laboratory features (see Tables 59-6 and 59-7). This life-threatening disorder is usually seen in older patients (mean age 61) and often occurs in previously undiagnosed diabetics; a gram-negative sepsis often underlies its onset. Dehydration tends to be

Table 59-6. Clinical Features and Physical Signs of Metabolic Disturbances in Diabetes Mellitus

Clinical state	Onset	History	Drug history	Physical signs
Hypoglycemia	Sudden	Sweating, faintness, personality changes, behavior disturbances	Insulin or oral hypoglycemic agent; alcohol ingestion	Dilated pupils, sweating, tachy-cardia
DKA	1–24 hr	Polyuria, polydipsia, nausea, vomiting, diarrhea, abdominal pain; average age 30	Insulin-requiring diabetes; 15% are new cases	Deep, sighing respirations; tachypnea; variable degrees of dehydration; confusion, to deep coma
NKHHC	24 hr–2 wk	↓ Fluid intake, increasing somno-lence, polyuria; average age 61	Forty percent new diabetes cases or noninsulin requiring; steroids, diazoxides, antimetab-olites, peritoneal dialysis	Rapid, *shallow* respirations, pro-found dehydration, obtunded to deep coma, often localizing neurologic signs (focal seizures)
Lactic acidosis	1–24 hr	Increasing obtundation; pre-existent liver, cardiac, or renal disease	Phenformin	Warm skin; vasodilation; deep, sighing respirations; deep coma
Alcoholic ketoacidosis	24 hr	Omission of solid food for 24–72 hr	Chronic alcoholism	Large liver, modest or no dehy-dration

Note: DKA = diabetic ketoacidosis; NKHHC = nonketotic hyperosmolar hyperglycemic coma.

Table 59-7. Laboratory Features of Diabetic Ketoacidosis, Nonketotic Hyperosmolar Hyperglycemic Coma, and Alcoholic Ketoacidosis

Laboratory test	Result		
	DKA[a]	NKHHC[b]	AKA[c]
Glucose (mg/100 ml)	675 ± 17 (SEM)	1,096 (400–2,760)	162 (25–235)
Serum ketones (by Acetest)	> 4$^+$ at 1:1 dilution	< 2$^+$ at 1:1 dilution	Up to 3$^+$ undiluted
Na$^+$ (mEq/L)	131 ± 0	144 (119–188)	140 (134–150)
K$^+$ (mEq/L)	5.3 ± 0.1 4% 3.5, 74% 3.5–6.0, 22% 6.0	5.0 (2.7–8)	4.9 (2.8–6.0)
Cl$^-$ (mEq/L)	....	99 (84–116)	94 (87–99)
HCO$_3^-$ (mEq/L)	6 ± 0	17 ± 5 (SD)	6.3 (5.0–8.0)
Arterial pH	7.07 (6.92–7.22)	7.26 (6.81–7.53)	7.16 (6.96–7.25)
Osmolarity (calculated)[d]	323 ± 1	405 (348–456)	299
Amylase (units/ml)	242 ± 52	....	346 (162–550)
Blood urea nitrogen (mg/100 ml)	35	87	48
Leukocytes/cu mm	18,387	↑ With infection	↑ With infection

[a]From Beigelman and Nabarro
[b]From Arrieff and McCurdy
[c]From Levy
[d]Calculated osmolarity = $2 \times (Na + K) + \dfrac{\text{glucose (mg/100 ml)}}{18}$

Note: DKA = diabetic ketoacidosis; NKHHC = nonketotic hyperosmolar hyperglycemic coma; AKA = alcoholic ketoacidosis; SEM = standard error of the mean; SD = standard deviation.

more severe in NKHHC than in DKA, and localizing neurologic signs, especially focal seizures, are seen in over 10 percent of patients in NKHCC. Severe acidosis is uncommon in NKHHC, whereas osmolarity and glucose levels are greater than in DKA and ketonemia is usually insignificant.

Lactic acidosis in diabetics can occur either in a pure form or mixed with ketoacidosis. Lactic acidosis mixed with DKA is a diagnosis of exclusion that should be suspected whenever a patient has a profound acidosis associated with a large, unexplained anion gap (see Chap. 54). Glucose concentrations are usually normal in pure lactic acidosis. In the differential diagnosis one should consider acidosis due to poisoning with salicylates, methanol, ethylene glycol, chloral hydrate, or paraldehyde. The history and toxicology studies on urine, blood, and gastric contents will help clarify the etiology. In nondiabetics, alcoholism associated with ketoacidosis (AKA) can easily be confused with DKA (see Tables 59-6 and 59-7).

In the present antibiotic era, DKA has been reported to be associated with an overall mortality rate of 3 to 10 percent. Prognosis worsens with increased duration of acidosis, increased age, and higher blood glucose concentrations. Loss of consciousness and hypotension are poor prognostic signs; myocardial infarction and septicemia are two major contributors to death. Fetal survival is extremely poor (70 percent fetal loss) during ketoacidosis in pregnancy; maternal survival is also threatened (10 percent mortality rate). Pancreatitis complicating DKA may be difficult to detect because of both the modest elevation of amylase and the abdominal pain that may occur commonly in DKA; severe acidosis and hyperglycemia are particularly ominous signs in hemorrhagic pancreatitis.

Diabetic ketoacidosis occurring in a uremic individual is extremely difficult to manage; death may occur quickly from fluid overload. Rarely, cerebral edema and electrolyte disturbances (either hypokalemia or hyperkalemia) may lead to death in DKA.

These are usually preventable and will be discussed below. Nonketotic hyperosmolar hyperglycemic coma has a considerably poorer prognosis than DKA, with a mortality rate of 40 to 70 percent. Most deaths are due to septicemia or other life-threatening disorders such as carcinoma or myocardial infarction. Gram-negative pneumonia is present in 15 percent of the fatalities. Death attributable to the hyperosmolar state per se has been reported in approximately 20 percent of patients, and the mortality increases with the duration of the hyperosmolarity. Pure lactic acidosis alone, even in the absence of circulatory insufficiency, is associated with a mortality rate in excess of 90 percent. Death usually results either from heart failure or hepatic insufficiency. Alcoholic ketoacidosis in the nondiabetic is a relatively benign disorder with a good outcome if the patient does not have underlying hemorrhagic pancreatitis or septicemia.

Initial Laboratory Tests

Initial laboratory tests of importance in differentiating DKA and NKHHC and estimating their severity include serum glucose, blood urea nitrogen, ketones, creatinine, and electrolytes; ECG; arterial blood gases; and serum amylase. After initial evaluation and therapy, the data base should be widened to include a complete blood count, urinalysis, chest x-ray, and liver function studies. Severe acidosis is indicated by a serum HCO_3 of 5 or less or a serum carbon dioxide at its lower limit of 10 to 12 mEq per liter. Hypokalemia and hyperkalemia should be looked for by direct measurement and by ECG evidence (see Chap. 32). A serum blood urea nitrogen-creatinine ratio of less than 10 should alert the physician that underlying renal disease may be contributing to the patient's problems or may complicate therapy. Marked elevation of serum amylase (> 500 units) suggests pancreatitis.

Serum ketone body concentrations should be estimated with serial dilutions of serum (using water or saline) and crushed nitroprusside tablets or powder. The reaction may be decreased in undiluted serum, and therefore testing at a $1:2$ dilution is mandatory. This reaction, as previously mentioned, measures primarily acetoacetate, not beta-hydroxybutyrate, the principal ketoacid.

Therapy

Regardless of the disorder, the first duty of the physician is to stabilize the patient's condition. As a routine, he should insert a large intravenous catheter, obtain initial laboratory studies, and begin a normal saline infusion; administer oxygen; and, if the patient is unconscious, empty the gastric pouch with a nasogastric tube. Bladder catheterization should be avoided unless the bladder becomes distended or unless urinary output must be monitored for therapy of shock. A carefully detailed flow sheet of laboratory results, vital signs, and therapy should be constructed for each patient. Patients with DKA associated with renal disease, pregnancy, cardiac disease, or hemorrhagic pancreatitis should be cared for in an intensive care unit. Because of the poor outlook and the often life-threatening nature of the underlying disorders, NKHHC should also be handled in the ICU. Patients with suspected cardiac or renal disease or those whose cardiovascular capacity is unknown should be monitored with a central venous pressure line or Swan-Ganz catheter in place.

Diabetic Ketoacidosis. There are eight principal steps in the therapy of diabetic ketoacidosis.

1. Initial insulin (conventional high-dose) therapy: This depends on clinical and biochemical estimates of the severity of the ketoacidosis (Table 59-8). Insulin should be given intravenously whenever circulatory insufficiency with decreased absorption of insulin is a possibility.

   Recent experimental low-dose insulin therapy in DKA has used (1) a constant infusion of 10 units of insulin per hour in saline to which 2 ml of 25% serum albumin is added to each 100 ml of infusate; (2) multiple IM injections of insulin beginning with 10 to 15 units and repeating 5 to 10 units hourly; or (3) multiple subcutaneous (SQ) injections of 5 units every 30 minutes. The first has gained the widest acceptance.

   High-dose therapy was based on clinical inferences that insulin resistance is common in DKA. However, it has now been shown that insulin resistance is an infrequent problem. The rate of fall of glucose levels is equivalent with either low-

Table 59-8. Therapy for Diabetic Ketoacidosis as Gauged by Clinical Severity

Clinical severity	Insulin, initial dose (units) and route	Serum acetone	Glucose (mg/100 ml)	Signs Neurologic	Vital
Mild	50–100 (½ SQ, ½ IV)	Strongly + at 1:2 dilution	300–600	Alert to confused	Within normal limits
Moderate	100–200 IV	Strongly + at 1:8	600–800	Obtunded	Within normal limits
Severe	200–300 IV	Strongly + at > 1:8	> 800	Comatose	Hypotension

or high-dose methods (50 to 150 mg/100 ml/hour). An infusion rate of 1 unit per hour results in insulin levels of 20 to 30 μU per milliliter. At 10 units per hour favorable insulin actions such as inhibition of lipolysis and ketogenesis and inhibition of glucose production are nearly maximal. Low-dose therapy may lead to a decrease in late complications of hypokalemia and hypoglycemia, provided glucose is also infused and insulin is stopped when glucose concentrations fall below 250 mg per 100 ml.

2. Initial fluid and electrolyte therapy: The safest initial fluid therapy in DKA is normal saline. Potassium and HCO_3^- should not be added unless serum K^+ is less than 3.0 mEq per liter or there is ECG evidence of hypokalemia. Four percent of individuals will have K^+ less than 3.5 mEq per liter, while 22 percent have K^+ of more than 6.0 mEq per liter. Bicarbonate causes a rapid shift of K^+ into cells in exchange with H^+, leading to an exaggeration of hypokalemia. The rapid infusion of K^+ in a hyperkalemic individual can lead to lethal K^+ intoxication. When hypokalemia is present initially, K^+ deficit is severe and requires replacing up to 100 mEq of KCl per hour (see below), constant ECG monitoring, and frequent determinations of serum K^+. Severe hypotension requires rapid volume repletion; as already mentioned, a central venous pressure line should be inserted and physiologic saline infused at 1 liter every 45 to 90 minutes until the venous pressure, blood pressure, and urinary output increase to the normal range. If rapid infusion of saline fails to increase the blood pressure when central venous pressure is rising, then pressor therapy should be instituted.

3. Repair of K^+ deficit (see Table 59-5): Potassium can safely be infused when urinary output is greater than 25 ml per hour. Actual levels of K^+ can be used only as an approximate indicator of the deficit. Patients who are treated with the large doses of insulin and HCO_3^- and sustain great falls in serum glucose are the likeliest candidates for hypokalemia. Potassium deficits should be replaced over 12 to 24 hours.

4. Correction of acidosis: Acidosis need not be corrected if HCO_3^- levels are above 10 mEq per liter. In modest acidosis the HCO_3^- space is 100 percent of the total body water (50 percent of the weight in kilograms). An HCO_3^- of 5 mEq per liter or less or a CO_2 of 10 to 12 mEq per liter indicates the presence of severe acidosis. This requires prompt, high-dose therapy with bicarbonate using a HCO_3^- distribution space equal to 200 percent of total body water. Only one-half of the HCO_3^- needed to replete HCO_3^- to 15 mEq per liter should be infused during the first 6 hours of therapy. It is essential to avoid overcorrection of acidosis; alkalosis resulting from infusion of unnecessarily large amounts of HCO_3^- can lead to respiratory depression and increased binding of oxygen by the hemoglobin.

5. Water deficit and repair (see Table 59-5): Dehydration in DKA can vary between 5 and 15 percent of total body water. A useful estimate of dehydration can be simply obtained by multiplying body weight (kg) $\times$ the average H_2O deficit in DKA (80 ml/kg); half of water deficit should be replaced in 12 hours, and the remainder can be replaced in the next 24 hours.

6. Insulin therapy: In moderately ill patients, insulin administration and laboratory follow-up studies

should be repeated every 2 hours; in the severely ill, they should be done every hour. If glucose levels and ketones increase, insulin resistance should be suspected. The initial dose of insulin (or rate of infusion) should then be doubled, and if necessary, redoubled hourly. When glucose concentrations fall to about 300 mg per 100 ml, insulin should be discontinued and 5% dextrose in water (D5W) infused. One must avoid decreasing serum glucose concentration to below 200 mg per 100 ml during the first 12 hours of therapy. Such drastic reductions in glucose levels cause cerebral edema in experimental DKA in rabbits and may explain the occasional occurrence of cerebral edema in man.

Long-acting insulin can be given on the second day of therapy.

7. Phosphate and Mg repair: As mentioned previously, phosphate and Mg deficits are substantial in DKA (see Table 59-5). Phosphate and K^+ may be replaced simultaneously by infusion of potassium phosphate (a mixture of dibasic and monobasic phosphates), 5 mmol per liter, in addition to KCl.

Magnesium cannot be replaced until urinary flow is adequate: then magnesium sulfate 2 gm (16.3 mEq) can be added to each liter of fluid when sodium bicarbonate is not needed. Up to 64 mEq of magnesium sulfate can be replaced in 24 hours.

8. Search for an underlying disorder: Resistance to therapy may be related to such underlying problems as septicemia, myocardial infarction, or pancreatitis.

Nonketotic Hyperosmolar Hyperglycemic Coma.
There are four principal steps in the treatment of this medical emergency.

1. Initial therapy: Since volume depletion is virtually universal in NKHHC, one should begin fluid therapy with saline. Effective osmolarity should then be calculated (see page 814) to identify individuals who are *not* hyperosmolar and may be extremely sensitive to the hypoglycemic actions of insulin (they usually have minimal to no neurologic deficit). Such patients require no more than 25 to 50 units of insulin administered every 2 to 4 hours. Too rapid a reduction of plasma glucose to normal in such a patient may lead to shock and renal insufficiency; these patients are also at special risk for water intoxication.

In *hyperosmolar* individuals initial insulin needs can be estimated simply by using Arrieff's formula of 10 percent of the plasma glucose as units of insulin to be given IV. For example, if plasma glucose is 2,000 mg per 100 ml, insulin need will be $2,000 \times 0.10 = 200$ units. Low-dose insulin therapy has not been reported for the treatment of NKHHC; however, this method should also prove effective in this disorder. If hypotension is present, saline should be infused until blood pressure and urine flow are restored or until central venous pressure begins to rise. If central venous pressure begins to rise without an increase in urine flow, pressor agents should be used. Severe acidosis is occasionally present in NKHHC and should be looked for. High-dose HCO_3^-, as outlined above, is then required.

2. Fluid and insulin therapy: Water deficit in NKHHC (see Table 59-5) can be estimated from body weight and the knowledge that the average water deficit is 25 percent of total body water (body water is 50 percent of the body weight in kilograms). The average amount of water required until osmolarity nears normal is 12 liters. No more than one-half of an estimated water deficit (plus urinary loss) should be replaced during the first 12 hours of therapy. Half-normal saline is the fluid of choice. Potassium chloride should be added to the regimen when urinary output increases to 25 ml per hour. Insulin can be safely administered, according to the given formula, every 2 hours IV with little risk of hypoglycemia. A rising blood glucose indicates insulin resistance and is handled as in DKA. When blood glucose concentrations fall to 300 mg per 100 ml, D5W should be infused so that plasma glucose concentrations are maintained between 200 and 300 mg per 100 ml.

3. Osmolar balance: A critical problem in NKHHC is the osmolar state itself. Persistence of (extreme) hyperosmolarity will lead to death. However, too rapid a reduction in hyperosmolarity may lead to

cerebral edema. Therefore osmolarity should be calculated every 2 hours. When plasma glucose falls below 300 mg per 100 ml or osmolarity falls below 310 to 320 mOsm per liter, D5W should be infused. Only half of the water deficit (plus urinary losses) should be replaced during the first 12 hours, and the remainder during the next 24 hours.

4. Potassium and sodium deficits (see Table 59-5): Hypokalemia is seldom a problem if KCl is added to fluids early in therapy (provided urine flow is adequate). A concentration of K^+ of 40 mEq per liter of fluid is sufficient. Potassium and sodium should be replaced over a period of 24 hours.

Alcoholic Ketoacidosis. Despite its similarities with DKA, alcoholic ketoacidosis differs markedly in the therapy required. This state requires modest replacement with fluids containing glucose and small amounts of HCO_3^-. Insulin therapy does not seem to improve recovery times. Recommended therapy in this disorder is 3 to 6 liters of D5W containing 44 mEq $NaHCO_3$ given IV every 90 minutes unless severe acidosis is present. Fluids should also contain KCl when urine flow is adequate. Twenty-five units (or less) of insulin can be administered every 4 hours if blood glucose concentrations are above 300 mg per 100 ml.

COMPLICATIONS OF DIABETES MELLITUS

Infection
In insulin-deficient patients, polymorphonuclear cells and macrophages migrate abnormally and are less than normally able to ingest and kill bacteria. Infections do not occur more frequently in diabetes, but they are often severe or may be in an atypical location. Diabetics out of metabolic control are susceptible to nosocomial infections, both bacterial and fungal.

Neuropathy
The characteristic lesion in diabetes is segmental demyelinization. Prolongation of muscle nerve conduction time and elevation in cerebrospinal fluid proteins is present in most patients very early in their disorders.

Peripheral Neuropathy (see Chap. 62). Most commonly the longest nerve trunks are involved most severely. Both reflexes and vibratory and position sense may be decreased or lost. There is some evidence that aggressive insulin therapy may reverse or stabilize early neurologic deficits. Chronic sensory loss may lead to Charcot joints, especially of the foot, ankle, or knee; or to neurotropic ulcers of the foot. Loss of tactile discrimination in the fingertips makes braille reading especially difficult for blind diabetics.

Mononeuritis. An acute, transient loss of function of a single nerve is presumed to be of vascular etiology and often involves the sixth, seventh, or third cranial nerves. When the third cranial nerve is involved, the pupil is characteristically spared. Spontaneous recovery usually ensues within 2 to 4 months.

Autonomic Neuropathy. Autonomic dysfunction may manifest itself as gastroenteropathy, vesiculopathy, orthostatic hypotension, or a combination of these. The gastroenteropathies include gastric dilatation, abnormal esophageal motility, and abnormal intestinal motility characterized by nocturnal diarrhea or constipation. Gastric dilatation may be seen acutely during diabetic ketoacidosis. However, occasionally this abnormality presents itself as a clinically difficult problem requiring treatment with multiple small meals, elevation of the head of the bed at night, and occasionally surgical intervention with drainage of the gastric pouch. All these measures are rather unsatisfactory. Approximately 10 percent of patients with diabetic diarrhea have bacterial overgrowth and can be treated by institution of antibiotics. Duodenal drainage and culture and small bowel biopsy should always be carried out in patients with diabetic diarrhea to find if a correctable lesion is present.

Vesiculopathy. In diabetics who have had their disease for more than 20 years, bladder denervation is common. This disorder has an insidious onset often marked by overflow incontinence. Such patients have large, dilated bladders with a decreased ability to detect bladder distention. A combination of cholinergic agents, bladder neck resection, and a program of frequent voiding is usually successful in reducing the residual volume of the bladder. Impotence after the age of 35 is also common in the diabetic population. Evidence of vesiculopathy or of an absent anal reflex is often associated with such impotence and indicates irreversible nerve damage.

Orthostatic Hypotension. Orthostatic hypotension is commonly associated with evidence of decreased sweating, atrophy of the skin and nails of the lower extremities, and peripheral neuropathy. Treatment with 9-α-fluorohydrocortisone is often effective in obliterating hypotensive symptoms.

Diabetic Amyotrophy. Diabetic amyotrophy is a rare disorder and primarily involves the pelvic girdle muscles. It is associated with muscular tenderness, a waddling gait, and difficulty arising from a stooped position. This is often unilateral and is usually self-limited.

Vascular Complications

Diabetes is associated with an increased incidence of large and small vessel disease (see Chap. 27). Seventy percent of diabetics die of coronary or cerebrovascular disease.

Microangiopathy. Microangiopathy involves primarily the muscular capillaries but has also been reported in other vessels of other tissues. As seen by the electron microscope, microangiopathy is characterized by irregular, thick deposits of endothelial basement membrane material.

Atherosclerosis. Atherosclerotic lesions in the diabetic are identical to those found in nondiabetics. However, they tend to be more advanced at an earlier age. For example, the difference in incidence between women and men of myocardial infarction prior to the menopause is not present in diabetics.

Diabetic Eye Disease

Ophthalmic lesions in diabetes include cataracts, so-called background retinopathy, and retinitis proliferans. The lesions of background retinopathy include venous dilatation, hard and soft exudates, hemorrhages, and microaneurisms. Background retinopathy begins first in the temporal fields; the earliest lesion generally is venous dilatation. For every microaneurism seen by direct ophthalmoscopy (appearing as tiny red dots), fluorescin angiography will reveal about 100. "Hard" exudates are well-defined yellow or white lesions; macular confluence of such lesions or an outright star figure may indicate macular edema and help explain decreased visual acuity. "Soft" exudates are indicative of capillary ischemia; these are poorly defined white patches superficial to the retinal vessels.

Hemorrhages may be associated with both retinitis proliferans and background retinopathy, but they seldom lead to permanent blindness. Background retinopathy may lead to macular edema with decreased vision, but it does not lead to blindness. Currently a national trial is under way to determine whether photocoagulation of areas of leaky capillaries will prevent progression of diabetic retinopathy to retinitis proliferans. Fluorescin angiography should be carried out in individuals who have progressive background retinopathy in hopes of detecting areas of capillary leakage. Retinitis proliferans is due to new vessel growth associated with fibrous tissue in the retina. This may lead to retinal detachment and permanent loss of vision. It is believed that angiogenic substances similar to those observed in tumors may leak from such areas of increased capillary permeability and ischemia and lead to the formation of new vessels.

Cataracts and glaucoma are also noted with increased frequency in diabetic patients. Cataracts may be associated with accumulation of sorbitol and dulcitol within the cells, but most are senile cataracts that occur prematurely. Transient fluctuations in visual acuity may occur secondary to osmotic changes in the lens following wide swings in serum glucose.

Diabetic Renal Disease

Accumulation of abnormal glomerular basement membrane material occurs early in diabetes. However, nephropathy is seldom an important clinical problem until the disease has been present for at least 20 years. Spiro and co-workers have demonstrated that this basement membrane material consists of increased amounts of glucosyl-galactose moieties associated with an increased content of hydroxylysine. This material traps many macromolecules such as immunoglobulins. Clinically important renal disease in the diabetic often manifests itself first as the nephrotic syndrome, followed by a long period of stability with slightly elevated creatinine concentrations (see also Chap. 53). After a period of 6 to 8 years, a period of hypertension may appear with progressive elevation of creatinine concentrations. It is followed by a terminal period lasting 2 or 3 years and marked by hypertension, progressive retinal lesions, and death due either to coronary artery disease or renal failure.

Pregnancy
Both maternal and infant mortality rates are higher in the diabetic than in the normal population. This problem can be minimized by aggressive control of blood glucose during the gestational period; diets should be aimed primarily at preventing excessive weight gain. However, starvation may cause ketonemia and may be associated with some abnormalities in fetal central nervous system development. Newborns of diabetic mothers are often large or edematous and have an increased incidence of respiratory distress syndrome. Such children have been exposed to high levels of glucose in utero and develop long-lasting beta cell hypertrophy which often results in hypoglycemic attacks during the first days or weeks of life.

Lipid Abnormalities
Lipid abnormalities are common in diabetes. Better metabolic control enables the body to properly activate lipoprotein lipase, thus reducing chylomicronemia. Diabetes and lipid abnormalities are independently inherited. See Chapter 26 for treatment.

Relation to Metabolic Abnormalities
to Diabetic Complications
Many complications of diabetes occur in tissues that do not require insulin for glucose transport. Hyperglycemia secondary to insulin deficiency leads to excessive accumulation of glucose in these tissues, and much of this glucose is shunted to alternate pathways of metabolism. In the polyol pathway, glucose is shunted to sorbitol and then to fructose. Sorbitol and fructose are osmotically active substances that

are metabolized slowly. It is postulated that toxic alterations in cells accumulating these substances may be responsible for complications in the renal medulla, peripheral nerves, central nervous system, and lens of the eyes. However, definite proof of this hypothesis is currently lacking. Abnormalities in basement membrane material have been found by Spiro and co-workers, as cited above. They have also been able to demonstrate that with insulin deficiency there is an increased activity of the enzyme linking glucose and galactose with a consequent formation of increased amounts of hydroxylysine. Experimentally these changes can be reversed in animals treated promptly with insulin, but they cannot be reversed in well-established diabetes. Thus the value of diabetic control in delaying or preventing the onset of complications of diabetes remains open at this point. Experimentally much animal data exists to show that lesions such as diabetic retinopathy, diabetic nephropathy, and diabetic neuropathy can be stabilized or even reversed by vigorous insulin therapy or by transplantation of diabetic tissues into normal animals. Exact metabolic control of diabetes is difficult to achieve in man, and no conclusive studies have yet been done to demonstrate its value in human disease.

LONG-TERM THERAPY OF DIABETES
Diet
In the insulin-secreting diabetic, the principal aim of diet therapy is to achieve ideal body weight. Restriction of total calories is more important than distribution of foods. Nevertheless, allotment of food evenly throughout the day, provision of protein along with carbohydrate, and the avoidance of free carbohydrate have proved useful. Diabetic diets should be simple and should approximate a normal dietary intake. A useful formula is 10 calories per pound of ideal body weight plus 30 percent. This will achieve weight maintenance in most patients. A caloric deficit of 500 calories per day will lead to about a 1-pound weight loss per week. Increased calories are required in very active patients. The usual food distribution is 50 percent of calories as carbohydrates, 25 percent as protein, and 25 percent as fat. In insulin-treated patients, the daily calories are distributed so that

hypoglycemia is avoided and ideal body weight is maintained.

Oral hypoglycemic Agents

Oral agents are used today mainly in patients unwilling or unable to take insulin and who require more than dietary management for metabolic and symptomatic control of diabetes.

Sulfonylureas. These several agents appear to act by a similar mechanism. They cannot be used in ketosis-prone diabetics with severe insulinopenia. In large bolus injections these agents stimulate beta cells to directly release insulin. With long-term use, this effect cannot be demonstrated. The sulfonylureas may act by sensitizing beta cells to rises in glucose, and they may also augment the actions of insulin on liver, muscle, and adipose tissue. The currently used drugs include those listed in Table 59-9.

Biguanides. Biguanides differ from the sulfonylureas in that their effect is not dependent on the presence of endogenous insulin. Because of the strong association of these drugs with excess cardiovascular mortality rates and the occasional occurrence of fatal lactic acidosis, these agents are reserved for patients who refuse insulin, are unsuccessfully maintained on sulfonylureas, and who have no liver or kidney dysfunction.

Side Effects and Toxicity. The acute side effects of the sulfonylureas are usually limited to hypoglycemic episodes and occasional gastrointestinal distress.

Renal or hepatic disease predisposes to hypoglycemia by prolonging the drugs' half-life. Alcohol not only potentiates hypoglycemia but may initiate an Antabuse (disulfiram) type of reaction in patients on oral agents. Three percent of patients on chlorpropamide develop hyponatremia that is related to a potentiating effect of the drug on the action of antidiuretic hormone. Long-term use of oral agents has recently come under scrutiny since the University Diabetes Group Program Study was published in 1970, in which the authors noted an increase in cardiovascular mortality rate in patients on tolbutamide and more strikingly in patients on phenformin, as compared with placebo- or insulin-treated groups. Although certain statistical and design problems have made this study controversial, at present the oral agents must be considered to have a limited role in diabetic therapy.

Insulin

Insulin therapy is used in ketosis-prone diabetics who remain symptomatic on dietary control. The dose required is highly variable in given individuals. In the absence of a metabolic crisis, therapy is usually begun with a dose of 15 to 20 units of an intermediate duration insulin each morning, and dose adjustment is made by following blood and urine glucose determinations. Various types of insulin are listed in Table 59-10.

Proper testing of double-voided urine specimens is essential if urine testing is to be used to gauge diabetic control. The physician should also assess the patient's renal threshold for glucose by obtaining

Table 59-9. Sulfonylureas Used in Long-Term Therapy of Diabetes

Name of drug	Dose form	Dose range per day	Duration of action (hr)	Site of metabolism
Tolbutamide	500-mg tablets	500 mg−3,000 mg	6	Liver
Acetohexamide	250-mg and 500-mg tablets	250 mg−1,500 mg	12	Kidney, liver
Tolazamide	100-mg and 250-mg tablets	100 mg−750 mg	12−16	Liver, kidney
Chlorpropamide	100-mg and 250-mg tablets	100 mg−750 mg	36	Kidney

Table 59-10. Insulin Preparations Used in Therapy of Diabetes

Type of insulin	Route	Peak hypoglycemia	Duration (hr)
Short duration			
Crystalline zinc (regular)	IV, IM, SQ	30–60 min	4–6
Semilente	SQ	60 min	6–8
NPH (neutral protamine hagedorn)	SQ	8–12 hr	22–24
Lente	SQ	8–12 hr	22–24
Long duration			
PZI (protamine zinc insulin)	SQ	12–18 hr	36
Ultralente	SQ	12–18 hr	36

concomitant urine and serum glucose measurements. Approximately 50 percent of patients will be maintained with good control on a single dose of intermediate duration insulin per day. In patients in whom a single A.M. dose does not give good control, dietary manipulation, the addition of a short or very long lasting insulin, and divided doses of insulin (two or more) may be useful.

Problems of Insulin Therapy. The following are some of the common problems in therapy of diabetes with insulin.

1. Diabetic edema: Edema is occasionally seen during the initial weeks of therapy of diabetes. It is self-limited, but it may be treated with diuretics.
2. Hypoglycemia: Hypoglycemia is the single most important problem associated with insulin therapy; all diabetic patients should be instructed in how to recognize its symptoms. They should carry an identification card at all times and an identification bracelet or necklace. A relative should be instructed in the administration of glucagon for hypoglycemic coma. Patients should be warned that alcohol, decreased caloric intake, or unusually vigorous exercise can precipitate hypoglycemia.
3. The Somogyi phenomenon: With wide swings of blood glucose from hyperglycemia to hypoglycemia or from very high glucose concentrations to less high glucose concentrations, the body responds by mustering various diabetogenic substances. This results in rebound hyperglycemia and transient insulin resistance. If this problem goes unrecognized, the patient and physician may respond by progressively increasing insulin dosage and increasing insulin resistance. If a good history cannot be obtained for hypoglycemia in patients who appear to have increasing insulin requirements over a short period of time, then one should proceed by testing early morning double-voided urine for glucose and adjusting the insulin dosage accordingly. If this is not helpful, the patient should be hospitalized for observation with frequent blood glucose measurements over a 24-hour period. In stable patients, a therapeutic trial of slowly decreasing doses of insulin may be tried at home.
4. Allergy: Approximately 10 percent of patients will have allergic phenomena associated with insulin, usually hives and pruritis. Allergy generally occurs within the first year of therapy, but it generally resolves in a few weeks on continued therapy. If necessary, the patient can be treated with antihistamines prior to insulin injection. Very rarely, more severe phenomena occur and desensitization may be required.
5. Insulin resistance: True insulin resistance is rare and results from multiple causes. Perhaps the most common is systemic infection, which can lead to profound resistance. There are certain syndromes characterized by insulin insensitivity, such as lipotrophic diabetes and a syndrome most often seen in women and associated with acanthosis nigricans. In the latter, there is a very severe deficiency in insulin receptors. All patients on insulin therapy for more than a few weeks at a time have antibodies directed against insulin. This is usually of no clinical importance. Occasionally high titers of antibodies directed against insulin

result in insulin insensitivity. Generally, patients on insulin bind less than 20 units of insulin per liter of plasma and require less than 150 units of insulin per day. In antibody-mediated resistance causing ketoacidosis, insulin dosage should be doubled every hour until a response occurs. This may require thousands of units per day. Treatment with glucocorticoids leads to a rapid reversal of this condition. At least 60 mg of prednisone per day is usually necessary, and great care must be exercised as the insulin requirement decreases.

Hypoglycemia

As a person passes from the fed to the fasting state, the metabolic set of the body switches from storing to generating glucose. While most of the body's energy production during a fast is a result of free fatty acid oxidation, adequate blood glucose levels are required for normal neural function. Early in a fast the brain uses almost exclusively glucose, but as the central nervous system accommodates to the fasting state, oxidation of ketone bodies by the brain increases in importance as an energy source. Initially the majority (75 to 85 percent) of glucose is supplied by glycogenolysis in the liver. Within 24 to 48 hours, however, hepatic glycogen stores are depleted and gluconeogenesis becomes the primary source of glucose. In a prolonged fast, the kidney can provide more than 25 percent of gluconeogenesis. However, the liver supplies virtually 100 percent of the glucose needed in a short fast.

In man, there are three major substrates for gluconeogenesis. Glycerol, derived from the breakdown of triglyceride, accounts for only a small portion of glucose production. Lactate is recycled to glucose by the liver (in resting man up to 30 percent of glucose used in anaerobic metabolism is recycled by this pathway). Probably the most important substrate in man for new glucose formation are the amino acids, especially alanine. A cycle has been proposed in which glucose is metabolized in muscle to pyruvate and then transaminated to alanine and returned to the liver for resynthesis to glucose. Alanine may also result from oxidation of other amino acids in muscle, and it may serve to bind ammonia, which is produced during exercise. Glucose synthesis is controlled by substrate levels and the effects of various hormones.

During a fast, glucose concentrations in the male will fall by about 15 mg to 60 to 65 mg per 100 ml and stabilize by 72 hours. In females, however, levels may reach 30 to 35 mg per 100 ml without any evidence of concurrent disease. Blood sugar levels of 40 to 50 mg per 100 ml in women should not be diagnosed as hypoglycemia unless they are associated with symptoms of epinephrine discharge, neurologic dysfunction, or both, and preferably there should be evidence of a biologic response to hypoglycemia such as elevations in the serum cortisol and glucagon. Sympathetic discharge is initiated by a rapid fall in the blood glucose, usually to levels below 40 mg per 100 ml. The autonomic symptoms include tachycardia, anxiety, sweating, and tremor. Central nervous system symptoms include confusion, bizarre behavior, seizures, or coma.

SPECIFIC CAUSES OF HYPOGLYCEMIA

It is useful to divide hypoglycemia into 3 large overlapping categories, as listed below.

I. Fasting hypoglycemia
  A. Nonpancreatic tumors
  B. Liver disease and renal disease
    1. Acquired
    2. Congenital
      a. Glycogen storage
      b. Galactosemia
  C. Alcohol and other hypoglycemic drugs
  D. Endocrine deficiencies
  E. Insulinomas
  F. Exercise, inanition
  G. Ketogenic hypoglycemia of childhood
II. Postprandial hypoglycemia
  A. Reactive functional
  B. Reactive — early diabetes
  C. Alimentary hypoglycemia
  D. Leucine sensitivity
  E. Hereditary fructose intolerance
III. Exogenous hypoglycemia
  A. Iatrogenic
  B. Factitious

Disorders that lead to fasting hypoglycemia are in general more serious than those that cause postprandial hypoglycemia.

Fasting Hypoglycemia

Maintenance of the blood glucose during a fast requires adequate substrate delivery, adequate hepatic function in terms of both gluconeogenesis and glycogenolysis, adequate hormonal set, and utilization of glucose matched by production rates. Any or all these steps may be defective in a fasting hypoglycemia.

Usually, inadequate substrate delivery leading to hypoglycemia is a problem of childhood and accounts for ketotic hypoglycemia of children. Children have a relatively low muscle mass and have been found to have decreased alanine levels during a fast accompanied by ketonemia; alanine infusion corrects this. In adults, inadequate substrate delivery may contribute to fasting hypoglycemia occasionally in pregnancy, and rarely in uremia.

Fasting hypoglycemia due to liver disease generally occurs in severe, diffuse liver disease such as a fulminant hepatitis. Congestive hepatomegaly can also be associated with hypoglycemia. Inherited causes of hepatic hypoglycemia will be discussed later. Because of the role of the liver as the major organ of glucose uptake after a meal as well as of glucose production during a fast, liver disease is associated with a pattern of fasting hypoglycemia and postprandial glucose intolerance.

Alcohol is the most common drug-related cause of hypoglycemia, especially when it occurs in a setting of poor nutrition. Gluconeogenesis is decreased by alcohol, at least partially, by increasing the NADH/NAD ratio, which inhibits phosphoenolpyruvate carboxykinase, a limiting enzymatic step in gluconeogenesis.

Cortisol deficiency is occasionally complicated by fasting hypoglycemia; much less frequently, growth hormone or thyroid deficiencies are associated with this problem (see Chaps. 56 and 58).

Tumors. About 50 percent of extrapancreatic tumors associated with hypoglycemia are mesenchymal tumors of the abdomen or thorax; these are generally larger than a kilogram in size. Other such hypoglycemic tumors include heptatoma, adrenocortical carcinoma, lymphoma, and gastrointestinal epithelial tumors as well as assorted other neoplasms. These tumors do not produce insulin, and hypoglycemia is associated with appropriately low insulin levels. Hypoglycemia in these patients is probably the result of a variety of causes. In some cases there is excessive glucose utilization by the tumor itself; in others, elevated levels of nonsuppressible insulin-like activity can be demonstrated. In most such cases these tumors seem to produce substances that inhibit gluconeogenesis.

Approximately 10 percent of pancreatic insulinomas are malignant, and 15 to 20 percent show diffuse nodules throughout the pancreas. These tumors often secrete unusual proportions of proinsulin, leading to much higher levels of immunoreactive insulin than the degree of hypoglycemia would indicate. This is rarely useful as a diagnostic test. Rarely bronchogenic, adrenal, or carcinoid tumors secrete insulin.

The diagnosis of hypoglycemia secondary to an insulin-secreting tumor (insulinoma) relies on a demonstration of an abnormal fasting insulin-glucose ratio, an increased responsiveness to various secretogogues, and a failure to decrease insulin levels while glucose concentrations are falling. A glucose tolerance test per se is not usually helpful in making this diagnosis. Approximately 50 percent of these individuals oversecrete insulin in response to glucose. Obesity even without insulinoma also causes hypersecretion. Any pattern of carbohydrate tolerance can be seen with insulinoma. If spontaneous fasting hypoglycemia is present in a nonobese individual, the demonstration of an insulin-glucose ratio of greater than 0.3 is strongly suggestive of insulinoma. Periodic observation of glucose and insulin levels while glucose concentrations are falling in obese as well as normal weight individuals usually demonstrates falling insulin levels.

Fish insulin injection can be used diagnostically to precipitate hypoglycemia. Since this insulin is biologically potent in man but is not measurable by the usual radioimmunoassay, the insulin concentrations which are then measured reflect endogenous insulin responses to the hypoglycemia. Insulinoma patients do not decrease their insulin levels appropriately. Intravenous tolbutamide testing serves to measure stimulated insulin secretion. (A positive test insulin increment is $>$ than 110 μU/ml.) Insulin levels during hypoglycemia can be monitored 30 to 120

Table 59-11. Glycogen Storage Disease

Type	Eponym	Organ involvement	Enzyme defect	Glycogen	Hypoglycemia	Clinical picture
I	Von Gierke	Liver; kidney	Glucose 6-phosphatase	Normal	++	Early onset, ↑ liver, xanthomas
II	Pompe	General	1,4-Glucosidase	Normal	0	Hypotonia, cardiomegaly
III	Cori	Liver, muscle, heart, RBC	Amylo-1,6-glucosidase	Abnormal	++	Similar to type I but milder
IV	Andersen's	Liver, WBC	1,4-Glucan 6-glycosyl transferase	Abnormal	0	Hypotonia, hepatosplenomegaly, cirrhosis
V	McArdle's	Muscle	Phosphorylase	Normal	0	Muscle cramps, with exercise, myoglobinuria
VI	Hers	Liver, WBC	Phosphorylase	Normal	+	Like I, less severe
VII	.....	Muscle, RBC	Phosphofructokinase	Normal	0	Like V
VIII	.....	Liver, WBC	Phosphoribosylkinase	Normal	0	Hepatomegaly

Note: RBC = red blood cells; WBC = white blood cells.

minutes after the injection of tolbutamide. Oral leucine, which does not produce hypoglycemia in normal individuals, raises insulin levels by greater than 15 μU per milliliter in 50 percent of insulinoma patients; obesity does not influence the leucine test. Glucagon, an insulin secretogogue, produces excess insulin release in 50 percent of such patients, but obesity may cause a false-positive result. One may have to resort to prolonged fasting (up to 72 hours) to precipitate hypoglycemia in insulinoma patients. The object of this study is to observe insulin regulation during hypoglycemia; mere demonstration of hypoglycemia alone is not sufficient.

Postprandial Hypoglycemia

Hypoglycemia commonly occurs postprandially, and it usually represents abnormalities in the timing of insulin release in relation to the absorption of foodstuffs. Rare patients are simply hypersensitive to the normal insulin-releasing activity of certain substrates such as leucine or have inhibited glucose production secondary to fructose ingestion. Hypoglycemia in the early part of a glucose tolerance test (occurring at 90 to 120 minutes) is associated with alimentary hypoglycemia. This occurs after gastrectomy or may be secondary to poorly defined abnormalities of the stomach and duodenum. Hypoglycemia occurring later (4 to 5 hours) in an individual with carbohydrate intolerance is occasionally an early sign of diabetes mellitus and is related to a delayed insulin release. The majority of patients with late hypoglycemia have no obvious cause. Functional hypoglycemia is a difficult diagnosis to make, because 17 percent of men and 15 percent of women will decrease their blood sugar to 50 mg per 100 ml at 4 hours during an oral glucose tolerance test. The diagnosis must rest on objective findings of signs and symptoms of hypoglycemia, preferably confirmed by a rise in catecholamines, human growth hormone, cortisol, or glucagon.

Treatment of reactive hypoglycemia generally starts with a low carbohydrate diet with at least six small feedings throughout the day. Propranolol (Inderal) therapy has been effective in some cases, and others have responded to anticholinergic agents.

Factitious hypoglycemia is a difficult problem.

In such cases a thorough room search will reveal insulin syringes or hypoglycemic agents. Since individuals not on insulin do not have circulating anti-insulin antibodies, detection of antibody is diagnostic of exogenous insulin administration.

Glycogen Storage Disease (see Table 59-11). Control of glycogen synthesis and catabolism is under tight hormonal and metabolic control.

$$\text{Glycogen} \underset{\substack{\text{glycogen} \\ \text{synthetase}}}{\overset{\text{phosphorylase}}{\rightleftharpoons}} \text{glucose 1-phosphate}$$

$$\longrightarrow \text{glucose 6-phosphate} \xrightarrow[\text{glucose 6-phosphatase}]{} \text{glucose}$$

Glycogen consists of a long chain of glucose molecules linked at the 1,4 position with periodic branches at the 1,6 position. Various diseases associated with a failure to break down glycogen, with the formation of an abnormal glycogen, or with the failure to release glucose into the bloodstream have all been described.

Bibliography

Alberti, K., Hockaday, T., and Turner, R. Small doses of intramuscular insulin in the treatment of diabetic coma. *Lancet* 2:515, 1973.

Arieff, A. I., and Carroll, H. J. Nonketotic hyperosmolar coma with hyperglycemia. *Medicine* 51:73, 1972.

Beigelman, P. M. Severe diabetic ketoacidosis (diabetic coma). *Diabetes* 20:490, 1971.

Bressler, R., and Galloway, J. A. Insulin treatment of diabetes mellitus. *Med. Clin. North Am.* 55: 861, 1971.

Broder, L. C., and Carter, S. K. Pancreatic islet cell carcinoma. *Ann. Intern. Med.* 79:101, 1973.

Butler, A. M., Talbot, N. B., Burnett, C. H., Stanberry, J. B., and MacLachlan, E. A. Metabolic studies in diabetic coma. *Trans. Assoc. Am. Physicians* 60:102, 1947.

Cooperman, M. T., Davidoff, F., Spark, R., and Palotta, J. Clinical studies of alcoholic ketoacidosis. *Diabetes* 23:433, 1974.

Fajans, S. S., and Sussman, K. E. (eds.). *Diabetes Mellitus: Diagnosis and Treatment*. Vol. 3.

New York: American Diabetes Association, Inc., 1971.

Felig, P. The glucose-alanine cycle. *Metabolism* 22:179, 1973.

Gabbay, K. H. Hyperglycemia, polyol metabolism, and complications of diabetes mellitus. *Annu. Rev. Med.* 26:521, 1975.

Howell, R. R. The Glycogen Storage Diseases. In J. B. Stanbury, J. B. Wyngaarden, and D. S. Fredrickson (eds.), *The Metabolic Basis of Inherited Diseases* (3rd ed.). New York: McGraw-Hill, 1972.

Kidson, W., Casey, J., Kraegen, E., and Lazarus, L. Treatment of severe diabetes mellitus by insulin infusion. *Br. Med. J.* 2:691, 1974.

Levy, L. F., Duga, M., Girgis, M., and Gordon, E. Ketoacidosis associated with alcoholism in nondiabetic patients with lactic acidosis. *Ann. Intern. Med.* 78:213, 1973.

McCurdy, D. K. Hyperosmolar hyperglycemic non-ketotic diabetic coma. *Med. Clin. North Am.* 54:683, 1970.

Nabarro, J. D. N., Spencer, A. G., and Stowers, J. M. Metabolic studies in severe diabetic ketoacidosis. *Q. J. Med.* 21:225, 1952.

Page, M. M., Alberti, K. G., Greenwood, R., Gumaa, K., et al. Treatment of diabetic coma with continuous low dose infusion of insulin. *Br. Med. J.* 2:687, 1974.

Roth, J., Prout, T., Goldfine, I., Wolfe, S. M., et al. Sulfonureas: Effects in vivo and in vitro. *Ann. Intern. Med.* 75:607, 1971.

Schein, P., Delellis, R., Kahn, C., Gorden, P., and Kraft, A. Islet cell tumors — current concepts and management. *Ann. Intern. Med.* 79:239, 1973.

Spiro, R. G. Biochemistry of the renal glomerular basement membrane and its alterations in diabetes mellitus. *N. Engl. J. Med.* 288:1337, 1973.

Steinke, J., and Taylor, K. Viruses and etiology of diabetes mellitus. *Diabetes* 237:631, 1974.

60

Disorders of Calcium Metabolism and the Parathyroid Glands

Robert M. Levin

Calcium Metabolism

Calcium plays a major role in many fundamental biologic processes such as nerve conduction, muscle contraction, enzyme activity, and blood coagulation; it also acts as the feedback mediator for the hormones parathormone and calcitonin. In addition, calcium is the essential structural component of the skeleton where most of the 1-Kg total of body calcium is located. The 4 to 6 gm of calcium contained in the rapidly exchangeable skeletal pool plays an important role in maintaining the serum calcium within its normal range of 8.8 to 10.5 mg per 100 ml, as measured by atomic absorption spectrophotometry. The normal diet in the United States contains about 1 gm of calcium daily, and of that amount, 25 to 35 percent is absorbed. However, this amount may vary considerably, depending on the dietary content of calcium and vitamin D, the patient's age, and even the season of the year. Despite the wide fluctuations that may occur in dietary calcium intake, the 24-hour urinary calcium excretion remains within rather narrow limits, 80 to 250 mg. Fecal calcium, on the other hand, is linearly related to calcium intake. The complex system whereby serum calcium is closely controlled will be described below.

Physiology of the Parathyroid Hormone and Vitamin D

The principal function of parathormone (PTH) is to maintain a normal blood calcium. Specifically, PTH prevents hypocalcemia by the following effects: (1) acceleration of bone resorption — there is evidence of a direct stimulating effect of PTH on both the proliferation of new osteoclasts and the metabolic activity of preexisting osteoclasts; (2) enhancement of renal reabsorption of calcium; and (3) promotion of gastrointestinal absorption of calcium, primarily in the duodenum. These three actions of PTH result from an activation of membrane-bound adenyl cyclase, and an intracellular increase in concentration of cyclic AMP (adenosine 3′:5′-cyclic phosphate); their regulation is related to the inter-relationship of PTH with vitamin D, as described below (see Fig. 60-1).

Ultraviolet irradiation of the 7-dehydrocholesterol in the skin converts it to vitamin D_3 (also called cholecalciferol). Vitamin D_3, whether derived from the skin or taken in the diet, must then undergo two enzymatic hydroxylations before it can produce its full biologic action at the target organs. In the liver, vitamin D_3 is converted to the polar metabolite 25-hydroxyvitamin (also called 25-hydroxy-cholecalciferol, hereafter referred to as 25-HCC). The 25-HCC is then transported to the kidney, where it undergoes a second hydroxylation and 1α,25-dihydroxycholecalciferol (hereafter referred to as 1,25-DHCC), the principal metabolically active form of vitamin D_3, is synthesized. This metabolite is much more active than 25-HCC in both mobilization of bone calcium and in intestinal calcium transport. Evidence of the importance of 1,25-DHCC in calcium metabolism is given in the demonstration that nephrectomized vitamin D-deficient animals show no intestinal calcium tranport response or bone calcium mobilization response to physiologic doses of 25-HCC, but such animals respond in a normal fashion to administered 1,25-DHCC.

The evidence noted above — that 1,25-DHCC is synthesized in the kidney and has its function in distant organs, the gut and bone — demonstrates that 1,25-DHCC should be regarded as a hormone. The synthesis of 1,25-DHCC is stimulated by several factors: PTH, hypocalcemia, and hypophosphatemia. Since PTH regulation is well known to be controlled by the level of the serum ionized calcium, PTH then represents the trophic hormone that stimulates the production of 1,25-DHCC in response to a decrease in the calcium level.

The production of 1,25-DHCC may be related to the renal tubular cell concentration of inorganic phosphorus. Renal tubular phosphate depletion, as reflected by a low serum phosphorus level, may directly stimulate the increased synthesis of 1,25-DHCC. Since PTH is a phosphate diuretic (blocks phosphate reabsorption by the kidney), this

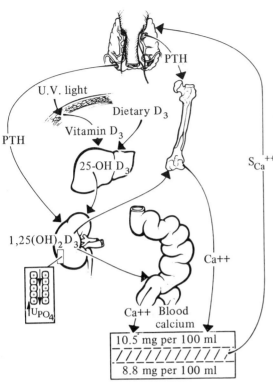

Figure 60-1. Interrelationship between vitamin D and parathyroid hormone.

may be the mechanism whereby PTH stimulates the increased production of 1,25-DHCC.

Calcitonin

In 1961 Copp perfused the thyroid and parathyroid glands of dogs with blood that had a high concentration of calcium and produced a fall in their serum calcium levels that was more rapid than that following a total parathyroidectomy. A calcium-lowering hormone called calcitonin and referred to here as CT was postulated and later was shown to be synthesized and secreted by the parafollicular cells (also called C cells) of the thyroid gland (see Chap. 58). Chemically, CT is a single-chain polypeptide made up of 32 amino acids. In comparing the amino acid sequences of CT from various species, the first nine amino acid residues appear to be necessary for biologic activity. However, the complete polypeptide is essential for full biologic activity.

It is still debatable whether CT has a physiologic role in man. Histologic examination of bone of patients treated with CT reveals a marked decrease in the number of osteoclasts, which explains the effectiveness of CT in the treatment of Paget's disease. Calcitonin has also been shown to be antagonistic to osteoclastic stimulators such as PTH. Factors affecting secretion of CT include calcium, magnesium, various gastrointestinal hormones, and the drug streptomycin and related compounds. However, the principal stimulus to CT production is clearly an elevated serum calcium, which increases both the synthesis and the secretion of CT. The following hormones have also been shown to raise the circulating levels of CT: gastrin, pancreozymin, glucagon, and pentagastrin.

SITE AND MECHANISM OF ACTION
Calcitonin acts primarily by inhibiting bone resorption; the mechanism is unknown. Although CT does inhibit PTH-induced bone resorption, its hypocalcemic effect is not due to this, because it is fully active even in parathyroidectomized rats. The gastrointestinal absorption of calcium and phosphate may be decreased by CT due to an inhibition of the conversion of 25-HCC to 1,25-DHCC by CT. On the other hand, CT causes increased jejunal secretion of sodium, potassium, chloride, and water. In the kidney, CT increases the urinary excretion of calcium, phosphate, sodium, and chloride. The physiologic significance of the natriuresis is not known. The kidney does, however, play a major role in the degradation of CT, which has a plasma half-life of only 15 minutes.

CLINICAL APPLICATION
Because of its calcium-lowering ability, CT has been tried in the treatment of hypercalcemia. However, it produces only a transitory decrease in serum calcium levels, its maximal effect is slowly reached, and the responses, in general, are quite variable. On the other hand, CT has been quite successful in the treatment of Paget's disease of bone (see Chap. 61). Serum levels of CT as measured by radioimmunoassay may be elevated in medullary carcinoma of the thyroid (see Chap. 58). Calcitonin levels may also be helpful in assessing the completeness of surgical removal of a thyroid medullary carcinoma and in diagnosing the

presence of recurrences. Basal levels of CT of thyroid origin have also been found to be elevated in bronchogenic carcinomas associated with bony metastases. Ectopic production of CT has also been reported in oat cell carcinoma of the lung.

Hypercalcemia

Considering that the extracellular fluid space normally contains only 0.1 percent of the total body calcium, it is not surprising that hypercalcemia may be produced by a large number of conditions, as listed below:

1. Excess parathyroid hormone
   a. Primary hyperparathyroidism
   b. Tertiary hyperparathyroidism
   c. Pseudohyperparathyroidism (ectopic PTH syndrome)
2. Excess vitamin D or abnormal sensitivity
   a. Vitamin D intoxication
   b. Sarcoidosis
   c. Idiopathic hypercalcemia of childhood
3. Increased bone turnover
   a. Malignancies with bone metastases (e.g., multiple myeloma, breast)
   b. Malignancies without bone metastases (e.g., hypernephroma producing prostaglandins)
   c. Thyrotoxicosis
   d. Immobilization (especially in patients with Paget's disease of bone)
   e. Tuberculosis
   f. Coccidioidomycosis
   g. Vitamin A intoxication
4. Miscellaneous
   a. Milk-alkali syndrome
   b. Adrenal insufficiency
   c. Thiazide diuretics
   d. Prolonged use of a tourniquet prior to drawing blood
   e. Rhabdomyolysis associated with acute renal failure

Elevated blood calcium levels are being increasingly recognized due to the multiphasic screening tests that are now being performed in many hospitals and clinics throughout the country. Patients with hypercalcemia may be totally asymptomatic, the blood test being done as part of a routine checkup, or they may present a varied assortment of symptoms, possibly including (1) general malaise, fatigue, lassitude, and weakness; (2) polydipsia, nocturia, and renal colic; (3) constipation, anorexia, epigastric pain, nausea, and vomiting; and (4) lethargy, drowsiness, confusion, psychosis, stupor, and coma. Although a history of recurrent kidney stones may alert the physician to order a serum calcium, many of the above symptoms may not readily suggest hypercalcemia. When the serum calcium exceeds 16 mg per 100 ml, a true medical emergency exists and treatment must be started immediately. This hypercalcemic crisis is characterized by intractable nausea and vomiting, abdominal pain, oliguria, circulatory collapse, myocardial necrosis, cerebral (and other) thromboses, progressive obtundation, and coma.

Although many conditions may cause hypercalcemia, metastatic cancer (especially breast cancer) in bone and multiple myeloma make up 55 percent of the cases; primary hyperparathyroidism, 20 percent; and pseudohyperparathyroidism (ectopic PTH syndrome), 15 percent; the remaining 10 percent are due to one of the conditions in the list above. A bone scan, skeletal x-rays, serum and urine electrophoresis studies, and a bone marrow aspiration will be of great value in making the proper diagnosis in most cases of hypercalcemia. The proper diagnostic tests to rule out conditions such as thyrotoxicosis, sarcoidosis, and adrenal insufficiency are relatively straightforward. An elevated level of serum immunoreactive PTH rules out metastatic disease to bone but may not differentiate primary hyperparathyroidism from pseudohyperparathyroidism.

Pseudohyperparathyroidism refers to the presence of nonparathyroid tumors that produce a PTH-like material. Hypernephromas and bronchogenic carcinomas account for 60 percent of these neoplasms, with many of the remaining 40 percent being tumors involving the urogenital tract, liver, pancreas, lymph nodes, esophagus, colon, and parotid gland. In attempting to distinguish pseudohyperparathyroidism from primary hyperparathyroidism, the following features strongly favor a diagnosis of pseudohyperparathyroidism: a rapidly progressive illness with marked weight loss, anemia, urinary calcium over 500 mg per day, a markedly elevated sedimentation rate, an increased alkaline phosphatase (in the presence of a normal bone scan), the presence of a metabolic alkalosis, and a serum calcium over 14 mg per 100 ml. These patients often fail to have a history of renal calculi, pancreatitis, or peptic ulcer disease because they do not live long enough to develop these complications, which actually are more characteristic of long-standing hypercalcemia. The clinical features of primary hyperparathyroidism will be discussed later in this chapter.

Management of Hypercalcemia. The treatment of hypercalcemia depends on the patient's serum calcium and clinical condition. If the patient does not appear acutely ill and the serum calcium is less than 13 mg per 100 ml, hydration with normal saline may be all that is necessary until the proper diagnostic tests are performed. However, moderate or severe hyper-calcemia in a symptomatic patient must be treated more aggressively and without delay. Volume de-pletion must be treated first. The polyuria produced by the hypercalcemia leads to excessive loss of salt and water, which is complicated by the patient's in-ability to take fluids by mouth due to the associated anorexia, nausea, and vomiting. This results in con-traction of the extracellular space and a further in-crease in the concentration of the calcium and phos-phorus in the blood. Precipitation of calcium phos-phate crystals (microthrombi) may then occur in small vessels throughout the body and produce pan-creatitis, pulmonary thromboses, or focal neurologic abnormalities. Therefore intravenous saline should be given rapidly while carefully monitoring the patient's central venous pressure and urinary output. A marked natriuresis should ensue, accompanied by a proportional increase in urinary calcium. Intravenous furosemide may also be given to produce further increases in urinary sodium and calcium. Urine volume and urinary sodium and potassium measure-ments should be made frequently in order to deter-mine the proper rate of fluid administration and electrolyte replacement.

Phosphate therapy may have to be added if the above regimen fails to lower the serum calcium. Phosphates are thought to promote the deposition of calcium into the skeleton and soft tissues. Oral phosphate therapy can be used (2 to 4 gm daily in divided doses) or, if necessary, intravenous phosphate (Inphos [disodium monopotassium phosphate] may be given). It is recommended that one begin with 50 mM Inphos (containing 1.55 gm phosphorus) intravenously. The serum calcium must be measured at frequent intervals, since there is no way of pre-dicting the response to phosphate therapy in a given patient. Complications of phosphate therapy include heart failure (due to a too-rapid drop in myocardial calcium with decreased myocardial contractility), phlebitis, and soft tissue and vascular calcifications. Hyperphosphatemia is a relative contraindication to phosphate therapy. However, if the patient is acutely ill, has a very high serum calcium, and has cardiac or kidney failure or both, intravenous phosphate therapy or hemodialysis or both may be required.

Steroids are beneficial in patients in whom the hypercalcemia is associated with vitamin D intoxica-tion, sarcoidosis, or certain malignancies. Up to 80 mg of prednisone per day in divided doses is required. However, the rate of response to steroids is so variable that in an emergency situation saline and phosphates are the preferred therapy.

Mithramycin, a cytostatic antibiotic useful in the treatment of testicular tumors, may be given as a single intravenous dose of 25 μg per kilogram of body weight. As with the steroids, the response to mithra-mycin is variable and unpredictable; one cannot predict either the onset or the duration of the hypo-calcemic effect of mithramycin. In addition, mithramycin is potentially a dangerous drug that is capable of causing bleeding problems.

Parathyroid and Related Diseases

The parathyroid glands are derived from the third and fourth branchial pouches. The total weight of the four glands is about 120 mg, with the mean size of a single gland being 5 x 5 x 3 mm. The glands are reddish or yellowish brown in color, each having a distinct stalk through which runs the supplying blood vessels and nerves. The parathyroid glands contain three types of cells: (1) chief cells, which produce PTH, (2) oxyphil (Hürthle) cells, which have no known function, and (3) *wasserhelle*, or water-clear, cells, which are present in small numbers in the normal gland but which may increase in number and produce

PTH in certain hyperplastic glands. The four para-thyroids are usually located on the posterior surface of the thyroid gland, but there may be as few as two and as many as ten in a given individual. It is important that the physician who does parathyroid surgery be aware that up to 10 percent of the parathyroid glands are situated in aberrant locations such as elsewhere in the neck or in the mediastinum.

Chemically, PTH is a single-chain polypeptide made up of 84 amino acids. There is a free alpha-amino group on the amino-terminal residue. It has been shown that the amino-terminal position is critical for biologic activity and that peptide fragments shorter than 2 to 27 amino acids have no biologic activity. Although a specific radioimmunoassay for bovine PTH cross reacts well albeit not completely with human PTH, it has been demonstrated that circulating immunoreactive PTH is heterogeneous, consisting of a family of related peptides of different sizes. The unavailability of sufficient human PTH to serve as a completely satisfactory reference standard (bovine and porcine PTH having been used in most immunoassays) has made clinicians somewhat wary of overinterpreting PTH values in a given patient. However, despite the problems of heterogeneity of the circulating PTH and the lack of a uniform standard of human PTH, certain clinical applications of the radioimmunoassay are useful: (1) Comparing the PTH levels obtained from selective catheterization of the right and left superior and inferior thyroidal veins may be helpful in locating an adenoma or in demonstrating the presence of so-called four-gland hyperplasia. (2) In hypercalcemic patients, a greater concentration of immunoassayable hormone found in the veins draining the thyroid as compared to the peripheral circulation favors a diagnosis of primary hyperparathyroidism rather than pseudohyperparathyroidism. (3) In the differential diagnosis of hypocalcemia, an elevated PTH level may help prove that the patient has a condition leading to secondary hyperparathyroidism such as chronic renal insufficiency and malabsorption. (4) Patients with hypercalcemia due to vitamin D intoxication, sarcoidosis, multiple myeloma, and many other tumors with bone metastases will have undetectable plasma PTH levels.

CLASSIFICATION OF HYPERPARATHYROIDISM

Hyperparathyroidism may be classified as a primary, secondary, or tertiary disorder. Primary or autonomous hyperparathyroidism refers to neoplasia of one or more of the parathyroid glands, that develops as a primary event for reasons not presently understood. Autonomy of the parathyroids is defined as the persistence of PTH secretion in the face of hypercalcemia; however, it does not necessarily imply that the rate of secretion has become totally unresponsive to changes in the serum calcium concentration. Secondary or compensatory hyperparathyroidism refers to hyperplasia of all four glands that occurs as a physiologically appropriate response to chronic hypocalcemia. The serum calcium is usually normal, or it may be slightly decreased in this condition. Occasionally secondary hyperplasia of the parathyroids may progress to autonomy as a result of either adenomatous change or a marked increase in the total mass of parathyroid tissue. In this instance the serum calcium becomes elevated and the condition is referred to as tertiary hyperparathyroidism.

Primary Hyperparathyroidism

Pathology, Etiology, and Incidence. Approximately 90 percent of patients with primary hyperparathyroidism have a single parathyroid adenoma. The remaining 10 percent have multiple adenomas, chief cell hyperplasia, clear cell hyperplasia, or carcinoma. The cause of parathyroid hyperplasia or adenoma is unknown, though occasionally there may be co-existent hyperplasia or adenomas of multiple endocrine glands, particularly of the pancreas and pituitary. Rarely, hyperparathyroidism is familial. It occurs in approximately 0.1 percent of patients seeking medical attention and is said to occur in as many as 5 to 10 percent of patients with calcium-containing renal stones. Primary hyperparathyroidism is two to three times as frequent in women as men and occurs most commonly between ages 30 and 60.

Clinical Features. The clinical manifestations of primary hyperparathyroidism may be exceedingly diverse. The patient may be totally asymptomatic;

more often, however, he has mild and nonspecific complaints such as fatigue, lassitude, and weakness that remain unappreciated, often for many years. Rarely, severe hypercalcemia develops rapidly, progressing to the hypercalcemic crisis already described. In order to summarize the clinical features of hyperparathyroidism in some sort of orderly fashion, the features are grouped in the following categories: hypercalcemia and symptoms directly related to the elevated blood calcium level; abnormal deposition of calcium in tissues; and the effects of increased bone resorption.

Hypercalcemia may give rise to a number of neuropsychiatric symptoms such as lassitude, irritability, depression, decreased recent memory, headaches, and personality change. Neuromuscular findings may include easy fatigability and weakness of the proximal muscles, particularly of the lower extremities. An increased calcium level has also been demonstrated to lead to gastric hypersecretion.

Abnormal deposition of calcium in tissues may be demonstrated in the kidney as calculi or nephrocalcinosis, either of which can lead to pyelonephritis, hypertension, and renal insufficiency. In the eye, macroscopic patches of calcium may be deposited in the conjunctiva and at the 3 o'clock and 9 o'clock positions in the exposed cornea adjacent to the limbus (band keratopathy). Calcification may also occur in joint capsules, tendons, and articular cartilages. Pancreatitis may result from an increased calcium content of the pancreatic secretions, which leads to calcium precipitation and duct obstruction.

Bone disease, both symptomatic and on x-ray, is less frequently being seen in primary hyperparathyroidism, probably because the diagnosis is being made earlier than was formerly the case. Radioisotopic techniques, however, reveal an increased bone resorption in nearly all patients. This increase in the rate of bone destruction may result in generalized demineralization (the skull gives a fuzzy appearance resembling ground glass), cyst formation (particularly in the hands, feet, ribs, pelvis, and jaw), and subperiosteal resorption of cortical bone. Subperiosteal resorption, the most specific x-ray abnormality, is best seen on the radial aspect of the middle phalanges of the middle and ring fingers. Vascular masses of osteoblasts and osteoclasts, called brown tumors, may mimic bone cysts on x-ray. And, in patients with good oral hygiene, absence of the lamina dura around the roots of the teeth is a helpful diagnostic finding. On bone biopsy, a single section may show evidence of excessive resorption (osteoporosis, osteitis fibrosa), excessive and disordered formation (osteosclerosis), and incomplete calcification (osteomalacia).

Carcinoma makes up less than 2 percent of functioning parathyroid tumors, but it may give rise to marked hypercalcemia. Whereas parathyroid adenomas are rarely palpable preoperatively, more than half of parathyroid carcinomas are sufficiently large to be palpable.

Diagnosis. Hyperparathyroidism can be suspected clinically, but the diagnosis requires laboratory confirmation. An elevated serum calcium is still the most important single diagnostic feature. However, the serum calcium may be minimal, even in patients with long-standing disease, and it may be elevated only intermittently; hence, repeated serum determinations must be made. The correct interpretation of calcium values requires knowledge of the serum protein concentration, since half of the total serum calcium is bound to protein. For every gram per 100 ml that the serum albumin is decreased below normal, the serum calcium will be spuriously lowered by 0.8 mg per 100 ml. Rarely, patients have been described with normal serum levels of calcium and protein but with elevated ionized calcium concentrations. However, measurement of ionized calcium is not really necessary in patients with unequivocal hypercalcemia.

When hypophosphatemia accompanies hypercalcemia, hyperparathyroidism is almost invariably present if other causes of phosphate depletion have been excluded. However, hypophosphatemia occurs in less than half the patients with normal renal function and is usually absent in patients with renal insufficiency. Hypercalciuria occurs when more than minimal hypercalcemia exists, except in patients with renal insufficiency. Alkaline phosphatase is elevated in patients with marked bone disease. Bone x-rays should include at least the hands, skull, clavicles, and lumbar spine.

The classic picture of primary hyperparathyroidism, with hypercalcemia, hypophosphatemia, hypercalciuria, elevated alkaline phosphatase, and x-ray evidence of subperiosteal bone resorption, is not usually seen until the disease is far advanced. Therefore the following additional diagnostic tests have been proposed, but of course they are least helpful when the hyperparathyroidism is mild and obscure.

1. Blood PTH level is elevated in over 90 percent of the patients, especially if one relates it to a simultaneously obtained serum calcium.
2. Steroid suppression (150 mg cortisone acetate daily for 10 days) usually will not lower the serum calcium in hyperparathyroidism but will lower the hypercalcemia associated with sarcoidosis, vitamin D intoxication, multiple myeloma, and a number of malignant diseases with bone metastases.
3. Reduction in the tubular reabsorption of phosphate and elevation of the renal phosphate clearance occurs in hyperparathyroidism provided renal function is normal.
4. Phosphate deprivation may exaggerate the hypophosphatemia, hypercalciuria, and occasionally the hypercalcemia of hyperparathyroidism.
5. Electrolyte abnormalities noted in hyperparathyroidism include serum chloride over 105 mEq per liter, chloride phosphate ratio over 33, and metabolic acidosis (PTH blocks the renal reabsorption of bicarbonate).
6. Elevation of the urinary cyclic-AMP level. This is particularly helpful when the cyclic AMP level is expressed in micromoles per gram of creatinine in the urine and is analyzed as a function of the serum calcium level. Under these circumstances, an elevated urinary cyclic AMP in the presence of an elevated serum calcium favors a PTH etiology.
7. Localization studies that may be helpful include x-ray examination of the esophagus during a barium swallow; selenium (^{75}Se)-labeled methionine scan of the parathyroid glands; selective arteriography; and PTH measurements made during selective sampling during retrograde catheterization of the major veins draining both the upper and lower poles of the thyroid lobes and the medias-

tinum. Venous sampling catheterization studies have provided the surgeon with invaluable assistance in rapidly locating a solitary adenoma, particularly in patients who have already been explored unsuccessfully.

Treatment. The treatment of primary hyperparathyroidism is surgical. Surgery may be difficult because, as previously noted, parathyroid glands may be atypical in number and location; an adenoma is difficult to distinguish (even histologically, at times) from hyperplasia; and the normal glands may be atrophied when an adenoma is present. Since extensive neck dissection or mediastinal exploration may be necessary, it is essential that the preoperative diagnosis be as certain as possible.

Most patients require no special preoperative preparation. However, those with severe hypercalcemia should be treated first with intravenous fluids and inorganic phosphate in order to lower the serum calcium, reverse coma or shock, and improve the general metabolic condition of the patient. Oral phosphate therapy, used as early as 1932 by Dr. Fuller Albright, may be given for prolonged periods in the management of hypercalcemia in selected patients with primary hyperparathyroidism in whom surgery must be deferred because of complicating problems such as (1) a recent myocardial infarction; (2) widely metastatic parathyroid gland carcinoma, or (3) recent unsuccessful neck exploration that makes immediate reoperation technically unsatisfactory until the inflammatory reaction in the neck subsides, which takes about 3 months.

The postoperative period after parathyroidectomy is often unremarkable, but it may be seriously complicated by the development of tetany within hours or days of surgery. Hypocalcemia may be either brief, due to atrophic or temporarily injured glands, or prolonged during the repair of osteitis fibrosa cystica and osteomalacia; it may be permanent due to irreparable damage to the remaining parathyroid tissue. Difficulties with severe postoperative hypocalcemia should be anticipated in patients with significant bone disease and an elevated serum alkaline phosphatase. Once active bone resorption ceases, the "hungry bones" will reheal and there may be a rapid deposition of calcium into the demineralized skeleton. Intravenous calcium should be given promptly as needed, and serum calcium levels should be measured frequently. If all the parathyroid glands have been injured or removed, long-term management of hypoparathyroidism then becomes necessary with oral calcium and vitamin D (see later in this chapter, under treatment of hypoparathyroidism).

Secondary Hyperparathyroidism

The parathyroid glands may become hyperplastic and secrete excessive amounts of hormone in conditions that cause hypocalcemia and osteomalacia. These conditions include renal insufficiency, malabsorption, vitamin D deficiency, renal tubular acidosis, and renal tubular defects with phosphate wasting. The chemical findings in secondary hyperparathyroidism depend on its cause, but usually they are distinct from those in primary hyperparathyroidism in that the serum calcium is not elevated above normal.

In the most common form of secondary hyperparathyroidism, that due to renal insufficiency, there is a normal or low serum calcium, elevated levels of serum phosphate and alkaline phosphatase, a metabolic acidosis, and osteomalacia as well as osteitis fibrosa. A number of factors may contribute to the parathyroid hyperplasia: Initially, a decrease in the glomerular filtration rate leads to hyperphosphatemia, which effects a lowering of the serum calcium and thereby stimulates the parathyroids; as the renal disease progresses, an altered metabolism of vitamin D and a decreased production of 1,25-DHCC occur. This deficiency of the active form of vitamin D results in a decreased intestinal absorption of calcium, thereby exaggerating the hypocalcemia and producing continued stimulation of the parathyroid glands. Thus the chronically elevated PTH levels combined with a low serum calcium and deficiency of the active form of vitamin D lead to the metabolic bone disease of renal insufficiency — renal osteodystrophy.

Secondary hyperparathyroidism is usually asymptomatic, but symptomatic bone disease may occur. A number of therapeutic suggestions have been made to correct the bone disease of renal insufficiency, including calcium administration, phosphate deprivation, vitamin D, and, in extraordinary instances,

subtotal parathyroidectomy. In attempting to arrive at the proper dose of vitamin D, frequent measurements of the serum calcium must be made to avoid vitamin D intoxication. The difference between the effective therapeutic dose and a dose producing hypercalcemia may be quite small.

Kaye and his colleagues reported the effectiveness of small doses of dihydrotachysterol in the treatment of renal osteodystrophy when equivalent doses of calciferol were ineffective. Doses as low as 0.25 mg daily of dihydrotachysterol have been shown to increase the intestinal absorption of calcium in patients with far-advanced kidney disease. Up to 1.0 mg daily has been required in some patients, but again, one must carefully follow the serum calcium levels to avoid hypercalcemia (1.0 mg dihydrotachysterol is biologically equivalent to 3.0 mg or 120,000 IU of vitamin D).

Hypoparathyroidism

Pathology, Etiology, and Incidence. Hypoparathyroidism, the inadequate production of PTH, is most commonly a complication of thyroid surgery; only rarely is it idiopathic. Three patterns of parathyroid dysfunction may be seen following thyroidectomy: (1) transient hypoparathyroidism, apparently due to edema, ischemia, or hemorrhage; (2) permanent parathyroid insufficiency, but with no spontaneous clinical or chemical abnormalities and demonstrable only by provocative testing; and (3) permanent clinical hypoparathyroidism, which occurs in approximately 1 percent of patients following subtotal thyroidectomy (even higher following total thyroidectomy). Additional rare causes of decreased parathyroid function include metastatic tumor infiltration of the parathyroid glands; radioactive iodine therapy for thyrotoxicosis; long-standing iron storage disease involving the parathyroids; and pseudohypoparathyroidism.

Idiopathic hypoparathyroidism is a rare disorder of unknown cause in which the parathyroid glands are partly or totally replaced by fat. Most patients are recognized during childhood, and occasionally the disorder is familial. A number of seemingly unrelated conditions occur with unusual frequency in patients with idiopathic hypoparathyroidism, including moniliasis (candidiasis), hypoadrenalism, hypothyroidism, hypogonadism, and pernicious anemia. Some patients have a number of these disorders and also antibodies to several tissues, hence an autoimmune etiology has been proposed. Congenital absence of both the parathyroids and the thymus is known as the Di George syndrome.

Pathophysiology. Hypoparathyroidism results in a decreased renal phosphate clearance and resultant hyperphosphatemia. Decreased bone resorption and decreased gastrointestinal calcium absorption result in hypocalcemia, which is responsible for the increased neuromuscular excitability in these patients. The increased neuromuscular excitability is the basis for most of the clinical manifestations of hypoparathyroidism. The mechanisms by which parathyroid insufficiency causes ectopic calcification and abnormalities of skin and teeth are not understood.

Clinical Manifestations. Tetany is the cardinal symptom of hypoparathyroidism. It may present as one of the many tetanic equivalents, such as muscle cramps and fatigue, paresthesias of the fingers and toes, carpopedal spasm, laryngeal spasm, bronchospasm, biliary colic, and focal or generalized seizures. Mental symptoms include anxiety, irritability, depression, delusions, and, in children, mental retardation. Episodes of tetany may be precipitated by menstruation, pregnancy, and lactation.

On examination, the skin may be dry and scaly, the nails brittle and transversely ridged, and the hair coarse and dry. Moniliasis is frequently seen in idiopathic hypoparathyroidism. Examination of the eyes may reveal lenticular opacities and papilledema. Dental signs, particularly in children, include hypoplasia, enamel defects, failure of eruption, and root defects of teeth. When a blood pressure cuff is inflated at greater than systolic pressure for as long as 3 minutes, the hand may be noted to assume a characteristic position: the thumb is adducted, and the fingers are pressed together and flexed at the metacarpophalangeal joints (Trousseau phenomenon). Neuromuscular irritability may also be demonstrated

by facial contraction elicited by percussion of branches of the facial nerve (Chvostek sign).

The major laboratory findings are hypocalcemia (as low as 4 mg/100 ml) and hyperphosphatemia (as high as 6 to 12 mg/100 ml). The serum alkaline phosphatase is normal or low, and the urinary calcium is low. The electrocardiogram may have a prolonged Q-T interval with a normal T wave (which is just the opposite of hypercalcemia, which has a short Q-T interval). X-ray films may demonstrate calcification of the basal ganglia and normal or slightly dense bones.

Differential Diagnosis. Hypoparathyroidism must be distinguished from other causes of hypocalcemia and tetany and from pseudohypoparathyroidism. Renal insufficiency closely simulates hypoparathyroidism, since it causes hyperphosphatemia as well as hypocalcemia and hypocalciuria. However, renal insufficiency is distinguished by azotemia, acidosis, and osteitis fibrosa. Hypoproteinemia is a common cause of hypocalcemia, but it does not cause tetany or hyperphosphatemia. Impaired intestinal absorption of calcium due to sprue, pancreatitis, or vitamin D deficiency causes hypocalcemia, tetany, and hypocalciuria, but these conditions may be distinguished from hypoparathyroidism by a low serum phosphate and by osteomalacia.

Tetany may occur in respiratory or metabolic alkalosis, in magnesium depletion, and in potassium depletion, but each of these causes is distinguished from hypoparathyroidism by lack of hypocalcemia or hyperphosphatemia. Idiopathic hypoparathyroidism is differentiated from pseudohypoparathyroidism primarily by an increased urinary excretion in the form of phosphate and cyclic AMP following the administration of parathyroid extract. Pseudohypoparathyroidism is also characterized by unique somatic abnormalities to be described below. Other causes of hypocalcemia are listed below.

1. Hypocalcemia related to parathyroid hormone
   a. Surgical hypoparathyroidism (following a thyroidectomy)
   b. Idiopathic hypoparathyroidism
   c. Pseudohypoparathyroidism

d. Infarction of a parathyroid adenoma
e. Hypomagnesemia
f. Parathyroid suppression in the newborn delivered of a mother with hyperparathyroidism
2. Hypocalcemia related to vitamin D
a. Renal insufficiency
b. Malabsorption
c. Vitamin D-deficient diet
3. Hypocalcemia related to therapeutic agents
a. Phenytoin (Dilantin) and phenobarbital
b. Phosphates
c. Ethylenediamine tetraacetic acid (EDTA)
d. Estrogen treatment of prostate cancer with bone metastases
e. Calcitonin
4. Miscellaneous causes of hypocalcemia
a. Acute pancreatitis
b. Hypoalbuminemia
c. Glucagonoma

Treatment. The aim of hypoparathyroidism therapy is to restore the serum calcium to normal in order to prevent tetany and the consequences of chronic hypocalcemia. Following thyroid or parathyroid surgery, particularly in patients who show evidence of marked skeletal demineralization preoperatively, the rapid development of hypocalcemia should be anticipated. Sufficient calcium should be given intravenously to control any symptoms or signs of neuromuscular instability that may develop. If tetany persists for more than several days, vitamin D and calcium should be started by mouth, as discussed under the management of secondary hyperparathyroidism. Therapy should be tapered slowly over the next several months to evaluate the possible return of parathyroid function. Regular determinations of the serum and urine calcium are necessary to ensure that the dosages of vitamin D and calcium are sufficient but not excessive. It is important to keep in mind that a fixed dose of vitamin D that has been successful in maintaining normocalcemia for years may suddenly be found to produce hypercalcemia. The majority of patients with hypoparathyroidism appear to need about 1 gm of elemental calcium and at least 50,000 units of vitamin D daily, but most patients will become hypercalcemic at some

point in their course on a vitamin D dosage exceeding 100,000 units per day.

Pseudohypoparathyroidism
Pseudohypoparathyroidism is a rare inherited disorder in which there are characteristic skeletal abnormalities in addition to the clinical and chemical manifestations of hypoparathyroidism. Pseudohypoparathyroidism is thought to be transmitted as an X-linked dominant trait with variable expression. It is called *pseudo*-hypoparathyroidism because the patient is clinically hypoparathyroid and yet has elevated serum levels of PTH. These levels of PTH are suppressible in a normal fashion by a calcium infusion. The manifestations of hypoparathyroidism are thought to be due to end-organ resistance to PTH, since the parathyroid glands have been found to be normal or even hyperplastic. This resistance may be demonstrated by a less-than-normal urinary phosphate excretion after intravenous injection of parathyroid extract (Ellsworth-Howard test), by minimal changes in serum calcium and phosphate after repeated daily intramuscular injections of parathyroid extract, and by the lack of increase in the urinary excretion of cyclic AMP following parathyroid extract. The Ellsworth-Howard test is of limited value, since the range of results reported for patients with hypoparathyroidism has shown too many instances of overlap with the results reported for normal subjects. The measurement of urinary cyclic AMP following the intravenous administration of parathyroid extract is the best test to distinguish pseudohypoparathyroidism from other forms of hypoparathyroidism.

Kooh and associates described the response of two children with idiopathic hypoparathyroidism and one with pseudohypoparathyroidism to the administration of 1,25-DHCC, the active polar metabolite of vitamin D. These patients responded to very small doses with a prompt rise in their serum calcium and an increase in intestinal calcium absorption, whereas it took 80 to 100 times as much 25-HCC to effect the same result. These data suggest that the underlying defect in these patients is an impairment in the renal conversion of 25-HCC to 1,25-DHCC. In pseudohypoparathyroidism, however, in which the levels of circulating PTH are often elevated, there is a resistance to the action of PTH that is thought to be caused by a defect in renal receptors or enzymes.

Actually, two types of pseudohypoparathyroidism have been described: type I, which is characterized by blunted urinary cyclic AMP and phosphaturic responses to parathyroid extract, and type II, which is characterized by a marked rise in the urinary excretion of cyclic AMP following the administration of parathyroid extract but without a phosphaturic or hypercalcemic response. The type II form suggests a defect in the intracellular reception of the cyclic AMP message.

All the clinical features of idiopathic hypoparathyroidism except for moniliasis may be present in patients with pseudohypoparathyroidism. However, the hyperphosphatemia, hypocalcemia, and tetany are usually less severe in pseudohypoparathyroidism, and fewer patients have cataracts or papilledema. Subcutaneous calcification and mental retardation occur more frequently in pseudohypoparathyroidism. The skeletal and developmental abnormalities of pseudohypoparathyroidism include a stocky build and short stature; round face; irregularly short metacarpals, metatarsals, and phalanges; and bony exotoses. Other endocrinopathies sometimes associated with pseudohypoparathyroidism include diabetes mellitus, the Turner syndrome, primary or secondary hypothyroidism, and abnormalities of smell and taste. The current therapy of pseudohypoparathyroidism is the same as that of hypoparathyroidism: vitamin D and calcium supplementation.

Pseudopseudohypoparathyroidism

Pseudopseudohypoparathyroidism is a very rare inherited disorder in which patients have all the features of pseudohypoparathyroidism except that the serum calcium and phosphorus are normal. This might suggest that there were two genetic defects in pseudohypoparathyroidism, one accounting for the skeletal abnormalities and the other accounting for the resistance to PTH. Possibly only one of these defects (that accounting for skeletal abnormalities) is inherited in pseudopseudohypoparathyroidism; however, both pseudohypoparathyroidism and pseudopseudohypoparathyroidism may occur in the same kinship; and finally, calcification of basal ganglia and lenticular opacities, which has been thought to be due to chronic hypocalcemia, may also occur in patients with pseudopseudohypoparathyroidism. All these facts suggest that there is a single genetic defect with complete expression in pseudohypoparathyroidism and only partial expression in pseudopseudohypoparathyroidism.

Bibliography

Avioli, L. V. The therapeutic approach to hypoparathyroidism. *Am. J. Med.* 57:34, 1974.

Bricker, N. S., Slatopolsky, E., Reiss, E., and Avioli, L. V. Calcium, phosphorus and bone in renal disease and transplantation. *Arch. Intern Med.* 123:543, 1969.

Boonstra, C. E., and Jackson, C. E. Serum calcium survey for hyperparathyroidism: Results in 50,000 clinic patients. *Am. J. Clin. Pathol.* 55:523, 1971.

Chase, L. R., and Slatopolsky, E. Secretion and metabolic efficacy of parathyroid hormone in patients with severe hypomagnesemia. *J. Clin. Endocrinol. Metab.* 38:363, 1974.

DeLuca, H. Vitamin D endocrinology. *Ann. Intern. Med.* 85:367, 1976.

Eisenberg, H., Pallotta, J., and Sherwood, L. M. Selective arteriography, venography and venous hormone assay in diagnosis and localization of parathyroid lesions. *Am. J. Med.* 56:810, 1974.

Frame, B., Jackson, C. E., Reynolds, W. A., and Umphrey, J. E. Hypercalcemia and skeletal effects in chronic hypervitaminosis A. *Ann. Intern. Med.* 80:44, 1974.

Kaye, M., Chatterjee, G., Cohen, M. B., and Sagar, S. Arrest of hyperparathyroid bone disease and dihydrotachysterol in patients undergoing chronic hemodialysis. *Ann. Intern. Med.* 56:225, 1970.

Kooh, S. W., Fraser, D., DeLuca, H. F., Holick, M. F., Belsey, R. E., Clark, M. B., and Murray, T. M. Treatment of hypoparathyroidism and pseudohypoparathyroidism with metabolites of vitamin D: Evidence for impaired conversion of 25-hydroxyvitamin D to 1α,25-dihydroxyvitamin D. *N. Engl. J. Med.* 293:840, 1975.

Lafferty, F. W. Pseudo-hyperparathyroidism.
  Medicine 45:247, 1966.

Lee, J. C., Catanzaro, A., Parthemore, J. G., Roach,
  B., and Deftos, L. Hypercalcemia in disseminated coccidioidomycosis. *N. Engl. J. Med.*
  297:431, 1977.

Lotz, M., Zesman, E., and Bartter, F. C. Evidence for
  a phosphorus depletion syndrome in man.
  N. Engl. J. Med. 278:409, 1968.

Mallette, L. E., Bilezikian, J. P., Heath, D. A., and
  Aurbach, G. D. Primary hyperparathyroidism:
  Clinical and biochemical features. *Medicine*
  53:127, 1974.

Potts, J. T., Jr., and Deftos, L. J. Parathyroid
  Hormone, Calcitonin, Vitamin D, Bone and Bone
  Mineral Metabolism. In P. K. Bondy (ed.),
  Duncan's Diseases of Metabolism. (7th ed.).
  Philadelphia: Saunders, 1974. Chap. 20.

Purnell, D. C., Smith, L. N., Schloz, D. A., Elveback,
  L. R., and Armand, C. D. Primary hyperpara-
  thyroidism: A prospective clinical study.
  Am. J. Med. 50:670, 1971.

Shai, F., Baker, R. K., Addruzzo, J. R., and Wallach,
  S. Hypercalcemia in mycobacterial infection.
  J. Clin. Endocrinol. Metab. 34:251, 1972.

Shaw, J. W., Oldham, S. B., Rosoff, L., Bethune, J. E.,
  and Fichman, M. P. Urinary cyclic AMP
  analyzed as a function of the serum calcium
  and parathyroid hormone in the differential
  diagnosis of hypercalcemia. *J. Clin. Invest.*
  59:14, 1977.

Silva, O. L., Becker, K. L., Primack, A., Doppman,
  J., and Snider, R. H. Ectopic production of
  calcitonin in oat cell carcinoma. *N. Engl. J.
  Med.* 290:1122, 1974.

The Third F. Raymond Keating, Jr., Memorial Symposium. Parathyroid hormone, calcitonin and
  vitamin D: Clinical considerations (Part II).
  Am. J. Med. 57:1, 1974.

Walser, M., Robinson, B., and Duckett, J. W., Jr.
  The hypercalcemia of adrenal insufficiency.
  J. Clin. Invest. 42:456, 1963.

61

Metabolic Bone Diseases

Daniel S. Bernstein

Diseases of the skeletal system have remained the same since antiquity, as has been demonstrated recently by pathologic studies using modern techniques for examining the bones of Egyptian mummies and early American Indians. New discoveries of the nature and physiology of parathyroid hormone, calcitonin, and vitamin D (see Chap. 60) are providing a better understanding of metabolic bone diseases. Bone is composed of an organic matrix of collagen and protein polysaccharide on which minerals are deposited as small crystals between and in the collagen fibers. The primary functioning unit of bone is the osteon, which is composed of a central haversian canal rimmed by osteoblasts that manufacture the collagen and protein polysaccharide matrix. The rate of production of this organic matrix by osteoblasts is modulated by hormonal factors, mechanical stress, age, and blood supply. As mineralization occurs on the organic matrix, the osteoblasts are trapped and become osteocytes, morphologically different but still capable of producing collagen and protein polysaccharide when properly stimulated. Osteocytes also can resorb bone and actually do carry on the majority of bone resorption. When resorption is increased (as in hyperparathyroidism), another cell form appears — the osteoclast, which is rarely found in normal mineralized bone but is thought to be derived from the osteocyte. Most bone histologists believe that osteocytes and osteoblasts under normal circumstances perform most of the normal bone processes of resorption and formation.

Calcium phosphate initially is deposited on the organic matrix in an amorphous form that rapidly recrystallizes into tiny crystals. The crystalline salt is mostly hydroxyapatite in which significant amounts of Na^+, Mg^{2+}, CO_3^-, and citrate^{2-} ions are incorporated. Fluoride, strontium, radium, plutonium, lead, and other such ions are readily bound to hydroxyapatite crystals. If, as in the case of fluorosis (see later in this chapter, under treatment of osteoporosis),

large amounts of these elements are incorporated into bone, the solubility and size of the crystal structure is altered; fluoride causes the hydroxyapatite crystal to increase markedly in size and "perfection" and to decrease in solubility.

Throughout life, bone is constantly remodeled through the processes of formation and resorption. Resorption in cortical bone is carried out by the osteoclastic formation of vascular channels (haversian canals), which later fill in by osteoblastic deposition of collagen and protein polysaccharide and eventual mineral deposition. Layer on layer of bone is remodeled in this fashion. In the entire skeleton at any one time, areas of resorption and formation occur at different rates, depending on a variety of physical, chemical, and hormonal stimuli. The axial skeleton metabolizes at approximately four times the rate of the appendicular skeleton.

The mechanisms of bone formation and resorption are dependent on a number of factors, some of which are only partially understood. Incompletely understood, for instance, is the fact that plasma and interstitial (bone) fluid is supersaturated with Ca^{2+} and PO_4^{2-} ions at a normal plasma pH. The bone cells, in some fashion, are able to maintain Ca^{2+} ions in the interstitial fluid above the level needed for bone mineral precipitation. It is probable that in the human the bone cells operate independently of overall calcium balance and separately from the metabolic rate of resorption and formation. In addition, bone cells produce collagenase, an enzyme that breaks down collagen, but the precise physiologic role of collagenase still requires much research. The blood supply to bone also plays a vital role in bone formation and resorption; about 5 percent of the cardiac output goes to bone, but under conditions of severe stress, bone blood flow drops to nearly zero. Paget's disease, on the other hand, is characterized by an increased bone blood flow associated with increased bone resorption.

Key hormonal factors in bone metabolism (parathyroid hormone, calcitonin, and vitamin D) are discussed in Chapter 60. Corticosteroids have been shown to inhibit protein synthesis in bone and in other connective tissues and therefore to diminish bone formation greatly. Thyroid hormone in excess, while accelerating bone formation, appears to increase bone resorption even more, with a resultant overall loss of bone tissue. However, little is known about the steady-state role of either cortisol or thyroid hormone in bone remodeling. Testosterone is involved in epiphyseal closure and may affect protein synthesis in bone, but it is generally thought to be less effective than estrogen in stimulating bone formation. Growth hormone stimulates cartilage growth, but interplay with other hormones also stimulated by growth hormone does not allow a precise interpretation of the role of growth hormone in bone metabolism.

Osteoporosis

Osteoporosis may be defined as an overall loss of bone mass. It may be a result of aging rather than a disease per se; certainly it is a skeletal disorder of the elderly and is more common in women. Numerous studies of the rate of loss of bone mass using x-ray techniques, photon densitometry, and radioactive isotopes have pointed out the following facts: From birth until the completion of adolescence there is an increase in bone density; from age 20 to 30 there is a plateau during which resorption and formation are approximately equal; and from age 30 on there is a gradual but definite loss of bone density. The rate of bone resorption with aging is highly variable, but perhaps because women generally have less bone than men, they have an earlier onset of clinically symptomatic osteoporosis than men.

Osteoporosis develops whenever bone resorption exceeds formation; trabecular bone is lost preferentially over cortical bone because of its greater surface-to-volume ratio and greater metabolic turnover. In the appendicular skeleton bone resorption takes place on the endosteal surfaces with a resultant expansion of the medullary cavity and a thinning of the cortex. Before there is visible x-ray evidence of diminished bone mass, at least 40 percent of the skeleton must be resorbed. All osteoporosis can be considered idiopathic except for the following conditions, in which there is a clear-cut etiology:

I. Parathyroid hormone hypersecretion (primary, secondary, tertiary hyperparathyroidism)

II. Osteomalacia
   A. Vitamin D deficiency
      1. Decreased production or conversion to active metabolites (chronic liver or kidney disease)
      2. Decreased intake (no sunlight exposure, dietary insufficiency)
      3. Decreased absorption (chronic diseases of stomach, pancreas, small intestine, or biliary system)
   B. Vitamin D resistance (genetic defect)
   C. Hypophosphatasia
III. Osteoporosis
   A. Idiopathic osteoporosis (postmenopausal, senile)
   B. Secondary osteoporosis (may affect development of idiopathic osteoporosis)
      1. Immobilization
      2. Cortisol excess
      3. Malnutrition
      4. Gonadal deficiency
      5. Hyperparathyroidism
      6. Acromegaly
      7. Vitamin C deficiency (scurvy)
      8. Metastatic carcinoma, especially multiple myeloma
   C. Heritable disorders of connective tissue
      1. Osteogenesis imperfecta
      2. Marfan syndrome

Osteoporotic Incidence. Idiopathic osteoporosis is rarely seen before the age of 40 in women or 50 in men. In the elderly the incidence is about equal between the sexes. It has been estimated that almost 20 percent of the people in the United States have osteoporosis, but how many of these have symptoms or have had an established diagnosis is not known.

Etiology. As already discussed, all patients with osteoporosis, whether their disease is of the idiopathic or the secondary variety, have an imbalance between the rate of bone formation and bone resorption, the resorption exceeding formation. A number of causal factors should be considered in every case of osteoporosis; none has a single etiology. For example, the calcium intake in many people may be lower than their metabolic needs, and this deficiency may be enhanced by various clinical states (cirrhosis; lactose intolerance, which may cause the person to stop drinking milk; malnutrition); on the other hand, most patients with osteoporosis have an adequate calcium intake, while certain individuals who do ingest low-calcium diets never develop clinical osteoporosis. Some people may have combined osteoporosis and osteomalacia proved by bone biopsy, which would indicate a deficiency of vitamin D. In some cases the combination of osteoporosis and osteomalacia approaches 10 percent of all bone biopsies. More recently, the possibility of dietary phosphate deficiency as an etiologic factor has been raised. Inorganic phosphate deficiency produced by prolonged antacid therapy for the treatment of duodenal ulcer can lead to osteomalacia in certain patients. It has been postulated that a combined deficiency of phosphate, calcium, and vitamin D is the prime factor in clinical osteoporosis.

Immobilization, especially when it is acute, as in a fractured limb, can lead to osteoporosis in the affected limb. Generalized osteoporosis is seen in patients who are immobile for periods of several months or more (as in spinal cord injury), and it is an important possibility in those who suffer debilitating arthritis.

Both estrogens and androgens have an effect on bone formation. It has been shown that osteoporosis is accelerated in women following the menopause, while men are not similarly affected when testosterone production falls off in later years. However, much experimental work indicates that gonadal deficiency is not the primary cause of osteoporosis, even though estrogens may be important in the therapy.

Diagnosis. The patient with idiopathic osteoporosis may present with a vertebral compression fracture after slight or insignificant trauma. Only rarely is the disease rapidly progressive; by far the majority of patients undergo long periods of remission with no further fractures, even if their osteoporosis remains untreated. Many patients with osteoporosis and multiple compression fractures have no clinical symptoms whatsoever. Acute back pain may be due to a vertebral fracture that is not demonstrable by x-ray (microfracture of the vertebra). Occasionally pain from a vertebral fracture can mimic myocardial infarction or an abdominal crisis because of irritation of the nerve roots near the site of fracture. When a vertebra collapses, it generally does so in the center, and the vertebrae most subject to fracture are in the lumbar and lower thoracic spine. Vertebral fractures generally result in kyphosis (dowager's hump) and in severe cases may compromise chest expansion. Hip fractures are the most common type of long bone fracture in osteoporosis.

The diagnosis of osteoporosis is easily established. The serum calcium, phosphate, and alkaline and acid phosphatases are normal, and the x-rays show generalized osteopenia often accompanied by one or more compression fractures of the vertebrae. The vertebrae may also show (by x-ray) increased vertical trabeculation of their centers with concavity and accentuation of the end plates. The long bone cortices are thinner than normal, and x-rays of the skull may show generalized osteopenia and thinning of the sella turcica.

The differential diagnosis of osteoporosis includes the disorders listed on page 843. Particular attention should be paid to malignant tumors (localized destructive lesions of bone, abnormal plasma proteins, and abnormal bone marrow morphology). Osteomalacia can be excluded by a careful history, no evidence of kidney or liver disease, and a normal serum alkaline phosphatase. Normal serum concentrations of calcium, phosphate, and alkaline and acid phosphatase on repeated determinations will exclude all of the other metabolic bone diseases. Thyroid function tests will exclude Graves' disease. A fasting plasma cortisol can be used as a screening test for Cushing's syndrome, but other measurements and tests of adrenal function should also be performed if indicated (see Chap. 56).

Treatment. Therapy of idiopathic osteoporosis is imprecise due to the multiple etiologic factors involved. Generally, a program of mild exercise to avoid immobilization, an optimal diet, and the use of pharmacologic agents are recommended. It should be understood at the outset that idiopathic osteoporosis probably develops over a period of many years to decades. By the time the diagnosis is established at least one-third to one-half of the skeleton has been resorbed; effective therapy will therefore require many years before there is demonstrable roentgenographic improvement. However, with the recent development of photon bone densitometric methods, improvements in bone density have been demonstrated over shorter periods with various therapeutic regimens. If a therapeutic agent induces positive calcium balance (retention), it has been assumed that this indicates the formation of new bone. This assumption has a moderate amount of experimental documentation, and hence one can assume in general that an agent that produces a positive calcium balance is efficacious in the treatment of osteoporosis.

Positive calcium balances have been induced by estrogen therapy of osteoporotic postmenopausal women. These positive balances are not maintained, however, despite the continued use of estrogens. Therapy with androgens in both men and women has little or no effect on osteoporotic bone, but it may promote anabolic changes in protein metabolism in patients with osteoporosis who have had a deficient diet.

Increasing the calcium intake to levels of 1,500 to 2,000 mg per day also causes a positive calcium balance, but the calcium balance usually reverts to pretreatment levels after a few months of sustained therapy. However, recent evidence indicates that increased oral calcium intake supplemented by small amounts of oral vitamin D (1,000 IU per day) promotes not only a positive calcium balance but also a slight increase in bone mass in some patients as measured by photon densitometry. Because photon densitometry allows an appreciation of small changes in bone mass as contrasted to ordinary x-ray techniques, it makes the demonstration of efficacious therapy for osteoporosis more practical.

Sodium fluoride (10 mg of fluoride ion or higher per day) will also produce a positive calcium balance in patients with osteoporosis. The fluoride is bound to the hydroxyapatite crystal of bone, converting it to a larger, less soluble crystal of fluoroapatite. At these dose levels fluoride increases not only bone formation, but also bone resorption; and hence it can cause increased osteomalacia (osteoid seams) followed by eventual osteosclerosis. Ordinary x-rays as well as photon densitometry may show an increase in bone mass on fluoride treatment; however, the use of fluoride at 10-mg or higher dose levels is precluded by the complex histologic features of fluorosis. Caution is advised until more evidence is available. On the other hand, it should be pointed out that in *naturally* fluoridated areas, where the average ingestion of fluoride ion ranges from 3 to 6 mg per day, there is a lowered incidence of osteoporosis and vertebral compression fractures, especially in women.

Phosphate supplementation has also been used therapeutically, and while positive calcium balances have been induced, it is too early to predict the efficacy of phosphate therapy. Calcitonin suppresses bone resorption, but it has been disappointing in its effect on osteoporosis; however, it has been quite useful in the treatment of Paget's disease, in which bone resorption is greatly increased.

Other general measures useful in the treatment of osteoporosis include support to the back muscles with a brace or strong corset; mild to moderate back strengthening exercises as tolerated; and a nutritious diet containing adequate protein and vitamins C and D.

SECONDARY OSTEOPOROSIS
As previously discussed, secondary osteoporosis is ascribed to known causes such as Cushing's syndrome, hyperthyroidism, and acromegaly. The relative rate of bone resorption always exceeds bone formation, even though bone formation may be either increased (as in hyperparathyroidism and acromegaly) or decreased (as in Cushing's syndrome). The end result of the imbalance between formation and resorption is osteoporosis that is indistinguishable from the idiopathic type.

Osteoporosis secondary to Cushing's syndrome, whether iatrogenic or spontaneous, usually progresses rapidly and is quite severe in its clinical presentation. Osteoporosis is a significant feature in almost 90 percent of patients with spontaneously occurring Cushing's syndrome (see Chap. 56). Glucocorticoids decrease gastrointestinal calcium absorption and increase urinary calcium excretion. Acromegaly (see Chap. 55) also produces an increase in the rate of both bone formation and resorption, frequently with osteoporosis. Osteoporosis is also associated with gonadal deficiency and has an earlier onset in castrates of either sex. It is not established whether gonadal insufficiency alone can produce osteoporosis. In hyperthyroidism (see Chap. 58) gastrointestinal calcium absorption is decreased, probably due in part to gastrointestinal hypermotility; urinary calcium excretion is increased secondary to the increased bone resorption, while bone formation is also increased, but not as much as resorption. In rare instances hypercalcemia can be found in Graves' disease, which also reverts to normal with adequate thyroid suppression.

Hyperparathyroidism (see Chap. 59) also produces osteoporosis; very occasionally hyperparathyroidism may present as clinical osteoporosis with collapsed vertebrae. Usually, however, the increased secretion of parathyroid hormone produces an accelerated rate of bone resorption largely carried out by osteoclasts, and it may result in the classic histologic picture of osteitis fibrosa cystica. The basic difference between idiopathic osteoporosis and hyperparathyroidism is the higher rate at which bone resorption proceeds in the latter.

Paget's Disease (Osteitis Deformans)

One of the commonest chronic bone disorders is Paget's disease, which may affect any part of the skeleton and often is widely dispersed. The basic pathophysiology is initiated by increased osteoclastic resorption of a bone (or section thereof), which is later replaced by fibrous connective tissue, characteristically quite vascular. The resorbed bone is slowly replaced by coarsely woven fibers of trabecular bone that are laid down in a disorganized fashion, giving rise to a "wooly" appearance on x-ray. It is not known what causes this course of events. The incidence of Paget's disease has been estimated at more than 3 percent in persons over 40, and it increases with age.

It should be emphasized that the basic disturbance in Paget's disease is a localized increased resorption of bone. This resorption is almost always accompanied by a compensatory increase in bone formation that is haphazard. When bone resorption predominates (osteoporosis circumscripta), the bones are prone to fracture; such fractures are most often visualized in the long bones. As formation begins to fill in new bone, the mixed phase ensues. As Paget's disease continues, bone resorption slows until eventually hard, dense bone predominates and gives rise to the sclerotic phase. The calcium balance is usually normal provided immobilization does not occur. The increase in the vascular spaces in pagetic bone causes both peripheral pooling of blood and increased cardiac output, rarely resulting in heart failure. There are no true arteriovenous shunts as was once believed; rather, india ink injections into pagetic bone show large venous pools or lakes.

The increase in both bone resorption and bone formation rates in Paget's disease correlates well with the rises in plasma acid and alkaline phosphatase, respectively. The serum calcium and phosphate levels are almost always normal, although there is a tendency for the serum phosphate to be slightly high. Hypercalcemia occurs rarely and only in immobilized patients with a large mass of bone involved with active Paget's disease. The urine hydroxyproline, which rises coincident with the increase in bone resorption, is a good general indicator of the activity of Paget's disease. The serum uric acid is also often elevated, and occasionally the frequent joint pains may be relieved by uricosuric agents and colchicine.

The roentgenographic findings in Paget's disease present as cystic radiolucencies (lytic phase), as increased density and expansion of the bone (sclerotic phase), or as a mixture of the two. The pelvis is most frequently involved in Paget's disease, followed by the femur, skull, spine, clavicles, and ribs. The bowing of the legs is due to the effects of stress and strain on structurally imperfect pagetic bones.

Most patients with Paget's disease are asymptomatic, and the diagnosis is made on a routine x-ray examination or by noting an increase in the serum alkaline phosphatase. An increase in hat size, indicative of an enlarging skull, often goes unnoticed by the patient. Pain in the femurs or tibiae is often secondary to incomplete fractures, and hip pain is not unusual. Deafness is frequent due to nerve involvement secondary to Paget's disease of the temporal bone. Platybasia is seen in some cases; it is secondary to involvement of the base of the skull and gradual compression of the brainstem. With pagetic involvement of the vertebrae, spinal cord compression and paraplegia may occur. Heat or warmth and occasionally a systolic bruit may be found over involved bones due to the increased blood supply.

Major complications of Paget's disease include (1) platybasia and brainstem compression; (2) spinal cord compression; (3) easy fractures, which may be spontaneous or secondary to minor trauma; (4) high cardiac output with failure (if over 50 percent of the skeleton is involved); (5) immobilization with coincident hypercalciuria (and stone formation), osteoporosis, and rarely, hypercalcemia; (6) osteogenic sarcoma. Of the above, the most serious complication is osteogenic sarcoma, which in various clinical studies ranges in incidence from 1 to 5 percent of all Paget's disease patients. Osteogenic sarcoma, along with the less frequently occurring fibrosarcoma and chondrosarcoma, usually arise in the long bones and skull and rarely in the vertebrae. The development of an osteogenic sarcoma is heralded by an increase in pain, a rapidly growing deformity in a pagetic bone, and a rapid, meteoric rise in the serum alkaline phosphatase. Because of the insidious onset of these tumors, treatment is limited, and the outcome is almost uniformly fatal.

Until recently there was no specific therapy for Paget's disease. Various therapies previously proposed include large amounts of acetysalicylic acid (3.0 to 4.0 gm) as tolerated; indomethacin, which may relieve pain and have a salutory effect on joint symptoms; large doses of corticosteroids to suppress bone resorption and formation, which have prohibitive side effects; and sodium fluoride in high doses (greater than 10 mg/day of fluoride ion) to suppress bone resorption, which has long-term effects not yet demonstrated to be beneficial.

In patients with severe Paget's disease manifested by moderately intractable pain, documented high-output cardiac failure, x-ray evidence of platybasia, or spinal cord compression, calcitonin therapy has been of demonstrable benefit. Calcitonin (see Chap. 58), a hormone elaborated by human thyroid C cells, is capable of reducing bone resorption markedly. The hormone is now available from commercial sources and is made from salmon ultimobranchial glands.

The peak action after intramuscular injection is 5 hours, and its action lasts about 8 hours. Therapy can be instituted at dose levels of 50 to 100 MRC (Medical Research Council) units per day, and some investigators have reported that injections of 50 to 100 MRC units every other day are also effective. Urinary hydroxyproline excretion and serum alkaline phosphatase levels decrease, and frequently bone pain is ameliorated. Improvement has not been demonstrated on x-ray as yet. The side effects (flushing of the face, tingling of the extremities, and dizziness) of calcitonin are minimal and are well tolerated. Secondary hyperparathyroidism has been reported, but therapy given every other day appears to reduce this effect. The long-range (in terms of years) benefits of calcitonin in Paget's disease have not been evaluated, since the hormone has been commercially available only since early 1975.

Osteogenesis Imperfecta
Osteogenesis imperfecta (fragilitas ossium) is a heritable disorder of connective tissue, the major manifestation of which occurs in bone. However, the connective tissue defect is generalized as exhibited by blue sclerae, deafness, hernias, and loose joints. There are two types of osteogenesis imperfecta, congenital and tarda (which occurs later in life), but in reality there is but one disease with a variety of systemic manifestations and a wide range of clinical severity; generalized osteopenia is a cardinal finding clinically and by x-ray. The skeleton is liable to fracture from even the most trivial trauma. Intrauterine and childhood fractures are common, but at pubescence the fractures decrease in frequency, only to exacerbate following menopause or in the sixth decade of life. Dwarfism secondary to femoral and tibial fractures is common; and a large, laterally bulging calvaria is often seen. Loose-jointedness often results in dislocation of joints, flat feet, and kyphoscoliosis. Deafness due to otosclerosis begins at puberty and usually is progressive.

Osteogenesis imperfecta is inherited as an autosomal dominant trait, although there is some evidence that a recessive mode of inheritance occurs in certain congenital forms of the disease. The pathologic defect in the bones is related to abnormal collagen maturation. The defective collagen produced by the osteoblasts does not permit calcification to proceed normally.

There is no treatment for osteogenesis imperfecta other than supportive. Fractures heal normally, but in some patients the healing is complicated by increased callus that does not calcify.

Miscellaneous Disorders of Bone and Cartilage

NEOPLASMS

There are two classifications of bone tumors, primary and metastatic (secondary). Primary tumors generally arise from one of the three cell types in bone: osteoblast, osteocyte, and osteoclast. Each of these cells produces a characteristic histologic pattern that affords a precise definition of the bone tumor. Although the mechanism is not clear, in almost all instances primary bone tumors seem to elaborate a substance that either resorbs bone locally or interferes with the normal blood supply. Some neoplasms cause a sclerotic reaction in the bone surrounding the tumor. Primary tumors of bone may be either benign or malignant; the commonest benign tumors are osteochondromas (exostoses), chondromas (Ollier's disease), fibromas, and benign giant cell tumors. The commonest primary malignant tumor is multiple myeloma (see Chap. 52), which arises from the plasma cells of the marrow. However, any benign tumor can become malignant. Osteogenic sarcoma is more common in patients with Paget's disease or in those who have received prior irradiation therapy, although it is also frequently seen in persons under 20 years of age. Other common bone malignancies are chondrosarcomas and Ewing's tumor (malignant sarcoma).

Metastatic tumors reflect the fact that bone is a common site for metastasis from carcinomas and sarcomas arising elsewhere in the body. Common locations of metastases are the vertebrae, femurs, pelvis, and ribs, and such metastases are generally suspected from the pain produced. There are two types of bone reaction to metastatic invasion, osteolytic and osteoblastic. Examples of the source of osteolytic metastases are thyroid, kidney, and bowel. Frequently carcinoma of the prostate (and rarely, of the breast) may produce osteoblastic metastases. Osteolytic metastases usually cause hypercalciuria and hypercalcemia, depending on the amount of bone involved by the tumor. Some osteoblastic metastases may also produce hypocalcemia. The serum alkaline and acid phosphatase levels reflect the osteoblastic and osteolytic behavior, respectively, of metastatic bone tumors.

The treatment of metastatic bone disease is usually palliative, depending on the type of tumor. Irradiation may decrease pain, while various hormonal therapies may also affect the growth of the tumor. The treatment of hypercalcemia and its consequences is discussed in Chapter 60.

OSTEOSCLEROTIC BONE DISEASES (OSTEOPETROSIS)

A rare disorder that is hereditary in nature, osteopetrosis (Albers-Schönberg disease) is known as marble bone disease. It is inherited as an autosomal recessive trait and has a varied expression. The malignant type originates in utero and is characterized by anemia, hepatosplenomegaly, hydrocephalus, visual nerve involvement, and death. The disease is also seen in a less severe form, with anemia and bone fractures as the major manifestations.

Normal bone remodeling is greatly decreased in osteopetrosis, which accounts for the great increase in bone mass that crowds out normal marrow. Osteoclasts are decreased, and there is little histologic evidence of bone resorption. Although dense, the bone fractures easily, and osteomalacia is often seen in osteopetrotic children. Because the entire skeleton is involved, extramedullary hematopoiesis occurs in the liver, spleen, and lymph nodes. Involvement of the cranial nerves occurs because of encroachment on the foramina by the dense bone.

The disease can also occur in a milder form in adults and is usually manifested by frequent fractures that usually heal normally, although union may be delayed. The serum calcium, phosphate, and alkaline phosphatase levels are normal in adults, although some children may have hypocalcemia and hypophosphatemia. Recently it has been postulated that persons affected with osteopetrosis may have an increase in calcitonin, since a process similar to osteopetrosis has been seen in so-called gray-lethal mice in which the C cells of the mouse thyroid are increased in number. However, evidence for increased calcitonin production in human osteopetrotic tumors is lacking. There is no treatment for the disease.

Pyknodysostosis is a disease resembling osteopetrosis in that the patients have increased bone density and frequent fractures. The other features of osteopetrosis (anemia, extramedullary hematopoiesis, cranial nerve involvement) are not seen; but short stature, separated cranial sutures, and dental hypoplasia are. The disease is inherited and recessive and does not affect longevity.

There are other varying types of osteosclerosis, generally benign, such as melorheostosis (sclerosis of one limb); progressive diaphyseal dysplasia (osteosclerosis of the diaphyses of the long bones); osteopoikilosis (spotty density in the trabecular bone in the epiphyses and adjacent parts of the metaphyses of long bones and pelvis); hyperostosis corticalis generalisata (osteosclerosis of the skull, jaw, clavicles, ribs, and diaphyses of the long bones); and hyperostosis frontalis interna (increased thickness of the inner table of the skull), which occurs almost exclusively in women as exostoses covered by dura projecting into the cranial cavity. This last condition is benign, although some women with it have been noted to be obese, hirsute, and to have a variety of psychiatric complaints.

OTHER BONE AND CARTILAGE DISORDERS
Fibrous dysplasia (Albright's syndrome) as originally described was a disease characterized by disseminated osteitis fibrosa, skin pigmentation, and endocrine imbalance with precocious puberty in girls. Since the original description it has been recognized that the fibrous dysplasia bony lesion may occur without the other manifestations described by Albright. The disease is not hereditary and is equally distributed in both sexes.

Skeletal lesions are either monostotic or polyostotic. In the monostotic form the lesions are usually confined to the craniofacial bones and ribs. Polyostotic lesions can occur in any bone and often involve over 50 percent of the skeleton; unilateral involvement is more common, although bilateral involvement occurs. Almost 50 percent of females with polyostotic fibrous dysplasia have abnormal skin pigmentation (café au lait spots, usually localized to

one-half of the body) and the very early onset of puberty (precocious puberty). Males have abnormal pigmentation in about 50 percent of the cases.

The bone lesions in both the monostotic and polyostotic forms of fibrous dysplasia consist of fibrous tissue appearing as fibromas imbedded in bone. On x-ray there are radiolucent areas in bones associated with thinning of the cortex. The involved bones may be deformed due to structural weakness caused by the fibrous dysplasia. In patients with precocious puberty, advanced bone age will be noted.

Clinically the course of fibrous dysplasia is variable; patients may present because of skeletal deformity and fractures or because of sexual precocity (girls). Levels of serum calcium and phosphate are normal, while serum alkaline phosphatase may be elevated. The cause of the sexual precocity in females is unknown, but it is believed that ovulation does not occur. Hyperthyroidism is frequently seen in the polyostotic form.

The differential diagnosis is not difficult. Normal serum calcium, areas of cutaneous pigmentation, and the age of the patient separate fibrous dysplasia from hyperparathyroidism. Neurofibromatosis (von Recklinghausen's disease) may involve bone and produce skin pigmentation and subcutaneous nodules; the skin pigmentation, however, is smooth (not rugged, so-called coast of Maine, as in fibrous dysplasia), and the pigmented maculae are more numerous. Treatment of the bone lesions of fibrous displasia is mainly orthopedic and consists in bone grafting and curettage.

There are many other dysplasias of bone and cartilage that for the most part are obscure. A few of the more common are achondroplasia, enchondromatosis, and the Tietze syndrome. Achondroplasia is a dysplasia of cartilage due to a decrease in the normal growth of cartilage cells at the zone of provisional calcification of the epiphyseal plate. This lesion produces one of the most common types of dwarfism characterized by short limbs, a normal trunk (vertebrae are not involved), a large skull, and a saddle nose. The disease is usually recognized at birth and is accompanied by normal development in all respects except skeletal. Its cause is unknown.

Enchondromatosis (Ollier disease) is a dysplasia affecting the epiphysis in which hypertrophic cartilage is not resorbed in the usual fashion (by blood vessel invasion) and therefore does not calcify. These pathophysiologic events produce masses of cartilage located in the metaphyses in proximity to the growth plate. The disorder is often recognized in childhood by the appearance of a skeletal deformity. The long bones are the most commonly involved. When cavernous hemangiomas are seen in association with enchondromas, the disorder is called the Maffucci syndrome.

The *Tietze syndrome* is a disorder of unknown etiology in which the costochondral junction becomes severely painful and slightly swollen. It is frequently misdiagnosed because the pain can mimic coronary artery insufficiency. The syndrome is evenly distributed between the sexes and occurs most frequently between the ages of 20 and 40 years. One or more costochondral junctions may be involved, and in some instances a palpable, exquisitely tender swelling of the costochondral junction may be found. Fever is absent, and all laboratory studies are negative. The condition may last from weeks to months, but the disorder is self-limited and requires no systemic treatment. Local nerve blocks or injections of corticosteroids into the painful junction may be of some benefit.

Bibliography

Barzel, U. S. *Osteoporosis.* New York: Grune & Stratton, 1970.

Fourman, P., Roger, P., Levell, M. J., and Morgan, D. B. *Calcium Metabolism and the Bone.* Oxford: Blackwell, 1968.

Frame, B., Parfitt, A. M., and Duncan, H. (eds.). *Clinical Aspects of Metabolic Bone Disease.* Amsterdam: Exerpta Medica, 1973.

Lutwak, L., Singer, F. R., and Urist, M. R. Current concepts of bone metabolism. *Ann. Intern. Med.* 80:630, 1974.

McKusick, V. A. *Heritable Disorders of Connective Tissue.* St. Louis: Mosby, 1966.

Paterson, C. R. *Metabolic Disorders of Bone.* Oxford: Blackwell, 1974.

Raisz, L. G. Physiologic and pharmacologic regulation of bone resorption. *N. Engl. J. Med.* 282: 909, 1970.

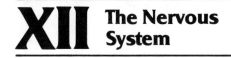

XII The Nervous System

62

Neurologic Diseases: A Symptomatic Approach

Robert G. Feldman

with

D. Frank Benson   (Neurobehavioral Disorders)
Jules Friedman   (Otoneurologic Disorders)
Simmons Lessell (Neurophthalmologic Disorders)
F. C. A. Romanul (Cerebrovascular and Related
                  Disorders)

Disturbed function of the nervous system may be signaled either by a loss of consciousness, movement, or sensation or by the appearance of sensations or involuntary movements. The physician must first determine where in the nervous system a lesion could be that would cause the symptoms and then decide what special techniques might be helpful in confirming his clinical impression. Specific therapeutic measures must be based upon clinicoanatomic correlations.

This chapter surveys the more common neurologic complaints. These symptoms are considered with respect to (1) their pathophysiologic mechanisms, (2) approaches to their further evaluation, (3) their differential diagnosis, and (4) their therapy.

Headache

When head pain interferes with daily activities and simple relief measures fail, a patient may seek a physician's help. An understanding of the quality of the pain, its location, and the pattern of onset and recurrence (temporal profile) is important in elucidating the cause of any headache. Family history and details regarding possible precipitating factors, such as fatigue, emotional stress, menstrual cycle, hunger, alcohol, or drugs, are necessary. Headaches may accompany intracranial disease or be caused by extracranial processes.

Quality of the Pain

Pain may be produced by irritation of nerve endings supplying either the larger arteries within the cranium or the extracranial arteries of the head and neck. Throbbing pain is caused by dilatation or distention of these blood vessels. Traction on the dura or the meninges produces a deep, constant, and often sharp pain. Muscle spasm secondary to local inflammation, trauma, or sprain results in cramplike discomfort. Muscle tension headache is described as a tight, aching sensation, often occurring in a "hatband" fashion.

Location of the Pain

It is of localizing value if the patient can tell where his pain is most intense. When *suboccipital,* the pain may be arising in the *posterior fossa* or in the *nuchal muscles. Retroorbital* pain may indicate a source in the *anterior fossa.* The afferent fibers of the trigeminal nerve mediate most of the pain sensations in the head, but the fibers of the glossopharyngeal, vagal, and upper cervical nerves can also mediate head pains. Because of the wide distribution and anastomoses of these nerve fibers, referred pain is common in headache syndromes.

Temporal Profile

Acute Headache. Superficial inflammatory processes, such as cellulitis of the scalp, periostitis, or osteomyelitis of the skull may cause head pain in an individual previously free of such discomfort. Other possible causes are acute sinusitis, glaucoma, temporal arteritis or early neuralgia associated with temporal arteritis, or trigeminal neuralgia. Sudden distention of a medium-sized artery occurring with an aneurysm or a stenotic occlusion may cause an acute headache.

Intracranial processes such as encephalitis or meningitis or intracranial bleeding are possible causes of an acute spasm of the extracranial muscles, which is a common cause of pain at the base of the skull and upper neck, often with radiation across the shoulders. Muscle spasm may be associated with osteoarthritis, localized lymphadenopathy, or extension (whiplash) injury of the neck, or it may be an acute anxiety reaction. An acute headache follows cerebral concussion or skull fracture. Abrupt obstruction in the flow of cerebrospinal fluid (CSF) by an intraventricular cyst or a mass in the posterior fossa produces severe acute headache. Hypoxia or hypercapnea may cause acute headache by vasodilation. Intoxication by carbon monoxide, carbon dioxide, lead, nitrites, glue, or methyl alcohol can bring on an acute headache. Various systemic illnesses, such as hypertensive crises with encephalopathy, hypoglycemia, uremia, or severe dehydration, may all present as headache.

Cyclic Headache. An example of this type of headache is *classic migraine.* Several people in a family may share a history of classic migraine, which usually affects one side of the head at a time, though not necessarily the same side each time the headache occurs. The headache often begins with a prodromal loss of vision, flashing lights, or other neurologic symptoms. Within an hour the pain intensifies and is accompanied by nausea and vomiting. Flare-up of these headaches during stress is common, while a decrease in their frequency and severity often occurs with older age.

Common migraine (sick headache) differs from classic migraine mainly in its symptom profile. This headache usually starts upon awakening, on one side of the head, and increases over several hours. Nausea, vomiting, polyuria, diarrhea, chills, and exhaustion often follow the headache. The annoying pain may persist until the patient is able finally to get to sleep, but it reappears daily upon awakening for as long as a week or more. Susceptible persons may also undergo mood changes, such as euphoria, depression, or irritability, preceding the pain.

In contrast to the relatively benign classic and common migraines, the recurring cephalalgias associated with cerebral angiomas, vascular anomalies, and aneurysms have a sudden onset and reach a peak within minutes. The latter headaches are usually located on the side of the vascular lesions. Neurologic disturbances associated with vascular malformations appear after the pain subsides and outlast it, instead of preceding it, like the prodromata in migraine. Often there is a history of convulsive seizures. A bruit may be heard through the cranium over the area of the vascular anomaly. Headaches due to vascular malformations occur more sporadically than true migraine and are never relieved by ergot preparations, which usually help migraine patients. If sub-

arachnoid bleeding has occurred, the headache is more acute and severe and often feels "explosive."

Cluster headaches occur with regularity, especially during resting periods. They may be preceded by a short, burning discomfort in the temple or eye followed by a steady or throbbing pain. Several acute episodes of this type may recur during the day, seldom lasting more than 2 hours. This form of headache is often associated with ipsilateral prominence of a temporal vessel, conjunctival vascular dilatation and lacrimation, salivation, blocking of the nasal passages, and, occasionally, unilateral sweating. The pain on the side of the forehead may spread bilaterally and be accompanied by deep pain in the neck. Use of alcohol, nitrites, nicotine, or other vasodilators may trigger an attack. Ergotamine results in dramatic relief, confirming the vascular nature of the headache.

Subacute and chronic forms of headache are often the most difficult to deal with. With this group of headaches it is important to note any changes in the severity of the pain and in the associated neurologic signs. Brain tumors can be overlooked when a chronic headache is accepted as psychoneurotic in origin without further diagnostic analysis. Headache associated with a brain tumor is usually an indolent discomfort with intermittent exacerbations, often precipitated by changes in position, coughing, or straining, or it may be a new complaint in a person never bothered by headache in the past. Initially, the pain occurs in a given place and has localizing value. The history may reveal that the headache fluctuated for a week or so, with a remission followed by exacerbation. Headache associated with brain tumor is not relieved by relaxation and often is not clearly related to emotional stress. The intervals between bouts of headache gradually shorten and neurologic signs appear as brain tissue is further affected by an enlarging neoplasm or increasing cerebral edema. Headache may be a late symptom of an infiltrative tumor and not occur until pain-sensitive structures are put under traction.

Muscle contraction headache is common in tense, anxious, or depressed people. These patients complain of a constant "tight band" sensation around the head. They claim that they have a headache all the time: "I get up with it and go to bed with it." Their discomfort is due to muscle tenseness. Severe pain develops, with radiation along muscles spreading across ligamentous attachments and insertions. Tenderness may be elicited by palpation at the sites of insertion of the frontalis muscles over the forehead, the cervico-occipital muscles over the mastoid prominences, or the nuchal muscles over the inion. Cramping and muscle spasm may be due to latent tetany resulting from chronic hyperventilation in some patients who are heavy cigarette smokers, and they react with further overbreathing; such patients have a gradual buildup of headache, a full feeling in the head, or light-headedness. Persistent contraction of the cervico-occipital muscles may induce ischemia by squeezing the local blood supply, resulting in a sensation of localized throbbing.

The widespread use of oral contraceptive preparations containing progestin and estrogen may produce constant dull headache in susceptible women. The actual mechanism of this headache is unknown; but it develops about 2 weeks after beginning a daily dose of The Pill. Cessation of medication eliminates the headache. Migraine-prone patients also have reported increased frequency of headache while receiving oral contraceptives.

DIAGNOSTIC STUDIES

To establish the cause of a headache, a careful history and physical examination must be followed by *x-rays* of at least the skull, chest, and cervical vertebrae. Displacement of a calcified pineal gland from the midline may indicate a shift of intracranial structures. Thinning of the inner table of the calvaria, or enlargement or erosion of the sella turcica may indicate chronic, slowly increased intracranial pressure. Hyperostosis of the sphenoid wing or inner table of the parietal bone may be the only finding to suggest a meningioma. Calcification of intracerebral blood vessels or flecks of calcium in certain slow-growing tumors, such as astrocytomas or oligodendrogliomas, may be seen on plain x-ray of the skull. Radiologic studies of the skull should be accompanied by studies of the chest to rule out the possibility of carcinoma of the lung with metastases to the brain. A helpful screening test for intracerebral lesions is the *radioisotope scan,* which can reveal unusual vascular areas,

meningiomas, or metastatic foci. Another noninvasive procedure, the *computerized axial tomography (CAT) scan,* has recently been introduced. The CAT scan can show intracranial lesions and in some cases it can differentiate between hemorrhages and tumors. A routine *electroencephalogram (EEG)* may show a preponderance of slow waves (4 to 6 cycles per second) or an actual spike focus in patients with brain tumor or brain abscess. The EEG of patients with migraines occasionally shows an increased sensitivity to photic stimulation.

A *lumbar puncture (LP)* should be performed to determine the resting opening pressure and the final pressure after several cubic milliliters of cerebrospinal fluid have been removed. A lumbar puncture should not be done if there is increased intracranial pressure, as indicated by papilledema, or suspicion of a mass in the posterior fossa. Under certain limited circumstances, however, such as when either a suppurative process or a subarachnoid hemorrhage is suspected, spinal fluid must be examined. Only the amount of fluid in the manometer plus a few more drops to equal a total of no more than 1 cubic milliliter should be removed slowly by means of a small (22-gauge) bore needle. Compression of the jugular vein (Queckenstedt's sign) is used to observe the intracranial pressure during a rise in cerebral venous pressure. When venous pressure in the head increases, the CSF pressure should increase. This test of dynamics may be helpful in determining a block in the subarachnoid space below the foramen magnum. However, testing by jugular compression carries a serious risk during lumbar puncture when intracranial disease is present. The increased venous pressure can precipitate obstruction when there is an already precarious posterior fossa lesion or impending cerebral edema. The cerebrospinal fluid should be examined microscopically for leukocytes and red cells in cases of suspected cerebral hemorrhage or meningitis. Early in viral infection a few polymorphonuclear cells may be present. Later the cell count includes predominantly lymphocytes. Similarly, chemical irritation from blood in the cerebrospinal fluid increases the number of neutrophils and lymphocytes in some acute cases following subarachnoid hemorrhage.

After centrifugation, supernatant CSF should be

crystal clear and colorless. Various pigments from the breakdown of red blood cells contribute to the xanthochromic appearance following intracranial bleeding. A high proportion of oxyhemoglobin is present with early bleeding, in contrast with the greater amount of bilirubin found in later specimens. For instance, a subacute or chronic subdural hematoma will cause greater amounts of methemoglobin and bilirubin than oxyhemoglobin to appear in the fluid. A new hemorrhage from an aneurysm should be suspected if the proportion of oxyhemoglobin in the xanthochromic specimens gradually increases while approximately the same degree of yellow appearance remains.

Increased amounts of CSF protein have been found following large infarctions of brain. A disturbance of the blood-brain barrier may occur in the presence of meningitis, with subsequent alteration in transport of sugar and proteins. An elevated protein concentration or a low sugar concentration may therefore be present. Neoplasm is usually associated with a moderate increase in CSF protein along with normal sugar. Carcinomatous meningitis is usually associated with low CSF sugar and high CSF protein, and cytologic study often reveals mitotic figures in neoplastic cells after centrifugation. In cases of cryptococcal meningitis, india ink stain may be valuable. The alcohol content of CSF was once thought useful in the diagnosis of cryptococcus, but recent experience has shown this to be an unreliable test. Acid-fast stain of cells in the spinal fluid must be done in suspected tuberculous meningitis. Routine bacteriologic cultures are usually sufficient for most infectious agents, but one should be prepared to plate the CSF in Sabouraud's agar to grow out fungal agents. Appropriate inoculations for virus cultures and studies for complement should be made.

Pneumoencephalography, in which filtered air is instilled into the subarachnoid space by lumbar puncture, and *arteriography,* in which radiopaque material is injected into the arterial system, are usually reserved for determining the presence and location of neurosurgically amenable lesions. Arteriography can be used to trace the normal or distorted course of intracerebral blood vessels and to reveal obstructions of flow or abnormal vasculature. A late phase film

taken when the deep cerebral veins have been filled outlines the size of the ventricles, giving an indication of possible hydrocephalus.

A pneumoencephalogram is done when a mass lesion or obstruction is suspected in the absence of lateralizing clinical signs. If a posterior fossa lesion is believed to be present, the neurosurgeon may choose to perform a *ventriculogram* by way of a small burr hole in the cranium through which air is instilled or contrast material is injected directly into the ventricular system.

Most patients with headache will not require these serious tests. However, when a definite negative answer will be helpful in the management of symptoms by reassurance, the physician may recommend these further studies.

THERAPY

Besides the appropriate neurosurgical treatment for neoplasm, intracerebral blood clot, or obstructive hydrocephalus, treatment of headache includes the use of adequate doses of analgesic, muscle relaxant, sedative, or specific vasoconstrictive drugs.

Muscle Contraction and Tension Headache. A clear, simple, and reassuring explanation of the nature of his headache is quite helpful to an anxious patient, who usually will be relieved to know that he does not have a life-threatening condition such as a brain tumor and that effective medicinal treatment is available. To be convinced, a patient may require a review of the results of various studies already done. It is necessary for the physician to break the cycle of anxiety and depression leading to headache, which in turn causes more anxiety, and to identify the underlying psychological conflicts and precipitating emotional events. Symptoms may be ameliorated with antidepressant or antianxiety drugs. A combination of analgesics, muscle relaxants, and sedatives has been found useful if administered soon after the onset of headache. There are several available combinations of aspirin (300 mg), meprobamate (400 mg), and amobarbital (15 mg). Some patients are unable to tolerate aspirin alone or in combination with caffeine and phenacetin, and require other analgesics, such as pentazocine or propoxyphene. To stop the development of pain early and prevent recurrence of headache for an 8- to 10-hour period, it is usually effective to administer a capsule containing propoxyphene hydrochloride (65 mg), aspirin (162 mg), and caffeine (32.4 mg) at the onset of the headache and repeat every 3 hours for 3 doses, whether the headache persists or not.

Tension headaches may linger because the patient is not given sufficient medication early enough in the development of the muscle spasm. If localized areas of tenderness are found in muscles, infiltration with 5 to 10 cubic milliliters of 2.0% procaine solution may abolish them. In severe, excruciating muscle contraction headaches, emergency treatment with amobarbital (0.2 to 0.5 gm) or large doses of sedatives given acutely, such as intramuscular chlorpromazine (50 mg) or diazepam (Valium) (10 to 20 mg), may be helpful. Prophylactic treatment to avoid the development of tension headache includes supportive psychotherapy in many instances. Appropriate intervention for depression may include the use of antidepressant medication, especially when the particular drug given improves the patient's quality of sleep. Avoidance of excessive fatigue and use of chloradiazepoxide hydrochloride (in doses of 10 to 25 mg three to four times per day) or a muscle relaxant-analgesic combination may prevent the sudden onset of muscle spasm due to increased emotional stress. Any method of relaxing muscles will be helpful. Heat applied to the involved muscles by hot packs is comforting and relaxing, as are prolonged warm tub soaks, including immersion of the neck and the back of the head in warm water. Careful massage of the involved area may give relief.

Migraines. Ergot derivatives, especially ergotamine tartrate, are the most useful drugs, but they must be administered in the prodromal period, or at least immediately after the onset of the headache. Oral use is desirable unless nausea and vomiting are present. The initial dose by mouth for each attack is 2 tablets (each containing 1 mg of ergotamine tartrate and 100 mg of caffeine), followed by 1 or more tablets at half-hour intervals to a total of no more than 5 or 6 until the necessary effect has been produced. A combination of ergotamine, caffeine,

and phenobarbital seems most helpful. The minimum effective dose must be determined for each patient. In some cases the effective dose may be 1 tablet; in others, 4 tablets may be necessary at the first sign of a headache. When there is nausea and vomiting, rectal suppositories are helpful. The suppositories, each containing ergotamine tartrate (2.0 mg), caffeine (100 mg), and phenobarbital (15 mg) are used every half hour for a total of 3 suppositories. The maximum dose of ergotamine tolerated before signs of ergotism (peripheral vasoconstriction, tingling of the hands and feet, muscle cramps, pains in the thighs and abdomen, and substernal pressure) appear is usually 6 to 8 mg in any one day. This maximum dose should not be given more than once a week. If it is necessary to use ergotamine tartrate by injection, not more than 0.5 mg subcutaneously or 0.25 mg intravenously should be administered in a single week. Some patients react poorly to ergotamine tartrate but can tolerate dihydroergotamine methanesulfonate, the usual dose of which is 1 mg intravenously or subcutaneously, repeated in 1 hour if necessary. As with ergotamine tartrate, dihydroergotamine methanesulfonate is contraindicated in the presence of peripheral vascular diseases, angina pectoris, impaired hepatic or renal function, septic states associated with intravascular clots, or pregnancy.

Any well-organized therapeutic plan tailored to the patient's needs will usually bring some favorable result. Adequate relaxation, improvement in restful sleep, and correction of any physiologic abnormalities are among the aids in reducing stress and, thus, the frequency of migraine attacks. Barbiturates and other sedatives have a limited but useful role in the treatment of migraine. Tranquilizer drugs may be of assistance in easing the concomitant tensions associated with migraine; moreover, in certain patients tranquilizers seem to reduce the frequency of headache. A small number of migraine patients respond to phenytoin (Dilantin) (100 mg given three times per day) as a prophylactic measure. Many common migrainous, or cluster-type, vascular headaches are markedly reduced in frequency and severity by methysergide (2.0 to 8.0 mg per day). Propranolol (Inderal) also has recently been found to be effective in preventing cluster headaches.

Epilepsy

Epileptic seizures are due to sudden, paroxysmal, and often recurrent discharges of electrical energy in neurons of the central nervous system, usually the cerebral cortex and the diencephalon. The diagnosis, prognosis, and prevention of seizures depend not only on understanding their causes, clinical manifestations, and trigger mechanisms but also on knowing what the electroencephalogram shows. Clinical analysis is best carried out by observing the patient's symptoms and signs in the preictal and postictal states. Some classifications of epilepsy are anatomic, as is indicated by such terms as *cortical* and *subcortical,* which denote the supposed origin of the epileptic discharge. A better classification is one that uses clinically descriptive terms.

In most patients the cause of seizures is unknown. In others, proper observation and tests yield a definite etiology. A seizure disorder for which no evident cause can be found in either the history or the physical examination is referred to as *primary,* or *idiopathic.* The seizure that appears to be a manifestation of underlying conditions, such as the residua of trauma or the effects of a brain tumor, vascular malformation, intracerebral bleeding, meningitis, encephalitis, hypoglycemia, hypoxia, or withdrawal from drugs or alcohol, is called *secondary* or *symptomatic* epilepsy.

Primary or Idiopathic Epilepsies

Generalized Type. Petit mal "absences," myoclonic seizures, akinetic attacks, and grand mal convulsions all exemplify generalized epilepsy. *Akinetic* seizures are characterized by a sudden brief loss of muscle tonus. Myoclonic seizures are accompanied by a sudden massive contraction of muscles. In these types of seizure there may simply be nodding or dropping of the head. Loud sounds or bright lights may precipitate either a myoclonic jerk or an akinetic seizure, and the EEG will reveal bilateral, synchronous, 3-cycles-per-second discharges. This form of generalized, nonfocal seizure disorder is usually seen in childhood, but it may persist after pubescence; the electrical pattern of 3-cycles-per-second spike and wave accompanies the clinical manifestations. In *petit mal epilepsy* the common feature is a lapse in attention, an arrest in speech, or only a momentary cloudiness in thinking or comprehension. The attacks consist of an absence of awareness lasting 5 to 8 seconds. Sometimes there is no other clinical sign or movement, but the electroencephalogram shows repetitive bursts for as long as 10 to 12 seconds. In a schoolchild one might easily attribute the blank stare and unresponsiveness to "daydreaming." A child in the classroom may hear his teacher say, "Two plus two is —," then *zap.* These repeated interruptions interfere with learning unless they are recognized and treated properly. Absence attacks may be precipitated by bright or flashing lights or loud sounds. As the patient with absence seizures reaches adolescence, the frequency of seizures decreases and an electroencephalogram may not show abnormal discharges except when provocative tests such as hyperventilation and photic stimulation are employed. The characteristic of the seizure may also change, with the appearance of automatisms, lip-smacking, and head-turning, all in the presence of characteristic EEG changes. As an adult the petit mal patient may experience an occasional grand mal seizure, a psychomotor seizure, or interspersed episodes of acute confusional states or depressions.

A *grand mal* convulsion is characterized by sudden loss of consciousness, with an initial tonic phase in which the patient falls to the ground, with or without vocalizations. The body remains tonic for a few moments with the eyelids and jaws clenched. Trembling develops into gross, clonic, irregular shaking of the extremities. A tonic-clonic phase may last 40 to 80 seconds, accompanied by a loss of sphincter control, hyperventilation, salivation, and sweating. A period of exhaustion follows, lasting from a few minutes to as long as several hours. The phase of recovery with prolonged sleep or stupor may last for hours.

The grand mal patient usually has no warning before a seizure. Sometimes he recognizes the premonitory period because of an unreal feeling of fear or excitement, odd sensations of smell or taste, headache, dizziness, or visual disturbance. Such pre-seizure phenomena or "aural" are actually part of the seizure itself, occurring before consciousness is lost. The seizure usually erases memory of these events. Onset of grand mal attacks is accompanied by nonfocal EEG features of high-amplitude, rapid synchronous bursts.

The group of seizures referred to as "partial seizures," in contrast with generalized seizures, arise from focal areas of the brain — those that subserve specific motor, sensory, or visceral functions — and are manifested clinically as specific, repeated patterns of activity. From the observed clinical manifestations of a given seizure the physician infers whether epileptic discharges are occurring in such a focus of the brain.

Focal motor seizures usually arise in the premotor cortex and cause movements of the contralateral limbs. The so-called *jacksonian seizure* is a focal motor attack consisting of involuntary movements beginning in the hand and spreading to the face, then to the leg, or beginning in the foot and spreading up the leg, down the arm, and to the face. This type of partial seizure may last 20 to 30 seconds without alteration in consciousness. It may spread over other cortical areas producing other movements, such as turning of the body or even a generalized convulsion. A focal motor seizure is sometimes followed by temporary weakening of the parts involved, in what is known as postictal paralysis. *Focal sensory seizures* are the result of epileptic discharges arising in the sensory cortex. The patient may describe a numbness or tingling, a coldness, or a sensation of water running over a part of the body. *Special sensory seizures* involving vision, hearing, and equilibrium have been described. Auditory and vertiginous seizures are frequently associated with further spread into temporal lobe structures.

Generalized seizures can occur at any time in a susceptible patient, but there is usually a definite precipitating event, both for the initial appearance and for the recurrence of these attacks. More than 90 percent of convulsive disorders have their onset in early life, and as many as 1 out of every 15 children admitted to hospital has a history of seizures. In the newborn, certain mechanisms that maintain stabilization of the nervous system in the adult are not completely developed. In immature infants, seizures are often associated with structural or metabolic disorders of the brain. Some children between the

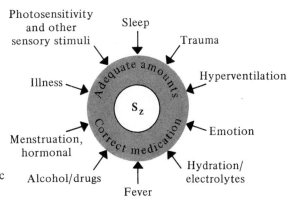

Figure 62-1. Factors that affect seizure control.

ages of 6 months and 3 years are susceptible to convulsions only during fever. Seizures are precipitated when there is an imbalance between the factors that tend to prevent seizures and those that are capable of triggering one (Fig. 62-1). Endocrine disturbances such as the growth spurts between the ages of 5 years and 7 years, the menarche, thyroid abnormalities, and fluctuations of the estrogen-progesterone levels during a menstrual cycle may lower the seizure threshold. Deprivation of sleep, fatigue, and emotional stress may be precipitating factors in a given patient. Hyperventilation (with or without exercise); intake of excessive amounts of water, alcohol, or certain antihistamine or sedative drugs; and superimposed infections — all are among the common occurrences a physician may find to be related to seizures in a particular patient.

The temporal lobe and its connections with the limbic system, which include the amygdala, hippocampus, thalamus, cingulum, and caudate nucleus, are the structures affected by seizure phenomena, which disturb awareness, perception, memory, and interpretation of environmental cues. Ictal emotional experiences associated with psychomotor epilepsy are very difficult to differentiate from psychiatric disturbances of nonorganic causes. A relatively high incidence of psychological abnormalities has been found in patients with diagnosed psychomotor epilepsy through observation during the interictal period (i.e., between the characteristic seizures). The known involvement of deep temporal, pararhinal, and diencephalic structures in psychomotor seizures can account for both affective disturbances and confusional states with minor alterations in consciousness.

Psychomotor epilepsy, arising in the temporal lobe, may be manifested as episodic, paroxysmal fluctuations in affect, memory, behavior, or attention. It can occur even in the absence of the more obvious concomitants of lip-smacking, loss of consciousness, or olfactory symptoms. Electroencephalographic correlates of these seizures may be absent on surface recordings. It may be necessary to use nasopharyngeal electrodes to detect abnormalities from ventromedial areas of the temporal lobes. When discharges are recorded from the surface, they appear as slow, paroxysmal waves in either the anterior temporal leads or the posterior temporal leads. Occasionally, bilateral synchronous spike-wave discharges are seen in the vertex and temporal leads. For special patients, for whom conventional electroencephalograms fail to reveal epileptic activity, depth electrodes surgically placed into the cerebrum have been used to obtain the information necessary to make a firm diagnosis.

Interictal personality disorders have been described as hysteric, obsessive-compulsive, or schizophreniclike. The paranoid states occurring in a true schizophrenic reaction and the paranoia of interictal confusional states of psychomotor epilepsy render the differential diagnosis quite difficult. Not uncommonly, psychogenic factors will aggravate an actual epileptic potentiality. It is known that some patients can abort seizures by distracting themselves or giving themselves a strong afferent stimulation, such as a pinch. A peculiar characteristic of many patients with long-standing psychomotor seizure problems coupled with an interictal personality disorder is that, once emotionally precipitated outbursts begin, the process becomes autonomous; that is, while the patient seems able to "turn on" a seizure in response to stress, he is unable to "turn it off." In some instances the seizure appears to be self-induced. A combined neurologic and psychiatric approach to therapy is needed once such an emotion-epileptic symptom complex is established.

If the patient has been well controlled on medication and there is exacerbation of the seizure tendency,

careful questioning may reveal that he is not receiving enough medication to balance the additional stress of a precipitating event. Usually there has also been an irregularity in his schedule of taking medications. The patient may have to adjust his sleep pattern to obtain sufficient rest, avoid alcoholic beverages, or undergo further study to uncover the presence of an otherwise unsuspected precipitating factor.

Secondary or Symptomatic Epilepsies
Posttraumatic epilepsy, arising from birth trauma, is due to shearing or tearing of intracranial blood vessels, with intracerebral damage from hypoxia of cortical neurons, or to the effects of subdural fluid collections. Almost one-half of all patients with epilepsy present a history of head trauma, although only about 5 percent of enclosed head injuries result in traumatic epilepsy. Among the injuries that penetrate the skull, the risk of epilepsy is as high as 50 percent. Posttraumatic seizures may occur immediately after the injury or after a lapse of 5 years or more. Although there is a greater risk of permanent posttraumatic epilepsy in those who have seizures during the first week after injury, the initial impact of a head injury in a child may produce a seizure without subsequent serious structural damage or epilepsy.

Epileptic attacks occurring as a result of an *intracerebral mass,* such as a tumor, are due to changes in the cortex following deprivation of its blood supply, traction on the cortex by the tumor, pressure from edema, or direct deformation of neural tissue by the tumor. The incidence of neoplasm presenting as seizures in adults has been reported to be 11.3 percent for patients 40 to 49 years old and 15.4 percent for those over 50 years old. The cell type of a cerebral tumor determines the incidence of seizures. Less malignant tumors of long duration are more likely to cause seizures than more rapidly growing ones. Tumors located deep in the white matter are likely to produce paralysis or other neurologic symptoms before manifesting themselves by a seizure. Meningiomas, usually located close to the cortex, are associated with seizures in as high as 67 percent of cases. Small meningiomas or indolent glial tumors are often incidental findings at autopsy or during an operation in patients considered to have long-standing primary or idiopathic epilepsy.

In 10 to 15 percent of the cases of *epilepsy associated with vascular disease,* onset follows cerebral infarction. Other causes are alteration in the blood supply to the cerebral cortex due to arteriosclerosis, inflammation of small blood vessels (arteritis), congenital heart disease, cardiac arrhythmias, and disturbed reflex circulatory control. Arteriovenous malformations are often associated with seizures that usually are focal and that begin during adolescence. Abnormal neuronal discharges are apt to occur whenever there is inadequate cerebral blood supply. Seizures that occur during the first week after a stroke, which are due to acute cerebral changes, rarely recur following recovery; but late-onset seizures months or years after a cerebral infarction tend to be recurrent and to require anticonvulsant therapy indefinitely. Epileptic attacks may occur during the night in elderly patients if their blood pressure declines to a critical level inadequate to maintain cerebral circulation. Similarly, postural hypotension may cause a seizure. A cerebral hemorrhage or a cortical infarction due to embolization by thrombi, fat, or air can cause a seizure.

Symptomatic epilepsy occurs when biochemical disturbances interfere with normal neuronal function. In such cases prompt therapy to restore normal metabolism may result in full functional recovery. *Hypoglycemia* and *hypoxia* cause seizures by depriving the brain of essential materials for oxidative metabolism. Lacking sufficient glucose, the brain oxidizes other noncarbohydrate substrates, such as lipids and amino acids, but none of these is adequate to maintain normal function for any significant length of time. After the stores of cerebral glucose and glycogen have been exhausted, the brain's own structural components are fed into the glycolytic and Krebs cycle pathways. Of the many causes of hypoglycemia that may lead to convulsions, overdoses of drugs such as insulin and tolbutamide are the most common. Excessive alcohol ingestion also results in lowered blood sugar. Hypoglycemia may be associated with hyperinsulinism due to tumors of the pancreas, with impaired glycogenolysis and glyconeogenesis resulting from hepatic disease, or with destructive or degenerative lesions of either the anterior lobe of the pituitary or the adrenal cortex, and so produce seizures. Physiologic hypoglycemia occurring after a large meal sometimes precipitates symptomatic epileptic attacks.

Acute uremia results in accumulation of protein breakdown products such as urea, creatine, and uric acid and in retention of inorganic and organic acids, including sulfate. The exact mechanism of interference with the function of the nervous system in uremia is not known, but the accumulation of abnormal substances, hypocalcemia, dehydration, acidosis, and hypokalemia may be contributory. Among the early neurologic symptoms of uremia are poor attention and a dull constant headache; among the later symptoms is neuromuscular and cerebral hyperexcitability. Finally, convulsions may develop along with stupor and coma. Epilepsy that persists after recovery from uremia suggests that damage to cortical neurons has occurred. An electroencephalogram early in renal failure shows nonfocal increases in slow wave activity. Spikes, usually in the range of 4 to 7 cycles per second, may appear as seizures become more of a problem.

Focal, generalized, or myoclonic seizures may occur in *hepatic portal-systemic encephalopathy.* Stupor and coma characterize the terminal stages of hepatic failure, which is accompanied by an increase in blood ammonia. Cerebral metabolism, either at the level of glutamine synthesis or in the reductive deamination of alpha-ketoglutarate, may be adversely affected by increased amounts of blood ammonia. The electroencephalogram may reflect increased ammonia by slow waves (2 to 3 cycles per second). The cause of the seizures in *hepatic failure* may be an interference in pyridoxal function, consequent disruption of glutamic acid-gamma amino butyric acid pathways, and resultant decreased cerebral oxygen consumption. Correction of hepatic dysfunction is the best means of treating these seizures. Phenytoin is less effective and diazepam only masks the problem by adding to the depressed nervous system.

Hyponatremic states may cause seizures with slow wave changes in the electroencephalogram. In animals with experimental seizures, a low epileptic threshold is related to a low level of serum sodium and a fall in the ratio of extracellular to intracellular sodium in the brain. Loss of sodium may occur as a result of diarrhea, excessive sweating, or increased excretion of sodium in the urine associated with renal disease or use of diuretics. Hyponatremia may also occur in association with CNS diseases such as encephalitis or third-ventricle tumors affecting hypothalamic structures. Reduced sodium levels may occur after parenteral administration of hyponatremic fluids, acute infections and fever, or acute expansion of extracellular fluid volume from retention of water. Convulsions due to water intoxication and hyponatremia are resistant to anticonvulsant drugs and can be controlled only by correcting the electrolyte imbalance. *Hypernatremic states* may result from CNS lesions that cause diabetes insipidus, or from dehydration, sodium retention, or excessive sodium intake. Ironically, too rapid a correction of hypernatremia may lead to seizures as a result of rebound hyponatremia.

Hypocalcemia, a condition of low ionic concentrations of calcium, may occur during treatment of hypernatremic states. When seizures occur in the presence of low serum calcium they are probably due to the effect of the low calcium on the permeability of cell membranes to potassium and sodium, with the fall in calcium leading to seizures only indirectly. Neonatal tetany, hypoparathyroidism, pseudohypoparathyroidism, rickets, steatorrhea, chronic renal disease, and treatment of acidosis by dehydration can all lead to seizures by an initial ionic hypocalcemic effect.

Drugs capable of affecting the nervous system as either sedatives, tranquilizers, or stimulants can be associated with a lowered seizure threshold. Patients who have continued use of relatively high levels of medication for periods of weeks or months followed by several days' abstinence may experience tremulousness, irritability, and often generalized convulsions. Barbiturates, heroin, meperidine, glutethimide, meprobamate, diazepoxide, and alcohol are a few of the drugs which, upon withdrawal, may induce seizures. In some individuals phenothiazines seem to potentiate an underlying seizure tendency but rarely cause

seizures of themselves. Stimulants such as amphetamines, pentylenetetrazol (Metrazol), caffeine, and ephedrine may also lower the seizure threshold. The common "rum fits" after heavy alcohol intake, which usually begin in adult life, occur when patients who have been chronically intoxicated decrease or stop their drinking. The exact mechanism is obscure, but hypomagnesemia and respiratory alkalosis have been suggested as important factors. The EEG pattern is usually normal except in immediate relationship to the seizure, and it often shows heightened sensitivity to photic stimulation (as in any other drug withdrawal state). Seizures may occur in drinkers, unassociated with either alcoholic intoxication or withdrawal, if a cerebral scar has been produced by either trauma or hypoxia in previous seizures.

FURTHER STUDIES

A search for evidence of injury, congenital abnormality, or family predisposition should be made in all seizure patients. An electroencephalogram is the only means to confirm the diagnosis of epilepsy. In the presence of an observed grand mal attack or repeated petit mal episodes, however, a normal tracing does not negate the diagnosis. Serial electroencephalograms and provocation techniques using hyperventilation, photic stimulation, or sleep deprivation may be useful in bringing out abnormalities in the EEG. Roentgen examinations of the skull and chest, isotope brain scans, and studies of CSF pressures, protein, cells, and bacteria are valuable both immediately and as bases for future observation. The new CAT technique may define the cause of the epilepsy or rule out certain other considerations without risk or discomfort to the patient. When clinical evidence is sufficient to warrant them, pneumoencephalography and arteriography should be done to rule out a surgically amenable situation.

THERAPY

Once it has been established that long-term control of the seizure tendency is the only appropriate therapy, each patient's problem must be approached on an individual basis, determined by the type of seizure and its severity. The age of the patient and the nature of his seizure disorder together with the

EEG characteristics will influence the type and dosage of medication to be prescribed.

Febrile convulsion is a tentative diagnosis made when a child has a generalized convulsion related to high fever. These seizures are often of brief duration and subside before any medication can be given. It is best therefore to anticipate the possible recurrence of convulsions during future acute systemic infections. Antipyretic drugs and specific antibiotic therapy should be given at the first sign of illness. Prophylactic doses of phenobarbital (7 to 10 mg/kg) are sometimes, but not always, helpful, if given early enough. If frequent seizures occur with slight febrile illnesses, or if the child has a convulsion not associated with fever, then daily antiepileptic therapy is indicated, especially when epileptic discharges are found in the EEG taken when the child is afebrile. Long-term prophylactic antiepileptic therapy is needed, with periodic adjustments of dosage with changes in age and size.

Grand Mal and Focal Seizures. Regardless of the cause of the seizure, the initial treatment for the generalized convulsion with tonic-clonic movements and loss of consciousness must be directed toward protecting the patient from bodily harm during the convulsion and providing an airway. The nose and mouth should remain uncovered. Objects such as padded tongue blades or spoons often cause injury to the mouth and teeth and produce insufficient airway. Ideally, a rubber or plastic mouthpiece for airway should be used during the seizure to allow for administration of oxygen if necessary. Excessive salivation may be present, requiring frequent suctioning to prevent aspiration. After the seizure, while the patient is in a postictal stupor or coma, antiepileptic medication should be administered to prevent recurrence of a seizure. An intravenous dose of phenytoin (7 to 10 mg/kg for children under the age of 10 years and up to 15 mg/kg for adolescents and adults) and phenobarbital (in similar dose per weight as for phenytoin) will usually achieve sufficient therapeutic blood and tissue levels to stop a seizure and prevent recurrence.

Serial seizures, with intervals of only 5 to 10 minutes between attacks, may occur after inadequate amounts of anticonvulsant medication. *Status epilepticus,* or seizure without interruption, is often difficult to control even by vigorous treatment. In an adult, intravenous sodium phenobarbital (300 mg) injected slowly over a period of 1 to 2 minutes usually stops a convulsion. Intravenous phenytoin (300 to 500 mg) given at the same time will provide both a "loading dose" and ongoing protection as the acute effects of the phenobarbital diminish. If the initial dose of phenobarbital does not stop the seizure, a second intravenous administration of 200 mg may be given 5 to 10 minutes after the first injection. Respiratory depression and hypotension should be watched for.

After the convulsive activity has subsided, it is necessary to continue medication, such as an additional 100 mg of phenobarbital every 6 hours and additional phenytoin (200 mg every 12 hours) for the next 24 to 36 hours. Ambulatory antiepileptic regimens to be maintained after discharge from the hospital should be instituted as soon as the acute seizures come under control. Other medications used to stop status epilepticus are paraldehyde, intravenous doses of diazepam, and general anesthesia. Diazepam must be used with care because it may be followed by cardiac or respiratory arrest, or by hypotension, if given too quickly. The usual intravenous dose of diazepam is 2 to 10 mg given over a 5-minute period. Shorter-acting barbiturates such as amobarbital and thiopental may suppress seizure activity, but their short action makes them less useful in controlling seizure activity.

A combination of phenytoin and phenobarbital may provide maximum protection against seizures with minimum side effects. The doses of anticonvulsant medications for a child are prescribed in proportion to the child's weight. However, small children very frequently require and are able to tolerate more medication per kilogram of body weight than can adolescents or adults. The reason for this is that both phenobarbital and phenytoin are eliminated from the body more rapidly in children than in adults. Adult dosage is regulated according to the patient's needs and also to the occurrence of side effects. It is best to begin with an oral dose of 100 mg of phenytoin twice per day. If neither rash nor ataxia develops, the average adult may receive an additional 100-mg dose. If on this amount of phenytoin seizures continue to occur, though reduced in severity and frequency, further protection may be provided by supplementation with phenobarbital in doses of 15 to 30 mg three or four times per day. Other medications, such as primidone (Mysoline) or mephobarbital, may be used when phenobarbital is not sufficient.

Petit mal seizures in children respond best to succinimide derivatives such as methyl-phenyl succinimide (Milontin), beginning with doses of 20 to 60 mg/kg per day. Methsuximide (Celontin), in 300-mg capsules, often gives a dramatic response in doses of 1 capsule two or three times per day, but after 18 to 24 months the dosage must be increased as tolerance becomes established. Ethosuximide (Zarontin) in doses of 250 mg two or three times per day is very effective. Acetazolamide (Diamox), 10 to 20 mg/kg/day for children or 125 mg three times per day for adults, has been a useful adjunct in decreasing the frequency of petit mal attacks. When grand mal seizures occur along with petit mal seizures, a combination of phenytoin or phenobarbital succinimides may be useful. In some cases of petit mal the use of phenytoin may aggravate seizure frequency rather than decrease it. Clonazepam (Clonopin) was recently introduced as an antiseizure medication for absence and akinetic seizures.

Psychomotor seizures are often controlled by the use of phenytoin, phenobarbital, or primidone. As has been stressed, for all seizures it is necessary to tailor the drug dosages for each patient. When anxiety is a precipitating factor, psychotherapy and the use of antianxiety medication are useful.

General Principles in Treating Epilepsy

The most common cause of recurrent seizures in otherwise "controlled patients" is a change in the amount of anticonvulsant drugs made available to the central nervous system, either because of the patients' neglect to take enough drugs or because of an increase in their need for drugs. Premenstrual tension, fluid imbalance, and hormonal changes are examples of periodic alterations in homeostasis that can decrease seizure threshold. Avoiding overfatigue

by regular sleeping habits may help to reduce the frequency of seizures. Because it may increase seizure frequency, alcohol intake should be discouraged. In some patients hard liquor itself may not be so troublesome as the volume of fluid taken in, as, for example, when a patient drinks a large quantity of beer.

Understanding by the patient, whether child or adult, and by the patient's family is absolutely essential to the proper management of epilepsy. This understanding requires a clear definition of the patient's capabilities as well as restrictions early in the course of the seizure disorder. Fear of a seizure coming at a possibly embarrassing time, such as at a job interview, can itself bring on an attack. In most cases children with epilepsy can grow up with a healthy self-image, provided their seizures are seriously treated and controlled. They should not tiptoe through life as fragile "eggshells" but should try to accept their condition, realizing that they can be free of seizures if they strictly maintain a regimen to prevent them.

Admittedly, the common emotional reaction to the word *epilepsy* is negative. For centuries epileptic attacks have been a mystery to humankind and social prejudice and discrimination have long made life difficult for epileptics. Misconceptions still exist, such as: "Epileptics have less intelligence than nonepileptics"; "Epilepsy is inherited"; "Epilepsy is a form of mental illness"; and "A common characteristic of the epileptic is a tendency to commit acts of violence." Archaic laws applicable to epileptics remain on the statute books of some states, although improvements have been made in recent years. Discoveries of effective antiepileptic therapy have brought social changes and concomitant increases in job opportunities for epileptics. In addition, active educational campaigns by organizations concerned with neurology and epilepsy have favorably affected public opinion. However, it is still usually considered a catastrophe when patients and their families experience a seizure. Therefore, early, careful counseling and continuing support of both patient and family are absolutely essential.

Control of seizures with modern prophylactic medication is now almost always assured. It may be necessary to ascertain by gas-liquid chromatography that a therapeutic blood level is being achieved by the amount of medicine the patient is taking by mouth. However, the blood level of medication should not be the sole criterion for dosages. It is also necessary to consider both the seizure threshold and the individual susceptibility of a patient to particular trigger mechanisms.

States of Consciousness

Consciousness consists of awareness of one's surroundings, clear perception of environmental cues, and appropriate responses to them. *Wakefulness* is the state of a person who is able to respond immediately, fully, and effectively to visual, auditory, or tactile stimulation. *Lethargy* means a condition of drowsiness, inaction, and indifference, in which the patient responds in an incomplete or delayed manner. *Obtundation* is a state of dulled indifference even when the patient is awake. *Stupor* is the condition of patients who are deeply obtunded but capable of being roused with vigorous stimulation, upon cessation of which they return to a state of unawareness. *Sleep* and *coma* resemble each other clinically. Sleep, however, can be interrupted by adequate stimulation; coma cannot be altered by even the strongest stimulation. Sleep has its basis in normal, active physiologic mechanisms, not abnormal processes, such as exist in coma, that prevent wakefulness. Disturbances of consciousness may arise from altered function of the cerebral cortex, the diencephalon, and the brainstem.

Supratentorial mass lesions produce altered consciousness by damaging the diencephalic and midbrain structures. Increased intracranial pressure causes the brain to be pushed downward toward the tentorial incisura, compressing the diencephalon. Shift of supratentorial structures laterally across the midline causes distortion of blood vessels, ischemia, and further edema. Progressive expansion of a supratentorial intracerebral mass manifests itself clinically by headache, lethargy, stupor, concomitant signs of paresis of the third and sixth cranial nerves, and, possibly, signs of papilledema. Supratentorial lesions, such as neoplasms, epidural hemorrhages, and subdural hematomas, may produce deep coma. As coma develops, respiratory and vasomotor irregularities may appear. Infiltration by glioma or encephalitic in-

volvement of the diencephalon may produce lethargy, obtundation, and coma. Rapidly developing cerebral edema following cerebral contusion usually produces irreversible coma and death. In children post-concussion stupor may last for 36 to 48 hours and then disappear without residue. About one-half of all cerebral hemorrhages produce unconsciousness. Severe swelling due to edema around a cerebral tumor, infarction, or empyema may cause altered consciousness or coma.

Subtentorial lesions within the brainstem can cause coma by invading the central core or by involving the blood supply to centers dealing with consciousness. Cerebrovascular disease may cause coma by occlusion of the paramedian branches of the basilar artery supplying the reticular formation. Nutritional deficiencies, sometimes associated with severe chronic alcoholism or with neoplastic diseases, may result in degeneration of the periaqueductal gray matter and so affect consciousness. Posterior fossa tumors and large aneurysms of the basilar artery may produce pressure on the tegmentum at the pontine level and affect consciousness by downward displacement and compression of the medulla. At the midbrain level, central brainstem lesions may not only produce coma but, in addition, interrupt pathways for pupillary light reflexes and damage the oculomotor nuclei. Damage at the lower pontine level may produce coma and also cause pinpoint pupils. Functional transection of the lower pons results in motor signs varying from flaccid quadriplegia to decerebrate rigidity. Occasionally, a lesion affecting the pons but sparing the central gray core may produce a "locked-in" syndrome, in which the patient, though fully alert, has no motor function whatsoever. This must be differentiated from the similar clinical picture of akinetic mutism, which is due to lesions in the diencephalon or midbrain.

Metabolic encephalopathy may result in disturbances of consciousness. Failures of neuronal metabolism can be divided into those arising from intrinsic disease of neurons and those due to secondary changes arising from systemic diseases or exogenous toxins. Neuronal degeneration, as in Alzheimer's, Pick's, and Jakob-Creutzfeld's diseases, results in obtundity, stupor, or coma. Certain cases of encephalopathy secondary to other problems may be reversed if the underlying problems are corrected. For example, in the early stages of acidosis, uremia, azotemia, hypoglycemia, hypertensive crisis, chronic carbon dioxide retention or pulmonary ventilatory failure, hypoxia, drug intoxication, or low sodium states, patients may also show drowsiness, stupor, dulled mental ability, and shortened attention span. The electroencephalogram is usually diffusely abnormal, with slow waves of high amplitude, 3 to 4 cycles per second.

DIAGNOSTIC STUDIES

Structural damage or metabolic disturbance as the cause of coma can be differentiated by a constellation of signs and by the history of the evolution of the clinical state. Preserved pupillary light reflexes despite concomitant respiratory depression, unresponsiveness to instillation of ice water into the external auditory canals (caloric testing), and decerebrate posture or flaccid paralysis suggest the diagnosis of metabolic coma. Except for the effects of the drug glutethimide and of asphyxia, complete absence of a pupillary light reflex implies a structural rather than a metabolic coma. When no history of previous systemic disease or of ingestion of exogenous material is available, laboratory tests are required. Blood should be drawn to provide sufficient serum for the appropriate chemical determinations. A lumbar puncture should be performed while the blood pH, bicarbonate, sodium, potassium, chloride, arterial oxygen saturation, carbon dioxide tension, ammonia, urea, and sugar are being determined and the peripheral white blood cell (WBC) count, differential count, and sedimentation rate are being studied. Most hospital laboratories can determine the blood levels of barbiturates, phenytoin, bromide, and chlordiazepoxide, but if all those substances are normal, a larger toxicology laboratory will often be required. CSF studies will be helpful in ruling out subarachnoid bleeding, meningeal irritation, or infection.

THERAPY

Treatment of coma includes maintenance of an adequate airway and sufficient oxygen supply. When the cause of the coma is unknown, immediate intravenous injection of glucose (50 mg) may be helpful if the patient is in hypoglycemic coma and will do little harm if he is not. An emergency electroencephalogram may aid by indicating the presence of drug intoxication before blood levels of the drug can be determined. The EEG may show changes consistent with a postseizure state or simply confirm the diagnosis of coma by showing high-amplitude, slow waves. Electrical asymmetries may suggest a subdural hematoma. Unless respiration is spontaneously maintained, intubation or tracheostomy and respiratory support may be necessary. In cases of overdosage of barbiturates or other drugs, it is best to encourage the patient's kidneys to excrete the material; but hemodialysis may be necessary. Use of counteracting CNS stimulants usually does not reverse the coma and may contribute to increased oxygen needs by the already stressed nervous system. N-allyl normorphine (Nalline) may be useful in cases of narcotic overdosage.

Coma from acute head injury with massive cerebral edema or from a cerebrovascular accident may respond to intravenous dexamethasone (16 mg) given immediately and followed with 4 to 8 mg every 4 to 6 hours. Osmotic diuretics such as mannitol given intravenously are helpful during the initial treatment. Correction of metabolic disturbances is the only method of treatment that will improve the patient — and then only if done quickly enough — when the coma is due to salt-and-water imbalance (see later in this chapter), to liver or kidney failure, or to asphyxia.

Diagnosis of irreversible coma, or "cerebral death," has become especially important with the increased use of organ donors. It should be emphasized that the nature of the coma — whether structural or metabolic — is important in deciding on the appropriate treatment and the prognosis for recovery. Obviously, coma due to structural damage from intracerebral hemorrhage or head injury will more likely be irreversible than a metabolic, diabetic coma. Asphyxia, anoxia, or hypoglycemia lasting more than 2 hours may produce devastating and lasting structural damage to the brain. A flat (isoelectric) electroencephalogram measured at maximum amplification with a standard machine, and using at least 18 electrodes placed over the scalp, is consistent with probable cerebral death, but only if it is so recorded on at least 2 consecutive days and if there are no reflexes, no spontaneous respirations, and no response to caloric tests or painful stimulation and the patient is receiving no drugs acting on the central nervous system.

Inability to maintain blood pressure without vaso-pressors is an additional bit of evidence of cerebral death. The decision to stop artificial respiration must be weighed in the light of all the facts in each case, not only the appearance of the electroencephalogram.

Neurobehavioral Disorders

D. Frank Benson

Behavior is a broad term, denoting any response of an organism to a stimulus. In a more restricted sense, *neurobehavior* refers to behavioral activity exclusive of primary motor and sensory responses of the central nervous system. Human beings exhibit a great number of abnormal neurobehavioral activities caused by brain disease.

Neurobehavioral disorders are identified and evaluated by the portion of the neurologic examination called the mental status review. Because the potential variety of behavioral manifestations is so vast, no battery of tests offers a comprehensive evaluation. Table 62-1 presents an outline of the major items in a mental status review.

The causes of neurobehavioral symptoms are almost as variable as the symptoms themselves. While drugs, toxic or metabolic influences, tumors, trauma, infectious processes, and vascular disorders are all likely to produce rather specific behavioral symptoms, there are many differences as well as similarities between the symptoms caused by various other etiologic processes. The particular portion of the central nervous system affected is just as important as the etiologic agent. Structural damage to one cortical or subcortical area may produce specific signs and symptoms that are readily distinguishable from abnormalities arising in a neighboring site. Study of neurobehavioral disorders therefore cannot center on either anatomic or etiologic factors, but on a combination of the two. The remainder of this section will reflect this interplay with discussions of some subjects as clinical syndromes and others as manifestations of anatomic involvement.

Clinical Syndromes

The State of Conscious Awareness. The first, and certainly a key, determination is the determination of awareness. Any aberration from normal will affect

Table 62-1. Mental Status Evaluation

1. State of Awareness
   a. Degree of alertness
   b. Attention
2. General Behavior and Appearance
   a. Neat
   b. Messy
3. Mood and Affect
   a. Objective
   b. Subjective
4. Verbal Function
   a. Spontaneous speech
   b. Comprehension
   c. Repetition
   d. Word-finding
   e. Reading and writing
5. Nonverbal Function
   a. Copy-drawing
   b. Designs
6. Memory
   a. Immediate recall
   b. Ability to learn
   c. Retrieval of old information
7. Manipulation of Knowledge
   a. Calculations
   b. Proverbs
   c. Similarities and differences
8. Mental Content
   a. Perception (hallucinations)
   b. Thought processes and content (delusions)
   c. Insight — judgment
   d. Personality
   e. Rapport
   f. Personal reaction to patient

behavior and therefore all the remaining portions of the mental status evaluation. The terms used to indicate abnormalities of conscious awareness include *clouding of consciousness, confusion, obtundation, lethargy, coma, stupor,* and *delirium.* Differentiation can be made between disorders of alertness (consciousness) and disorders of attention.

Although highly significant to clinicians, fluctuations in degree of alertness are difficult to evaluate and quantify. Thus, while *coma, stupor, semicoma, lethargy, obtundation, drowsiness,* and similar terms are intended to indicate degrees of depressed consciousness, it is often more helpful to record disturbances of consciousness on a behavioral basis, using tests of stimulus-response. For any patient with less than fully normal alertness, this state will be quantified by description of the degree of stimulus (e.g., verbal coaxing, pinching, strong pain) that was necessary to produce a degree of response (e.g., verbalization, moaning, grimacing, body movement). While this stimulus-response description is at best crude, any alteration it documents in the level of consciousness from one examination to the next has obvious significance.

Variations in attention are also noteworthy, but difficult to evaluate. Two major variations are inattention associated with decreased alertness and inattention despite full alertness. In the first, patients can be alerted, but attention then wanes and they drift back into a somnolent state. The patients apparently falls asleep — a state that can be described as "failing attention." While these patients can be alerted, there is an abnormality of background alertness producing the disturbance of attention. The usual cause is pathologic involvement of the midbrain or diencephalic portions of the reticular activating system as a result of intoxication (drugs, metabolic disturbances), pressure (tumors), vascular insufficiency (stroke), or trauma.

In the second variety of disturbed attention, patients appear to be fully alert and attempt to be cooperative, but they have great difficulty maintaining concentration on the immediate task. Almost any external stimulus will distract their attention. Such disturbance may be described as "wandering attention," which may result from either focal or widespread brain disease. The focal pathologic condition (tumor, vascular infarction, trauma, or CNS syphilis) usually involves subfrontal or frontal structures, higher in the neuraxis than the structures undergoing the disorders that produce failing attention.

The test of digit span, or one of its many modifications, can be used to quantify attention. "Normal" can be considered the span of 7 plus or minus two digits. If letter span is used, subtract one, and if words are used, subtract two. Tests of span are not fully reliable, however, and clinical suspicion and careful observation are often necessary to discover a symptomatically significant disturbance of attention.

Akinetic mutism may be defined as a state of limited responsiveness in the absence of gross alteration of the primary sensory-motor mechanisms. Two varieties are recognized, an active type (coma vigil) and an apathetic type (somolent mutism). In coma vigil the patient lies immobile but appears alert because of free movement of the eyes in following visual stimuli. In somnolent mutism the patient is immobile but with eyes closed, apparently asleep; and, even with sufficient stimulus to produce eye-opening, ophthalmoplegia or extraocular palsy of some variety is usually noted. The two variations of akinetic mutism reflect different anatomic lesions. The apathetic variety results from abnormality in the mesencephalic-diencephalic junction; the vigilant variety, from abnormality in the subfrontal or septal area.

Language Syndromes. In human beings the primary motor, sensory, auditory, and visual cortices have connections with subcortical regions. The main afferent and efferent connections of each of these primary motor and sensory areas are with the association cortex lying immediately adjacent. The three cortical areas subserving language association pathways are (1): *Broca's area* (2 in Fig. 62-2), anterior to the lower end of the motor cortex (1 in Fig. 62-2), which is concerned with movements of cranial musculature; (2) *Wernicke's area* (4 in Fig. 62-2), which includes the cortex of the postero-superior temporal region, lying adjacent to the primary auditory cortex (the transverse temporal gyrus, concealed within the lateral (Sylvian) fissure (Wernicke's area is probably involved in the learning patterns of auditory signals); and (3) the *angular gyrus region* (5 in Fig. 62-2), located at the junction of the visual, somesthetic, and auditory association cortices. A knowledge of these anatomic areas as the basis of speech is necessary for clinical localization of lesions in the aphasias.

Although much more is known about abnormal language function (generally called *aphasia*) than any other neurobehavioral disorder, language disturbances are difficult to diagnose and manage. Aphasia can be defined most simply as a loss or impairment of language caused by brain damage. This definition excludes nondevelopment of language (language

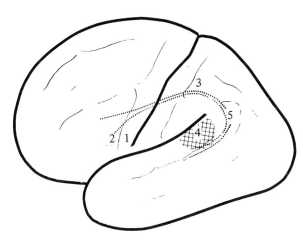

Figure 62-2. Cortical areas subserving language: (1) motor area, (2) Broca's area, (3) arcuate fasciculus, (4) Wernicke's area, (5) angular gyrus region. These areas and their connections serve as the anatomic basis of speech.

retardation of childhood) and pure speech disturbances (bulbar palsy, parkinsonian dysarthria). Aphasia usually results from damage to one cerebral hemisphere (the dominant hemisphere, which in the majority of humans is the left). Crude figures suggest that more than 99 percent of the right-handed individuals and more than 60 percent of the left-handed who suffer aphasia have a left-hemisphere insult.

Aphasia, then, indicates left-hemisphere abnormality in over 95 percent of instances.

Table 62-2 gives the classification currently used at the Boston Veterans Administration Aphasia Research Center. The more common and more striking varieties of aphasia are described here, but for greater detail the reader is advised to consult the references.

Broca's aphasia (also called motor aphasia, cortical dysarthria, and verbal aphasia) has recognizable characteristics. Conversational speech is nonfluent (dysarthric, sparse, dysprosodic, and effortful, with disturbed repetition and word-finding), yet comprehension of spoken language is comparatively well preserved. Writing is abnormal, and reading comprehension is often disturbed. The causative lesion almost invariably involves the posteroinferior portion of the third frontal convolution (Fig. 62-2). Most patients with Broca's aphasia have a right hemiplegia, and apraxia often interferes with the motor performance of the apparently normal left limbs.

Wernicke's aphasia (sensory aphasia, receptive aphasia) differs strikingly from Broca's aphasia. Although conversational speech is fluent (well articulated, displaying normal melody and phrase length, effortless), it is often contaminated by paraphasic substitution of syllables or entire words. If the output is rapid and full of paraphasia, it is incomprehensible; it is called jargon aphasia. There is a severe disturbance

Table 62-2. Clinical Varieties of Aphasia

1. Aphasia with repetition disturbance
   a. Broca's aphasia
   b. Wernicke's aphasia
   c. Conduction aphasia
2. Aphasia without repetition disturbance
   a. Isolation of the speech area
   b. Transcortical motor aphasia
   c. Transcortical sensory aphasia
   d. Anomic aphasia
3. Disturbance primarily affecting reading and writing: Alexia with agraphia
4. Total aphasia: Global aphasia
5. Syndromes with disturbance of a single language modality
   a. Alexia without agraphia
   b. Aphemia
   c. Pure word deafness
6. Nonaphasia misnaming

of comprehension and of repetition, and usually word-finding is deficient. Both reading and writing are abnormal. Most patients with Wernicke's aphasia have no paralysis or other overt neurologic signs. The site of the abnormality producing Wernicke's aphasia is the posterosuperior portion of the temporal lobe (Fig. 62-2).

Conduction aphasia. A lesion located between the temporal and frontal language areas produces a distinctive abnormality called conduction aphasia (central aphasia, repetition aphasia) (Fig. 62-2). Conversational speech is fluent, but with paraphasias; comprehension is good, but repetition is strikingly abnormal. Word-finding and writing are usually disturbed, but reading comprehension is often maintained. The most frequent pathologic site is in the white matter deep to the supramarginal gyrus.

Isolation syndrome. If the perisylvian area remains intact but there is widespread damage to the remaining cortex, as in a border-zone infarction, an unusual and distinctive aphasia occurs. Patients can repeat with ease items such as complex sentences, foreign phrases, and nonsense syllables, but they can neither initiate nor comprehend speech; they cannot name anything nor read or write. The speech area necessary for repetition is effectively isolated from the remainder of the cortex. This rare syndrome is usually the result of severe anoxia or acute left carotid occlusion, but incomplete degrees of the condition (called transcortical motor aphasia or transcortical sensory aphasia) are not uncommon.

Anomic aphasia. Aphasia consisting primarily of word-finding problems is very common. Usually anomic aphasia is accompanied by a writing abnormality, and in some cases by reading problems or difficulty with comprehension. Many loci of pathologic conditions can produce anomic aphasia; indeed, widespread degenerative disease such as presenile dementia (Alzheimer's disease) produces a significant anomia. Table 62-3 offers the language features of the major varieties of aphasia.

Aphasia can result from any insult to the brain that involves the appropriate cortical site. Vascular infarctions, traumas, or tumors are responsible for most cases of aphasia, with occasional cases caused by infections, degenerative diseases, or metabolic processes. A lengthy and often frustrating experience, rehabilitation of the aphasic is successful frequently enough to warrant great effort. A complete rehabilitation program includes aphasia therapy (by a specially trained speech pathologist), physical therapy, social and vocational counseling, and a great deal of support and reassurance. Obviously, treatment of the underlying cause must be carried on along with rehabilitation measures.

Table 62-3. Clinical Features of Aphasia

	Spontaneous speech	Comprehension	Repetition	Naming	Reading	Writing
Broca's aphasia	Nonfluent	+	−	±	Aloud − Comp. ±	−
Wernicke's aphasia	Fluent	−	−	−	−	−
Conduction aphasia	Fluent	+	−	±	Aloud − Comp. +	−
Isolation syndrome	Fluent	−	+	−	−	−
Transcortical motor aphasia	Fluent	+	+	−	Aloud − Comp. +	−
Transcortical sensory aphasia	Fluent	−	+	−	−	−
Anomic aphasia	Fluent	+	+	−	±	±
Alexia with agraphia	Fluent	+	+	+	−	−
Alexia without agraphia	Fluent	+	+	+	−	+

Memory. *Memory* and *amnesia* (loss of memory) are much-used, much-abused terms that need careful definition. Memory cannot be considered a single, unitary function. For diagnostic purposes, most clinicians apply three distinctly different techniques for outlining memory disturbance. These are (1) tests of serial repetition, as typified by the digit span; (2) tests of ability to learn new material; and (3) tests of ability to retrieve old learned information. Occasionally all three tests will show abnormality, but often only one technique will demonstrate a defect. The terms suggested for memory disturbances remain unsettled, and they are often used in a variable and confusing manner. In particular, the experimental psychologist's division of memory function into two types — short-term memory and long-term memory — fails to encompass the memory disturbances seen in clinical practice. For present purposes, older terms are used to describe failure according to the three major testing techniques: (1) immediate recall — for immediate repetition span; (2) recent memory — for ability to learn new material; and (3) remote memory — for ability to retrieve old information.

The amnesic syndrome is characterized by an inability to acquire new information despite adequate intellectual functioning and no clouding of consciousness. The classic example of the amnesic syndrome is alcoholic psychosis (Korsakoff's psychosis), secondary to thiamine deficiency. A similar mental state may be seen following head trauma (posttraumatic amnesia), cerebral surgery, brain tumor, cerebral vascular disease, encephalitis, and electroshock therapy.

Korsakoff's psychosis is often called the amnestic-confabulatory syndrome, emphasizing its two most conspicuous features. Patients have excellent (often above-normal) immediate recall but fail to retain information for even a few minutes. The ability to retrieve old information is relatively well preserved, but there is often a period of several years preceding the onset of illness about which they remember nothing (retrograde amnesia). Confabulation is not constant, but it is dramatic when present. When asked questions, the patient volunteers answers that are obviously wrong and often bizarre. If investigated closely, however, most of the confabula-

tions are found to be items from the patient's earlier experiences. The confabulatory state has been described as one in which patients cannot remember that they cannot remember; thus they answer questions with the best information available from their stock of old information. Confabulation is seen only in the early stages. As patients begin to understand that they are suffering a memory loss, confabulation decreases and then disappears.

Recovery from Korsakoff's psychosis is variable, ranging from almost no improvement to a total return of learning ability. There is usually a striking personality pattern accompanying alcoholic psychosis, a state characterized by passivity, indifference, apathy, and contentment.

The pathologic state in Korsakoff's psychosis is reported to be bilateral degeneration of the mammillary bodies. Other causes of the amnesic syndrome, such as trauma, tumor, and cerebrovascular accident, usually involve the medial temporal lobes bilaterally. The ability to learn new material appears to be dependent upon the intactness of the central core of the limbic system, at least on one side.

Cognition. The ability to use one's store of information in a creative manner — that is, to manipulate old knowledge — is one of the major aspects of cognition. Testing cognitive function is done best by specialized psychological methods, but several simple tests, particularly proverb interpretation and arithmetic calculation, help the clinician to gauge intellectual competency. Problem-solving demands manipulation of old, overlearned arithmetic, while proverb interpretation is dependent upon the ability to comprehend the meaning of language and to alter that meaning through metaphor formation. Both represent high-level intellectual activities.

Dementia may be characterized as a loss or impairment of intellectual function, usually accompanied by some memory loss and personality change. An almost limitless number of disorders can produce dementia, seriously complicating etiologic diagnosis. Many dementing states are reversible, but specific therapy is necessary and depends upon an accurate etiologic diagnosis. For practical purposes, dementias can be divided into those with and those without hydrocephalus; and the hydrocephalic dementias can be subdivided into obstructive and nonobstructive varieties.

Dementia without hydrocephalus, which is most often due to metabolic, fluid, or electrolyte disturbances, should be investigated vigorously because many of the causative conditions are amenable to treatment. The clinician should also remember that emotional or functional disorders may produce the appearance of dementia. Both depressive and hysterical pseudodementias are reported, and a syndrome of "approximate answers" (Ganser's syndrome) is sometimes based on pseudodementia.

Hydrocephalic dementia without objective sign of obstruction, as demonstrated by pneumoencephalogram, CAT scan, or isotope cysternography, usually indicates a degenerative process — for example, Alzheimer's disease, Pick's disease, Jakob-Creutzfeldt disease, subcortical sclerosis, and senile dementia. At present there is no specific treatment for any of these conditions.

Obstructive hydrocephalus can be studied by radiographic or isotope techniques. Obstruction of the ventricular outflow channels usually produces signs of increased intracranial pressure, along with depressed intellect. Treatment is usually by surgical extirpation, or, if that is not possible, by shunting of CSF from the ventricles to the subarachnoid space. Obstruction of CSF flow through the cortical-subarachnoid channels — so-called normal pressure hydrocephalus — can be corrected by shunting CSF away from the subarachnoid space to the peritoneum or into the right atrium. In some patients shunting procedures produce dramatic improvements in intellectual status.

Frontal Lobe

The *frontal lobes,* which are very large in human beings, affect many aspects of behavior, particularly motor response patterns. The principal symptoms of frontal damage are changes in movement, aphasia, and even disturbances in attention to sensory stimuli. In addition, however, damage to the frontal lobes often produces a characteristic behavioral pattern, the so-called frontal lobe syndrome.

The frontal lobe syndrome is a collection of be-

havioral aberrations that may be seen in patients with frontal disorders. In full sway, these behavioral patterns may be characterized as irritability with euphoric apathy — an unusual combination, indicating advanced frontal abnormality. Careful study of frontal cases produced by head injury, psychosurgery, brain tumor, and neurosyphilis suggests four major components of the frontal lobe syndrome: (1) some degree of poor judgment and lack of foresight; (2) shallow affective state; (3) disinhibition, tactlessness, and inappropriate social acts; and (4) reduced drive and loss of self-concern.

While trauma, tumor, and psychosurgery are the most frequent sources of the frontal lobe syndrome, there is a common variant produced by vascular disease involving the upper motor neuron pathways. It is called pseudobulbar palsy, because of abnormality in bulbar motor activities (dysphagia, drooling, expressionless face, hoarseness), but the most striking sign is an excessive response to emotional stimuli. Thus, slightly sad remarks may produce uncontrollable weeping, while a mild joke can cause almost hysterical laughter. Though appropriate for the stimulus, the response is excessive (disinhibited); it has been termed lability of emotional expression and is strongly suggestive of bilateral upper motor disease.

Temporal Lobe

Like the frontal lobe, the temporal lobe has many facets, and disease can produce a multiplicity of symptoms, the most common being disturbances of auditory perception and memory. The temporal lobe contains the most epileptogenic tissues in the brain, and seizures are a common manifestation of temporal lobe dysfunction. Temporal lobe seizures more than seizures arising from other areas are liable to be associated with behavioral disorders, as either ictal, preictal, or postictal manifestations. Temporal lobe disorders frequently produce fear as an aura. Abnormality of the temporal lobe often accounts for abnormality of perception, too, as part of a seizure picture. Thus, illusions such as micropsia, macropsia, metamorphopsia, and feelings of depersonalization suggest pathologic findings in the temporal lobe. Déjà vu — the feeling of familiarity or reexperiencing, which everyone has occasionally — is much more common in temporal lobe disease states. Hallucinations (both auditory and visual), thought blocking, and disorders in the sense of time have all been reported as part of temporal lobe seizure patterns. While usually associated with the motor manifestations of a seizure, each of these behavioral changes may occur alone, causing problems in diagnosis.

Parietal Lobe

The *parietal lobe* receives somesthetic stimuli and through its association areas integrates those stimuli with other sensory inputs. The tests of parietal function include those of position sense, graphesthesia, stereognosis, and two-point discrimination. Disturbances of parietal association-area function may produce many behavioral abnormalities, which for the sake of brevity will be considered under two broad categories, unilateral neglect and disturbances of body image.

While many parietal lesions produce actual sensory loss, patients with cortical damage may show adequate sensory perception but they may neglect, or actually be unaware of, stimuli coming to one side. Thus, if auditory, visual, or somesthetic stimuli are given to only one side at a time, the response is correct; but if bilateral stimuli are offered simultaneously, the patient responds only to the stimulus from the side contralateral to the lesion. Of the various explanations that have been offered for this phenomenon, one suggests a change in perceptual rivalry between the hemispheres. Normally, each hemisphere receives stimuli from one-half of external space. These signals are carefully balanced by years of practice. With damage to one of the signal systems, the message in the other becomes so overwhelming that it drowns out its rival. This can be observed clinically in the patient who ignores or even denies the existence of his affected side. If cortical denial or neglect is present, there is always an additional factor, such as memory loss or confusional state.

In somewhat the same manner, disturbances may occur in the recognition of one's body image in space. Many clinical variations of this disorder are seen. One of the more common is the combination of finger agnosia, right-left disorientation, acalculia, and agraphia (Gerstmann's syndrome) that indicates dominant-hemisphere parietal disturbance. Constructional disturbances (such as difficulties in drawing and making block designs and stick constructions) may occur with any significant cerebral damage, but they are particularly prevalent after parietal lesions of either hemisphere. Disturbances of orientation in space (topographagnosia) also occur much more frequently after parietal damage.

Occipital Lobe

The major neurologic abnormality occurring after occipital damage is unilateral disturbance of vision (homonymous hemianopia). In addition, several specific behavioral syndromes may occur. A very distinct one is seen after infarction of the left calcarine area together with the splenium of the corpus callosum. This produces a right homonymous hemianopia and an inability to read, despite quite normal ability to write. The clinical situation is the consequence of the patient's ability to see with his left visual field, but inability of this visual input to reach the left-hemisphere language area. Writing remains normal because the entire left-hemisphere language area is intact.

Visual hallucinations may occur with occipital disturbances. If the disorder is posterior, involving primarily the occipital lobe, the hallucinations are likely to be formless (stars, zigzags, sprinkled dots of color). If the damage is more anterior in the temporal-occipital axis, well-formed images (animals, humans) occur. Often the hallucinated images occur in the blind or visually deficient half-field. Denial of blindness (Anton's syndrome) usually suggests some disturbance (memory loss, confusion) in addition to visual loss.

DISTURBANCES OF MOVEMENT

The patient may first notice proximal muscle weakness when he has difficulty climbing stairs, and distal weakness when he is unable to hold a glass properly or to guide a pen without strain. He may also notice muscular atrophy, such as wasting of the first dorsal interosseous space or the thenar eminence. Sometimes the main complaint is described as progressive weakness following exercise, as a dysphagia or a diplopia, which recovers after rest. A freak accident of a broken leg may be the first sign of weakness of muscular stabilization of the hip. The doctor must consider whether a patient's inability to perform motor functions is due to a lesion of the brain, the spinal cord pathways, or the motor nerves and their connections with muscles, or whether it arises in the muscle itself.

The anterior horn cell, its axon, and its neuromuscular junction together comprise a *motor unit.* A peripheral nerve is made up of the axons of many motor units. Knowledge of the segmental arrangement of nerves is helpful in relating a given muscle paralysis to a lesion of a particular nerve, nerve root, or level of spinal anterior horn cells.

Selective electromyographic techniques may help by revealing fibrillation potentials in an affected muscle. These indicate a neurogenic defect, with spontaneous firing of muscle-fiber membranes that have been separated from the trophic effects of the anterior horn cell in a particular motor unit, as may occur when the neuron is diseased (e.g., in poliomyelitis); when the axon is injured or severed by trauma; or when the myelin sheath cannot conduct properly because of infectious, degenerative, or abnormal metabolic processes. Fibrillation potentials in a group of muscle fibers lacking complete innervation appear about 21 days after denervation and persist as long as the fiber is viable, disappearing only when the fiber becomes atrophic or fibrotic. (Polyphasic potentials, which indicate regeneration of nerve fibers, can also be recorded electromyographically in affected muscles.)

Weakness of muscles occurs whenever nerve impulses fail to cross the neuromuscular junction and initiate a meaningful contraction. Disturbances of neuromuscular transmission can be produced by various drugs, such as curare or succinylcholine, or they may occur in patients with myasthenia gravis, or as the result of poisoning by botulin toxin or as an effect of certain neoplasms. The muscle itself may be diseased, inflamed, or degenerating, and thus be weakened. Such myopathies can be differentiated from diseases of the motor unit by their appearance

on biopsy, as well as by their electrical pattern of low-amplitude, short-duration potentials, firing rapidly from all fibers upon contraction, despite muscle weakness.

Anterior Horn Cell Diseases. When upper motor neurons become affected, the initial clinical effect on muscle tone is spasticity. When lower motor neuron lesions predominate, there is mainly progressive muscle weakness, and, later, atrophy. Primary involvement of motor neurons occurs in several conditions, one of which is *amyotrophic lateral sclerosis* (also known as *progressive muscular atrophy* and *progressive bulbar palsy*). In amyotrophic lateral sclerosis, upper as well as lower motor neurons are affected. The concurrent progression of this disease in motor neurons at all levels results in a combined picture of amyotrophy and spasticity due to lateral corticospinal tract involvement (Lou Gehrig's disease). When the spastic paraparesis is first noted, the physician looks for a surgically remediable lesion in the cervical region, such as spondylosis or tumor; then he considers vitamin B_{12} deficiency, and demyelinating diseases of the spinal cord such as multiple sclerosis and transverse myelopathy. Dysarthria, dysphagia, or both may be the earliest symptoms when the process begins in the bulbar nuclei. Weakness of the hands and fingers leads to clumsiness of movement. Not uncommonly, the process begins asymmetrically and goes on for 2 to 5 years, rarely longer. The patient usually experiences sudden, large involuntary movements of groups of muscle fibers before atrophy is recognized beneath the subcutaneous fat and skin. The spontaneous muscle movements, sometimes accentuated by exercise, which are known as fasciculations, can be recorded by electromyography as large, high-amplitude, multiphasic potentials of moderate duration occurring at random frequency. When only the hands are affected, especially unilaterally, the difficulty is often attributed to a peripheral nerve lesion or to a cervical radiculopathy. Further observation of the patient will often reveal spreading muscular wasting. Early in the process the shoulder girdle and upper arms are involved. The palate is affected shortly after the tongue, which shows fasciculations on its surface.

Acute anterior poliomyelitis produces asymmetric flaccid paralysis by poliovirus infection and destruction of motor cells in the spinal cord and brainstem. Following systemic infection by the virus, paralysis develops 2 to 5 days after the appearance of meningeal signs. Progression of motor weakness may continue for another 3 to 5 days; then the clinical picture stabilizes. The paralytic cases fan be subdivided into spinal and bulbar forms. Respiratory paralysis often results in death when the medullary nuclei are affected. The CSF reveals lymphocytosis and normal to moderately elevated protein. The prognosis is poor when the paralysis becomes extensive. Partially denervated muscles may have some recovery of function. The degree of residual motor paralysis depends on the total number of ventral horn cells that have been permanently destroyed.

Syringomyelia can produce muscle atrophy following initial weakness and fasciculations and, differing from amyotrophic lateral sclerosis, sensory deficits. Similarly, *spinal cord tumors* involving the cervical region are likely to cause both muscle wasting of the shoulders and upper extremities and local sensory losses. There may also be spasticity in the lower extremities, due to corticospinal-tract involvement. A neurogenic bladder occurs, with spinal cord compression (this is extremely unusual in cases of amyotrophic lateral sclerosis until very late in the illness). In *syphilitic amyotrophy* and *diabetic amyotrophy,* early weakness and wasting is accompanied by pain and usually occurs in a radicular distribution. Following nonspecific viral illnesses or after injection of vaccines, isolated motor neuropathy may develop. *Postinfectious polyneuropathy* (Guillain-Barré syndrome) is often preceded by sudden radicular pain.

Recognition of the treatable motor unit diseases is very important. Sometimes surgical aspiration of a cyst associated with syringomyelia or decompression of the spinal cord by removal of a tumor or spondylotic protrusion will ameliorate the symptoms.

Radiculopathies

Cervical spondylosis, producing impingement on nerve roots and entrapment syndromes of peripheral nerves, may simulate motor neuron disease when associated with muscle wasting. Fasciculations with no sensory loss may occur. Cervical vertebrae may undergo degenerative changes at their articulating surfaces as a response to repeated trauma and aging. Incidental radiologic findings of degenerative arthropathic changes with spur formation are found without symptoms in many people over 50 years old. The changes involve degeneration of the intervertebral disks and secondary changes in the vertebral bodies and in the neurocentral and apophyseal joints. Pathologic changes also appear in the anulus fibrosus and in the region of the intervertebral foramina. Symptoms arise when the spinal cord is impinged upon directly by a spondylotic bar, when its blood supply is interfered with, or when nerve roots are compressed or impinged upon by a spur. Varied symptoms may result from a combination of root and spinal cord involvement.

The pain associated with cervical radiculopathy is presumably due to traction upon nerve roots and upon the dural sleeves. Cervical muscle spasm may contribute to the pain, although it also serves as a natural "splinting" of the cervical spines. The muscle spasm associated with cervical radiculopathies may be so severe as to eliminate the normal lordosis of the cervical spine on x-ray examination. Symptoms of referred pain and abnormalities of the deep tendon reflexes will be helpful in determining which segmental spinal level is involved, and whether or not the pain is due to root involvement. Radiculopathy at the fifth and sixth cervical levels often presents as a burning sensation in the ipsilateral suprascapular region, by way of the dorsal scapular nerve; a C7 root impingement may cause an ache in the elbow associated with pain in the lower neck. When the sensory fibers are affected, pain may radiate from lesions in the middle cervical region (C5 to C6) to the middle or index fingers or to the lateral aspect of the arm; with low cervical lesions (C7 to C8), the pain may be referred to the hypothenar region and to the fourth and fifth fingers. Movement of the neck or percussion of an involved cervical spine may reproduce the discomfort radiating into the arm. Careful muscle testing will be useful when weakness is present. The combination of weakness in the biceps muscle and a reduced biceps tendon reflex suggests a C6 involvement. The differential diagnosis of neck-arm pain should include other nerve entrapment syndromes with referred pain, such as thoracic outlet or median nerve compression, ulnar group involvement, or lesions of the radial nerve at the humerus level. Angina pectoris has often been mistaken for cervical radiculopathy, and vice versa.

Lumbosacral radiculopathies have the same mechanisms as the cervical root syndromes. Pain in the gluteal region and in the area of the greater trochanter may be due to L5 radiculopathy or to intertrochanteric bursitis. Spasm of the piriform muscle may be part of the mechanism of sciatic pain. Radiation of pain from the sciatic notch down the back of the leg may also occur with L5 root compression. Because the physician must also keep in mind pain due to intrapelvic encroachment upon the lumbar plexus or the sciatic nerve, rectal and pelvic examinations should be a part of the workup for back pain. Sprains of the low back muscles and ligaments may cause pain in the paravertebral regions, with radiation down the back of the leg. In such cases the pain is due in part to hamstring muscle spasm. Lateral leg pain spreading to the dorsum of the foot may occur with sprain syndromes associated with spasm of the tensor fasciae latae. The recurrent back pain associated with menstruation has been attributed by some to psoas muscle spasm.

A burning pain in the knee, with reduced knee jerk and quadriceps reflexes and weakness of the anterior thigh muscles, suggests involvement of lumbar root levels (L3 to L4), while a reduced Achilles tendon reflex and dysesthesia in the heel indicate S1 root compression. Weakness of the extensor hallucis and the extensor digitorum brevis muscles is usually present with L5 and S1 radiculopathies. Aggravation of low back pain on motion with referred pain down the legs occurs with root syndromes, but these are also signs of intraspinal processes. *Cauda equina tumors* may produce bilateral leg pain and a perianal burning sensation. As was mentioned above, intrapelvic masses must be ruled out by rectal examination in every case of low back pain. In some cases, sigmoidoscopy and barium enema examinations are necessary. Intravenous pyelography may reveal a pelvic mass, as with endo-

metriosis, that can produce symptoms of lumbar radiculopathy by traction on the lumbar plexus. Most of the effects of so-called whiplash injuries are due to acute muscle strain and stretching with minor tearing in the musculoligamentous attachments along the spinous processes. Transient contusion of the spinal cord rarely occurs. Spinal nerve roots may be damaged, or the intravertebral disks may be ruptured, disturbing the adjacent nerve roots. Similar pathologic processes may occur in the lumbar region, although they are less frequent than in the cervical region.

FURTHER DIAGNOSTIC STUDIES
The differential diagnosis of cervical or lumbar radiculopathy may be difficult if considered only on a clinical basis. Pain may be present without objective signs of muscle weakness or reflex changes. The possibility of secondary gain (e.g., legal compensation) accentuates underlying but otherwise tolerable discomfort in many patients complaining of low back or neck-arm pain. Underlying depression reduces a patient's tolerance for discomfort. *Electromyography* (EMG) may reveal denervation in some cases of subacute radiculopathy; however, atrophy and weakness are already present by the time the EMG is helpful. Occasionally, fibrillations may be found in the extensor digitorum brevis muscles (D1) or in the triceps (C7) and biceps (C5) muscles. Reduced numbers of motor units are often the only finding. A corresponding change in deep tendon reflexes is the most convincing evidence of a particular root injury. *Myelography* has become the best confirmatory test in localizing an impinged nerve root, a spinal cord compression, or other intraspinal abnormality. In some cases myelography may be negative, but clinical signs and persistent pain may justify an exploration at the appropriate root level.

THERAPY
Treatment of radicular syndromes requires relief of the associated muscle spasm and reduction of the irritation of the nerve root, both of which produce pain. Pain results in more muscle spasm, and a vicious cycle ensues. If we exclude cases due to acute protrusions that cause cord or cauda equina compres-

sion and require emergency laminectomy, radicular syndromes are managed best by conservative measures in 90 percent of patients, especially for the first attack. Treatment consists in bed rest on a firm mattress or bed boards for 2 to 3 weeks. Hot soaks, mild hyperextension, and analgesics may help. Leg traction is not specifically useful, but it does help keep the patient at rest. For acute cervical disk protrusions, gentle cervical traction (5 to 12 pounds for 20 to 30 minutes, four times per day) with the neck slightly flexed and the patient sitting semi-upright is the treatment of choice. This may be followed by physical therapy and use of a supporting towel or plastic collar around the neck. For severe spondylosis, with or without a ruptured disk, conservative treatment may not suffice. After study of the patient by myelography, appropriate surgical procedures should be considered.

Peripheral Neuropathies

The symptoms may include *paresthesias* (numbness, tingling, or other spontaneous sensations in the absence of an actual applied stimulus); *dysesthesias* (painful, unpleasant distortions of actual sensation); *hyperesthesias* (excessive reactions, or persistence of sensation, to a given stimulus); and *hypoesthesias* (reduced sensibilities to a stimulus). Signs of dysfunction of peripheral nerves reflect the location and degree of damage to nerve fibers and their myelin sheaths. The longest peripheral fibers are usually affected earliest; this is the reason for the "stocking-glove" pattern of sensory loss in polyneuropathy. Motor signs after denervation are hypotonia and muscle weakness, hyporeflexia, and muscle atrophy. In systemic illnesses with polyneuropathy, usually all nerves are affected, and they show prolonged conduction velocities, distally more than proximally. In the presence of severe polyneuropathy, with dense loss of all sensation in an extremity, patients may experience curious symptoms during periods of sensory deprivation, especially when the lights are off and no sound is heard. Their fingers may show "dancing" movements (pseudoathetosis) — spontaneous movement that is attributed to patients' attempts to localize their extremities in space by use of joint sensation.

Peripheral Nerve Lesions (Traumatic and Entrapment Syndromes)

Injuries to several divisions within the cervical plexus or within the lumbar plexus are approached clinically as in root syndromes, although the signs are usually more obvious. For example, weakness of both the anterior and posterior muscles of the leg would be more suggestive of a plexus lesion than a simple foot drop due to the weakness of the extensor muscles alone. Therefore the differential diagnosis of peripheral nerve lesions from plexus lesions requires careful physical examination and thorough knowledge of the anatomy and innervation of the muscles involved. In a region of localized injury and inflammation of a peripheral nerve, delay in conduction caused by damage to the myelin sheath produces weakness in the muscles subserved. Localized pain and distal sensory disturbances may be earlier symptoms than weakness and atrophy. Exogenous damage, such as a contusion or a chronic entrapment of the nerve, may produce dysfunction at the point of injury. Repeated trauma from movement of the nerve within an entrapment area usually leads to an inflammatory response, with formation of adhesions and obstruction of blood supply.

Examples of mononeuropathies due to entrapment are described below.

Occipital Nerve Syndrome. A chronic ache, a burning sensation, and tenderness over the mastoid area may be the effect of repeated traction on the occipital nerve on the same side. Recurrent muscle spasm and headache can also occur. Xylocaine injection of the nerve may give some relief, but occipital neurectomy is often necessary for complete elimination of the symptoms.

Thoracic Outlet Syndromes (Costoclavicular Syndrome, Scalenus Syndrome). Symptoms of pain in the arm, local tenderness in the costoclavicular region, and a full, engorged feeling in the arm may occur with these syndromes. There may be episodes of coldness in the fingers and of numbness along the distribution of the ulnar nerve. Motor weakness may develop in the small muscles of the hand. The diagnosis of thoracic outlet syndrome may be suspected from the history and will be strengthened if the physician hears an arterial bruit on auscultation over the anterior cervical triangle. The bruit is usually accentuated by abducting and extending the arm. Turning the head to the side opposite to the lesion may exaggerate the symptoms. The radial pulse will usually disappear as the symptoms are brought out. The inferior cord of the brachial plexus along with the subclavian artery and vein constitute the neurovascular bundle, which has an intimate relationship with the scalenus anterior muscle and tendon and with an enlarged cervical transverse process or a fibrous band uniting such a process to the first rib. The mutual relationships of the various structures of the upper thoracic outlet are continually being altered, both by respiratory movements and by movements of the arms. Repeated trauma of the neurovascular bundle from a stretch injury to the arm, from changes in posture due to pregnancy or weight gain, or from wearing a heavy pack with shoulder straps may lead to compression entrapment of the nerve, artery, and vein. Nerve conduction studies may be of little help in making this diagnosis except in instances of prolonged compression of the nerve; then, ulnar and median nerve conduction velocities may be slowed. Plethysmographic studies of the vascular physiology or brachial arteriography may be needed to establish convincing bases for an operation (see Chap. 27).

Dorsal Scapular Nerve Syndrome. A burning pain in the scapular region may result from impingement of the dorsal scapular nerve. This nerve, which is derived from the distal portion of the fifth cervical root, passes through the body of the scalenus medius muscle and proceeds inferoposteriorly to reach the rhomboid muscles and a portion of the levator scapulae muscle. Overactivity of the scalenus medius muscle with unremitting pressure on the dorsal scapular nerve may set up chronic irritation and inflammation. Eventually, weakness and atrophy of the affected muscles leads to winging of the scapula. Treatment by surgical section of the scalenus medius muscle to give the nerve more freedom of movement will usually relieve pain and, when the muscles regain strength, lead to proper fixation of the scapula against the chest wall when the arm is abducted.

Long Thoracic Nerve Syndrome. Winging of the scapula due to dorsal scapular nerve entrapment and rhomboid paralysis must be differentiated from entrapment of the long thoracic nerve, which also travels through the scalenus medius muscle. The long thoracic nerve supplies the serratus anterior muscle, which fixes the scapula when forward pressure is exerted with the arm. Winging of the scapula may be greater with serratus anterior paralysis than with rhomboid paralysis. The appropriate treatment is surgical exploration and sectioning of the scalenus medius muscle.

Radial Nerve Syndrome. The radial nerve passes from the axilla down the arm, spiraling posteriorly from the medial to the lateral side of the humerus between the origins of the lateral and medial heads of the triceps muscle. It pierces the lateral intramuscular septum to occupy a position in front of the lateral condyle of the humerus between two other muscles, the brachialis and the brachioradialis. After bifurcation, the deep branch passes under a fibrous edge of the extensor carpi radialis muscle and then through a slit in the supinator muscle. At any of the various points of close relationship to muscle edges, slow compression of the fibers may occur. Development of a lesion such as a lipoma within the supinator muscle may cause extensor paralysis and atrophy without pain. However, the radial nerve syndrome usually consists of pain in the elbow region with slight weakness and atrophy in the extensor muscles. Dorsiflexion or supination of the wrist or extension of the fingers will aggravate the pain. Extension of the middle finger while the elbow is extended is especially painful. The superficial branch of the radial nerve runs down the forearm under the brachioradialis, lying on the extensor carpi radialis longus muscle. Entrapment of the superficial branch occurs in patients in whom the nerve penetrates the extensor carpi radialis brevis before emerging to supply the skin in the region of the metacarpal multangular joints. This area becomes dysesthetic when the superficial branch is compressed or becomes injured, as during removal of a ganglion at that location. When the posterior interosseous branch is entrapped as it passes through the interosseous ligament in the forearm there is paralysis of the indicis proprius, making the patient unable to extend his index finger.

Ulnar Nerve Syndromes. The ulnar nerve passes through an opening in the medial intermuscular septum of the upper arm to reach a groove behind the medial epicondyle of the elbow. The nerve is held in the groove behind the medial epicondyle by a fibrous expansion of the origin of the common flexor muscle. Trauma may be the result of a single blow (on the "funny bone"), with subsequent scarring, or of repeated tightening of the nerve within the cubital tunnel, brought about by a disturbed angle of the elbow following fracture, dislocation, or infection. Localization of a block in the ulnar nerve is based on the degree of hypalgesia in the sensory distribution of the nerve and on the extent of weakness of the flexor carpi ulnaris and flexor digitorum profundus muscles. Nerve conduction velocity studies may reveal prolonged latencies across the cubital tunnel, with normal conduction velocity above the elbow and slow conduction below the elbow. Cubital tunnel syndromes, with an inadequate relationship between the taut nerve and the fibrous roof of the tunnel, are often bilateral. *Tardy ulnar nerve palsy,* a neuropathy arising months or years after an earlier trauma, is usually unilateral. Occupational hazards may be responsible, as in a taxi driver who rests his elbow on an armrest or a traffic policeman who makes frequent flexing and extending movements at the elbow, pulling the taut nerve against the wall of the canal. A too freely moving ulnar nerve may slide in and out of the groove if the fascial covering over the tunnel is inadequate or if the bone groove is shallow. Complete dislocation of the nerve may occur with extreme movements of the elbow. The nerve is often palpable as it is moved over the medial epicondyle. The best treatment for a freely moving ulnar nerve is surgical transposition of the nerve anteriorly. *Entrapment of the palmar branch* of the ulnar nerve may occur as the nerve passes into the hand or through a shallow opening between the pisiform bone and the hook of the hamate. Trauma to the pisiform bone or fracture of the hamate may lead to entrapment of the ulnar

nerve at this point. Complaints of burning dysesthesia in the fourth and fifth fingers will accompany the onset of entrapment of the palmar trunk or of its superficial branches. Later, weakness of fine movements of the fingers and atrophy of the interosseous muscles are noted. When only the deep branch is involved, there are signs of weakness and atrophy without sensory defect. Radiologic examination of the hand may reveal a small fracture or dislocation of the pisiform-hamate tunnel. Electromyography may confirm the diagnosis, and surgical exploration of the hand may be necessary.

Median Nerve Syndromes. The median nerve passes through the pronator teres muscle and dips under the edge of the flexor digitorum sublimis muscle to reach its midforearm position between that muscle and the flexor digitorum profundus muscle. The nerve can be traumatized by the fibrous edge of the sublimis bridge or lifted up by the ulnar head of the pronator. The main complaints are numbness and dysesthesia over the radial side of the palm and the palmar side of the first, second, and third digits and half of the fourth digit. The patient is unable to pronate or to flex the wrist and has partial loss of flexion of the fingers and loss of apposition of the thumb. Sudden, direct trauma is unusual as a cause, but constant pressure on the inner aspect of the arm is common, as from carrying a heavy load, resting a partner's head on the upper forearm ("honeymoon paralysis"), or bearing pressure from the strap of a heavy purse at the susceptible point. In the pronator syndrome, deep palpation of the median nerve in the proximal portion of the forearm will reproduce the patient's complaints of numbness and tingling. Nerve conduction studies may be helpful in differentiating pronator entrapment from the more distal carpal tunnel syndrome. Radiographic examination of the humerus may reveal a supracondylar process predisposing to entrapment. Surgical exploration may be indicated.

A diagnosis of *carpal tunnel syndrome* can be made when the patient has severe pain in the hand that appears during sleep and intensifies upon awakening. After several such episodes of nocturnal pain, the patient learns that shaking the hand downward or holding it over the side of the bed or running cold water over the hand and wrist will give relief. A woman may tell her physician that the pain is worse premenstrually. She may relate it to dish-washing, gardening, crocheting, or any other activity requiring exertion of the wrists. Both wrists may have aching or pain, but the one used more will show the symptoms first. Not uncommonly, a woman in the seventh month of pregnancy may complain of such hand pain, which will intensify until term and then subside after delivery. Rarely is it necessary to relieve entrapment of the median nerve during pregnancy, unless the pain becomes very severe. Other patients may develop wrist and hand pain later in life after other precipitating circumstances, such as hypothyroidism, rheumatoid arthritis, diabetes, weight gain, or simply wearing a tight bracelet or watchband. Various industrial maneuvers too may bring on symptoms of the carpal tunnel syndrome.

The carpal tunnel consists of the transverse carpal ligament, the fibrous sheath over the carpal bones, and their interosseous ligaments. The thick and relatively inelastic transverse carpal ligament forming the roof extends from the wrist forward to the medial convexity of the thenar eminence. The motor branch of the median nerve is damaged at the distal edge of the ligament. Entrapment at the wrist causes dys-esthesia in the index and middle fingers and some-times in all the fingertips, weakness of the abductor pollicis brevis muscle, and variable degrees of weak-ness of the opponens muscle. Tenderness is present at the wrist, where gentle tapping will evoke an electric-shocklike sensation in the fingers (Tinel's sign). Latency of median nerve conduction across the wrist is the best finding to make a positive diagnosis of carpal tunnel syndrome — latency being determined as the time for a stimulus applied to the median nerve below the carpal ligament to produce a motor response in the abductor pollicis brevis muscle. If the latency is greater than 5.0 msec in the affected hand and less than that in the unaffected one, and if, in addition, the ulnar latencies across the wrist are normal — that is, less than 5.0 msec — the lesion is likely to be in the median nerve at the wrist. Often the latency times are prolonged as much

as 12 to 17 msec. Motor responses may be completely absent when there has been significant atrophy. An evoked sensory latency — namely, one recorded over the nerve at the wrist after a stimulus sufficient to produce a conducted impulse in the sensory fibers of the index and middle fingers — may show a pro-longation when the motor response either is normal or cannot be elicited at all. Palliation may be afforded by injecting hydrocortisone into the carpal tunnel, but definitive sectioning of the transverse carpal ligament high into the base of the hand is usually necessary to relieve the entrapment.

Lateral Femoral Cutaneous Syndrome. Burning dysesthesia along the lateral aspect of the upper thigh is called *meralgia paresthetica*. Composed of fibers derived from the L2 and L3 roots, the lateral femoral cutaneous nerve emerges from the lateral border of the psoas major muscle and runs within the lateral wall of the pelvis to reach the iliacus fascia, enters the fascia, and goes through an opening in the lateral attachment of the inguinal ligament. After coursing through the deep fascia of the upper thigh, the lateral femoral cutaneous nerve pierces through to superficial tissues. Entrapment may occur at the anterior superior spine, where the nerve passes through the lateral end of the inguinal ligament. The nerve may also be tensed against its surrounding muscle and fascia when the leg is abducted, with sudden shifts in trunk posture, after leg or back injuries, or after a marked increase in subcutaneous fat. Direct trauma to the nerve may occur at its site of exit or following a fracture of the anterior portion of the ilium. Rarely, a neuroma may form on the nerve at the point of exit from the pelvis under the inguinal ligament. Intrapelvic neoplasia is oc-casionally associated with meralgia paresthetica. Treatment is conservative in most cases. Weight reduction, posture correction by shoe lifts, or im-proved walking habits may be sufficient to decrease the traction on the nerve at points of entrapment. Occasionally, surgical exploration at the site of en-trapment must be done to give relief.

Ilioinguinal Nerve Syndrome. This nerve arises from the L1 to L2 roots and runs within the wall of the pelvis through and between the transversalis and internal oblique muscles to reach the round ligament or spermatic cord under the external oblique muscle. Pain may arise at the entrapment point in the region of the anterior spine. Radiation of pain or dull ache to the groin from this cause is often attributed to intrapelvic disease or to disturbances in the genitalia.

Obturator Nerve Syndrome. Trauma to the pelvis, an obturator hernia, or osteitis pubis may irritate this nerve and produce severe groin pain radiating down the inner side of the thigh. As the nerve passes from the psoas muscle, the posterior division goes through the obturator externus muscle, where hip motions may cause pain. Adductor weakness may also develop. The entrapment usually occurs in the obturator membrane as it forms a canal against the pubic bone. Numbness may be found on the inner aspect of the thigh. Adhesions within the pelvis following rupture of an ovarian cyst can produce obturator nerve entrapment and damage. Intrapelvic exploration of the nerve is the only definitive treatment.

Sciatic Nerve Syndrome. The large sciatic nerve, which is made up of contributions by L4, L5, and S2 roots, leaves the pelvis by way of the greater sciatic notch. External trauma to the sciatic nerve is unusual, but traction on the nerve against the rim of the notch, as in a sudden, severe fall on the buttocks, may result in local damage to it. Ischemia of the sciatic nerve from prolonged sitting, as on a toilet seat, that compresses the nerve against the rim of the notch may cause local neuropathy. Endometrial cysts may be found binding down the nerve at the sciatic notch. Mechanical trauma can occur during delivery from the fetus's compressing the nerve against the rim of the sciatic notch. Premonitory signs during pregnancy are leg pain and paresthesias in the distribution of the external popliteal and peroneal nerves. Bilateral foot drop may be a residual of puerperal sciatic neuropathy.

Femoral Nerve Syndrome. The femoral nerve passes through the psoas muscle and the pelvis, exiting beneath the inguinal ligament, lateral to the femoral sheath and femoral blood vessels. In the femoral canal it is surrounded by subcutaneous fat. Most of the intrapelvic entrapments are associated with mass lesions such as abscesses or tumors. Entrapment under the inguinal ligament occurs when there is a concomitant femoral-triangle hernia. Femoral neuropathy may be produced by a tight pantie gridle or as a complication of hysterectomy. The clinical features include weakness of extension of the knee, absent knee jerk, and hypalgesia over the anterior inferior portion of the thigh. In a differential etiologic diagnosis of femoral neuropathy, the physician would consider — besides entrapment — metabolic causes such as diabetes, uremia, and thiamine deficiency, the remote effects of cancer, and vascular infarction of the nerve. Treatment is usually conservative, with progressive resistance exercises. Occasionally, to maintain tone and strength in the quadriceps muscle, surgical exploration of the femoral canal may be warranted.

Common Peroneal Nerve Syndrome. The lateral position of the common peroneal nerve as it courses around the fibular neck allows it to be easily bruised. Slender people who bump into the corner of a desk drawer or sit with their legs tightly entwined frequently compress the nerve against the bone beneath. The common peroneal nerve is a branch of the sciatic that leaves the posterior tibial nerve to divide anteriorly into the superficial peroneal, deep peroneal, and recurrent nerves. Entrapment may also occur along the fibrous edge of the peroneus longus muscle, over which the deep and superficial branches must pass. The nerves may be damaged in a person wearing an ill-fitting boot or a short leg brace or cast, or in a patient whose legs are held in lithotomy position by improperly placed stirrups. Weakness of eversion of the foot and sensory changes over the dorsum of the foot and the lateral aspect of the lower leg are findings in this syndrome. A complete foot drop with paralysis of dorsiflexion due to peroneal nerve involvement must be differentiated from that due to sciatic nerve of L5 to S1 root involvement. Ruling out root involvement will be of value in preserving function of the posterior tibial nerve, since it too is supplied by the same roots. Nerve conduction-velocity studies will locate the block in the common peroneal nerve at the head of the fibula.

Peripheral Neuropathies (Parenchymatous and Interstitial

Peripheral neuropathies may develop and cause disability in the absence of any known trauma or evidence of mechanical entrapment. The manifestations are similar whether the neuron, its axoplasm, and the myelin sheath are affected *(parenchymatous neuropathy)* or the nerves are involved secondarily to disease in the perineurium and surrounding connective tissue and blood vessels *(interstitial neuropathy).*

Parenchymatous Neuropathies

<u>Nutritional and Alcoholic Neuropathies.</u> Changes in nerves' myelin sheath, swelling of the internodal segments, and droplet formation in the myelin, with subsequent disturbances of nerve conduction, occur in patients with inadequate intake of thiamine and related B complex vitamins. Both motor and sensory nerves are affected, but the sensory fibers may show damage first, as indicated by the patient's complaints of "burning feet" paresthesias. Chromatolysis in the ganglion cells of both the anterior horn and dorsal root ganglia occurs in severe cases. Weakness and atrophy of muscles are common signs, as are hypalgesia and hypoactive reflexes. Treatment consists in large doses (100 mg) of thiamine administered intramuscularly each day for 10 days and B complex vitamins, including vitamin B_{12}, given parenterally indefinitely to circumvent lack of absorption through the gut. In the absence of adequate thiamine, mental changes (Korsakoff's syndrome) may develop abruptly in a patient with a chronic nutritional neuropathy. Emergency treatment with replacement vitamins must be used to reverse polyneuritic psychosis (Korsakoff's syndrome). Short leg braces and cock-up splints may be needed for patients with motor weaknesses. Physical therapy is usually helpful.

<u>Toxic Neuropathies.</u> Parenchymatous changes in peripheral nerves may result from exposure and absorption of toxic substances, such as heavy metals (lead, arsenic, mercury, bismuth), triorthocresyl-phosphate, trichlorethylene, hexanes, acrylamide, streptomycin, nitrofurantoin, isoniazid, thalidomide, and certain of the *Vinca* derivatives used in treating malignancies (e.g., vincristine). Histologically, toxic neuropathies are characterized by myelin destruction, damage to axis cylinders and, sometimes, neuronal chromatolysis. The symptoms are the same as in the nutritional neuropathies, but the history of exposure should be helpful in making the differential etiologic diagnosis. Chelating agents are useful in the treatment of heavy metal intoxication.

<u>Carcinomatous Neuropathy.</u> This type of complication of neoplasia, which may precede any actual signs of cancer, occurs in about 16 percent of patients with carcinoma of the lung and 4.4 percent of those with carcinoma of the breast. Whether the destruction of myelin is related to nutritional factors or to neoplastic toxic substances that interfere with the metabolism of the Schwann's cell is as yet unknown.

<u>Acute Porphyric Neuropathy.</u> Painful paresthesias are often seen in patients who have *acute porphyria,* associated with vomiting, constipation, fever, tachycardia, hypertension, and leukocytosis. During the symptoms the urine contains increased amounts of uroporphyrin. Shortly after the abdominal cramps, a flaccid paralysis may appear involving the arms and legs. Bulbar paralysis is responsible for the 50 percent mortality in porphyric neuropathy. Pathology studies have shown that the spinal cord is spared, but that varying degrees of segmental myelin degeneration and axon degeneration may occur in the more peripheral parts of the nerves. The actual pathogenesis of porphyric neuropathy is thought to be directly toxic, but this is uncertain. Treatment is symptomatic. Barbiturates should be avoided, since they exacerbate symptoms. Corticotropin (ACTH) and cortisone have been used, with variable results.

<u>Uremic Neuropathy.</u> Patients with chronic uremia may experience neuropathy of insidious onset, progressively involving sensory and motor functions in a symmetric distribution in both feet and legs, and in some instances hands and forearms. The most important pathologic change is the disappearance,

in a segmental fashion, of large medullated fibers in both the myelin sheaths and the axis cylinders. Uremic neuropathy has been found to worsen after renal dialysis. The pathogenesis has been attributed to a specific uremic disorder of the nerves rather than to an associated nutritional deficiency.

Allergic and Postinfectious Peripheral Neuropathies. These neuropathies include instances of interstitial infiltration with inflammatory cells following serum therapy, typhoid inoculation, or smallpox vaccination. Sometimes called acute idiopathic polyneuritis, the syndrome of acute infective polyneuritis, or *Guillain-Barré syndrome,* is characterized by ascending motor weakness, areflexia, and distal sensory impairment. The cerebrospinal fluid shows a unique change in an albuminocytologic dissociation; that is, the acute cerebrospinal fluid may have four to five white blood cell counts (WBCs) and moderately elevated protein, but after 6 to 10 days the CSF protein may reach remarkably elevated levels (150 to 300 mg per 100 ml), with only two or three WBCs or none. The CSF protein may stay elevated throughout the entire course of the illness, returning to normal 4 to 6 months after recovery. The CSF sugar content is not abnormally high or low.

The signs and symptoms usually appear within a week to 10 days following an acute febrile illness, most commonly an upper respiratory infection. Over a period of several days weakness progresses to involve the trunk, upper extremities, face, and bulbar muscles. Urinary retention may occur. If the patient survives the initial acute phase, and especially respiratory and vasomotor collapse, which occurs in 30 percent of cases, the prognosis is good for complete recovery within 4 to 6 months. In uncomplicated cases the prognosis is usually good. Treatment with steroids has no significant effect on the course of the illness, or on the mortality rate. Supportive measures, tracheostomy if necessary, and respiratory assistance are the main means of management.

Leprosy (Hansen's Disease). Initially, leprous infection is confined to the sheaths of the small nerves in the dermis, where there are foci of infiltration with lymphocytes, histiocytes, and a few epithelioid cells. Sparse numbers of *Mycobacterium leprae* may be found in and around the nerve cells or in the cellular exudate in the surrounding connective tissue. From its early state the disease may progress, either to form subcutaneous lepromatous lesions or to spread up the nerve and produce the neural or maculo-anesthetic type of the disease. In the lepromatous type, nodules begin around the nerves and sweat glands but soon destroy the nerve fibers. These lesions are often described as perivascular. Subcutaneous nodules occur characteristically on the extensor surfaces of the limbs and on the face, where they may cause a leonine appearance. Cutaneous ulcers too may form. In the neural type, the infection may be confined to nerves or it may be combined with florid skin lesions. The posterior auricular, ulnar, and peroneal nerves — said to be the most often impaired — may be palpable as thickened cords. Secondary degeneration of myelin and axis cylinders occurs. The neural lesions are usually irreversible. Treatment consists in the use of sulfones, arsenicals, and stilbamidine.

Vascular and Ischemic Neuropathies. Thrombosis of a popliteal artery, an anterior spinal artery, or a femoral or other artery may result in infarction of the area supplied by that particular vessel, and damage to, if not destruction of, the peripheral nerves subserved. Disease of small arteries, such as periarteritis nodosa or vasculitis, may also cause ischemia in the peripheral nerves. In such conditions either single or multiple nerves may be involved, with secondary necrosis of the myelin and axis cylinders.

Diabetic Neuropathy. This condition in patients with diabetes mellitus may be due in part to vascular abnormalities, to some obscure metabolic abnormality in the neuron itself, or to a combination of these factors. The incidence of neuropathy in patients with diabetes increases with the duration of the disease and the age of the patient. Patients with diabetes have a high incidence of intraneural vascular lesions, consisting of hyalinization, stenosis, and thickening of the small arterial walls. The neuropathy seems to be unrelated to the degree of therapeutic control of the diabetes. The most common neurologic syndrome in diabetes is involvement of the lower extremities, often bilaterally, and usually in a predominantly sensory impairment. Isolated cranial nerve palsies such as third-, seventh-, and fifth-nerve paralyses are not uncommon, and in fact they may give warning of previously unsuspected diabetes. There may also be autonomic or visceral involvement leading to vasomotor instability, pilomotor or sudomotor abnormalities, postural hypotension, sexual impotence, and bladder dysfunction. Skin atrophy and pain, paresthesias, absence of deep tendon reflexes, decreased vibration sense, and elevation of CSF protein are common clinical findings.

Muscle Weakness

The terminus of the functional motor unit is the myoneural junction. Disorders of transmission of the nerve impulse may develop when the release of acetylcholine is opposed by low ionic calcium; when the acetylcholine must compete with a curarelike substance for the receptor site; when the end plate is rendered unresponsive to acetylcholine by methonium compounds of certain snake venoms; or when either a deficiency or an excess of potassium ion renders the muscle unable to propagate an action potential adequately and to contract effectively.

Myasthenia gravis is the prototype of clinical myoneural disorders. It may occur at any age from infancy to old age, but the common, chronic form rarely begins in either young children or the elderly. Two subtypes are seen: a *relapsing form,* which usually occurs in young women and is associated with germinal follicles in the thymus gland; and a *progressive form,* which usually affects older men and is often associated with thymoma. The commonest symptoms are ptosis, diplopia, dysphagia, dysarthria, rapid fatigability, and weakness, which initially are relieved by rest. There is a striking tendency toward involvement of ocular and bulbar muscles, although the axial and appendicular muscles may also be affected, but with normal peripheral sensation, preservation of tendon reflexes, and absence of muscular atrophy. The defect can usually be relieved by anticholinesterase drugs, such as neostigmine (Prostigmin) or edrophonium chloride (Tensilon). Although a history of progressive weak-

ness following repetitive movements of an extremity, or of increasing difficulty in maintaining the focus of one's eyes as the day progresses, is highly suggestive, confirmatory tests using the physiologic principles of neuromuscular transmission are available. For example, repetitive stimulation of a peripheral nerve, such as the ulnar, while the responses of a small muscle in the hand (abductor digiti minimi) are being recorded may reveal a declining amplitude of muscle response as the stimulations are repeated at a constant shock strength. When the muscle responses have been reduced significantly and increases in shock strength do not alter their amplitude, administration of 1 ml of edrophonium hydrochloride containing 10 mg of drug will restore the muscle responses. Edrophonium must be administered intravenously in fractional doses, as 0.2 ml (2 mg) initially, with a lapse of 30 seconds allowed before additional amounts are given, up to the total dose of 10 mg over a 3-minute period to avoid arterial hypotension and cardiac irregularities, which otherwise might occur as side effects of the drug. Increased lacrimation, salivation due to the muscarinic effects of edrophonium and neostigmine, and explosive diarrhea may occur.

Neostigmine can be used therapeutically in similar fashion, in doses of 1.5 mg (prostigmine methyl sulfate) administered subcutaneously or intramuscularly (never intravenously). Clinical improvement should be anticipated only after 15 to 20 minutes, but the effect should last as long as 40 minutes. By contrast, edrophonium hydrochloride is rapidly metabolized, and its effect therefore is usually gone within 1 to 2 minutes. The muscle weakness associated with chronic thyrotoxic myopathy or polymyositis or the myasthenic syndrome associated with oat cell carcinoma of the lung may also respond to these drugs, but in a variable way. In true myasthenia gravis the electromyographic recordings of fatigue of muscles on repeated stimulation differ from the muscle responses recorded in patients with the myasthenic syndrome, in that myasthenia gravis patients fail to exhibit an initial facilitation, while those displaying the myasthenic syndrome show muscle responses increasing in amplitude for several contractions; then fatigue sets in.

Other features help to differentiate the myasthenic syndrome associated with occult neoplasm from myasthenia gravis. For example, the myasthenic syndrome tends to affect the larger, more proximal muscles. Further, myasthenia may be encountered in association with other diseases, many of which seem to have an autoimmune basis.

The degree of severity of myasthenia gravis can be described clinically according to the following groups: group I, ocular involvement only; group II(a), mild, generalized weakness, including ocular involvement; group II(b), moderate severity, including ocular and mild bulbar involvement; group III, acute, severe myasthenia gravis developing over a period of weeks to months, usually requiring tracheostomy and respirator because of severe bulbar involvement; group IV, late, severe condition, requiring respiratory support; group V, complete remission, leaving only mild muscle atrophy.

Treatment of myasthenia gravis requires careful titration of anticholinesterase medication to suit the activities of the patient and the severity of the illness. Initially, neostigmine bromide may be given as 15-mg tablets throughout the day, especially at times to anticipate fatigue, as half an hour before meals, when chewing might become difficult. As few as 4 or as many as 20 tablets per day may be needed. A longer-acting but somewhat less potent preparation than neostigmine, pyridostigmine bromide (Mestinon), may be used (60-mg tablets, 3 to 6 tablets per day) and a dose of 60 to 180 mg may be given at night to maintain a patient's respiratory muscle function. Combinations of the long-acting form and shorter-acting doses can be given throughout the day after the patient's individual requirements have been established. Periodic intravenous edrophonium hydrochloride tests are useful in determining additional need for medication; if the patient shows no further improvement, there is no need for more medication. In fact, edrophonium tests will help differentiate a cholinergic crisis (i.e., overtreatment) from a myasthenic crisis (insufficient anticholinesterase medication).

Patients with severe cases of *myasthenic crisis* should be admitted to the hospital for supportive care, which may include tracheostomy and respira-

tory support while medications are being readjusted. There is often substantial improvement of symptoms and reduced need for anticholinesterase medication after thymectomy. This is especially true if the operation is performed within 5 years of the onset of symptoms, particularly in young women who have no evidence of thymoma and no other associated illnesses. The prognosis is poor if a thymoma is allowed to remain, though radiotherapy may be beneficial. Although variable in effect, prednisone has been used in patients with myasthenia gravis to produce a remission of symptoms, or at least to reduce the amount of anticholinergic medication needed to control the symptoms. Usually the patient's condition seriously worsens on 40 to 80 mg per day of prednisone for the first 10 to 14 days; thereafter a remarkable improvement is seen. The improvement persists for months to years on small maintenance doses of steroids.

Hypokalemic periodic paralysis is a form of muscle weakness that occurs both sporadically and in families. In the latter instance, the condition is believed to be transmitted as an autosomal dominant with a complete penetrance.

The liberation of acetylcholine at the myoneural junction excites muscle contraction by initiating an electrical charge in the muscle membrane, which is influenced by the level of blood potassium. Muscular contractility is impaired by either an abnormally low or an abnormally high level of potassium in the blood. Attacks of periodic paralysis in which blood potassium is low begin in the teenage years, usually in males; often they occur at night. They may appear after heavy carbohydrate intake, after resting, or during emotional stress or vigorous exercise. The proximal muscles of the limbs and trunk are affected more often than the distal muscles. Reflexes are lacking. During an attack there is a marked positive balance of potassium, which presumably moves out of the serum and into the muscle cells. The electrocardiogram shows T-wave changes characteristic of low serum potassium (see Chap. 21). Serum inorganic phosphate and cocarboxylase levels fall in parallel, while blood pyruvate and lactate increase. In many patients the condition can be prevented by a diet high in potassium and low in carbohydrate and sodium. Once the serum potassium has been shown to be low during an attack, 10 gm of potassium chloride followed by 5 gm in 1 hour will usually abort an attack that otherwise might last up to 24 hours. Hydrochlorothiazide or spironolactone may also alleviate a severe attack.

In certain families *hyperkalemic periodic paralysis* has been reported in which attacks can be precipitated by giving potassium. A mild weakness of the proximal musculature of the pelvis and shoulder girdle may be continuously present, with slow progression. Increased weakness and even flaccid paralysis may occur following a period of rest after exercise. Delayed relaxation after contraction (myotonia) is demonstrable in the muscles of the eyelids or tongue or upon percussion of the thenar eminence.

Myopathies

Muscular dystrophy includes a group of disorders characterized by no evidence of disease of the nervous system, weakness and wasting of the striated muscle, a progressive clinical course, and often a hereditary background. Although most patients have their first symptoms early in life, onset may be at any age, if one considers the various forms of the disease.

The *pseudohypertrophic type (Duchenne muscular dystrophy)* appears in the preschool years and affects boys almost exclusively. The progression is steady, usually necessitating a wheelchair before the end of the patient's first decade, with death in most instances resulting from respiratory or cardiac defects before the late teens. The early symptoms of difficult gait and difficult running or toe-walking are rarely recognized as caused by muscular dystrophy unless the disease has been known in other members of the family. Enlargement of the calves may precede noticeable weakness by many months and actually can be mistaken for unusually good muscular development. The so-called climbing up the thighs (Gowers' sign) indicates weakness of proximal muscles. The patient places his hands upon his thighs and pushes his trunk up to a standing position. In *hypertrophic muscular dystrophy* the blood levels of creatine phosphokinase (CPK) are grossly elevated early in the disease, even before clinical symptoms become evident. As the

disease progresses the CPK gradually declines toward normal values. (This test is sufficiently specific to cast doubt on a diagnosis of early Duchenne muscular dystrophy when the CPK values are not elevated.)

Muscle biopsy and electromyography can be important diagnostic aids in muscular dystrophy. The typical histologic changes are size variation and hyaline degeneration of muscle fibers, with infiltration of fat between muscle bundles. The electromyograph shows short-duration, low-amplitude, rapidly firing potentials in the presence of a weak muscle contraction. This form of muscular dystrophy is transmitted by a sex-linked recessive mechanism. Occasionally a girl may show some symptoms, but they are almost always mild and nonprogressive. Treatment is supportive, with attempts to prevent contractures. Sometimes surgical procedures to lengthen the Achilles tendon allow additional months of ambulation before the child is confined to a wheelchair.

The *limb-girdle type of muscular dystrophy* has a later onset, affects the pelvic and shoulder girdle muscles, and displays a benign, slow course. Genetic transmission here is by an autosomal mechanism. Symptoms may occur during the first three decades. Muscle biopsy and serum enzyme studies are less valuable in the diagnosis of limb-girdle muscular dystrophy than in pseudohypertrophic muscular dystrophy. The *facioscapulohumeral form of muscular dystrophy* is inherited by an autosomal dominant mechanism and both sexes are affected with equal frequency. The illness appears early in puberty, and the clinical course is relatively slow and sometimes abortive. It is not unusual for patients to remain ambulatory until an advanced age. The muscles earliest affected are those of the face, shoulder, girdle, and upper arms. Involvement of the lower extremities may follow after a decade or two.

Myotonic muscular dystrophy is characterized by symptoms of weakness and wasting, delayed relaxation of muscles after an initial contraction (myotonia), and certain extramuscular changes consisting of frontal baldness, bilateral lens opacities and, in males, testicular atrophy. Inheritance is autosomal dominant.

It is not uncommon for children and adults with

polymyositis to be diagnosed initially as having muscular dystrophy. Therefore it is of prime importance to differentiate between the two, because in muscular dystrophy there is no specific or satisfactory therapy, while in polymyositis some reasonably definitive treatment is available. The signs and symptoms of polymyositis, as in certain forms of muscular dystrophy, are predominantly those of proximal muscle weakness of the pelvic and shoulder girdles. Systemic signs and symptoms are rarely present early in the disease. Typically, the onset is insidious, with weakness of the proximal muscles of the lower and upper limbs and defective swallowing mechanisms gradually appearing over weeks to months. Moderate fluctuations in the intensity of the clinical disease are characteristic. Muscular pain and tenderness are more common in the acute form than in subacute or chronic cases. Raising the arms over the head and, especially, maintaining them in an overhead position, as in combing the hair, becomes difficult. In severe or advanced cases the weakness may be extreme and the patient is then bedridden. Muscle atrophy is a late occurrence.

The link between polymyositis and certain of the connective tissue diseases can be observed in the similarities of the skin manifestations of systemic lupus erythematosus, scleroderma, and polymyositis (see Chap. 35). Furthermore, mild or transitory arthritis occurs in about one-third to one-half of the cases of polymyositis. The diagnosis may be confirmed when the serum glutamic oxaloacetic transaminase and serum aldolase are significantly elevated. These enzymes, which are released as a result of the destructive myopathy, are increased in the acute and subacute stages. Electromyography in polymyositis shows abnormal potentials in nearly all stages of the disease. During rest there are small potentials that are indistinguishable from spontaneous fibrillations; upon voluntary movement, a complex, polyphasic pattern of motor unit potentials may be observed. Short bursts of rapidly repeating action potentials that fade away after a brief initial period (pseudomyotonia) have been described. Muscle biopsy will disclose changes if the sample is taken from an affected muscle, the best choice in general being a proximal muscle that is partially but not completely weakened.

The histologic features include either primary focal or extensive degeneration of muscle fibers, sometimes with vacuolization; evidence of regeneration, as demonstrated by sarcoplasmic basophilia and the presence of large nuclei and prominent nucleoli; necrosis of a part or the whole of one or more fibers, with phagocytosis; interstitial infiltration of inflammatory cells, and, in long-standing cases, interstitial fibrosis. Treatment for acute polymyositis should include methylprednisolone (50 to 70 mg by mouth per day, in divided doses given every 6 to 8 hours). Serial analyses of one or more serum enzymes will provide the best therapeutic and prognostic guides. Once the enzyme levels have returned toward normal, a lowering of dosage can be attempted. Maintenance therapy should be continued for months or years with a methylprednisolone dosage ranging from 7.5 to 20 mg per day. The usual cause of death is bronchopneumonia associated with aspiration; but about 1 patient in 3 will be found to have an underlying malignant disease heralded by the onset of polymyositis.

Disturbances of Tone, Posture, and Movement

The localization of a lesion in the central nervous system is based partly upon careful analysis of any disorders of movement. If movement is totally absent, there must be a primary defect in the pyramidal system; if there is an abnormal movement, it is likely that the extrapyramidal system is involved. The pyramidal system includes the cortex and its corticobulbar and corticospinal pathways; the extrapyramidal system includes the extrapyramidal cortex, the basal ganglia, the cerebellum, and their connections with each other and with the spinal cord. The nature of a central lesion will determine both the pattern of motor deficits and the possible associated sensory defects.

All cortical neurons are organized for special functions. In the frontal areas, anterior to the central gyrus, the neurons are responsible for voluntary movements. The motor cortex has a topographic arrangement in which the knee, trunk, shoulder, and elbow movements are located predominantly on the convexity of the brain. Lower down on the motor strip are the areas dealing with movements of the hand, face, mouth, and tongue, swallowing, and speech. Parietal lobe structures are involved in the processes of perception, association, and conceptualization. Temporal lobe neurons are concerned with auditory perception, memory, and emotions. The occipital cortex deals with visual perception and the association of visual images with names. Stimulation of one of these areas will usually produce a predictable experience, and ablation or destruction of a certain area will result in loss of a particular ability. Similarly, interruption of the pathway from upper motor neuron to lower motor neuron in the internal capsule or in the corticospinal tract will produce a disorder of movement. Many abnormal movements and postures seen in patients after lesions of the central nervous system resemble the normal movements of infants with a developing nervous system. For example, a newborn infant is expected to show the tonic neck reflex, a sign of an intact labyrinthine component of a body-on-body reflex needed to orient the organism in relationship to gravity. No motor act can be accomplished without sensory feedback to regulate its accuracy, amplitude, and force. Separation of the spinal reflex mechanisms from the higher centers dealing with muscle tone results in decerebrate states. Derangements resulting from imbalance of proprioceptive or righting reflexes are seen in the dyskinesias.

Examination of a muscle at rest, whether it is of a limb, the trunk, or the neck, reveals a sense of tension that can be felt when the limb is passively moved. This is called *tone. Hypotonia* is a decreased resistance to passive motion, seen in disorders of the cerebellum and posterior columns and early in Huntington's chorea; it is associated with a feeling of flabbiness of the muscle and, on occasion, increased extensibility of muscles and limbs. *Hypertonia* is an increased resistance to passive motion, which is seen in such disorders as parkinsonism, paraplegia, and hemiplegias of many different kinds. There are three types of hypertonia: spasticity, rigidity, and gegenhalten (paratonia). *Spasticity,* which follows lesions of the corticospinal tract, is an increased resistance on passive stretch that suddenly melts or gives way (the lengthening reaction of the muscle); it is often

associated with hyperreflexia and clonus. *Rigidity* is an increased resistance through the full range of motion, both in flexion and extension; it is seen in disorders of basal ganglia, in particular putamenal and pallidal lesions. *Gegenhalten* is a resistance that increases as the limb is passively moved; superficially, the patient seems uncooperative. Though not always present, it is seen in disorders of the parietal lobe. In extreme degree it results in hyperextensibility at all the joints and can lead to the bizarre postures of a "plastic man," as may be seen in tabes dorsalis.

Dystonia is defined as a tendency toward, or an abnormal degree of, fixity of any attitude or posture owing to sustained muscular contraction. *Segmental dystonia* is an abnormality of posture that results when special parts of the body are involved. Spasmodic torticollis is an example of segmental dystonia (see below in this section). *Hemiplegic dystonia* is a posture in which the paralyzed side of the body displays flexion of the upper extremity at the elbow, wrist, and fingers, extension of the leg, and plantar flexion of the foot. In general appearance it resembles hemiplegic spasticity. Such postures are seen also in hepatolenticular degeneration (Wilson's disease), in which condition they usually involve both sides and early in the course of the illness are associated with plastic rigidity. As the disorder progresses, the lengthening reaction (i.e., the ability of a muscle to increase in length on stretching) is lost and the limbs assume a fixed posture. *Flexion dystonia* results in a persistent attitude of flexion in all the limbs, with the wrists overflexed and pronated, the fingers eventually flexed (though initially extended), the legs flexed upon the abdomen, and the feet plantarflexed. It may be seen in the end stage of parkinsonism and related disorders. Early in the course of the disorder the posture can be modified by body surface contact or labyrinthine stimulation, such as headturning.

Disorders manifested by alterations in muscle tone and posture, such as parkinsonism, may also be associated with inability to initiate movement, even though there is no weakness. In its most severe form, called *akinesia,* there eventually is reduction of all spontaneous movement. *Bradykinesia* is very slow movement. During the evolution of bradykinesia to akinesia there can be freezing or halting into a fixed posture in the midst of a muscular movement.

There are other types of involuntary movements. *Ballism* is an involuntary violent flinging movement of a limb or limbs secondary to lesion of the subthalamic nucleus. When only one side of the body is involved it is called hemiballismus. *Spasmodic torticollis* is an intermittent and often painful involuntary turning of the head that is associated with abnormal activity of the sternocleidomastoid muscle on one side, though usually other neck and head muscles are involved. A static form can be seen in the maldevelopment of the neck in children that is secondary to sternocleidomastoid fibrosis or to an ocular imbalance. In many situations the spasmodic type is considered to be a fragment of a torsion dystonia. *Akathisia* is a condition in which an individual has "restless legs" and cannot sit still for any period. It is seen as a concomitant of tardive dyskinesia, or following massive dosages of phenothiazine, or as a side effect of high doses of L-dopa used in the treatment of parkinsonism. *Tics* are stereotyped, sudden, brief movements that recur at irregular intervals in precisely the same manner. They can take any form, such as eye-blinking, shrugging, coughing, or twitching of various parts of the body. A tic is peculiar to the patient and can be reproduced at will or suppressed momentarily. *Oculogyric crises* are sustained spasms of conjugate deviation of the eyes, usually upward or to the right or left. A feature of postencephalitic parkinsonism, they are seen as a reaction to phenothiazines.

Paralysis or *plegia* is the inability to perform a movement at all. *Paresis* is a condition of weakness in performing a task. If half the body is involved, as in lesions of the corticospinal or pyramidal tracts above the foramen magnum or high cervical region, a *hemiplegia* or *hemiparesis* results. If only one extremity is involved, then a *monoparesis* or *monoplegia* is said to be present. A paralysis or weakness can also be present as a result of emotional disorders, as, for example, in conversion hysteria.

Apraxia is the failure to perform a given motor act upon request, although the individual retains the ability to make the necessary component movements and understands the request. Such a phenomenon, which is seen in diffuse cerebrocortical disorders, will be elaborated upon later in discussions of higher neuron functions.

Just as there can be little movement when there is either weakness or fixity of posture, there can also be too much movement, as in chorea, tremor, or ataxia. *Chorea* refers to quick, continued, fleeting, and unpredictably random movements of the limbs, lips, face, tongue, or body, along with a loss of posture. It must be differentiated from *athetosis,* in which there can be slow, writhing movements and an alternation of hyperextension with pronation and flexion with supination of the arms. Two diseases to be noted here are progressive hereditary chorea (Huntington's disease) and Sydenham's chorea, the former associated with cell loss and atrophy of the caudate nuclei and the latter with no known pathologic process, since it is usually a self-limiting process and spontaneously resolves. Sydenham's chorea is usually associated with rheumatic fever or a collagen disease.

Tremor is a rhythmic alternation in movement, faster than one per second, which tends to be consistent in pattern, amplitude, and frequency; it is usually due to the reciprocal contraction of a muscle group and its antagonist. A *static tremor* is a tremor present at rest; an *action tremor* occurs during movement; and an *intention tremor,* seen in cerebellar hemispheral disorders, is one that is accentuated toward the end of a purposeful movement. *Ataxia* is a disturbance of coordination that is independent of any motor weakness. *Cerebellar ataxia* is characterized by a combination of disturbances (1) in amplitude of individual movements (hypermetria or dysmetria); (2) in combining of elementary movements (asynergia); (3) in speed of alternating movements (adiadodyskinesis); (4) in continuity of contractions (akinetic and static tremor); and (5) in speed of initiation and arrest of movement (dyschronometria). In cerebellar disorders the uncoordinated movement maintains the intended direction and orientation, and it is not aggravated on closing the eyes. Often there is hypotonia and increased range of passive motion of the limb.

Labyrinthine ataxia is characterized by disturbances of equilibrium in standing and walking and does not affect isolated limb movements, though past pointing is present. It has features in common with cerebellar ataxia (i.e., broad-based gait, staggering, leaning over backward or to one side, and deviation from direction of gait); but, in contrast, it is often associated with nystagmus and vertigo (see later in this chapter, under Otoneurologic Disorders).

Sensory ataxias, as seen in tabes dorsalis or in subacute combined degeneration of the spinal cord, usually follow loss of position sensation, worsen on eye closure, and are both kinetic and static in type. Sensory ataxias secondary to decreased deep sensibility can also be seen in peripheral neuropathies and in posterior thalamic and parietal lobe lesions. These ataxias, however, are usually not so severe as those seen in tabes or combined systems disease.

Differential Diagnosis

The differential diagnosis of disorders of movement must include various processes that destroy the cerebral cortex and its pathways in the hemispheres and cause disturbances of function in the integration of control of postural reflexes. Traumatic lesions to the central nervous system may produce all combinations of pyramidal and extrapyramidal disorders. Cerebrovascular accidents may destroy gray and white matter within specific areas of vascular supply. Multiple sclerosis affects primarily white-matter pathways. Degenerative diseases may select either primarily white matter or gray nuclear masses.

Cerebrovascular And Related Disorders
C. A. Romanul

Cerebrovascular Disease

The brain becomes infarcted at sites where circulation of the blood falls below a critical level, producing anoxic crises. Blood flow depends on cardiac output and systemic blood pressure and on the patency of the arteries and veins. The territory supplied by an artery that becomes occluded proximally must derive its blood flow entirely through anastomotic channels. Preservation of cerebral tissue then depends on the effectiveness of the collateral circulation: Poor flow may allow extensive brain infarction to occur, whereas good collateral circulation may prevent any cerebral

damage. However, if the flow through the anastomoses is later decreased as a result of a fall in the systemic blood pressure, the brain may then become infarcted in the territory normally supplied by the occluded artery.

Occlusion of a Major Cerebral Artery. When the lumen of one of the major cerebral arteries, such as the middle cerebral artery, becomes occluded, blood can come only through the pial anastomoses with the adjacent major cerebral arteries — in this instance, the anterior and posterior cerebral arteries. Stenosis of a major cerebral artery may or may not result in infarction of brain. If two adjacent major cerebral arteries are stenotic, the brain is infarcted in the border zone between the territories of the two vessels (Figs. 62-3, 62-4). Thus the blood flow is most severely reduced in the pial anastomoses uniting the two arteries and in the most distal arterial branches from which those anastomoses originate. Occlusion of a large artery in the neck is less likely to cause infarction of brain than occlusion of a major cerebral artery, because two additional levels of arterial communication exist: the circulus arteriosus cerebri (circle of Willis) and the extracranial anastomoses. If the occlusion of the neck artery is rapid, considerable collateral flow is available through the circle of Willis, but only small amounts of blood can be obtained through the extracranial anastomoses because time is needed for them to increase in size. In humans, sudden occlusion of a neck artery without prior stenosis is a rare occurrence. The neck arteries are most frequently affected by atherosclerosis, which usually causes slow occlusion of the lumen, giving the extracranial anastomoses ample time to increase in caliber and to become valuable pathways of collateral blood flow.

Occlusion of the Internal Carotid Arteries. If an internal carotid artery is occluded in the neck, blood flow distal to the occlusion is obtained both through the ophthalmic artery from the external carotid and through the anterior and posterior communicating arteries from the other large vessels. The collateral circulation is often sufficient to prevent any ischemic damage to the brain. When it is less adequate, the

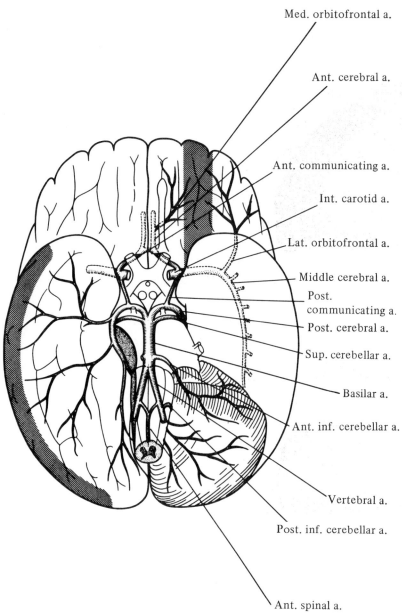

Med. orbitofrontal a.

Ant. cerebral a.

Ant. communicating a.

Int. carotid a.

Lat. orbitofrontal a.

Middle cerebral a.

Post. communicating a.

Post. cerebral a.

Sup. cerebellar a.

Basilar a.

Ant. inf. cerebellar a.

Vertebral a.

Post. inf. cerebellar a.

Ant. spinal a.

Figure 62-3. The arterial system of the brain viewed from the base. The border zones of arterial supply are shaded. [Figures 62-3 through 62-8 from F. C. A. Romanul, Examination of the Brain and Spinal Cord, in C. Tedeschi (ed.), Neuropathology: Methods and Diagnosis. *Boston: Little, Brown, 1970.]*

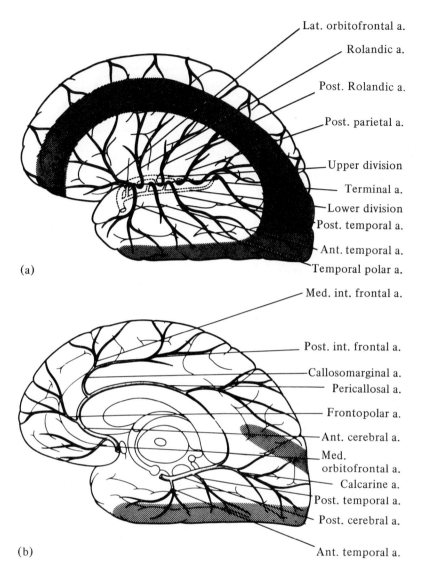

Lat. orbitofrontal a.

Rolandic a.

Post. Rolandic a.

Post. parietal a.

Upper division

Terminal a.

Lower division

Post. temporal a.

Ant. temporal a.

Temporal polar a.

(a)

Med. int. frontal a.

Post. int. frontal a.

Callosomarginal a.

Pericallosal a.

Frontopolar a.

Ant. cerebral a.

Med. orbitofrontal a.

Calcarine a.

Post. temporal a.

Post. cerebral a.

(b)

Ant. temporal a.

Figure 62-4. The arteries viewed from the lateral (a) and medial (b) aspects.

brain becomes infarcted in the border zone between the territories of the anterior and middle cerebral arteries, the two large branches of the internal carotid (Fig. 62-5a–c). If the area of infarction is small, it is usually located in the anatomic border zone between the two vessels. At other times it may be shifted toward the territory of either the anterior or the middle cerebral artery by a more pronounced

atheromatous stenosis of the respective vessel. When the area of infarction is wider, it affects also the adjacent portions of the territories of the anterior and middle cerebral arteries. The infarct frequently extends more into the field of supply of the middle cerebral artery, since there is greater reduction of flow in this vessel because of the small caliber of the posterior communicating artery.

A different localization of the infarct is found as a result of occlusion of the internal carotid artery in the neck if the homolateral side of the circle of Willis

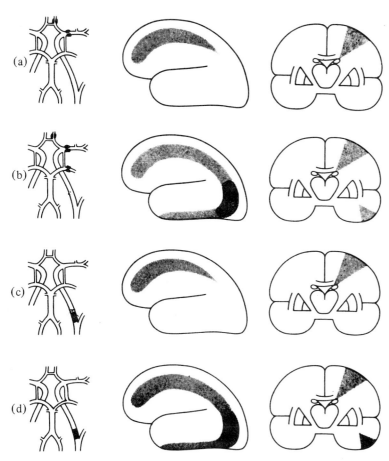

Figure 62-5. Patterns of arterial occlusion and cerebral infarction (see text).

has retained an embryonic configuration, namely, one with the posterior cerebral artery receiving most of its blood flow from the internal carotid. Under these circumstances the blood flow is decreased in the respective anterior, middle, and posterior cerebral arteries, and the brain is infarcted in the border zones between the territories of all three of these vessels (Fig. 62-5d). The most valuable area is the parieto-occipital region of the cerebral convexity, where the territories of all three arteries meet. In patients with thrombosis of both internal carotid arteries in the neck, the findings in the two cerebral hemispheres depend on the time elapsed between the occlusions of the two vessels. When an internal carotid artery is the first to become thrombosed, an infarction in the

described location may occur in the corresponding cerebral hemisphere. When both internal carotid arteries are occluded slowly by atheroma, anastomoses usually have time to develop bilaterally, and there may be minimal infarction, if any, in both cerebral hemispheres.

Occlusion of the Vertebral Arteries. When occlusion of a vertebral artery in the neck causes an infarction in the brain, it is practically impossible to predict the extent of the damage. For one thing, there is great variability in the branches of the vertebral and basilar arteries. A more important reason is that any of the penetrating arteries supplying the brainstem may be narrowed at its origin by atheromatous changes in the basilar artery. Occasionally, when the posterior communicating arteries are very small and there is minimal atherosclerosis of the basilar, the infarction occurs in the border zone between the territories of the cerebellar arteries. In such a case there may be additional damage in the pons at the junction of the base with the tegmentum (Fig. 62-6a–c). This region represents the border zone between all the penetrator branches supplying the pons. If the vertebral artery is occluded near its upper end, the decrease in blood flow is more severe because the anastomotic connections in the neck are no longer useful. Occlusion of both vertebral arteries causes more severe impairment of circulation in the vertebrobasilar system.

Occlusion of the Basilar Artery. In the vertebrobasilar system, occlusion of the basilar artery has an effect on blood flow somewhat similar to that caused by occlusion of both vertebral arteries near their upper ends (Fig. 62-7a, b). The important difference be-

Figure 62-6. Patterns of arterial occlusion and cerebral infarction in the border zone between the territories of the cerebellar arteries (a); one or more penetrator arteries (b); lateral portions of medulla due to obstruction of origin of posterior inferior cerebellar artery (c).

tween the two situations is that occlusion of the basilar artery usually obstructs the origin of some of the branches supplying the brainstem and cerebellum. Above the occlusion the blood flow is provided mostly by the internal carotids through the posterior communicating arteries.

In cases of basilar artery thrombosis there is always infarction of the brainstem in the territories of the penetrator branches that have their origins blocked by the clot. If the thrombus obstructs one of the cerebellar arteries at its origin, the infarction may be minimized in its field of supply because of the existence of pial anastomoses over the surface of the cerebellum (Fig. 62-7c).

When both a vertebral and an internal carotid artery are occluded in the neck, the brain usually becomes infarcted in the border zone between the territories of the three major cerebral arteries on the side of the occluded carotid (Fig. 62-7d).

Transient Cerebrovascular Insufficiency. A transient neurologic deficit is usually due to a temporary impairment of blood flow in some part of the brain. An episode of neurologic dysfunction may occur only

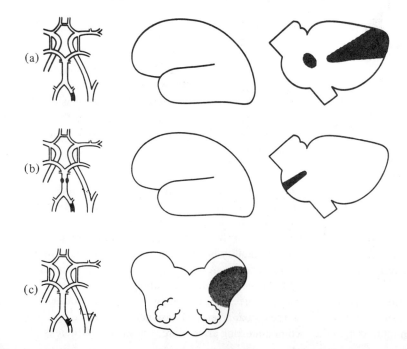

(a)

(b)

(c)

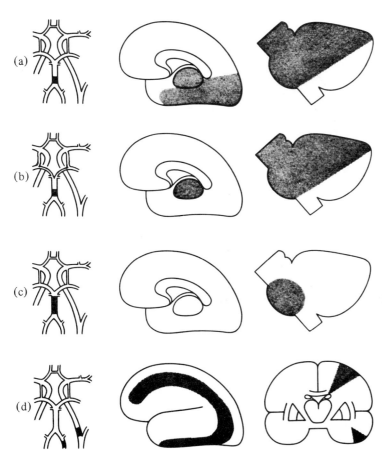

Figure 62-7. Patterns of arterial occlusion and cerebral infarction (see text).

once or on repeated occasions. The cause of a single episode is seldom clear clinically but it may become apparent on pathologic examination. Multiple episodes are usually due to either repeated embolism or recurrent vascular insufficiency. Emboli are scattered in an unpredictable manner in the brain, and no preferential distribution has ever been convincingly demonstrated. Recurrent bouts of insufficiency occur when the blood flow in some portion of the brain is precariously balanced and then is repeatedly lowered to a critical level, as by fluctuations in blood pressure or cardiac output. On rare occasions the insufficiency is brought about by a specific physical activity — which indicates a shunting of blood away from the brain. For example, exercise of an upper

extremity may induce symptoms of vertebrobasilar insufficiency. This process, which occurs with occlusion of the homolateral subclavian artery proximal to the origin of the vertebral, is known as the *subclavian steal syndrome*. Hypertensive and diabetic patients, owing to predominant disease of small arteries, are more likely to have insufficiency in penetrator branches. With poor flow through the main trunk of the middle cerebral artery (Fig. 62-8 a, b), the mildest insufficiency affects the perisylvian region, to be manifested clinically by recurrent episodes of weakness and numbness of the contralateral face. When this disturbance occurs in the dominant cerebral hemisphere, there is, in addition, global dysphasia. In cases of severe ischemia in the middle cerebral territory, weakness and numbness may affect the entire contralateral half of the body.

In cases of stenosis of all the large arteries in the

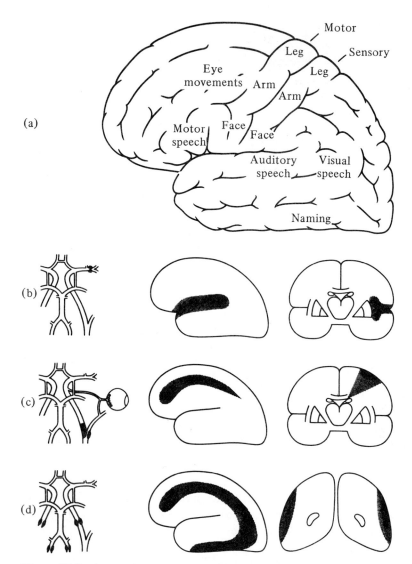

Figure 62-8. Anatomic correlates of symptoms associated with transient ischemic attacks (see text).

neck, the blood flow is likely to become inadequate first in the parietooccipital regions of both cerebral hemispheres (Fig. 62-8c, d) in the border zone between the territories of the three major cerebral arteries. The resulting complex clinical picture includes disorientation in space and regarding one's own body, visual agnosia, alexia, agraphia, acalculia, and apraxia, which are seldom distinguishable from a nonspecific confusional state. When the insufficiency

is caused by hypotension during major surgery, the neurologic deficit in temporal-parietal lobe function — as the patient demonstrates aphasia, confusion, or spatial disorientation — is sometimes mistakenly thought to represent a psychiatric disorder. In some patients a combination of occlusive disease of the large vessels in the neck and cardiac disease results in repeated ischemia in these same portions of the brain.

A stabilized disturbance of movement following a brain lesion due to vascular disease is treated by physical therapy, depending on the muscle tone and the strength remaining in the affected extremity. Leg braces, walkers, and canes should be used whenever applicable. Range-of-motion exercises, which prevent contractures of paretic limbs and improve strength in the remaining normal muscles, should be instituted as soon as possible following a stroke or head trauma. Other occupational and physical rehabilitative measures should be pursued. Acute treatment of *cerebrovascular accidents* should be directed toward assisting in establishment of collateral circulation and improvement of cerebral blood flow. Anticoagulation has been thought to be of value for some patients with transient ischemic attacks, but it has no place in long-term prophylactic treatment or in the face of a completed stroke. Prophylactic use of aspirin or dipiridamole (persentine) to decrease platelet stickiness is unproved but theoretically interesting. Thus far, surgical treatment of extracranial cerebrovascular stenosis and occlusion has been shown of value for patients with the combination of unilateral stenosis and transient ischemic attacks. Therapeutic measures toward control of hypertension and of serum lipid concentrations may be the most important aspect of long-term prevention of cerebrovascular disease.

Parkinsonism. A very common extrapyramidal syndrome is paralysis agitans (Parkinson's disease). In this disease, a tremor characterized by the opposed thumb beating against the first finger may be associated with tremor of the lips and tongue before tremor occurs in other parts. The soft, yielding plastic rigidity appears first in the flexors of the upper limbs and is associated with delay in initiation of movement, though the relative degrees of bradykinesia and objective rigidity are variable. As the disease progresses the wrists become flexed and pronated, with fingers extended, and the ankles become plantar-flexed. Any attempt to displace any part from this attitude meets with resistance. In some cases there is a more symmetric involvement, with more behavioral disorders, and often these are oculogyric crises associated with autonomic disturbances such as excessive oiliness of the skin. The neuropathologic course of parkinsonism is characterized by severe loss of cell pigment in the substantia nigra. In sections stained for myelin the globus pallidus presents a diffuse pallor. The significance

of dopamine as a neurohumeral transmitter substance affecting the nigrostriatal pathways has recently been emphasized. It is believed that in Parkinson's disease there is a deficiency of dopamine — a belief that is the basis for clinical use of large oral doses of L-dopa to try to improve synthesis of brain dopamine. Experience of this therapy may shed much light on the pathogenesis of the disease. The pharmacologic treatments of Parkinson's disease include, besides L-dopa, a variety of anticholinergic medications that affect certain aspects of parkinsonism. It is believed that a combination of both types of drugs benefits the patient. The side effects of trihexyphenidyl (Artane), benztropine mesylate (Cogentin), and amantadine (Symmetrel) are dry mouth, blurred vision, and confusion. The doses of L-dopa must be carefully regulated for each patient, and modified frequently, since too much L-dopa produces dyskinesia, increased rigidity, increased salivation, and confusion. Carbidopa increases the CNS concentrations of L-dopa, but sometimes it also increases the incidence of side effects when the combination of carbidopa and L-dopa (Sinemet) is used. Often the physician mistakes the increased rigidity or akinesia that is due to excess dopamine as a call for more medication; and, as is obvious, increased dosage of L-dopa in such cases causes more trouble. Reduction of dosage leads to improvement.

Progressive hereditary chorea (Huntington's disease) is a progressive extrapyramidal disorder occurring in members of a family as an autosomal dominant. The pathologic changes are those of diffuse neuronal degeneration in the frontal cortex, caudate nucleus, and putamen. Clinically, patients show chorea and athetosis, progressive dementia, and personality disturbances. Pneumoencephalograms and CAT scans reveal enlargement of the superior lateral aspects of the lateral ventricles with profound atrophy of the caudate nucleus. Recent studies have shown a deficiency in the concentration of gamma-aminobutyric acid (GABA) in the basal ganglia.

Hepatolenticular degeneration (Wilson's disease) is due to a disturbance of copper metabolism. This rare familial disorder, which is carried through autosomal recessive genes, may appear either in childhood or as late as the fourth decade of life. A constant sign is a circumcorneal brownish discoloration seen with tangential illumination or by slit-lamp examination. Patients show increased urinary excretion of copper (more than 100 μg per 24 hours) and depression of serum ceruloplasmin (below 20 mg per 100 ml). The neuropathologic changes seen in advanced Wilson's disease are atrophy and cavitation of the putamen, together with a striking hyperplasia of the astrocytes and a loss of nerve cells. Treatment has been directed toward the use of chelating agents to remove the excess copper. Penicillamine has been preventive in members of certain families with this disease.

Multiple sclerosis is a frustrating disease to treat, since its causes are still unknown. The pathologic findings are known to be irregular areas of degenerated white matter. Subsequent glial scar formation replaces the areas of demyelination and axonal degeneration. The symptoms and signs are the result of damage in the myelin and axons in a particular location. When there are many areas of demyelination, in many different areas of the nervous system, the constellation of neurologic symptoms and signs are difficult to tie together into a single anatomic diagnosis. Often the inconsistencies between the patient's complaints and the findings on examination raise the possibility of psychogenic causes for the disability — a conclusion that can be avoided by a careful review of the symptoms, signs, and tempo of the illness. If there are a variety of complaints that have had exacerbations and remissions over a period of months or years, and the findings are mainly those of dysfunction within white-matter systems, then a diagnosis of multiple sclerosis is justified. If the CSF protein is normal or minimally elevated and contains 18 percent or more of the protein in the form of gamma globulin, the diagnosis is even more likely to be correct.

In making a diagnosis of multiple sclerosis, the differential diagnosis must include all possible remediable conditions. A foramen magnum meningioma or a cerebellar pontine angle tumor (acoustic neuroma) may produce brainstem signs of cranial neural dysfunction, ataxia, and weakness, which could be blamed on demyelination in the brainstem. Sudden onset of impotence or sensory and motor signs attributable to spinal cord dysfunction may

indeed be due to a large demyelinative lesion, but one must consider also the possibility of compression by arthritic spondylosis or a tumor within the spinal canal. Pain syndromes such as trigeminal neuralgia or radiculopathic pains may be the consequence of an attack of demyelination, but local entrapment or inflammation of these nerves can produce the same symptoms. Retrobulbar optic neuritis causing visual disturbance in one eye may be associated with subsequent attacks or exacerbations of symptoms affecting other areas of myelin within the central nervous system. Multiple sclerosis is sometimes a diagnosis of exclusion, and one that should be made with the greatest care and suspicion, since the prognosis is so variable from patient to patient and there is no specific therapy yet available.

The course of the illness is unpredictable and may follow several patterns, incorporating signs and symptoms from various parts of the central nervous system, so that even controlled studies are difficult to evaluate. Some patients recover from acute exacerbations without any medication. Others seem to be relieved of their acute symptoms — for example, weakness or dysconjugacy of gaze — when given a short course of corticosteroids and adrenocorticotropic hormone (ACTH). Still other patients appear to have fewer exacerbations on continued dosage of vitamin B_{12} (1,000 μg IM per month) or ACTH (20 units IM per month). Muscle spasm may be severe and contraction may develop in the flexor groups. Range-of-motion exercises and muscle relaxant drugs are often needed. Diazepam (Valium) (10 mg three to four times per day) may decrease spasticity; however, in some patients it may cause the "spastic crutch" effect to be lost, making the patient even less able to stand than when untreated. Newer medications show promise of reducing spasticity and offering some functional support for gait-training purposes.

Neuro-ophthalmologic Disorders
Simmons Lessell

Six of the cranial nerves are associated with the eye or its accessory structures, and a large portion of the sensory input of the brain passes through the visual system. Therefore it is not surprising that ocular symptoms and signs are frequently encountered in diseases of the nervous system. The following is a brief discussion of the differential diagnosis of the ocular manifestations of neurologic disease.

Disorders of Ocular Motility

Diplopia. Diplopia (double vision) is usually due to a lesion of the eye muscles or of their nerves that causes a misalignment of the visual axes of the two eyes. Diplopia is of neurologic significance only if present when both eyes are open, and most patients with such diplopia keep one of their eyes closed or covered. Monocular diplopia (double vision when the patient is using only one eye), a much rarer symptom, reflects local ocular disease rather than a neurologic lesion. It is most frequently due to refractive problems or to early opacification of the lens. While many ophthalmologists and neurologists regard monocular diplopia as a hysteric symptom, it usually has an organic basis.

Diplopia that begins abruptly is usually the result of a lesion of the third, fourth, or sixth cranial nerve or its nucleus. Sudden third-nerve palsies with involvement of the pupil are most commonly due to aneurysms of the circle of Willis. Headache is a common accompaniment. Third-nerve palsies also occur in diabetics, presumably from occlusion of vasa nervosa; they are often painful but usually spare the pupil, and they tend to recover completely within 3 months. Other painful third-nerve palsies can occur from herpes zoster, tumors, temporal arteritis, migraine, and mucoceles of the sphenoid sinus. A sudden, painless third-nerve palsy with contralateral hemiplegia indicates a unilateral midbrain infarction on the side of the ophthalmoplegia. Transtentorial herniation of the brain and expansion of intracranial masses or clots can produce a third-nerve palsy that evolves rapidly, with early pupil involvement. Slowly evolving third-nerve palsies are seen in basal tumors, granulomas, and infiltrating neoplasms of the midbrain.

Isolated sixth-nerve palsies can occur from diabetes, intracavernous (subclinoid) aneurysms of the carotid artery, basal tumors (especially metastatic lesions, tumors extending from the nasopharynx, cordomas, and meningiomas), herpes zoster, temporal arteritis, migraine, spontaneous dural fistulas, and increased intracranial pressure. Abducens neuropathies that develop in patients with increased intracranial pressure are usually due to the pressure per se and not to the underlying cause of the pressure. Therefore, in the presence of increased intracranial pressure a sixth-nerve palsy has no localizing significance. Sudden lateral rectus palsies with homolateral facial paralysis (and sometimes internuclear ophthalmoplegia or gaze palsy) indicate infarction of the pontine tegmentum. The progressive appearance of such signs is typical of pontine gliomas. A significant minority of patients with abducens palsies recover without any cause having been established. "Benign" palsies of this type are more common in children than in adults.

Fourth-nerve palsies, which are rarer than third- or sixth-nerve palsies, most commonly are due to trauma. Other causes are diabetes, tumor (intramedullary or extramedullary), and mesencephalic infarcts. A significant number of patients with trochlear nerve palsy experience spontaneous recovery, and the cases are never explained.

Combinations of eye muscle palsies may occur with orbital masses, inflammations, or infections; infraclinoid aneurysms; basal tumors; carotid-cavernous fistulas; cavernous sinus tumors, granulomas, or inflammations; basilar meningitis; herpes zoster; and brainstem infarcts or tumors. Patients with thiamine deficiency (particularly alcoholics) may present with Wernicke's encephalopathy, a disease characterized by rapid development of ophthalmoplegia in a setting of nystagmus, ataxia, and Korsakoff's psychosis. The ophthalmoplegia generally responds to parenteral thiamine therapy within hours. Since Wernicke's disease can be fatal if untreated, it is important to diagnose and treat it without delay. Sudden painful ophthalmoplegia, often with headache and visual loss, can be an indication of infarction of a pituitary adenoma. Painful ophthalmoplegia, associated with periorbital edema, malaise, myalgia, and fever, occurs in some patients with trichinosis. Orbital infections can produce proptosis, pain, and ophthalmoplegia, and one should be particularly alerted when those symptoms occur in a diabetic. Diabetics seem particularly susceptible to orbital cellulitis due to mucormycosis or related fungi; mucormycotic infections of the orbit are fatal if untreated.

An important orbital cause of diplopia is endocrine exophthalmos. Patients can have unilateral or bilateral involvement. The manifestations are progressive exophthalmos, conjunctival injection and congestion, and ophthalmoplegia. There is frequently retraction of the upper lid, and the orbits feel "tight" when one attempts to reposition the globe. The most prominent defect in eye movement is in upward gaze.

Many patients with myasthenia gravis have ophthalmoplegia, with or without ptosis (see below in this section). The ophthalmoplegia generally involves more than one muscle and increases as the day wears on. Spontaneous remissions may occur. Even if ptosis is not present spontaneously, it can often be induced by having the patient gaze upward for several minutes. This causes the lid gradually to ptose. Usually weakness of eye closure is also present. Administration of short-acting anticholinesterase agents such as edrophonium hydrochloride may reverse the ophthalmoplegia and establish the diagnosis, but, unfortunately, false-negative reactions may occur.

The eye muscles can become involved in certain muscular dystrophies (see above in this chapter). Ptosis may appear, and eventually the disease, which slowly progresses over a period of months or years, may leave the patient with completely immobile eyes. Clinical involvement may appear limited to the muscles of the eye, the lids, and the face, but biopsy of limb muscles frequently reveals pathologic findings. It has recently been suggested that not all these diseases are primary myopathies. Some may represent neuropathies or even supranuclear defects in eye movement.

Lesions of the medial longitudinal fasciculi, a small paired tract that integrates the vestibular and ocular motor systems in the brainstem, may produce a unique disturbance of ocular motility — internuclear ophthalmoplegia. Patients with internuclear ophthalmoplegia generally have straight eyes when they look straight ahead. However, on gaze to the side opposite the lesion, the eye on that side fails to adduct. The contralateral eye abducts but has a coarse, horizontal nystagmus. However, both medial recti may perform normally when the patient is asked to converge. Bilateral internuclear ophthalmoplegia is usually due to multiple sclerosis, and it is the most characteristic disturbance of ocular motility in that disease. Unilateral cases are most often due to vascular disease.

There is only one important supranuclear cause of diplopia — skew deviation, a form of acquired vertical strabismus. In this condition one eye is higher than the other, usually in all fields of gaze. Sometimes it is difficult to differentiate skew deviation from eye muscle palsy due to lesions of the lower motor neruon. Skew deviation indicates disease in the cerebellum or brainstem, and lesions in the vicinity of the middle cerebellar peduncle seem particularly likely to produce it. Multiple sclerosis, vascular lesions, and neoplasms of the brainstem or cerebellum are the commonest causes.

Gaze Disturbances. The inability of both eyes to look synchronously in a particular direction is a *gaze palsy*. The centers for horizontal gaze in the cerebral hemispheres can be damaged by vascular, traumatic, neoplastic, infectious, and inflammatory lesions, and they may discharge as a facet of a focal seizure. In the acute stages of damage to these centers, the eyes remain deviated to the same side as the lesions and cannot look in the opposite direction. When the patient becomes alert, the gaze palsy usually disappears. Pontine lesions produce gaze palsies that have a direction opposite to those due to cerebral lesions. Thus, patients with pontine lesions cannot look to the same side of the lesion. They also differ from patients with cerebral gaze palsies in that they do not improve when they become alert. Pontine gaze paresis is encountered in multiple sclerosis, Wernicke's encephalopathy, tumors, and vascular lesions.

Vertical gaze movements appear to be mediated through the pre-tectum. Lesions of the rostral mesencephalon and the posterior portion of the third ventricle characteristically affect vertical gaze. Impaired upward gaze together with fixed pupils, known as Parinaud's syndrome, is classically associated with pineal tumors. Parkinsonism and Huntington's chorea, as well as other disorders of the basal ganglia, can also produce defects in upward gaze. In some cases of postencephalitic parkinsonism and in phenothiazine intoxication, transient uncontrollable upward deviation of the eyes (oculogyric crisis) may occur.

Most disorders of vertical gaze affect upward gaze predominantly. There are exceptions; for example, in a disease called progressive supranuclear palsy there is sometimes selective or predominant involvement of downward gaze early in the course of the illness. Later, all vertical movements are affected. The disease is sporadic, occurs in middle and late life, and is associated with progressive dementia, extrapyramidal signs and symptoms, and gait disturbance. Downgaze paralysis may also be a prominent feature in Huntington's chorea.

In some patients who have a profound degree of gaze paralysis in all directions, it may be difficult to distinguish between central paralysis of gaze and ophthalmoplegia due to disease of the peripheral cranial nerves or of the eye muscles themselves. In central gaze paralysis, called pseudo-ophthalmoplegia, the true cause can be demonstrated by suddenly turning the patient's head to one side, then to the other. The eyes will have a full range of motion in the direction opposite to that in which the head is turned (doll head movements). These movements occur because the higher centers of gaze have been disconnected from the appropriate cranial nerve nuclei, and the more primitive vestibular mechanisms are in control (see later in this chapter, under Otoneurologic Disorders). One also can show that the lower motor neurons in the oculomotor system are intact by demonstrating deviation of the eyes when the auditory canal is irrigated with cold water (caloric test).

Nystagmus. *Nystagmus* refers to the rhythmic alternating movement of the eyes that can occur under both physiologic and pathologic circumstances. It may have either a distinct rapid and a distinct slow component (jerk type) or no distinct rapid and slow phases (pendular type).

Nystagmus can be induced in normal individuals by stimulation of the semicircular canals (labyrinths), either by rotation of the patient (as in Bárány's test) or by irrigation of the external auditory canal with cold (or hot) water (caloric test). Another form of physiologic nystagmus is opticokinetic nystagmus, which is induced by having the patient look at a repeating pattern (e.g., stripes) passed in a horizontal or vertical direction in front of his eyes. The patient develops nystagmus with a slow component in the direction toward which the stimulus is being moved, followed by a fast corrective movement back toward the midline. Opticokinetic nystagmus testing has many uses in neurology and ophthalmology. Since the nystagmus cannot be voluntarily suppressed, the test is a good one for hysteric or feigned blindness. One can demonstrate opticokinetic nystagmus in such cases, indicating objectively that there is some visual function. By using targets with different intervals between the stripes, it is possible to gauge the visual acuity of infants and other persons not testable by conventional methods. Defects in opticokinetic nystagmus are typically encountered in lesions of the posterior half of the cerebral hemispheres, especially of the parietal lobe. A diminished or absent response is noted when the target is rotated toward the side of the lesion. The impairment is not dependent upon the presence of a hemianopia. In the presence of a hemianopia, normal opticokinetic responses strongly suggest a nonparietal locus of the lesion. An exception may be porencephalic cysts of the parietal lobe. Abnormal opticokinetic nystagmus in the presence of an occipital lesion should be suggestive of neoplasm.

Pendular nystagmus is most commonly seen in individuals who lost their central vision in both eyes within the first 5 years of life. Optic atrophy, congenital cataract, optic nerve hypoplasia, hydrocephalus, uveitis, and albinism are some of the more common causes of significant visual impairment in early childhood. In a disorder called spasmus nutans, pendular nystagmus, often asymmetric in amplitude in the two eyes, develops within the first 2 years of life and is frequently associated with head-nodding, head-banging, or unusual head postures. The prognosis for recovery is generally good, and there are usually no associated lesions of the nervous system. The cause of the condition has not been established.

Jerk nystagmus may be present as a congenital abnormality, in which case it is rarely vertical. It is also seen with peripheral vestibular disorders such as labyrinthitis and Ménière's disease. In these circumstances the nystagmus is frequently rotary, and usually it is most severe at the onset and then gradually improves. There is often also impaired hearing and tinnitus. In diseases of the brainstem, the characteristic sign is an upbeating vertical nystagmus, with or without a horizontal component, on up-gaze. Barbiturates and phenytoin (Dilantin) commonly produce nystagmus of this type. In multiple sclerosis, jerk nystagmus, with the fast component in the direction of gaze, along with intention tremor and scanning speech form Charcot's triad. Jerk nystagmus may be produced by vascular accidents in the distribution of the basilar artery and by neoplasms in the brainstem or in the cerebellum pressing down from above. Upbeating, small-amplitude vertical nystagmus in the primary position of gaze is thought to indicate lesions, particularly tumors, of the anterior vermis of the cerebellum. Nystagmus that is downbeating is typical of lesions involving the cervicomedullary junction (e.g., Arnold-Chiari malformation).

Certain forms of nystagmus have great localizing value. Nystagmus in which the eyes rhythmically converge or rhythmically contract into the orbit (retractory nystagmus) indicates disease of the mesencephalon. Seesaw nystagmus, in which one eye moves up while the other eye moves down, is associated with chiasmatic and suprasellar lesions (especially craniopharyngiomas). Acquired discordant nystagmus, in which the two eyes move in different directions or in which the nystagmus is of different amplitude in the two eyes, points to disease of the brainstem.

Ptosis. Any process that produces damage to the third nerve or its nucleus may result in *ptosis*. Myasthenia gravis frequently causes ptosis (see above in this section). Oculopharyngeal muscular dystrophy results in marked bilateral ptosis, which begins in middle life. Some patients with myotonic dystrophy have ptosis, but in that disease nonophthalmic symptoms predominate. In many patients the cause of ptosis remains unidentified; the condition may be due to an abiotrophic disorder. Familial occurrences of this type, usually inherited as a dominant

trait, are well recognized. Interruption of the sympathetic innervation to the orbital structures results in Horner's syndrome — ptosis with miosis and anhidrosis — which is usually caused by lesions in the chest or neck, with trauma and malignant neoplasms the commonest causes. The Horner syndrome can also result when there is occlusive disease of the carotid artery or a degenerative disease, neoplasm, or syrinx of the spinal cord. Lateral medullary infarction can cause a homolateral Horner's syndrome.

Defects in Accommodation. Any lesion that produces damage to the third nerve can produce paralysis of accommodation along with pupillary dilatation, ptosis, and external ophthalmoplegia. In Adie's syndrome, defects in accommodation occur together with a large, sluggish pupil. Paralysis of accommodation may be seen as an isolated finding in diphtheria, and also as part of the characteristic neuro-ophthalmic picture of botulism. Spasm of accommodation and convergence is encountered in structural disease of the nervous system, but is most typically seen in psychoneurotic persons (when such patients are refracted they appear to be myopic, due to the spasm of accommodation; however, if, on correct diagnosis, they are given a cycloplegic agent, such as topical atropine, their ciliary muscle relaxes and the myopia vanishes).

Disturbances of Pupillary Motility. With unilateral blindness the patient does not show the direct pupillary response to light but there is an intact consensual reaction. Visual loss in one eye does not produce unequal pupils. The presence of a normal pupillary response to light in a totally blind patient points to a cortical (or geniculocalcarine) origin for the blindness.

A fixed, dilated pupil may accompany any lesion of the third cranial nerve, but it is seen most characteristically with aneurysms and shifts in the cranial contents. In cases of subdural hematoma with pressure on the third nerve, the abnormal pupil is usually on the side of the lesion. In perplexing cases of fixed, dilated pupils without other evidence of disease of the nervous system, one should consider the possibility that the patients are instilling a mydriatic agent into their own eyes or that they have had accidental contact with such a drug. Blunt trauma to the globe may also produce a fixed, dilated pupil; often after a period of weeks there is recovery from such traumatic mydriasis, but in some cases it can be permanent.

The occurrence of a small pupil in Horner's syndrome has already been noted. Pontine hemorrhages produce bilateral fixed miosis. In the so-called paratrigeminal syndrome, miosis is seen along with homolateral facial pain and tearing, but with sweating preserved over the whole face. When unaccompanied by other neurologic signs, this syndrome almost always indicates a benign process.

Pupils fixed in the midposition are seen in Parinaud's syndrome (see above in this chapter) and in combined sympathetic and parasympathetic denervation of the globe. The Argyll Robertson pupil is small and does not react to light; it does react on convergence. The condition is usually bilateral, but the two pupils are unequal. Classic Argyll Robertson pupils are usually due to syphilis of the central nervous system, but similar pupillary abnormalities can result from diabetes, trauma, or herpes zoster. In Adie's syndrome, the pupil is unilaterally dilated and shows an unusually slow or apparently absent response to light stimulation. This may be associated with paralysis of accommodation (see above in this section). The pupil is unusually sensitive to parasympathomimetic drugs. Miosis of the involved pupil will be produced by 2.5% metacholine (Mecholyl) or 0.25% pilocarpine applied topically, with no effect on the other eye. Both parasympathetic and sympathetic denervation of the pupils may be seen in familial dysautonomia.

Diseases of the Optic Nerve

Papilledema. Swelling of the optic nerve head is an important sign of disease of the nervous system. It is essential to differentiate papilledema (swelling of the optic nerve due to increased intracranial pressure) from pseudopapilledema (nonpathologic disc elevation). No hemorrhage, exudate, or venous congestion is seen in pseudopapilledema, whereas in true papilledema there is always congestion of the veins, and often there are hemorrhages and exudates on and around the disc. Visual acuity is the prime means of distinguishing between papilledema and optic neuritis or other primary diseases of the optic nerve in which disc swelling may occur: Patients with optic neuritis or other optic neuropathies have alterations in visual function, while acuity remains good in papilledema.

Any condition that produces increased intracranial pressure can produce papilledema. This includes all space-occupying lesions in the cranial cavity. Papilledema is most pronounced and occurs earliest in tumors of the posterior fossa. It is also seen in pseudotumor cerebri, hypertensive encephalopathy, carbon dioxide retention, meningitis, and subarachnoid hemorrhage. Occasionally it is encountered in hypocalcemic states and when the spinal fluid protein is markedly elevated. Swelling of the optic nerve can occur in local ocular disorders such as occlusion of the central retinal vein, infarction of the optic nerve, uveitis, and severe ocular hypotonia.

The *Foster Kennedy syndrome* consists of papilledema in one eye and optic atrophy in the other. Encountered in sphenoidal and olfactory groove meningiomas, it is commonly mimicked by sequential bilateral ischemic optic neuropathy (infarction of the optic nerve head). Swelling of the optic nerve may also occur from direct infiltration of the nerve metastatic tumors or primary gliomas. Optic nerve gliomas generally develop in childhood, and many are associated with neurofibromatosis (von Recklinghausen's disease). Disc swelling also occurs with primary optic nerve sheath meningiomas.

Optic Neuritis. The optic nerve can be involved by inflammation at any point in its course from the nerve head back to the chiasm. When the most peripheral portion of the nerve is involved — a condition known as papillitis — the optic nerve head is swollen. When only the portion behind the globe is affected, the condition is known as retrobulbar neuritis, and there is little or no visible abnormality in the optic nerve head. Both conditions are characterized by impairment of visual acuity and alterations in the visual fields. There is also impairment of color perception, sometimes out of proportion to the amount of visual loss. In most cases optic neuritis is rapid in onset, with the maximum visual deficit apparent within several weeks. There is often pain on movement or palpation of the globe.

Optic neuritis is most characteristic of multiple sclerosis. Involvement of the optic nerve probably occurs at some time in the majority of patients with multiple sclerosis. While the prognosis for vision is usually good after a single episode, the patient is often left with a small sector of atrophy in the temporal part of the optic nerve head (temporal pallor). About 15 percent of multiple sclerosis cases begin with an attack of optic neuritis; but subsequent signs of multiple sclerosis may be long delayed. Between 10 and 40 percent of patients with apparently uncomplicated optic neuritis in the first four decades of life will eventually develop other symptoms and signs of multiple sclerosis. The majority of the remaining cases never receive an etiologic diagnosis. Optic neuritis can also occur as an inherited defect, usually in males (Leber's disease).

Optic neuritis may accompany various forms of viral encephalitis, including those due to the childhood exanthems. Occlusion of the nutrient vessels of the optic nerve (ischemic optic neuropathy), as in temporal arteritis, produces sudden visual loss and disc swelling. Temporal arteritis should be suspected whenever a patient over the age of 50 develops an acute optic neuropathy. The temporal arteritis may be occult; that is, there may be no fever, leukocytosis, or headache. The erythrocyte sedimentation rate is usually elevated, and biopsy of the temporal artery usually shows the characteristic lesions. However, negative biopsy does not rule out the diagnosis. Steroid therapy will protect the fellow eye if started early and in high doses.

Although some cases of optic neuropathy are ascribed to the combined effects of tobacco and alcohol, there are no conclusive data to support this hypothesis. The optic neuropathy that may complicate chronic alcoholism probably results from malnutrition. It is questionable whether there is such a thing as tobacco amblyopia. However, some investigators believe that tobacco amblyopia is a real entity, and that it is somehow related to a defect in the metabolism of exogenous cyanide. Numerous other toxins — for example, the organic arsenicals, ethambutol, organic solvents, chloramphenicol, isoniazid, streptomycin, sulfonamides, and thallium —

have also been considered to be implicated in optic neuropathies.

Some patients originally thought to have optic neuritis are ultimately found to have compression of the optic nerve by a neoplasm or an aneurysm. These patients usually have a history of slowly progressive visual loss. Such a history makes the diagnosis of optic neuritis unlikely. Therefore, while patients with optic neuritis or optic atrophy should have careful plain x-ray studies of the skull, those with a history of slowly progressive visual failure deserve more intensive neurologic and neuroradiologic investigations.

Optic Atrophy. Optic atrophy may be conveniently divided into three types, based upon ophthalmoscopic appearance — glaucomatous, primary, and secondary.

Glaucomatous optic atrophy is characterized by cupping or excavation of the nerve head. This change usually occurs on the temporal side, just above or below the horizontal meridian. In this area the disc margin loses its normal pink color and becomes gray or yellow. The usual cause is a prolonged elevation of intraocular pressure. Typical glaucomatous optic atrophy is occasionally seen in patients without abnormally high intraocular pressures. If it is unilateral one should suspect interference with the blood supply to the optic nerve. Some patients who present with glaucomatous optic atrophy but without elevated pressures or progression of their deficit have a history of previous vasomotor collapse and shock. Unilateral atherosclerotic narrowing of an internal carotid artery may cause acceleration of glaucomatous optic atrophy on the same side as the narrowing.

Primary optic atrophy is manifested by a flat white or pale yellow optic nerve head with unusually distinct borders. The number of fine vessels crossing the optic margin of the disc is reduced. Primary optic atrophy may result from trauma, pressure on the optic nerve or chiasm (as with pituitary adenomas), infarction of the optic nerve or retina, or optic neuritis. Optic atrophy of this type is also seen in CNS syphilis.

Secondary optic atrophy is manifested by a dirty-white or gray optic disc that is slightly elevated. It is usually the sequel of neglected chronic papilledema, optic neuritis, or ischemic optic neuropathy.

Defects in the Visual Fields

Lesions anywhere in the visual pathway may result in visual field defects. When a visual field defect is limited to one eye, the responsible lesion must (with rare exceptions) be situated between the cornea and the chiasm. Central scotomas (areas of depressed vision located at the patient's point of fixation) are most characteristic of optic neuritis. They also occur in diseases of the macular zone of the retina. Monocular sector field defects often are due to local retinal vascular disease. Ring scotomas are characteristic of pigmentary retinopathies. Bilateral centrocecal scotomas (involving the blind spot and the fixation point) may be due to toxic conditions or deficiency disorders of the optic nerve. Lesions of the optic nerve adjacent to the chiasm may produce a central scotoma or blindness in the homolateral eye and a superior temporal field defect in the contralateral eye. This occurs because the inferior nasal retinal fibers from each eye dip into the opposite optic nerve after crossing at the anterior angle of the chiasm. Altitudinal field defects (upper or lower) are caused by infarction of the optic nerve, glaucoma, or retinal detachment.

Lesions of the chiasm usually produce bitemporal field defects. The commonest cause is tumor of the pituitary. In pituitary tumors the defects typically start in the superior temporal fields. If, however, the lesion involves the posterior angle of the chiasm, bitemporal central hemiscotomas may occur.

Lesions posterior to the chiasm produce homonymous field defects (i.e., the defect is on the same side in both eyes). The closer the lesion is to the occipital pole, the more likely it is for the defect to be congruous (of similar size, shape, and density in both eyes). Even in complete homonymous hemianopias (with splitting of fixation) the visual acuity is normal. Superior quadrantanopias are characteristic of temporal lobe lesions and inferior quadrantanopias are most characteristic of parietal lesions. The value of opticokinetic nystagmus testing in the presence of a hemianopia has been noted above.

Alterations in Vision

Amaurosis. Transient blurring or loss of vision in older patients is frequently due to atherosclerosis of the carotid or vertebral arteries, with consequent insufficiency of blood flow. Transient unilateral blurring (amaurosis fugax) suggests insufficiency of the internal carotid artery. Ophthalmodynamometry in such cases reveals lowered pressures in the central retinal artery on the side of the narrowing. A bruit may be elicited over the homolateral carotid artery or the contralateral eye. Transient bilateral visual blurring implicates the vertebrobasilar arterial system and suggests ischemia of both occipital lobes. Symptoms or signs of brainstem dysfunction that are frequently present help to confirm the clinical diagnosis. Similar symptoms can occur in occlusive arteritis of the aortic arch.

Visual Hallucinations. Migraine sufferers may present predominantly visual symptoms. Transient hemianopias, scotomas, and monocular amaurosis are not uncommon, and visual hallucinations in the form of scintillating colored lights, balls, or patterns are common. The visual symptoms precede the onset of headache in given attacks and presumably reflect cerebral or retinal vasoconstriction. Similar visual hallucinations may result from cortical lesions. Temporal lobe foci tend to produce formed pictures. Hallucinations of occipital origin are usually simple photisms — flashes of light or color. These may occur as isolated phenomena in focal seizures or form part of the symptom complex in occipital lobe or temporal lobe tumors or vascular accidents.

Geniculocalcarine Blindness. *Geniculocalcarine* (cortical or cerebral) *blindness* refers to bilateral loss of vision from disease of the visual system "behind" the optic tract. The pupils react normally to light, and the optic discs do not show atrophy. Opticokinetic nystagmus cannot be elicited. Such blindness can result from any bilateral geniculate or retrogeniculate lesion. Bilateral occipital lobe infarction from vertebrobasilar occlusive disease is the commonest cause in adults. Trauma, perinatal anoxia, anesthesia accidents, hypoglycemia, progressive subcortical encephalopathy (Schilder's disease), angiography, mercury intoxication, and tumors can all produce the syndrome.

Changes in the Fundus Oculi in Nervous System Diseases

Lipidoses and Related Disorders. The lipidoses are inherited disorders of lipid metabolism in which the storage of lipids occurs to an abnormal degree in many organs, including the brain and the eye. In lipid histiocytosis (Niemann-Pick disease) and the infantile form of amaurotic familial idiocy (Tay-Sachs disease), storage of lipid in the perifoveal ganglion cells produces the appearance of a cherry-red spot. Victims of Tay-Sachs disease become blind and show optic atrophy. In the late infantile form (Bielschowsky-Jansky or Spielmeyer-Vogt disease) and the juvenile form (Batten-Mayou disease) of amaurotic family idiocy (which are neuronal lipofuchsinoses rather than lipidoses), the cherry-red spot is not seen; but pigmentary degeneration of the retina is present. This may involve either only the central portion or all of the retina. The adult form of amaurotic family idiocy (Kufs' disease) usually has no retinal changes.

Phakomatoses. There is an abundance of ocular lesions in neurofibromatosis (von Recklinghausen's disease). The commonest fundus manifestations are neurofibromas of the optic disc, optic atrophy from tumors of the optic nerve or chiasm, and papilledema secondary to intracranial neoplasms. About 15 percent of all primary tumors of the optic nerve and chiasm are associated with neurofibromatosis. Retinal tumors are found in tuberous sclerosis. The tumors appear like mulberries on the disc or, less commonly, in the peripheral retina, or as superficial oval or circular light-colored lesions. Since brain tumors are frequent in tuberous sclerosis, papilledema can occur. In cerebroretinal angiomatosis (Lindau-von Hippel disease), retinal angiomas are seen in conjunction with cerebellar hemangioblastomas. Vitreous hemorrhages and retinal detachments may occur in association with these vascular tumors. Glaucoma is frequent in the Sturge-Weber-Dimitri syndrome; therefore, glaucomatous optic atrophy may be seen. Choroidal hemangioma may be present on the same side as the facial vascular nevus.

Pigmentary Degeneration of the Retina. Retinitis pigmentosa, which is manifested by clumping of pigment, primarily in the equatorial region of the fundus, is associated with narrowing of the retinal vessels and pallor of the optic nerve head. It most often occurs as a disorder of unknown cause, with abnormalities limited to the eyes. Many cases are familial, and several modes of inheritance have been identified. Fundus pictures similar to those in retinitis pigmentosa may be seen in association with disorders of the nervous system. In the Laurence-Moon-Biedl syndrome, retinitis pigmentosa is associated with mental retardation, hypogenitalism, polydactylia, and obesity. In the Bassen-Kornzweig syndrome, retinitis pigmentosa occurs with spinocerebellar degeneration and misshapen red blood cells (acanthocytes). In Refsum's syndrome, pigmentary degeneration of the retina is associated with polyneuropathy and ataxia, and deafness is usually present. The occurrence of pigmentary retinal degeneration in the late infantile and juvenile forms of amaurotic family idiocy has been commented on above.

Otoneurologic Disorders
Jules Friedman

Vertigo and Dizziness

Dizziness is one of the most common symptoms clinicians encounter. Some patients use *dizziness* to describe light-headedness or faintness. The sensation may be caused by hypotension resulting from vasovagal and orthostatic reflexes or by more serious cardiovascular conditions. Metabolic dysfunction, especially hypoglycemia, may cause such complaints. Hyperventilation syndrome, usually associated with anxiety or depression, produces light-headedness, which may be followed by circumoral and distal extremity paresthesias, unsteadiness, precordial pain, and even tetany or syncope. Patients will often describe the tightness or fullness in the head stemming from common tension-related cranial or cervical muscle spasm as dizziness. Visual disturbances such as blurred vision or diplopia can also be so described. Toxic agents, especially sedatives, tranquilizers, narcotics, and tobacco, can produce such symptoms. Patients with any combination of bilateral visual dysfunction, proprioceptive dysfunction, or vestibular dysfunction (multiple sensory deficits) may experience spatial disorientation, which they describe as dizziness or unsteadiness. This is quite common in older age groups, and especially so in diabetics. Only a minority of those complaining of "dizziness" are actually experiencing vertigo. *Vertigo* is an illusion of movement of self or surroundings and, although most commonly rotary, it may also involve a sensation of rocking, tilting, or pulsion. It indicates dysfunction of the vestibular system, which is anatomically a paired system, consisting of the vestibular labyrinth, the vestibular nerve, the vestibular nuclear complex in the brainstem, and vestibular connections to other CNS centers.

As in evaluation of disease of other parts of the nervous system, the differential diagnosis of dysfunction of the vestibular system depends on precise localization of the site of the lesion and determination of the pathologic process responsible for the lesion at that locus. Localization is accomplished by recognition of the symptoms and physical findings characteristic of lesions at a given locus in the vestibular system. One makes a determination by selecting, according to characteristic clinical profiles, the appropriate process from among those pathologic processes known to occur at a given locus.

Localization of Lesions

A *unilateral vestibular lesion* of acute onset is invariably characterized by one or more of the following symptoms and signs. There is a persistent sensation of movement of self or surroundings, known as vertigo. In acute unilateral lesions, vertigo is spontaneous; that is, although exacerbated by movement, it can begin and persist with the patient at rest. There are rhythmic eye movements, known as nystagmus, which consists of a slow, tonic deviation of the eyes in one direction followed by a fast, jerklike return in the opposite direction. These alternating slow and fast components together form the rhythmic oscillations of nystagmus. It should be noted that it is the lesion of the vestibular system that produces the slow, tonic ocular deviation, whereas the fast jerk return is merely a compensatory reflex reaction originating elsewhere in central nervous system. By convention, however, the direction of nystagmus is described according to the direction of the fast component. Thus, nystagmus

with the slow component to the left and the fast component to the right is a "right-beating nystagmus."

Associated symptoms secondary to excitation of the parasympathetic nervous system (vegetative symptoms) may be present. Nausea, vomiting, pallor, and diaphoresis are common. On occasion diarrhea or even hypotension with syncope may occur. The extent of vegetative symptoms in a given vestibular lesion varies greatly from patient to patient.

Signs of abnormal station and gait include past pointing, a positive Romberg test, and gait ataxia. In the test of *past pointing* the patient extends both arms forward and places the index finger of each hand on the palm of the examiner's hand. With eyes closed, the patient raises both arms over his head and then slowly returns them to the original position. This is repeated several times, and past pointing is said to be present if the position of the arms deviates and the finger falls laterally upon return to the original position on the examiner's hand. In the *Romberg test* the patient stands with both feet together, first with eyes open and then with eyes closed. Patients in the acute phase of unilateral vestibular lesions and patients with cerebellar lesions manifest a definite tendency to fall, both with eyes open and with eyes closed. Cerebellar lesions can often be differentiated by testing of the extremities (heel-to-shin test, finger-to-nose test; rapid alternating movements), which results in intention tremor or dysmetria. Patients with subacute or longstanding lesions of the vestibular system or with lesions of the proprioceptive system tend to fall only with eyes closed. Lesions of the proprioceptive system can be differentiated by direct testing of position sense in the distal extremities. *Gait ataxia* – a staggering gait, usually with a tendency to fall to one side – may be noted in patients with acute unilateral lesions of the vestibular system. With less acute or mild lesions, gait is usually wide-based with occasional staggering and a tendency to drift toward a particular side. Ataxia due to cerebellar lesions may be difficult to distinguish from ataxia due to vestibular lesions, but the latter are often characterized by a striking increase in gait difficulties when the patient's eyes are closed or when it is dark. As this characteristic also holds in ataxia due to lesions of the proprioceptive system, position testing of the extremities should be performed to differentiate vestibular from proprioceptive (sensory) ataxia. When unilateral lesions are slowly progressive, rather than acute, the striking clinical manifestations described above may not be present (see discussion of motion-induced dysfunction on p. 911). The unilaterality of the lesion must then be determined by recognition of associated unilateral auditory or CNS dysfunction and by clinical testing.

Bilateral vestibular lesions display few symptoms and signs. The clinical manifestations observed in unilateral vestibular dysfunction result from an imbalance in the neural activity of one side over the other side of the system. In bilaterally equal and synchronous vestibular dysfunction no such imbalance occurs and clinical manifestations result from a greater dependence upon other compensatory systems needed for spatial orientation, such as vision and proprioception. Thus, ataxia occurring in circumstances of reduced vision (such as in a darkened room) is characteristic of reduced bilateral vestibular function. The most common cause of bilateral vestibular lesions is ototoxicity, produced by certain antibiotics. Streptomycin sulfate, kanamycin, gentamicin, and ethacrynic acid are ototoxic. The site of damage is the neuroepithelium of the labyrinth itself, and usually the damage is irreversible. Rarely, basal skull fractures will extend bilaterally and involve the labyrinths equally.

The next task in localization consists in differentiating *peripheral* and *central* vestibular lesions. *Peripheral vestibular lesions* (acute unilateral lesions) produce vertigo, ataxia, and nystagmus. These symptoms are relatively proportional in intensity. The reason for this is that impairment of neural activity in the peripheral system is reflected in all the more central parts of the system. Nausea, vomiting, and diaphoresis are often present. In peripheral lesions, even those that are irreversible or of very long duration, there is a predictable, rather limited duration of the above symptom complex. Spontaneous vertigo will resolve within 3 to 7 days, although momentary vertigo provoked by rapid head movements (motion-induced vertigo) may persist. Spontaneous nystagmus will also resolve in 3 to 7 days, although, again, vigorous head movements may provoke momentary recurrence. Ataxia resolves gradually over several weeks, but it may present a persistent problem when the patient's eyes are closed or when it is dark. The somewhat limited duration of clinical manifestations in peripheral lesions results from a process called *accommodation* that occurs in the vestibular nuclear complex. This mechanism reestablishes the neural balance between both sides of the central vestibular system, thus eliminating the cause of spontaneous nystagmus (Table 62-4).

Many lesions of the peripheral vestibular system will be manifested by nystagmus that does not occur spontaneously, but only with positional change. *Positional nystagmus* may be induced by performing special positional testing. In this useful maneuver (Nylen-Bárány test) the patient, who is seated near the end of a table, is rapidly placed in the supine position with the head extended over the edge of the table and rotated to one side. The patient fixes his eyes at a point several feet ahead. Observations are made for 60 seconds and the patient is then rapidly returned to the sitting position, where he again fixes. The maneuver is repeated in the same fashion with the

Table 62-4. Spontaneous Nystagmus in Vestibular Lesions and the Differentiation of Peripheral and Central Vestibular Lesions

1. Central or Peripheral Vestibular Lesions
   a. Nystagmus direction is not altered by position of gaze (direction fixed).
   b. Intensity of nystagmus increases with gaze in the direction of the fast component.

2. Peripheral Vestibular Lesions
   a. Nystagmus increases with eyes closed or in darkness (reduced ocular fixation).
   b. Nystagmus is proportional in degree to vertigo and ataxia.
   c. Nystagmus is a mixture of rotary and oblique components.
   d. Nystagmus (spontaneous) resolves within 3 to 7 days.

3. Central Vestibular Lesions
   a. Nystagmus may not increase and may even decrease with reduced ocular fixation.
   b. Nystagmus intensity may be out of proportion to vertigo or ataxia.
   c. Nystagmus may be purely horizontal, vertical, or rotary.

Table 62-5. Positional Nystagmus
in Differentiation of Peripheral
and Central Vestibular Lesions

1. Peripheral Vestibular Lesions
   a. Nystagmus begins after a delay (latency) of several seconds.
   b. Nystagmus is a mixture of horizontal, vertical, and rotary components.
   c. Vertigo is prominent.
   d. Nystagmus and vertigo resolve within 60 seconds.
   e. The entire sequence of events recurs with resumption of the sitting position, except that the direction of nystagmus reverses.
   f. Repetition of the maneuver results in progressive diminution of the response (fatiguing).
   g. The response varies in intensity from exam to exam and on many occasions may not be manifested at all.
2. Central Vestibular Lesions
   a. Nystagmus begins immediately; there is no latency.
   b. Nystagmus is purely horizontal or vertical.
   c. Vertigo is absent or minimal.
   d. Nystagmus persists beyond 60 seconds.
   e. No response occurs upon resumption of the sitting position.
   f. No fatiguing occurs.
   g. The response is consistently reproducible from exam to exam.

head rotated to the opposite side and once again with the head straight. Two patterns of pathologic responses can be identified, one due to lesions of the labyrinth, and the other due to lesions of central vestibular connections or other brainstem or cerebellar connections, or both (Table 62-5).

Central vestibular lesions may produce only a portion of the potential symptom complex of vertigo, ataxia, and nystagmus. The reason for this is that the lesion may be so situated as to interfere with neural transmission in only one of the central vestibular connections. Transmission between the intact peripheral system and all the remaining central connections remains unimpaired. One may have nystagmus alone, with no vertigo or ataxia, in lesions

that affect only vestibulo-ocular pathways. Central lesions may be so situated as to interfere with the process of accommodation (see above), thus resulting in clinical manifestations lasting much longer than with peripheral lesions.

Central lesions can cause positional vertigo and nystagmus. The positional test should be performed and the central pattern of response sought (Table 62-5). As with peripheral lesions, evaluation of spontaneous nystagmus may give valuable localizing information (see Table 62-4). Lesions of the central vestibular system often involve other CNS structures, giving associated symptoms and signs of cerebral, cerebellar, or brainstem dysfunction. Peripheral vestibular lesions present with no such CNS manifestations unless they have spread centrally, as occurs with tumors.

Clinical Profiles of Vestibular Lesions
In vestibular lesions there are four commonly encountered clinical profiles: (1) acute paroxysmal, (2) those of acute onset with gradual resolution, (3) motion-induced, and (4) position-induced.

The acute paroxysmal profile is characterized by symptoms and signs of vestibular dysfunction that appear acutely and persist unremittingly for periods ranging from several minutes to several hours. Such a pattern is indicative of a reversible lesion. Of the lesions of the peripheral vestibular system manifested by the acute paroxysmal profile, *Ménière's disease* (endolymphatic hydrops) is the most common. This disease classically involves both the vestibular and auditory end organs (labyrinth and cochlea); it presents classically with unilateral sensorineural hearing loss, tinnitus, feelings of blocking or plugging in the ear, and episodes of spontaneous vertigo and ataxia lasting several minutes to several hours. Hearing loss and tinnitus may be exacerbated during episodes of vestibular dysfunction. Associated vegetative symptoms are common, but they vary in both degree and duration. The clinical course can be marked by significant periods of remission, in which episodes of vestibular dysfunction and even hearing loss and tinnitus may significantly resolve for weeks or months. In approximately 10 to 20 percent of cases, the involvement becomes bilateral by 10 years after the original onset. Another peripheral lesion with an acute paroxysmal profile is the *perilymphatic fistula,* which is a rupture of either the round or oval labyrinthine windows. This lesion, which commonly follows head trauma or barotrauma or as a known complication of stapedectomy, frequently occurs spontaneously, presenting with hearing loss that may be slowly progressive or of sudden onset. The loss of hearing may, as in Ménière's disease, have significant fluctuations. Tinnitus and a blocking or plugging feeling of the ear are common. The vestibular manifestations include episodes of acute paroxysmal vertigo, ataxia, and vegetative symptoms lasting minutes to hours. In addition, episodes of positional vertigo, sometimes lasting nearly a minute, may occur with major changes in position. Patients may manifest ataxia that is independent of their episodes of vertigo. The findings in patients with perilymphatic fistula are sensorineural and conductive hearing loss (as documented by audiometry), positional nystagmus of the peripheral type (see Table 62-5), ataxia made more manifest when their eyes are closed, and a positive *fistula test.* The fistula test is performed by compressing a column of air in the ear canal with a pneumatic otoscope. A positive response consists in forced deviation of eyes and head away from the stimulated side followed by brief nystagmus and accompanied by momentary vertigo. *Infectious processes* involving middle and inner ear, or both, uncommonly cause paroxysmal vestibular manifestations, and may do so especially if they involve the bony structures contiguous with the otic capsule. When secondary *cholesteatoma* develops, an acute paroxysmal profile is common with eventual development of a fistula into the lateral semicircular canal. This finding can be documented with adequate otoscopic or microscopic examination of the ear, with the fistula test, and with adequate radiography. Syphilitic involvement of the peripheral vestibular system can also present with a similar clinical picture.

Of those lesions of the *central vestibular system* presenting with an acute paroxysmal profile, transient ischemia in the distribution of the vertebrobasilar arterial system is most common. *Transient vertebrobasilar insufficiency* is a diagnosis that should be made with great hesitancy when the sole manifestation is vertigo. However, the diagnosis becomes much more likely when vertigo is accompanied by any other manifestation of brainstem ischemia (e.g., diplopia, dysarthria, facial paresthesias, obscuration of vision). On rare occasions, vertebrobasilar insufficiency may be secondary to compression in one vertebral artery by spondylotic spurs on one or more cervical vertebrae and occurs with rotation and hyperextension of the neck. *Demyelinating disease* (multiple sclerosis) involving the central vestibular connections may present this profile. The diagnosis rests upon those criteria outlined earlier in this chapter. *Seizure disorders* may be manifested with acute paroxysmal episodes of well-defined vertigo if the cortical representation of the vestibular system in superior temporal and inferior parietal lobes are involved. Less well defined dizziness may be one of the manifestations of mesial temporal lobe seizures. Often manifestations of seizure activity in other cortical areas will precede or follow the vertigo. Loss of consciousness following vertigo or dizziness is suggestive of seizure disorder.

The profile of *acute onset with gradual resolution* of clinical manifestations is characterized by resolution of symptoms and signs over days to weeks and results from an irreversible or slowly reversible lesion with the process of central accommodation superimposed. As previously discussed, in *peripheral lesions* the process of accommodation results in a rather abbreviated clinical course. Spontaneous vertigo will resolve within 3 to 7 days, although momentary vertigo provoked by rapid head movements may persist (motion-induced vertigo). Spontaneous nystagmus will resolve in 3 to 7 days, although vigorous head movements may provoke momentary recurrences. Ataxia subsides gradually over several weeks, although it may present a persistent problem in darkness or with eyes closed. Of the lesions of the peripheral vestibular system manifested by this profile, viral and bacterial infections are quite common. *Viral inflammations* may involve labyrinth (labyrinthitis) or nerve (neuritis), but these respective entities are difficult to distinguish clinically, although labyrinthitis is more likely to extend to involve cochlea and auditory functions. Commonly, a viral upper respiratory infection type prodrome occurs within 1 or 2 weeks of the acute onset. *Bacterial labyrinthitis* occurs as an extension of acute or chronic otitis media and, unlike viral disease, commonly involves auditory as well as vestibular functions. The presence of bacterial disease is reflected in the finding of otitis media on otoscopic examination.

Head trauma results in symptoms with acute onset and gradual resolution through labyrinth involvement in temporal bone fracture. Almost invariably, the cochlea is also involved, with concurrent impairment of auditory function.

Infarctions of the peripheral vestibular system, which can occur with thrombosis of the anterior inferior cerebellar artery (AICA), the internal auditory artery, or its branches, are not commonly found and, with the exception of AICA thromboses in which other CNS structures are also infarcted, they are clinically difficult to distinguish from inflammatory peripheral lesions. Acute onset of both auditory and vestibular dysfunction in a patient in an older age group with other findings indicative of vascular disease is suggestive.

Brainstem infarctions account for the majority of central lesions presenting with this clinical profile. These vascular lesions may be large when due to atheromatous or embolic involvement of large vessels, such as the vertebral or basilar artery or the posterior inferior cerebellar artery. In such cases the deficits include many other manifestations of brainstem dysfunction (e.g., lateral medullary syndrome). When infarcts are due to compromise of small penetrating brainstem arteries secondary to hypertension or diabetic cerebrovascular disease, the deficits may be quite limited (see above in this chapter, under Cerebrovascular and Related Disorders).

Motion-induced dysfunction is characterized by momentary symptoms of vertigo and ataxia that occur only with rapid movements of head or body (even if the movements are quite limited). This state, which occurs when unilateral vestibular lesions exist but have been accommodated, results from acute processes with gradual resolution as described above. It can also exist with no prior symptoms of acute

dysfunction in lesions that are slowly progressive. In such cases of slowly progressive impairment of vestibular function, accommodation keeps pace and minimizes acute symptoms. The most common such lesion is acoustic neurinoma in the cerebellopontine angle. This benign tumor initially causes progressive sensorineural hearing loss. Its most common presenting symptom is tinnitus. Its vestibular manifestations are usually confined to brief episodes of motion-induced vertigo and unsteadiness together with ataxia, which may appear when the patient is walking in darkness or has his eyes closed. When the tumor becomes larger, other cranial nerves (i.e., fifth, seventh), the cerebellum, and the brainstem may be compromised.

Position-induced dysfunction is characterized by vertigo, ataxia, and vegetative symptoms produced only with major positional change, such as lying back, sitting up, turning over, stooping over, or hyper-extending and rotating the neck. Perilymphatic fistula is one lesion of the peripheral vestibular system that often produces this profile, usually with other subsequent manifestations of auditory and vestibular dysfunction that have been described in detail above. When this profile is the only clinical manifestation and positional testing indicates peripheral localization (see Table 62-5), the patient often receives the clinical diagnosis of "benign positional vertigo" — rather a "wastebasket" category, representing any one of a number of minor structural lesions of the labyrinth that usually have a self-limited course of weeks to months, with occasional recurrences.

When the position-induced dysfunction profile is observed and positional testing indicates *central localization* (see Table 62-5), the cause may be vascular, demyelinating, or mass lesion involving brainstem or cerebellum. The physician should evaluate the associated symptoms and signs together with the clinical course to localize the lesion further and narrow the possible differential diagnoses.

DIAGNOSTIC STUDIES IN VESTIBULAR DISORDERS
Specific testing of the function of each side of the vestibular system can be performed. The ice water caloric test can be performed easily at the bedside

or in an office setting. With the patient's head tilted to one side, 0.4 ml of ice water is instilled by syringe against the tympanic membrane of the upper ear. After 20 seconds all the water is decanted out by tilting the head in the opposite direction. The head is then immediately extended back 60 degrees if the patient is seated or flexed forward 30 degrees if the patient is supine. This will produce observable horizontal nystagmus beating away from the stimulated ear. The duration of the nystagmus can then be noted. After a 5-minute rest an identical stimulus can be applied to the contralateral ear and the duration of the two responses compared. If one ear responds with a nystagmus duration 20 to 30 seconds less than for the other ear, vestibular dysfunction on that side is to be suspected.

More sensitive testing of vestibular function can be performed with electronystagmography (ENG). This type of testing — recording eye movements by means of surface electrodes applied around each orbit — provides a much more accurate measurement of caloric responses than the minimal caloric test. Further, it provides a record and evaluation of spontaneous and positional nystagmus under eyes-closed conditions (which intensify all forms of vestibular nystagmus).

Documentation of associated auditory dysfunction provides valuable localizing and etiologic information that is helpful in evaluating vestibular dysfunction. A sophisticated *audiogram* is thus a necessary part of any such evaluation and should always be included in the preliminary battery of tests. Modern audiometry can often differentiate lesions of the cochlea from those of nerve and thus help to localize the underlying lesion more precisely.

X-rays of the skull with special attention to the temporal and mastoid portions are invaluable in evaluating traumatic, infectious, and mass processes. In suspected acoustic neurinoma it is essential to obtain plain and polytomographic views of the internal auditory canal. Should they be positive, *posterior fossa myelography* is the means of choice for study of the lesion. For other posterior fossa vascular or mass lesions, CAT *scans, arteriography,* or *pneumoencephalography* or all three may be indicated.

The electroencephalogram is invaluable in documenting and localizing seizure disorders. In suspected temporal lobe epilepsy, special nasopharyngeal leads are often used diagnostically.

THERAPY

Vertigo and associated vegetative symptoms are often treated symptomatically with agents such as meclizine (Antivert) or dimenhydrinate (Dramamine), with varying degrees of success. Since drowsiness is a common side effect, patients should be duly cautioned.

Bacterial labyrinthitis requires appropriate antibiotic intervention and, if necessary, surgery. Secondary cholesteatoma requires surgery. *Viral labyrinthitis* or neuritis is self-limited and requires, at most, only symptomatic treatment.

Ménière's disease is often treated only symptomatically, but with rather poor results. Attempts at specific therapy, such as administration of oral diuretic or salt restriction, or both, are far from definitive. Corrective surgical procedures such as endolymphatic shunts are, again, less than definitive. Destructive labyrinthectomy, if complete, will permanently halt episodes of paroxysmal vestibular dysfunction in the affected ear, but it entails sacrifice of hearing in one ear and should be considered only in severe, prolonged incapacitation. Moreover, since 10 to 20 percent of the cases will eventually involve the contralateral ear, even this radical therapy may not give permanent relief. Fortunately, significant spontaneous remissions in the disease are common, and efforts should be directed at tiding patients over with symptomatic treatment and encouragement until such remissions occur. Although *perilymphatic fistulas* can be definitively diagnosed and treated by exploratory tympanotomy with repair of the fistula, many fistulas will heal spontaneously and a trial of several weeks should be given, especially if auditory function appears stable. The syndrome of *benign positional vertigo* can be treated best by utilizing the vestibular system's intrinsic process of accommodation. Patients should be encouraged to position themselves several times each day to hasten accommodation and thus shorten the clinical course. Episodes of *transient vertebral basilar ischemia* may require anticoagulation, after the physician has given due consideration to the many contraindications of the potentially dangerous therapy. *Acoustic neurinomas* must be resected surgically. Early diagnosis significantly reduces morbidity. *Seizure disorders* can be managed with anticonvulsant therapy, once it has been determined that no progressive structural lesion underlies the seizure focus.

Auditory Dysfunction

The symptoms of dysfunction of the auditory system are hearing loss and tinnitus. In a great many cases the cause is found to be relatively benign (e.g., aging or excessive noise exposure), but there may be a significant pathologic condition involving the middle ear or the peripheral or central auditory neuraxis.

Hearing Loss

It can be misleading to evaluate hearing loss solely on the basis of the patient's history. Patients often complain of hearing difficulties when there are none or recognize no difficulties when they are indeed present. Even when correct about the presence of hearing loss, patients commonly fail to distinguish unilateral from bilateral difficulties and may even err in identifying which ear is involved in a unilateral loss. Although not many patients present such inaccuracies, the errors are common enough to demand that the examiner always rely upon clinical testing for reliable determination and localization of hearing impairment.

Although definitive documentation of hearing loss requires audiometry, adequate screening for hearing loss can be performed as part of the routine physical examination. This is most easily done using the high-frequency sound of a ticking watch held several inches from each ear and the midfrequency sound of bisyllabic words whispered several feet from each ear. The greatest pitfall in such testing is failure to test each side of the auditory system independently. In order to do this effectively, the examiner must present a masking noise in the contralateral ear — as by rubbing the ear with his hand — in order to insure that the test sounds are indeed being perceived by the ear being tested.

Once hearing loss has been confirmed, the clinician must attempt to localize the lesion to a given portion of the auditory system, which is an anatomically paired system, consisting of the middle ear, cochlea, cochlear nerve, cochlear nuclei, brainstem connections (with important waystations at inferior colliculi and medial geniculate bodies), and auditory cortex.

Conductive hearing loss results from lesions of the middle ear. The middle ear functions as an amplifier of sound to the cochlea, which can also receive sound, although much less efficiently, by direct conduction through the bones of the skull. When the middle ear "amplifier" is malfunctioning, the patient can no longer hear sound better by air conduction (i.e., through the middle ear) than by bone conduction.

Documentation of conductive hearing loss by the Rinne and Weber tests can also be performed as part of the physical examination. In the *Rinne test*, a vibrating tuning fork (512 Hz and 256 Hz are the best screening frequencies) is placed on the mastoid process. When the patient no longer appreciates the sound, the fork is placed near the external ear canal. The patient with conductive hearing loss cannot hear the sound when the fork is placed in the latter position. This response — described as a negative Rinne test — indicates that air conduction is no better than bone conduction. When the patient has either normal hearing or a lesion of cochlea or nerve, the sound is appreciated anew when shifted from mastoid (bone conduction) to external ear (air conduction). This response (a positive Rinne test) indicates that air conduction is better than bone conduction and that the middle ear is functioning normally.

One caution to the examiner is that there is potential for error in interpretation of the Rinne test when the patient has severe nonconductive hearing loss in one ear. When the test is for bone conduction in that ear, the sound is transmitted through the skull to the intact contralateral cochlea and is perceived but poorly localized by the patient. Then, when air conduction is tested, the patient perceives nothing (in this instance, air conduction to the contralateral ear being much less efficient than bone conduction). The patient appears to be describing bone conduction greater than air conduction, indicating a conductive loss. In actuality, he has a severe nonconductive loss, such that he perceives nothing at all by the tested ear. This is called the "false-negative" Rinne test. In many cases the danger of incorrect diagnosis can be overcome by presenting a very loud masking noise in the intact ear while testing the impaired ear.

The *Weber test* is performed by placing the vibrating tuning fork against the center of the forehead. The patient is then asked whether the sound is lateralized to one side or appears to be midline. If it is midline, this indicates equal acuity in both ears. If it lateralizes to the side of the hearing loss, this indicates a conductive loss. If it lateralizes to the side opposite to the hearing loss, this indicates a nonconductive hearing loss. The reason for the response of lateralizing to the side opposite to the hearing loss is obvious, in that both air and bone conduction are impaired on one side and therefore the sound is heard better on the intact side. The reason for the response of lateralizing to the side of the hearing loss is that, with a conductive loss, interfering external background noise is not well amplified to the cochlea on the involved side. Bone conduction is normal to both ears, however, and the tuning fork sound appears louder in the impaired ear, with diminished air-conducted background noise.

Sensory hearing loss results from lesions of the cochlea, whch is the sensory receptor of the auditory neuraxis located in the inner ear. Lesions of the cochlea can be suggested but not precisely localized by the Rinne and Weber tests, which merely differentiate conductive losses from nonconductive (sensory or neural) losses. Precise localization depends upon identification and localization of associated vestibular lesions, and upon the site of lesion audiometric testing.

Presbycusis, or senile hearing loss, which is secondary to aging, results from changes in the cochlea and other portions of the auditory system and produces high-frequency nonconductive hearing loss that is essentially symmetric. *Ménière's disease* produces sensory hearing loss that begins in one ear (but in a minority of patients may come to involve the contralateral ear). The loss can involve any portion of the auditory frequency range, but classically it begins with low-frequency and midfrequency loss. The most striking feature of this disease is a potential for significant fluctuations in hearing loss (the clinical profile of Ménière's disease is further described above in this section, under Clinical Profiles of Vestibular Lesions). *Perilymphatic fistula* commonly produces nonconductive or mixed conductive and nonconduc-tive hearing loss in the affected ear. The hearing loss may be sudden or progressive, and there may be significant fluctuations. *Labyrinthitis,* especially if nonviral, may have associated nonconductive hearing loss. If the infectious process has spread from the middle ear, the loss may be mixed conductive and nonconductive. *Head trauma,* with or without fracture of the temporal bone, commonly causes nonconductive hearing loss by direct damage to the cochlea. Of the pathologic processes involving the cochlea, one of the most common is *noise trauma.* Prolonged exposure to high-level noise produces high-frequency nonconductive hearing loss, which is usually symmetric. *Congenital lesions,* which can be hereditary or the result of prenatal infections such as rubella and syphilis, are manifested as sensory hearing loss. *Ototoxic agents* such as streptomycin sulfate, dihydrostreptomycin, kanamycin, and gentamicin cause cochlear damage, which is most always symmetric and usually is irreversible.

Neural hearing loss, resulting from lesions involving the cochlear nerve, is a nonconductive hearing loss. Mass lesions of the posterior fossa (abscess, meningioma, carcinoma) may extend to involve cochlear or vestibular nerves, or both. Cerebellopontine angle lesions may involve cochlear as well as vestibular portions of the eighth cranial nerve. *Acoustic neurinoma* is the most common. *Granulomatous meningitis* will also involve the eighth as well as other cranial nerves around the basal portion of the brain. *Syphilitic meningovasculitis* may occur at this locus. *Diabetic neuropathy* may involve cranial nerves, including the cochlear or vestibular portions, or both, of the eighth cranial nerve. *Demyelinating disease* (multiple sclerosis) can produce unilateral or bilateral neural hearing loss.

Hearing loss resulting from lesions of the *cochlear nuclei and central connections* is much less common, because of the rich crossover of the auditory neural network existing in the brainstem. Audiometric testing is much less reliable in its ability to localize such lesions. Rather, the clinician must depend on associated symptoms of brainstem dysfunction for such localization. *Infarctions* and mass lesions in the brainstem can also produce hearing loss on a central basis.

Tinnitus

Tinnitus is the subjective appreciation of noise. It can be of any frequency, and it may be localized to one ear or in both ears. When tinnitus is pulsatile, one must suspect either a vascular lesion in the ear in the intracranial or extracranial cerebrovascular tree or a transmitted precordial murmur. Not uncommonly, pulsatile tinnitus is spurious, representing only recognition of normal vascular sounds by an overly attentive patient. Nonpulsatile tinnitus represents either a psychoneurotic symptom or an auditory lesion. Although diagnosis of the former is a process of exclusion, it must be considered in the depressed, anxious, and hyperalert person.

Tinnitus can result from a lesion anywhere in the auditory system and, since there is little if anything in the symptom itself to aid in localization, one must depend on evaluation of associated hearing loss and other deficits to determine the site of the pathologic process.

Treatment

Medical treatment of hearing loss is directed at specific therapy for underlying lesions. The rule is *antibiotics* for infectious processes and *surgical intervention* for mass lesions. When no specific therapy exists, use of amplification (hearing aids) may be useful.

There is no reliable treatment, medical or surgical, for tinnitus, but reassurance and sedatives may make the disturbance more tolerable.

Bibliography

Baker, A. B., and Baker, L. H. *Clinical Neurology.* Vol. 1 (1955) and Vol. 2 (1975). Hagerstown, Md.: Harper & Row.

Barber, H. O. Head injury: Audiological and vestibular findings. *Ann. Otol. Rhinol. Laryngol.* 78:239, 1969.

Cogan, D. G. *Neurology of the Ocular Muscles* (2nd ed.). Springfield, Ill.: Thomas, 1956.

Drachman, D., and Hart, C. W. An approach to the dizzy patient. *Neurology (Minneap.)* 22:323, 1972.

Dyck, P. J., Thomas, P. K., and Lambert, E. H. (eds.). *Peripheral Neuropathy.* Vols. I and II. Philadelphia: Saunders, 1975.

Feldman, R. G., Pincus, J. H., and McEntee, W. J. Cerebrovascular accident or subdural fluid collection? *Arch. Intern. Med.* 112:966, 1963.

Friedman, A. P. Drug treatment of a migraine. In P. J. Vinken and G. W. Bruyn (eds.), *Handbook of Clinical Neurology.* Vol. 5. Amsterdam: N. Holland Publ. Co., 1968.

Grant, W. M. *Toxicology of the Eye* (2nd ed.). Springfield, Ill.: Thomas, 1974.

Harbert, F., and Young, I. M. Audiologic findings in Ménière's syndrome. *Acta Otolaryngol. (Stockh.)* 57:145, 1964.

Healey, G. B., and Strong, M. S. Ataxia, vertigo and hearing loss. *Arch. Otolaryngol.* 100:130, 1974.

Jerger, J. Audiological manifestations of lesions in the auditory nervous system. *Laryngoscope* 70:417, 1960.

Lance, J. W., and McLeod, J. G. *A Physiological Approach to Clinical Neurology* (2nd ed.). London: Butterworth, 1975.

Newell, F. W. *Ophthalmology: Principles and Concepts.* St. Louis: Mosby, 1965.

Plum, F., and Posner, J. B. *Diagnosis of Stupor and Coma* (2nd ed.). Philadelphia: Davis, 1972.

Pulec, J. L., Hocise, W. F., Britton, B. H., Jr., and Hitselberger, W. E. A system of management of acoustic neuroma based on 364 cases. *Trans. Am. Acad. Ophthalmol. Otolaryngol.* 75:48, 1971.

Romanul, F. C. A. Examination of the Brain and Spinal Cord. In C. Tedeschi (ed.), *Neuropathology: Methods and Diagnosis.* Boston: Little, Brown, 1970.

Thiel, R. *Atlas of Diseases of the Eye: Typical Ocular Diseases with Diagnosis, Differential Diagnosis and Histopathology* (1st English ed.). New York: Elsevier, 1963.

Walsh, F. B., and Hoyt, W. F. *Clinical Neuro-Ophthalmology* (3rd ed.). Baltimore: Williams & Wilkins, 1969.

Wolfson, R. J. (ed.). *The Otolaryngologic Clinics of North America.* Vol. 6. Philadelphia: Saunders, February, 1973.

63

Infections of the Nervous System

William R. McCabe and Nelson M. Gantz

Infections of the Central Nervous System

Infections of the central nervous system (CNS) are produced by bacteria, viruses, and fungi and, rarely, even by protozoal parasites. The availability of anti-microbial therapy effective against pyogenic bacteria, *Mycobacterium tuberculosis,* and fungi makes it essential to distinguish these infections from those caused by viruses, and to identify each etiologic agent accurately. Accurate diagnosis and prompt therapy with appropriate antibiotics are imperative in CNS infections, which rank among the most urgent medical emergencies.

CNS infections may involve the meninges (meningitis), the brain (brain abscess or encephalitis), or perimeningeal foci (e.g., epidural abscess). Meningitis is by far the most frequent of these infections; it is produced by pyogenic bacteria, mycobacteria, fungi, or viruses. Viral infections of the central nervous system most often produce evidence of meningeal inflammation, but they can also cause cerebral dysfunction (altered consciousness, seizures, or abnormal mentation) and encephalitis. Specific clinical syndromes tend to occur with infections at various sites or with infections produced by specific microorganisms. The patient's age, congenital or acquired structural abnormalities, and immunologic factors also may influence the type of infection. Table 63-1 lists the most frequent types of CNS infections and the most frequent etiologic agents. In general, these infections can be recognized on the basis of symptoms and clinical findings. Examination of the cerebrospinal fluid (CSF), however, is essential for identification of the type of infection, determination of the most likely etiologic agent, and selection of appropriate antimicrobial therapy. Lumbar puncture for examination of the spinal fluid is a necessary part of the initial evaluation of any patient with suspected CNS infection, except possible cases of brain abscess. Brain abscess with increased intracranial pressure may constitute a contraindication to lumbar puncture, because

removal of spinal fluid under increased pressure can result in downward displacement of the brain into the foramen magnum, with cardiorespiratory failure. Herniation of the brain is an emergency requiring prompt neurosurgical decompression.

As Table 63-2 shows, the characteristics of the cerebrospinal fluid usually allow distinction between acute bacterial and viral infections and chronic meningitis caused by *M. tuberculosis* or *Cryptococcus neoformans.* Bacterial meningitis is characterized by marked pleocytosis in the cerebrospinal fluid. The white blood cell (WBC) count usually exceeds 1,000 with more than 85 percent consisting of polymorphonuclear leukocytes. The CSF sugar is markedly decreased, less than 40 percent of concomitant blood sugar levels; and the protein content is increased. Gram-stained smears and cultures of the cerebrospinal fluid usually demonstrate the etiologic agent; but both smears and cultures may be negative in meningitis that is caused by *Neisseria meningitidis,* in contrast to the high frequency of positive cultures in other types of meningitis. In viral meningitis the CSF white cell count is lower than in bacterial meningitis, and the cells are almost exclusively mononuclear leukocytes; the total white cell count rarely exceeds 1,000 per cubic millimeter and usually is considerably lower. Although early in the course of viral meningitis a preponderance of polymorphonuclear leukocytes may be seen, within a few hours this gives way to a preponderance of mononuclear cells. The CSF sugar in viral meningitis usually is normal, with a modest elevation of protein. The characteristics of the CSF in chronic meningitis caused by tubercle bacilli and fungi are similar to those seen in viral meningitis, in that a predominance of mononuclear cells is found; in contrast, however, the sugar content is usually decreased. (Although a decreased sugar content may not be observed on the first analysis, sequential examination of the CSF will demonstrate a fall in sugar concentration in ample time to allow initiation of effective antituberculous therapy.) Smears and cultures are frequently negative in tuberculous meningitis; they are usually positive in fungal meningitis. In brain abscesses, the CSF findings are extremely variable. A slight elevation of the protein concentration is the most frequent abnormality.

Table 63-1. Most Frequent Types of Central Nervous Systems Infections and Etiologic Agents

Type of infection	Pathogenesis	Most frequent etiologic agent
Acute bacterial infections		
Abscesses Brain Subdural Epidural Septic sinus thrombosis	Direct extension (sinuses, ears, trauma, and neurologic or orthopedic surgery) or metastatic (lung, skin, heart valves, gastrointestinal tract)	*Bacteroides* sp. Peptostreptococci Staphylococci Streptococci
Meningitis Neonates (< 2 months)	Metastatic (intestinal, genitourinary, or from birth canal contamination)	Streptococci, group B *E. coli*, K1 serotype Other gram-negative bacilli
Children (2 months–8 years)	Metastatic	*H. influenzae*, type B *N. meningitidis* *S. pneumoniae*
Adults	Metastatic	*S. pneumoniae* *N. meningitidis* Rarely others
All ages	Direct extension secondary to head trauma, congenital anomalies, neurologic diagnostic procedures, and neurosurgical, orthopedic, and ENT surgery	*S. pneumoniae* Streptococci, group A Staphylococci *P. aeruginosa* Other gram-negative bacilli
Chronic meningitis (All ages)		
Tuberculous	Metastatic (lungs)	*M. tuberculosis*
Cryptococcal	Metastatic (lungs)	*C. neoformans*
Others	Metastatic	*H. capsulatum* *Candida* sp. *C. immitis*
Acute viral meningitis or encephalitis		
"Aseptic" or viral meningitis	Metastatic	Enteroviruses Mumps virus Measles Rubella Varicella Poliomyelitis Lymphocytic choriomeningitis
Viral encephalitis	Metastatic	Arboviruses Mumps virus Herpes virus Enteroviruses Poliomyelitis Rabies

Table 63-2. Cerebrospinal Fluid Changes in Nervous System Infections

Type of infection	Cell count and cell type	Glucose	Protein	Stained smear	Culture
Abscesses	Normal to 100 Occasional PMN[a]	Normal	Often elevated slightly	Negative	Negative
Bacterial meningitis	⩾ 1,000 85% PMNs[a]	Very low (5–40 mg per 100 ml)	Elevated	Usually positive	Usually positive
Tuberculous meningitis	20–500 85% L[b]	Low (20–40 mg per 100 ml)	Elevated	Usually negative	Often negative
Fungal meningitis	20–1000 85% L[b]	Low (20–40 mg per 100 ml)	Elevated	Often negative	Usually positive
Viral meningitis or encephalitis	< 1,000 85% L[b]	Normal (50–80 mg per 100 ml)	Slightly elevated	Negative	Negative

[a]Granulocytic polymorphonuclear leukocytes.
[b]Lymphocytes.

Although the white cell count is usually normal, there may be a slight increase in polymorphonuclear leukocytes, even with a normal total count.

LOCALIZED INFECTIONS OF THE NERVOUS SYSTEM AND ADJACENT STRUCTURES

Brain Abscess

Brain abscesses result either by direct extension of infection from the middle ear or the paranasal sinuses or by hematogenous dissemination from infections at distal sites. Metastatic brain abscesses secondary to suppurative pulmonary disease, which once were common, have become rare over the past few decades. Today, middle ear and sinus diseases are the most frequent sources of brain abscesses. Bacterial endocarditis and staphylococcal bacteremia also may cause brain abscess. There is an increased frequency of brain abscess in patients with cyanotic heart disease, even without bacterial endocarditis. Brain abscesses can also result from penetrating wounds of the brain, but they may not become apparent until months or even years after the injury.

Invasion of nervous tissue leads to an advancing inflammatory reaction that produces necrosis and liquefaction accompanied by surrounding edema, termed *suppurative encephalitis.* This is followed by accumulation of purulent material that is enclosed in a thick, fibrous capsule. The temporal lobe, the lateral cerebellar lobe, and the frontal lobe are the most frequent sites of involvement. Clinical symptoms and physical findings may vary considerably. Fever is not prominent and meningeal signs are minimal or absent. Yet in some instances a characteristic sequence of events strongly suggesting brain abscess may be observed. For example, cessation of an aural discharge in a patient with known chronic otitis, followed by headache, vomiting, and confusion, should suggest brain abscess. In hematogenous abscesses the onset is often abrupt, with headache, focal seizures, and localized neurologic symptoms. A substantial number of patients with brain abscesses, however, present only with focal neurologic manifestations.

Anaerobic bacteria, peptostreptococci, peptococci, and species of Bacteroides and other anaerobic gram-negative bacilli, are the microorganisms most fre-quently isolated from brain abscesses, but the etiologic agents vary with the underlying cause, as, for example, in staphylococcal bacteremia, bacterial endocarditis, pneumococcal otitis, or mastoiditis.

A number of procedures are helpful in diagnosing and determining the site of brain abscess. CSF examination is often of value, but, as noted previously, it must be carried out with extreme caution because of the hazard of herniation of the brainstem. Electroencephalography and ventriculography were once of great diagnostic importance, but the development of brain scanning, arteriography, and computer-assisted axial tomographic (CAT) scans and the ease of performing these procedures have proved them to be of greatest value in recent years.

Once the diagnosis has been established, prompt surgical intervention is indicated. Although antibiotic therapy may hasten the localization of suppurative cerebritis, surgical drainage or removal remains the cornerstone of effective therapy. Discussion of the differences of opinion concerning the relative merits of drainage or surgical extirpation is beyond the scope of this presentation. Current antibiotic treatment most often consists of penicillin used in combination with chloramphenicol prior to receipt of reports of the causal bacteria and their antibiotic sensitivities.

Extradural and Subdural Abscesses. These abscesses usually result from cranial or vertebral osteomyelitis due to the spread of infection from an adjacent sinus, or from the middle ear, or from a distal site by lymphangitic or hematogenous routes. Purulent subdural accumulations may also follow bacterial meningitis, especially in children. Spinal epidural abscesses result from hematogenous vertebral osteomyelitis or, more rarely, from extension of a retropharyngeal abscess or a mediastinal infection. Although headache and fever are common with cranial epidural or subdural abscesses, the focal neurologic signs may be minimal. In spinal epidural abscess there is a rapid progression from localized spinal pain to tenderness, fever, and evidence of nerve root pain. This is soon followed by motor weakness and sensory changes, which progress to motor paralysis. Gallium and technetium scanning are often of diagnostic assistance.

Immediate surgical drainage and appropriate antibiotic therapy are required.

Septic Thrombophlebitis. Cavernous sinus thrombosis, which usually is secondary to skin infection of the face, is most often caused by *Staphylococcus aureus.* Homolateral headache and facial pain followed by eyelid edema, chemosis, and paralysis of the oculomotor nerves are the usual manifestations.

Lateral sinus thrombosis usually results from otitic infections. Focal neurologic signs are generally absent but papilledema sometimes occurs. Signs and symptoms of systemic infection usually predominate. Superior longitudinal sinus thrombophlebitis produces headache, papilledema, and edema and engorgement of the scalp over the vortex. Monoplegia of one leg or paraplegia may develop.

Vigorous antibiotic therapy, usually with an antistaphylococcal penicillin, is the primary method of treatment of cavernous sinus thrombosis. Although heparin has been used for anticoagulation, its value is uncertain. Surgical drainage of the lateral sinus or ligation of the internal jugular vein may be required if antibiotic treatment is unsuccessful.

GENERALIZED INFECTIONS OF THE CENTRAL NERVOUS SYSTEM

The clinical manifestations of meningitis are relatively similar irrespective of the etiologic agent, but the rapidity of onset, progression of symptoms and physical findings, and severity of illness may differ markedly, depending on the nature of the etiologic agent. Bacterial meningitis is more rapidly progressive and is associated with more severe symptoms and manifestations than viral meningitis. Meningitis caused by either *M. tuberculosis* or the fungus *C. neoformans* characteristically has an insidious onset and a slowly progressive course, and is often termed *chronic* or *granulomatous* meningitis.

The clinical manifestations of meningeal inflammation are fever, severe headache, nuchal rigidity, nausea, vomiting, and varying degrees of disorientation, stupor, or agitation. The headache is usually severe and often is more intense than any headache previously experienced. A few days of fever may precede the onset of meningeal signs, especially when the

meningeal infection is secondary to infection in other sites. Nuchal rigidity, pain and resistance to dorsiflexion of the head, is a hallmark of meningeal infection. Other indications of meningeal inflammation include positive Kernig's and Brudzinski's signs. Cranial nerve palsies also may occur and are especially prominent when there is extensive meningeal involvement of the base of the brain — for example, in tuberculous meningitis. The evolution of meningeal signs is more gradual with tuberculous infection, but rarely do more than 4 weeks elapse between the first indications of meningeal tuberculosis and the full picture of meningitis. The course of cryptococcal meningitis is even more insidious, and various complaints or neurologic abnormalities may arise over a period of months before meningeal inflammation becomes apparent. Other findings in meningitis may be the result of the initial disease process (parotitis-mumps meningitis, lobar pneumonia-pneumococcal meningitis), and they may provide clues to the specific etiologic agent.

The clinical features of meningitis may vary considerably. This is especially true for the extremes of age — the very young and the very old. Meningitis in the newborn is notoriously difficult to recognize because of the lack of clinical findings. Fever and nuchal rigidity are usually of low order or absent in newborns. Extreme irritability, "failure to thrive," or bulging of the fontanelles due to increased intracranial pressure may be the only indications of meningitis in newborn infants. For this reason, lumbar puncture is performed almost routinely in the evaluation of any illness in the newborn (see below). The diagnosis of meningitis and the distinction between bacterial and viral meningitis are based almost exclusively on the clinical features of the illness and examination of the cerebrospinal fluid (see Tables 63-1 and 63-2). The discussion below will follow the format of Table 63-2, with more detailed consideration given to individual types of meningitis under the age group most frequently involved.

Acute Bacterial Meningitis

Neonatal Meningitis. The causative factors of meningitis occurring in infants less than 2 months old differ strikingly from those of meningitis at all other ages. This difference can be attributed, in part, to the immunologic immaturity of the newborn, whose IgG antibodies have been received solely through transplacental passage or from colostrum and whose IgM antibodies are almost completely absent due to nonpassage through the placenta. The relative paucity of immunoglobulins in newborns coupled with their more limited potential exposure to the usual causes of meningitis (*Haemophilus influenzae,* pneumococci, and meningococci) explain why a unique group of bacteria are responsible for meningitis in neonates: The bacteria producing neonatal meningitis are almost always normal inhabitants of the female genital or gastrointestinal tract that colonize the infant's skin or gastrointestinal tract following delivery. *Escherichia coli* and streptococci of Lancefield group B are the most frequent causes of neonatal meningitis, but *Klebsiella pneumoniae, S. aureus, Enterobacter aerogenes, Pseudomonas aeruginosa,* and species of *Proteus* have occasionally been implicated.

As mentioned previously, the manifestations of meningitis in the newborn are extremely subtle and difficult to recognize and has led to the almost routine performance of lumbar puncture in neonates when there is any suspicion of illness. In neonatal meningitis the cellular response tends to be less intense with a lower total white cell count and a lower proportion of polymorphonuclear leukocytes than in meningitis in older patients.

Treatment of neonatal meningitis is usually initiated with ampicillin or penicillin and gentamicin until culture reports and sensitivity results become available, as shown in Table 63-3. After culture and antibiotic sensitivity results have been received, therapy is altered to utilize the most effective and least toxic agents. Despite the availability of effective antibiotics, death rates in neonatal meningitis remain high, and residual neurologic and intellectual defects have been observed in as many as 20 to 50 percent of surviving infants. The fact that aminoglycoside antibiotics penetrate poorly into the cerebrospinal fluid even in the presence of marked meningeal inflammation may partially explain these unsatisfactory therapeutic results; and intrathecal administration of gentamicin does not bring about a material improvement in therapeutic

response. For this reason it is often preferable to change to an antibiotic other than an aminoglycoside if the organism is susceptible, to ensure better antibiotic levels in the CSF.

Childhood Meningitis. The manifestations and clinical course of meningitis in children differ little from those of meningitis in adults, but there is a striking difference in the prevalence of the various etiologic agents; for example, *H. influenzae* type B, which is the most frequent cause of meningitis in children, rarely produces meningitis in adults. *Neisseria meningitidis* and *S. pneumoniae* are less frequent causes of meningitis in children (hence, these are described below under Meningitis in Adults).

The almost exclusive limitation of infections of *H. influenzae* type B to children between 2 months and 8 years old has been explained by lack of antibody to *H. influenzae* during this time. Maternally transmitted antibody to *H. influenzae* lasts only the first few months of life and then disappears. Almost all children have developed antibody by 6 to 8 years of age as a result of exposure to *H. influenzae*. It is during the period between the disappearance of maternal antibody and production of autologous antibody to *H. influenzae* that this organism becomes the most frequent cause of meningitis.

H. influenzae Meningitis. *H. influenzae* is an encapsulated organism for which six polysaccharide capsular types — A, B, C, D, E, and F — have been identified. Meningitis is caused almost exclusively by type b. *H. influenzae* is a natural inhabitant of the upper respiratory tract, and signs and symptoms of upper respiratory tract infection often precede meningitis. Bacteremia, which is found in approximately 70 percent of cases of influenzal meningitis, results in dissemination to the central nervous system. Headache, vomiting, and stiff neck herald the occurrence of meningitis. Skin petechiae are occasionally seen, but they tend to be small and much less numerous than in meningococcal disease. Other clinical features differ little from those observed in other types of meningitis produced by pyogenic bacteria. Concomitant pharyngitis, epiglottitis, otitis media, or pneumonia may be present.

The death rates from *H. influenzae* meningitis have varied from 3 to 8 percent in several large series treated in major medical centers. The incidence of residual neurologic damage is greater. For a discussion of diagnosis and treatment, see below (pp. 923–925).

Meningitis in Adults

Meningococcal Meningitis. The meningococcus is the most frequent cause of meningitis beyond the age of 8 years. Males are affected approximately twice as often as females. Meningococcal disease may be manifested as fulminant meningococcemia, meningococcemia that rapidly progresses to meningitis, or meningitis in which the phase of meningococcemia is not clinically apparent. For this reason, a more detailed description of meningococcemia is given in Chapter 6.

Nasopharyngeal complaints frequently precede the development of meningitis. The signs and symptoms of meningeal involvement do not differ from those seen in meningeal infections caused by other bacteria except that petechial or purpuric skin lesions occur in 50 to 75 percent of patients with meningococcal meningitis.

The death rates from meningococcal meningitis in civilian populations range from 7 to 10 percent, with most of the fatalities occurring in the elderly and the very young (epidemics among military personnel have been associated with death rates of less than 5 percent). Palsies of cranial nerves VI, III, IV, I, VII, and VIII are infrequent occurrences. Pyogenic arthritis, pericarditis, and myocarditis are other infrequent complications. For diagnosis and treatment, see below (pp. 923–925).

Pneumococcal Meningitis. The pneumococcus *Streptococcus* (Diplococcus) *pneumoniae* is the third most frequent cause of meningitis, but pneumococcal meningitis is associated with a higher death rate than either meningococcal or influenzal meningitis. Pneumococcal meningitis occurs most frequently in infants and the elderly. In the young, pneumococcal meningitis is often secondary to otitis media, mastoiditis, or pneumonia. A considerably increased incidence of pneumococcal meningitis is found in patients with

sickle cell anemia, and in alcoholics. Pneumonia, otitis, and mastoiditis are the most frequently identified primary sites of infection, although no primary site can be found in 40 to 50 percent of adults with pneumococcal meningitis. Acute bacterial endocarditis may occur concomitantly with pneumococcal meningitis.

The death rates from pneumococcal meningitis — which are higher than with other bacterial meningitides — are rarely lower than 20 to 25 percent. The complications are similar to those observed in other types of meningitis.

Other Types of Pyogenic Meningitis. Microorganisms either are introduced mechanically into the subarachnoid space or they arrive there by direct invasion. In these circumstances, almost all bacterial species can produce meningitis. Trauma to the skull, congenital malformations such as spina bifida and meningomyeloceles, pneumoencephalography, lumbar puncture, spinal anesthesia, neurosurgical or ear, nose, and throat (ENT) procedures, or orthopedic surgery involving the nervous system or contiguous bony structures have all been followed by the development of meningitis. Fractures that involve the petrous portion of the temporal bone or the cribriform plate provide access to the subarachnoid space for bacteria residing in the middle ear, mastoid cells, or sinuses. The pneumococcus is the most frequent cause of meningitis following skull fracture, although a variety of other bacteria have also been implicated. Staphylococci and gram-negative bacilli are relatively more frequent causes of meningitis secondary to meningomyeloceles, lumbar puncture, neurodiagnostic procedures, and surgery.

Recurrent meningitis, with as many as ten to twelve episodes, has occurred in some patients, again with the pneumococcus the most frequent etiologic agent. Previously unrecognized skull fracture is the most common cause, but dermal sinuses and undetected meningomyeloceles can also be responsible. Careful radiographic examination and injection of radioactive isotopes are used to localize these defects and thus permit surgical correction. Recurrent episodes of meningitis have also occurred in patients with agammaglobulinemia.

Diagnosis

It is usually easy to make the distinction between bacterial and viral meningitis on the basis of history, physical findings, white cell count, differential cell count, and examination of the CSF. It is often assumed that prior antibiotic therapy can materially influence the characteristics of the CSF constituents, but careful studies have indicated that such treatment has surprisingly little effect. Thus, prior antibiotic therapy in patients whose illness subsequently progresses to evident meningitis rarely masks the cellular response typical of bacterial meningitis. Gram's stains of the sediment of centrifuged CSF promptly demonstrate the etiologic agent in 50 to 80 percent of patients with bacterial meningitis. On occasion, difficulty may be encountered in distinguishing *H. influenzae* and *N. meningitidis*. The quellung or "capsular-swelling" reaction with type-specific pneumococcal or *H. influenzae* antiserum may be utilized for immediate identification of the specific etiologic agent when positive spinal fluid Gram's stains are obtained. Cultures of the cerebrospinal fluid are often positive when stained CSF preparations are negative, but such results are never immediately available, and treatment should not be delayed until cultures have been completed.

Regrettably, the value of Gram-stained smears and cultures from sites other than the CSF is often neglected. Positive blood cultures are found in 50 to 80 percent of patients with bacterial meningitis; hence, two to three blood cultures should be obtained from all patients with suspected meningitis. Similarly, smears and cultures of petechial skin lesions yield *N. meningitidis* in 50 percent of patients.

More recently, countercurrent immunoelectrophoresis has proved to be valuable as a rapid diagnostic method to identify bacterial meningitis caused by *H. influenzae, S. pneumoniae,* or *N. meningitidis.* This technique allows identification of the capsular polysaccharides of these bacteria in both serum and cerebrospinal fluid. In addition, evidence suggests that quantitative measurement of the capsular antigen is of prognostic value.

Treatment

Every effort should be made to initiate antibiotic treatment as early as possible, to eliminate infection rapidly and minimize permanent neurologic damage. Obviously, therapy cannot be delayed until receipt of culture reports; it must be undertaken on the basis of assessment of the most likely etiologic agent — an assessment derived from knowledge of the patient's age and history, physical findings, and microscopic examination of stains of the sediment of centrifuged CSF. In most instances, especially in adults, an etiologic diagnosis can be made and treatment initiated with a high degree of certainty. There is a greater problem in determining initial therapy in neonatal meningitis, or in meningitis in children when CSF Gram's stains are negative. Table 63-3 lists recommended initial treatment regimens, both for meningitis in which the etiologic agent has not yet been established and for meningitis of proved cause. After the etiologic agent has been determined and the sensitivity results are known, the initial therapeutic regimen is altered to utilize more appropriate or less toxic agents, as shown at the bottom of Table 63-3.

Few antibiotics diffuse well into the cerebrospinal fluid, even in the presence of marked meningeal inflammation. For this reason, antibiotics used in the treatment of meningitis should always be administered intravenously. Use of extremely large IV doses provides adequate CSF levels of most antibiotics. The aminoglycosides, streptomycin, kanamycin, gentamicin, tobramicin, and amikacin, and the polymyxin antibiotics, polymyxin B, and colistin, do not achieve therapeutic levels in the cerebrospinal fluid even with maximal tolerated doses; they must be given intrathecally when required for the treatment of meningitis caused by gram-negative bacilli. In contrast, chloramphenicol diffuses well into the cerebrospinal fluid and brain tissue, even in the absence of meningeal inflammation, and this property makes chloramphenicol extremely useful in the treatment of meningitis. Diffusion of antibiotics into the cerebrospinal fluid also decreases as the patient

Table 63-3. Recommended Treatment Regimens for Meningitis

Meningitis of uncertain etiology	Meningitis of proved etiology
Neonatal meningitis *First week of life.* Ampicillin (50 mg/kg) or penicillin G (50,000 units/kg) and gentamicin (2.5 mg/kg) every 12 hours *Two weeks of age.* Ampicillin (70 mg/kg) or penicillin G (70,000 units/kg) and gentamicin (2.5 mg/kg) every 8 hours **Meningitis in children** *Two months–8 years.* Penicillin G (50,000 units/kg) every 4 hours and chloramphenicol (25 mg/kg) every 6 hours or ampicillin* (25–33 mg/kg) every 4 hours **Meningitis in adults** Penicillin G (50,000 units/kg) every 4 hours	**Pneumococcus** Penicillin G (50,000 units/kg) every 4 hours (alternatives – erythromycin [4–6 gm/day] or chloramphenicol [25 mg/kg] every 6 hours) **Meningococcus** Penicillin G (50,000 units/kg) every 4 hours (alternatives – chloramphenicol [25 mg/kg] every 6 hours or tetracycline [10 mg/kg] every 6 hours) *Haemophilus influenzae* Chloramphenicol (25 mg/kg) every 6 hours or, if organism proved sensitive, ampicillin (25–33 mg/kg) every 4 hours. See below* (alternative – tetracycline [10 mg/kg] every 6 hours) *Staphylococcus aureus* Oxacillin or Nafcillin (33 mg/kg) every 4 hours or methicillin (45 mg/kg) every 4 hours. Change to penicillin only after organism *proved* not to be penicillin-sensitive.

*The recent recognition and apparently increasing frequency of ampicillin-resistant *H. influenzae* have made the combination of penicillin G and chloramphenicol the currently recommended therapeutic regimen for the initial treatment of bacterial meningitis of uncertain etiology in children.

improves and meningeal inflammation diminishes, making it necessary to continue full IV dosages. Treatment should be continued until the temperature has been normal for 5 days and clinical signs of meningitis have disappeared. The spinal fluid WBC count should be below 100 per cubic millimeter and the CSF glucose concentration should be normal. The duration of treatment averages 7 to 10 days for meningococci and 10 to 14 days for pneumococci and *H. influenzae.* Neonatal meningitis should be treated for 3 weeks.

The treatment regimens listed in the upper portion of Table 63-3 for meningitis of undetermined cause are based on the most likely etiologic agent for the age groups shown. Until recently, ampicillin was the treatment of choice in childhood meningitis because of its effectiveness against *H. influenzae, N. meningitidis,* and *S. pneumoniae;* but reports of ampicillin-resistant *H. influenzae* appearing in recent years have resulted in recommendations for combined treatment of childhood meningitis with penicillin and chloramphenicol until the etiologic agent has been isolated and its sensitivity determined. Penicillin G remains

the preferred therapeutic agent in meningitis of uncertain cause in adults because of the almost exclusive roles of the meningococcus and pneumococcus as etiologic agents. Table 63-3 also lists alternative therapeutic agents when allergic reactions or other contraindications preclude use of the agent of first choice.

A second examination of spinal fluid after 24 to 36 hours of therapy provides an in vivo test of therapeutic efficacy. Bacteria should have disappeared from the sediment and a slight increase in glucose concentration should have occurred after 24 hours of treatment.

Acute cerebral edema may complicate meningitis. Attempts at correction should be limited to patients with marked papilledema, respiratory irregularity, decreasing heart rate, and increased blood pressure. Glycerol, 2.0 gm per kilogram administered every six hours by nasogastric tube, or mannitol, 2 gm per kilogram given intravenously over 30 minutes, may be used several times over a 24-hour period, but creatinine levels and electrolyte values should be followed closely. Use of corticosteroids for cerebral edema has been recommended, but controlled studies of this treatment in bacterial meningitis have failed to demonstrate increased survival rates. Phenobarbital is given if seizures occur.

One occasionally sees persistence of fever after evidence of improvement in meningitis. Common causes of continued fever are phlebitis at the site of IV infusions, subdural effusions (in infants and children), urinary tract infection, pneumonitis, and drug fever. Metastatic infections, endocarditis, pericarditis, and arthritis can complicate meningococcal and pneumococcal meningitis. Persistent unresolved mastoid infection can also cause persistent fever in patients with meningitis originating from an otitic focus.

Tuberculous Meningitis

Hematogenous dissemination of tubercle bacilli to form intracranial caseous foci may occur with primary pulmonary tuberculosis. Meningitis arises either from direct extension to the meninges of intracranial foci or as part of miliary tuberculosis. Involvement is greatest at the base of the brain, where a fibrinous exudate often compresses the adjacent cranial nerves, with subsequent paralysis. Obstruction of the aqueducts may produce hydrocephalus.

In young children tuberculous meningitis has a peak incidence from 1 to 3 years of age. Onset is usually within 6 to 12 months of the primary infection. Although meningitis in adults may also closely follow the primary infection, it usually represents reactivation of a latent infection.

Patients typically present with 2 to 3 weeks of symptoms, but the duration of illness before a physician's examination can range from 2 days to several weeks. Headache, lethargy, and low-grade fever are prominent initial complaints. After several weeks, progression of disease may include weight loss, confusion, diplopia, stiff neck, hemiplegia, seizures, and coma. Cranial nerve palsies, particularly of the sixth nerve, are common, as well as meningismus, altered mental status, and focal neurologic signs.

Tuberculin skin testing using either intermediate-strength purified protein derivative (PPD) of tuberculin (5 TU) or second-strength material (250 TU) is positive in over 80 percent of patients. An abnormal chest x-ray occurs in 50 percent and shows pulmonary calcification in adults or a primary lung lesion in children. Liver and bone marrow biopsies for histologic study and culture are useful because of the frequent coincidence of miliary and meningeal infection. The diagnosis is made by an examination of the cerebrospinal fluid, with the typical results shown in Table 63-2. An early case may have an atypical CSF with polymorphonuclear leukocyte predominance and normal glucose, but serial taps will reveal lymphocyte pleocytosis and, almost always, low sugar. CSF smears for acid-fast tubercle bacilli are positive in 10 to 22 percent, and cultures are positive in 60 to 85 percent. Positive sputum or gastric washings provide supporting evidence. Since CSF smears for tubercle bacilli are usually negative, antituberculous therapy is begun on the presumptive diagnosis, pending bacteriologic confirmation. Suggestive criteria include the clinical picture, CSF cell count under 1,000 cells per cubic meter with 30 to 100 percent lymphocytes, CSF sugar less than 40 mg per 100 ml, and evidence of miliary disease on chest x-ray. History of household exposure to tuberculosis is often helpful. Irreversible damage may occur if therapy is delayed 6 weeks for a culture result. Treatment should include at least three drugs: isoniazid (10 mg/kg body weight/day), ethambutol (25 mg/kg/day for the first 6 to 8 weeks, then 15 mg/kg), and rifampin (600 mg for adults, and 15 to 20 mg/kg, not to exceed 600 mg/day, for children). In addition, streptomycin and pyrazinamide may be of benefit. Intrathecal therapy is not indicated. Treatment of cerebral edema may be required.

Response to treatment is slow. The CSF glucose may not become normal for several weeks, and protein and WBC count may remain elevated for several months. Fever usually subsides within 1 month. The poorest prognosis is for patients admitted in coma and for those less than 3 years old. The possible neurologic sequelae are organic brain syndrome, seizures, blindness, hemiplegia, and cranial nerve palsies. Complete recovery may occur.

Cryptococcal Meningitis

Cryptococcus neoformans, a yeastlike fungus with a thick polysaccharide capsule, is the most common cause of fungal meningitis. The fungus exists as a saphrophyte in nature and is often associated with pigeon droppings. Infection results from inhalation of the organism followed by hematogenous spread to the meninges and brain. Human-to-human transmission does not occur. The disease strikes susceptible individuals, both normal hosts and, especially, those with impaired cellular immunity, such as patients with Hodgkin's disease or renal transplants.

The symptoms and signs are gradual onset of headache, nausea, and vomiting, lethargy, diplopia, low-grade fever, mild neck stiffness, and altered mental status with disorientation, confusion, and personality changes. Cranial nerve involvement is common, with loss of hearing, ocular nerve paralysis, and decreased visual acuity. Papilledema occurs in one-third of cases. Skin papules, ulcers, and subcutaneous nodules occur in 10 percent.

Table 63-2 presents the typical findings on lumbar puncture, which resemble those in tuberculous meningitis. An india ink examination of the spun CSF will show the encapsulated yeast in 50 percent of cases. When examining the CSF it should be noted that artifacts and, especially, lymphocytes may be mistaken for yeast. Diagnosis can be established either by a positive CSF culture for cryptococci or by detection of cryptococcal polysaccharide antigen in the serum or CSF according to the latex agglutination technique (the height of the latex agglutination titer reflects the severity of the infection and is a useful prognostic indicator). Urine, blood, and sputum cultures for cryptococci may also be of value.

Intravenous amphotericin B (0.6 mg/kg body weight), either alone or at half the dose in combination with oral 5-fluorocytosine (150 mg/kg body weight) is the therapy of choice. Combination therapy is given for 6 weeks. Intrathecal amphotericin B is reserved for those who fail to respond or those who are unable to tolerate systemic therapy. About 75 percent of patients recover. Toxic reactions to the drugs are common and require close monitoring of renal and bone marrow function. Complications such as hydrocephalus and cerebral edema should be managed appropriately.

Coccidiodal Meningitis

Coccidiodes immitis is a dimorphic fungus capable of causing chronic meningitis. The organism is frequently inhaled in endemic areas but only rarely (in less than 1 percent of cases) disseminates to involve the meninges. The key to diagnosis — usually made on the basis of the clinical picture and the CSF findings, which resemble those in cryptococcal meningitis — is discovering previous residence in or travel to an endemic area, such as Southern California. Cutaneous or pulmonary involvement may be present. A positive CSF complement fixation test for antibody to the organism will confirm the clinical diagnosis. The fungus can be cultured from CSF, and the spherules are on rare occasions visible on smear. Skin tests with coccidioidin are usually negative. Intrathecal and intravenous administration of amphotericin B is required, but, despite therapy, the disease has a prolonged morbidity and high mortality. Miconazole nitrate, a new antifungal agent, may be of value in treatment.

Candida Meningitis

Candida is an unusual cause of CNS infection, even in immunosuppressed patients. Involvement of the brain and meninges may occur in disseminated candidiasis. Cerebrospinal fluid smears and cultures are usually positive for *Candida*. Administration of amphotericin B intravenously, with or without 5-fluorocytosine, is the therapy of choice.

Histoplasma Meningitis

Histoplasma can involve the meninges in patients with generalized histoplasmosis and, although very rarely, in the absence of disseminated infection. The illness clinically resembles other fungal types of chronic meningitis. Diagnosis is very difficult because CSF cultures and serologic tests may be negative. Amphotericin B is an effective therapeutic agent.

Viral Meningitis and Encephalitis

Viral infections of the central nervous system can produce either meningitis or encephalitis. Either syndrome may be produced by any of the neurotropic viruses, but certain viruses are more likely to produce meningitis than encephalitis. *Meningitis* indicates inflammation limited to the meninges and characterized by headache and stiff neck; *encephalitis* indicates extension of the inflammatory process to brain tissue, with clinical evidence of cerebral dysfunction (seizures, altered mentation, and variations in consciousness). Clinical distinction between these two syndromes may be difficult, especially early in the illness.

The incidence of viral meningitis is probably greater than is usually recognized, since CSF examination is not often performed on patients with viral syndromes and mild meningeal symptoms. With the disappearance of poliomyelitis as a disease, mumps virus, Coxsackie virus B, echovirus, and Coxsackie virus A have become the most frequent causes of viral meningitis in the United States; the mumps virus, herpes simplex virus, arboviruses (St. Louis, Western equine, Eastern equine, and California viruses), and Coxsackie virus B have been reported as the most frequent causes of encephalitis. The relative incidence of various etiologic agents varies from year to year, and also seasonally. In the United States, enteroviral and arbovirus infections occur primarily in the summer. Mumps occurs throughout the year but has a peak incidence in winter and spring.

The site of entrance varies with individual agents — for example, the respiratory tract for mumps and the gastrointestinal tract for enteroviruses. Skin inoculation is the means of entry by arthropod vectors.

The onset of illness is usually gradual, with a few days of fever, malaise, and anorexia; but with severe encephalitis it may be more abrupt. Headache, often severe, and moderate nuchal rigidity follow. Exanthems may be seen in children with some enteroviral infections. After somewhat similar initial manifestations, gradual improvement occurs in patients with meningitis, while more severe symptoms and signs develop in those with encephalitis (e.g., coma, convulsions, abnormal reflexes, and cranial nerve palsies). Herpes simplex infection tends to involve the orbital region of the frontal lobe and the inferior and medial portions of the temporal lobe; it may result in a relatively characteristic clinical syndrome. Death rates and residual neurologic defects tend to be greater with encephalitis caused by herpes simplex virus and arboviruses than with encephalitis caused by other viruses.

Diagnosis

Examination of the CSF provides a basis for distinguishing CNS infection of viral origin from acute bacterial meningitis. Differentiation from tuberculous or cryptococcal meningitis may be more difficult but can usually be accomplished on the basis of clinical features and repeated CSF examinations for a lowered glucose concentration or the presence of *C. neoformans.* Leptospiral meningitis also produces a lymphocytic pleocytosis, but the concomitant occurrence of severe myalgia, jaundice, conjunctivitis, and evident renal injury should suggest this possibility.

Identification of the specific virus by serologic methods and isolation of the virus from stool, throat, and CSF specimens has met with variable success. According to various reports, successful identification of the specific cause of viral meningitis ranges from 25 to 75 percent.

Treatment

At present, treatment of viral meningitis and encephalitis is only supportive. Treatment of herpes encephalitis with 5-iodo-2′-deoxyuridine (idoxuridine) and 1-beta-D-arabinofuranosylcytosine (cytosine arabinoside) has been associated with severe toxic reaction and has yielded no clinical benefit. Another purine nucleoside, 9-beta-D-arabinofuranosyladenine (adenine arabinoside) appears to be less toxic and to display in vitro activity. Clinical evaluation of this agent has indicated therapeutic efficacy.

Bibliography

Barrett-Connor, E. Tuberculous meningitis in adults. *South Med. J.* 60:1061, 1967.

Butler, W. T., Alling, D. W., Spickard, A., and Utz, J. P. Diagnostic and prognostic value of clinical and laboratory findings in cryptococcal meningitis. *N. Engl. J. Med.* 270:59, 1964.

Chernik, N. L., Armstrong, D., and Posner, J. B. Central nervous system infections in patients with cancer. *Medicine* 52:563, 1973.

DeVita, V. T., Utz, J. P., Williams, T., and Carbone, P. P. Candida meningitis. *Arch. Intern. Med.* 117:527, 1966.

Digmond, R. D., and Bennett, J. E. Prognostic factors in cryptococcal meningitis. *Ann. Intern. Med.* 80:176, 1974.

Ellner, J. J., and Bennett, J. E. Chronic meningitis. *Medicine* 55:341, 1976.

Falk, A. U.S. Veterans Administration-Armed Forces Cooperative Study on the Chemotherapy of Tuberculosis. XIII. Tuberculous meningitis in adults with special reference to survival, neurologic residuals, and work status. *Am. Rev. Respir. Dis.* 91:823, 1965.

Feldman, H. A. Meningococcal disease. *J.A.M.A.* 196:391, 1965.

Lepper, M. H., and Spies, H. W. The present status of the treatment of tuberculosis of the central nervous system. *Ann. N.Y. Acad. Sci.* 106:106, 1963.

Tomek, M. O., Starr, S. E., McGowan, J. E., Jr., Terry, P. M., and Nahmias, A. G. Ampicillin-resistant haemophilus influenzae type B infection. *J.A.M.A.* 229:295, 1974.

Utz, J. P., Garriques, I. L., Sande, M. A., Warner, J. F., Mandell, G. L., McGehee, R. F., Dumas, R. J., and Shadomy, S. Therapy of cryptococcosis with a combination of flucytosine and amphotericin B. *J. Infect. Dis.* 132:368, 1975.

Wehrle, P. F., Mathies, A. W., Leedom, J. M., and Ivler, D. Bacterial meningitis. *Ann. N.Y. Acad. Sci.* 145:488, 1967.

Winn, W. C. Coccidiodal meningitis: A follow-up report. In L. Ajello (ed.), *Coccidiomycosis.* Tucson: University of Arizona Press, 1967.

Index

Index

Abducens nerve, palsy of, 899
Abetalipoproteinemia, 438–439
  liver in, 498
Abreaction, in psychotherapy, 27
Abscess
  of brain, 916, 919
    in nocardiosis, 162
  extradural, 919
  of liver, 494–496
  of lung, 148–149
    treatment of, 149
  subdural, 919
  subphrenic, 217
Absidia, and phycomycosis, 165
Absorption, intestinal, 434
  and malabsorption, 434–442.
    See also Malabsorption
Acanthosis nigricans, 65–66
Accommodation
  defects in, 902
  in vestibular lesions, 908, 909
Acetanilid, hemolysis from, in G-6-
  PD deficiency, 630
Acetazolamide
  acidosis from, 729
  in seizures, 864
Acetylsalicylic acid. *See* Aspirin
Achalasia, 409–411
  compared to diffuse esophageal
    spasm, 412
  diagnosis of, 408, 410
  differential diagnosis of, 410
  pathophysiology of, 410
  symptoms of, 407, 409
  treatment of, 411
Achlorhydria, 421
Achondroplasia, 849
Acid-base balance, 726–733
  and acidosis, 726, 727–731
  and alkalosis, 726, 731–732
  mixed disorders in, 732–733
Acid secretion, gastric
  in gastroduodenal disorders, 421,
    423
  hypoglycemia induction for test
    of, 427
  in Zollinger-Ellison syndrome,
    428
Acidemia, electrocardiogram in,
  381
Acidosis, 726
  alcoholism with ketoacidosis,
    816, 820
  in cardiogenic shock, 347
  diabetic, 728, 813–817
  drug-induced, 728–729
  hyperchloremic, 728, 729

Acidosis – *Continued*
  lactic acid, 728
  metabolic, 726, 727–730
    treatment of, 729–730
  renal tubular, 728
  respiratory, 726, 730–731
    treatment of, 730–731
  in uremia, 721
Aciduria, paradoxical, 732
Acne
  rosacea, 70
  vulgaris, 69
Acoustic neurinoma, hearing loss
  in, 914
Acrocyanosis, 270
Acromegaly, 749–750
  hypothalamic neuroendocrine
    secretion in, 748
  osteoporosis in, 845
Acrosclerosis, 593
ACTH, 747, 751
  big ACTH, 761, 773
  and cortisol secretion, 766
  ectopic production of, 751
    by tumors, 762, 773
  plasma levels of, 751
    in Cushing's disease, 776
  release after metyrapone, 760
  secretion in bronchogenic
    carcinoma, 190
  tests with, in adrenocortical
    failure, 771
Actinomyces israelii, 162
Actinomycosis, 162–163
  skin lesions in, 70
Adaptation
  phases in, 9–11
  and psychiatric symptoms,
    17
Addiction
  to alcohol. *See* Alcoholism
  to drugs. *See* Drug dependence
Addison's disease, 770–773
  pigmentation in, 68
Adenocarcinoma
  of small intestine, 443
  of stomach, 430–431
Adenohypophyseal hormones,
  749–762. *See also* Pituitary
  gland, anterior
Adenoma
  adrenocortical, solitary, 779
  bronchial, 192
  of colon, villous, 456
  gastric, mucosal, 431
  of liver, 517
  parathyroid, 834
  pituitary, 760–761
Adenomatosis, multiple
  endocrine, 807

Adenomatous polyps, of colon,
  455–456
Adenopathy, inguinal, disorders
  with, 104
Adenosine diphosphate (ADP), and
  platelet aggregation, 667
  defects in, 678–679
Adenosine triphosphate (ATP), in
  erythrocytes, 629
Adenovirus infections, of respiratory
  tract, 127, 141
  pneumonia, 140
Adie's syndrome, 902, 903
Adipocytes, in obesity, 57
Adolescence, and puberty, 783
Adrenal glands, 765–781
  aldosterone secretion, 766–767
  aldosteronism, 777–781
  androgen secretion, 767–768
  cortical hyperfunction, 773–777
  cortical insufficiency, 770–773
    chronic, 770–771
    primary, 770
    secondary, 771–772
    treatment of, 772–773
  cortisol secretion, 766
  disorders of
    in cortex, 766–777
    in medulla, 765–766
    in histoplasmosis, 159
  hyperplasia of, congenital, 768
  inborn errors of steroid synthesis,
    768–770
  pheochromocytoma, 765–766
  tumors of, cutaneous manifesta-
    tions of, 64
α-Adrenergic agents, in cardiogenic
  shock, 346
β-Adrenergic agents
  in asthma, 552, 557
  in cardiogenic shock, 347
β-Adrenergic blockade theory, and
  allergy development, 552
β-Adrenergic blocking agents
  in angina pectoris, 281
  in hyperthyroidism, 801
  in pheochromocytoma, 765–766
Aerosol therapy, in chronic bronchitis,
  205
Agammaglobulinemia
  and bronchiectasis, 168
  gastrointestinal symptoms in, 440
Aganglionosis, and megacolon, 449
Aging
  and degenerative joint disease, 596
  responses to, 11
  sideroblastic anemia in, 622
Agranulocytosis, 651–652
  leukocyte transfusions in, 640
Ahumada-del Castillo syndrome, 758

Cyanosis – *Continued*
  in pulmonary edema, 343
  in Raynaud's disease and phe-
    nomenon, 269
  in respiratory acidosis, 730
  in tetralogy of Fallot, 299
Cyclic AMP
  intracellular, bronchodilating
    action of, 170
  and release of mediators from
    mast cells, 547–548, 557
  urinary levels
    in hyperparathyroidism, 836
    in hypertension, 238
Cycloserine
  side effects of, 155
  sideroblastic anemia from, 622
Cyproheptadine, in Cushing's
    disease, 748, 777
Cyst
  of kidney, 720
  polycystic disease
    of kidney, 719–720
    of liver, 514–515
  ovarian, 790
  pulmonary, in eosinophilic
    granuloma, 177
Cystic duct stone, clinical features
    of, 471
Cystic fibrosis, 169, 527
  bronchiectasis in, 168
Cystine stones, renal, 717
Cystourethrogram, voiding, 694
Cytology
  in esophageal neoplasms, 408–409
  in gastric cancer, 431
  in gastroduodenal disorders, 420
Cytomegalovirus infection, 87–88
  as opportunistic infection, 97
  pneumonia in, after immuno-
    suppression, 140
  from transfusions, 645–646
  urethritis in, 101

Danazol, in angioneurotic edema,
  545
Deafness, 913–914. *See also*
  Hearing loss
Death
  attitudes toward, 11, 16
  cerebral, 866
  sudden, in coronary artery
    disease, 276, 288
Defibrillation, ventricular, 383
Degenerative joint disease, 595–597
Dehydration, 733
  in diabetic ketoacidosis, 818
  in uremia, 721
Dehydroepiandrosterone, 766, 767
Del Castillo syndrome, 788

Delirium
  management of, 24–25
  tremens, 40
Delusions, in acute schizophrenia, 25
Dementia, 871–872
Denial of illness, mechanisms in, 16
Dependency, and hospitalization, 15
Depressants of CNS
  addiction to, 32, 35–37
  overdose of, 36–37
Depression, management of, 21–22
DeQuervain's thyroiditis, 808
Dermacentor
  andersoni, 81
  variabilis, 81
Dermatitis
  atopic, 71
  contact, 71, 550, 562
    patch tests in, 551–552
  eczematous, 63
  factitial, 67
  herpetiformis, 73
  seborrheic, 70
Dermatographia, in urticaria, 559
Dermatology. *See* Skin
Dermatomyositis, 65, 594–596
  esophagus in, 418
Dermatophytosis, 70
Dermopathy, diabetic, 63
20,22-Desmolase deficiency, 768,
  769
Dexamethasone
  in nasal spray, for allergic rhinitis,
    555
  test in Cushing's syndrome, 774,
    775
Dextran, affecting platelets, 679
Diabetes insipidus, 763–764
  treatment of, 764
Diabetes mellitus, 811–825
  amyotrophy in, 875
  and atherosclerosis, 255
  blood vessels in, 821
  and candidiasis, 164
  in carcinoma of pancreas, 526
  clinical features of, 812–813, 815
  complications of, 820–822
  and cryptococcosis, 161
  cutaneous manifestations of, 63
  diet in, 822
  etiology of, theories in, 812
  eye disease in, 821
  glucose tolerance in, 811–812
  and hemochromatosis, 507
  hypertension in, 249–250
  infections in, 820
  insulin therapy in, 823–825
  ketoacidosis in, 728, 813–817
    treatment of, 817–819
  lipid abnormalities in, 822

Diabetes mellitus – *Continued*
  liver in, 498
  long-term therapy of, 822–825
  neuropathies in, 820, 883–884
    hearing loss in, 914
  nonketotic hyperosmolar hyper-
    glycemic coma in, 813–817
    treatment of, 819–820
  and obesity, 58
  oral hypoglycemic agents in, 823
  and osteomyelitis, 96
  in pancreatitis, 524
  and phycomycosis, 165
  in pregnancy, 822
  renal disease in, 821–822
  Somogyi phenomenon in, 824
Diagnosis
  in clinical medicine, 3–4
  of psychiatric problems, 16–18
Dialysis
  in acute renal failure, 698
  in hyperkalemia, 743
  long-term, 723–724
  peritoneal, peritonitis after,
    530–531
Diamox. *See* Acetazolamide
Diaphragm, 216–217
  eventration of, 216–217
  flutter of, 216
  hernias of, 217
  motion disorders of, 216–217
  paralysis of, 216
  "stitch" in, 216
  in subphrenic abscess, 217
Diarrhea, 465–469
  acidosis in, 728
  in amebiasis, 467
  in cholera, 466
  in colonic disease, 445
  in Crohn's disease, 460, 461
  diagnostic techniques in, 467–468
  in eosinophilic gastroenteritis, 440
  from *Escherichia coli,* 467
  in folic acid deficiency, 624
  in gastroenteritis, acute non-
    bacterial, 438
  in hepatitis, chronic, 493
  in immunoglobulin deficiency
    syndromes, 440
  in irritable colon syndrome, 447,
    448
  in ischemic colitis, 462
  in lactase deficiency, 438
  in pseudomembranous entero-
    colitis, 467
  in Reiter's syndrome, 582
  in salmonellosis, 465–466
  in scleroderma, 593
  in shigellosis, 466
  in small bowel disease, 434